First Aid Clinical Algorithms for the USMLE Step 2 CK

Jonathan Kramer-Feldman, MD
Department of Psychiatry
University of California, San Francisco
San Francisco, California

Linda Jiang, MD
Department of Internal Medicine
University of Pittsburgh Medical Center
Pittsburgh, Pennsylvania

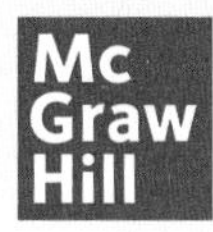
Mc
Graw
Hill

New York Chicago San Francisco Athens London Madrid
Mexico City Milan New Delhi Singapore Sydney Toronto

First Aid Clinical Algorithms for the USMLE Step 2 CK

1 2 3 4 5 6 7 8 9 LWI 28 27 26 25 24 23

ISBN 978-1-264-27013-2
MHID 1-264-27013-5

Notice

Medicine is an ever-changing science. As new research and clinical experience broaden our knowledge, changes in treatment and drug therapy are required. The authors and the publisher of this work have checked with sources believed to be reliable in their efforts to provide information that is complete and generally in accord with the standards accepted at the time of publication. However, in view of the possibility of human error or changes in medical sciences, neither the authors nor the publisher nor any other party who has been involved in the preparation or publication of this work warrants that the information contained herein is in every respect accurate or complete, and they disclaim all responsibility for any errors or omissions or for the results obtained from use of the information contained in this work. Readers are encouraged to confirm the information contained herein with other sources. For example and in particular, readers are advised to check the product information sheet included in the package of each drug they plan to administer to be certain that the information contained in this work is accurate and that changes have not been made in the recommended dose or in the contraindications for administration. This recommendation is of particular importance in connection with new or infrequently used drugs.

This book was set in Minion Pro and LucidCharts by KnowledgeWorks Global Ltd.
The editors were Bob Boehringer and Kim J. Davis.
The production supervisor was Catherine Saggese.
Project management was provided by Revathi Viswanathan of KnowledgeWorks Global Ltd.

This book is printed on acid-free paper.

Library of Congress Control Number: 2022951629

Jonathan: for my fiancée Elizabeth, my parents Jane and Mitch, my sister Nina, her husband Adam and their children, Isaac and Zoe. Thank you for your support, patience, and joy you bring into my life.

Linda: for my parents, Ning Jiang and Qin Wang, and my brother, Henry. Thank you for your love, care, and support. You inspire me every day to chase my dreams.

Contents

Acknowledgments

This book would not have been possible without the tireless efforts of a number of medical students, as well as resident, fellow, and attending physicians who spent countless hours on this book on top of their full-time clinical and academic responsibilities. Our deepest gratitude is offered to Carson Quinn, MD, Gaurang Gupte, MD, and Matthew Williams, MD, MBA, for their creative energy and dedication to this book. We thank Bob Boehringer for his expert guidance and sense of humor, Revathi Viswanathan, Kim Davis, Kay Conerly, Lior Raz-Farley, and everyone else at McGraw Hill who helped make this book a reality.

Editors

Associate Editor

Carson Quinn, MD
Department of Neurology
Harvard Medical School
Massachusetts General Hospital
Brigham and Women's Hospital
Boston, Massachusetts

Project Manager

Gaurang Gupte, MD
Department of Anesthesiology
Washington University School of Medicine in St. Louis
Barnes–Jewish Hospital
St. Louis, Missouri

Section Editors

Medicine

Karly Hampshire, BS
University of California, San Francisco School of Medicine
San Francisco, California

Jessica Meng Jia Hao, MD
Combined Family Medicine and Psychiatry
University of Pittsburgh Medical Center
St. Margaret Hospital, Western Psychiatric Hospital
Pittsburgh, Pennsylvania

Valentina Jaramillo-Restrepo, MD
Department of Internal Medicine
University of Pittsburgh Medical Center
Pittsburgh, Pennsylvania

Mitchell Lynn, MD, MBA
Department of Radiology
University of Missouri–Kansas City
Kansas City, Missouri

Surgery

Chelsie Anderson, MD
Department of General Surgery
University of California, San Francisco
San Francisco, California

Edward Andrews, MD
Department of Neurosurgery
University of Pittsburgh Medical Center
Pittsburgh, Pennsylvania

Nicolás Matheo Kass, BA
University of Pittsburgh School of Medicine
Pittsburgh, Pennsylvania

Jorge Zarate Rodriguez, MD
Department of General Surgery
Washington University School of Medicine in St. Louis
Barnes–Jewish Hospital
St. Louis, Missouri

Michael Sadighian, MD
Department of Urology
University of Southern California
Los Angeles, California

Neurology

Carson Quinn, MD
Department of Neurology
Harvard Medical School
Massachusetts General Hospital
Brigham and Women's Hospital
Boston, Massachusetts

Prashanth Rajarajan, MD, PhD
Department of Neurology
Harvard Medical School
Massachusetts General Hospital
Brigham and Women's Hospital
Boston, Massachusetts

Obstetrics and Gynecology

Christina N. Schmidt, BS
Department of Obstetrics and Gynecology
University of California, San Francisco School of Medicine
San Francisco, California

Psychiatry

Jimmy He, MD
Department of Psychiatry
Kaiser Permanente Oakland Medical Center
Oakland, California

Pediatrics

Florence Lambert-Fliszar, MD
Department of Pediatrics
University of Washington School of Medicine
Seattle Children's Hospital
Seattle, Washington

Divya Kalyani Natarajan, MD, MPhil
Department of Pediatrics
University of Washington School of Medicine
Seattle Children's Hospital
Seattle, Washington

Faculty Editors

Rachel Bratlie, DO, PMH-C
Adult and Perinatal Psychiatrist
Director of Residency Education
Department of Psychiatry
Kaiser Permanente Oakland Medical Center
Oakland, California

Dennis Chang, MD
Associate Professor of Medicine
Department of Internal Medicine
Washington University School of Medicine in St. Louis
Barnes–Jewish Hospital
St. Louis, Missouri

Steven Cheng, MD
Professor of Medicine
Department of Internal Medicine (Nephrology)
Washington University School of Medicine in St. Louis
Barnes–Jewish Hospital
St. Louis, Missouri

David Daniels, MD
Assistant Professor of Psychiatry
Department of Psychiatry
Washington University School of Medicine in St. Louis
Barnes–Jewish Hospital
St. Louis, Missouri

Casey Duncan, MD, MS
Assistant Professor of Surgery, General Surgery, and Surgical Oncology
Department of Surgical Oncology
UT Health Sciences Center at Houston
Houston, Texas

Gerome V. Escota, MD, FIDSA
Section of Infectious Disease and Travel Medicine
Park Nicollet Clinic and Specialty Center
St. Louis Park, Minnesota

Maria Farooq, MD
Fellow
Department of Hematology-Oncology
National Cancer Institute
National Institutes of Health
Bethesda, Maryland

Francesca Galbiati, MD
Fellow
Department of Endocrinology
Harvard Medical School
Brigham and Women's Hospital
Boston, Massachusetts

Tanmay Gokhale, MD, PhD
Fellow
Department of Cardiology
University of Pittsburgh Medical Center
Pittsburgh, Pennsylvania

G. Kyle Harrold, MD
Instructor in Neurology
Department of Neurology
Harvard Medical School
Brigham & Women's Hospital
Boston, Massachusetts

Jennifer Jo, MD
Fellow
Department of Gastroenterology
Icahn School of Medicine at Mount Sinai
Mount Sinai Medical Center
New York, New York

Ilana Roberts Krumm, MD
Fellow
Department of Pulmonary & Critical Care
University of California, San Francisco
San Francisco, California

Randall Lee, MD
Fellow
Department of Urology
University of Southern California
Los Angeles, California

Kathryn Leyens, MD
Fellow
Department of Medicine-Pediatrics
University of Pittsburgh Medical Center
Pittsburgh, Pennsylvania

Brianna Rossiter, MD, MS
Assistant Professor of Medicine
Department of Internal Medicine
University of Pittsburgh Medical Center
Pittsburgh, Pennsylvania

Joseph Sleiman, MD
Fellow
Department of Gastroenterology, Hepatology and Nutrition
University of Pittsburgh Medical Center
Pittsburgh, Pennsylvania

Jeffrey Stepan, MD, MSc
Assistant Professor of Orthopedic Surgery and Rehabilitation Medicine
Department of Orthopedic Surgery
The University of Chicago Medical Center
Chicago, Illinois

Eric Strand, MD
Chief, General Obstetrics and Gynecology
Professor, Department of Obstetrics and Gynecology
Associate Program Director, Residency, Obstetrics and Gynecology
Washington University School of Medicine in St. Louis
Barnes–Jewish Hospital
St. Louis, Missouri

Timothy Yau, MD
Associate Professor of Medicine
Department of Internal Medicine (Nephrology)
Washington University School of Medicine in St. Louis
Barnes–Jewish Hospital
St. Louis, Missouri

Resident Editors

Teresa Chen, MD
Department of Ophthalmology
UCLA Jules Stein Eye Institute
Los Angeles, California

Ryan Halvorson, MD
Department of Orthopedic Surgery
University of California, San Francisco
San Francisco, California

Sarah Mohamedaly, MD, MPH
Department of General Surgery
University of California, San Francisco
San Francisco, California

Christopher Puchi, MD
Department of Otolaryngology – Head & Neck Surgery
Northwestern University Feinberg School of Medicine
Northwestern Medicine
Chicago, Illinois

Susrutha Puthanmadhom-Narayanan, MD
Department of Internal Medicine
University of Pittsburgh Medical Center
Pittsburgh, Pennsylvania

Matthew Williams, MD, MBA
Department of Psychiatry
University of California, San Francisco
San Francisco, California

David Xiong, MD
Department of Dermatology
University Hospitals Cleveland Medical Center/Case Western Reserve University
Cleveland, Ohio

Contributors

Uzoma Ahiarakwe, MS
Eastern Virginia Medical School
Norfolk, Virginia

Austin Anthony, MA
University of Pittsburgh School of Medicine
Pittsburgh, Pennsylvania

Ellen Barry, MD
University of Pittsburgh Medical Center (St. Margaret Hospital)
Pittsburgh, Pennsylvania

Hannah Beaman, MD
New York University Langone Health
New York, New York

Tierra Bender, BS
University of Pittsburgh School of Medicine
Pittsburgh, Pennsylvania

Kathryn Bennett-Brown, MD
Kaiser Permanente Oakland Medical Center
Oakland, California

Ninad Bhat, MD
University of California, San Francisco School of Medicine
San Francisco, California

Anika Binner, MD
University of Pittsburgh Medical Center
Pittsburgh, Pennsylvania

Shaila Bonanno, MD
University of Washington School of Medicine
Seattle Children's Hospital
Department of Pediatrics
Seattle, Washington

Sonny Caplash, MD
University of Pittsburgh Medical Center
Pittsburgh, Pennsylvania

Luis Carrete, BS
University of California, San Francisco School of Medicine
San Francisco, California

Henry Clay Carter, BS
University of California, San Francisco School of Medicine
San Francisco, California

Chloe Cattle, MD
University of California, San Francisco
San Francisco, California

Ingrid Lynn Chen, MD
Kaiser Permanente Oakland Medical Center
Oakland, California

Shulei Shelley Chen, MD, MS
San Mateo County Behavioral Health and Recovery Services
San Mateo, California

Sarah Cohen, BS, MPH
Washington University in St. Louis
St. Louis, Missouri

Prisca C. Diala, BA
University of California, San Francisco
San Francisco, California

Ronaldo C. Fabiano Filho, MD
University of Pittsburgh Medical Center
Pittsburgh, Pennsylvania

Lauryn M. Falcone, MD, PhD
University of Pittsburgh Medical Center
Pittsburgh, Pennsylvania

Oluleke Falade, BS
University of Pittsburgh School of Medicine
Pittsburgh, Pennsylvania

Vanessa F. Fernanda Ferreira, MD
Massachusetts General Hospital
Harvard Medical School
Boston, Massachusetts

Emily Flaherty, BA
University of Pittsburgh School of Medicine
Pittsburgh, Pennsylvania

David Fogg, BS
University of Pittsburgh School of Medicine
Pittsburgh, Pennsylvania

Jose V. Forero, MD
The Ohio State University Wexner Medical Center
Columbus, Ohio

Dylan Fortman, MD
University of Pittsburgh Medical Center
Pittsburgh, Pennsylvania

Gio Gemelga, MD
St. Joseph's Medical Center
Stockton, California

Natalie Griffin, MD
University of Pittsburgh Medical Center
Pittsburgh, Pennsylvania

Inderpreet Hayer, MS
University of California, Berkeley-San Francisco Joint Medical Program
Berkeley, California

Alex Hedeya, MD
Heersink School of Medicine
The University of Alabama at Birmingham
Birmingham, Alabama

Alexander Hedaya, MD
The University of Alabama at Birmingham
Birmingham, Alabama

Zachary Hier, MD
University of Louisville
Louisville, Kentucky

Nuzhat Islam, MD
University of California, San Diego Health
San Diego, California

Elizabeth Kairis, BS
University of Pittsburgh School of Medicine
Pittsburgh, Pennsylvania

Daniel Kim, MD
Cedars-Sinai Medical Center
Los Angeles, California

Anisha Konanur, MD
University of Washington Medical Center
Department of Otolaryngology–Head and Neck Surgery
Seattle, Washington

Alan Kong, MD
University of California, Los Angeles
Los Angeles, California

Arthur Lenahan, MD, MPH
University of Washington School of Medicine
Seattle Children's Hospital
Department of Pediatrics
Seattle, Washington

Liza Leykina, BA
University of California, San Francisco School of Medicine
San Francisco, California

Carrie Li, MD
Massachusetts General Hospital
Harvard Medical School
Boston, Massachusetts

Audrey Lim, MD
University of Pittsburgh Medical Center
Pittsburgh, Pennsylvania

Brandon Lippold, MD
Washington University School of Medicine in St. Louis
Barnes-Jewish Hospital
St. Louis, Missouri

Grace Lisius, MD
University of Pittsburgh Medical Center
Pittsburgh, Pennsylvania

Sarah Lowenstein, MD
University of Washington School of Medicine
Seattle Children's Hospital
Department of Pediatrics
Seattle, Washington

Maxwell Marlowe, MD
University of Washington School of Medicine
Seattle Children's Hospital
Department of Pediatrics
Seattle, Washington

Asher Mirvish, BA
University of Pittsburgh School of Medicine
Pittsburgh, Pennsylvania

Alicia Mizes, MD
Memorial Sloan Kettering Cancer Center
New York, New York

Eider Moreno, MD
Mayo Clinic
Phoenix, Arizona

Arman Mosenia, MD
University of Texas, Austin Dell Medical School
Austin, Texas

Snehal Murthy, MD, MS
University of California, San Francisco
San Francisco, California
Benioff Children's Hospital Oakland
Oakland, California

Jennifer Meylor, MD
University of Washington School of Medicine
Seattle Children's Hospital
Department of Pediatrics
Seattle, Washington

Fiona Miller, BA
University of California, San Francisco
San Francisco, California

Blair Mockler, MD
University of Washington School of Medicine
Seattle Children's Hospital
Department of Pediatrics
Seattle, Washington

Joshua Norman, MD
Stanford University
Stanford, California

Ryan Norris, MD
Kaiser Permanente Oakland Medical Center
Oakland, California

Breanna Nyugen, BA
University of Pittsburgh School of Medicine
Pittsburgh, Pennsylvania

India Perez-Urbano, BA
University of California, San Francisco
San Francisco, California

Michael Raver, BS
University of Pittsburgh School of Medicine
Pittsburgh, Pennsylvania

Camille Rogine, MD
University of California, San Francisco School of Medicine
San Francisco, California

Harriet Rothschild, BA
University of California, San Francisco
San Francisco, California

Nikhil Sharma, MS
University of Pittsburgh School of Medicine
Pittsburgh, Pennsylvania

Monica Stretten, MD
University of California, Los Angeles
Los Angeles, California

Fritz Steuer, BS
University of Pittsburgh School of Medicine
Pittsburgh, Pennsylvania

Sukruth Shashikumar, SB
Washington University School of Medicine in St. Louis
St. Louis, Missouri

Raisa Lomanto Silva, MD
University of Pittsburgh Medical Center
Pittsburgh, Pennsylvania

Scott Swartz, MS
University of California, San Francisco School of Medicine
San Francisco, California

Alice Tang, BS
University of California, San Francisco School of Medicine
San Francisco, California

Avery Thompson, MD
Brigham and Women's Hospital
Boston, Massachusetts

Christopher Thompson, MD
University of Pittsburgh Medical Center
Pittsburgh, Pennsylvania

Hannah Tierney, MPH
University of California, San Francisco School of Medicine
San Francisco, California

Savannah Tollefson, BS
University of Pittsburgh School of Medicine
Pittsburgh, Pennsylvania

Adrienne Visani, MD
Washington University School of Medicine in St Louis
Barnes-Jewish Hospital
St. Louis, Missouri

Nathan Vengalil, MD
Washington University School of Medicine in St. Louis
Barnes-Jewish Hospital
St. Louis, Missouri

Jordan Wallace, MD
University of Washington School of Medicine
Seattle Children's Hospital
Department of Pediatrics
Seattle, Washington

Lucas Weiser, MD
Cedars Sinai Medical Center
Los Angeles, California

Yael Wollstein, BA
University of Pittsburgh School of Medicine
Pittsburgh, Pennsylvania

Toby Zhu, BS
University of Pittsburgh School of Medicine
Pittsburgh, Pennsylvania

Valerie Zike, BS
Washington University School of Medicine in St. Louis
St. Louis, Missouri

Introduction

Why should I use this book?

We are excited to introduce *First Aid Clinical Algorithms for the USMLE Step 2 CK*, a new and improved study tool to help you excel on the Step 2 CK. Unlike other textbooks that present diseases by shared pathology, this book organizes material by presenting symptoms in algorithms meant to demonstrate the clinical reasoning that should be used to answer the questions on test day.

Many chief complaints have broad differentials that are often not helpful to consider in their entirety for any given patient. Instead, a clinician or test-taker should notice a few initial clues to narrow the differential from, say, dizziness to vertigo or a cardiac arrhythmia. Before developing a differential diagnosis. In this book, this step is organized by "meta-algorithms" that show the steps to reach a more specific chief complaint, for which there is an algorithm/HYF page from the broader chief complaint (dizziness to vertigo). These pages serve to describe frameworks for a chief complaint and the initial salient features to note.

Algorithms present in a visually clear way the most vital information needed to discriminate between similarly presenting diagnoses and the correct timing of different management steps. The benefit of this format is that it helps the reader to distill the "information overload" often present in Step 2 question stems to the salient information that is needed to answer the questions quickly and correctly without being bogged down in unnecessary details.

The book is comprised of paired algorithms and "**High-Yield Facts**" (HYF) pages so that, for a given chief complaint, the diseases that should be on your differential will be included in an algorithm that provides a step-by-step method to guide you from the chief complaint to the correct diagnosis and initial treatment. Accompanying each algorithm will be the HYF page, which lists the diseases from the algorithm and includes pertinent *high-yield* information that is not present in the algorithm, in particular, a brief clinical vignette, management steps, and potential complications.

How should I use this book?

- It will be most helpful to begin using this book early in your clinical education as you prepare for and start clerkships. The specialty-specific chapters are designed to be study tools for the shelf exams and will also provide frameworks for the patients and diseases you encounter on the wards and in clinic. As you work through the chapters on each clerkship, you will be well prepared to review the book as a whole when studying for the Step 2 CK exam.
- This book will help you to answer the **6 primary types of questions** on the Step 2 CK (and shelf) exams:
  1. **"Diagnosis" questions** simply ask you to diagnose the condition based on a question stem and set of data. The algorithm, as well as the clinical vignette on the HYF page, should be studied to answer these questions.
  2. **"Treatment" questions** ask you to identify the appropriate treatment for the described condition. Often you must first identify the condition based on the question stem. Studying the algorithms (and potentially further treatment steps on HYF pages) should prepare you well for these questions.
  3. **"Best next step" questions** ask you to (implicitly) form a differential and then decide the next step in either diagnosis or treatment. Oftentimes the specific diagnosis is not clear, but a management step must be chosen anyway. The algorithm format is ideal for thinking through these questions.
  4. **"Complications" questions** ask you to predict the treatment complication the patient is at risk for developing based on the drug or procedure indicated once you know a diagnosis or treatment. Use the algorithm to determine the diagnosis and then the complications are listed in the HYF page.
  5. **"Differentiate" questions** ask what essential diagnostic test will differentiate one diagnosis from another, closely related diagnosis. The algorithm format is designed to focus on these essential diagnostic steps.
  6. **"Facts" questions** ask for specifics on a disease once you have identified it, such as epidemiology (often what populations are at risk) and pathophysiology. The highest-yield facts are covered in the HYF page.
- The algorithms are best used alongside practice questions. After you finish a practice exam or question set, use this book as you review incorrect (and correct) answers. Identify the chief complaint and turn to the corresponding meta-algorithm or primary algorithm. Alternately, as you glance through the answer choices, identify the algorithm that best includes these. Work your way down the algorithm using the data provided in the question stem. If you made a mistake in the workup or sequence of management, it should be clear where that mistake was made based on the algorithm. If you answered correctly, tracing your steps down the algorithm will help to reinforce your reasoning.
- The algorithms can also be used to help to understand clinical decision-making on the wards or to provide guides for brief on-rounds teaching on the management of specific complaints. However, it should be noted that in instances of conflict, this book favors the "test correct" approach, and occasionally this approach may differ from usual clinical practice.

Anatomy of an Algorithm:

- The algorithms are designed to follow a similar structure across the book. Information is embedded via the written text, as well as through colors, symbols, and shapes. As the reader becomes more familiar with the format throughout the course of the book, the meanings of these non-textual signifiers will become second nature and not require frequent referencing of the key included below.

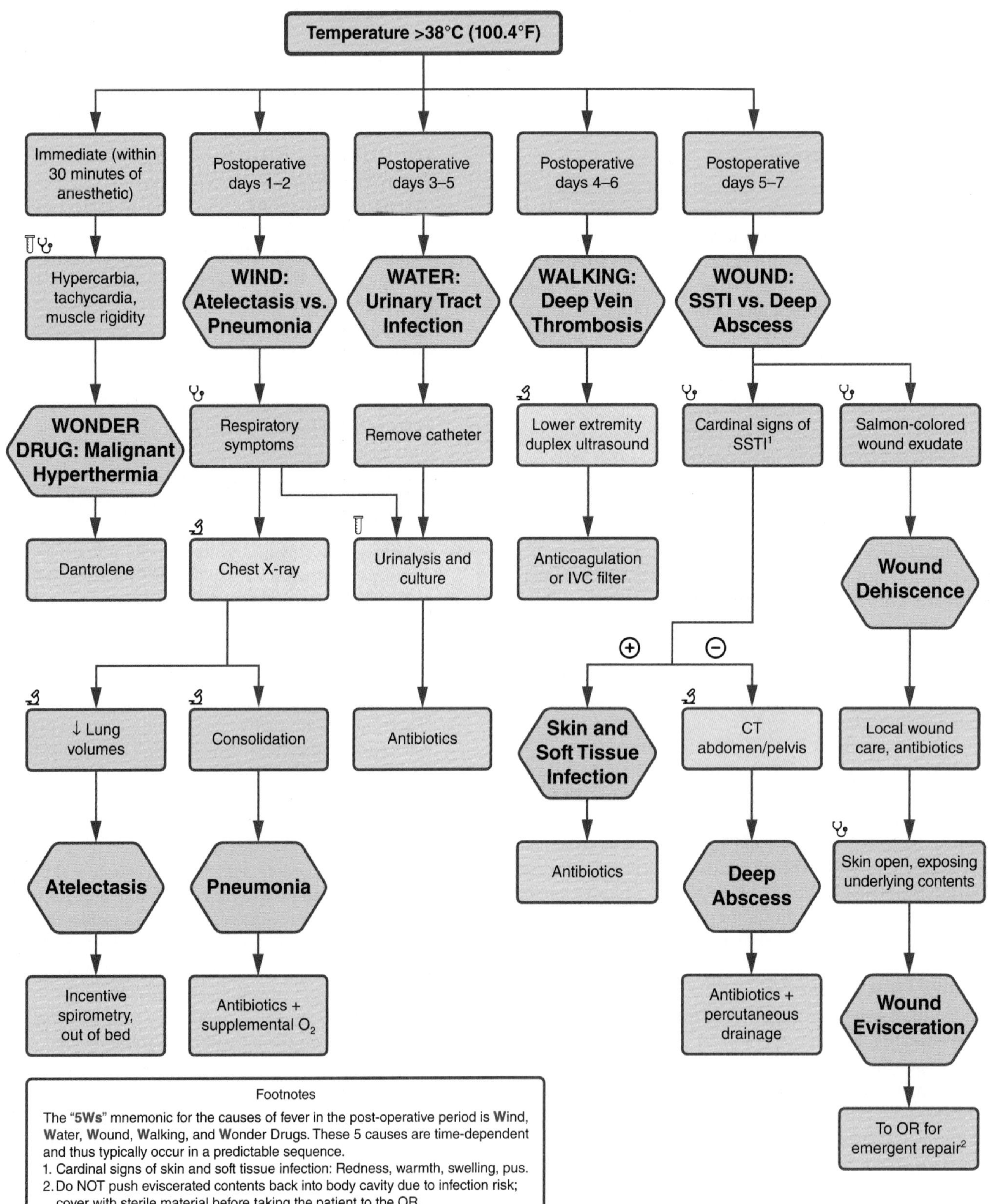

Temperature >38°C (100.4°F)
Immediate (within 30 minutes of anesthetic)
Postoperative days 1–2
Postoperative days 3–5
Postoperative days 4–6
Postoperative days 5–7
Hypercarbia, tachycardia, muscle rigidity
WIND: Atelectasis vs. Pneumonia
WATER: Urinary Tract Infection
WALKING: Deep Vein Thrombosis
WOUND: SSTI vs. Deep Abscess
WONDER DRUG: Malignant Hyperthermia
Respiratory symptoms
Remove catheter
Lower extremity duplex ultrasound
Cardinal signs of SSTI[1]
Salmon-colored wound exudate
Dantrolene
Chest X-ray
Urinalysis and culture
Anticoagulation or IVC filter
Wound Dehiscence
↓ Lung volumes
Consolidation
Antibiotics
Skin and Soft Tissue Infection
CT abdomen/pelvis
Local wound care, antibiotics
Atelectasis
Pneumonia
Antibiotics
Deep Abscess
Skin open, exposing underlying contents
Incentive spirometry, out of bed
Antibiotics + supplemental O2
Antibiotics + percutaneous drainage
Wound Evisceration
To OR for emergent repair[2]
Footnotes
The "5Ws" mnemonic for the causes of fever in the post-operative period is Wind, Water, Wound, Walking, and Wonder Drugs. These 5 causes are time-dependent and thus typically occur in a predictable sequence.
1. Cardinal signs of skin and soft tissue infection: Redness, warmth, swelling, pus.
2. Do NOT push eviscerated contents back into body cavity due to infection risk; cover with sterile material before taking the patient to the OR.

Chief complaint: All algorithms start with a chief complaint that brings you to that algorithm. It can be either a symptom (cough), sign (macular rash), or lab value (hyponatremia).

Workup: Gray box. Next will be a box with an element of the workup that will help to discriminate the different pathways that will take you to the correct and alternate diagnoses. This can be a lab test, imaging test, physical exam finding, or element of the history.

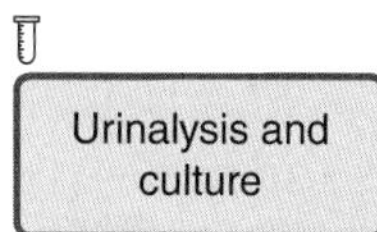
Urinalysis and culture

Positive and negative branches: If that element of the workup is positive, follow the + sign. If it is negative, follow the – sign. All branches have arrows to indicate the direction of the clinical reasoning from chief complaint to diagnosis.

Findings: Green box. Often, the element of the workup does not have a binary answer (+/–). In this case, the finding from that workup step will be the next box below.

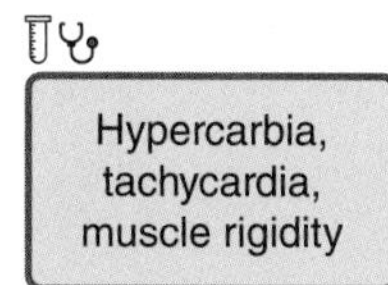
Hypercarbia, tachycardia, muscle rigidity

Diagnosis: Gold hexagon. After several steps, you will have reached the diagnosis. These are in a bright color and larger font, so you can immediately see all the diagnoses present on a given algorithm (ie, the differential diagnosis for that chief complaint).

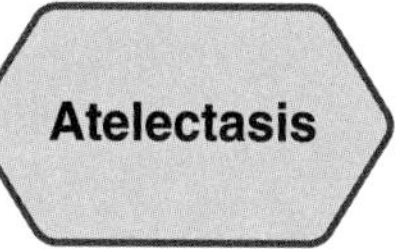
Atelectasis

Treatment: Blue box. Treatment steps will stand out from the workup by the blue color of their boxes. They can be empiric treatment steps before you have reached the diagnosis or directed treatment that are below/after the diagnosis.

Antibiotics + supplemental O_2

Symbols: In Workup and Findings boxes, the stethoscope symbol indicates a physical exam maneuver or finding, the test tube symbol indicates a lab test, and the microscope symbol indicates an imaging study.

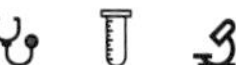

Footnotes: Detailed information that is necessary for understanding the algorithm but too lengthy to be suited for the graphic algorithm is included in the footnotes with numbered superscripts to link it to the appropriate place in the algorithm.

Images: Images are included when they are likely to show up on test questions as important pieces of data to narrow a differential, such as classic radiology, pathology, or physical exam findings.

1
Internal Medicine: Cardiology

1-1 Chest Pain

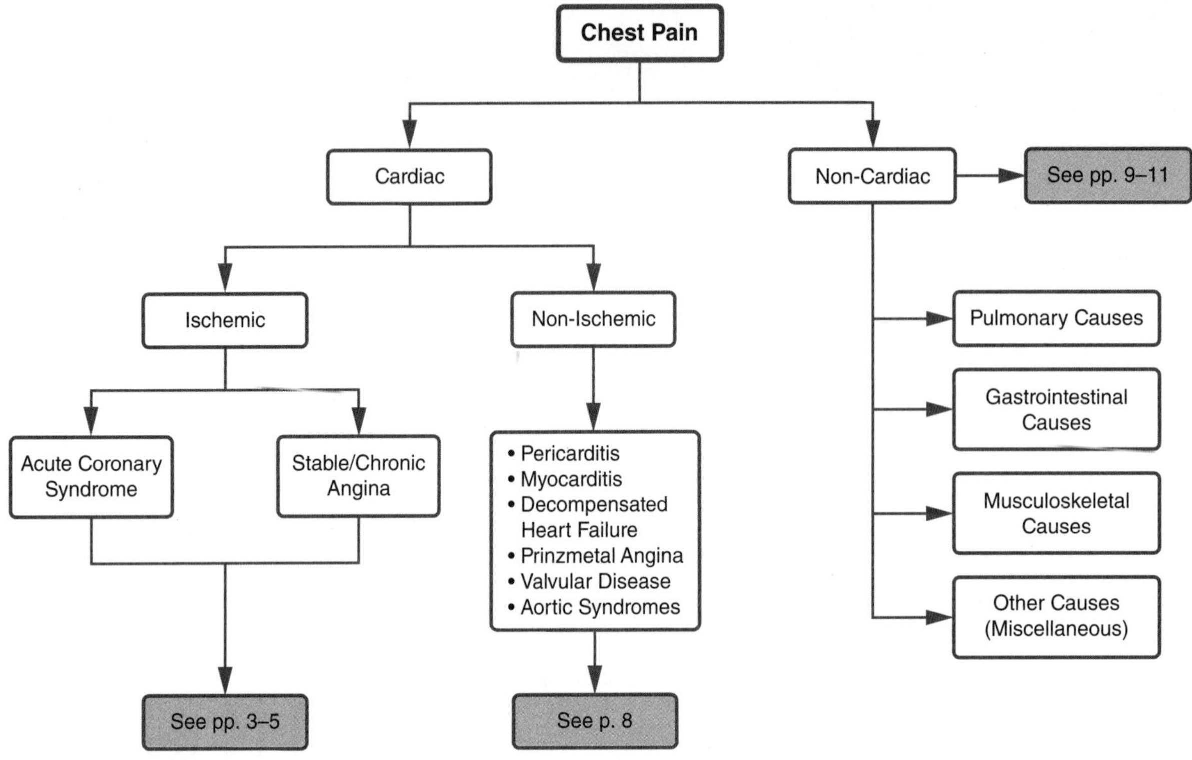
Chest Pain
Cardiac
Non-Cardiac
See pp. 9–11
Ischemic
Non-Ischemic
Pulmonary Causes
Gastrointestinal Causes
Acute Coronary Syndrome
Stable/Chronic Angina
• Pericarditis
• Myocarditis
• Decompensated Heart Failure
• Prinzmetal Angina
• Valvular Disease
• Aortic Syndromes
Musculoskeletal Causes
Other Causes (Miscellaneous)
See pp. 3–5
See p. 8

Chest pain is one of the most common reasons in which a patient presents for medical care. There are many etiologies of chest pain or discomfort, and certain life-threatening pathologies cannot be missed. Acute chest pain or discomfort can be framed into 3 primary categories: Myocardial ischemia, non-ischemic cardiac chest pain, and non-cardiac chest pain.

Myocardial ischemia usually presents with typical chest pain, which often consists of chest, arm, and/or jaw pain described as dull, heavy, tight, or crushing. It may be accompanied by dyspnea, nausea, vomiting, abdominal pain, diaphoresis, as well as a sense of anxiety or uneasiness, and can be triggered or exacerbated by physical exertion and stress. If ongoing myocardial ischemia is suspected, the patient should be evaluated with basic diagnostic tools like EKG and cardiac biomarkers for acute coronary syndrome, a spectrum of clinical presentations caused by plaque disruption or coronary vasospasm leading to inadequate oxygen delivery to meet the heart's metabolic demands. If myocardial ischemia is severe or prolonged in duration, irreversible ischemic injury occurs, leading to myocardial infarction.

Both non-ischemic cardiac chest pain and non-cardiac chest pain usually present with atypical chest pain, which is frequently described as epigastric or back pain or pain that is sharp, stabbing, burning, or suggestive of indigestion. If the chest pain has these non-ischemic qualities, there is a 95% negative predictive value. Non-ischemic causes of cardiac chest pain include acute inflammatory or infectious processes (eg, infective endocarditis), pericardial disease, aortic dissection, valvular pathologies, and heart failure. The majority of patients that present with chest pain will have a non-cardiac etiology. The most common etiologies of chest pain are pulmonary (eg, pulmonary embolism, pneumothorax), gastrointestinal (eg, GERD, dyspepsia), and musculoskeletal (eg, costochondritis). We will discuss these etiologies in more depth in the following pages. In addition, some patients that present with acute chest discomfort may have an underlying psychiatric condition (eg, panic disorder) and experience chest tightness associated with difficulty breathing, anxiety, and heart palpitations.

When a patient presents with chest pain, the first step in management is obtaining vital signs, including pulse oximetry, and a thorough cardiopulmonary examination. If the patient is hemodynamically unstable, follow the ACLS protocol. If hemodynamically stable, obtain a thorough history on the quality, location (including radiation), and pattern (including onset, duration, and provoking or alleviating factors) of the pain. Obtaining a description of associated symptoms (eg, dyspnea, palpitations, hemoptysis) and the patient's prior medical history (eg, coronary artery disease, connective tissue disease, malignancy) is also helpful. Pulmonary etiologies (eg, pulmonary embolism) are usually associated with dyspnea and/or an ↑ oxygen requirement, and the chest pain is often pleuritic in nature. Acute aortic dissection often presents with a terrible, tearing chest pain. Musculoskeletal pain is often reproduced with certain movements or upon palpation of a specific area. A burning quality or exacerbation with eating can be suggestive of a gastrointestinal etiology. All together, the patient's demographics and chest pain characteristics, as well as basic diagnostic tools like EKG, chest x-ray, and cardiac biomarkers, narrow the differential and help guide management.

FIGURE 1.1

1-2 Ischemic Chest Pain

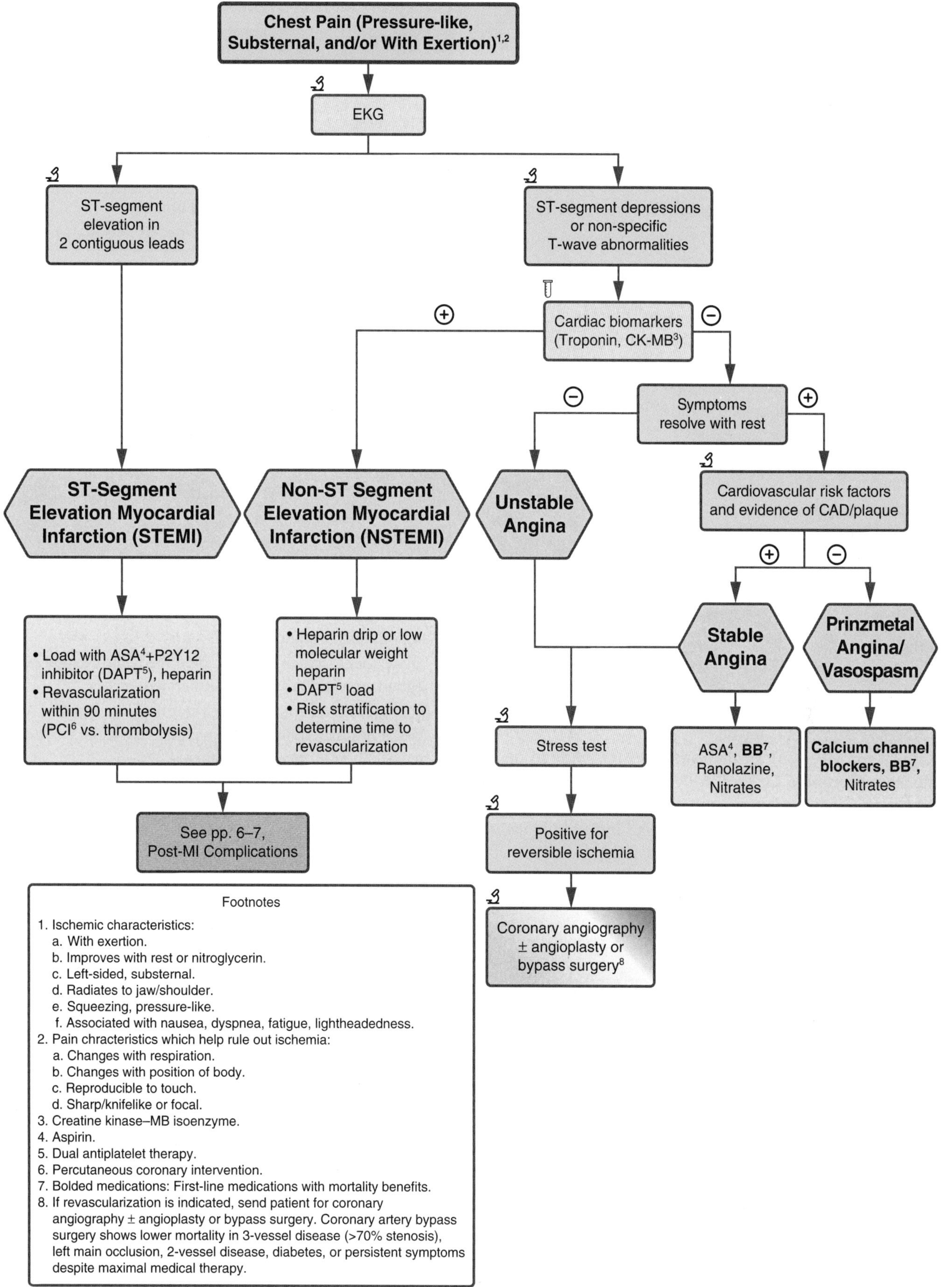
Chest Pain (Pressure-like, Substernal, and/or With Exertion)[1,2]
EKG
ST-segment elevation in 2 contiguous leads
ST-segment depressions or non-specific T-wave abnormalities
Cardiac biomarkers (Troponin, CK-MB[3])
Symptoms resolve with rest
Cardiovascular risk factors and evidence of CAD/plaque
ST-Segment Elevation Myocardial Infarction (STEMI)
Non-ST Segment Elevation Myocardial Infarction (NSTEMI)
Unstable Angina
Stable Angina
Prinzmetal Angina/ Vasospasm
• Load with ASA[4]+P2Y12 inhibitor (DAPT[5]), heparin
• Revascularization within 90 minutes (PCI[6] vs. thrombolysis)
• Heparin drip or low molecular weight heparin
• DAPT[5] load
• Risk stratification to determine time to revascularization
Stress test
ASA[4], **BB[7]**, Ranolazine, Nitrates
Calcium channel blockers, BB[7], Nitrates
See pp. 6–7, Post-MI Complications
Positive for reversible ischemia
Coronary angiography ± angioplasty or bypass surgery[8]

Footnotes

1. Ischemic characteristics:
   a. With exertion.
   b. Improves with rest or nitroglycerin.
   c. Left-sided, substernal.
   d. Radiates to jaw/shoulder.
   e. Squeezing, pressure-like.
   f. Associated with nausea, dyspnea, fatigue, lightheadedness.
2. Pain chracteristics which help rule out ischemia:
   a. Changes with respiration.
   b. Changes with position of body.
   c. Reproducible to touch.
   d. Sharp/knifelike or focal.
3. Creatine kinase–MB isoenzyme.
4. Aspirin.
5. Dual antiplatelet therapy.
6. Percutaneous coronary intervention.
7. Bolded medications: First-line medications with mortality benefits.
8. If revascularization is indicated, send patient for coronary angiography ± angioplasty or bypass surgery. Coronary artery bypass surgery shows lower mortality in 3-vessel disease (>70% stenosis), left main occlusion, 2-vessel disease, diabetes, or persistent symptoms despite maximal medical therapy.

FIGURE 1.2

1-2 Ischemic Chest Pain

ST-SEGMENT ELEVATION MYOCARDIAL INFARCTION (STEMI)

A 55-year-old M with PMH of diabetes and hypertension presents with crushing substernal chest pain, improving with rest and sublingual nitroglycerin. The pain radiates to his neck and arm and is associated with dyspnea, nausea, vomiting, diaphoresis, and lightheadedness. **Exam:** Blood pressure 86/50, heart rate 120, SpO_2 88% on room air. He has bilateral crackles and elevated JVP and is cold and clammy. **Labs/Imaging:** EKG shows ST-segment elevation in 2 contiguous leads.

Management:

1. Revascularization is key. Emergent angiography and PCI should be performed, if possible. If PCI cannot be performed within 90 minutes, perform thrombolysis (tPA, reteplase, streptokinase) if there are no contraindications. While awaiting revascularization, load with DAPT and start heparin drip.
2. If cardiogenic shock is present, consider mechanical support devices.
3. Give patient oxygen support, pain medications, and nitrates (eg, nitroglycerin) as needed/tolerated.
4. During hospital course, start statin, β-blocker and ACE/ARB. Optimize other cardiovascular risk factors: hypertension, hyperlipidemia, smoking, diabetes.

Complications: Cardiogenic shock, heart failure, bradyarrhythmias, ventricular arrhythmias (See pp. 6–7, Post-MI Complications).

HYF:

- Treatment for MI: Don't let the patient **B MOAN**ing in pain: **β**-**B**lockers, **M**orphine, **O**xygen, **A**SA + **A**dditional antiplatelet agent (ie, clopidogrel, prasugrel, or ticagrelor), **N**itrates.
- In inferior wall MI (ie, right ventricular infarction), avoid nitrates due to risk for hypotension (preload-dependent).
- Contraindications to thrombolytics: Major GI or brain bleed, recent surgery (last 2 weeks), severe hypertension (>180/110), non-hemorrhagic stroke in the last 6 months.
- ASA and β-blocker: Medications that decrease mortality.
- Commonly occluded coronary arteries: LAD > RCA > circumflex. Ischemia can come from different pathophysiologic processes: Plaque rupture (type I MI), demand ischemia (type II MI), coronary artery dissection. Coronary angiography is the gold standard for diagnosing acute coronary syndrome.
- Women, the elderly, diabetics, and post–heart transplant patients may have clinically silent or atypical presentations of MIs.
- SCAD (spontaneous coronary artery dissection): Young women, other collagen/mixed connective tissue diseases.

EKG Localization of STEMI

Location	Vessel	EKG leads with ST elevations or Q waves
Anteroseptal	LAD	V1–V2
Anteroapical	LAD	V3–V4
Anterolateral	LAD, LCX	V5–V6
Lateral	LCX	I, aVL
Inferior	RCA	II, III, aVF
Posterior	PDA	V7–V9, ST depression in V1–V3

NON–ST-SEGMENT ELEVATION MYOCARDIAL INFARCTION (NSTEMI)

A 55-year-old M with PMH of diabetes and hypertension presents with crushing substernal chest pain, improving with rest and sublingual nitroglycerin. The pain radiates to his neck and arm and is associated with dyspnea, nausea, vomiting, diaphoresis, and lightheadedness. **Exam:** Blood pressure 160/80, heart rate 98, SpO_2 94% room air. **Labs/Imaging:** EKG shows ST depressions in V2–V4 that were not previously present. Troponin is elevated.

Management:

1. Load with DAPT and start heparin drip. Risk-stratification for when to revascularize. If persistent pain, hemodynamic instability, or electrical instability, take to cath lab for coronary angiography ± angioplasty.
2. Give patient oxygen support, pain medications, and nitrates (eg, nitroglycerin) as needed/tolerated.
3. During hospital course, start a statin, β-blocker, and ACE/ARB. Optimize other cardiovascular risk factors: hypertension, hyperlipidemia, smoking, diabetes.

Complications: Refer to STEMI.

HYF:

- Refer to STEMI.
- EKG differentiates STEMI from NSTEMI. With STEMI, EKG shows ST-segment elevations. With NSTEMI, EKG does not show ST-segment elevations but can show ST changes (eg, ST depression, T-wave inversions, nonspecific changes). Both NSTEMI and STEMI are associated with elevated cardiac enzymes (indicating myocardial necrosis).

UNSTABLE ANGINA

A 55-year-old M with PMH of diabetes and hypertension presents with crushing substernal chest pain, improving with rest and sublingual nitroglycerin. **Exam:** Blood pressure 160/80, heart rate 98, SpO_2 94% room air. **Labs/Imaging:** EKG shows ST depressions in V2-V4 that were not previously present. Serial troponins are negative.

1-2 Ischemic Chest Pain

Management:

1. Load with DAPT and start heparin drip. Risk stratification for revascularization vs. stress testing.
2. If persistent pain, hemodynamically unstable, or electrical instability, take to cath lab for coronary angiography ± angioplasty.
3. During hospital course, start a statin and β-blocker. Optimize other cardiovascular risk factors: hypertension, hyperlipidemia, smoking, diabetes.

Complications: Progression to myocardial infarction.

HYF:

- Medications that decrease mortality: ASA and β-blocker. Hormone replacement therapy is not protective in post-menopausal women.
- Stress testing: Functional assessment with exercise stress testing is preferred over pharmacological stress testing if the patient is able to exercise. Resting EKG abnormalities that preclude a stress EKG: Left bundle branch block, pacemaker, on digoxin, left ventricular hypertrophy with strain pattern. Pharmacological stress testing involves dipyridamole/adenosine or dobutamine. Dipyridamole/adenosine can worsen bronchospasm. Avoid in severe or active asthma. Before any stress test, avoid caffeine and β-blockers.

STABLE ANGINA

A 55-year-old M with PMH of diabetes and hypertension presents with recurrent episodes of chest pain for the past 6 months that worsen with exertion and resolve with nitroglycerin or rest. **Exam:** Blood pressure 160/80, heart rate 98, SpO_2 94% room air. **Labs/Imaging:** EKG does not show any new or concerning changes. Serial troponins are negative.

Management:

1. β-blockers, ASA.
2. Other antianginals: Nitrates (nitroglycerin, isosorbide dinitrate, mononitrate), ranolazine.
3. Stress testing to risk-stratify coronary artery disease.
4. Optimize other cardiovascular risk factors: Hypertension, hyperlipidemia, smoking, diabetes.

Complications: With time, plaques can worsen, and patients can develop acute coronary syndrome/myocardial infarction.

HYF:

- Refer to Unstable Angina.
- Patient history distinguishes stable from unstable angina. Stable angina presents with substernal chest pain that is precipitated by exertion and relieved by rest or nitrates. In contrast, unstable angina presents with chest pain that is 1) new onset, 2) progressive (triggered with less exertion, lasts longer, less responsive to medications), or 3) occurs at rest. Both stable and unstable angina do not have elevated cardiac enzymes.

PRINZMETAL ANGINA/CORONARY VASOSPASM

A 35-year-old F with PMH of hypertension and tobacco use disorder presents with recurrent episodes of chest pain, usually at rest, which last <10 minutes and resolve with nitroglycerin. She is not currently experiencing chest pain. **Exam:** Blood pressure 120/80, heart rate 98, SpO_2 94% on room air. **Labs/Imaging:** EKG without any new or concerning changes. Serial troponins are negative.

Management:

1. Nitrates, calcium channel blockers.
2. Counsel on smoking cessation (if applicable).
3. Stress testing to risk-stratify coronary artery disease.

Complications: This condition is difficult to treat, and many patients have recurring symptoms. Episodes of coronary vasospasm are associated with development of arrhythmias (ventricular fibrillation) and sudden cardiac death.

HYF:

- Classically affects young women at rest (instead of with activity) in the early morning and is associated with transient ST-segment elevation.
- Tobacco smoking is a risk factor.
- Common triggers: Illicit drugs (especially cocaine), alcohol, triptans.
- Avoid β-blockers because they can ↑ vasospasm.

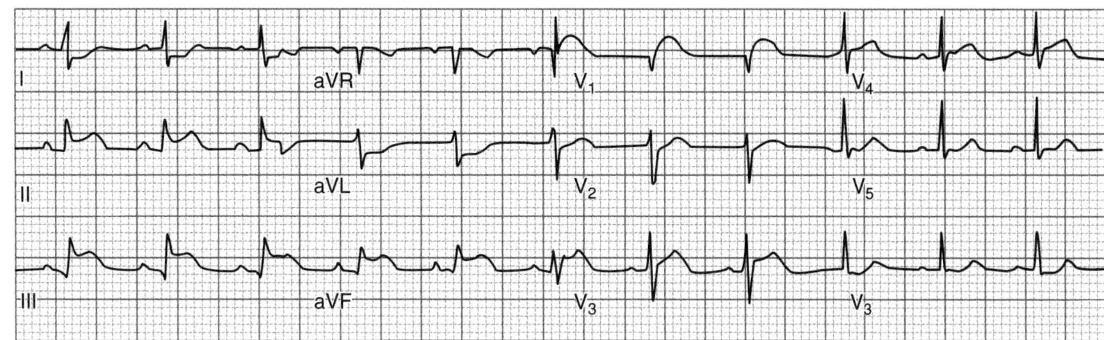
I
aVR
V1
V4
II
aVL
V2
V5
III
aVF
V3
V3

ST-segment elevation myocardial infarction. EKG showing inferior ST-segment elevation myocardial infarction and ST-segment elevation in lead V1 consistent with right ventricular infarction.

1-3 Post-MI Complications

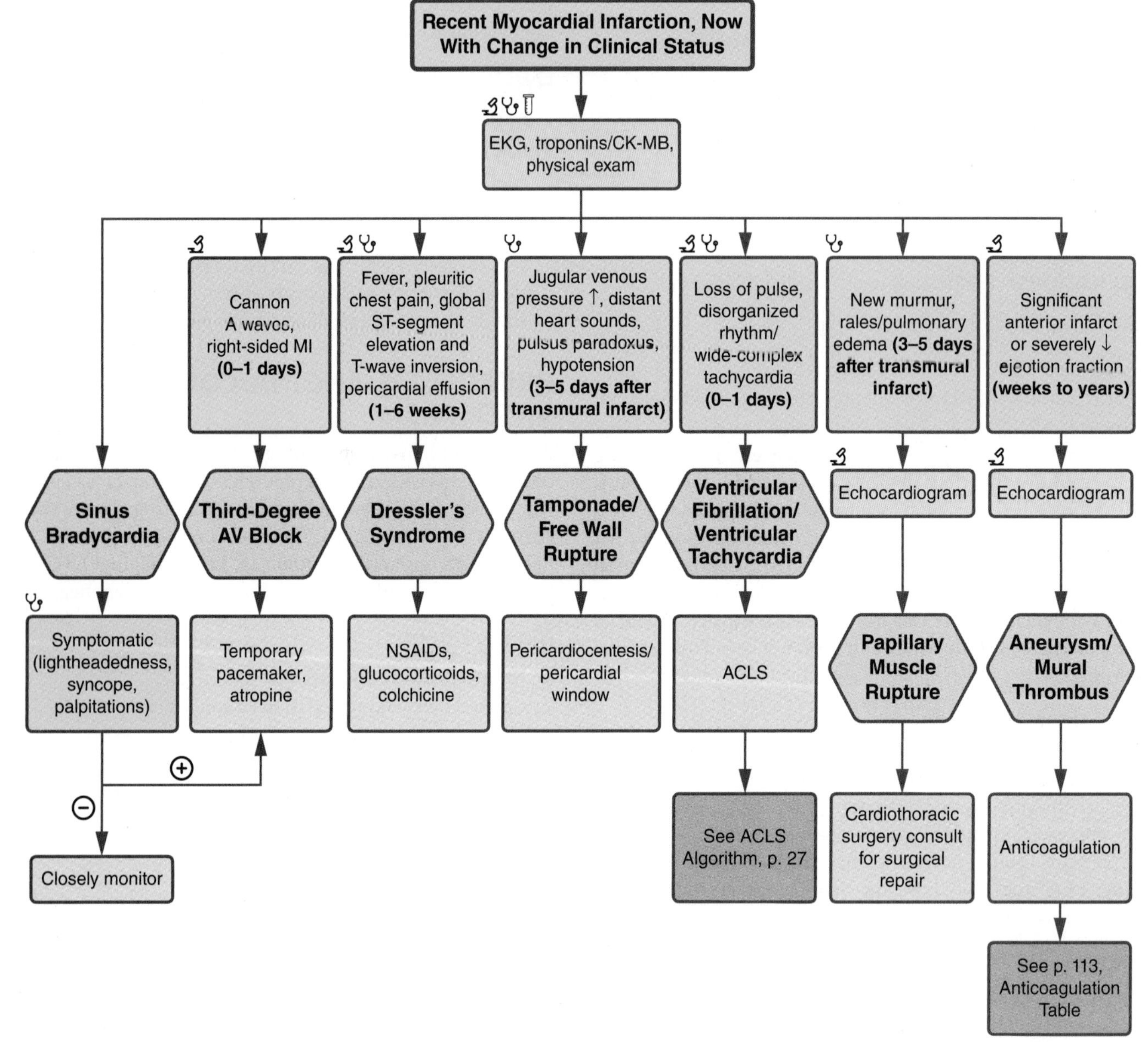
Recent Myocardial Infarction, Now With Change in Clinical Status
EKG, troponins/CK-MB, physical exam
Cannon A waves, right-sided MI (0–1 days)
Fever, pleuritic chest pain, global ST-segment elevation and T-wave inversion, pericardial effusion (1–6 weeks)
Jugular venous pressure ↑, distant heart sounds, pulsus paradoxus, hypotension (3–5 days after transmural infarct)
Loss of pulse, disorganized rhythm/ wide-complex tachycardia (0–1 days)
New murmur, rales/pulmonary edema (3–5 days after transmural infarct)
Significant anterior infarct or severely ↓ ejection fraction (weeks to years)
Sinus Bradycardia
Third-Degree AV Block
Dressler's Syndrome
Tamponade/ Free Wall Rupture
Ventricular Fibrillation/ Ventricular Tachycardia
Echocardiogram
Echocardiogram
Symptomatic (lightheadedness, syncope, palpitations)
Temporary pacemaker, atropine
NSAIDs, glucocorticoids, colchicine
Pericardiocentesis/ pericardial window
ACLS
Papillary Muscle Rupture
Aneurysm/ Mural Thrombus
⊕
⊖
Closely monitor
See ACLS Algorithm, p. 27
Cardiothoracic surgery consult for surgical repair
Anticoagulation
See p. 113, Anticoagulation Table

FIGURE 1.3

1-3 Post-MI Complications

DRESSLER'S SYNDROME

A 55M with PMH of recent MI s/p PCI 4 weeks ago presents with pleuritic chest pain, fever, palpitations, dyspnea, and malaise. **Exam:** Fever of 102.2, tachycardic with a pericardial friction rub heard on auscultation. **Labs/Imaging:** ↑ WBCs with left shift, ↑ ESR and CRP, and high-titer of anti-heart antibodies. EKG shows global ST-segment elevations and T-wave inversions. TTE shows a small pocket of pericardial fluid.

Management:

1. Aspirin + colchicine. Avoid glucocorticoids and NSAIDs if within 4 weeks of MI, as they may impair the healing process and cause ventricular rupture.
2. In severe cases (eg, significant pericardial effusion, symptoms indicate imminent cardiac tamponade or constrictive pericarditis), pericardiocentesis with subsequent catheter drainage (generally 24–48 hours) and concomitant initiation of anti-inflammatory treatment.

SYMPTOMATIC BRADYCARDIA OR AV BLOCKS

A 68-year-old M with PMH of hypertension and diabetes presents with sudden onset of retrosternal chest pain. **Exam:** Bradycardic, nausea, active emesis, diaphoretic. **Labs/Imaging:** EKG with 2nd degree Mobitz II AV block, ST-segment elevations in II, III, aVF.

Management

1. Temporary pacemaker.
2. If persistent after appropriate revascularization, permanent pacemaker. (See pp. 30–31, Bradyarrhythmias.)

PAPILLARY MUSCLE RUPTURE – FLAIL LEAFLET/VSD

A 68-year-old M with PMH of hypertension and diabetes, admitted 2 days ago for acute STEMI, now reports acute onset shortness of breath. **Exam:** Abrupt pulmonary edema, hypotension, loud holosystolic murmur. **Labs/Imaging:** TTE shows new anatomic defect (acute severe mitral regurgitation or new ventricular septal defect).

Management

1. Cardiac surgery consult STAT.
2. Manage cardiogenic shock. (See pp. 15–26, Cardiomyopathy/Cardiogenic Shock.)

TAMPONADE/FREE WALL RUPTURE

A 68-year-old M with PMH of hypertension and diabetes, admitted 2 days ago for acute anterior STEMI, is found to be unresponsive by his nurse. **Exam:** Pulseless electrical activity. **Labs/Imaging:** Emergent point-of-care ultrasound while running ACLS protocol shows new LV free wall rupture and severe pericardial effusion with right ventricular diastolic collapse.

Management:

1. Follow ACLS protocol.
2. Pericardocentesis and cardiac surgery consult STAT.

VENTRICULAR FIBRILLATION/ VENTRICULAR TACHYCARDIA

A 68-year-old M with PMH of hypertension and diabetes, admitted 2 hours ago for acute STEMI now status post PCI, is found to have a new rhythm on telemetry. **Exam:** Tachycardic, diaphoretic, hypotensive. **Labs/Imaging:** telemetry and 12-lead EKG show sustained monomorphic VT, which quickly degenerates into ventricular fibrillation.

Management

1. Follow ACLS protocol.
2. Look for persistent underlying ischemia and electrolyte derangements. Usually, take the patient back to the cath lab, given risk of reocclusion of coronary artery.
3. Implantable cardioverter/defibrillator (ICD) indicated if LVEF <35%, at least 40 days after unrevascularized MI, or 90 days after PCI/CABG.

ANEURYSM/MURAL THROMBUS

A 68-year-old M with PMH of hypertension and diabetes, admitted 3 days ago for acute anterior STEMI now status post PCI, is currently feeling well. **Exam:** BP 110/80, heart rate 70, SPO_2 98% on room air, no other findings. **Labs/Imaging:** TTE with LVEF severely decreased to 10%, ventricular aneurysm cavity, and mural thrombus.

Management:

1. Treat heart failure (diuretics, GDMT) and start anticoagulation.

Sinus Bradycardia: See p. 30.

1-4 Non-Ischemic Chest Pain (Cardiac)

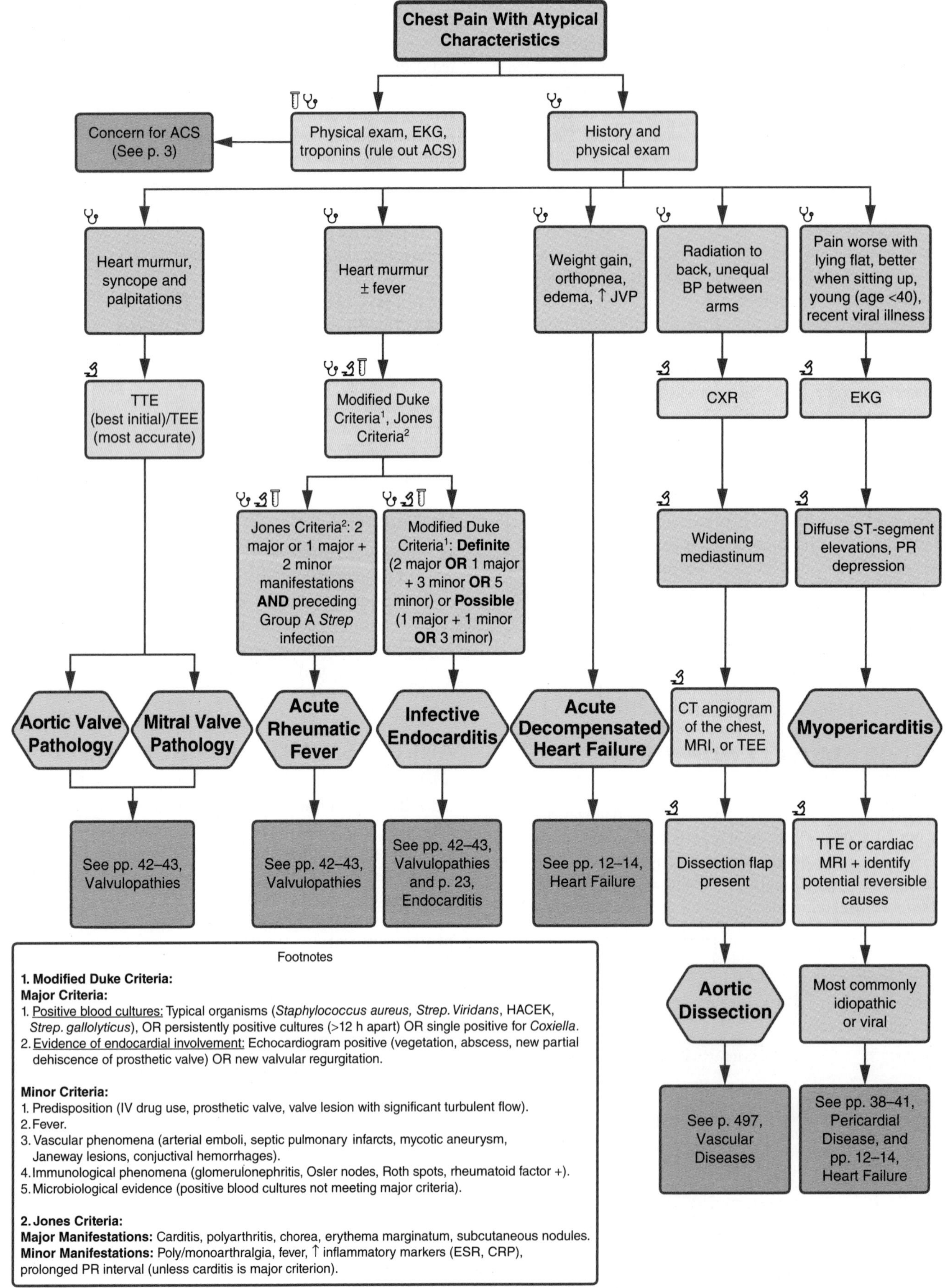
Chest Pain With Atypical Characteristics
Physical exam, EKG, troponins (rule out ACS)
Concern for ACS (See p. 3)
History and physical exam
Heart murmur, syncope and palpitations
Heart murmur ± fever
Weight gain, orthopnea, edema, ↑ JVP
Radiation to back, unequal BP between arms
Pain worse with lying flat, better when sitting up, young (age <40), recent viral illness
TTE (best initial)/TEE (most accurate)
Modified Duke Criteria[1], Jones Criteria[2]
CXR
EKG
Jones Criteria[2]: 2 major or 1 major + 2 minor manifestations AND preceding Group A Strep infection
Modified Duke Criteria[1]: Definite (2 major OR 1 major + 3 minor OR 5 minor) or Possible (1 major + 1 minor OR 3 minor)
Widening mediastinum
Diffuse ST-segment elevations, PR depression
Aortic Valve Pathology
Mitral Valve Pathology
Acute Rheumatic Fever
Infective Endocarditis
Acute Decompensated Heart Failure
CT angiogram of the chest, MRI, or TEE
Myopericarditis
See pp. 42–43, Valvulopathies
See pp. 42–43, Valvulopathies
See pp. 42–43, Valvulopathies and p. 23, Endocarditis
See pp. 12–14, Heart Failure
Dissection flap present
TTE or cardiac MRI + identify potential reversible causes
Aortic Dissection
Most commonly idiopathic or viral
See p. 497, Vascular Diseases
See pp. 38–41, Pericardial Disease, and pp. 12–14, Heart Failure

Footnotes

1. Modified Duke Criteria:

Major Criteria:

1. Positive blood cultures: Typical organisms (*Staphylococcus aureus, Strep. Viridans*, HACEK, *Strep. gallolyticus*), OR persistently positive cultures (>12 h apart) OR single positive for *Coxiella*.
2. Evidence of endocardial involvement: Echocardiogram positive (vegetation, abscess, new partial dehiscence of prosthetic valve) OR new valvular regurgitation.

Minor Criteria:

1. Predisposition (IV drug use, prosthetic valve, valve lesion with significant turbulent flow).
2. Fever.
3. Vascular phenomena (arterial emboli, septic pulmonary infarcts, mycotic aneurysm, Janeway lesions, conjuctival hemorrhages).
4. Immunological phenomena (glomerulonephritis, Osler nodes, Roth spots, rheumatoid factor +).
5. Microbiological evidence (positive blood cultures not meeting major criteria).

2. Jones Criteria:

Major Manifestations: Carditis, polyarthritis, chorea, erythema marginatum, subcutaneous nodules.
Minor Manifestations: Poly/monoarthralgia, fever, ↑ inflammatory markers (ESR, CRP), prolonged PR interval (unless carditis is major criterion).

FIGURE 1.4

1-5 Non-Ischemic Chest Pain (Pulmonary)

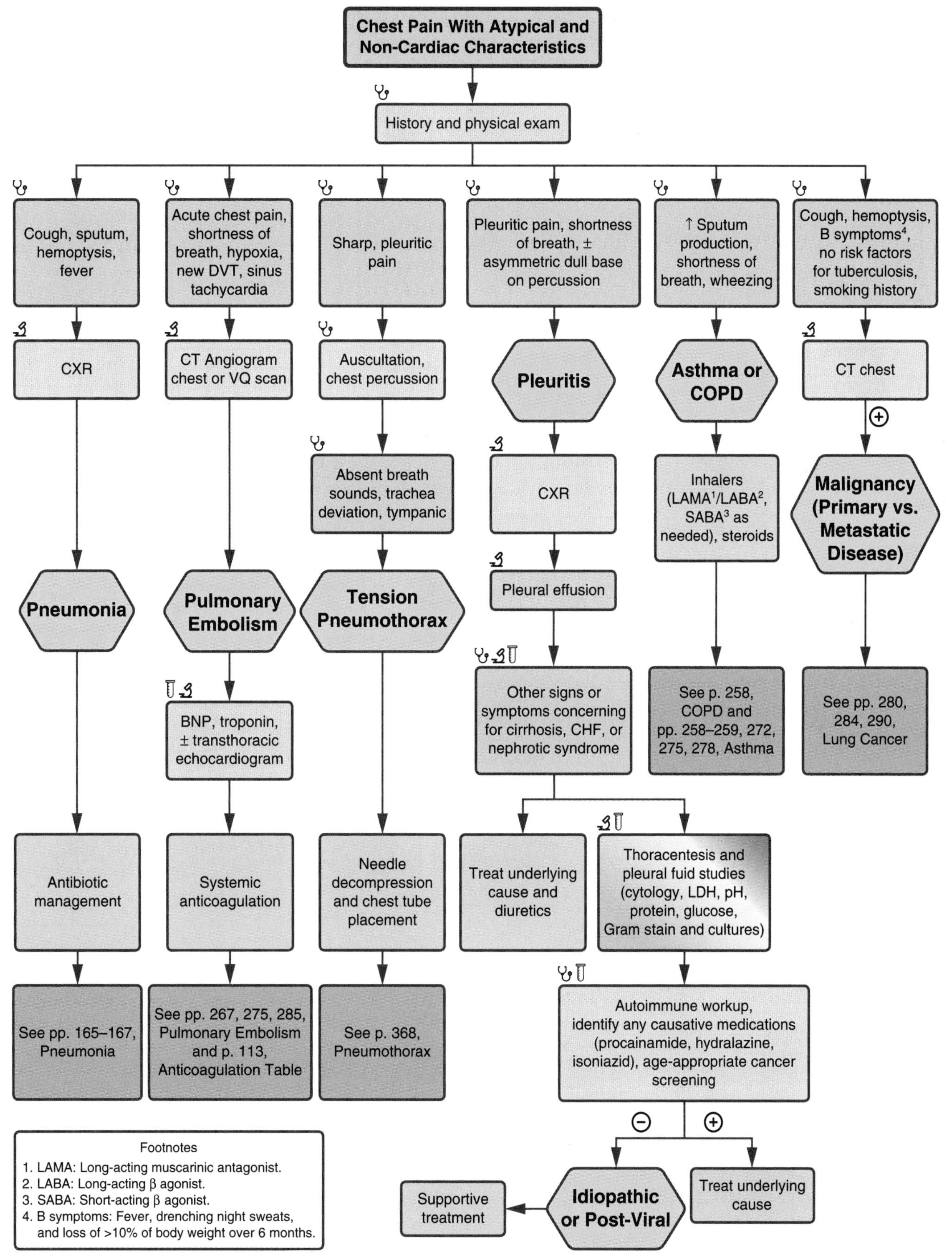
Chest Pain With Atypical and Non-Cardiac Characteristics
History and physical exam
Cough, sputum, hemoptysis, fever
CXR
Pneumonia
Antibiotic management
See pp. 165–167, Pneumonia
Acute chest pain, shortness of breath, hypoxia, new DVT, sinus tachycardia
CT Angiogram chest or VQ scan
Pulmonary Embolism
BNP, troponin, ± transthoracic echocardiogram
Systemic anticoagulation
See pp. 267, 275, 285, Pulmonary Embolism and p. 113, Anticoagulation Table
Sharp, pleuritic pain
Auscultation, chest percussion
Absent breath sounds, trachea deviation, tympanic
Tension Pneumothorax
Needle decompression and chest tube placement
See p. 368, Pneumothorax
Pleuritic pain, shortness of breath, ± asymmetric dull base on percussion
Pleuritis
CXR
Pleural effusion
Other signs or symptoms concerning for cirrhosis, CHF, or nephrotic syndrome
Treat underlying cause and diuretics
Thoracentesis and pleural fuid studies (cytology, LDH, pH, protein, glucose, Gram stain and cultures)
Autoimmune workup, identify any causative medications (procainamide, hydralazine, isoniazid), age-appropriate cancer screening
Idiopathic or Post-Viral
Supportive treatment
Treat underlying cause
↑ Sputum production, shortness of breath, wheezing
Asthma or COPD
Inhalers (LAMA1/LABA2, SABA3 as needed), steroids
See p. 258, COPD and pp. 258–259, 272, 275, 278, Asthma
Cough, hemoptysis, B symptoms4, no risk factors for tuberculosis, smoking history
CT chest
Malignancy (Primary vs. Metastatic Disease)
See pp. 280, 284, 290, Lung Cancer
Footnotes
1. LAMA: Long-acting muscarinic antagonist.
2. LABA: Long-acting β agonist.
3. SABA: Short-acting β agonist.
4. B symptoms: Fever, drenching night sweats, and loss of >10% of body weight over 6 months.

FIGURE 1.5

1-6 Non-Ischemic Chest Pain (GI)

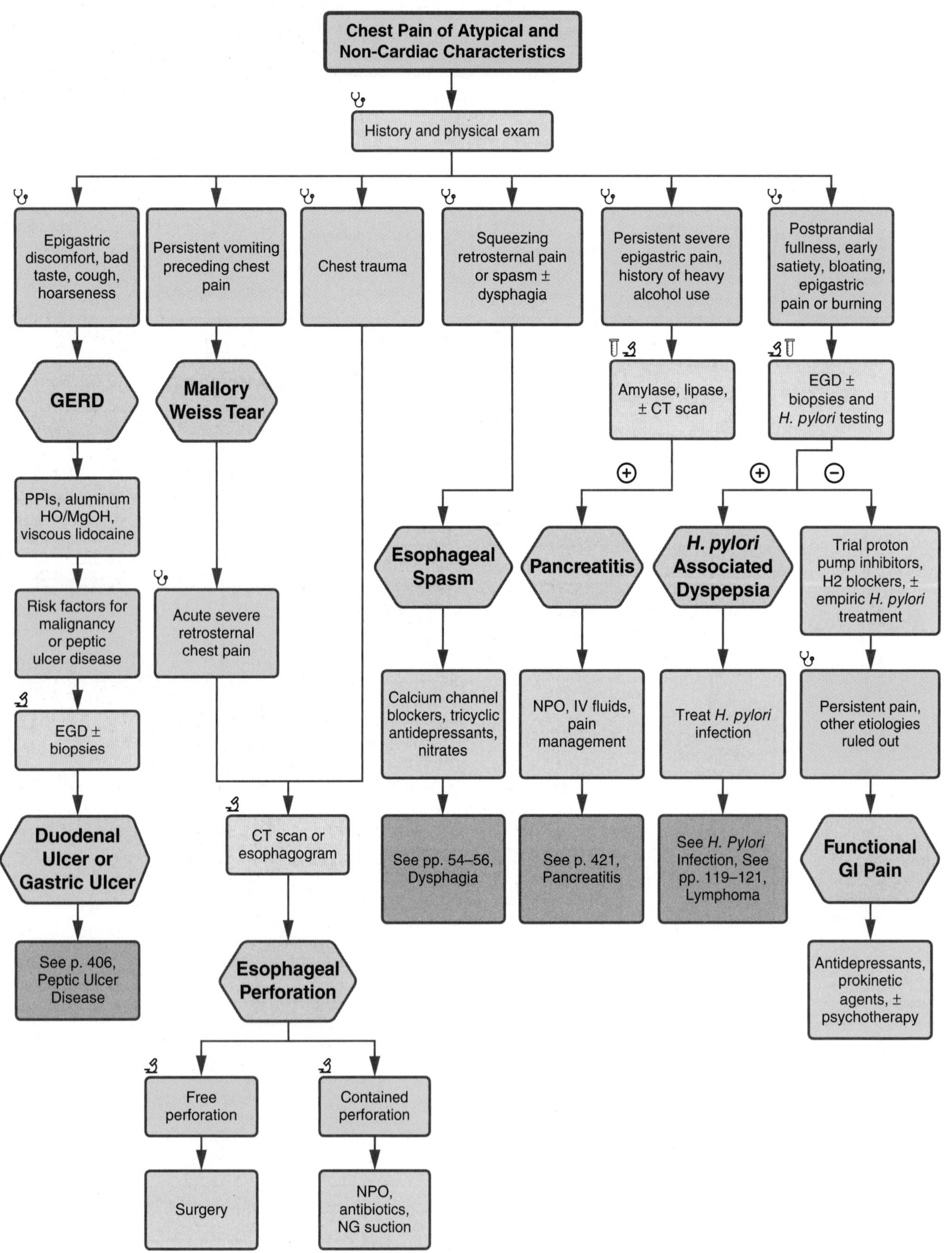
Chest Pain of Atypical and Non-Cardiac Characteristics
History and physical exam
Epigastric discomfort, bad taste, cough, hoarseness
Persistent vomiting preceding chest pain
Chest trauma
Squeezing retrosternal pain or spasm ± dysphagia
Persistent severe epigastric pain, history of heavy alcohol use
Postprandial fullness, early satiety, bloating, epigastric pain or burning
GERD
Mallory Weiss Tear
Amylase, lipase, ± CT scan
EGD ± biopsies and H. pylori testing
PPIs, aluminum HO/MgOH, viscous lidocaine
Esophageal Spasm
Pancreatitis
H. pylori Associated Dyspepsia
Trial proton pump inhibitors, H2 blockers, ± empiric H. pylori treatment
Risk factors for malignancy or peptic ulcer disease
Acute severe retrosternal chest pain
Calcium channel blockers, tricyclic antidepressants, nitrates
NPO, IV fluids, pain management
Treat H. pylori infection
Persistent pain, other etiologies ruled out
EGD ± biopsies
Duodenal Ulcer or Gastric Ulcer
CT scan or esophagogram
See pp. 54–56, Dysphagia
See p. 421, Pancreatitis
See H. Pylori Infection, See pp. 119–121, Lymphoma
Functional GI Pain
See p. 406, Peptic Ulcer Disease
Esophageal Perforation
Antidepressants, prokinetic agents, ± psychotherapy
Free perforation
Contained perforation
Surgery
NPO, antibiotics, NG suction

FIGURE 1.6

1-7 Non-Ischemic Chest Pain (Musculoskeletal)

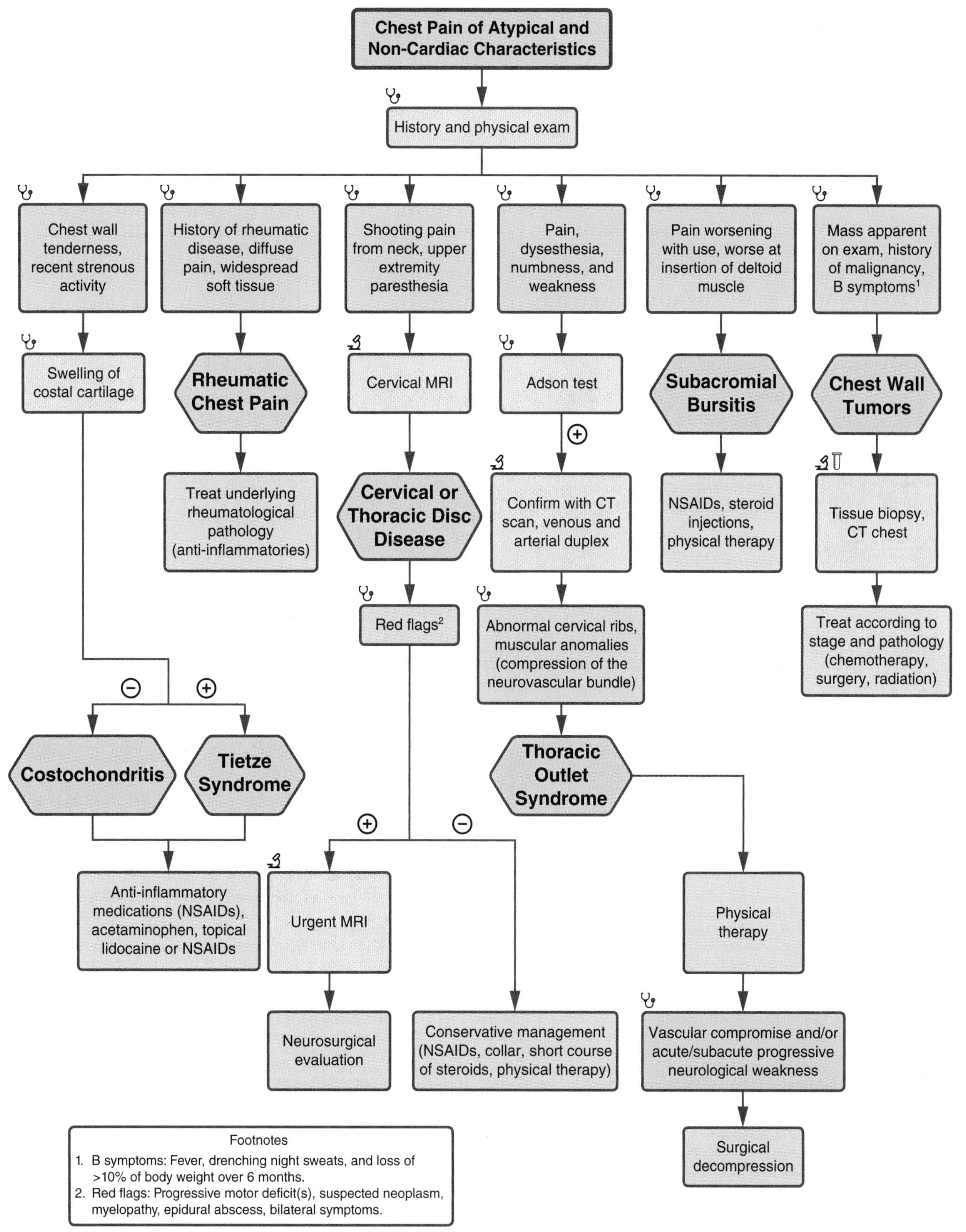

Chest Pain of Atypical and Non-Cardiac Characteristics
History and physical exam
Chest wall tenderness, recent strenous activity
History of rheumatic disease, diffuse pain, widespread soft tissue
Shooting pain from neck, upper extremity paresthesia
Pain, dysesthesia, numbness, and weakness
Pain worsening with use, worse at insertion of deltoid muscle
Mass apparent on exam, history of malignancy, B symptoms1
Swelling of costal cartilage
Rheumatic Chest Pain
Cervical MRI
Adson test
Subacromial Bursitis
Chest Wall Tumors
Treat underlying rheumatological pathology (anti-inflammatories)
Cervical or Thoracic Disc Disease
Confirm with CT scan, venous and arterial duplex
NSAIDs, steroid injections, physical therapy
Tissue biopsy, CT chest
Red flags2
Abnormal cervical ribs, muscular anomalies (compression of the neurovascular bundle)
Treat according to stage and pathology (chemotherapy, surgery, radiation)
Costochondritis
Tietze Syndrome
Thoracic Outlet Syndrome
Anti-inflammatory medications (NSAIDs), acetaminophen, topical lidocaine or NSAIDs
Urgent MRI
Physical therapy
Neurosurgical evaluation
Conservative management (NSAIDs, collar, short course of steroids, physical therapy)
Vascular compromise and/or acute/subacute progressive neurological weakness
Surgical decompression
Footnotes
1. B symptoms: Fever, drenching night sweats, and loss of >10% of body weight over 6 months.
2. Red flags: Progressive motor deficit(s), suspected neoplasm, myelopathy, epidural abscess, bilateral symptoms.

FIGURE 1.7

1-8 Congestive Heart Failure

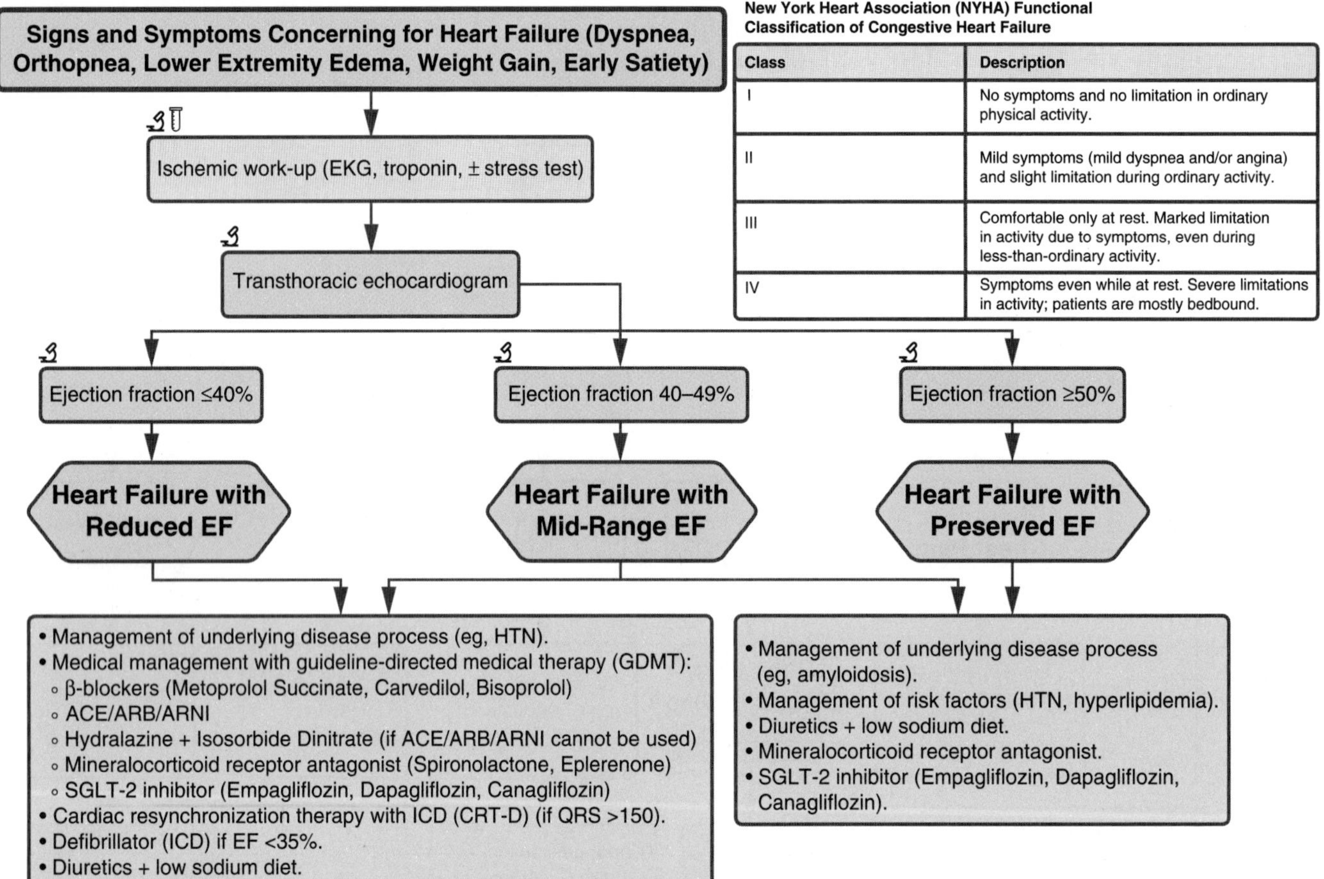
Signs and Symptoms Concerning for Heart Failure (Dyspnea, Orthopnea, Lower Extremity Edema, Weight Gain, Early Satiety)
Ischemic work-up (EKG, troponin, ± stress test)
Transthoracic echocardiogram
Ejection fraction ≤40%
Ejection fraction 40–49%
Ejection fraction ≥50%
Heart Failure with Reduced EF
Heart Failure with Mid-Range EF
Heart Failure with Preserved EF
• Management of underlying disease process (eg, HTN).
• Medical management with guideline-directed medical therapy (GDMT):
∘ β-blockers (Metoprolol Succinate, Carvedilol, Bisoprolol)
∘ ACE/ARB/ARNI
∘ Hydralazine + Isosorbide Dinitrate (if ACE/ARB/ARNI cannot be used)
∘ Mineralocorticoid receptor antagonist (Spironolactone, Eplerenone)
∘ SGLT-2 inhibitor (Empagliflozin, Dapagliflozin, Canagliflozin)
• Cardiac resynchronization therapy with ICD (CRT-D) (if QRS >150).
• Defibrillator (ICD) if EF <35%.
• Diuretics + low sodium diet.
• Management of underlying disease process (eg, amyloidosis).
• Management of risk factors (HTN, hyperlipidemia).
• Diuretics + low sodium diet.
• Mineralocorticoid receptor antagonist.
• SGLT-2 inhibitor (Empagliflozin, Dapagliflozin, Canagliflozin).

New York Heart Association (NYHA) Functional Classification of Congestive Heart Failure

Class	Description
I	No symptoms and no limitation in ordinary physical activity.
II	Mild symptoms (mild dyspnea and/or angina) and slight limitation during ordinary activity.
III	Comfortable only at rest. Marked limitation in activity due to symptoms, even during less-than-ordinary activity.
IV	Symptoms even while at rest. Severe limitations in activity; patients are mostly bedbound.

Congestive heart failure (CHF) is a clinical diagnosis based on a constellation of signs and symptoms. In other algorithms, we discuss etiologies of heart failure, including ischemic heart disease, valvulopathies, and cardiomyopathies. In this next series of algorithms, we discuss the nature of heart failure progression, from acute decompensated heart failure to cardiogenic shock.

Heart failure patients often present with ↑ dyspnea on exertion (DOE) or at rest, orthopnea, paroxysmal nocturnal dyspnea (PND), cough, and/or peripheral edema. The physical exam can show ↑ (>8 cm) jugular venous pressure (JVP), hepatojugular reflux, parasternal lift, abnormal heart sounds (S3: systolic left-sided heart failure, S4: hypertensive heart disease, loud P2: pulmonary hypertension), rales on lung auscultation, and bilateral lower extremity edema. Due to ↑ dyspnea, a chest x-ray is often obtained upon initial evaluation, which can show alveolar edema ("bat's wings"), pleural effusions, interstitial edema (Kerley B lines), cephalization of pulmonary vessels, and cardiomegaly. Labs will often show ↑ brain natriuretic peptide (BNP), ↑ creatinine (due to cardiorenal syndrome), mild troponin elevation due to ↑ cardiac demand, and mild hyponatremia. Treatment generally consists of managing acute decompensated heart failure and addressing volume overload (eg, diuresis with furosemide or bumetanide ± metolazone) and, if applicable, guideline-directed medical therapy (GDMT) to slow progression of chronic heart failure (eg, β-blockers, ACE/ARB/ARNI, mineralocorticoid receptor antagonists, SGLT-2 inhibitors). Risk factors for CHF include coronary artery disease, HTN, diabetes, cardiomyopathy, valvular heart disease, and pulmonary disease (*cor pulmonale*).

Heart failure often only affects the left or right side of the heart but can affect both. **Left-sided heart failure** (most common) results from inability of the left ventricle to pump blood through the systemic circulation. Blood builds up in the pulmonary veins, leading to dyspnea and coughing. Left-sided heart failure is usually caused by ischemic heart disease or longstanding, poorly controlled hypertension. Right-sided heart failure results from inability of the right ventricle to pump blood to the lungs. Blood builds up in the veins that carry blood from organs and tissues back to the heart. ↑ pressure in the veins pushes fluid into the surrounding tissue, leading to peripheral edema in the legs and, if severe, the genital area and abdomen. **Right-sided heart failure** generally develops from advanced left-sided heart failure but can also be due to pulmonary hypertension, pulmonary embolism, or lung diseases such as COPD. **Biventricular heart failure** causes the same symptoms as both left- and right-sided heart failure, including dyspnea and volume overload.

One of the most frequently used heart failure classification systems is the **New York Heart Association (NYHA) Functional Classification**, which classifies heart failure based on a patient's functional status during exertion. The American College of Cardiology (ACC) and the American Heart Association (AHA) developed a different classification system for heart failure that complements the NYHA system by identifying a patient class not present in the NYHA Classification: patients who do not have heart failure yet but are at high risk for developing the condition. Based on ejection fraction, heart failure is classified into 3 types: heart failure with reduced ejection fraction (HFrEF), heart failure with mid-range ejection fraction (HFmEF), and heart failure with preserved ejection fraction (HFpEF). For each stage/class of heart failure, there are guideline-directed medical therapies that can halt or slow disease progression.

The ACC/AHA[1,2] Stages of Heart Failure

Class	Description
A	At high risk for heart failure but without structural heart disease or symptoms of heart failure.
B	Structural heart disease but without signs or symptoms of heart failure.
C	Structural heart disease with prior or current symptoms of heart failure.
D	Refractory heart failure requiring advanced interventions (eg, biventricular pacemakers, left ventricular assist device, transplantation).

[1]The American College of Cardiology (ACC). [2]The American Heart Association (AHA).

FIGURE 1.8

1-9 Acute Decompensated Heart Failure

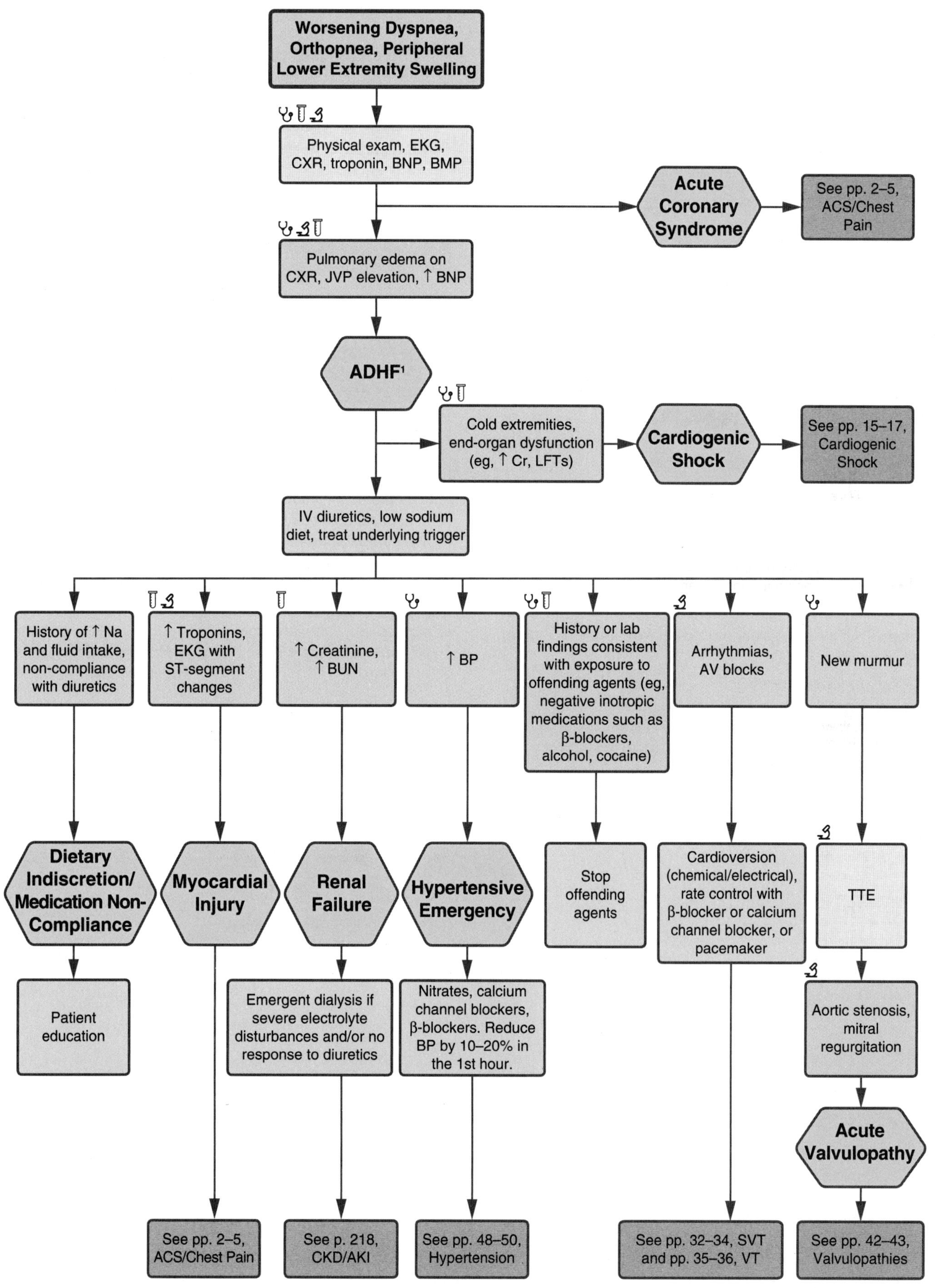
Worsening Dyspnea, Orthopnea, Peripheral Lower Extremity Swelling
Physical exam, EKG, CXR, troponin, BNP, BMP
Acute Coronary Syndrome
See pp. 2–5, ACS/Chest Pain
Pulmonary edema on CXR, JVP elevation, ↑ BNP
ADHF[1]
Cold extremities, end-organ dysfunction (eg, ↑ Cr, LFTs)
Cardiogenic Shock
See pp. 15–17, Cardiogenic Shock
IV diuretics, low sodium diet, treat underlying trigger
History of ↑ Na and fluid intake, non-compliance with diuretics
↑ Troponins, EKG with ST-segment changes
↑ Creatinine, ↑ BUN
↑ BP
History or lab findings consistent with exposure to offending agents (eg, negative inotropic medications such as β-blockers, alcohol, cocaine)
Arrhythmias, AV blocks
New murmur
Dietary Indiscretion/ Medication Non-Compliance
Myocardial Injury
Renal Failure
Hypertensive Emergency
Stop offending agents
Cardioversion (chemical/electrical), rate control with β-blocker or calcium channel blocker, or pacemaker
TTE
Patient education
Emergent dialysis if severe electrolyte disturbances and/or no response to diuretics
Nitrates, calcium channel blockers, β-blockers. Reduce BP by 10–20% in the 1st hour.
Aortic stenosis, mitral regurgitation
Acute Valvulopathy
See pp. 2–5, ACS/Chest Pain
See p. 218, CKD/AKI
See pp. 48–50, Hypertension
See pp. 32–34, SVT and pp. 35–36, VT
See pp. 42–43, Valvulopathies

FIGURE 1.9

1-9 Acute Decompensated Heart Failure

ACUTE DECOMPENSATED HEART FAILURE

A 55-year-old M with PMH of ischemic cardiomyopathy presents with progressive dyspnea for the past 3 days. He also reports orthopnea, paroxysmal nocturnal dyspnea, and increased swelling in his legs to the point that he cannot put on his shoes. He states he has not been taking his diuretics or tracking his salt or fluid intake. **Exam:** JVP elevated, bibasilar crackles, hypoxic, 2+ pitting edema in bilateral lower legs. **Labs/Imaging:** BNP elevated 3× ULN, troponin mildly elevated. EKG without ischemic changes. CXR shows diffuse interstitial opacities concerning for pulmonary edema.

Management

1. IV loop diuretics.
2. Consider cardiogenic shock when a patient has hypotension, cold extremities, decreased mentation, nausea, vomiting, and/or abdominal pain and labs are concerning for poor organ perfusion (elevated AST/ALT, creatinine, lactate). If so, start positive inotropic agents (milrinone, dobutamine) and transfer to ICU.
3. Guideline-directed medical therapy (GDMT) according to patient's ACC/AHA stage for chronic HF:
   a. A = consider ACE/ARBs if they have HTN or DM.
   b. B = GDMT if reduced EF, ICD if EF <30%, CRT (resynchronization) if QRS >150 ms.
   c. C = diuretics for symptom management + all measures for Stage B. Can add digoxin, nitrate, or hydralazine if symptoms are not well-controlled.
   d. D = all measures for Stages A–C, consider IV inotropes, ventricular assistance device, or transplant.

Complications: Cardiogenic shock, acute respiratory insufficiency, hyponatremia, arrhythmias, acute renal failure.

HYF:

- The most common cause of heart failure and decompensation is ischemic heart disease.
- Interventions that decrease mortality in HFrEF: β-blocker, ARB/ACE/ARNI, mineralocorticoid receptor antagonist, SGLT2i, CRT, and ICD (when indicated).

Classification of Diuretics

Drug Class	Adverse Effects/Toxicities
Osmotic diuretics (eg, mannitol, isosorbide)	Dehydration, pulmonary edema
Loop diuretics (potassium-wasting) (eg, furosemide, torsemide, bumetanide, ethacrynic acid)	Hypokalemia, hypocalcemia, hyperuricemia, ototoxicity
Thiazide diuretics (eg, hydrochlorothiazide, amiloride, chlorthalidone, metolazone)	Hypokalemia, hyponatremia, metabolic alkalosis, hyperglycemia, hyperlipidemia, hypercalcemia, hyperuricemia
Potassium-Sparing agents (eg, mineralocorticoid receptor antagonists [spironolactone, eplerenone], Na^+ channel inhibitors [amiloride, triamterene])	Hyperkalemia, sexual dysfunction, gynecomastia (not eplerenone)
Carbonic anhydrase inhibitors (eg, acetazolamide, dorzolamide)	Paresthesias, hyperchloremic metabolic acidosis, hyperammonemia, sulfa allergy reaction

1-10 Cardiogenic Shock

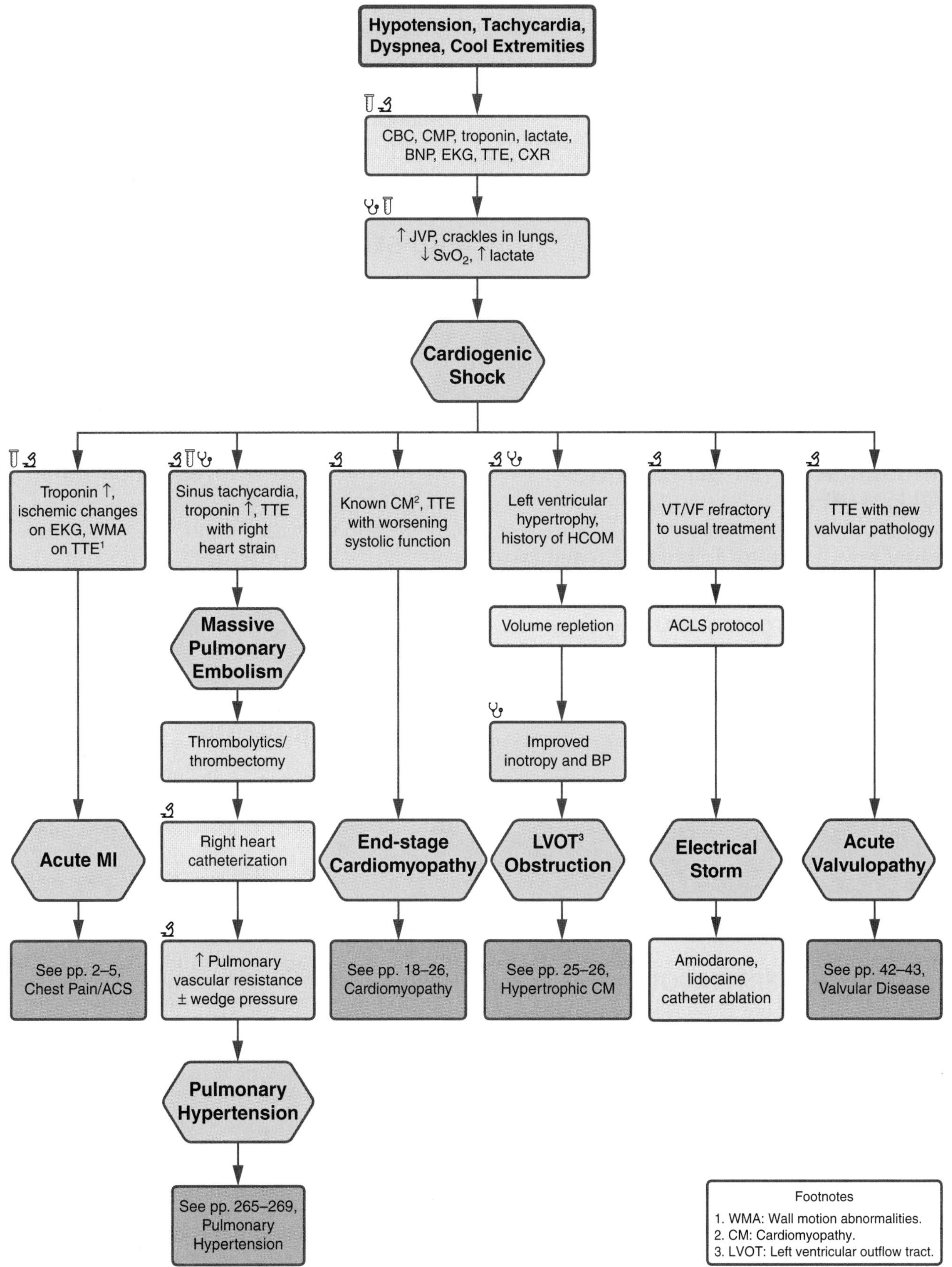
Hypotension, Tachycardia, Dyspnea, Cool Extremities
CBC, CMP, troponin, lactate, BNP, EKG, TTE, CXR
↑ JVP, crackles in lungs, ↓ SvO_2, ↑ lactate
Cardiogenic Shock
Troponin ↑, ischemic changes on EKG, WMA on TTE[1]
Sinus tachycardia, troponin ↑, TTE with right heart strain
Known CM[2], TTE with worsening systolic function
Left ventricular hypertrophy, history of HCOM
VT/VF refractory to usual treatment
TTE with new valvular pathology
Massive Pulmonary Embolism
Volume repletion
ACLS protocol
Thrombolytics/ thrombectomy
Improved inotropy and BP
Right heart catheterization
Acute MI
End-stage Cardiomyopathy
LVOT[3] Obstruction
Electrical Storm
Acute Valvulopathy
See pp. 2–5, Chest Pain/ACS
↑ Pulmonary vascular resistance ± wedge pressure
See pp. 18–26, Cardiomyopathy
See pp. 25–26, Hypertrophic CM
Amiodarone, lidocaine catheter ablation
See pp. 42–43, Valvular Disease
Pulmonary Hypertension
See pp. 265–269, Pulmonary Hypertension
Footnotes
1. WMA: Wall motion abnormalities.
2. CM: Cardiomyopathy.
3. LVOT: Left ventricular outflow tract.

FIGURE 1.10

1-10 Cardiogenic Shock

ACUTE MI

A 54-year-old M with PMH of hyperlipidemia and T2DM presents with chest pain radiating down the left arm. **Exam:** Hypotension, cool clammy extremities, diaphoresis. **Labs/Imaging:** Elevated troponin, lactate, and LFTs; EKG with ST segment elevation in contiguous leads (eg, II, III, aVF) and corresponding hypokinetic segment on TTE.

Management:

1. Support perfusion with pressors, inotropes, and/or mechanical circulatory support.
2. Coronary artery reperfusion (PCI, CABG).

Complications: Cardiac rupture (ventricular septum, papillary muscle, cardiac wall), valvular regurgitation.

HYF: Acute MI is caused by plaque rupture causing transmural infarct.

HIGH-RISK/MASSIVE PULMONARY EMBOLISM (PE)

A 39-year-old F G1P0 GA 28W with PMH of antiphospholipid syndrome and recent overseas travel presents with acute dyspnea and presyncope. **Exam:** Hypotension, tachycardia, cool clammy extremities, SpO_2 92% with new O_2 requirement of 4L O_2. **Labs/Imaging:** Elevated troponin, Cr, BNP, and LFTs; right heart strain on EKG (S1Q3T3), flattening of the intraventricular septum, and RV dysfunction with sparing of the apex on TTE (McConnell sign); perfusion defect on CTA chest.

Management

1. TPA or surgical/IR thrombectomy.

Complications: Acute RV failure, hypoxia, eventual LV failure, cardiac arrest.

HYF: PEs are considered massive (high-risk) if there is hemodynamic compromise. The Wells' score and Geneva score are 2 scoring systems to quantify the risk of PE.

PULMONARY HYPERTENSION

A 50-year-old M with PMH of severe obstructive sleep apnea presents with acute dyspnea and altered mental status. **Exam:** JVD, Kussmaul sign, peripheral edema. **Labs/Imaging:** EKG showing RV hypertrophy and dilation; TTE with elevated pulmonary artery pressures (mPAP >20 mmHg or sPAP >30 mmHg), RV septal flattening, non-compressible IVC.

Management:

1. Aggressive oxygenation and treatment of hypercapnia for maximal pulmonary vasodilation (avoid intubation; if intubated, avoid excess airway pressures), maintain mean arterial pressure.
2. Consider inhaled pulmonary vasodilators for refractory hypoxemia (contraindication = LV failure). See Pulmonary Hypertension, pp. 265–269 for further management outside of acute shock.

Complications: Cardiac arrest from right ventricular failure or hypoxia.

HYF: Pulmonary hypertension will lead to right ventricular failure.

END-STAGE CARDIOMYOPATHY

A 74-year-old M with PMH of HFrEF (EF 20%) 2/2 ischemic cardiomyopathy presents with worsening lower extremity edema, weight gain, anuria, and persistent nausea. **Exam:** Hypotension, altered mental status, cool and clammy extremities, bilateral lower extremity edema. **Labs/Imaging:** Elevated lactate, creatinine, LFTs (ie, end-organ damage due to hypoperfusion).

Management:

1. Support perfusion with pressors, inotropes and/or mechanical circulatory support.

Complications: Sudden cardiac death/arrhythmias/cardiac arrest.

HYF: Consider palliative care consult given that end-stage cardiomyopathy without options for transplantation or other advanced therapies has an extremely high mortality.

LEFT VENTRICULAR OUTFLOW TRACT (LVOT) OBSTRUCTION

A 26-year-old M with family history of sudden cardiac death presents with lightheadedness and dyspnea after a 20-mile hike. **Exam:** Harsh crescendo-decrescendo systolic murmur, heard best at the apex and lower left sternal border, which decreases in intensity with passive leg raise and worsens with Valsalva maneuver. **Labs/Imaging:** Elevated lactate, creatinine, and LFTs; EKG shows left ventricular hypertrophy; TTE shows LV outflow tract obstruction.

Management

1. Increase preload with IV fluids, support perfusion with pressors. Avoid inotropes to allow for increased diastolic filling and preload to maximize stroke volume and cardiac output.
2. Specific management for the cause of LVOT: For example, the patient here has HOCM, which is managed with nodal blocking agents and potentially alcohol septal ablation (See Cardiomyopathy, pp. 18–24). In patients with LVOT obstruction due to other etiologies (eg, severe aortic stenosis), treatment would be valve replacement (see Valvular Heart Disease on pp. 42–43 and Hypertrophic CM on pp. 25–26).

Complications: Sudden cardiac death, arrhythmias.

1-10 Cardiogenic Shock

HYF:

- Vasodilators and diuretics should be used with caution or avoided in patients with significant LVOT obstruction (preload-dependent).
- Genetically determined heart muscle disease is most often caused by mutations in one of several sarcomere genes, which encode components of the contractile apparatus. Genetic counseling is offered to these patients and their relatives.

ELECTRICAL STORM

A 74-year-old M with PMH of HFrEF (EF 20%) 2/2 ischemic cardiomyopathy is brought by EMS after an episode of syncope. He was noted to be in unstable ventricular tachycardia when EMS arrived and he was given 2 shocks. **Exam:** Hypotension, altered mental status, cool and clammy extremities, bilateral lower extremity edema. **Labs/Imaging:** Cardiac monitor shows sustained VT. Elevated lactate, liver function tests, creatinine (ie, end-organ damage due to hypoperfusion).

Management:

1. Antiarrhythmics (amiodarone, lidocaine).
2. Consider ischemia as a triggering factor and activate the cath lab.
3. Catheter ablation.
4. Placement of implantable cardiac defibrillator (ICD).

Complications: Cardiac arrest/sudden cardia death.

HYF:

- Common triggers: Drug toxicity, electrolyte disturbances, new or worsened heart failure, and acute myocardial ischemia.

1-11 Cardiomyopathy

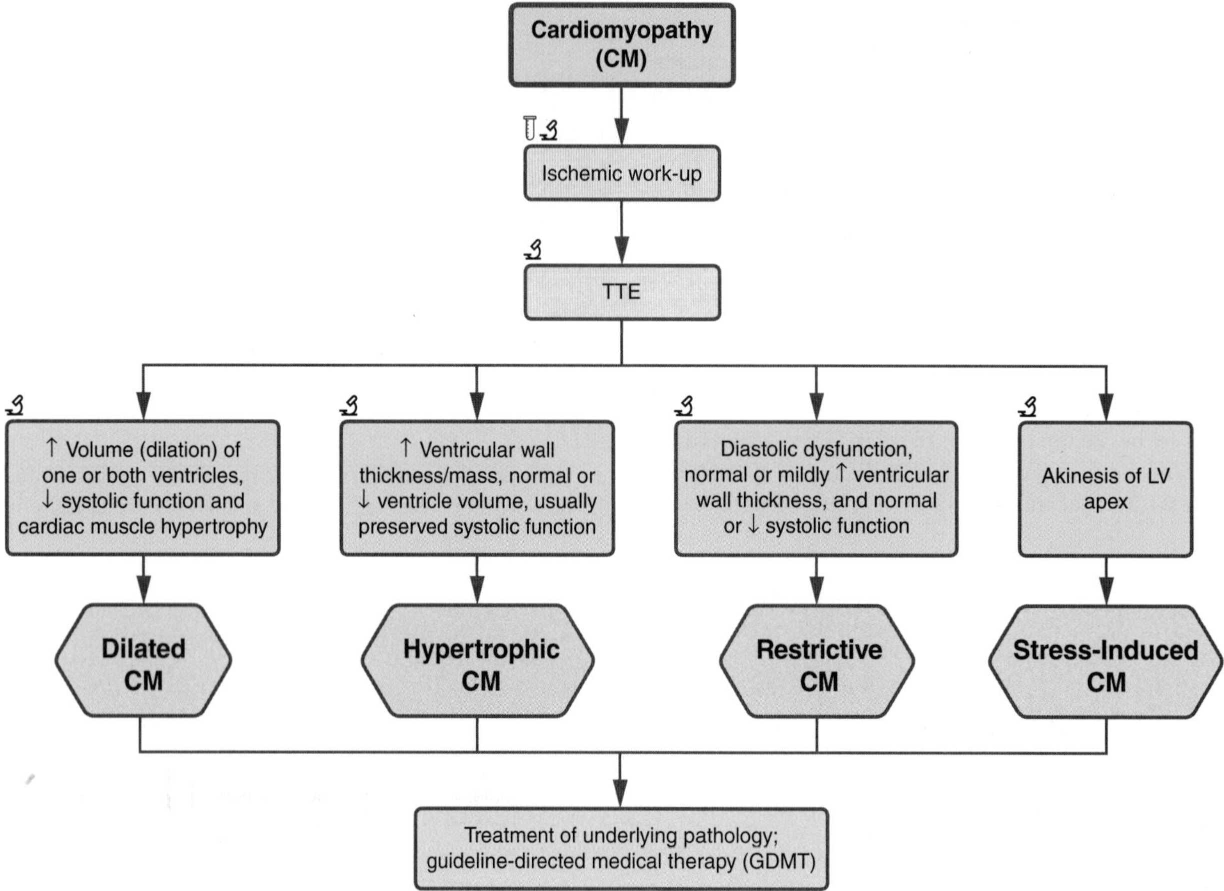
Cardiomyopathy (CM)
Ischemic work-up
TTE
↑ Volume (dilation) of one or both ventricles, ↓ systolic function and cardiac muscle hypertrophy
↑ Ventricular wall thickness/mass, normal or ↓ ventricle volume, usually preserved systolic function
Diastolic dysfunction, normal or mildly ↑ ventricular wall thickness, and normal or ↓ systolic function
Akinesis of LV apex
Dilated CM
Hypertrophic CM
Restrictive CM
Stress-Induced CM
Treatment of underlying pathology; guideline-directed medical therapy (GDMT)

Cardiomyopathy (CM) is an acquired or hereditary disease of the myocardium that reduces the heart's ability to pump blood, often leading to development of arrhythmias and heart failure. Ischemic CM is the most common cause of CM in the United States. Due to the prevalence of ischemic CM and its potential to be treated with revascularization, the first step whenever a patient has a new diagnosis of CM or presents with new heart failure symptoms is almost always an evaluation for ischemic heart disease (eg, EKG, serial troponins, stress testing, coronary angiogram). Exceptions can be made for specific cases of young adults with classic presenting symptoms suggestive of other etiologies. After that initial step, based on history, labs, and findings on transthoracic echocardiogram (TTE), CM can be classified into dilated, hypertrophic, restrictive, or lastly stress-induced CM.

Dilated CM is characterized by systolic dysfunction and is the most common cause of CM. It displays eccentric hypertrophy (sarcomeres added in series) and is most often idiopathic or familial (mutation of *TTN* gene encoding the sarcomeric protein titin). Known 2° causes include ischemic heart disease (most common), poorly controlled longstanding HTN, alcohol, post-infectious myocarditis, drugs (doxorubicin, zidovudine, cocaine), peripartum status, radiation, infection (coxsackievirus, HIV, Chagas disease, parasites), endocrinopathies (thyroid disease, acromegaly, pheochromocytoma), and nutritional disorders (wet beriberi). Classic findings include S3 and systolic regurgitant murmur on auscultation, balloon appearance of heart on CXR, and dilated heart on TTE.

Hypertrophic CM is characterized by diastolic dysfunction due to impaired left ventricular relaxation and filling as a result of thickened ventricular walls. It displays concentric hypertrophy (sarcomeres added in parallel). Etiologies include longstanding hypertension (most common cause), aortic stenosis, and Friedrich's ataxia. The congenital variant is hypertrophic obstructive cardiomyopathy (HOCM), which is characterized by hypertrophy that involves the interventricular septum. Asymmetric septal hypertrophy and systolic anterior motion of the mitral valve leads to left ventricular outflow tract obstruction (LVOT) and impaired ejection of blood, leading to heart failure, possible syncope during exercise, and sudden death due to ventricular arrhythmias. Classic findings of hypertrophic CM include S4, systolic murmur on auscultation, and mitral regurgitation due to impaired mitral valve closure on TTE. EKG may be normal or show signs of left ventricular hypertrophy; in HOCM, septal Q waves in the inferolateral leads are common.

Restrictive CM is characterized by diastolic dysfunction without significant systolic dysfunction (a normal or near-normal EF) due to ↓ myocardial elasticity. Etiologies include infiltrative disease (eg, amyloidosis, hemochromatosis, sarcoidosis), scleroderma, Loeffler eosinophilic endocarditis (associated with hypereosinophilic syndrome), endomyocardial fibrosis, and radiation leading to scarring and fibrosis. Classic findings include signs and symptoms of right-sided heart failure (JVD, peripheral edema, ascites) that often predominate over left-sided heart failure, left bundle branch block and low voltages on EKG (especially in amyloidosis), rapid early filling and normal to near-normal EF on TTE, and fibrosis or evidence of infiltrative disease on cardiac biopsy. The mainstay of management of restrictive CM (besides treatment of the underlying disorder) involves management of volume status without excessive diuresis due to preload dependence, optimization of hemodynamics and heart failure symptoms, and management of arrhythmias.

Stress-induced CM (otherwise known as Takotsubo's CM or broken heart syndrome) is characterized by ventricular apical ballooning likely due to ↑ catecholamine stimulation in the setting of physical or emotional stress (eg, critical illness, death of loved one). Patients can present with chest pain typical of an MI, and there is often also evidence of ischemia based on EKG (eg, ST-elevation, T-wave inversions in the anterior precordial leads) and ↑ troponins, but coronary angiography would not show evidence of obstructive coronary artery disease. Classically, TTE shows impaired contractility and left ventricular dysfunction with mid- and apical hypokinesis and basilar hyperkinesis leading to a distinctive balloon shape.

Generally, once there is an established diagnosis of CM and heart failure, the treatment will be largely based on guideline-directed medical therapy, diuretics for symptom control, and individualized interventions depending on the specific etiology.

FIGURE 1.11

1-12 Dilated Cardiomyopathy

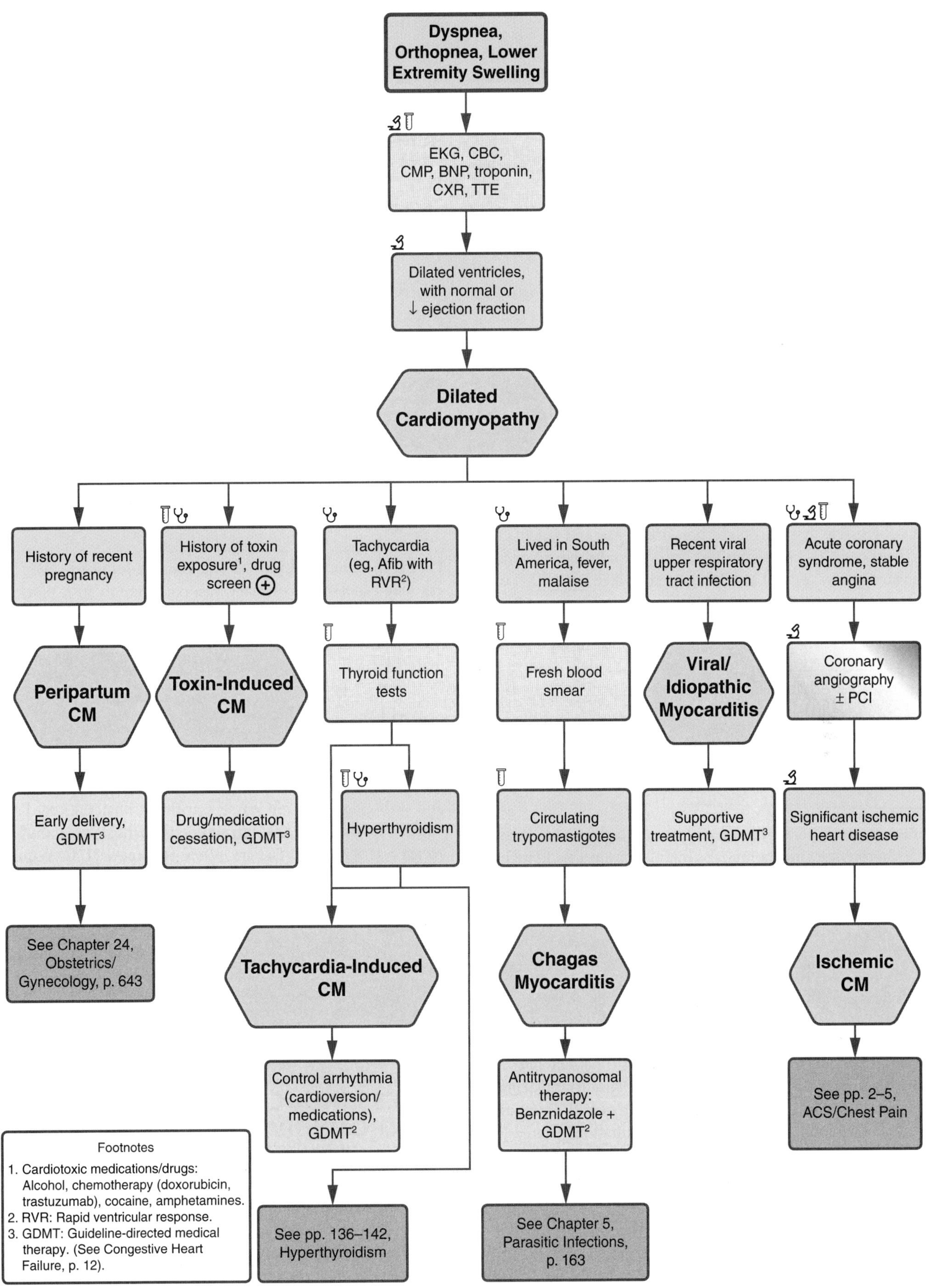
Dyspnea, Orthopnea, Lower Extremity Swelling
EKG, CBC, CMP, BNP, troponin, CXR, TTE
Dilated ventricles, with normal or ↓ ejection fraction
Dilated Cardiomyopathy
History of recent pregnancy
History of toxin exposure[1], drug screen ⊕
Tachycardia (eg, Afib with RVR[2])
Lived in South America, fever, malaise
Recent viral upper respiratory tract infection
Acute coronary syndrome, stable angina
Peripartum CM
Toxin-Induced CM
Thyroid function tests
Fresh blood smear
Viral/ Idiopathic Myocarditis
Coronary angiography ± PCI
Early delivery, GDMT[3]
Drug/medication cessation, GDMT[3]
Hyperthyroidism
Circulating trypomastigotes
Supportive treatment, GDMT[3]
Significant ischemic heart disease
See Chapter 24, Obstetrics/ Gynecology, p. 643
Tachycardia-Induced CM
Chagas Myocarditis
Ischemic CM
Control arrhythmia (cardioversion/ medications), GDMT[2]
Antitrypanosomal therapy: Benznidazole + GDMT[2]
See pp. 2–5, ACS/Chest Pain
See pp. 136–142, Hyperthyroidism
See Chapter 5, Parasitic Infections, p. 163
Footnotes
1. Cardiotoxic medications/drugs: Alcohol, chemotherapy (doxorubicin, trastuzumab), cocaine, amphetamines.
2. RVR: Rapid ventricular response.
3. GDMT: Guideline-directed medical therapy. (See Congestive Heart Failure, p. 12).

FIGURE 1.12

1-12 Dilated Cardiomyopathy

PERIPARTUM CARDIOMYOPATHY

A 32-year-old F who is 2 months postpartum presents with subacute dyspnea on exertion, bilateral lower extremity swelling, and orthopnea. **Exam:** Hypoxic with 2L O_2 requirement, 2+ pitting edema on bilateral lower extremities, JVD elevated to 12 cm. **Labs/Imaging:** Elevated BNP, CXR with pulmonary edema, normal EKG, newly reduced LVEF of 40% on TTE.

Management:

1. Delivery (C-section) should be considered for antepartum patients with acute heart failure.

Complications: Heart failure, cardiogenic shock.

HYF: Diagnosed between 1 month antepartum to 5 months postpartum. Avoid ACE/ARBs and MRAs in antepartum patients due to teratogenicity.

TACHYCARDIA-INDUCED CARDIOMYOPATHY

A 58-year-old M with PMH of hyperthyroidism presents with palpitations, progressive dyspnea on exertion, orthopnea, and weight gain. **Exam:** Heart rate 120–130, 2+ pitting edema to mid-thigh bilaterally, JVP elevated to 10–12 cm. **Labs/Imaging:** Elevated BNP, CXR with pulmonary edema, EKG with atrial fibrillation and frequent PVCs, TTE with dilated LV without hypertrophy.

Management: Management of tachyarrhythmia (eg, β-blocker, calcium channel blocker, amiodarone). See Arrhythmia on pp. 32–36 for further details.

Complications: Heart failure, cardiogenic shock.

HYF:

- Common conditions that may lead to tachycardia include hyperthyroidism and anemia; the initial workup should include TFTs and CBC.
- Diagnosis is confirmed by recovery of EF ~1–6 months after treatment of tachycardia and management of HF.

GIANT CELL MYOCARDITIS

A 22-year-old F with PMH of Crohn's disease presents with acute onset bilateral lower extremity swelling, chest pain, and dyspnea; within several hours of arrival to the ED, the patient becomes altered with worsening hypoxia. **Exam:** Irregularly irregular heart rhythm with HR 120s, BP 90/52, SpO_2 90% with new 2L O_2 requirement, crackles in bilateral lung bases on auscultation, elvated JVP to 12 cm, pitting edema to mid-shins bilaterally. **Labs/Imaging:** Elevated BNP and lactate, CXR with pulmonary edema, EKG with atrial fibrillation and frequent PVCs, TTE with biventricular dilation and no evidence of hypertrophy. Endomyocardial biopsy shows myocyte necrosis and a diffuse inflammatory cell infiltrate composed of T lymphocytes, multinucleated giant cells, plasma cells, and eosinophils.

Management:

1. Immunosuppressive therapy.
2. Cardiac transplant if immunosuppressive therapy is ineffective.

Complications: Acute heart failure, cardiogenic shock. Recurrence in ~25% of transplanted hearts.

HYF: Usually acute and fulminant presentation with poor prognosis. Strong association with autoimmune disorders and tumors of immune cells such as thymoma or lymphoma.

TOXIN-INDUCED CARDIOMYOPATHY

A 42-year-old F with PMH of alcohol use disorder presents with progressive lower extremity swelling, dyspnea on exertion, and palpitations. **Exam:** 2+ lower extremity pitting edema to shins, coarse crackles in bilateral lung fields. **Labs/Imaging:** Elevated BNP, serum ethanol level 159 mg/dL. TTE is notable for dilated and hypokinetic ventricles.

Management: Stop exposure to offending substance.

Complications: Heart failure, cardiogenic shock.

HYF: If stimulant-induced (eg, cocaine-induced CM), β-blockers may exacerbate coronary vasoconstriction so β-blockers with α activity (eg, labetolol) are preferred for GDMT. Associated with alcohol and illicit drug use (eg, cocaine, amphetamines), as well as various medications including anthracyclines (eg, **d**oxorubicin, **d**aunorubicin; prevent with **d**exrazoxane) and trastuzumab.

VIRAL/IDIOPATHIC MYOCARDITIS

A 24-year-old M with PMH of recent upper respiratory infection presents with progressive DOE, bilateral lower extremity swelling, and orthopnea. **Exam:** Coarse crackles at bilateral lung bases, elevated JVP, symmetrical 2+ pitting edema to the knees. **Labs/Imaging:** Heart rate 85, BP 90/58, SpO_2 90% with new 3L O_2 requirement, enlarged cardiac silhouette and pulmonary edema on CXR, LV dilation and global hypokinesis on TTE.

Management: Supportive measures.

Complications: Heart failure, cardiogenic shock.

HYF: Low utility of anti-viral therapy, as patient often presents days to months after acute viral infection.

STRESS-INDUCED (TAKOTSUBO) CARDIOMYOPATHY

A 68-year-old F with multiple traumatic injuries s/p surgical repair after falling down 2 flights of stairs was found to have chest pain and acute signs and symptoms of volume overload on post-op day 2. **Exam:** Multiple facial lacerations and diffuse ecchymoses, coarse crackles in bilateral lung fields. **Labs/Imaging:** ST-elevations in the anterior precordial leads on EKG, modest elevation in troponin. Coronary angiogram does not show any obstructive coronary

1-12 Dilated Cardiomyopathy

lesions but does reveal apical ballooning on left ventricular angiography. TTE confirms apical ballooning seen on angiogram.

Management: Supportive measures, as condition self-resolves in several weeks.

Complications: Heart failure, cardiogenic shock.

HYF: Takotsubo CM is a diagnosis of exclusion. Characterized by a transient systolic dysfunction of the apical and/or mid-segments of the left ventricle with hyperkinesis of the basal segments, leading to a "balloon-like" appearance of the left ventricle. Patients often present with chest pain suggestive of MI and/or symptoms of decompensated heart failure. EKG can show evidence of ischemia in the anterior precordial leads, and cardiac enzymes can be elevated. However, coronary angiography would rule out obstructive coronary artery disease. It is seen predominantly in post-menopausal women who have experienced severe physical or emotional stress (eg, critical illness, new cancer diagnosis). Patients who recover from Takotsubo CM have a 2% per year risk of recurrence.

1-13 Restrictive Cardiomyopathy

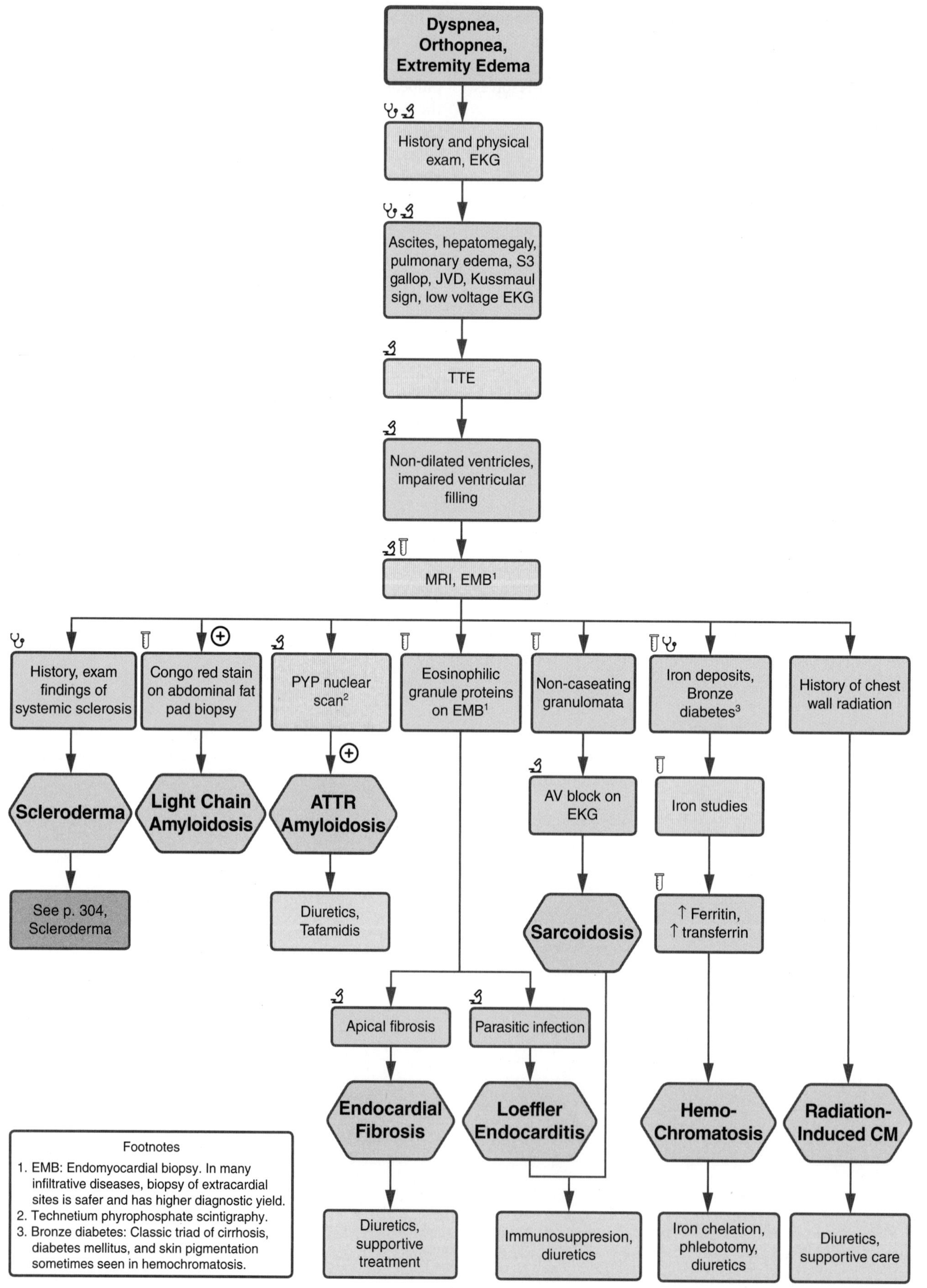
Dyspnea, Orthopnea, Extremity Edema
History and physical exam, EKG
Ascites, hepatomegaly, pulmonary edema, S3 gallop, JVD, Kussmaul sign, low voltage EKG
TTE
Non-dilated ventricles, impaired ventricular filling
MRI, EMB1
History, exam findings of systemic sclerosis
Congo red stain on abdominal fat pad biopsy
PYP nuclear scan2
Eosinophilic granule proteins on EMB1
Non-caseating granulomata
Iron deposits, Bronze diabetes3
History of chest wall radiation
Scleroderma
Light Chain Amyloidosis
ATTR Amyloidosis
AV block on EKG
Iron studies
See p. 304, Scleroderma
Diuretics, Tafamidis
Sarcoidosis
↑ Ferritin, ↑ transferrin
Apical fibrosis
Parasitic infection
Endocardial Fibrosis
Loeffler Endocarditis
Hemo-Chromatosis
Radiation-Induced CM
Diuretics, supportive treatment
Immunosuppresion, diuretics
Iron chelation, phlebotomy, diuretics
Diuretics, supportive care
Footnotes
1. EMB: Endomyocardial biopsy. In many infiltrative diseases, biopsy of extracardial sites is safer and has higher diagnostic yield.
2. Technetium phyrophosphate scintigraphy.
3. Bronze diabetes: Classic triad of cirrhosis, diabetes mellitus, and skin pigmentation sometimes seen in hemochromatosis.

FIGURE 1.13

1-13 Restrictive Cardiomyopathy

SCLERODERMA/SYSTEMIC SCLEROSIS (SSC)

A 42-year-old F with PMH of Reynaud disease, GERD, and recurrent angina presents with worsening dyspnea on exertion and LE swelling. **Exam:** Irregularly irregular rate and rhythm, paradoxical JVD on inspiration, and ulcers on fingertips, 1+ pitting edema to knees bilaterally. **Labs/Imaging:** (+) ANA, anti-Scl-70 antibody. Troponins are WNL. EKG shows new atrial fibrillation. TTE shows normal EF and diastolic dysfunction. Cardiac MRI shows diffuse subendocardial interstitial fibrosis.

Management:

1. Start immunosuppressive therapies (eg, glucocorticoids) to prevent disease progression. See Scleroderma on p. 304.

Complications: Pulmonary hypertension, heart failure.

HYF: Cardiac involvement in SSc is often due to recurrent coronary microvascular ischemia, which leads to myocardial inflammation, necrosis, and eventual fibrosis.

AMYLOIDOSIS

A 83-year-old M with PMH of neuropathy presents with syncopal episodes. **Exam:** Irregularly irregular HR, anasarca, hepatomegaly, diffuse ecchymoses. **Labs/Imaging:** Protein gap (total protein – albumin >4), elevated spot urine protein: creatinine ratio, low-voltage EKG with 2nd-degree Mobitz II block. TTE reveals biventricular diastolic dysfunction and dilated atria. Technetium phyrophosphate scintigraphy (PYP scan) is suggestive of cardiac amyloidosis. Diagnosis is confirmed with abdominal fat pad aspiration showing apple-green birefringence on Congo red stain.

Management:

1. Treatment of amyloidosis. For transthyretin (TTR) amyloidosis, specific agents include tafamidis or inotersen. For light chain (AL) amyloidosis, treatment includes chemotherapy agents and/or bone marrow transplant.

Complications: Heart failure, cardiogenic shock, extra-cardiac complications of amyloidosis (eg, multi-organ failure).

HYF:

- Amyloidosis is the most common cause of restrictive CM in the US. AL amyloidosis is the most common overall cause of amyloidosis. Wild-type transthyretin is most commonly found in elderly individuals.
- In patients with restrictive cardiomyopathy and a protein gap, consider sending serum protein electrophoresis (SPEP) and urine protein electrophoresis (UPEP) to work up light chain amyloidosis.

LOEFFLER ENDOCARDITIS

A 58-year-old F with PMH of eosinophilic esophagitis presents with progressively worsening dyspnea and lower extremity edema. **Exam:** JVD, hepatomegaly, 2+ pitting edema. **Labs/Imaging:** Elevated absolute eosinophil count. EKG with 1st-degree AV block and left atrial enlargement. TTE shows severe left atrial enlargement and diastolic dysfunction. Cardiac MRI shows diffuse endocardial late gadolinium enhancement consistent with fibrosis. EMB shows eosinophilic infiltrate.

Management:

1. High-dose steroids for immunosuppression.

Complications: Heart failure, cardiogenic shock.

HYF: Loeffler endocarditis is a cardiac manifestation of hypereosinophilic syndromes.

SARCOIDOSIS

A 47-year-old F presents with subacute onset of palpitations. **Exam:** Heart rate irregularly irregular, tender raised nodules on the shins. **Labs/Imaging:** Mild anemia, hypercalcemia. CXR shows prominent bilateral hilar adenopathy. EKG shows low voltage QRS complexes, 1st-degree AV block, and frequent PVCs. TTE shows EF 55–60% and diastolic dysfunction. Cardiac MRI shows multifocal areas of late gadolinium enhancement. Biopsy of hilar lymph nodes shows non-caseating granulomas.

Management:

1. Treat conduction abnormalities. Consider pacemaker/defibrillator implantation if indicated for heart block.
2. Start immunosuppressive therapies (eg, glucocorticoids) to prevent disease progression.

Complications: Arrhythmias, heart failure, cardiogenic shock.

HYF: Sarcoidosis can manifest as restrictive or dilated cardiomyopathy. Females > Males. A typical question stem will suggest bilateral hilar lymphadenopathy, possible pulmonary reticular opacities, as well as skin, joint, or eye lesions. Cardiac involvement is suggested by the presence of arrhythmias, conduction abnormalities, or symptoms of heart failure. Though biopsy of extra-cardiac sites (eg, hilar lymph nodes) is preferred, EMB is reasonable if there are isolated cardiac manifestations and high suspicion of cardiac sarcoidosis.

HEMOCHROMATOSIS

A 35-year-old F with PMH of T2DM presents with subacute lower extremity swelling and dyspnea on exertion. **Exam:** Hyperpigmented skin, 2+ pitting edema to the knees, S3 gallop, hepatomegaly. **Labs/Imaging:** Elevated AST and ALT, transferrin saturation of 65%, serum ferritin of 403. EKG with low-voltage QRS. TTE with preserved EF and diastolic dysfunction.

Management:

1. Therapeutic phlebotomy if patients do not have anemia or severe heart failure. Iron (**Fe**) chelation (with **de**fera**s**irox, **de**feroxamine, **de**feri**p**rone); low-iron diet.
2. Eventual heart transplant for patients refractory to medical therapy.

(Continued)

1-13 Restrictive Cardiomyopathy

Complications: Heart failure, cardiogenic shock extra-cardiac manifestations of iron overload (eg, liver, thyroid).

HYF: Autosomal recessive. Mutation in ***HFE*** gene (chromosome 6) → ↑ intestinal **iron** absorption (↑ ferritin, ↑ iron, ↓ TIBC → ↑ transferrin saturation). Patients can present with bronze diabetes, a classic triad of cirrhosis, diabetes mellitus, and skin pigmentation. Cardiac involvement in hemochromatosis can manifest as restrictive or dilated cardiomyopathy.

RADIATION-INDUCED CARDIOMYOPATHY

A 55-year-old M with PMH of Hodgkin lymphoma s/p chemotherapy and radiation presents with subacute bilateral lower extremity swelling and DOE. **Exam:** 2+ pitting edema to the knees, elevated JVP. **Labs/Imaging:** Elevated BNP. EKG with low-voltage QRS. TTE with preserved EF and diastolic dysfunction.

Management:

1. Eventual heart transplant for end-stage cardiomyopathy.

Complications: Heart failure, cardiogenic shock.

HYF: Radiation leads to fibrosis of the myocardium and epicardium, leading to restrictive cardiomyopathy with diastolic dysfunction. Clinical presentation may occur decades after radiation exposure.

1-14 Hypertrophic Cardiomyopathy

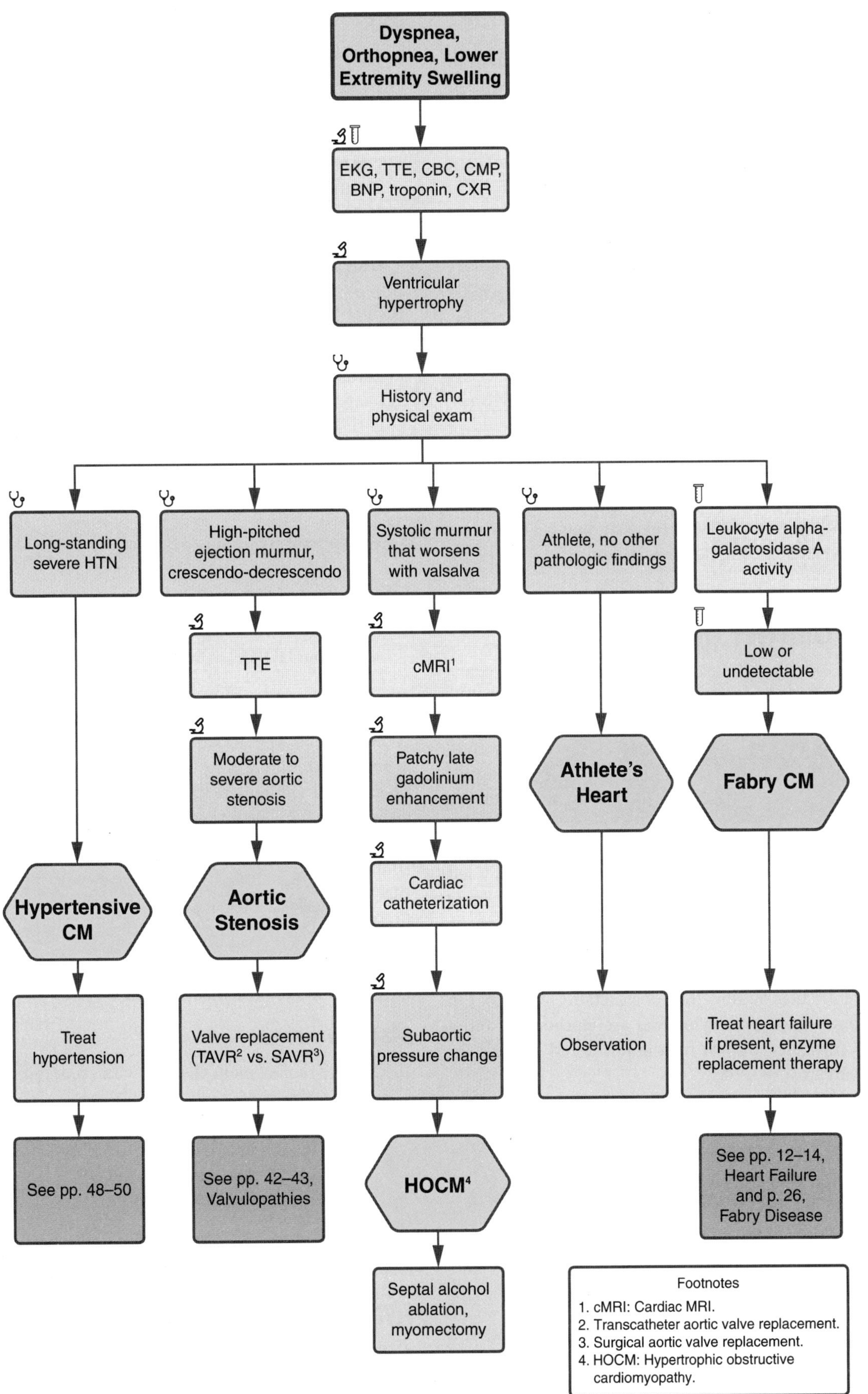
Dyspnea, Orthopnea, Lower Extremity Swelling
EKG, TTE, CBC, CMP, BNP, troponin, CXR
Ventricular hypertrophy
History and physical exam
Long-standing severe HTN
High-pitched ejection murmur, crescendo-decrescendo
Systolic murmur that worsens with valsalva
Athlete, no other pathologic findings
Leukocyte alpha-galactosidase A activity
TTE
cMRI[1]
Low or undetectable
Moderate to severe aortic stenosis
Patchy late gadolinium enhancement
Athlete's Heart
Fabry CM
Cardiac catheterization
Hypertensive CM
Aortic Stenosis
Treat hypertension
Valve replacement (TAVR[2] vs. SAVR[3])
Subaortic pressure change
Observation
Treat heart failure if present, enzyme replacement therapy
See pp. 48–50
See pp. 42–43, Valvulopathies
HOCM[4]
See pp. 12–14, Heart Failure and p. 26, Fabry Disease
Septal alcohol ablation, myomectomy
Footnotes
1. cMRI: Cardiac MRI.
2. Transcatheter aortic valve replacement.
3. Surgical aortic valve replacement.
4. HOCM: Hypertrophic obstructive cardiomyopathy.

FIGURE 1.14

1-14 Hypertrophic Cardiomyopathy

HYPERTENSIVE CARDIOMYOPATHY

A 52-year-old M with PMH of CKD and resistant hypertension presents with a 2-day course of worsening dyspnea. **Exam:** BP 180/110 HR 90, S3 on auscultation, 2+ bilateral lower extremity pitting edema to the knees. **Labs/Imaging:** EKG shows left ventricular hypertrophy (tall R waves in V6–aVL or S waves on V3) and left axis deviation. EKG shows LVH (tall R waves in V5/V6). TTE shows normal LVEF and LV hypertrophy.

Management: Optimize anti-hypertensive regimen.

Complications: Heart failure. Patients are also at risk of developing Sympathetic Crashing Acute Pulmonary Edema (SCAPE), characterized by sudden-onset severe dyspnea, hypoxemia, and diffuse rales in the setting of uncontrolled HTN; treat with CPAP/BiPAP and aggressively reduce BP with vasodilators (nitroglycerin) ± nicardipine or clevidipine drip.

HYF:

- Seen in long-standing, uncontrolled hypertension. Often seen in conjunction with other sequelae of longstanding HTN, such as CKD already written in complications section.

HYPERTROPHIC OBSTRUCTIVE CARDIOMYOPATHY (HOCM)

A 25-year-old M with no significant PMH presents with dyspnea on exertion and atypical chest pain. He states he fainted today while he was in the gym. His family history includes an uncle who passed suddenly while swimming. **Exam:** Harsh crescendo-decrescendo systolic murmur that begins slightly after S1, is heard best at the apex and lower left sternal border, increases with Valsalva and standing up a from squatting/sitting position, and decreases with handgrip and passive leg elevation. Diffuse, forceful LV apical impulse. S3–S4 in younger patients. EKG shows left ventricular hypertrophy, left axis deviation, and right atrial enlargement, as well as prominent Q waves in the inferior and lateral leads and deeply inverted T waves in the mid-precordial leads (V2-V4). TTE shows left ventricular hypertrophy, LVEF normal, systolic anterior motion of the mitral valve, and left ventricular outflow tract obstruction (LVOTO). On exercise stress test, the patient's symptoms are reproduced, and a worsening left ventricular outflow tract gradient and exercise-induced hypotension are observed.

Management:

1. β-blockers. If β-blocker is contraindicated or not tolerated, then consider non-dihydropyridine calcium channel blocker (verapamil).
2. Disopyramide as 2nd-line agent in patients with LVOTO.
3. If refractory symptoms or severe obstruction, septal ablation or myomectomy.

Complications: Arrhythmias, syncope, sudden cardiac death, heart failure.

HYF:

- HOCM is most commonly inherited in an autosomal dominant pattern and is the most common cause of sudden death in young, healthy athletes in the United States. Most cases are inherited in an autosomal dominant pattern and caused by mutations in 1 of several sarcomere genes (myosin binding protein C, β-myosin heavy chain). Upon diagnosis, patient and family members should be offered genetic counseling.
- Vasodilators and diuretics should be used with caution in patients with significant LVOT obstruction (preload dependent).

ATHLETE'S HEART

A 30-year-old M with no significant PMH is being evaluated for an annual physical in the primary care office. He has no complaints. **Exam:** S4 on auscultation, otherwise unremarkable. **Labs/Imaging:** EKG shows sinus bradycardia, increased QRS voltage, tall-peaked T wave, J point elevation. TTE shows left ventricular hypertrophy.

Management: Observation.

Complications: None identified.

HYF:

- Cardiac MRI is the most accurate way to differentiate athlete's heart from HOCM.

FABRY DISEASE

A 29-year-old M is evaluated in the emergency department for syncope. Additionally, he reports a painful burning sensation in his toes and feet for the past few years, particularly after he exercises at the gym. He takes no medications. Family history is notable for maternal grandfather and maternal granduncle who had similar burning symptoms for years and died from strokes in their early 40s. **Exam:** blood pressure is 170/98, irregular heart rate, presence of several angiokeratomas around umbilical area. **Labs/Imaging:** EKG with left ventricular hypertrophy. TTE with concentric LVH and normal LVEF. BUN and creatinine are elevated. Urinalysis shows protein and blood.

Management:

1. Enzyme replacement therapy with recombinant human α-galactosidase A.
2. If there is presence of ventricular arrhythmias, the patient qualifies for an implantable cardiac defibrillator. If symptomatic, bradycardia qualifies for a permanent pacemaker.

Complications: Myocardial fibrosis, arrhythmias, valve diseases (atrial and mitral regurgitation most commonly), heart failure, aortic dilation.

HYF:

- Fabry disease is an X-linked recessive inborn error of glycosphingolipid metabolism caused by deficiency of α-galactosidase A. Unexplained LVH is the hallmark of the cardiac manifestation of Fabry disease.

1-15 Adult Cardiac Arrest (VF/pVT/Asystole/PEA) (ACLS Protocol)

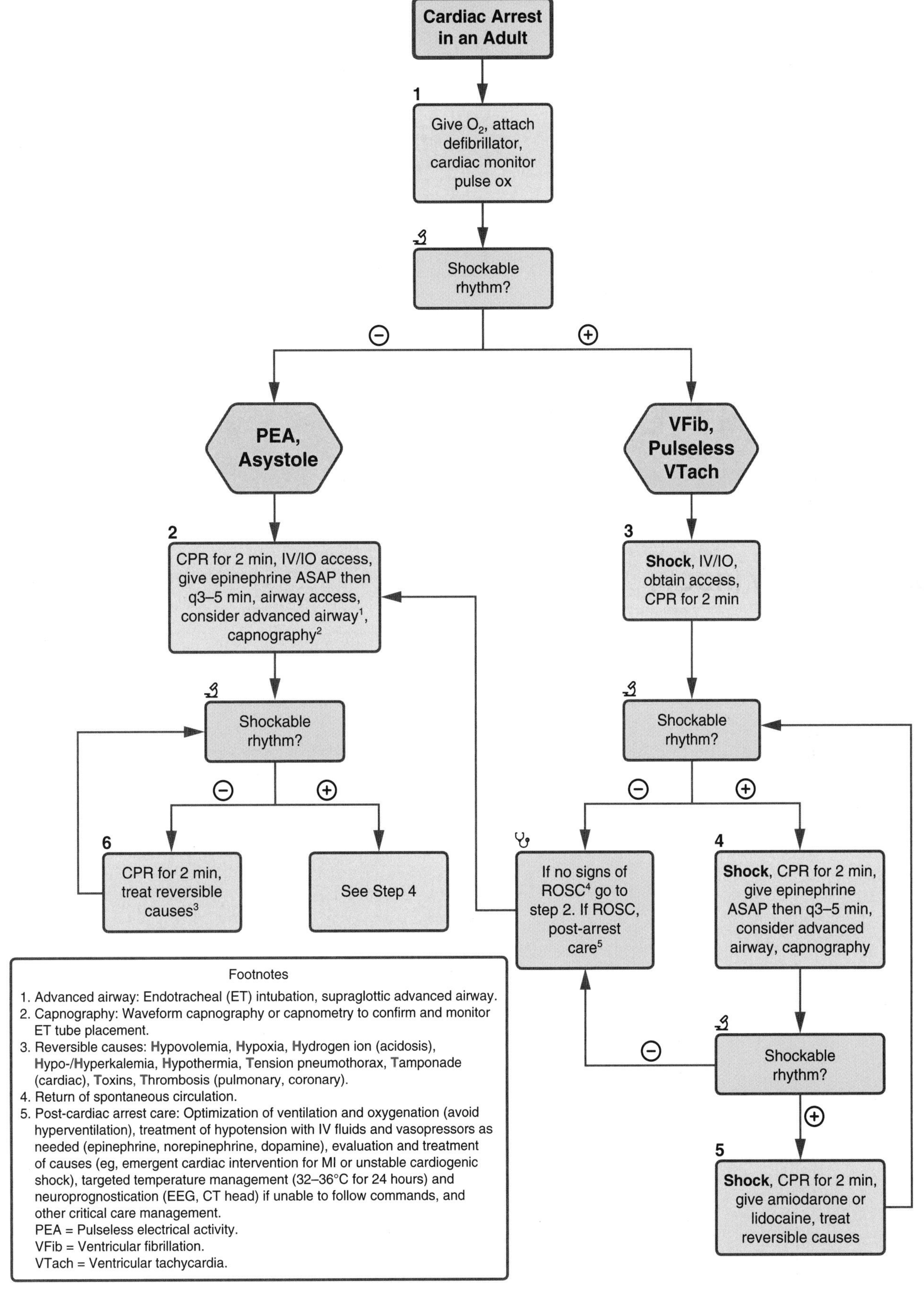
Cardiac Arrest in an Adult
1
Give O_2, attach defibrillator, cardiac monitor pulse ox
Shockable rhythm?
⊖
⊕
PEA, Asystole
VFib, Pulseless VTach
2
CPR for 2 min, IV/IO access, give epinephrine ASAP then q3–5 min, airway access, consider advanced airway[1], capnography[2]
3
Shock, IV/IO, obtain access, CPR for 2 min
Shockable rhythm?
Shockable rhythm?
6
CPR for 2 min, treat reversible causes[3]
See Step 4
If no signs of ROSC[4] go to step 2. If ROSC, post-arrest care[5]
4
Shock, CPR for 2 min, give epinephrine ASAP then q3–5 min, consider advanced airway, capnography
Shockable rhythm?
5
Shock, CPR for 2 min, give amiodarone or lidocaine, treat reversible causes

Footnotes

1. Advanced airway: Endotracheal (ET) intubation, supraglottic advanced airway.
2. Capnography: Waveform capnography or capnometry to confirm and monitor ET tube placement.
3. Reversible causes: **H**ypovolemia, **H**ypoxia, **H**ydrogen ion (acidosis), **H**ypo-/**H**yperkalemia, **H**ypothermia, **T**ension pneumothorax, **T**amponade (cardiac), **T**oxins, **T**hrombosis (pulmonary, coronary).
4. Return of spontaneous circulation.
5. Post-cardiac arrest care: Optimization of ventilation and oxygenation (avoid hyperventilation), treatment of hypotension with IV fluids and vasopressors as needed (epinephrine, norepinephrine, dopamine), evaluation and treatment of causes (eg, emergent cardiac intervention for MI or unstable cardiogenic shock), targeted temperature management (32–36°C for 24 hours) and neuroprognostication (EEG, CT head) if unable to follow commands, and other critical care management.

PEA = Pulseless electrical activity.
VFib = Ventricular fibrillation.
VTach = Ventricular tachycardia.

FIGURE 1.15a

1-15 Adult Bradyarrhythmia (ACLS protocol)

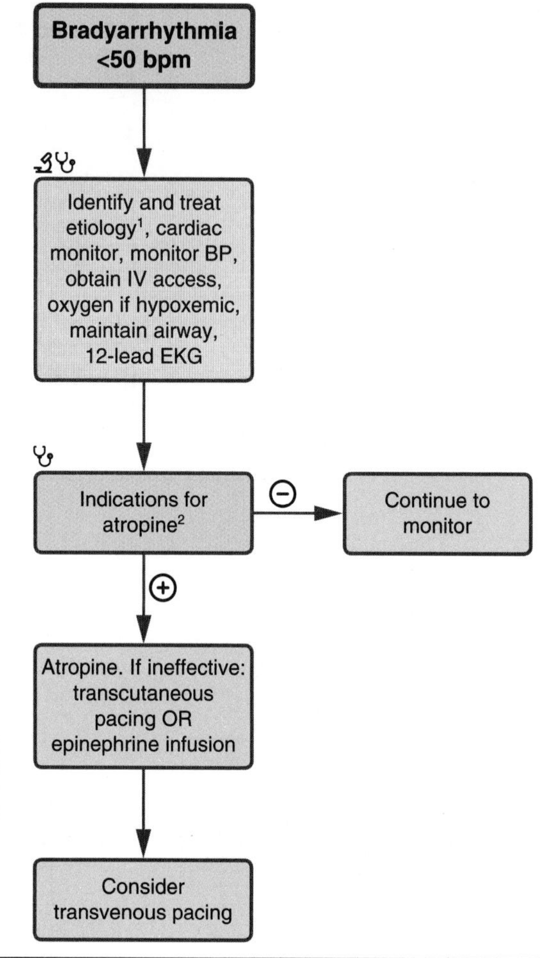
Bradyarrhythmia
<50 bpm
Identify and treat etiology1, cardiac monitor, monitor BP, obtain IV access, oxygen if hypoxemic, maintain airway, 12-lead EKG
Indications for atropine2
Continue to monitor
Atropine. If ineffective: transcutaneous pacing OR epinephrine infusion
Consider transvenous pacing

Footnotes

1. Potential causes: Electrolyte abnormalities (severe hyperkalemia), toxicologic/ medication-induced (eg, β blockers, calcium channel blockers), myocardial infarction.
2. Signs of shock, altered mental status, chest pain, hypotension acute heart failure.

FIGURE 1.15b

1-15 Adult Tachyarrhythmia with a Pulse (ACLS Protocol)

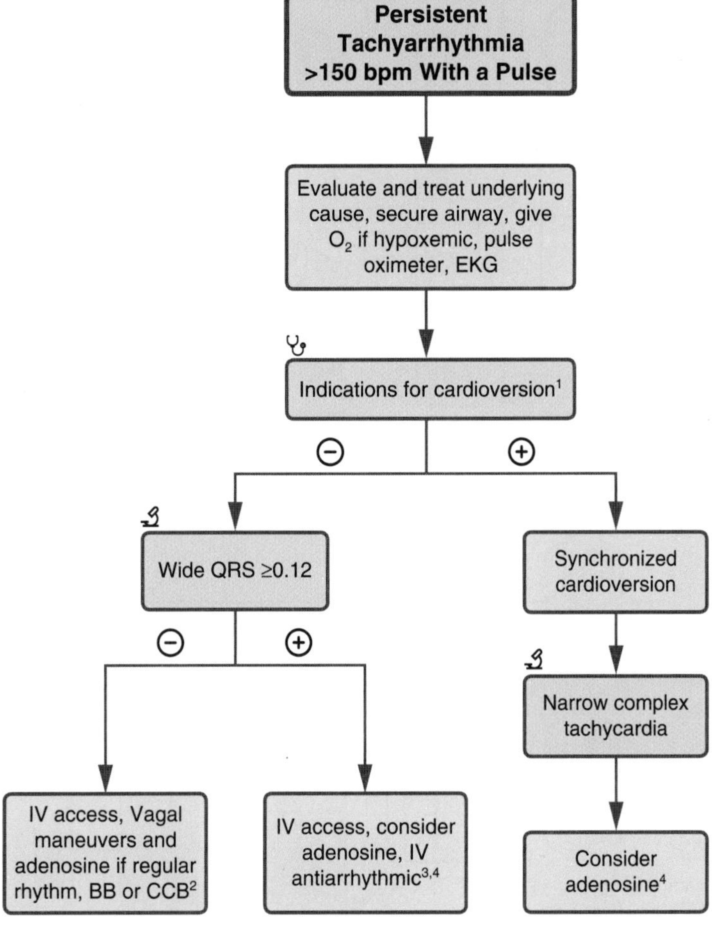
Persistent Tachyarrhythmia >150 bpm With a Pulse
Evaluate and treat underlying cause, secure airway, give O_2 if hypoxemic, pulse oximeter, EKG
Indications for cardioversion[1]
Wide QRS ≥0.12
Synchronized cardioversion
Narrow complex tachycardia
IV access, Vagal maneuvers and adenosine if regular rhythm, BB or CCB[2]
IV access, consider adenosine, IV antiarrhythmic[3,4]
Consider adenosine[4]

Footnotes

1. Hypotension, signs of end organ dysfunction, chest pain, heart failure, altered mental status.
2. BB: β blocker.
   CCB: Calcium channel blocker.
3. Procainamide, amiodarone, sotalol.
4. If refractory to the above measures, consider addition of an anti-arrhythmic agent, ↑ energy level for the next cardioversion, and evaluation and treatment of any potential underlying causes.

FIGURE 1.15c

1-16 Bradyarrhythmias

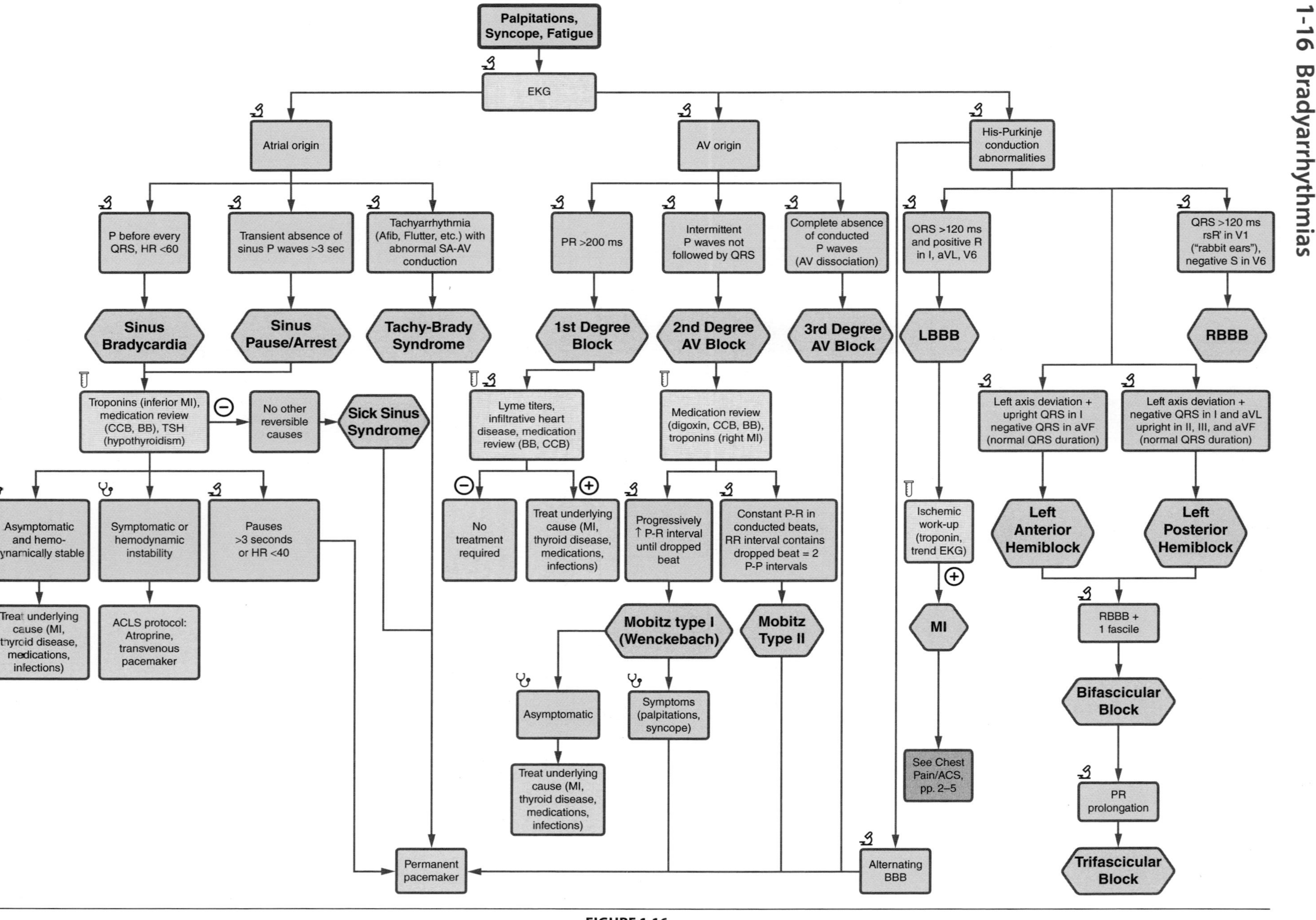
Palpitations, Syncope, Fatigue
EKG
Atrial origin
AV origin
His-Purkinje conduction abnormalities
P before every QRS, HR <60
Transient absence of sinus P waves >3 sec
Tachyarrhythmia (Afib, Flutter, etc.) with abnormal SA-AV conduction
PR >200 ms
Intermittent P waves not followed by QRS
Complete absence of conducted P waves (AV dissociation)
QRS >120 ms and positive R in I, aVL, V6
QRS >120 ms rsR' in V1 ("rabbit ears"), negative S in V6
Sinus Bradycardia
Sinus Pause/Arrest
Tachy-Brady Syndrome
1st Degree Block
2nd Degree AV Block
3rd Degree AV Block
LBBB
RBBB
Troponins (inferior MI), medication review (CCB, BB), TSH (hypothyroidism)
No other reversible causes
Sick Sinus Syndrome
Lyme titers, infiltrative heart disease, medication review (BB, CCB)
Medication review (digoxin, CCB, BB), troponins (right MI)
Left axis deviation + upright QRS in I negative QRS in aVF (normal QRS duration)
Left axis deviation + negative QRS in I and aVL upright in II, III, and aVF (normal QRS duration)
Asymptomatic and hemo-dynamically stable
Symptomatic or hemodynamic instability
Pauses >3 seconds or HR <40
No treatment required
Treat underlying cause (MI, thyroid disease, medications, infections)
Progressively ↑ P-R interval until dropped beat
Constant P-R in conducted beats, RR interval contains dropped beat = 2 P-P intervals
Ischemic work-up (troponin, trend EKG)
Left Anterior Hemiblock
Left Posterior Hemiblock
Treat underlying cause (MI, thyroid disease, medications, infections)
ACLS protocol: Atroprine, transvenous pacemaker
Mobitz type I (Wenckebach)
Mobitz Type II
MI
RBBB + 1 fascile
Asymptomatic
Symptoms (palpitations, syncope)
Bifascicular Block
Treat underlying cause (MI, thyroid disease, medications, infections)
See Chest Pain/ACS, pp. 2–5
PR prolongation
Permanent pacemaker
Alternating BBB
Trifascicular Block

FIGURE 1.16

1-16 Bradyarrhythmias

BRADYARRHYTHMIAS

A 65-year-old M with PMH of coronary artery disease presents with chest pain and hypotension. **Exam:** He is diaphoretic, bradycardic with HR <60 bpm, and hypotensive with BP 75/40. **Labs/Imaging:** EKG shows bradycardia with ST elevations in the R leads and ST depressions in the anterior leads.

Management:

- Acute inferior MI: Re-vascularization, IV fluids, avoid nitroglycerin.
- AV block:
  - First-degree and Type 1 second-degree: Observation, if asymptomatic.
  - Type II second-degree and third-degree (complete heart block): Permanent pacemaker.
  - If symptomatic: Atropine, pacemaker.
  - All hemodynamically unstable patients: ACLS protocol (atropine/dopamine/epinephrine, emergent transcutaneous pacing to stabilize the patient, transvenous pacing).

Complications: Cardiac arrest, syncope.

HYF:

- Permanent pacing is indicated for symptomatic bradycardia with no underlying reversible cause and in asymptomatic patients who have AV and infranodal conduction disturbances that have a high risk for progression to complete heart block or asystole.

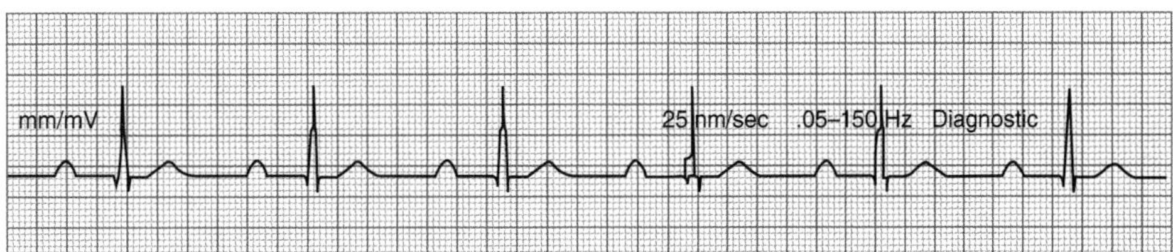
mm/mV
25 mm/sec
.05–150 Hz
Diagnostic

Sinus rhythm with 1st-degree atrioventricular block.

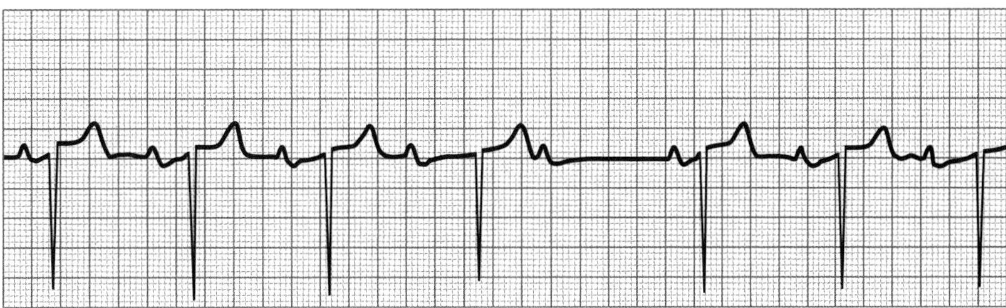

Second-degree AV block: Mobitz type I AV block with Wenckebach phenomenon.

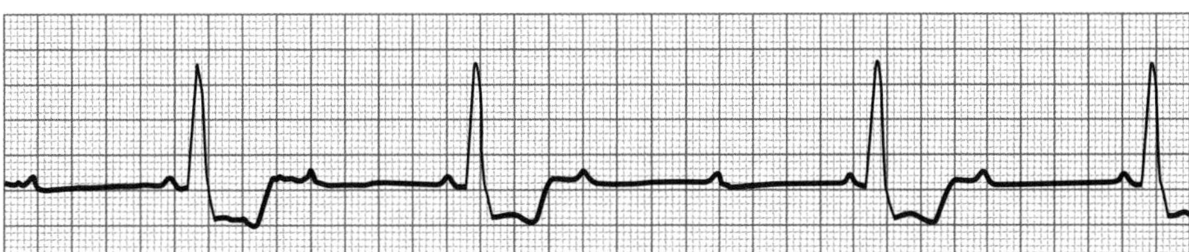

Second-degree AV block: Mobitz type II with a 2:1 to 3:1 AV block.

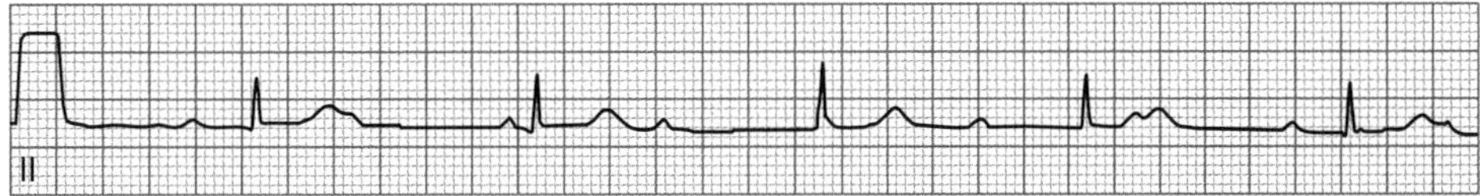
II

Complete or third-degree AV block.

1-17 Supraventricular Tachyarrhythmias

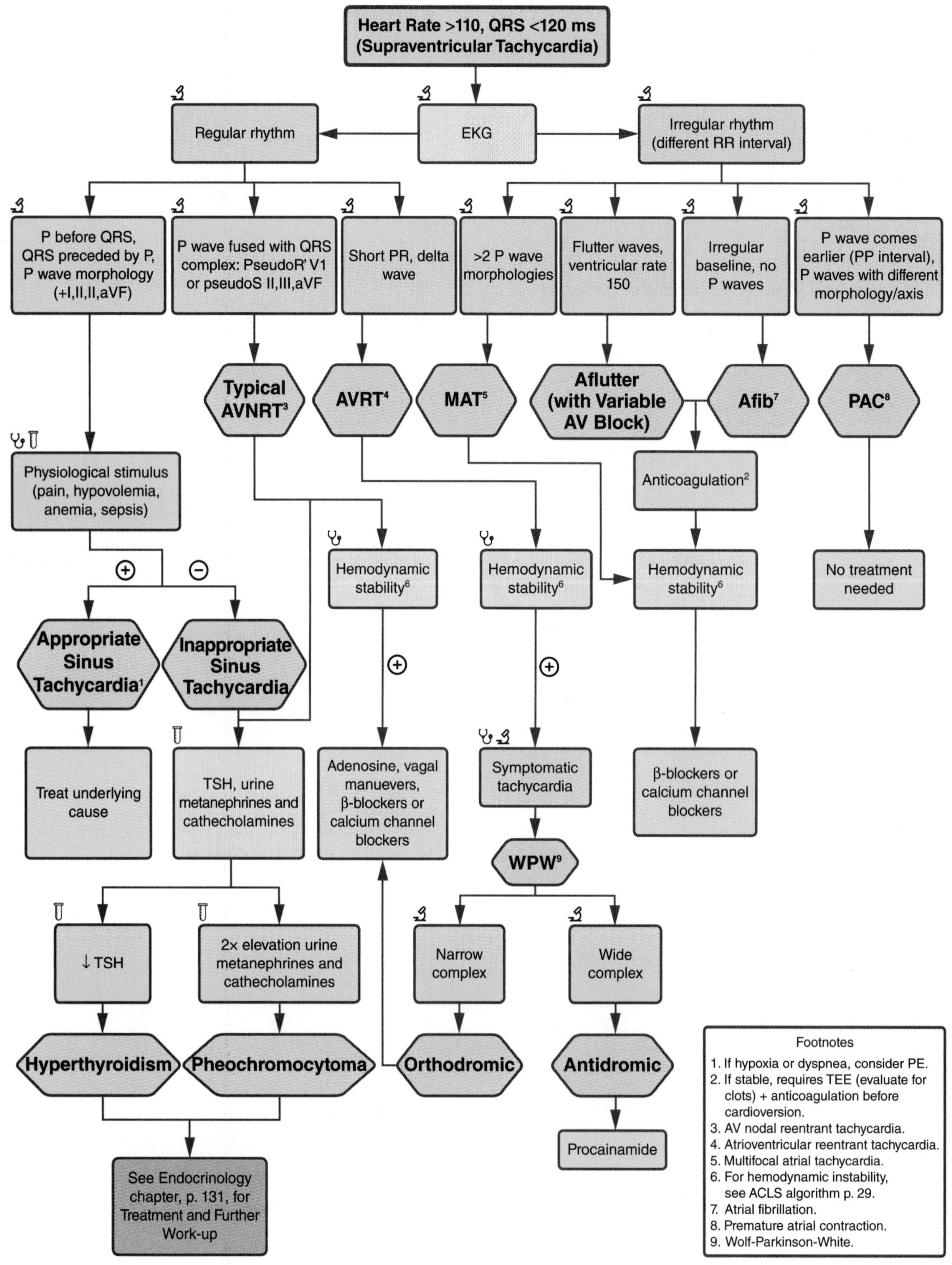
Heart Rate >110, QRS <120 ms (Supraventricular Tachycardia)
EKG
Regular rhythm
Irregular rhythm (different RR interval)
P before QRS, QRS preceded by P, P wave morphology (+I,II,II,aVF)
P wave fused with QRS complex: PseudoR' V1 or pseudoS II,III,aVF
Short PR, delta wave
>2 P wave morphologies
Flutter waves, ventricular rate 150
Irregular baseline, no P waves
P wave comes earlier (PP interval), P waves with different morphology/axis
Typical AVNRT3
AVRT4
MAT5
Aflutter (with Variable AV Block)
Afib7
PAC8
Physiological stimulus (pain, hypovolemia, anemia, sepsis)
Anticoagulation2
Hemodynamic stability6
Hemodynamic stability6
Hemodynamic stability6
No treatment needed
Appropriate Sinus Tachycardia1
Inappropriate Sinus Tachycardia
Treat underlying cause
TSH, urine metanephrines and cathecholamines
Adenosine, vagal manuevers, β-blockers or calcium channel blockers
Symptomatic tachycardia
β-blockers or calcium channel blockers
WPW9
↓TSH
2× elevation urine metanephrines and cathecholamines
Narrow complex
Wide complex
Hyperthyroidism
Pheochromocytoma
Orthodromic
Antidromic
Procainamide
See Endocrinology chapter, p. 131, for Treatment and Further Work-up
Footnotes
1. If hypoxia or dyspnea, consider PE.
2. If stable, requires TEE (evaluate for clots) + anticoagulation before cardioversion.
3. AV nodal reentrant tachycardia.
4. Atrioventricular reentrant tachycardia.
5. Multifocal atrial tachycardia.
6. For hemodynamic instability, see ACLS algorithm p. 29.
7. Atrial fibrillation.
8. Premature atrial contraction.
9. Wolf-Parkinson-White.

FIGURE 1.17

1-17 Supraventricular Tachyarrhythmias

Supraventricular tachycardia (SVT) arises in the atria or AV junction. Paroxysmal supraventricular tachycardia (PSVT) usually arises in patients who are young with healthy hearts and is often caused by abnormal reentry pathways (AVNRT, AVRT); EKG shows normal QRS. SVTs also include atrial fibrillation, atrial flutter, and multifocal atrial tachycardia; EKG shows irregular QRS.

SINUS TACHYCARDIA (APPROPRIATE AND NOT APPROPRIATE)

A 34-year-old F with no PMH presents with nausea, right flank pain, dysuria and fever. **Exam:** Tachycardia (>100), BP 90/65, temperature 101.1, and costovertebral angel tenderness on the right. **Labs/Imaging:** CBC with leukocytosis; UA with many bacteria, pyuria, hematuria. Urine culture positive for *Escherichia coli*. EKG with normal sinus rhythm and tachycardia.

Management:

1. If appropriate: Treat underlying cause that triggers physiologic tachycardic response (eg, if sepsis, give fluids and start antibiotics).
2. If inappropriate: β-blockers, calcium channel blocker.

Complications: Depending on the underlying cause. Can lead to hemodynamic instability and shock.

HYF: If unclear physiologic trigger, consider inappropriate sinus tachycardia. This should always be a diagnosis of exclusion.

PREMATURE ATRIAL CONTRACTION (PAC)

A 30-year-old F with family history of sudden cardiac death presents to primary care clinic to establish care. She denies any symptoms. **Exam:** Vital signs and complete physical exam are normal. **Labs/Imaging:** EKG shows a P wave followed by normal QRS complex with a different PP interval (shorter than previous interval).

Management:

1. Asymptomatic: No interventions needed.
2. Symptomatic: Consider β-blockers.

Complications: Very rare. Atrial fibrillation, ischemic stroke.

HYF: Isolated PACs (without premature ventricular complexes) are not associated with increase risk of sudden cardiac death.

ATRIOVENTRICULAR NODAL REENTRY TACHYCARDIA (AVNRT) / ATRIOVENTRICULAR REENTRANT TACHYCARDIA (AVRT)

A 30-year-old F with no PMH presents with palpitations or syncope, mostly when exercising. **Exam:** Tachycardia (>100), BP 100/65. **Labs/Imaging:** EKG with narrow complex tachycardia, normal QRS.

Management:

1. If unstable, cardioversion.
2. If stable, consider vagal maneuvers (eg, Valsalva, carotid massage), IV adenosine.
3. For long-term control, consider AV nodal blockade (BB, CCB) or catheter ablation of accessory conduction pathway. Of note, if there is concern that AVRT is due to rapid AFib in patient with WPW, avoid BB and CCB.

Complications: Tachycardia-induced cardiomyopathy.

HYF:

- AVNRT is due to the presence of both slow and fast conduction pathways in the AV node, creating a reentry circuit in the AV node that depolarizes the atrium and ventricle almost simultaneously. On EKG, the P wave is hidden in the QRS or seen shortly after. It is the most common SVT and presents commonly in a patient's thirties and forties. Female > male.
- AVRT is due to a separate accessory conduction pathway between the atrium and ventricle that causes a reentry circuit. On EKG, a retrograde P wave is often seen after a normal QRS. Seen in WPW (below).

MULTIFOCAL ATRIAL TACHYCARDIA (MAT)

An 80-year-old M with PMH of COPD presents with palpitations, dizziness, and chest pain. **Exam:** HR 135 and irregular, SpO_2 of 86%. **Labs/Imaging:** EKG shows an irregularly irregular rhythm with ≥3 different P-wave morphologies that have irregular intervals.

Management

1. Treat the inciting disease.
2. Electrolyte repletion for hypomagnesemia or hypokalemia.
3. Calcium channel blockers (verapamil, diltiazem) are often 1st-line.
4. If no concurrent heart failure or bronchospasm, can use β-blockers (metoprolol).

HYF: MAT is associated strongly with pulmonary disease, most often COPD. Renal failure, hypomagnesemia, and hypokalemia are also common contributing factors. While the pathophysiology remains unclear, it is thought to be related to right atrial distention from pulmonary hypertension, leading to multiple competing sites of atrial activity.

ATRIAL FIBRILLATION

A 65-year-old F with PMH of obstructive sleep apnea and alcohol use disorder presents with palpitations and dizziness. **Exam:** HR >100 with irregular pulse, BP 80/50. **Labs/Imaging:** EKG with narrow complex tachycardia and irregularly irregular rhythm with no discernible P waves.

Management:

1. If unstable, cardioversion.
2. If stable, rate control with β-blocker, calcium channel blocker, or digoxin.
3. If already on anticoagulation or new-onset AF <2 days, consider chemical (amiodarone) or electrical cardioversion.
4. If onset >2 days or unclear duration, obtain TEE to rule out presence of atrial thrombus. If no thrombus, cardiovert. If atrial thrombus is seen, start anticoagulation and wait 3–4 weeks before cardioversion.

(Continued)

1-17 Supraventricular Tachyarrhythmias

5. Alternative therapies include rhythm control with antiarrhythmics or catheter ablation, or AV node ablation with pacemaker implantation.
6. Anticoagulation for patients with CHA2DS2-VASc score ≥2.

Complications: Tachycardia-induced cardiomyopathy if rapid ventricular response is sustained. Cardioembolic phenomena (stroke, limb ischemia).

HYF: Usually due to ectopic foci within the pulmonary veins. Patients can be asymptomatic or present with dyspnea, chest pain, dizziness, or palpitations. Sustained rapid ventricular response can induce tachycardia-mediated cardiomyopathy, leading to heart failure and cardiogenic shock. Poor atrial contraction can lead to formation of mural thrombi in the left atrium (most commonly the left atrial appendage), which can cause strokes. Etiologies of Afib: **PIRATES** (**P**ulmonary disease, **I**schemia, **R**heumatic heart disease, **A**nemia/**A**trial myxoma, **T**hyrotoxicosis, **E**thanol, **S**epsis).

ATRIAL FLUTTER

A 50-year-old F with PMH of COPD and mitral valve prolapse presents with 2 days of palpitations and dizziness. **Exam:** HR is 150 bpm. **Labs/Imaging:** EKG shows narrow complex tachycardia with sawtooth waves in II, III, and AVF.

Management:

1. Management of atrial flutter is similar to that of atrial fibrillation. Mainstays of treatment are rate control and anticoagulation for patients with CHA2DS2-VASc score ≥2. Catheter ablation is often the definitive treatment.
2. For inconclusive EKGs, adenosine administration can briefly block AV nodal conduction and reveal the classic "sawtooth" waves that may be hiding behind the QRS.

Complications: Thromboemboli, heart failure.

HYF: Atrial flutter is usually a regularly regular rhythm (ie, consistently rapid rate) unless there is variable AV block, as opposed to atrial fibrillation, which is irregularly irregular. EKG will reveal a narrow complex tachycardia of 150 bmp with "sawtooth" waves in leads II, III, and aVF. Patients often have a history of cardiac or pulmonary disease.

WOLFF-PARKINSON-WHITE (WPW) SYNDROME

A 20-year-old M with no PMH presents with syncope after playing soccer. He had no prodromal symptoms. **Exam** is normal. **Labs/Imaging** EKG shows a slurred upstroke of the QRS consistent with a delta wave.

Management:

1. Observation for asymptomatic patients.
2. In setting of acute irregular tachycardia from atrial fibrillation/flutter in patient with WPW, administer amiodarone or procainamide. Avoid CCBs or digoxin.
3. Radiofrequency catheter ablation is curative.

Complications: Sudden cardiac death (rare).

HYF: This type of AVRT is caused by an abnormal fast accessory conduction pathway from atria to ventricle (Bundle of Kent). Delta waves are characteristic.

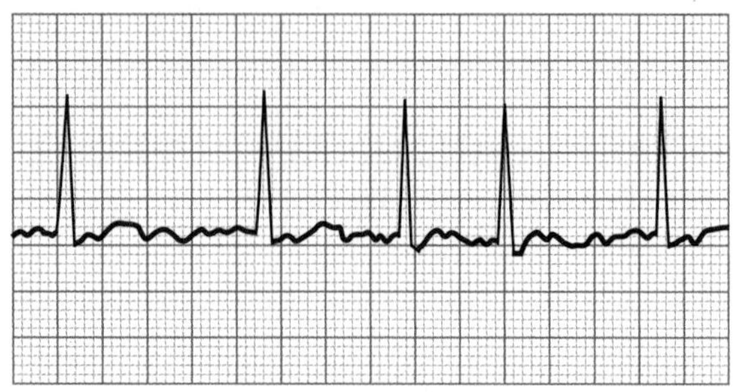

Atrial fibrillation.

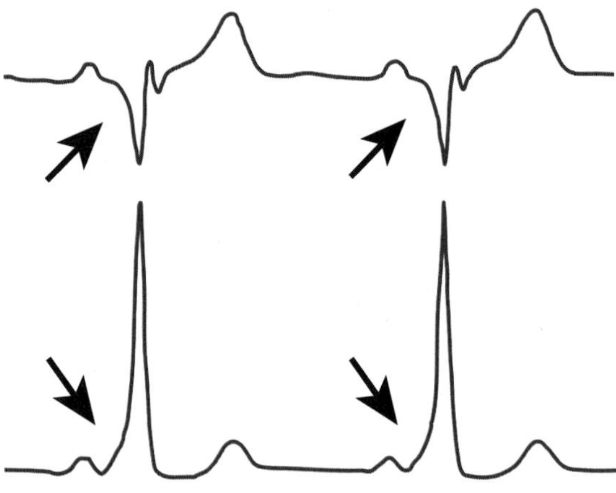

Delta wave in Wolff–Parkinson–White syndrome.

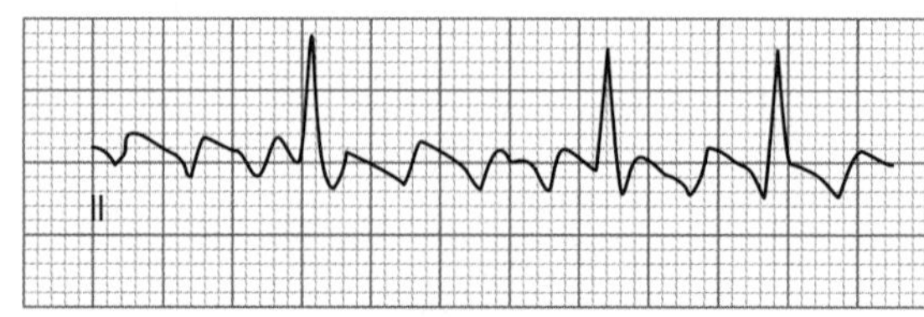
II

Atrial flutter with variable block.

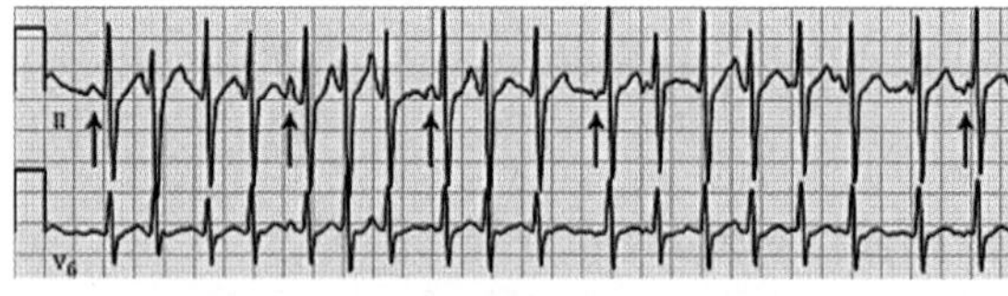

Multifocal atrial tachycardia (MAT) with varying P-wave morphologies and P-P intervals.

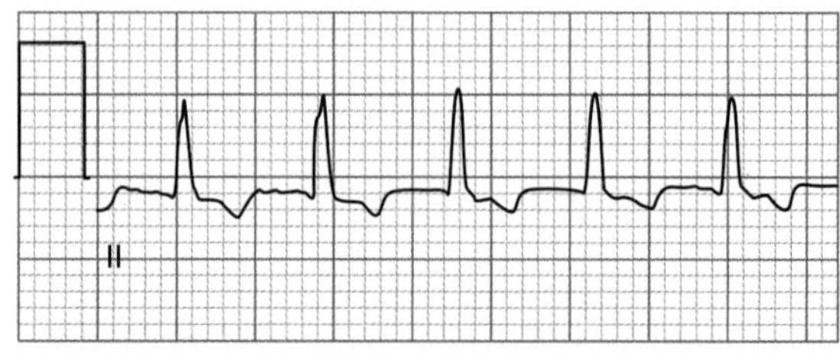
II

Atrioventricular nodal reentrant tachycardia (AVNRT).

1-18 Ventricular Tachyarrhythmias

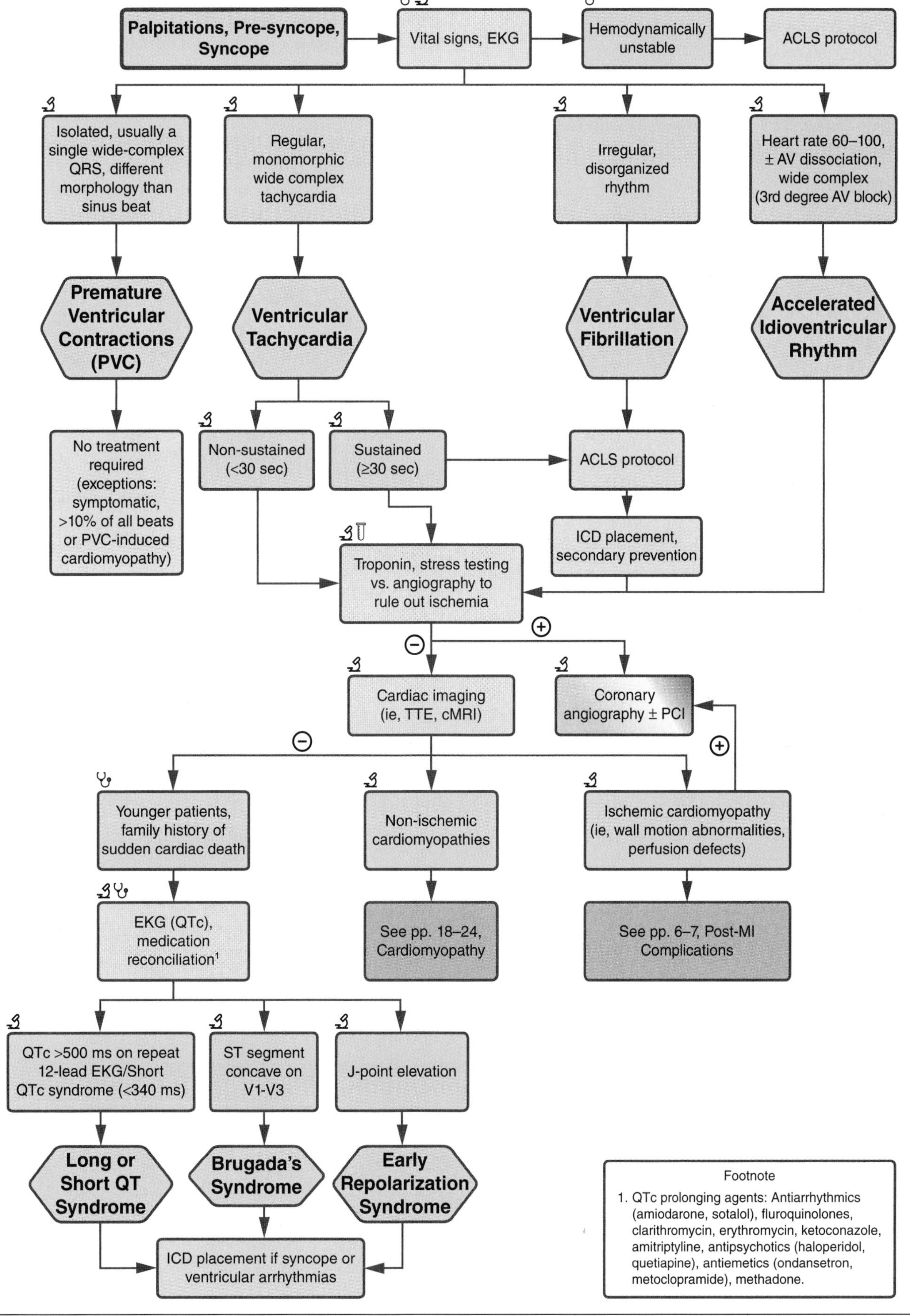
Palpitations, Pre-syncope, Syncope
Vital signs, EKG
Hemodynamically unstable
ACLS protocol
Isolated, usually a single wide-complex QRS, different morphology than sinus beat
Regular, monomorphic wide complex tachycardia
Irregular, disorganized rhythm
Heart rate 60–100, ± AV dissociation, wide complex (3rd degree AV block)
Premature Ventricular Contractions (PVC)
Ventricular Tachycardia
Ventricular Fibrillation
Accelerated Idioventricular Rhythm
No treatment required (exceptions: symptomatic, >10% of all beats or PVC-induced cardiomyopathy)
Non-sustained (<30 sec)
Sustained (≥30 sec)
ACLS protocol
ICD placement, secondary prevention
Troponin, stress testing vs. angiography to rule out ischemia
Cardiac imaging (ie, TTE, cMRI)
Coronary angiography ± PCI
Younger patients, family history of sudden cardiac death
Non-ischemic cardiomyopathies
Ischemic cardiomyopathy (ie, wall motion abnormalities, perfusion defects)
EKG (QTc), medication reconciliation[1]
See pp. 18–24, Cardiomyopathy
See pp. 6–7, Post-MI Complications
QTc >500 ms on repeat 12-lead EKG/Short QTc syndrome (<340 ms)
ST segment concave on V1-V3
J-point elevation
Long or Short QT Syndrome
Brugada's Syndrome
Early Repolarization Syndrome
ICD placement if syncope or ventricular arrhythmias

Footnote

1. QTc prolonging agents: Antiarrhythmics (amiodarone, sotalol), fluroquinolones, clarithromycin, erythromycin, ketoconazole, amitriptyline, antipsychotics (haloperidol, quetiapine), antiemetics (ondansetron, metoclopramide), methadone.

FIGURE 1.18

1-18 Ventricular Tachyarrhythmias

VENTRICULAR TACHYCARDIA (VT)

A 66-year-old M with PMH of T2DM, tobacco use disorder, non-ischemic cardiomyopathy, and HFrEF (EF 25%) presents with palpitations and lightheadedness. **Exam:** HR 180, BP 90/65, SpO_2 92% on room air. **Labs/Imaging:** EKG shows wide-complex tachycardia with no discernible P waves, troponin mildly elevated, hypomagnesemia and hypokalemia.

Management:

1. If sustained VT or hemodynamically unstable: Treat based on ACLS protocol (defibrillation, epinephrine, amiodarone).
2. If non-sustained VT:
   a. Medications for non-sustained VT: β-blocker, antiarrhythmics (class IA, IB, II, or III).
   b. If refractory to medications: Catheter ablation.
   c. Evaluate for and treat reversible causes of arrhythmia: Electrolyte imbalances (replete K, Mg), myocardial ischemia (troponin, stress test vs. coronary angiography), hypoxia, adverse drug effects, anemia.
3. Consider ICD for secondary prevention.

Complications: Ventricular fibrillation, sudden cardiac death, cardiogenic shock.

HYF: Torsades de Pointes is VT with a characteristic morphology of a 'twisting' QRS with increasing and decreasing amplitude. It is usually triggered by QTc prolongation, either due to medications, electrolyte abnormalities, or congenital long QT syndromes. Has a poor prognosis, as it can rapidly convert to ventricular fibrillation. Give magnesium and cardiovert if unstable.

VENTRICULAR FIBRILLATION (VFib)

A 65-year-old M with PMH of T2DM, tobacco use disorder, and HTN is brought by EMS after he lost consciousness in the supermarket and bystanders called 911. CPR was started. He was found to be in a shockable rhythm by AED and received 2 shocks before return of spontaneous circulation. **Exam:** BP 100/65, HR 103, SpO_2 92% on room air, diaphoretic. **Labs/Imaging:** Rhythm strip on the field shows ventricular fibrillation that broke after 2 shocks. Current EKG shows normal sinus rhythm, troponin elevated.

Management:

1. ACLS protocol (defibrillation, epinephrine, amiodarone).
2. Once stabilized, evaluate for coronary artery disease (eg, left heart catheterization).
3. Consider ICD for secondary prevention.

Complications: Sudden cardiac death, cardiogenic shock.

HYF: EKG for ventricular fibrillation shows no P waves or QRS; the irregular deflections represent ventricular quivering, which may be fine or coarse.

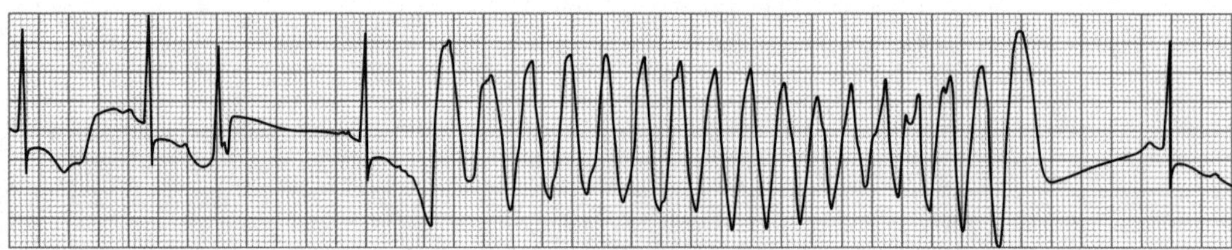

Torsade de Pointes ventricular tachycardia (VT).

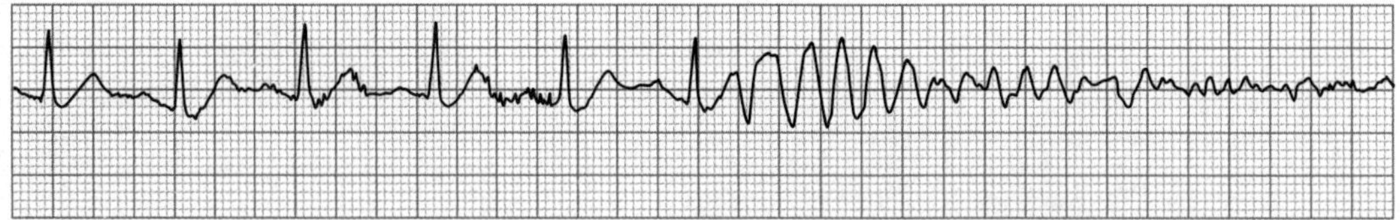

Ventricular fibrillation. After 6 beats, sinus rhythm degenerates into ventricular fibrillation.

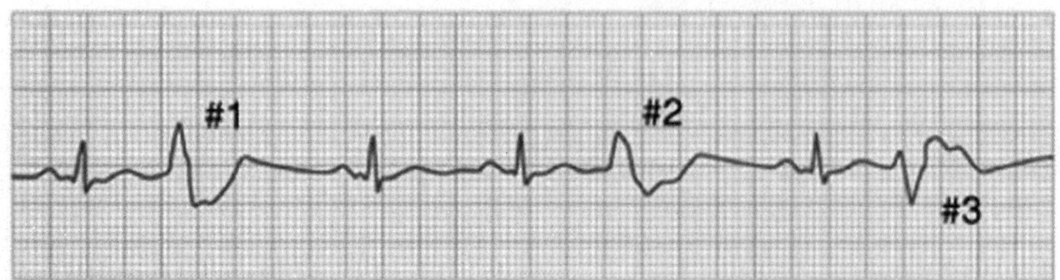
#1
#2
#3

Multifocal PVCs: 2nd, 6th, and 9th beats are PVCs.

1-19 Antiarrhythmic Drugs

Antiarrhythmic Drugs

Class	Mechanism of Action	Agents	Effects	Use	Side Effects	Contraindications
IA	Na channel blockade, some K channel blockade	1. Dysopyramide 2. Procainamide 3. Quinidine	Slows down depolarization, prolongs repolarization	Brugada, WPW, SVT, Afib, ventricular arrhythmias	Anticholinergic effects, lupus-like syndrome (procainamide)	Ischemic or structural heart disease, prolonged QT, advanced kidney disease
IB	Na channel blockade	1. Lidocaine 2. Mexiletine 3. Phenytoin	Slows down depolarization	Ventricular arrhythmias	Headaches, dizziness, other neurologic symtpoms. Seizures with lidocaine toxicity	Advanced liver disease
IC	Na channel blockade	1. Flecainide 2. Propafenone	Slows down depolarization, shortens repolarization	Afib, SVT, ventricular arrhythmias	Headaches, dizziness, other neurologic symtpoms	Ischemic or structural heart disease, heart block without pacemaker
II	β adrenergic blockade	1. Atenolol 2. Bisoprolol 3. Metoprolol 4. Propranolol	Decrease sympathetic tone	Rate control atrial arrhythmias, SVT, ventricular arrhythmias	Fatigue, drowsiness, dizziness, depression, erectile dysfunction, bronchospams	Severe asthma, cardiogenic shock, 2nd-3rd degree block, pre-excitation
III	K channel blockade	1. Dofetilide 2. Ibutilide 3. Sotalol	Prolongs action potential duration	Afib, Aflutter, ventricular arrhythmias, pharmacological cardioversion	Headaches, dizziness, bradycardia, fatigue, dyspnea (sotalol). Rarely Torsades de Pointes (dofetilide)	CrCl <40, QTc >440s, sinus bradycardia <50, heart block without pacemaker
IV	Ca channel blockade	1. Diltiazem 2. Verapamil	Suppresses sinoatrial and AV conduction	SVT, rate control of atrial arrhthymias, outflow tract VTs	Dependent edema, dizziness, constipation	Sginificant sinus node dysfunction, AV block without pacemaker, pre-excitation
Multichannel Blockers	Several mechanisms (Na, K, Ca)	1. Amiodarone 2. Dronedarone	Principally extends repolarization	Atrial arrhthymias, ventricular arrhythmias	Fatigue, dizziness, nausea, vomiting, constipation or diarrhea, tremor. Amiodarone is associated with QT prolongation, pulmonary toxicity (cough, fever, dyspnea), hypo/hyperthyroidism, elevated LFTs, photosensitivity to UV light, blue-gray skin discoloration, optic neuropathy, and corneal microdeposits. Routine serial monitoring with EKGs, CXR, TFTs, and LFTs is required.	Advanced lung, liver or thyroid disease (amiodarone). Advanced liver disease, permanent Afib, recent decompensated heart failure (NYHA III-IV) (dronedarone)
Late Na channel blockers	Late Na channel blockade	1. Ranolazine	Shortens action potential, prevents Ca overload	Afib and ventricular arrhthymias	Dizziness, nausea, headaches, constipation, hypoglycemia	Advanced liver disease, use of strong CYP3A4 inhibitor/inducer
Adenosine receptor agonists	A1 receptor agonism	1. Adenosine	Slows or blocks sinoatrial or AV node conduction	Termination of SVT	Flushing, dyspnea, chest pain, hypotension, dizziness, nausea	Severe asthma, cardiac transplant
Cardiac glycoside	Increase vagal activity	1. Digoxin	Slows AV node conduction	Rate control for Afib	Nausea, vomiting, dizziness, blurry vision and yellow halos, thrombocytopenia	Advanced kidney disease (dose adjustment)
Hyperpolarization-activated cyclic nucleotide-gated (HCN) channel blockers	Selectively inhibits pacemaker current (If)	1. Ivabradine	Reduced depolarization rate of sinoatrial node, decreased cell automaticity	Stable angina, chronic heart failure	Bradycardia, hypertension, visual brightness	Acute decompensated heart failure, heart block without pacemaker, severe bradycardia or hypotension, advanced liver disease, use of strong CYP3A4 inhibitors

FIGURE 1.19

1-20 Pericardial Disease

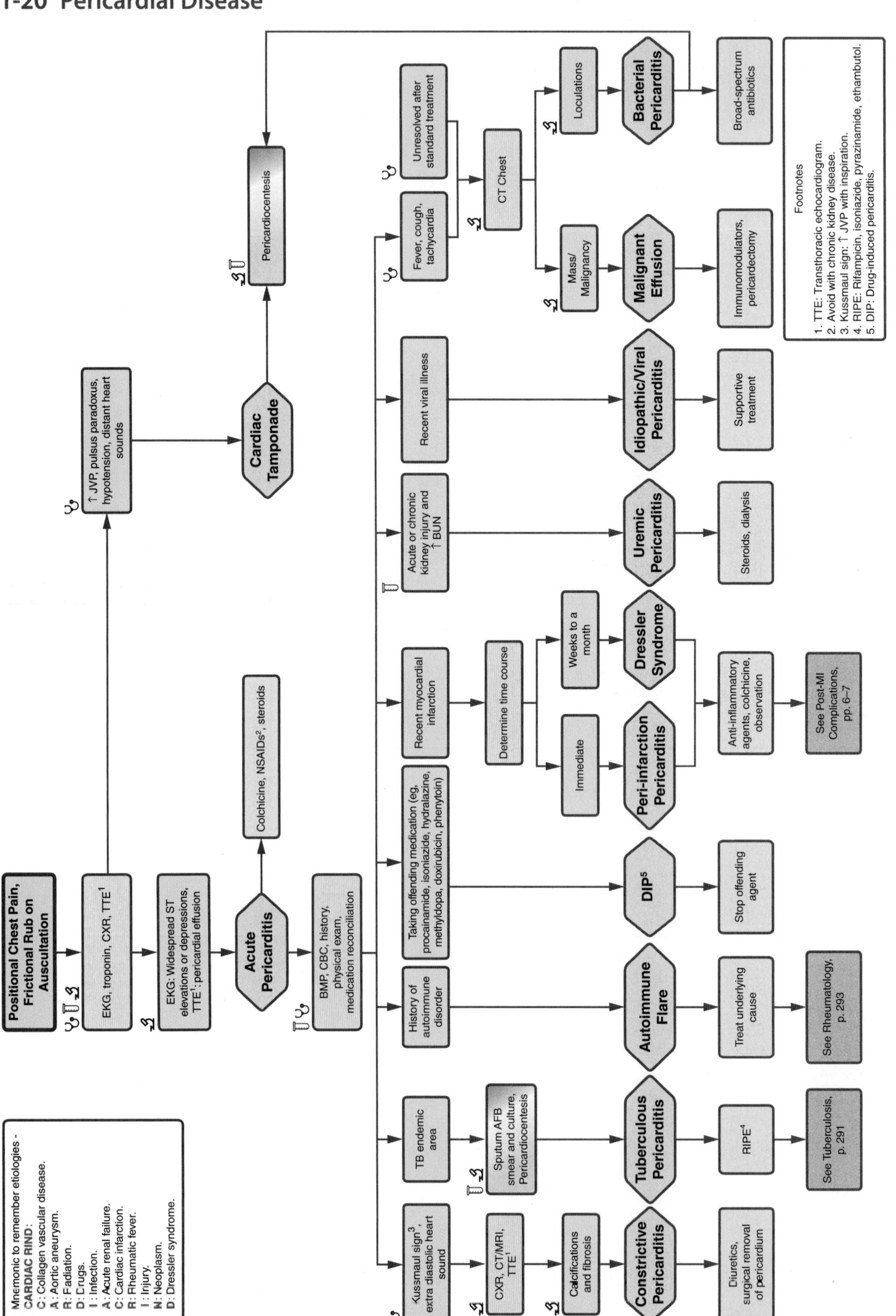
Mnemonic to remember etiologies - CARDIAC RIND:
C: Collagen vascular disease.
A: Aortic aneurysm.
R: Radiation.
D: Drugs.
I: Infection.
A: Acute renal failure.
C: Cardiac infarction.
R: Rheumatic fever.
I: Injury.
N: Neoplasm.
D: Dressler syndrome.
Positional Chest Pain, Frictional Rub on Auscultation
EKG, troponin, CXR, TTE¹
EKG: Widespread ST elevations or depressions, TTE¹: pericardial effusion
Acute Pericarditis
Colchicine, NSAIDs², steroids
↑ JVP, pulsus paradoxus, hypotension, distant heart sounds
Cardiac Tamponade
Pericardiocentesis
BMP, CBC, history, physical exam, medication reconciliation
Kussmaul sign³, extra diastolic heart sound
CXR, CT/MRI, TTE¹
Calcifications and fibrosis
Constrictive Pericarditis
Diuretics, surgical removal of pericardium
TB endemic area
Sputum AFB smear and culture, Pericardiocentesis
Tuberculous Pericarditis
RIPE⁴
See Tuberculosis, p. 291
History of autoimmune disorder
Autoimmune Flare
Treat underlying cause
See Rheumatology, p. 293
Taking offending medication (eg, procainamide, isoniazide, hydralazine, methyldopa, doxirubicin, phenytoin)
DIP⁵
Stop offending agent
Recent myocardial infarction
Determine time course
Immediate
Weeks to a month
Peri-infarction Pericarditis
Dressler Syndrome
Anti-inflammatory agents, colchicine, observation
See Post-MI Complications, pp. 6–7
Acute or chronic kidney injury and ↑ BUN
Uremic Pericarditis
Steroids, dialysis
Recent viral illness
Idiopathic/Viral Pericarditis
Supportive treatment
Fever, cough, tachycardia
Unresolved after standard treatment
CT Chest
Mass/ Malignancy
Loculations
Malignant Effusion
Bacterial Pericarditis
Immunomodulators, pericardectomy
Broad-spectrum antibiotics
Footnotes
1. TTE: Transthoracic echocardiogram.
2. Avoid with chronic kidney disease.
3. Kussmaul sign: ↑ JVP with inspiration.
4. RIPE: Rifampicin, isoniazide, pyrazinamide, ethambutol.
5. DIP: Drug-induced pericarditis.

FIGURE 1.20

1-20 Pericardial Disease

IDIOPATHIC/VIRAL PERICARDITIS

A 60-year-old F with PMH of recent viral respiratory infection presents with sharp, positional chest pain that radiates to her left shoulder and neck. The pain worsens that worsens with inhalation and improves when she sits up and leans forward. **Exam:** She has a low-grade fever and a friction rub on heart auscultation. **Labs/Imaging:** Mildly ↑ troponin, ↑ ESR, ↑ CRP. EKG shows widespread ST-segment elevation and PR-depression in the precordial leads. TTE shows a small pericardial effusion.

Management:

1. NSAIDs, colchicine, or glucocorticoids.
2. Treat underlying condition if applicable (eg, dialysis for uremic pericarditis).

Complications: Pericardial effusion, cardiac tamponade.

HYF: Acute pericarditis is characterized by acute inflammation of the pericardium. Patients present with positional, sharp chest pain that worsens with inhalation and improves with sitting up and leaning forward. Patients can also have referred shoulder pain, as the pericardium is innervated by the phrenic nerve. Friction rub on heart auscultation is pathognomonic. Most cases are idiopathic (presumed viral) and usually self-limited. Coxsackievirus (types A and B) and echovirus are common viral culprits.

CARDIAC TAMPONADE

A 50-year-old M has been admitted for the past 4 days for myocardial infarction and underwent coronary angiogram angioplasty a few hours ago. The patient has suddenly become unresponsive. **Exam:** Hypotensive, tachycardic, pulsus paradoxus present, JVP elevation, no distant heart sounds. **Labs/Imaging:** Stat CXR shows a large cardiac silhouette with a "water bottle" appearance. EKG shows sinus tachycardia, low-amplitude QRS complexes, and electrical alternans. TTE shows a severe circumferential effusion, with right ventricle and right atrial collapse in diastole.

Management: IV fluids (preload-dependent), pericardiocentesis, and later pericardial window.

Complications: Obstructive shock, cardiac arrest.

HYF:

- Tamponade is a clinical diagnosis. Diagnostic tools can aid with diagnosis but should not delay treatment. Classically presents with Beck triad: hypotension, distant heart sounds, and JVD. Pulsus paradoxus (exaggerated ↓ systolic BP with inspiration) and EKG with electrical alternans are also strongly suggestive of the diagnosis.

CONSTRICTIVE PERICARDITIS

A 50-year-old M with PMH of sarcoidosis presents with bilateral lower extremity edema and scrotal edema slowly worsening for the past 4–6 months. **Exam:** Pulsus paradoxus present, JVP elevation, ↑ jugular venous distention on inspiration (Kussmaul sign), pericardial knock. **Labs/Imaging:** Pericardial fibrosis and calcifications on CT chest or cardiac MRI. Increase pericardial thickness and pronounced respiratory variation in ventricular filling on TTE.

Management:

1. Initial conservative management is similar to the treatment of acute pericarditis (anti-inflammatory medications).
2. Chronic or persistent symptoms: Pericardiectomy.

Complications: Heart failure, cardiogenic shock, pulmonary edema, anasarca, cachexia, atrial fibrillation, hepatic dysfunction, or pericardial calcification.

HYF:

- Constrictive pericarditis can occur after virtually any pericardial disease process.
- Patients with chronic constrictive pericarditis or signs of progressive systemic congestion should undergo earlier surgical intervention.

TUBERCULOUS PERICARDITIS

A 40-year-old F who moved from India 2 months ago presents with subjective fever, cough, and dyspnea. **Exam:** Fever, tachycardia, ↑ jugular venous pressure, hepatomegaly, ascites, peripheral edema, pericardial friction rub. **Labs/Imaging:** TTE shows calcified pericardium and pericardial effusion. Sputum AFB smear is positive. CXR is clear. CT chest also shows calcified and thickened pericardium. Pericardiocentesis yields exudative fluid, characterized by high protein content and ↑ WBCs with a predominance of lymphocytes and monocytes. ADA is positive on fluid.

Management:

1. Anti-TB therapy (See Chapter 7, p. 291, Tuberculosis).

Complications: Constrictive pericarditis, cardiac tamponade, heart failure.

HYF:

- Tuberculous pericarditis should be considered in patients with pericarditis who do not have a self-limited course and have risk factors for TB exposure.
- Diagnosis: Detection of bacilli in smear or culture of pericardial fluid and/or by detection of tubercle bacilli or caseating granulomata on histological examination of the pericardium.
- Very high risk for constrictive pericarditis.

AUTOIMMUNE FLARE

A 50-year-old F with PMH of SLE presents with dyspnea and chest pain improved by leaning forward. **Exam:** Friction rub on cardiac auscultation. Otherwise, vital signs are unremarkable. **Labs/Imaging:** EKG without significant changes. TTE with presence of new pericardial effusion. Elevated creatinine and anti-DS antibodies.

Management:

1. Treat underlying rheumatological disorder.

Complications: Constrictive pericarditis, cardiac tamponade, heart failure.

(Continued)

1-20 Pericardial Disease

HYF:

- The most common types of pericardial involvement with systemic inflammatory diseases (SLE, rheumatoid arthritis) are acute pericarditis and asymptomatic pericardial effusions.

DRUG-INDUCED PERICARDITIS

A 58-year-old M with PMH of HTN on hydralazine presents with constant sharp chest pain that improves when he leans forward and is progressively after onset several days ago. **Exam:** BP and HR WNL, friction rub on cardiac auscultation. **Labs/Imaging:** EKG with diffuse ST-elevation and PR-depression, troponins minimally elevated.

Management:

1. NSAIDs and colchicine.
2. Stop the offending agent.

Complications: Constrictive pericarditis, cardiac tamponade, heart failure.

HYF:

- Drugs associated with DIP:
  - Lupus-like syndrome: Hydralazine, procainamide, isoniazid, phenytoin, and methyldopa.
  - Penicillin: A hypersensitivity reaction.
  - Minoxidil: Idiosyncratic reaction.
  - Chemotherapy: Most commonly anthracyclines (eg, doxorubicin).

UREMIC PERICARDITIS

A 42-year-old M with PMH of end-stage renal disease currently on hemodialysis presents with worsening mental status and constant chest pain after missing several HD sessions. **Exam:** BP 188/90, HR 80, anasarca, friction rub on cardiac auscultation. Patient is confused but does not have focal neurological deficits. **Labs/Imaging:** BUN 100, potassium 5.6, bicarbonate 16. EKG without major changes. TTE with concentric moderate pericardial effusion, no signs of tamponade.

Management:

1. Steroids, emergent/urgent hemodialysis.

Complications: Constrictive pericarditis, cardiac tamponade, heart failure.

HYF:

- Uremic pericarditis can occur in the setting of acute or chronic renal failure. Pericarditis in the setting of chronic kidney disease is usually an indication for initiation of dialysis. Classic EKG signs of acute pericarditis may be absent in uremic pericarditis.

MALIGNANT PERICARDITIS

A 46-year-old F with newly diagnosed breast cancer presents with worsening dyspnea and chest pain for the past 2 weeks. Her chest pain is constant and positional, worsening with deep breaths or lying down. **Exam:** BP 135/80, HR 90, SpO_2 89% on room air, friction rub on cardiac auscultation, and ↓ breath sounds in the left lower lung field. **Labs/Imaging:** EKG with diffuse ST elevation. CXR with big cardiac silhouette and left-sided pleural effusion. TTE reveals moderate pericardial effusion. Cytology of the pericardial fluid reveals malignant cells.

Management:

1. NSAIDs and colchicine.
2. Therapeutic drainage (pericardiocentesis). Malignant pericarditis is frequently accompanied by malignant pleural effusions, so may consider thoracentesis ± pigtail drainage.

Complications: Constrictive pericarditis, cardiac tamponade, heart failure.

HYF:

- Most common primary tumor involving the pericardium is the lung. Other common tumors: breast, esophagus, melanoma, lymphoma, and leukemia.

BACTERIAL PERICARDITIS

A 68-year-old M with PMH of end-stage renal disease on hemodialysis presents with chest pain for the past week, subjective fever, and cough. **Exam:** BP 100/70, HR 79, temperature 101.0, SpO_2 98% on room air, friction rub on cardiac auscultation, HD fistula slightly erythematous. **Labs/Imaging:** CBC shows leukocytosis with neutrophil predominance. EKG with diffuse ST elevation and PR depression. CXR WNL. Blood cultures positive for *Staphylococcus aureus*. TTE with moderate-to-severe pericardial effusion with loculations within the fluid, no valvular vegetations. Pericardiocentesis reveals frank pus (elevated PMNs).

Management:

1. Broad-spectrum antibiotics and pericardial window.
2. Treat underlying bloodstream infection.

Complications: Constrictive pericarditis, cardiac tamponade, heart failure.

HYF:

- Most common organisms include *Staphylococcus, Pneumococcus, Streptococcus* (rheumatic pancarditis), *Haemophilus*.
- Mechanisms: Direct spread from an intrathoracic focus of infection, hematogenous spread, extension from a myocardial focus, direct contamination from trauma or surgery, and extension from a subdiaphragmatic suppurative focus.

Dressler's Syndrome: See Post-MI Complications, pp. 6–7.

1-20 Pericardial Disease

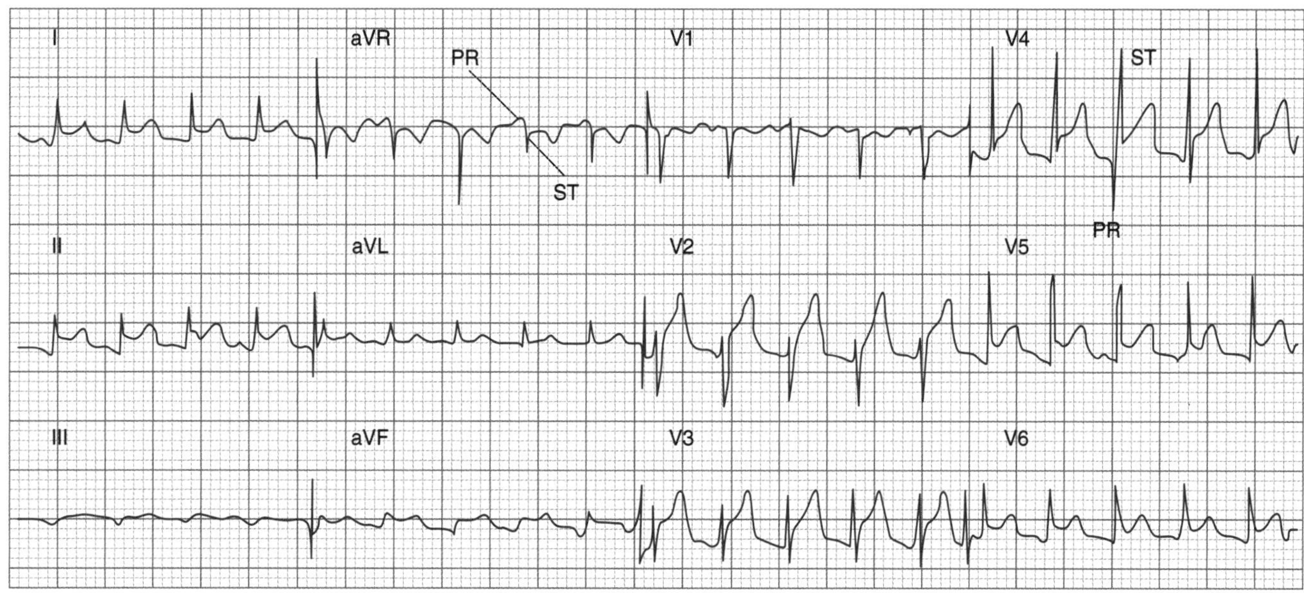
I
aVR
PR
ST
V1
V4
ST
PR
II
aVL
V2
V5
III
aVF
V3
V6

Acute pericarditis.

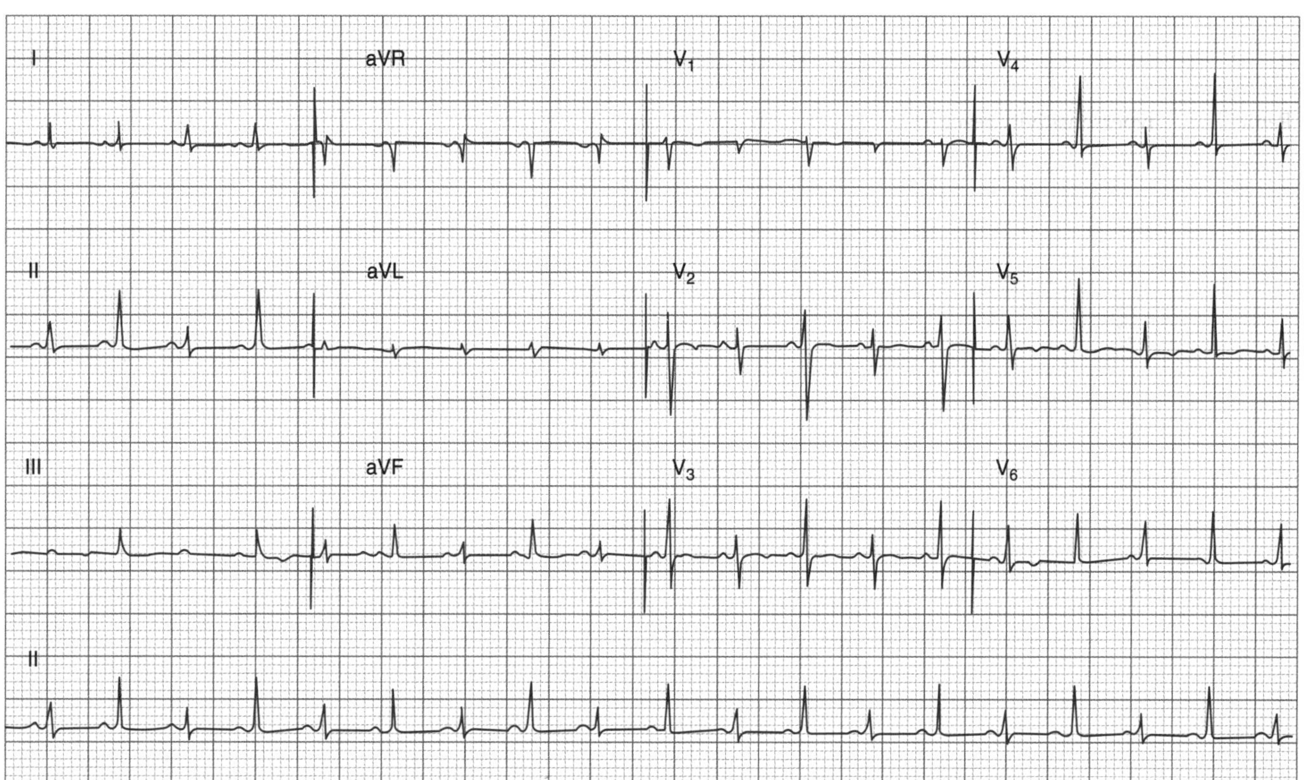
I
aVR
V_1
V_4
II
aVL
V_2
V_5
III
aVF
V_3
V_6
II

Electrical alternans in the setting of cardiac tamponade.

1-21 Valvulopathies

AORTIC STENOSIS (AS)

An 80-year-old M with PMH of coronary artery disease, HTN, and extensive smoking history presents with dyspnea on exertion and lightheadedness when walking up a flight of stairs. **Exam:** He has a slow-rising carotid pulse, loud mid- to late-peaking systolic ejection murmur in the right intercostal space ("crescendo-decrescendo"), a single 2nd heart sound, and an S4. The murmur increases with passive leg raise and decreases with Valsalva or standing. **Labs/Imaging:** TTE shows aortic leaflets are generally thickened and calcified with reduced systolic motion and a small aortic orifice during systole.

Management

1. Aortic valve replacement (surgical or transcatheter): Indicated for severe stenosis with symptoms, asymptomatic and low EF, asymptomatic with severe features and going for another cardiac surgery (ie, CABG).
2. As a temporizing measure, consider valvulotomy with balloon as a bridge to valve replacement.
3. Medical management: Careful diuresis (preload-dependent), control hypertension.

Complications: Heart failure, cardiomyopathy, syncope.

HYF:

- Younger patients with AS may have a bicuspid (as opposed to tricuspid) valve. If there is an ejection click, think of bicuspid AS (younger patients).
- In more severe AS, patients have a late-peaking murmur, paradoxically split S2, small and delayed carotid pulse (*pulsus parvus et tardus*).

AORTIC REGURGITATION (AR)

A 73-year-old M with PMH of peripheral vascular disease, extensive smoking history, and transient ischemic attack presents with 2 weeks of worsening dyspnea on exertion and orthopnea. **Exam:** He has wide pulse pressure (SBP–DBP) and an early diastolic murmur. The murmur is high-pitched, decrescendo, and blowing in quality with a mid-to-late diastolic rumble (Austin Flint murmur); it increases by sitting forward and with handgrip. **Labs/Imaging:** TTE with AR and concomitant ascending aorta dilation.

Management:

1. If heart failure: Treat with diuretics and GDMT (see pp. 12–14, Heart Failure).
2. Aortic valve replacement if symptomatic or severe LV dysfunction: Surgical valve replacement is treatment of choice.

Complications: Heart failure/cardiomyopathy.

HYF:

- Chronic AR: Classic signs include water hammer pulse (rapid rise/fall), head-bobbing with heartbeat (De Musset sign). Caused by disease of the valve leaflets or enlargement of the aortic root. Most common etiology in developing countries is rheumatic heart disease. Most common etiologies in developed countries are aortic root dilation, congenital bicuspid aortic valve, and calcific valve disease.
- Acute AR: Caused by endocarditis, aortic dissection, traumatic leaflet rupture.

MITRAL REGURGITATION (MR)

A 45-year-old F with PMH of SLE presents with fevers and chills after a major dental procedure 1 week ago. Additionally, she is complaining of dyspnea on exertion, orthopnea, and mild constant chest pain. **Exam:** Apical holosystolic or mid-to-late systolic murmur. Murmur increases with hand grip and decreases with Valsalva. Diastolic rumble present, hyperdynamic PMI, obscured S1, widely split S2, and brisk carotid upstroke. **Labs/Imaging:** Visualization of the valve on TTE is suboptimal. TEE is performed, which shows severe MR.

Management

1. Acute: Consider ischemia or endocarditis as primary causes. Start vasodilators (nitrates) and diuretics to relieve vascular congestion, and consider mechanical support (intra-aortic balloon pump) or inotropes as a bridge to surgical valve replacement.
2. Chronic, severe primary MR: MV replacement if symptomatic and EF >30%, or if symptomatic and EF 30–60% or LV dilated.
3. Non-operative patients (high-risk): Mitral clip.

Complications: Heart failure, pulmonary edema, arrhythmias, clot formation, and stroke.

HYF: One cause of MR is mitral valve prolapse, whose murmur is a high-pitched, mid-systolic click. Etiologies include sporadic or familial myxomatous degeneration of MV apparatus, trauma, endocarditis, congenital, connective-tissue disease (Marfan). Standing (decreased preload) will increase the murmur; squatting (increased preload) will decrease the murmur. If symptomatic, consider trial of β-blockers.

MITRAL STENOSIS (MS)

A 40-year-old F who moved to the US 3 years ago from Colombia presents with exertional dyspnea and decreased exercise tolerance for the past month. During her last PCP visit a week ago, she was also found to be anemic and started iron supplements. **Exam:** Irregularly irregular heart rhythm and diastolic murmur best heard in left lateral decubitus during expiration that increases with exertion. **Labs/Imaging:** EKG shows atrial fibrillation and left atrial enlargement. TTE shows mitral valve stenosis and fusion of commissures.

Management

1. Consider mitral balloon valvotomy vs. surgical repair for symptomatic patients with severe MS (depending on degree of severity and surgical risk).
2. If rheumatic MS, give antibiotic prophylaxis for secondary prevention of rheumatic fever.
3. If valvular atrial fibrillation, anticoagulation indicated with vitamin K antagonist (warfarin).

Complications: Heart failure, left atrial enlargement, arrhythmias, clot formation, and stroke.

1-21 Valvulopathies

HYF:

- Precipitants: Exercise, fever, anemia, infection, pregnancy. The most common cause of MS is rheumatic heart disease with mitral commissural fusion ("fish mouth valve").
- Ortner syndrome: Hoarseness from left atrium (LA) compression of recurrent laryngeal nerve (LA enlargement due to severe stenosis).
- EKG: *P mitrale* due to LA enlargement.
- Associated with atrial fibrillation: Very common embolic events (eg, stroke).

PROSTHETIC HEART VALVES

A 68-year-old M with no PMH presents with dyspnea on exertion that has worsened over the past few days. He is active at home mowing the lawn, chopping wood, and gardening. **Exam:** BP 120/70, mid-systolic murmur at the right upper sternal boarder that radiates to the carotids. **Labs/Imaging:** TTE shows diffuse hypokinesis and LVEF ~30%. Aortic valve cusp is heavily calcified with decreased mobility, with increase transvalvular gradient.

Management

1. For this patient, given symptoms, implications of untreated valvulopathy (ie, cardiomypathy), and low surgical risk (no comorbidities, young, good functional status), consider surgical aortic replacement > transaortic valve replacement (TAVR).
2. Anticoagulation in patient with bioprosthetic vs. mechanical valves:
   a. Bioprosthetic: Direct oral anticoagulation or warfarin for 3–6 months plus ASA; then, if no contraindications, can either continue both or only ASA.
   b. Mechanical: Lifelong oral anticoagulation with warfarin plus ASA.
3. Refer to other vignettes under "Valvulopathies" for additional information.

Complications: Clot formation, stroke, arterial embolic phenomena, hemolysis, prosthetic valve infective endocarditis.

HYF:

- Long term anticoagulation is only strictly necessary for mechanical valves; warfarin is superior to direct oral anticoagulants (dabigatran, rivaroxaban, apixaban).
- Mechanical valves have more risk of hemolysis and stroke if INR is not therapeutic. They last longer than bioprosthetic valves.
- All types of prosthetic valves have higher risks of endocarditis.
- Suspect prosthetic valvular dysfunction if new cardiac symptoms, hemolytic anemia, new murmurs, or embolic phenomena.

TRICUSPID REGURGITATION

A 65-year-old M with PMH of pulmonary hypertension presents with increased dyspnea on exertion and peripheral edema. **Exam:** Rales on lung auscultation, hepatosplenomegaly, ascites, bilateral lower extremity pitting edema, increased jugular venous distension with inspiration (Kussmaul's sign), and S3. There is a blowing holosystolic murmur heard best in the left lower sternal border that increases with inspiration and leg raising and decreases with standing and Valsalva maneuver. **Labs/Imaging:** BNP, creatinine, and LFTs are elevated. CXR shows marked cardiomegaly, pleural effusions, and pulmonary venous congestion. EKG shows right axis deviation indicating RV hypertrophy and tall R waves in V1 to V2. TTE shows tricuspid leaflet prolapse and dilated right atrium and right ventricle in the presence of moderate-severe tricuspid regurgitation.

Management:

1. Diuretics (reduce preload) for volume overload.
2. If symptomatic and severe TR, tricuspid valve surgery.

Complications: Arrhythmias (atrial fibrillation), thrombus formation and embolization, cardiac cirrhosis.

HYF: Can be 2/2 pulmonary HTN leading to *cor pulmonale*, tricuspid endocarditis, RV infarction, inferior wall MI, or RV dilation. May be present in up to 70% of normal adults; patients typically remain asymptomatic unless they develop pulmonary HTN or right-sided heart failure.

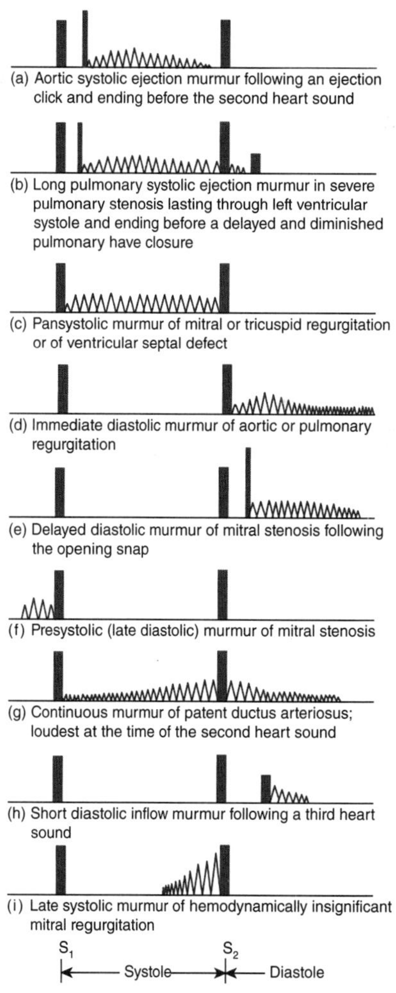
(a) Aortic systolic ejection murmur following an ejection click and ending before the second heart sound
(b) Long pulmonary systolic ejection murmur in severe pulmonary stenosis lasting through left ventricular systole and ending before a delayed and diminished pulmonary have closure
(c) Pansystolic murmur of mitral or tricuspid regurgitation or of ventricular septal defect
(d) Immediate diastolic murmur of aortic or pulmonary regurgitation
(e) Delayed diastolic murmur of mitral stenosis following the opening snap
(f) Presystolic (late diastolic) murmur of mitral stenosis
(g) Continuous murmur of patent ductus arteriosus; loudest at the time of the second heart sound
(h) Short diastolic inflow murmur following a third heart sound
(i) Late systolic murmur of hemodynamically insignificant mitral regurgitation
S1
S2
Systole
Diastole

Timing and intensity of cardiac murmurs.

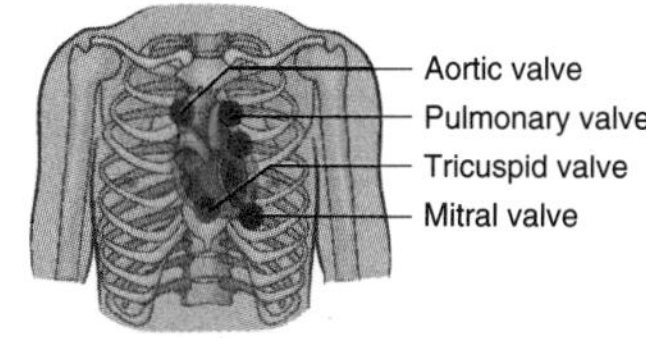
HEART AUSCULTATION POINTS
Aortic valve
Pulmonary valve
Tricuspid valve
Mitral valve

1-22 Syncope

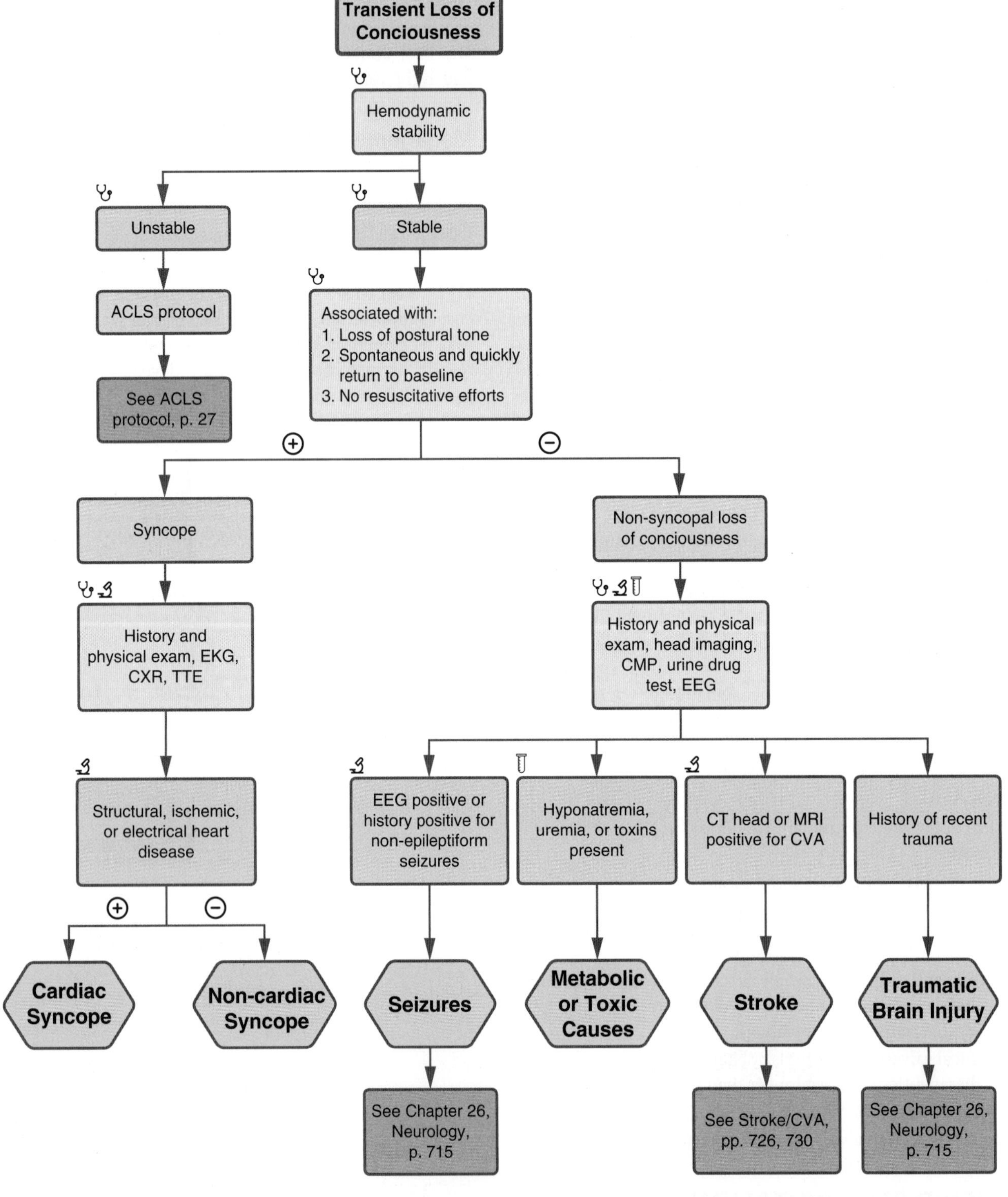
Transient Loss of Conciousness
Hemodynamic stability
Unstable
Stable
ACLS protocol
See ACLS protocol, p. 27
Associated with:
1. Loss of postural tone
2. Spontaneous and quickly return to baseline
3. No resuscitative efforts
+
−
Syncope
Non-syncopal loss of conciousness
History and physical exam, EKG, CXR, TTE
History and physical exam, head imaging, CMP, urine drug test, EEG
Structural, ischemic, or electrical heart disease
+
−
Cardiac Syncope
Non-cardiac Syncope
EEG positive or history positive for non-epileptiform seizures
Hyponatremia, uremia, or toxins present
CT head or MRI positive for CVA
History of recent trauma
Seizures
Metabolic or Toxic Causes
Stroke
Traumatic Brain Injury
See Chapter 26, Neurology, p. 715
See Stroke/CVA, pp. 726, 730
See Chapter 26, Neurology, p. 715

When presented with syncope, it is important to first assess hemodynamic stability and then distinguish true syncope vs. non-syncopal loss of conciousness. True syncope is a transient loss of conciousness due to inadequate cerebral blood flow. A thorough history, including associated symptoms prior to, during, and after the event; past medical history; medication reconciliation; social history; triggers; and collateral informaton from bystanders will offer clues. Alternative non-syncopal etiologies of loss of consciousness include epileptic seizure or nonepileptic spell (see Seizures, p. 761), stroke (see Stroke, pp. 726, 730), toxic or metabolic causes, and traumatic brain injury. This chapter will focus on syncope, approaching causes related directly to the heart (cardiac syncope) separately from primarily non-cardiac causes that more directly involve the peripheral vasculature (non-cardiac syncope). Additionally, the clinician should be aware of sequela of syncope, including falls leading to an epidural or subdural hematoma, concussion, fracture, or bleeding.

FIGURE 1.22

1-23 Syncope (Cardiac)

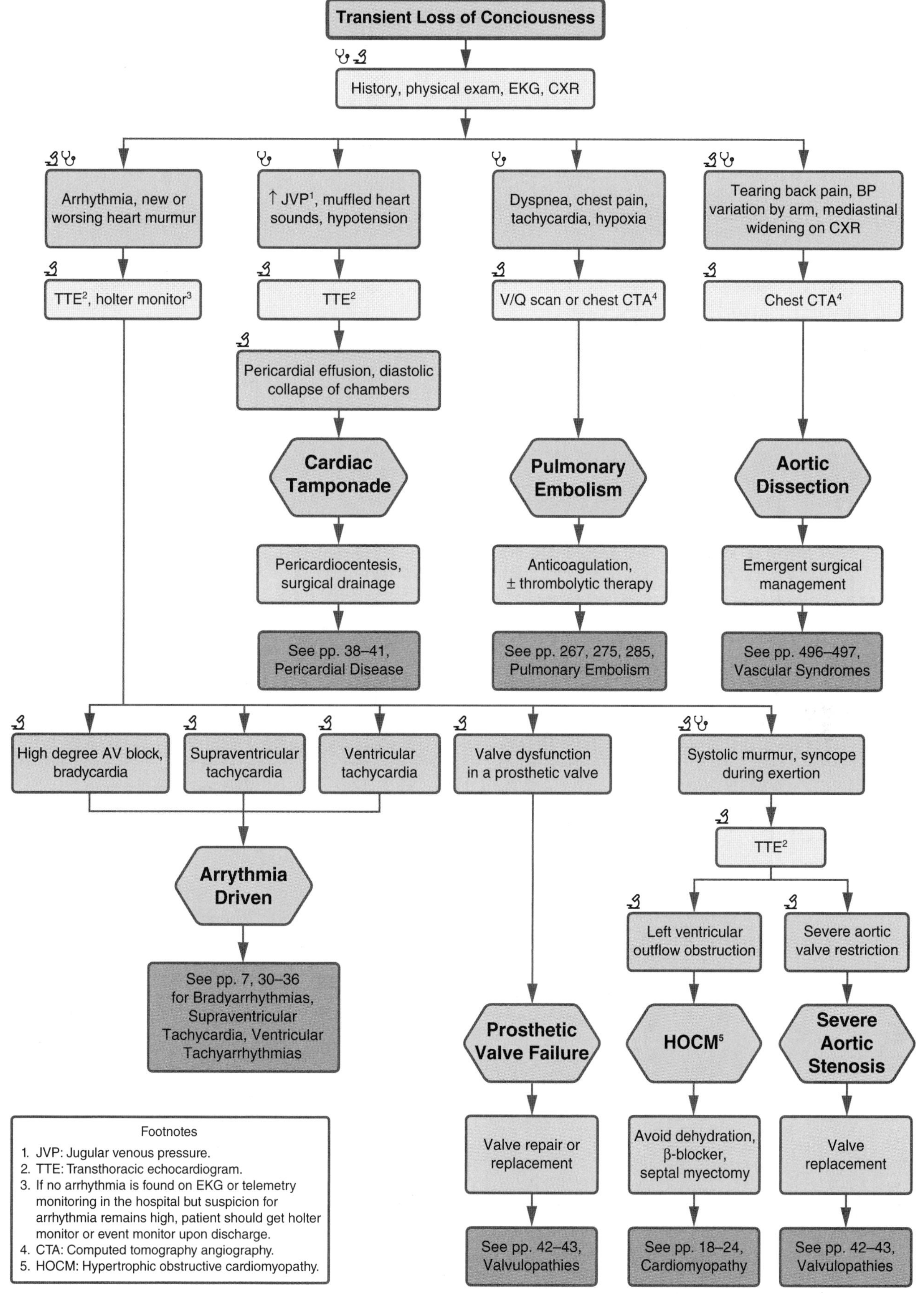
Transient Loss of Conciousness
History, physical exam, EKG, CXR
Arrhythmia, new or worsing heart murmur
↑ JVP¹, muffled heart sounds, hypotension
Dyspnea, chest pain, tachycardia, hypoxia
Tearing back pain, BP variation by arm, mediastinal widening on CXR
TTE², holter monitor³
TTE²
V/Q scan or chest CTA⁴
Chest CTA⁴
Pericardial effusion, diastolic collapse of chambers
Cardiac Tamponade
Pulmonary Embolism
Aortic Dissection
Pericardiocentesis, surgical drainage
Anticoagulation, ± thrombolytic therapy
Emergent surgical management
See pp. 38–41, Pericardial Disease
See pp. 267, 275, 285, Pulmonary Embolism
See pp. 496–497, Vascular Syndromes
High degree AV block, bradycardia
Supraventricular tachycardia
Ventricular tachycardia
Valve dysfunction in a prosthetic valve
Systolic murmur, syncope during exertion
TTE²
Arrythmia Driven
Left ventricular outflow obstruction
Severe aortic valve restriction
See pp. 7, 30–36 for Bradyarrhythmias, Supraventricular Tachycardia, Ventricular Tachyarrhythmias
Prosthetic Valve Failure
HOCM⁵
Severe Aortic Stenosis
Valve repair or replacement
Avoid dehydration, β-blocker, septal myectomy
Valve replacement
See pp. 42–43, Valvulopathies
See pp. 18–24, Cardiomyopathy
See pp. 42–43, Valvulopathies
Footnotes
1. JVP: Jugular venous pressure.
2. TTE: Transthoracic echocardiogram.
3. If no arrhythmia is found on EKG or telemetry monitoring in the hospital but suspicion for arrhythmia remains high, patient should get holter monitor or event monitor upon discharge.
4. CTA: Computed tomography angiography.
5. HOCM: Hypertrophic obstructive cardiomyopathy.

FIGURE 1.23

1-24 Syncope (Non-Cardiac)

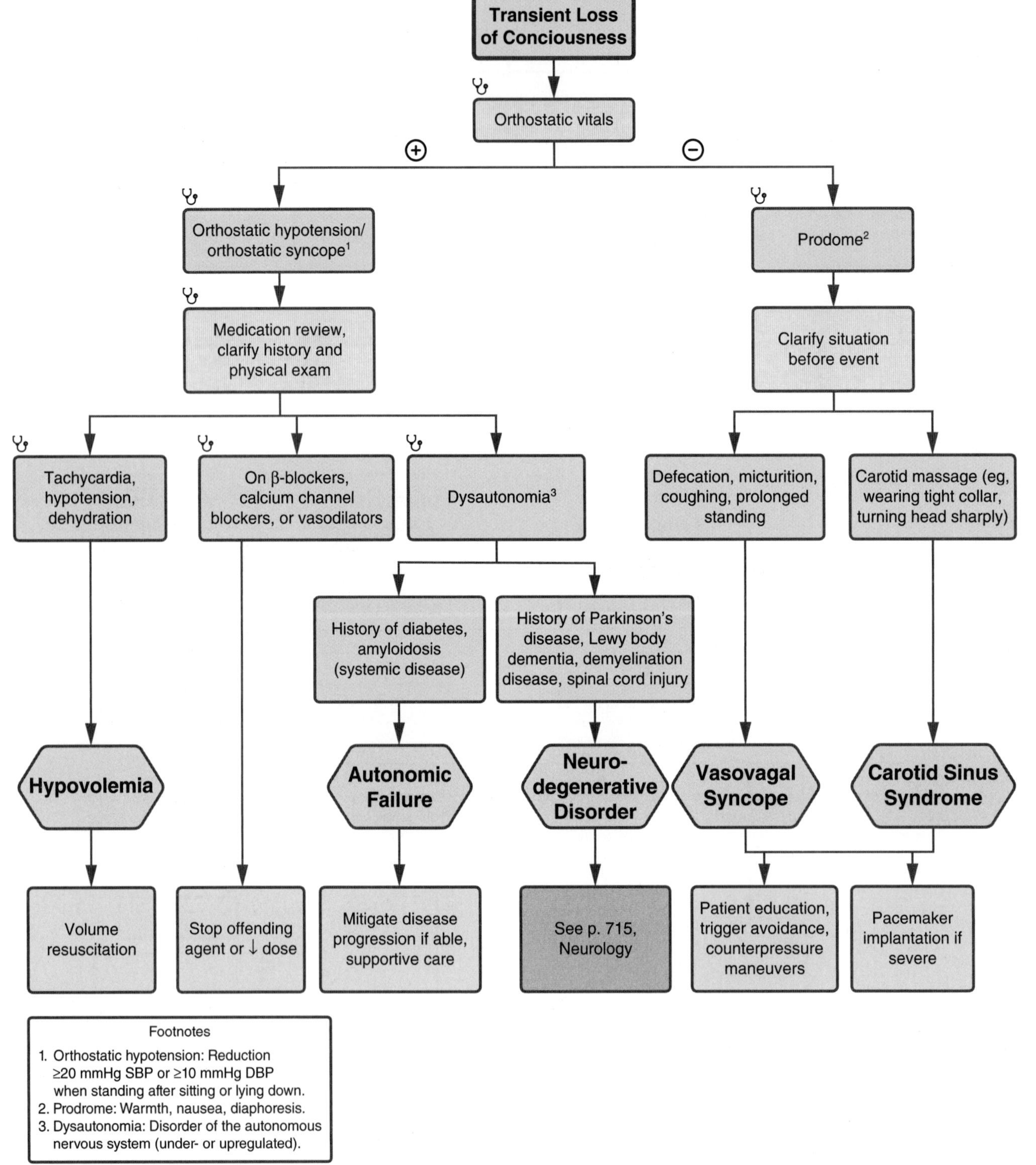

Transient Loss of Conciousness
Orthostatic vitals
⊕
⊖
Orthostatic hypotension/ orthostatic syncope1
Medication review, clarify history and physical exam
Tachycardia, hypotension, dehydration
On β-blockers, calcium channel blockers, or vasodilators
Dysautonomia3
History of diabetes, amyloidosis (systemic disease)
History of Parkinson's disease, Lewy body dementia, demyelination disease, spinal cord injury
Hypovolemia
Autonomic Failure
Neuro-degenerative Disorder
Volume resuscitation
Stop offending agent or ↓ dose
Mitigate disease progression if able, supportive care
See p. 715, Neurology
Prodome2
Clarify situation before event
Defecation, micturition, coughing, prolonged standing
Carotid massage (eg, wearing tight collar, turning head sharply)
Vasovagal Syncope
Carotid Sinus Syndrome
Patient education, trigger avoidance, counterpressure maneuvers
Pacemaker implantation if severe

Footnotes

1. Orthostatic hypotension: Reduction ≥20 mmHg SBP or ≥10 mmHg DBP when standing after sitting or lying down.
2. Prodrome: Warmth, nausea, diaphoresis.
3. Dysautonomia: Disorder of the autonomous nervous system (under- or upregulated).

FIGURE 1.24

1-24 Syncope (Non-Cardiac)

HYPOVOLEMIC HYPOTENSION

A 67-year-old M with PMH of HTN on carvedilol presents with recent loss of consciousness. For the past 4 days, he has been having viral gastroenteritis and endorses nausea, vomiting, and diarrhea. **Exam:** BP initially 120/80 while sitting that then drops to 80/60 when he stands, HR 103. Dry mucous membranes and poor skin turgor. **Labs/Imaging:** Elevated hematocrit, elevated BUN and creatinine, low sodium.

Management: Volume resuscitation and hold antihypertensive agents.

Complications: Falls leading to traumatic injury (eg, subdural hematomas in the elderly).

HYF:

- Hypovolemia leading to orthostatic syncope can arise from, among other things, blood loss, insufficient volume repletion after exercise or heat exposure, diarrhea/vomiting, or impaired thirst drive in older adults.

AUTONOMIC FAILURE

A 78-year-old M with PMH of uncontrolled diabetes and Parkinson's disease presents with a witnessed episode of loss of consciousness. **Exam:** BP initially 140/80 while sitting that then drops to 100/65 when he stands up, HR 110. No signs of hypovolemia. **Labs/Imaging:** Chemistry and CBC WNL.

Management:

1. Mitigate progression of the underlying disease if possible, encourage salt/fluid intake, abdominal binder, may benefit from sympathomimetics or mineralocorticoids.

Complications: Falls leading to traumatic injury.

HYF:

- Risk factors: Poorly controlled diabetes, alcohol use disorder, degenerative neurological diseases (eg, Parkinson's disease).
- Mechanism: Postganglionic sympathetic neurons do not release norepinephrine appropriately. Blood pressure falls progressively after standing because the gravitational pooling of blood in the legs cannot be compensated by sympathetic vasoconstriction.

VASOVAGAL

A 17-year-old F with no significant PMH presents with what is described by bystanders as "having a seizure" before giving blood at the local blood drive. She reports binocular vision loss and then loss of consciousness after getting stuck by the nurse; she was witnessed to have stereotyped movements during the episode and then returned to full consciousness 20 seconds later. **Exam:** Diaphoretic, pale, and anxious-appearing, but exam is otherwise unremarkable. **Labs/Imaging:** Spot EEG and brain MRI are both unremarkable. No other abnormal labs noted.

Management:

- Reassurance and patient education, trigger avoidance, and countermeasure maneuvers such as leg crossing or hand grip.

Complications: Falls leading to traumatic injury.

HYF:

- Vasovagal is the most common type of syncope. Convulsive motor activity, which may be confused for epileptic convulsions, can occur during vasovagal syncope.

CAROTID SINUS SYNDROME/ CAROTID SINUS HYPERSENSITIVITY

An 80-year-old M with PMH of peripheral arterial disease, coronary artery disease, and previous left carotid endarterectomy presents after a ground-level fall when he was at home. His wife mentioned he was shaving his neck when suddenly he lost consciousness and fell. **Exam:** Vital signs are stable; when performing carotid massage he has a 4-second sinus pause, and this reproduces his symptoms. **Labs/Imaging:** EKG and Holter monitor without evidence of any arrhythmias when he is not getting a carotid sinus massage.

Management: If symptoms are very significant, refer for pacemaker placement.

Complications: Falls leading to traumatic injury, arrhythmias triggered by pauses/bradycardia.

HYF:

- Treatment is only warranted if CSH is deemed responsible for symptoms of syncope, lightheadedness, or unexplained falls.

Arrhythmias: See Supraventricular Arrhythmias, pp. 32–34, Bradyarrhythmias, pp. 30–31, and Ventricular Arrhythmias, pp. 35–36.

Cardiac Tamponade: See Cardiac Tamponade, p. 39.

Pulmonary Embolism: See Pulmonary Embolism, pp. 267, 275, 285.

Aortic Dissection: See Aortic Dissection, p. 497.

Hypertrophic Cardiomyopathy: See Cardiomyopathy, pp. 25–26.

Aortic stenosis/Valvulopathies: See Valvulopathies, pp. 42–43.

1-25 Hypertension

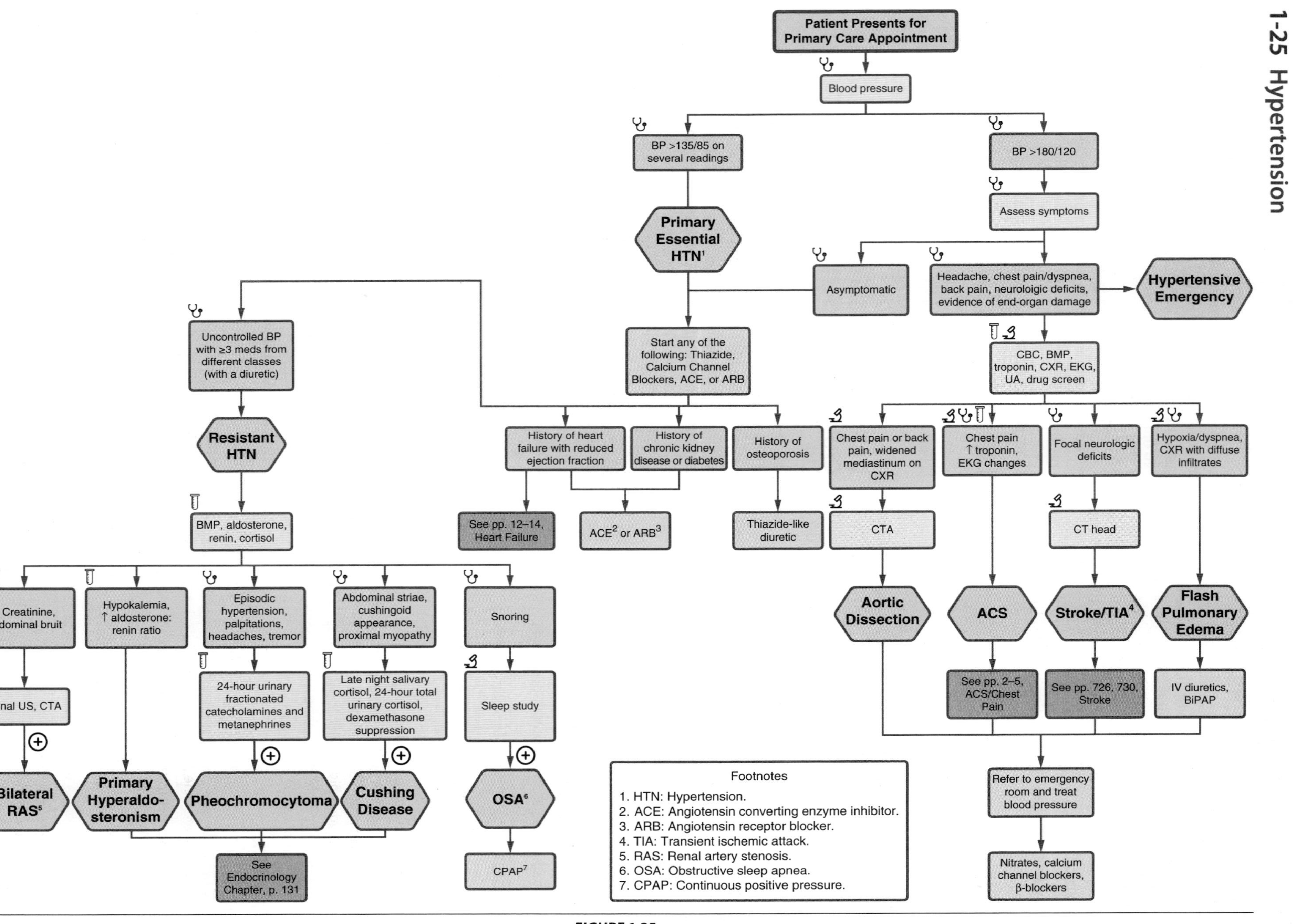

Patient Presents for Primary Care Appointment
Blood pressure
BP >135/85 on several readings
BP >180/120
Assess symptoms
Primary Essential HTN1
Asymptomatic
Headache, chest pain/dyspnea, back pain, neuroloigic deficits, evidence of end-organ damage
Hypertensive Emergency
Uncontrolled BP with ≥3 meds from different classes (with a diuretic)
Start any of the following: Thiazide, Calcium Channel Blockers, ACE, or ARB
CBC, BMP, troponin, CXR, EKG, UA, drug screen
Resistant HTN
History of heart failure with reduced ejection fraction
History of chronic kidney disease or diabetes
History of osteoporosis
Chest pain or back pain, widened mediastinum on CXR
Chest pain ↑ troponin, EKG changes
Focal neurologic deficits
Hypoxia/dyspnea, CXR with diffuse infiltrates
BMP, aldosterone, renin, cortisol
See pp. 12–14, Heart Failure
ACE2 or ARB3
Thiazide-like diuretic
CTA
CT head
↑ Creatinine, abdominal bruit
Hypokalemia, ↑ aldosterone: renin ratio
Episodic hypertension, palpitations, headaches, tremor
Abdominal striae, cushingoid appearance, proximal myopathy
Snoring
Aortic Dissection
ACS
Stroke/TIA4
Flash Pulmonary Edema
Renal US, CTA
24-hour urinary fractionated catecholamines and metanephrines
Late night salivary cortisol, 24-hour total urinary cortisol, dexamethasone suppression
Sleep study
See pp. 2–5, ACS/Chest Pain
See pp. 726, 730, Stroke
IV diuretics, BiPAP
+
Bilateral RAS5
Primary Hyperaldo-steronism
Pheochromocytoma
Cushing Disease
OSA6
Refer to emergency room and treat blood pressure
See Endocrinology Chapter, p. 131
CPAP7
Nitrates, calcium channel blockers, β-blockers
Footnotes
1. HTN: Hypertension.
2. ACE: Angiotensin converting enzyme inhibitor.
3. ARB: Angiotensin receptor blocker.
4. TIA: Transient ischemic attack.
5. RAS: Renal artery stenosis.
6. OSA: Obstructive sleep apnea.
7. CPAP: Continuous positive pressure.

FIGURE 1.25

1-25 Hypertension

ESSENTIAL HYPERTENSION

A 59-year-old M presents to primary care for the first time to establish care. He has a history of coronary artery disease, type 2 diabetes, and obesity. **Exam:** BP 180/79, HR 75. After >5 minutes sitting comfortably, repeat blood pressure is 182/78. The rest of the physical exam is within normal limits. **Labs/Imaging:** Ambulatory blood pressure monitor for ≥ 24 hours confirms sustained hypertension.

Management:

1. Rule out end-organ damage when BP is significantly high (>160/80): hypertension urgency vs. emergency.
2. Non-pharmacological interventions: DASH diet (reduces BP by 11 mmHg), weight loss (reduces BP by 5 mmHg), aerobic physical activity (reduces BP by 5–8 mmHg), decrease alcohol consumption (reduces BP by 4 mmHg).
3. Start any of the following: thiazide, calcium channel blocker, ACE, or ARB. If BP >160/80, likely will require ≥2 agents.

Complications: Left ventricular hypertrophy, stroke, heart failure, ischemic heart disease, chronic kidney disease, retinopathy.

HYF:

- Defined as systolic blood pressure (SBP) ≥130 mm Hg and/or diastolic blood pressure (DBP) ≥80 mm Hg.
- When selecting an anti-hypertensive medication, consider the patient's comorbidities:
  - HFrEF: Choose between β-blocker and ACE/ARB.
  - CKD (proteinuria): ACE/ARBs.
  - Diabetes: ACE/ARBs.

HYPERTENSIVE EMERGENCY

A 56-year-old woman with PMH of poorly controlled HTN presents with a severe headache and blurry vision. **Exam:** Her BP is 220/120 and HR 90. Her neurologic exam is unremarkable. On **imaging:** CT head without contrast does not show evidence of ischemic stroke or intracranial hemorrhage. Funduscopic exam shows arteriolar narrowing, arteriovenous nicking, and cotton wool spots. She is given IV labetalol.

Management:

1. For hypertensive emergency, reduce BP by 10–20% within the 1st hour and another 5-15% within the next 24 hours. Exceptions to gradual reduction in BP include ischemic stroke and aortic dissection. Agents of choice include IV β-blockers (labetalol, esmolol), calcium channel blockers (nicardipine, clevidipine), and nitrates (nitroprusside, nitroglycerin).

Complications: Sequalae of end-organ damage (vision loss, stroke, acute kidney injury), death.

HYF:

- *Hypertensive emergency* is defined as severely elevated BP (SBP ≥180 and/or DBP ≥120) with end-organ damage. In contrast, *hypertensive urgency* is defined as severely elevated BP without end-organ damage. Hypertensive emergency requires gradual reduction in BP as outlined above, as there is a risk of stroke from decreased cerebral perfusion if BP reduction occurs too quickly. Hypertensive urgency requires chronic management of BP (eg, oral thiazide or calcium channel blocker); there is no need to immediately reduce BP.
- Posterior Reversible (Leuko) Encephalopathy Syndrome (PRES) is a clinical and radiologic syndrome in which a patient often presents with acutely altered mentation, headache, visual impairment, and/or seizures in the setting of a hypertensive emergency. Brain MRI shows vasogenic edema as a hyperintense signal on T2, most commonly in the parieto-occipital lobes. Pathophysiology is poorly understood, but PRES is often associated with HTN, renal disease requiring dialysis, cancer, organ transplantation, autoimmune disorders, and certain medications (immunosuppressants, chemotherapy). Management involves treating the underlying etiology if possible, in addition to careful management of HTN.

Summary of Antihypertensive Drugs

Class	Drug	Mechanism of Action	Clinical Presentation With Toxicity
Diuretics	Chlorothiazide, Chlorthalidone, Hydrochlorothiazide, Metolazone	Inhibition of distal tubule sodium chloride absorption	Hypokalemia, hypercalcemia
	Bumetanide, Furosemide	Inhibition of sodium-potassium-chloride symporter in renal loop of Henle	Hypocalcemia, hypokalemia, hypomagnesemia
	Amiloride, Triamterene	Inhibition of sodium absorption and potassium elimination in renal distal collecting duct	Hyperkalemia
	Eplerenone, Spironolactone	Mineralocorticoid antagonist	Hyperkalemia
Sympatholytics	Doxazosin, Prazosin, Tamsulosin, Terazosin	α_1-Adrenergic receptor antagonist	
	Clonidine	α_2-Adrenergic receptor agonist, Imidazoline receptor agonist, μ-Receptor opioid agonist	Bradycardia, neurologic depression
	Oxymetazoline, Tetrahydrozoline	Imidazoline receptor agonist	Bradycardia, neurologic depression
	Guanadrel, Methyldopa, Reserpine	Decreased norepinephrine release	Bradycardia, hemolytic anemia (idiosyncratic reaction to methyldopa)

(Continued)

1-25 Hypertension

Summary of Antihypertensive Drugs (Continued)

Class	Drug	Mechanism of Action	Clinical Presentation With Toxicity
Angiotensin-converting enzyme inhibitors	Benazepril, Captopril, Enalapril, Quinapril	Inhibition of ACE, Inhibition of bradykininase	Hyperkalemia, angioedema (idiosyncratic), cough (idiosyncratic)
Angiotensin receptor blockers	Candesartan, Irbesartan, Losartan, Valsartan	Angiotensin II receptor antagonist	Hyperkalemia, angioedema (less common than with ACE inhibitors)
Vasodilators	Hydralazine	Arteriolar vasodilation	Hypotension, lupus-like syndrome
	Minoxidil	Arteriolar vasodilation	Tachycardia, increased myocardial oxygen demand
	Sodium nitroprusside	Arteriolar and venous vasodilation (via nitric oxide release)	Hypotension, tachycardia, thiocyanate toxicity, cyanide toxicity (very rare)

Abbreviations: ACE = angiotensin-converting enzyme; ARB = angiotensin II receptor blocker; ACEI = angiotensin-converting enzyme inhibitors.

RESISTANT HYPERTENSION (HTN)

A 62-year-old F presents to primary care for a regular follow-up visit. She has a history of diabetes, obesity, and long-standing hypertension. Currently, she is taking 4-medications to treat her HTN at maximal doses, including a diuretic. **Exam:** BP is 180/90. Other vitals and remaining physical exam are within normal limits. **Labs/Imaging:** Ambulatory BP monitor for at least 24 hours confirms sustained hypertension.

Management:

1. Address medication non-adherence; stop medications that can increase BP (eg, NSAIDs).
2. Rule out end-organ damage when BP is significantly high (>160/80): hypertension urgency vs. emergency.
3. Non-pharmacological interventions, as above.

Complications: Left ventricular hypertrophy, stroke, heart failure, ischemic heart disease, kidney disease.

HYF:

- In young patients or patients with resistant hypertension, investigate causes of secondary hypertension (renin/aldosterone levels, renal artery ultrasound, sleep study, catecholamine levels).

1-26 Hyperlipidemia

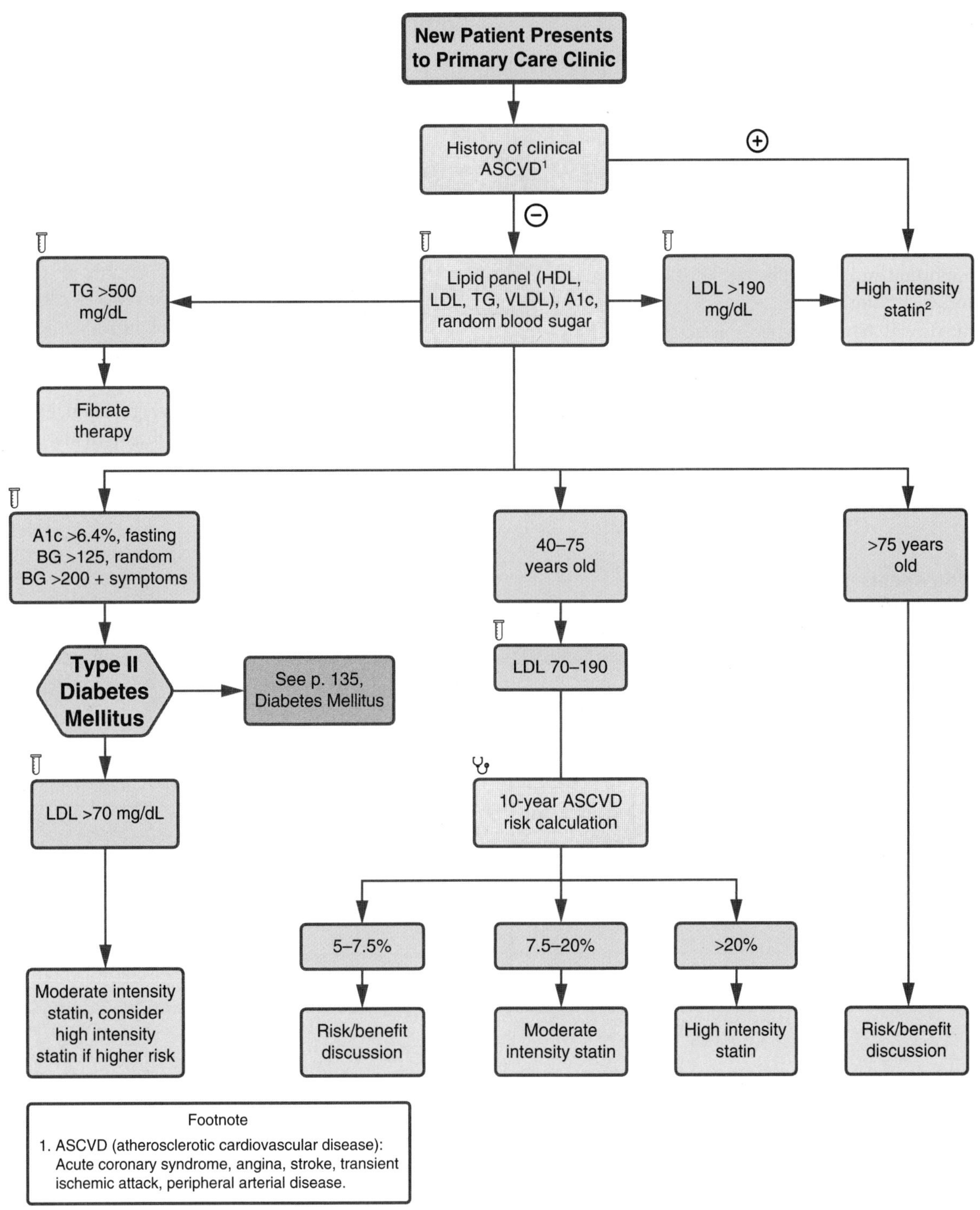
New Patient Presents to Primary Care Clinic
History of clinical ASCVD[1]
⊕
⊖
Lipid panel (HDL, LDL, TG, VLDL), A1c, random blood sugar
TG >500 mg/dL
Fibrate therapy
LDL >190 mg/dL
High intensity statin[2]
A1c >6.4%, fasting BG >125, random BG >200 + symptoms
Type II Diabetes Mellitus
See p. 135, Diabetes Mellitus
LDL >70 mg/dL
Moderate intensity statin, consider high intensity statin if higher risk
40–75 years old
LDL 70–190
10-year ASCVD risk calculation
5–7.5%
Risk/benefit discussion
7.5–20%
Moderate intensity statin
>20%
High intensity statin
>75 years old
Risk/benefit discussion
Footnote
1. ASCVD (atherosclerotic cardiovascular disease): Acute coronary syndrome, angina, stroke, transient ischemic attack, peripheral arterial disease.

FIGURE 1.26

1-26 Hyperlipidemia

HYPERLIPIDEMIA

A 55-year-old M with no PMH presents to establish care with a primary care physician. **Exam:** BP 120/70, BMI 25%, no other positive findings. **Labs/Imaging:** Lipid panel with LDL 210. Otherwise, A1c is 5.6% and there are no other lab abnormalities.

Management:

1. Lifestyle modifications (exercise, weight loss, diet).
2. Medications:
   a. Most important and most effective: HMG-CoA reductase inhibitors (ie, statins).
   b. For patients with familial hypercholesterolemia: PCSK9 inhibitors: alirocumab, evolocumab.
   c. Other agents (less effective): Ezetimibe, fibrates, niacin, bile acid sequestrants.
   d. Hypertriglyceridemia: Fibrates.

Complications: Coronary artery disease, stroke, peripheral vascular. Severe hypertriglyceridemia (>500) increases risk for pancreatitis.

HYF:

- ASCVD risk calculator: Takes into account the patient's age, BP, lipid panel, smoking history, and comorbidities (HTN, diabetes).
  - High intensity statin: Daily dose reduces >50% LDL.
  - Moderate intensity: Daily dose reduces 30–49% LDL.
  - Low intensity statin: Daily dose reduces <30% LDL.
- Patients who will almost always require a statin: 40–75 years old with risk score >7.5%, have T2DM, and/or have clinical ASCVD (eg, history of MI, angina, stroke).
- Baseline labs and monitoring: Liver function test and lipid panel. Monitor transaminases and CPK only if the patient develops symptoms of hepatic and/or muscle disease.
- Severe hypertriglyceridemia increases risk for pancreatitis.

Lipid-Lowering Agents

Drug	Effect on LDL	Effect on HDL	Effect on Triglycerides	Side Effects
HMG–CoA reductase inhibitors (atorvastatin, rosuvastatin)	↓↓	↑	↓	Increased LFTs, myositis (monitor transaminases and CPK if the patient develops symptoms of hepatic and/or muscle disease)
PCSK9 inhibitors (alirocumab, evolocumab)	↓↓	↑	↓	Flu-like illness, nasopharyngitis, myalgia, arthralgia, injection site reaction
Cholesterol absorption inhibitors (ezetimibe)	↓	–	–	Myalgias
Fibrates (gemfibrozil, fenofibrate)	↓	↑	↓↓	Increased LFTs, myositis
Bile acid sequestrants (colestipol, colesevalam, cholestyramine)	↓	–	–/↑	GI upset
Niacin	↓	↑	↓	Increased LFTs, facial flushing, GI upset, gout flares, insulin resistance

2

Internal Medicine: Gastroenterology

2-1 Dysphagia

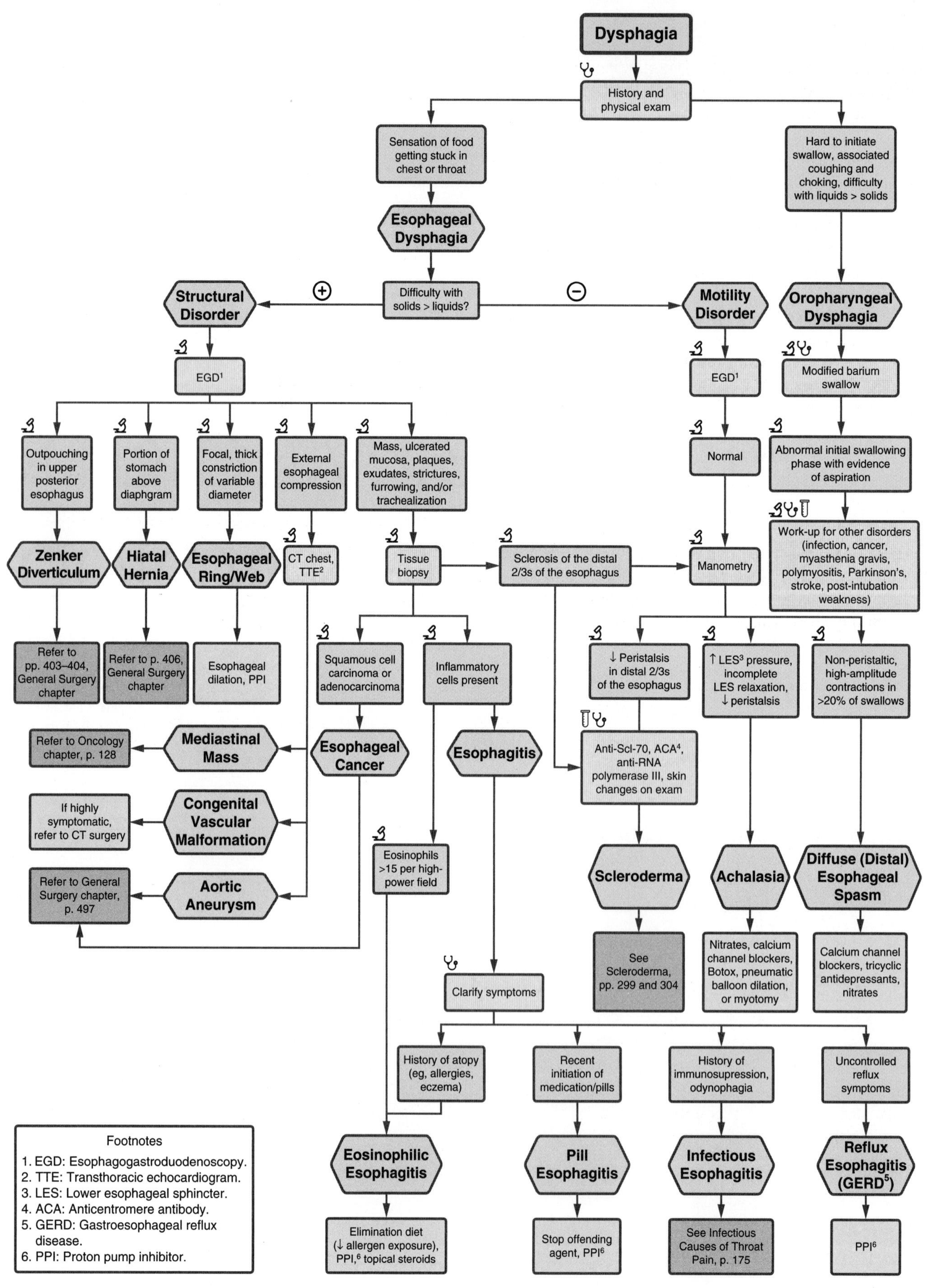

Dysphagia
History and physical exam
Sensation of food getting stuck in chest or throat
Hard to initiate swallow, associated coughing and choking, difficulty with liquids > solids
Esophageal Dysphagia
Difficulty with solids > liquids?
⊕
⊖
Structural Disorder
Motility Disorder
Oropharyngeal Dysphagia
EGD[1]
EGD[1]
Modified barium swallow
Outpouching in upper posterior esophagus
Portion of stomach above diaphgram
Focal, thick constriction of variable diameter
External esophageal compression
Mass, ulcerated mucosa, plaques, exudates, strictures, furrowing, and/or trachealization
Normal
Abnormal initial swallowing phase with evidence of aspiration
Work-up for other disorders (infection, cancer, myasthenia gravis, polymyositis, Parkinson's, stroke, post-intubation weakness)
Zenker Diverticulum
Hiatal Hernia
Esophageal Ring/Web
CT chest, TTE[2]
Tissue biopsy
Sclerosis of the distal 2/3s of the esophagus
Manometry
Refer to pp. 403–404, General Surgery chapter
Refer to p. 406, General Surgery chapter
Esophageal dilation, PPI
Squamous cell carcinoma or adenocarcinoma
Inflammatory cells present
↓ Peristalsis in distal 2/3s of the esophagus
↑ LES[3] pressure, incomplete LES relaxation, ↓ peristalsis
Non-peristaltic, high-amplitude contractions in >20% of swallows
Refer to Oncology chapter, p. 128
Mediastinal Mass
Esophageal Cancer
Esophagitis
Anti-Scl-70, ACA[4], anti-RNA polymerase III, skin changes on exam
If highly symptomatic, refer to CT surgery
Congenital Vascular Malformation
Eosinophils >15 per high-power field
Scleroderma
Achalasia
Diffuse (Distal) Esophageal Spasm
Refer to General Surgery chapter, p. 497
Aortic Aneurysm
See Scleroderma, pp. 299 and 304
Nitrates, calcium channel blockers, Botox, pneumatic balloon dilation, or myotomy
Calcium channel blockers, tricyclic antidepressants, nitrates
Clarify symptoms
History of atopy (eg, allergies, eczema)
Recent initiation of medication/pills
History of immunosupression, odynophagia
Uncontrolled reflux symptoms
Eosinophilic Esophagitis
Pill Esophagitis
Infectious Esophagitis
Reflux Esophagitis (GERD[5])
Elimination diet (↓ allergen exposure), PPI,[6] topical steroids
Stop offending agent, PPI[6]
See Infectious Causes of Throat Pain, p. 175
PPI[6]
Footnotes
1. EGD: Esophagogastroduodenoscopy.
2. TTE: Transthoracic echocardiogram.
3. LES: Lower esophageal sphincter.
4. ACA: Anticentromere antibody.
5. GERD: Gastroesophageal reflux disease.
6. PPI: Proton pump inhibitor.

FIGURE 2.1

2-1 Dysphagia

Dysphagia refers to difficulty swallowing, while odynophagia refers to pain with swallowing. Dysphagia can usually be classified into 2 main categories: Oropharyngeal dysphagia and esophageal dysphagia. Oropharyngeal dysphagia refers to problems with initiation of swallowing, which can lead to aspiration events. Patients can be observed choking or coughing when they swallow, or they may present recurrently with aspiration pneumonia. Patients classically present with more difficulty swallowing liquids than solid foods. The etiology is usually neuromuscular (eg, stroke, myasthenia gravis, Parkinson's disease). Esophageal dysphagia refers to issues with transit of food in the esophagus and may be due to structural or motility disorders of the esophagus. Patients may report a sensation of food getting stuck in their throat ("globus sensation") or chest pain. Patients with a structural disorder (eg, esophageal strictures, webs, carcinoma) tend to have more difficulty with swallowing solids than liquids. Patients with motility disorders (eg, achalasia, esophageal spasm, scleroderma) tend to have difficulty with swallowing both solids and liquids.

OROPHARYNGEAL DYSPHAGIA

A 68-year-old M with PMH of recent stroke is brought in by family who are worried that he has difficulty swallowing his meals since the stroke. On **exam**, vitals are normal. He has dysarthric speech and focal weakness on the right upper extremity and right lower extremity. When he starts drinking fluids, he immediately starts coughing. On **imaging**, modified barium swallow study shows an abnormal initial swallowing phase with evidence of aspiration.

Management:

1. If possible, treat underlying condition.
2. Speech-language-pathology therapy and aspiration precautions.

Complications:

- Aspiration event leading to aspiration pneumonia or severe hypoxia.

HYF: Oropharyngeal dysphagia is characterized by difficulty initiating swallowing as opposed to esophageal dysphagia, which is characterized by difficulty swallowing for several seconds after initiating a swallow. Oropharyngeal dysphagia is classically associated with neuromuscular disease.

ESOPHAGEAL WEB OR RING

A 45-year-old F with PMH of iron deficiency anemia and gastroesophageal reflux disease (GERD) presents with several months of intermittent difficulty with swallowing solid foods. She describes a sensation of food getting stuck in her throat and has no issue with swallowing liquids. **Exam** is unremarkable. **Labs** show iron deficiency anemia. EGD reveals an esophageal ring in the distal esophagus.

Management:

1. EGD with esophageal dilation.
2. Acid suppression with a proton pump inhibitor.

Complications:

- Recurrent dysphagia: Treat with repeat esophageal dilation and indefinite acid suppression with PPI.

HYF: Esophageal rings and webs are structures that partially occlude the esophageal lumen. Most patients are asymptomatic. Associated with eosinophilic esophagitis and Plummer-Vinson syndrome (triad of atrophic glossitis, upper esophageal webs, and iron deficiency anemia), which can lead to squamous cell carcinoma of the esophagus.

PILL ESOPHAGITIS

A 25-year-old M with recent diagnosis of cellulitis presents with 1 week of progressive odynophagia and dysphagia with solids and liquids. His symptoms are triggered even with swallowing saliva, but he is still able to manage secretions. He recently started a course of antibiotics, which he takes right before bed. **Exam** and **labs** are unremarkable.

Management:

1. Discontinue offending medication.
2. Proton pump inhibitor (PPI) until symptoms resolve.
3. If symptoms persist >1 week after medication cessation, perform EGD.
4. Supportive care.

Complications:

- Symptom recurrence.

HYF: Usually caused by prolonged contact of the medication with the esophageal mucosa due to delayed esophageal transit. High-risk medications: antibiotics (especially tetracyclines), bisphosphonates, potassium chloride, and NSAIDs.

EOSINOPHILIC ESOPHAGITIS (EoE)

A 25-year-old M with PMH of asthma, eczema, and multiple food allergies presents with several months of dysphagia with solid foods. **Exam** and **labs** are unremarkable. EGD shows a proximal esophageal stricture, white papules, trachealization, and linear furrows.

Management:

1. EGD with biopsy. Treat stricture with esophageal dilation.
2. Acid suppression with PPI.
3. Swallowed glucocorticoids (eg, fluticasone, budesonide).
4. Discussion of elimination diet.
5. Gastroenterologists may also discuss biologic therapy (eg, dupilumab, an inhibitor of IL-4 and IL-13) on a case-by-case.

Complications:

- Esophageal strictures.
- Food impaction leading to esophageal perforation.

HYF: Associated with food allergies and atopy. EoE can present with dysphagia, heartburn, food disimpaction, and/or epigastric

(Continued)

2-1 Dysphagia

pain. EGD findings can reveal a variety of features in the esophagus, and endoscopic appearance alone has limited utility in diagnosis. Criteria for diagnosis of EoE: Symptoms related to esophageal dysfunction, eosinophil-predominant inflammation on esophageal biopsy (≥15 eosinophils per high-power field), and exclusion of other causes that may contribute toward symptoms.

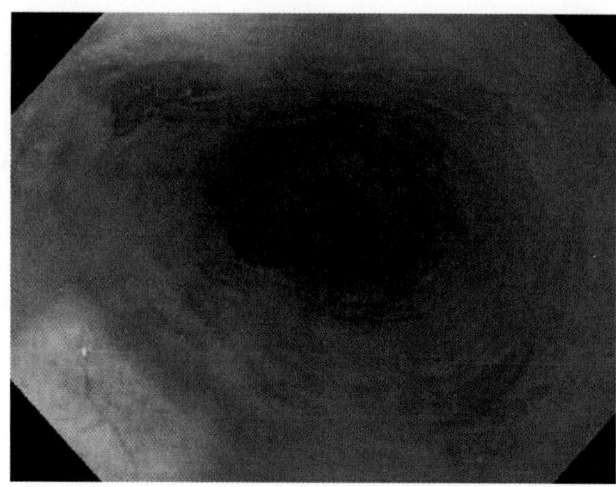

Eosinophilic esophagitis with mucosal lacerations.

DIFFUSE (DISTAL) ESOPHAGEAL SPASM

A 50-year-old F with PMH of GERD presents with intermittent episodes of dysphagia with solids and liquids, odynophagia, and mid-sternal chest pain triggered by drinking hot or cold liquids. During one such episode, she took her husband's nitroglycerin and experienced symptom relief. **Labs** including troponin are unremarkable. EGD is unremarkable. Esophageal manometry reveals high-amplitude, simultaneous non-peristaltic contractions in 25% of swallows.

Management:

1. Calcium channel blockers (eg, diltiazem), tricyclic antidepressants, or nitrates.
2. If refractory symptoms, consider botulinum toxin injection or esophageal myotomy.

Complications:

- ~5% of patients develop achalasia (eg, worsening dysphagia, regurgitation).

HYF: Associated with emotional stress and functional GI disorders. Symptoms can resemble hypercontractile esophagus (formally called "nutcracker esophagus"), in which manometry shows high pressure but normal sequential contractions in the smooth muscle esophagus.

Hiatal Hernia: See Gastrointestinal Surgery, p. 406.

Mediastinal Mass: See Oncology, p. 128.

Aortic Aneurysms: See Vascular Surgery, p. 497.

Esophageal Cancer: See Gastrointestinal Surgery, p. 403.

Infectious Esophagitis: See Infectious Diseases, p. 175.

Scleroderma: See Rheumatology, p. 304.

GERD/Reflux Esophagitis: See Abdominal Pain, p. 80.

Achalasia: See Gastrointestinal Surgery – Esophagus, p. 403.

Zenker Diverticulum: See Gastrointestinal Surgery – Esophagus, pp. 403–404.

2-2 Diarrhea

Approach to Diarrhea

	Inflammatory	Non-Inflammatory
Acute	Acute Inflammatory Diarrhea (see pp. 189–191)	Acute Non-Inflammatory Diarrhea (see pp. 192–193)
Chronic	Chronic Inflammatory Diarrhea (see pp. 58–60)	Chronic Non-Inflammatory Diarrhea (see pp. 61–63)

Diarrhea is defined as passing >3 loose or watery stools in a 24-hour period. There are many etiologies of diarrhea, including infectious, neoplastic, endocrine, and structural causes. In general, when approaching a patient with diarrhea in a vignette, we recommend asking 2 questions: 1. Is the diarrhea acute (lasting <2–4 weeks) or chronic (lasting >2–4 weeks)? and 2. Is the diarrhea inflammatory or non-inflammatory? Inflammatory diarrhea is suggested by fever, blood in the stool (hematochezia), and/or lab markers such as ↑ fecal leukocytes, fecal lactoferrin, and fecal calprotectin. Once you have established the answer to those questions, you can construct your differential diagnosis using other epidemiologic risk factors (eg, travel history and food exposure), clinical clues (eg, concomitant weight loss), or the nature of the diarrhea (eg, fatty vs. malabsorptive vs. secretory).

The vast majority of acute diarrhea is infectious and self-limited, not warranting diagnostic work-up or targeted treatment in an immunocompetent host. However, as diarrhea persists and becomes chronic, noninfectious etiologies such as inflammatory bowel disease, irritable bowel syndrome, and cancer become more likely. Though those diagnoses are referenced in the algorithms in this chapter, you can find more detail elsewhere.

FIGURE 2.2

2-3 Chronic Inflammatory Diarrhea

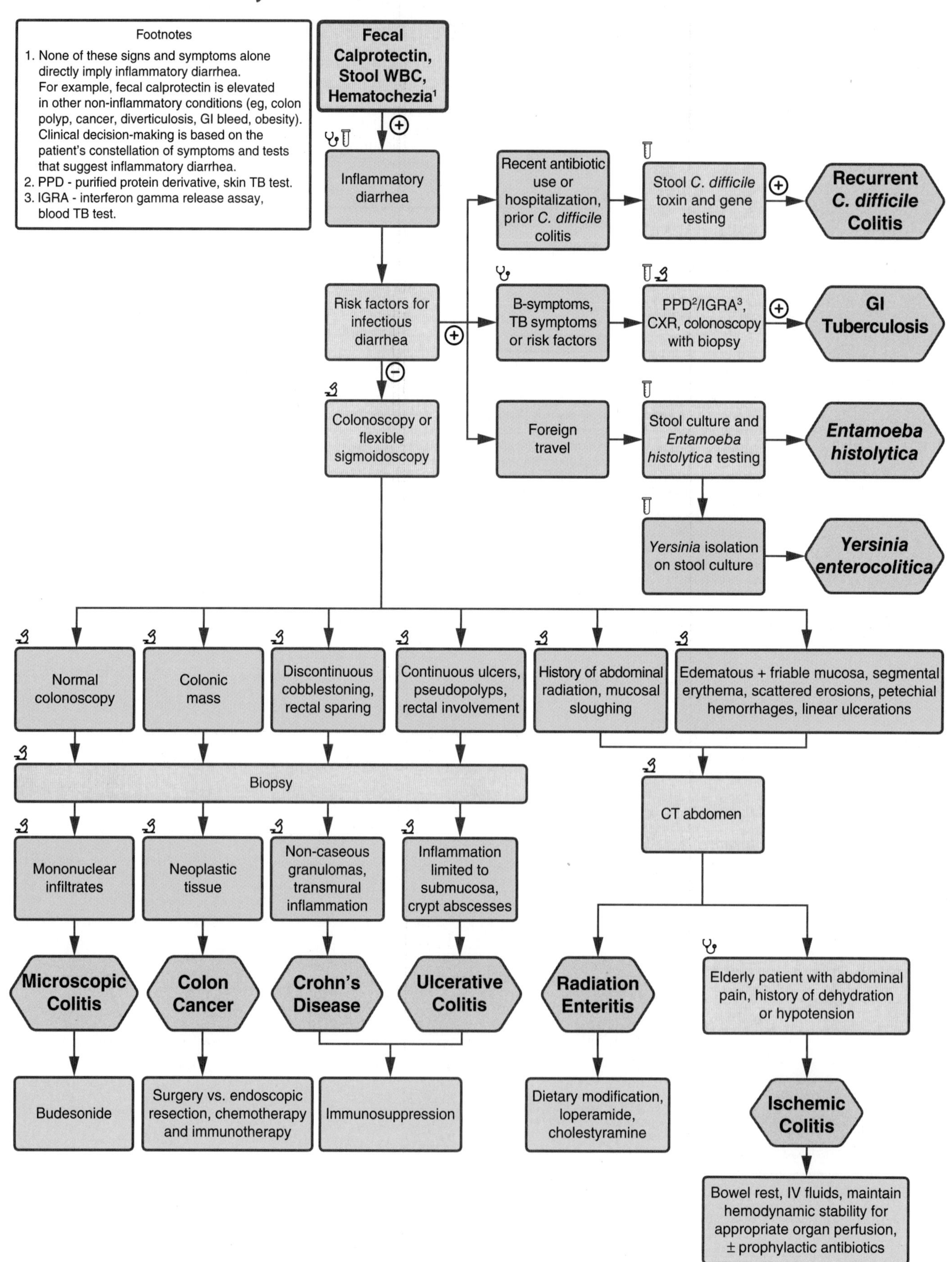
Footnotes
1. None of these signs and symptoms alone directly imply inflammatory diarrhea. For example, fecal calprotectin is elevated in other non-inflammatory conditions (eg, colon polyp, cancer, diverticulosis, GI bleed, obesity). Clinical decision-making is based on the patient's constellation of symptoms and tests that suggest inflammatory diarrhea.
2. PPD - purified protein derivative, skin TB test.
3. IGRA - interferon gamma release assay, blood TB test.
Fecal Calprotectin, Stool WBC, Hematochezia[1]
Inflammatory diarrhea
Risk factors for infectious diarrhea
Recent antibiotic use or hospitalization, prior C. difficile colitis
Stool C. difficile toxin and gene testing
Recurrent C. difficile Colitis
B-symptoms, TB symptoms or risk factors
PPD[2]/IGRA[3], CXR, colonoscopy with biopsy
GI Tuberculosis
Foreign travel
Stool culture and Entamoeba histolytica testing
Entamoeba histolytica
Yersinia isolation on stool culture
Yersinia enterocolitica
Colonoscopy or flexible sigmoidoscopy
Normal colonoscopy
Colonic mass
Discontinuous cobblestoning, rectal sparing
Continuous ulcers, pseudopolyps, rectal involvement
History of abdominal radiation, mucosal sloughing
Edematous + friable mucosa, segmental erythema, scattered erosions, petechial hemorrhages, linear ulcerations
Biopsy
CT abdomen
Mononuclear infiltrates
Neoplastic tissue
Non-caseous granulomas, transmural inflammation
Inflammation limited to submucosa, crypt abscesses
Microscopic Colitis
Colon Cancer
Crohn's Disease
Ulcerative Colitis
Radiation Enteritis
Elderly patient with abdominal pain, history of dehydration or hypotension
Ischemic Colitis
Budesonide
Surgery vs. endoscopic resection, chemotherapy and immunotherapy
Immunosuppression
Dietary modification, loperamide, cholestyramine
Bowel rest, IV fluids, maintain hemodynamic stability for appropriate organ perfusion, ± prophylactic antibiotics

FIGURE 2.3

2-3 Chronic Inflammatory Diarrhea

ISCHEMIC COLITIS

A 75-year-old F with PMH of HFrEF presents with sudden LLQ cramping and subsequent bloody diarrhea after aggressive diuresis causing hypotension. **Exam** reveals LLQ pain and bright red blood per rectum. **Labs** show Cr 3.4 and lactate 5.4.

Management:

1. Bowel rest, IV fluids, maintain hemodynamic stability for appropriate organ perfusion, prophylactic antibiotics in moderate to severe cases.
2. If bowel is necrotic, surgical resection.

Complications:

- Fulminant colitis, gangrenous bowel.

HYF: Due to mesenteric artery hypoperfusion with intermittent ischemia in watershed areas, which are located at the edge of the region supplied by the superior mesenteric artery and the inferior mesenteric artery and frequently dependent upon collateral circulation. There are 2 classic watershed areas that are vulnerable to ischemia: The splenic flexure and the rectosigmoid junction. Differentiate from acute mesenteric ischemia (complete vascular occlusion) and chronic mesenteric ischemia (due to ASCVD, think "GI angina").

RECURRENT C. *DIFFICILE* COLITIS

A 67-year-old M with PMH of recent cellulitis treated with clindamycin and prior *C. difficile* infection presents with 4 weeks of watery diarrhea, >3 stools/day. **Exam** reveals fever, dry mucous membranes, and diffuse abdominal pain. **Labs** show leukocytosis and positive *C. difficile* stool PCR and toxin.

Management:

1. Oral vancomycin or fidaxomicin ± metronidazole for fulminant colitis.
2. Consider fecal microbiota transplant if recurrent *C. difficile* colitis.
3. Volume repletion if large-volume diarrhea.

Complications:

- Fulminant colitis, toxic megacolon, bowel perforation.

HYF: Mechanism of action: Ingestion of spores → convert to GPRs in the colon → colonization in the colon → pathogenic strains produce exotoxins ("toxins A and B") → watery diarrhea. Risk factors: Recent antibiotic use, gastric acid suppression (eg, PPIs), recent hospitalization, elderly. Two-step verification for diagnosis: NAAT PCR (most sensitive) only shows *C. difficile* colonization and that the *C. difficile* can produce toxin; EIA/ELISA for toxins (most specific) proves that the toxin has been produced and there is a true infection. Classic finding on colonoscopy is pseudomembranous colitis: Bowel wall erythema, edema, and friability. Treat toxic megacolon with bowel rest, NG tube, aggressive antibiotic therapy (PO and rectal vancomycin or fidaxomycin ± IV metronidazole), and cessation of antimotility agents (eg, anticholinergics, opiates); if clinical deterioration, may require colectomy.

GASTROINTESTINAL TUBERCULOSIS

A 34-year-old M recent immigrant presents with fever, abdominal pain, and chronic diarrhea. **Exam** shows diffuse abdominal tenderness. **Labs** show positive IGRA. Colon biopsy shows acid-fast bacilli on culture.

Management:

1. Rifampin, isoniazid, pyrazinamide, ethambutol (refer to Infectious Disease chapter, p. 169).

Complications:

- Bowel obstruction, perforation, abscess, fistula.

HYF: Abdominal tuberculosis can cause ascites associated with abdominal pain, fever, and night sweats (due to TB reactivation). TNF-α inhibitors can cause reactivation of latent TB. TB is a granulomatous disease → hypercalciuria → kidney stones. GI TB is the most common mimicker of Crohn's disease in underdeveloped countries.

ENTAMOEBA HISTOLYTICA

A 30-year-old F from Guatemala presents with 3 months of chronic bloody diarrhea. **Exam** shows diffuse abdominal pain. Stool ova and parasite (O&P) and antigen are positive for *Entamoeba histolytica* antigen.

Management:

1. Metronidazole or tinidazole for colitis, paromomycin for intraluminal cysts.

Complications:

- Fulminant colitis, bowel necrosis, toxic megacolon.
- Liver abscess → liver capsule rupture into peritoneum.

HYF: Transmitted via fecal-oral route (food, water, fecal-oral sexual transmission). Most infections are asymptomatic; treat asymptomatic cases to prevent spread to household contacts. Bloody diarrhea occurs due to colon wall invasion. Liver abscesses can form several months after initial infection due to spread to the liver from the colonic mucosa via the portal vein. They classically present with RUQ pain, elevated LFTs, positive *E. histolytica* serology, and imaging (RUQ US, CT) showing a single subcapsular cyst in the right hepatic lobe.

YERSINIA ENTEROCOLITICA

A 6-year-old M, otherwise healthy, presents with 3 weeks of fever and bloody diarrhea. **Exam** is unremarkable. **Labs** show a positive serum *Yersinia* IgM and stool culture growing *Yersinia*.

Management:

1. Supportive care.

Complications: Pseudo-appendicitis syndrome, reactive arthritis.

HYF: Yersiniosis is associated with a pseudo-appendicitis syndrome with RLQ pain. Reactive arthritis (conjunctivitis, urethritis, oligoarthritis, skin findings such as balanitis circinata) can follow after the acute GI infection. Hereditary hemochromatosis increases infection risk.

(Continued)

2-3 Chronic Inflammatory Diarrhea

CROHN'S DISEASE

A 30-year-old F with presents with weeks of crampy abdominal pain, low-grade fever, weight loss, watery diarrhea, anal pain, oral aphthous ulcers, and joint pain. On **exam**, she has perianal fissuring. **Labs** show positive fecal calprotectin, elevated ESR/CRP, and anemia.

Management:

1. Colonoscopy with mucosal biopsies of terminal ileum.
2. Acute flare: 5-ASA (if mild) or steroids based on colonoscopy findings.
3. Maintenance therapy: Non-steroidal immunomodulators (AZA, 6MP, MTX). Consider advanced therapy: Biologics (anti-TNF-α inhibitors, anti-integrin, anti-IL-12/23), and small molecules (upadacitinib).
4. Bowel resection in complicated cases of fistulizing disease and abscesses, obstructive strictures, and malignancy.

Complications:

- Bowel obstruction, abscess, perforation, fistulae, strictures, increased risk for colon and small bowel cancer.

HYF: Can occur anywhere from mouth to anus (most commonly ileocecal) with rectal sparing. Characterized by skip lesions, linear ulcerations, cobblestoning, transmural inflammation, and non-caseating granulomas. Extraintestinal symptoms: Erythema nodosum, pyoderma gangrenosum, uveitis, seronegative arthritis (waxes/wanes with bowel symptoms), and interstitial lung disease. Associated with nutrient deficiencies (vitamin B_{12}, fat-soluble vitamins, niacin, zinc), fat malabsorption, cholesterol gallstones (due to ↓ enterohepatic bile acid recycling), and calcium oxalate kidney stones. Smoking is strongly associated with poor prognosis.

ULCERATIVE COLITIS (UC)

A 26-year-old F presents with 6 weeks of fever, fatigue, weight loss, rectal urgency, tenesmus, and bloody diarrhea. **Exam** shows abdominal tenderness. **Labs** show anemia and elevated ESR. Colonoscopy reveals pseudopolyps and submucosal inflammation, with biopsy showing crypt abscesses but no non-caseating granulomas.

Management:

1. 5-ASA (eg, mesalamine, sulfasalazine, balsalazide).
2. Corticosteroids (topical or systemic) for flares or severe disease.
3. For maintenance: Non-steroidal immunomodulators (6MP, AZA). Consider advanced therapy: TNF-α inhibitors (eg, adalimumab, infliximab, golimumab) and other biologics (eg, vedolizumab, ustekinumab), small molecules (eg, tofacitinib, upacitinib).
4. For severe, refractory UC, total proctocolectomy with either ileoanal anastomosis or end ileostomy.

Complications:

- Colon cancer, toxic megacolon.

HYF: Continuous inflammation of colon starting in rectum up to ileocecal valve is more consistent with UC than Crohn's disease. See Crohn's Disease for extraintestinal associations of inflammatory bowel disease (IBD). Associated with primary sclerosing cholangitis (PSC). Colonoscopy is indicated immediately for colon cancer screening if diagnosed with PSC concomitantly. Otherwise, begin colon cancer screening 8 years after diagnosis and then repeat screening every 1–2 years. GI symptoms can worsen during pregnancy; UC patients have lower fertility rates.

RADIATION ENTERITIS

A 68-year-old F with PMH of uterine cancer presents with bloody diarrhea and abdominal pain 3 weeks after pelvic radiation therapy. **Exam** shows diffuse abdominal tenderness with normal **labs**. On **imaging**, CT A/P with thickened bowel loops.

Management:

1. Dietary modification, loperamide, cholestyramine.
2. In some cases, surgery is required.

Complications:

- Malabsorption, abscess, bowel obstruction and strictures.

HYF: GI epithelium has increased radiation sensitivity causing inflammation and mucosal denudation (hematochezia) and decreased absorptive capacity (diarrhea).

MICROSCOPIC (LYMPHOCYTIC) COLITIS

A 72-year-old F with PMH of tobacco use disorder presents with nocturnal, watery diarrhea. **Exam** and **labs** are unremarkable. Endoscopy and stool cultures are also normal. Colon biopsy shows intraepithelial lymphocytes and subepithelial collagen bands.

Management:

1. Stop offending agent.
2. Budesonide. For milder cases, can alternatively consider cholestyramine or loperamide for symptom management.
3. For resistant cases, consider infliximab.

Complications: None.

HYF: Associated with smoking and drugs (SSRIs, NSAIDs).

2-4 Chronic Non-Inflammatory Diarrhea

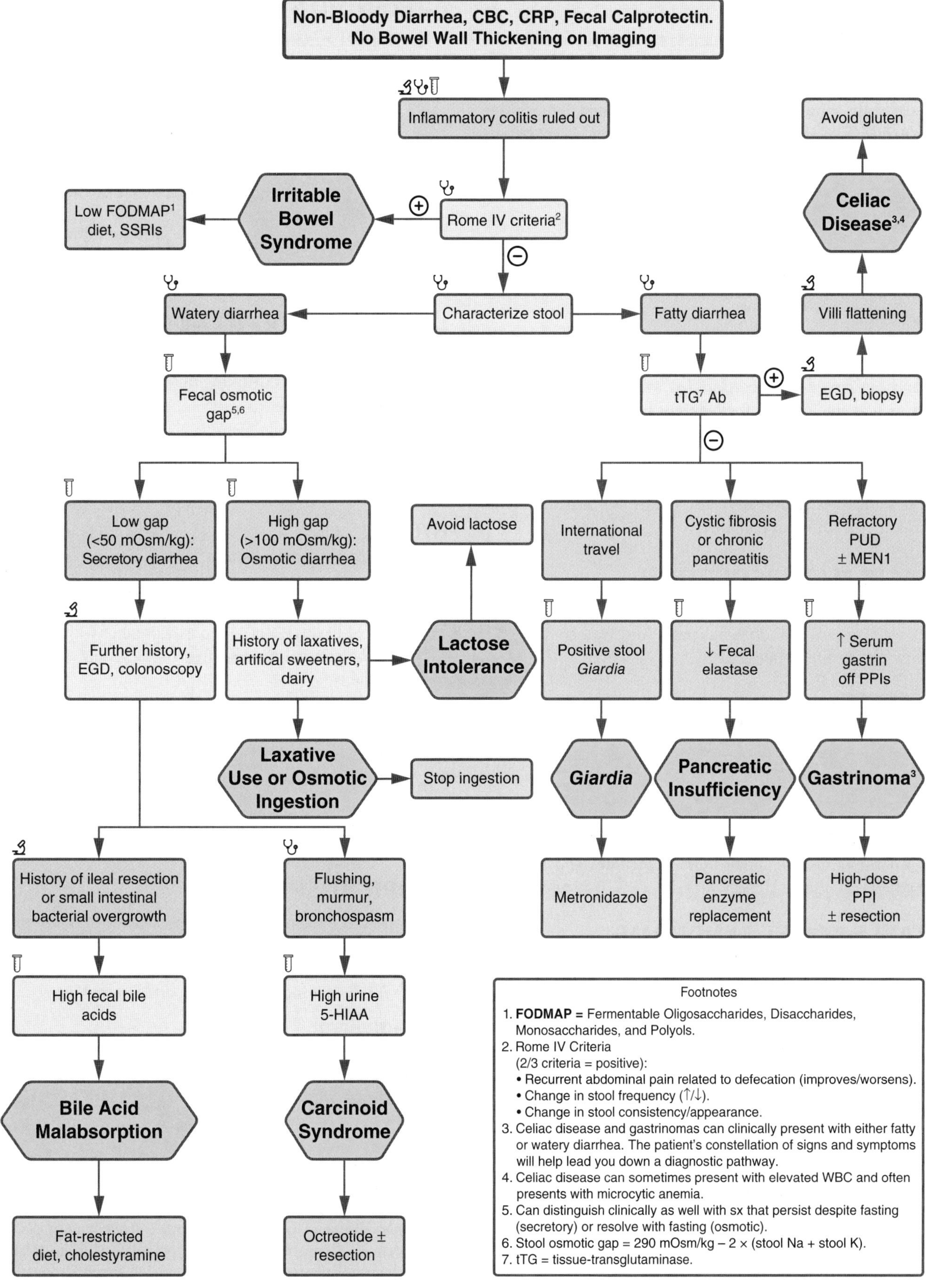
Non-Bloody Diarrhea, CBC, CRP, Fecal Calprotectin. No Bowel Wall Thickening on Imaging
Inflammatory colitis ruled out
Rome IV criteria[2]
Irritable Bowel Syndrome
Low FODMAP[1] diet, SSRIs
Characterize stool
Watery diarrhea
Fatty diarrhea
Fecal osmotic gap[5,6]
tTG[7] Ab
EGD, biopsy
Villi flattening
Celiac Disease[3,4]
Avoid gluten
Low gap (<50 mOsm/kg): Secretory diarrhea
High gap (>100 mOsm/kg): Osmotic diarrhea
Avoid lactose
International travel
Cystic fibrosis or chronic pancreatitis
Refractory PUD ± MEN1
Further history, EGD, colonoscopy
History of laxatives, artifical sweetners, dairy
Lactose Intolerance
Positive stool Giardia
↓ Fecal elastase
↑ Serum gastrin off PPIs
Laxative Use or Osmotic Ingestion
Stop ingestion
Giardia
Pancreatic Insufficiency
Gastrinoma[3]
History of ileal resection or small intestinal bacterial overgrowth
Flushing, murmur, bronchospasm
Metronidazole
Pancreatic enzyme replacement
High-dose PPI ± resection
High fecal bile acids
High urine 5-HIAA
Bile Acid Malabsorption
Carcinoid Syndrome
Fat-restricted diet, cholestyramine
Octreotide ± resection

Footnotes

1. **FODMAP =** Fermentable Oligosaccharides, Disaccharides, Monosaccharides, and Polyols.
2. Rome IV Criteria (2/3 criteria = positive):
   - Recurrent abdominal pain related to defecation (improves/worsens).
   - Change in stool frequency (↑/↓).
   - Change in stool consistency/appearance.
3. Celiac disease and gastrinomas can clinically present with either fatty or watery diarrhea. The patient's constellation of signs and symptoms will help lead you down a diagnostic pathway.
4. Celiac disease can sometimes present with elevated WBC and often presents with microcytic anemia.
5. Can distinguish clinically as well with sx that persist despite fasting (secretory) or resolve with fasting (osmotic).
6. Stool osmotic gap = 290 mOsm/kg – 2 × (stool Na + stool K).
7. tTG = tissue-transglutaminase.

FIGURE 2.4

2-4 Chronic Non-Inflammatory Diarrhea

CELIAC DISEASE

A 34-year-old F with PMH of Hashimoto thyroiditis presents with 4 months of foul-smelling diarrhea fat droplets and an itchy rash on her buttocks. Exam shows erythematous papules/excoriations on buttocks. Labs show anemia, vitamin D deficiency, and positive serum IgA/IgM TTG. EGD shows villi flattening and crypt hyperplasia on duodenal biopsy.

Management:

1. Avoid gluten.

Complications: Dermatitis herpetiformis (IgA skin deposition), GI lymphoma, iron/folate/B12 deficiency, osteoporosis, small bowel adenocarcinoma.

HYF: Celiac disease is an immune reaction to gliadin, found in gluten, and can commonly be associated with other autoimmune disorders such as autoimmune thyroiditis or type 1 diabetes. Testing must be done while the patient is on a gluten-containing diet, and treatment consists of eliminating gluten in the diet. If IgA deficient, tTG IgA can be false negative → test for IgG. Dermatitis herpetiformis can sometimes accompany celiac disease as a pruritic inflammatory rash of the forearms and knees.

BILE ACID MALABSORPTION

A 43-year-old M with PMH of cholecystectomy and Crohn's disease presents with urgency, abdominal pain, and watery diarrhea. Labs show elevated fecal bile acids.

Management:

1. Fat-restricted diet, cholestyramine.

Complications: Malabsorption.

HYF: Issue with enterohepatic bile circulation (ileal pathology/bile excess) causes diarrhea. Can be due to cholecystectomy, ileal disease in Crohn's disease, small bowel resections, and bacterial overgrowth.

IRRITABLE BOWEL SYNDROME

A 26-year-old F presents with 3 months of abdominal cramping relieved with stooling that is loose, mucusy, and non-bloody. Exam and labs are normal.

Management:

1. Low FODMAP diet, TCAs, SSRIs, symptomatic treatment with antispasmodics and cholestyramine.

Complications: Chronic constipation may cause anal fissures.

HYF: IBS subtypes: Constipation, diarrhea, and mixed. The patient above has IBS-diarrhea, which can be managed with a low FODMAP diet, SSRIs, anti-diarrheal agents, cholestyramine, fiber, and/or rifaximin. New agents include eluxadoline and alosetron. IBS-constipation can be managed with diet and fiber supplementatino. New agents include linactolide, lubiprostone, tenapanor, and plecanatide.

CARCINOID SYNDROME

A 63-year-old presents with flushing, wheezing, and diarrhea. Exam reveals an audible tricuspid regurgitation. Labs reveal ↑ urine 5-HIAA.

Management:

1. Octreotide and tumor resection.

Complications: Metastases, right-sided valvular disease.

HYF: Functional carcinoid tumors produce hormones including serotonin. Symptoms result from inability to convert serotonin to 5-HIAA due to liver metastases.

LACTOSE INTOLERANCE

A 15-year-old M from China presents with diarrhea, abdominal pain, and bloating after drinking milk. Exam and labs are normal.

Management:

1. Avoid lactose.

Complications: None.

HYF: Lack of lactase enzyme expression leads to osmotic diarrhea/gut fermentation of lactose.

LAXATIVE ABUSE/INGESTIONS

A 32-year-old F with PMH of anorexia presents with chronic watery diarrhea. She eats many sugar-free candies daily. Labs show high stool osmolality.

Management:

1. Laxative screening and stop offending agent.

Complications: Electrolyte/acid-base issues.

HYF: Associated with eating disorders. Artificial sweeteners are osmotically active.

TROPICAL SPRUE

A 53-year-old F from Puerto Rico presents with 6 months of fatty diarrhea. Exam is normal. Labs show megaloblastic anemia, negative tTg IgM/IgG, and negative infectious diarrhea work-up. EGD shows villi shortening and crypt hyperplasia on biopsy.

Management:

1. Antibiotics (tetracyclines).

Complications: Folate/B12 deficiency.

HYF: Lived for >1 month in tropical area. Possibly infectious, as it improves with antibiotics, but no causative pathogen has been discovered.

*__Whipple's disease:__ Due to infection with *Tropheryma whipplei* (intracellular Gram ⊕). Characterized by PAS⊕ granules in intestinal lamina propria on biopsy. Patients present with arthralgias, lymphadenopathy, cardiac symptoms, and neurologic symptoms, followed by diarrhea/steatorrhea later in the disease course. Most common in older men. Treat with antibiotics (eg, trimethoprim/sulfamethoxazole, penicillin, cephalosporins).

2-4 Chronic Non-Inflammatory Diarrhea

GIARDIA

A 37-year-old M presents with fatty stools and weight loss after drinking lake water in Mexico. On **exam**, he has diffuse abdominal TTP. **Labs** show + *Giardia* stool antigen, NAAT, and stool O&P with cysts.

Management:

1. Metronidazole.

Complications: Stunted growth in children.

HYF: Diarrhea is not bloody (no mucosal invasion). Associated with river/lake exposure or travel to developing countries. Fecal-oral transmission.

PANCREATIC INSUFFICIENCY

A 20-year-old M with PMH of cystic fibrosis presents with fatty stools, bloating, cramping, and weight loss. **Labs** show elevated fecal fat and decreased fecal elastase.

Management:

1. Pancreatic enzyme replacement.

Complications: Malabsorption.

HYF: Associated with chronic pancreatitis and cystic fibrosis.

GASTRINOMA (ZOLLINGER-ELLISON SYNDROME)

A 54-year-old M with PMH of refractory PUD despite maximum PPI therapy presents with weight loss and chronic diarrhea with steatorrhea. On **exam**, he has epigastric TTP. **Labs** show a serum gastrin of 1354.

Management:

1. Fasting serum gastrin levels >1000 pg/mL with normal gastric pH. If non-diagnostic serum gastrin level, obtain secretin stimulation test. If serum stimulation test is negative but there is strong suspicion for gastrinoma, get calcium infusion study.
2. EGD, which will typically show erosive esophagitis as well as peptic ulcer disease beyond the ligament of Treitz.
3. CT/MRI, somatostatin scintigraphy for tumor localization.
4. Resect tumor if possible and screen for MEN1.
5. High-dose PPI.

Complications: Small bowel perforation, GI bleed.

HYF: Stomach acid inactivates pancreatic enzymes, causing steatorrhea and malabsorption. Ulcers can often be seen in the duodenum and jejunum. Stop PPI prior to secretin stimulation test. Secretin ↑ gastrin production from gastrinoma but ↓ gastrin production from normal G-cells (eg, autoimmune gastritis/achlorhydria). Gastrinoma is the most common GI neuroendocrine tumor in MEN1.

2-5 Jaundice

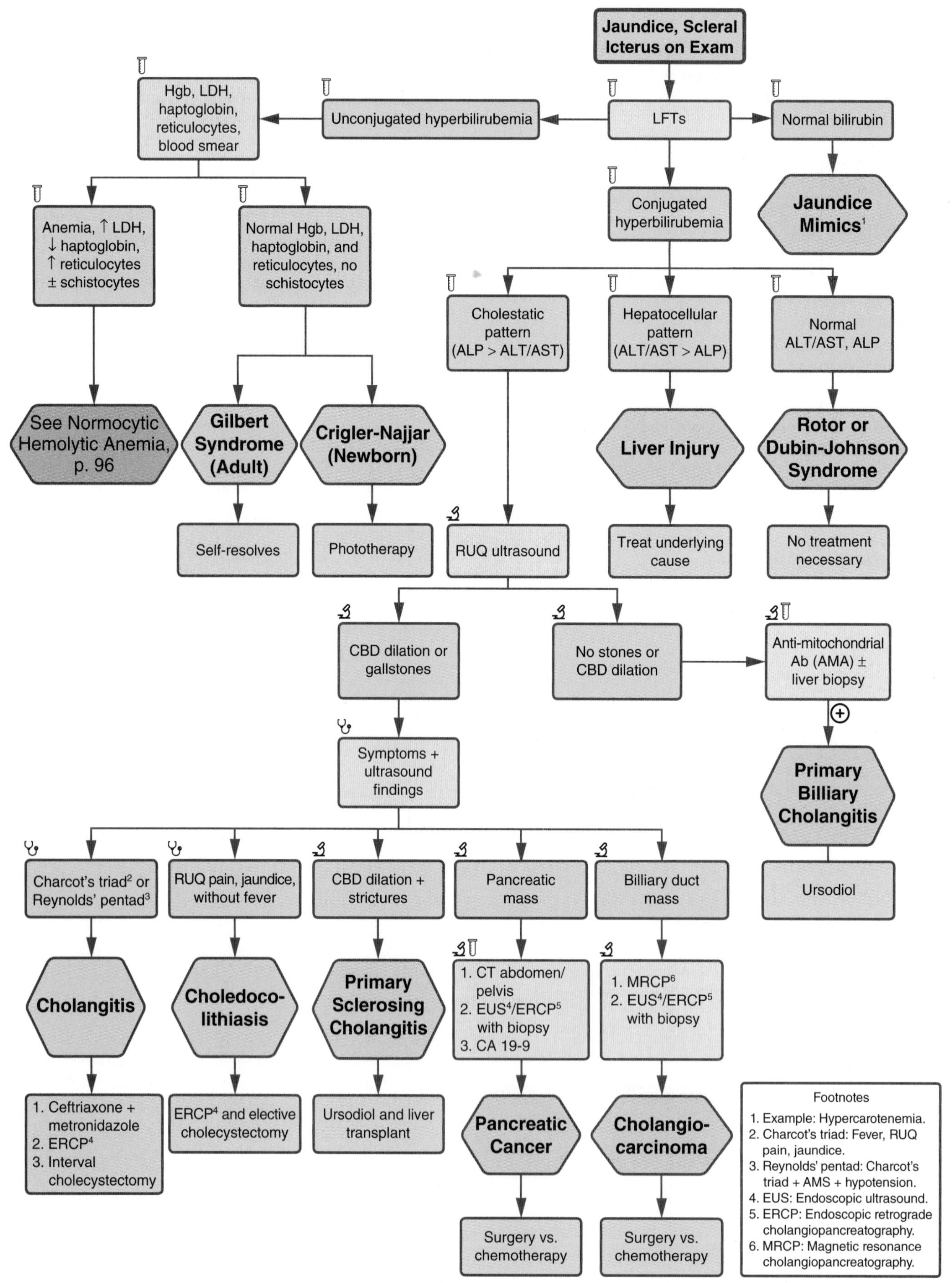
Jaundice, Scleral Icterus on Exam
LFTs
Unconjugated hyperbilirubemia
Normal bilirubin
Jaundice Mimics[1]
Hgb, LDH, haptoglobin, reticulocytes, blood smear
Anemia, ↑ LDH, ↓ haptoglobin, ↑ reticulocytes ± schistocytes
Normal Hgb, LDH, haptoglobin, and reticulocytes, no schistocytes
See Normocytic Hemolytic Anemia, p. 96
Gilbert Syndrome (Adult)
Crigler-Najjar (Newborn)
Self-resolves
Phototherapy
Conjugated hyperbilirubemia
Cholestatic pattern (ALP > ALT/AST)
Hepatocellular pattern (ALT/AST > ALP)
Normal ALT/AST, ALP
Liver Injury
Treat underlying cause
Rotor or Dubin-Johnson Syndrome
No treatment necessary
RUQ ultrasound
CBD dilation or gallstones
No stones or CBD dilation
Anti-mitochondrial Ab (AMA) ± liver biopsy
+
Primary Billiary Cholangitis
Ursodiol
Symptoms + ultrasound findings
Charcot's triad[2] or Reynolds' pentad[3]
RUQ pain, jaundice, without fever
CBD dilation + strictures
Pancreatic mass
Billiary duct mass
Cholangitis
Choledoco-lithiasis
Primary Sclerosing Cholangitis
1. CT abdomen/pelvis
2. EUS[4]/ERCP[5] with biopsy
3. CA 19-9
1. MRCP[6]
2. EUS[4]/ERCP[5] with biopsy
1. Ceftriaxone + metronidazole
2. ERCP[4]
3. Interval cholecystectomy
ERCP[4] and elective cholecystectomy
Ursodiol and liver transplant
Pancreatic Cancer
Cholangio-carcinoma
Surgery vs. chemotherapy
Surgery vs. chemotherapy
Footnotes
1. Example: Hypercarotenemia.
2. Charcot's triad: Fever, RUQ pain, jaundice.
3. Reynolds' pentad: Charcot's triad + AMS + hypotension.
4. EUS: Endoscopic ultrasound.
5. ERCP: Endoscopic retrograde cholangiopancreatography.
6. MRCP: Magnetic resonance cholangiopancreatography.

FIGURE 2.5

2-5 Jaundice

GILBERT SYNDROME

A 29-year-old, otherwise healthy surgery resident on her first 28-hour call has not eaten for 16 hours and was noticed by her co-resident to have scleral icterus. **Labs** notable for an isolated unconjugated hyperbilirubinemia.

Management:

1. Clinical diagnosis requiring no treatment if patient otherwise has normal LFTs with isolated, unconjugated hyperbilirubinemia.

Complications: Increased risk of cholelithiasis.

HYF: Mutation of *UGT1A1* causes decreased enzymatic activity and impaired bilirubin glucuronidation. Jaundice can be triggered by fasting, restrictive diet, illness, stress, or menstruation.

PRIMARY BILIARY CHOLANGITIS (PBC)

A 47-year-old F presents with several months of worsening fatigue and itching. On **exam**, she has mild jaundice, diffuse excoriations, eyelid xanthelasmas, and hepatosplenomegaly. **Labs** show ALP 532, AST 111/ALT 99, Tbili 2.8, and positive antimitochondrial antibody. She was also noted to have a serum cholesterol of 823 with 750 HDL. On **imaging**, RUQ US suggests intrahepatic cholestasis (no biliary tract dilation). Liver biopsy shows granulomatous destruction of the bile ducts.

Management:

1. Ursodeoxycholic acid.
2. Liver transplant.

Complications: Malabsorption, fat-soluble vitamin deficiencies, osteomalacia, cirrhosis, hepatocellular carcinoma.

HYF: T-cells destroy intrahepatic bile ducts causing cholestasis. Occurs almost always in middle-aged women.

CHOLANGITIS

A 42-year-old F with PMH of gallstones presents with right-sided abdominal pain. On **exam**, she has hypotension, jaundice, RUQ abdominal pain, and altered mental status. **Labs** show WBC 13.2, Tbili 3.4, Dbili 2.8, AST 111, ALT 123. On **imaging**, RUQ US shows a dilated common bile duct.

Management:

1. Antibiotics (ceftriaxone plus metronidazole OR piperacillin-tazobactam).
2. ERCP (both diagnostic and therapeutic).
3. Interval cholecystectomy.

Complications:

- Septic shock.
- Pancreatitis (post-ERCP).

HYF: A stone in the bile duct (choledocholithiasis) causes bile stasis, allowing gut bacteria (*E. coli, Klebsiella*) to ascend the bile duct and cause infection. Classic presentations include Charcot's triad (fever, abdominal pain, and jaundice) and Reynolds' pentad (Charcot's triad plus altered mental status and hypotension).

CHOLEDOCHOLITHIASIS

A 40-year-old F with no significant PMH presents with nausea, vomiting, abdominal pain, and jaundice for the past 12 hours. On **exam**, she is afebrile and jaundiced with RUQ tenderness to palpation. **Labs** show ALP 923, AST 99, ALT 63, WBC 6.5. On **imaging**, RUQ US shows a dilated common bile duct.

Management:

1. ERCP.

Complications:

- Cholangitis.
- Pancreatitis.
- Gallstone ileus.

HYF: Presence of stones in the common bile duct causing cholestasis without superimposed infection. In comparison with biliary colic, the pain associated with choledocholithiasis is constant and prolonged. On RUQ US, bile duct dilation is more important than stone visualization, which may not be present. If RUQ US is indeterminate, order MRCP. Risk factors include obesity, female sex, middle age, and multiparity.

PRIMARY SCLEROSING CHOLANGITIS (PSC)

A 32-year-old M with PMH of ulcerative colitis presents with fatigue and generalized itching. On **exam**, he has jaundice, hepatosplenomegaly, and excoriations. **Labs** show ALP 438, Tbili 3.2, Dbili 2.8, and AST 120/ALT 134. On **imaging**, MRCP shows stricturing of intra- and extra-hepatic bile ducts resembling beads on a string. Liver biopsy shows fibrous obliteration of small bile ducts with replacement by connective tissue resembling an "onion-skin" pattern.

Management:

1. Ursodiol for symptomatic treatment.
2. Liver transplant as definitive management.

Complications: Cirrhosis and liver failure, gallbladder carcinoma, cholangiocarcinoma, hepatocellular carcinoma. Cholesterol or pigment gallstones. Osteoporosis and decreased absorption of fat-soluble vitamins due to cholestasis.

HYF: Most patients with ulcerative colitis (UC) do not have PSC, but most patients with PSC have ulcerative colitis (UC). Characterized by inflammation and fibrosis of the intra- and extra-hepatic biliary ducts. Associated with increased serum IgM levels, p-ANCA, and ANA. Monitor for multiple possible malignancies as above.

(Continued)

2-5 Jaundice

PANCREATIC CANCER

A 54-year-old M with PMH of alcohol use disorder presents with 3 months of painless jaundice, unintentional weight loss, and greasy stools. On **exam**, he has mild scleral icterus and a non-tender, palpable gallbladder (Courvoisier's sign). **Labs** show ALP 343, AST 130, ALT 150, Tbili 4.3, WBC 3.2. On **imaging**, RUQ US shows simultaneous dilatation of the common bile and pancreatic ducts (double duct sign). CT A/P with contrast shows a mass in the pancreatic head. Endoscopic ultrasound (EUS) with biopsy confirms a diagnosis of pancreatic adenocarcinoma. Ca 19–9 levels are elevated.

Management:

1. Cross-sectional imaging (CT) for staging.
2. Whipple procedure (pancreaticoduodenectomy) if resectable.
3. Chemotherapy and immunotherapy if unresectable.

Complications:

- Complete bile duct obstruction (may require palliative ERCP with stenting).
- Gastric outlet obstruction.

HYF: Risk factors include smoking (#1 risk factor), M > F, age >45 years, African American, obesity, diabetes, alcohol use disorder, and chronic pancreatitis. There is a subset of diagnoses associated with familial syndromes like BRCA1/2, Lynch's syndrome, and Peutz-Jeghers syndrome. Most pancreatic cancers are adenocarcinomas in the head of the pancreas and present with painless jaundice. On imaging, the presence of simultaneous dilatation of the common bile and pancreatic ducts (double duct sign) represents a malignant etiology until proven otherwise. Pancreatic cancer can also present without jaundice if the tumor is not located in the pancreatic head and does not compress the CBD. Patients may have an associated migratory thrombophlebitis (Trousseau's syndrome) or palpable, non-tender gallbladder (Courvoisier sign). Ca 19–9 is an associated tumor marker but is neither sensitive nor specific. Highly fatal, ~1-year prognosis.

CHOLANGIOCARCINOMA

A 62-year-old F presents with RUQ abdominal pain, painless jaundice, and weight loss. On **exam**, she has RUQ abdominal pain. **Labs** show ALP 443, AST 200/ALT 231, normal AFP, and elevated Ca 19–9. On **imaging**, RUQ US shows bile duct dilation without a stone and an intra-hepatic mass.

Management:

1. RUS US or CTAP to exclude gallstones and detect mass.
2. EUS or ERCP for biopsy.
3. Rarely resectable, primarily chemotherapy and immunotherapy.

Complications: Local invasion and metastasis, biliary obstruction.

HYF: Bile duct cancer originating from intra- or extra-hepatic bile ducts, excluding the gallbladder or ampulla of Vater. Risk factors include age >40, PSC, chronic cholecystitis leading to porcelain gallbladder, parasitic liver fluke (*Clonorchis sinensis*), especially in Southeast Asia from eating undercooked fish. Associated with Ca 19–9 and CEA, which can be used for screening of patients with PSC in conjunction with RUQ US. Differentiate intrahepatic cholangiocarcinoma (↑ CEA/Ca 19–9, normal AFP) from hepatocellular carcinoma (normal CEA and Ca 19–9, sometimes ↑ AFP). Can transform from biliary cysts that were not surgically resected.

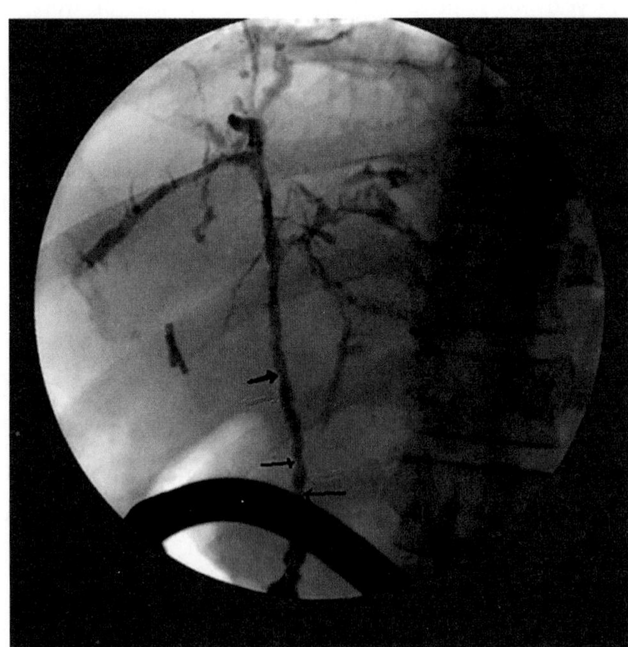

"Beads on a string" appearance of intrahepatic and extrahepatic ducts in primary sclerosing cholangitis.

2-6 Elevated Transaminases

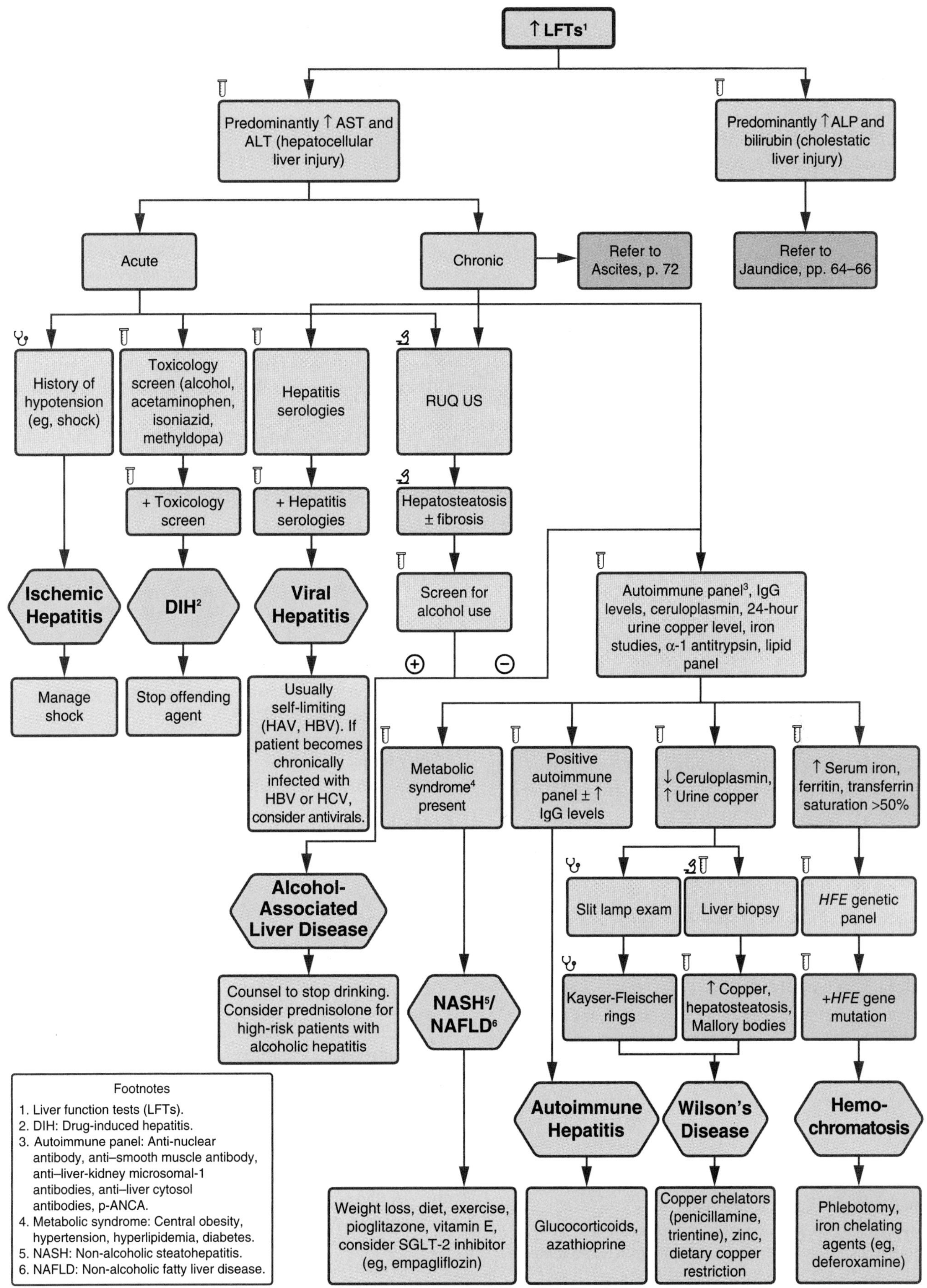
↑ LFTs[1]
Predominantly ↑ AST and ALT (hepatocellular liver injury)
Predominantly ↑ ALP and bilirubin (cholestatic liver injury)
Acute
Chronic
Refer to Ascites, p. 72
Refer to Jaundice, pp. 64–66
History of hypotension (eg, shock)
Toxicology screen (alcohol, acetaminophen, isoniazid, methyldopa)
Hepatitis serologies
RUQ US
+ Toxicology screen
+ Hepatitis serologies
Hepatosteatosis ± fibrosis
Screen for alcohol use
Ischemic Hepatitis
DIH[2]
Viral Hepatitis
Autoimmune panel[3], IgG levels, ceruloplasmin, 24-hour urine copper level, iron studies, α-1 antitrypsin, lipid panel
+
−
Manage shock
Stop offending agent
Usually self-limiting (HAV, HBV). If patient becomes chronically infected with HBV or HCV, consider antivirals.
Metabolic syndrome[4] present
Positive autoimmune panel ± ↑ IgG levels
↓ Ceruloplasmin, ↑ Urine copper
↑ Serum iron, ferritin, transferrin saturation >50%
Alcohol-Associated Liver Disease
Slit lamp exam
Liver biopsy
HFE genetic panel
Counsel to stop drinking. Consider prednisolone for high-risk patients with alcoholic hepatitis
NASH[5]/ NAFLD[6]
Kayser-Fleischer rings
↑ Copper, hepatosteatosis, Mallory bodies
+HFE gene mutation
Autoimmune Hepatitis
Wilson's Disease
Hemo-chromatosis
Weight loss, diet, exercise, pioglitazone, vitamin E, consider SGLT-2 inhibitor (eg, empagliflozin)
Glucocorticoids, azathioprine
Copper chelators (penicillamine, trientine), zinc, dietary copper restriction
Phlebotomy, iron chelating agents (eg, deferoxamine)
Footnotes
1. Liver function tests (LFTs).
2. DIH: Drug-induced hepatitis.
3. Autoimmune panel: Anti-nuclear antibody, anti–smooth muscle antibody, anti–liver-kidney microsomal-1 antibodies, anti–liver cytosol antibodies, p-ANCA.
4. Metabolic syndrome: Central obesity, hypertension, hyperlipidemia, diabetes.
5. NASH: Non-alcoholic steatohepatitis.
6. NAFLD: Non-alcoholic fatty liver disease.

FIGURE 2.6

2-6 Elevated Transaminases

ALCOHOLIC HEPATITIS

A 50-year-old M with PMH of alcohol use disorder presents with RUQ pain, anorexia, nausea, and vomiting. He reports drinking a 6-pack of beer every day for the past 20 years. On **exam**, he has a fever and tenderness to palpation in the RUQ. **Labs** show elevated AST and ALT (in a >2:1 ratio), serum bilirubin, gamma-glutamyl transferase (GGT), and INR, as well as leukocytosis with neutrophil predominance and thrombocytopenia. On **imaging**, RUQ US shows hepatosteatosis without evidence of cirrhosis or ascites.

Management:

1. Alcohol cessation.
2. Rule out infection (eg, blood and cultures, sputum sample).
3. Supportive care: IV fluids, nutritional support (eg, thiamine, vitamin B_{12}, and folate supplementation).
4. If severe alcoholic hepatitis, give glucocorticoids. If failure to respond to treatment, consider liver transplant or palliative therapy.

Complications:

- Renal failure.
- Gastric ulcers if critically ill.
- Cirrhosis and its sequelae (eg, hepatic encephalopathy, coagulation dysfunction).
- Death.
- Alcohol use disorder is associated with vitamin B_{12}/folate deficiency (leading to megaloblastic anemia), vitamin B_1 deficiency (Wernicke's encephalopathy), and hypomagnesemia.

HYF: Excessive alcohol use is associated with a spectrum of hepatic diseases (eg, alcoholic fatty liver disease, alcoholic hepatitis, cirrhosis). Alcoholic hepatitis is used to describe the acute onset of symptomatic hepatitis in the setting of alcohol use and usually presents as jaundice, tender hepatomegaly, and labs associated with impaired liver function (eg, coagulation abnormalities). Depending on disease severity, mortality can be high.

DRUG-INDUCED HEPATITIS (ACETAMINOPHEN)

A 25-year-old M with PMH of depression is brought in by family after being found vomiting in the bathroom. They found an empty pill bottle in his room. Upon questioning, he says he took the entire bottle of pills last evening in a suicide attempt. On **exam**, he is lethargic with mild tenderness to palpation in the RUQ. **Labs** are remarkable for mildly elevated LFTs, and serum acetaminophen level is high.

Management:

1. Secure airway, breathing, and circulation (ABCs) as needed.
2. Give activated charcoal.
3. Use nomogram to determine treatment with N-acetylcysteine (NAC) based on acetaminophen levels.
4. Supportive care: IV fluids, antiemetics.
5. In cases of massive poisoning or renal failure, consider hemodialysis. Dialysis removes acetaminophen and toxic metabolites (NAPQI).
6. If fulminant liver failure, refer for liver transplant.

Complications:

- Acute liver failure: Encephalopathy + LFT derangements + synthetic liver dysfunction (eg, increased PT, INR).
- Acute renal failure due to acetaminophen's direct renal tubular toxicity vs. hepatorenal syndrome.
- Death.

HYF: Acetaminophen causes liver necrosis due to overproduction of N-acetyl-p-benzoquinone imine (NAPQI), which is usually detoxified via glucuronidation. In acetaminophen overdose, this pathway becomes overwhelmed. NAC increases glutathione levels and binds to NAPQI, preventing hepatic injury if administered early after ingestion. Signs and symptoms of hepatic necrosis (eg, elevated transaminases) usually occur within 24–48 hours after ingestion. The clinical course for acetaminophen toxicity is divided into 4 phases: 1) 30 min to 24 hours: May be asymptomatic or have emesis, 2) 18–72 hours: Emesis + RUQ pain + hypotension, 3) 72–96 hours: Significant liver dysfunction with renal failure, coagulopathies, metabolic acidosis, and encephalopathy (death most commonly occurs at this stage), and 4) 4 days to 3 weeks: Recovery, if possible.

DRUG-INDUCED HEPATITIS (ISONIAZID)

A 40-year-old F with a recent diagnosis of latent tuberculosis, now undergoing treatment, presents with nausea, vomiting, and abdominal pain. She was started on isoniazid (INH) 2 months ago. On **exam**, she has mild tenderness in the RUQ. **Labs** show AST 415, ALT 376, INR 1.2, ALP 165, and total bilirubin 1.8.

Management:

1. Discontinue isoniazid and other hepatotoxic agents (eg, acetaminophen, alcohol).
2. Most cases are self-limited. Obtain serial transaminases until they normalize.
3. If severe liver failure, refer for liver transplant.

Complications:

- Liver failure.
- Isoniazid is also associated with pyridoxine deficiency (leading to peripheral neuropathy).

HYF: Clinical symptoms usually present within 2–3 months after starting isoniazid and can include malaise, nausea, flu-like symptoms, jaundice, and RUQ pain. Timely discontinuation of isoniazid and other hepatotoxins is key. Most cases are self-limited, but cases of severe hepatitis may lead to fulminant liver failure requiring liver transplantation.

VIRAL HEPATITIS

A 65-year-old M with PMH of IV drug use in remission presents for follow-up of abnormal routine labs. His AST and ALT were elevated by ~3× the upper limit of normal. He denies recent alcohol or drug use and is not taking any medications. **Exam** shows no signs of jaundice, hepatosplenomegaly, or findings suggestive of portal hypertension. As part of the work-up, **labs** including viral hepatitis serologies are sent, which are positive for anti-hepatitis C virus antibody (HCV) and detectable HCV viral level. On **imaging**, RUQ US does not show any evidence of cirrhosis.

2-6 Elevated Transaminases

Management:

1. Treat HCV with direct-acting antivirals based on genotype and patient factors (eg, presence of cirrhosis, renal failure). Typically, treatment consists of 2 direct-acting antivirals (DAAs) or 1 DAA plus ribavirin. DAAs include:
   a. NS3/4A protease inhibitors (eg, glecaprevir, grazoprevir).
   b. NS5A inhibitors (eg, daclatasvir, elbasvir).
   c. NS5B RNA-dependent RNA polymerase inhibitors: Nucleoside/nucleotide analogues (NPIs) (eg, sofosbuvir), non-nucleoside analogues (NNPIs) (dasabuvir).
2. Assess for sustained virologic response (SVR), defined as an undetectable RNA level 12 weeks after therapy. If patient has a SVR and no fibrosis or cirrhosis, no further follow-up is needed. If patient fails to achieve a SVR, re-treat for HCV infection. Regardless of treatment response, patients with fibrosis or cirrhosis require serial monitoring (eg, RUQ US) for hepatocellular carcinoma and other complications.
3. In addition to standard vaccinations, HCV-infected patients who are not immune to hepatitis A virus (HAV) and hepatitis B virus (HBV) should receive those vaccines. Patients with chronic liver disease should also receive pneumococcal vaccination.

Complications:

- Cirrhosis and its sequelae.
- Increased risk of hepatocellular carcinoma leukoclastic vasculitis, mixed cryoglobulinemia syndrome, membranous nephropathy.

HYF:

Virus	Mode of Transmission	Serologic Markers	HYF
HAV	Enteral (fecal-oral)	Antigen: HAV. Antibodies: –Anti-HAV IgM (acute). –IgG anti-HAV (prior infection).	Acute hepatitis that is self-limited. Can cause fulminant liver failure. Most common cause of viral hepatitis globally. Watch for history of restaurant outbreaks.
HBV	Bodily fluids	Antigens: HBsAg (found on surface of HBV; presence indicates carrier state), HBcAg (associated with core of HBV), HbeAg. –Acute: HBsAg, IgM anti-HBc. –Chronic: IgG anti-HBc (indicates current or prior infection), HBsAg. –Markers of replication: H**Be**Ag (indicator of transmissibility [**Be**ware!], HBV DNA. –Anti-HBs appears following infection (protective antibody, indicates immunity to HBV).	High rate of transmission. May present as viral prodrome and/or jaundice. HBV post-exposure prophylaxis: Non-immunized individuals require vaccination and immunoglobulins. HBV-immunized individuals don't require post-exposure prophylaxis. Can cause fulminant liver failure requiring treatment with antivirals or liver transplantation. Most infections in adults are self-limited. Most vertically transmitted cases become chronic.
HCV	Bodily fluids	Antigen: HCV core antigen. Antibodies: –Acute diagnosis: Anti-HCV, HCV RNA. –Chronic diagnosis: Anti-HCV, HCV RNA.	Most cases become chronic. May present with mild acute phase (ie, asymptomatic, viral prodrome, and/or jaundice). Rarely causes fulminant liver failure. Associated with cryoglobulinemia (ie, palpable purpura, arthralgia, low complement levels).
HDV	Bodily fluids	Antigen: HbsAg, HDAg. Antibodies: Anti-HBs, Anti-HDV.	Defective RNA virus that requires HBV surface antigen. Seen in co-infections with HBV or superinfection in patients with prior HBV. **HDV is Dependent on HBV.**
HEV	Enteral (fecal-oral)	Antigen: HEV antigen. Antibodies: Anti-HEV.	High mortality in pregnant women. Usually presents as self-limited acute hepatitis but can become chronic in immunosuppressed patients.

NONALCOHOLIC STEATOHEPATITIS/ FATTY LIVER DISEASE

A 55-year-old F with PMH of morbid obesity, T2DM, and HLD is found to have elevated AST and ALT on routine labs. **Labs** including viral hepatitis panel and autoimmune hepatitis panels are negative. On **imaging**, RUQ US shows increased hepatic echogenicity. Liver biopsy shows hepatic steatosis and lobular inflammation.

Management:

1. Weight loss, diet, exercise, alcohol abstinence, vitamin E.
2. Thiazolidinediones (eg, pioglitazone), GLP-1 receptor agonists (eg, semaglutide), SGLT2 inhibitors (empagliflozin, licogliflozin).

Complications:

- Cirrhosis and its sequelae.
- Increased risk of hepatocellular carcinoma.

HYF: Nonalcoholic steatohepatitis is an obesity-related cause of chronic liver disease and cirrhosis. Risk factors: Diabetes, HLD, and HTN.

(Continued)

2-6 Elevated Transaminases

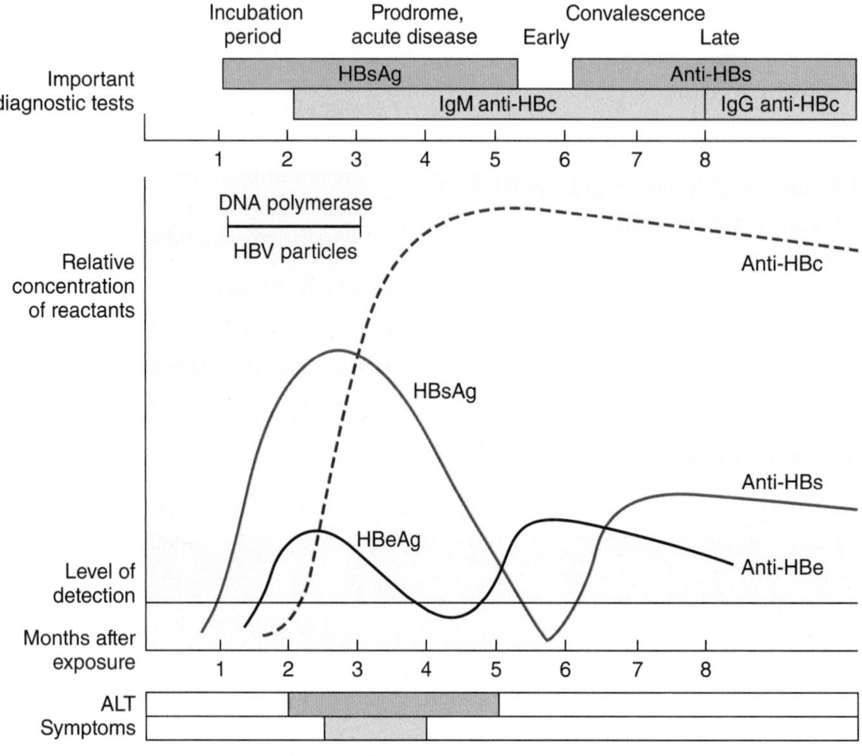
Incubation period
Prodrome, acute disease
Convalescence
Early
Late
Important diagnostic tests
HBsAg
Anti-HBs
IgM anti-HBc
IgG anti-HBc
1 2 3 4 5 6 7 8
DNA polymerase
HBV particles
Relative concentration of reactants
Anti-HBc
HBsAg
Anti-HBs
HBeAg
Anti-HBe
Level of detection
Months after exposure
ALT
Symptoms

Timeline of HBV infection with serologic markers.

AUTOIMMUNE HEPATITIS

A 35-year-old F with PMH of celiac disease is found to have transaminitis on routine labs. **Exam** shows hepatomegaly and mild tenderness in the RUQ. **Labs** show elevated AST 425 and ALT 376, as well as (+) ANA and smooth muscle antibody. IgG levels are elevated. On **imaging**, RUQ US shows liver fibrosis. Liver biopsy shows fibrotic changes and multi-lobular necrosis.

Management:

1. Corticosteroids ± azathioprine.
2. If refractory to 1st-line agents, consider mycophenolate, cyclosporine, or tacrolimus.
3. If refractory to medical therapy, consider liver transplant.

Complications:

- Cirrhosis and its sequelae, increased risk of HCC.
- Associated with other autoimmune conditions.
- Relapse is common.

HYF: T-cell mediated disease. Type 1 autoimmune hepatitis is associated with anti–nuclear and anti–smooth muscle antibodies, while type 2 is associated with anti–liver-kidney microsomal-1 and anti–liver cytosol antibodies. Patients may also have elevated serum immunoglobulins (IgG) and p-ANCA. Risk factors: Female > male, viral hepatitis, measles, AIRE gene mutation. If antimitochondrial antibody is positive, primary biliary cholangitis should be considered.

WILSON'S DISEASE

A 25-year-old F with PMH of depression presents with worsening tremor. On **exam**, she has ataxia, tremor, increased rigidity, and hepatomegaly. Slit lamp exam shows Kayser-Fleischer rings (see below). **Labs** show slightly increased AST and ALT, decreased serum ceruloplasmin level, and increased 24-hour urinary copper after giving penicillamine. Liver biopsy shows increased hepatic copper deposits.

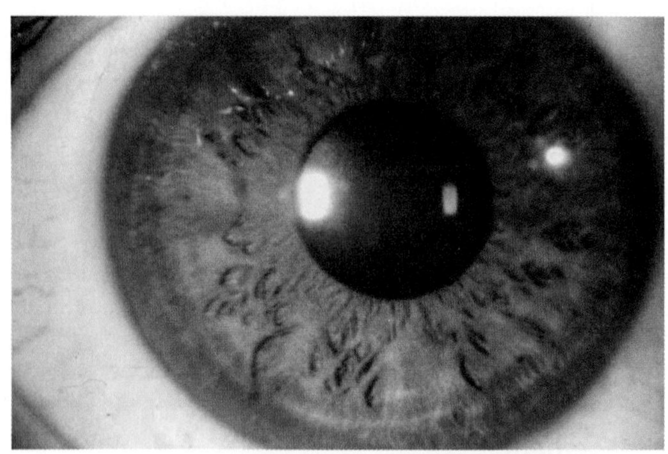

Kayser-Fleischer rings seen in Wilson's disease.

2-6 Elevated Transaminases

Management:

1. Trientine or penicillamine for copper chelation.
2. Zinc for maintenance therapy.
3. Dietary copper restriction.
4. Vitamin B_6 supplementation.
5. Liver transplantation is curative.

Complications:

- Fulminant liver failure.
- Hemolysis
- Cirrhosis.
- Death.

HYF: AR mutation of *ATP7B* leads to defective copper transport → copper accumulation and deposition in the liver and brain. Kayser-Fleischer rings can be seen on the slit lamp exam of the eyes due to copper deposition in Descemet's membrane. Typically presents in patients age <30. Liver disease precedes neurologic symptoms.

HEMOCHROMATOSIS

A 45-year-old F with PMH of T2DM is found to have mildly elevated AST and ALT on routine lab work. **Exam** reveals hepatomegaly. **Labs** show elevated AST and ALT, ↑ serum iron, % saturation of iron, and ferritin with ↓ serum transferrin. Transferrin saturation (serum iron divided by TIBC) is >50%. Liver biopsy shows a high hepatic iron index. *HFE* gene mutation screen (C282Y/H63D) is positive.

Management:

1. Serial phlebotomy to normalize iron levels.
2. Iron chelating agents (eg, deferoxamine).

Complications:

- Cirrhosis and its sequelae, increased risk of HCC.
- Skin hyperpigmentation.
- Diabetes.
- Hypopituitarism, secondary hypogonadism.
- Arthropathy, pseudogout, chondrocalcinosis.
- Cardiomyopathy, arrhythmias.
- Increased susceptibility to infections by *Vibrio vulnificus, Listeria monocytogenes*, and *Yersinia enterocolitica* infections.

HYF: Hemochromatosis is an iron-overload state in which hemosiderin accumulates in the liver, heart, and other organs. Hereditary (primary) hemochromatosis is due to an AR mutation in the *HFE* gene → excessive absorption of dietary iron. Patients receiving chronic transfusions (eg, sickle cell anemia) can develop secondary hemochromatosis.

2-7 Liver Cirrhosis and its Sequelae

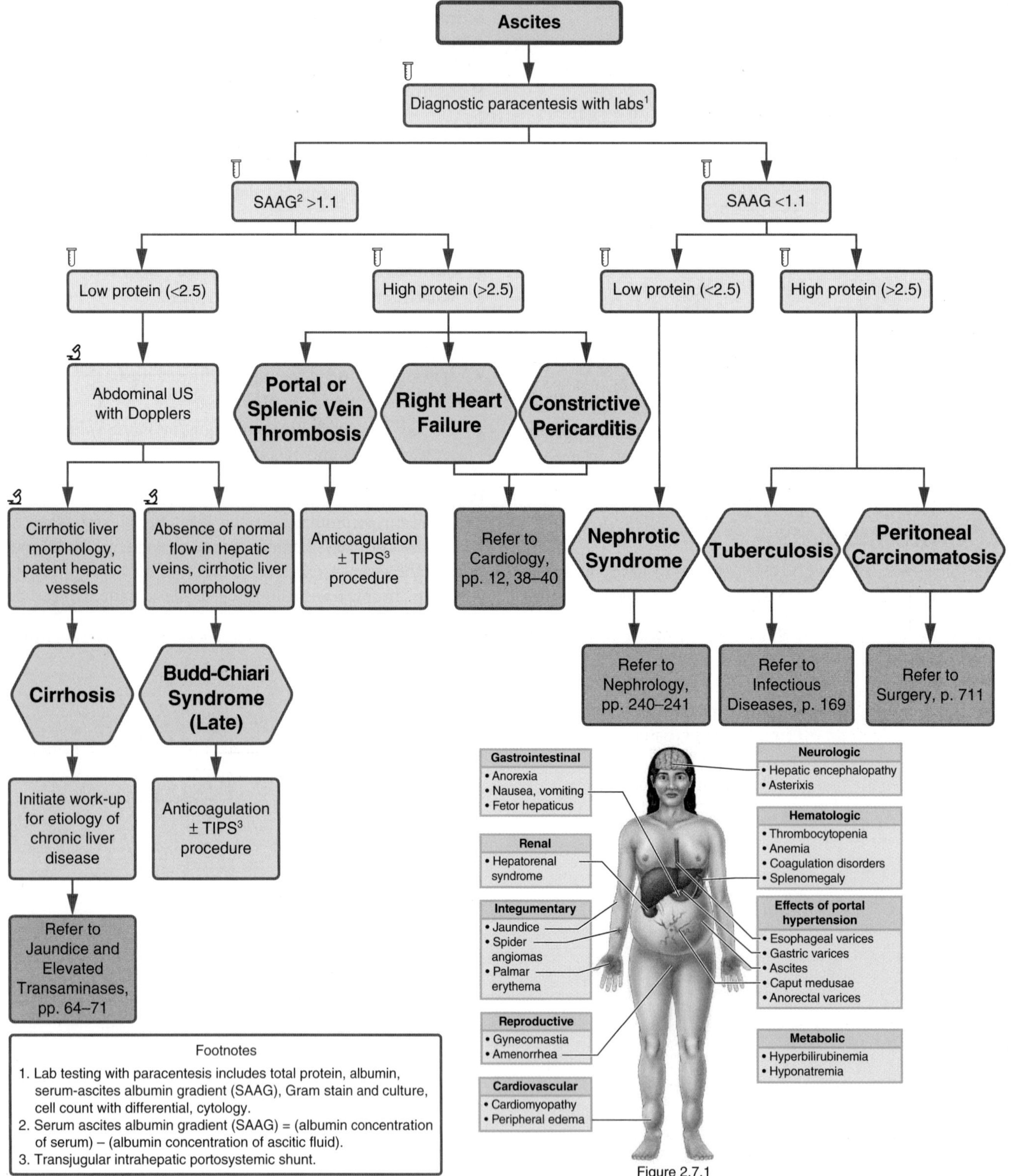

Ascites
Diagnostic paracentesis with labs[1]
SAAG[2] >1.1
SAAG <1.1
Low protein (<2.5)
High protein (>2.5)
Low protein (<2.5)
High protein (>2.5)
Abdominal US with Dopplers
Portal or Splenic Vein Thrombosis
Right Heart Failure
Constrictive Pericarditis
Cirrhotic liver morphology, patent hepatic vessels
Absence of normal flow in hepatic veins, cirrhotic liver morphology
Anticoagulation ± TIPS[3] procedure
Refer to Cardiology, pp. 12, 38–40
Nephrotic Syndrome
Tuberculosis
Peritoneal Carcinomatosis
Cirrhosis
Budd-Chiari Syndrome (Late)
Refer to Nephrology, pp. 240–241
Refer to Infectious Diseases, p. 169
Refer to Surgery, p. 711
Initiate work-up for etiology of chronic liver disease
Anticoagulation ± TIPS[3] procedure
Refer to Jaundice and Elevated Transaminases, pp. 64–71
Gastrointestinal
• Anorexia
• Nausea, vomiting
• Fetor hepaticus
Renal
• Hepatorenal syndrome
Integumentary
• Jaundice
• Spider angiomas
• Palmar erythema
Reproductive
• Gynecomastia
• Amenorrhea
Cardiovascular
• Cardiomyopathy
• Peripheral edema
Neurologic
• Hepatic encephalopathy
• Asterixis
Hematologic
• Thrombocytopenia
• Anemia
• Coagulation disorders
• Splenomegaly
Effects of portal hypertension
• Esophageal varices
• Gastric varices
• Ascites
• Caput medusae
• Anorectal varices
Metabolic
• Hyperbilirubinemia
• Hyponatremia

Footnotes

1. Lab testing with paracentesis includes total protein, albumin, serum-ascites albumin gradient (SAAG), Gram stain and culture, cell count with differential, cytology.
2. Serum ascites albumin gradient (SAAG) = (albumin concentration of serum) – (albumin concentration of ascitic fluid).
3. Transjugular intrahepatic portosystemic shunt.

Figure 2.7.1

Ascites is the accumulation of fluid in the abdominal cavity. Patients usually present with abdominal distension. Physical exam can reveal a fluid wave or shifting dullness. Imaging such as abdominal ultrasound can help confirm the presence of ascites. Etiologies for ascites include portal hypertension (eg, cirrhosis, Budd-Chiari syndrome, portal vein thrombosis), hypoalbuminemia leading to loss of oncotic pressure (eg, nephrotic syndrome, severe malnutrition), or various peritoneal diseases (eg, malignancy, infection, inflammation). Assessment of ascites should begin with a diagnostic paracentesis with labs: serum-ascites albumin gradient (SAAG), total protein, albumin, Gram stain and culture, cell count with differential, and cytology. SAAG is calculated as serum albumin – ascitic fluid albumin. SAAG >1.1 g/dL suggests portal hypertension, whereas SAAG <1.1 g/dL indicates lack of portal hypertension as the cause of ascites. Total protein >2.5 g/dL suggests sufficient synthetic function of protein by the liver, so we would consider non-hepatic causes of ascites (eg, right-sided heart failure, constrictive pericarditis, schistosomiasis, portal or splenic vein thrombosis, tuberculosis, ovarian cancer leading to peritoneal carcinomatosis). Total protein <2.5 g/dL suggests poor liver synthetic function or excessive protein loss (eg, cirrhosis, nephrotic syndrome, malnutrition, enteropathy). We cover numerous etiologies of ascites in other algorithms. In the next page, we will focus on liver cirrhosis and its sequelae.

FIGURE 2.7

2-7 Liver Cirrhosis and its Sequelae

Cirrhosis results from chronic liver injury and inflammation. The most common etiologies in the US are alcohol, chronic HCV, and non-alcoholic steatohepatitis (NASH). Patients may be asymptomatic or present with jaundice, easy bruising due to coagulopathy, and complications of portal hypertension (eg, ascites, hepatic encephalopathy, gastroesophageal varices, thrombocytopenia). Exam may reveal an enlarged liver and other signs of portal hypertension and liver failure. Labs may show synthetic dysfunction (eg, ↓ albumin, ↑ PT/INR, and ↑ bilirubin) and thrombocytopenia (due to hypersplenism, platelet sequestration in the liver, and ↓ thrombopoietin production). Abdominal US would show hepatic atrophy and nodularity. Liver biopsy (the most accurate test) would show bridging fibrosis and nodular regeneration. The goal of treatment is to prevent progression of cirrhosis and episodes of acute decompensated cirrhosis (variceal bleeding, hepatic encephalopathy, or ascites). All cirrhotic patients require HAV, HBV, and PPSV-23 (pneumonia) vaccinations.

ACUTE DECOMPENSATED CIRRHOSIS WITH ASCITES

A 50-year-old M with PMH of alcohol use disorder and chronic HCV presents with progressive abdominal distension and lower extremity edema. On **exam**, he has scleral icterus and jaundice, as well as abdominal distension with a fluid wave, numerous spider angiomas, several ecchymoses on his extremities, and 2+ pitting edema to the upper thighs. **Labs** show elevated AST and ALT (in a >2:1 ratio), serum bilirubin, gamma-glutamyl transferase (GGT), and INR, as well as thrombocytopenia. Creatine is elevated. WBC is normal. On **imaging**, abdominal US with Doppler shows large-volume ascites and cirrhotic liver morphology, patent hepatic vessels, and no liver lesions. HCV antibody and HCV RNA PCR are positive. Diagnostic and therapeutic paracentesis is done with 10 L of straw-colored ascites drained and labs showing SAAG >1.1, total protein 2.0, albumin 1.2, and cell count 356 (27% neutrophils).

Management:

1. Alcohol cessation, low-salt diet.
2. Treat underlying cause of cirrhosis (eg, alcohol cessation, direct-acting antiviral therapy for HCV, antiviral therapy for HBV that will suppress viral replication and reduce liver inflammation).
3. Diuretics (eg, furosemide, spironolactone).
4. Avoid hepatotoxins and nephrotoxins. Stop medications that cause decreased renal perfusion (eg, NSAIDs, β-blockers, ACEi/ARBs).
5. If refractory ascites, consider serial therapeutic paracentesis and/or trans-jugular intra-hepatic portosystemic shunts (TIPS).
6. Consider liver transplantation once stable.

Complications:

- Renal failure due to hepatorenal syndrome.
- Sequelae of cirrhosis: Gastroesophageal varices, hepatic encephalopathy.
- Spontaneous bacterial peritonitis.
- Umbilical hernia, hepatic hydrothorax due to tense ascites.
- Portal vein thrombosis.

HYF: Baclofen and naltrexone are often used to decrease alcohol cravings and improve alcohol abstinence in cirrhotic patients. Placement of a TIPS addresses portal hypertension by creating a low-resistance channel between the hepatic vein and an intrahepatic branch of the portal vein, allowing blood to return to systemic circulation; it is contraindicated in cases of severe hepatic encephalopathy, portal vein thrombosis, and thrombocytopenia with platelets <20,000.

SPONTANEOUS BACTERIAL PERITONITIS (SBP)

A 65-year-old F with PMH of alcoholic cirrhosis presents with diffuse abdominal pain, nausea, and vomiting. **Exam** reveals a fever of 38.5°C, HR 105, RR 12, and BP of 90/60 mmHg. She has scleral icterus, jaundice, and abdominal distension with a fluid wave and rebound tenderness. On **imaging**, abdominal US shows large-volume ascites. Diagnostic paracentesis shows >250 PMNs/mL. Fluid cultures are pending.

Management:

1. IV antibiotics (3rd-generation cephalosporins to cover Gram negatives) *after* paracentesis.
2. Prophylaxis with a fluoroquinolone to prevent recurrence.

Complications:

- Variceal bleeding, death if not detected and treated early.

HYF: In all patients with cirrhosis who are hospitalized, paracentesis should be done on admission if ascites is present to rule out SBP and expedite antibiotics. Due to gut translocation of enteric bacteria into ascitic fluid. Most common pathogens are gut bacteria (eg, *E. coli* and *Klebsiella*), followed by *Streptococcus* and *Staphylococcus*. Diagnosis is established with ascitic fluid PMN count >250 cells/mL. To increase yield of ascitic fluid cultures, administer antibiotics after paracentesis, if possible. If prior upper GI bleeding, start SBP prophylaxis (eg, fluoroquinolone, trimethoprim-sulfamethoxazole).

HEPATOCELLULAR CARCINOMA

A 68-year-old M with PMH of alcohol use disorder complicated by cirrhosis presents with several months of malaise, unintentional weight loss, and worsening abdominal distension. **Exam** reveals scleral icterus and severe abdominal distension. **Labs** reveal elevated transaminases and alpha fetoprotein (AFP). On **imaging**, triple-phase CT of the abdomen and pelvis shows a liver mass with arterial phase enhancement and delayed phase washout. Liver biopsy confirms the diagnosis.

Management:

1. Partial hepatectomy or liver transplant, if able.
2. If localized disease and/or unable to undergo resection or transplant, consider radioembolization, trans-arterial chemoembolization (TACE), and systemic chemotherapy. Sorafenib for metastatic disease.
3. Screen for recurrence with serial AFP levels and surveillance imaging (eg, abdominal US, CT).

(Continued)

2-7 Liver Cirrhosis and its Sequelae

Complications:

- Budd-Chiari syndrome, portal vein obstruction, liver failure.
- Poor prognosis.

HYF: Most common liver malignancy. Risk factors: Cirrhosis (from alcohol, NASH, HCV) and HBV (with or without cirrhosis) in the US; HBV and aflatoxins from food in developing countries. In all cirrhotic patients, perform HCC screening with serial imaging and AFP. Paraneoplastic syndromes: Hypercalcemia, watery diarrhea, hypoglycemia, erythrocytosis, skin lesions. Most liver masses are from metastatic disease (breast, lung, or colon cancer) rather than primary liver cancer.

ACUTE DECOMPENSATED CIRRHOSIS WITH GASTROESOPHAGEAL VARICES

A 55-year-old F with PMH of alcoholic cirrhosis presents with hematemesis and melena. **Exam** reveals HR 105, RR 18, and BP 80/50, as well as jaundice and a firm, palpable liver. She has a large, tarry bowel movement during the interview. **Labs** reveal mildly elevated transaminases, increased INR, and Hgb 8.0.

Management:

1. Stabilize patient (airway, breathing, circulation). Give blood transfusions as needed.
2. Start prophylactic antibiotics (eg, ceftriaxone).
3. Initiate vasoactive agent (eg, octreotide, somatostatin, vasopressin, terlipressin).
4. Urgent upper endoscopy (EGD) with band ligation or sclerotherapy of varices.
5. If refractory bleeding, refer for urgent TIPS.
6. Prophylaxis for recurrent variceal bleed: EGD with band ligation and/or non-selective β-blockers (propranolol, nadolol).

Complications:

- Bacterial infections (aspiration pneumonia, SBP, UTI).
- Hepatic encephalopathy.
- Renal failure.

HYF: Esophageal varices are portosystemic anastomoses that develop due to portal hypertension. Variceal bleeds can be exacerbated by underlying coagulopathy in the setting of impaired synthetic liver function (ie, impaired synthesis of all clotting factors *except* factor VIII); in cases of acute bleed in liver patients, consider administration of fresh frozen plasma. TIPS may be offered as preemptive therapy to prevent rebleeding after a first GI bleed, but it is often used in variceal bleeds that are refractory to banding attempt. All cirrhotic patients require endoscopic surveillance for development of esophageal varices.

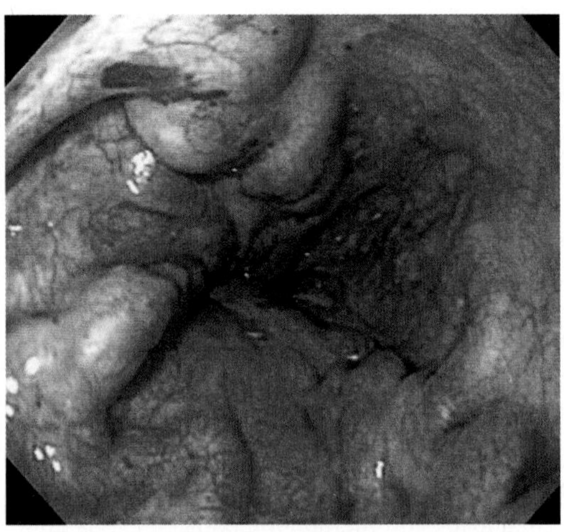

Esophageal varices on EGD in a patient with liver cirrhosis.

Main Sites of Portosystemic Anastomoses

Location	Portal Component	Systemic Component	Clinical Presentation
Distal esophagus	Left gastric vein	Esophageal veins → azygos and hemiazygos veins	Esophageal varices
Umbilicus	Paraumbilical veins	Superior and inferior epigastric veins	Caput Medusae
Rectum	Superior rectal vein	Middle rectal veins and inferior rectal veins	Hemorrhoids
Retroperitoneum	Splenic, pancreatic, colic, etc. veins	Left renal, lumbar, retroperitoneal, etc. veins	—
Bare area of liver	Branches of the portal vein	Diaphragmatic veins	—

2-7 Liver Cirrhosis and its Sequelae

ACUTE DECOMPENSATED CIRRHOSIS WITH HEPATIC ENCEPHALOPATHY

A 55-year-old M with PMH of alcoholic cirrhosis and recent bout of gastroenteritis presents with altered mental status. On **exam**, he is difficult to arouse, slow to answer questions, and jaundiced with asterixis. He also appears dehydrated, with dry mucous membranes and delayed capillary refill. **Labs** reveal elevated transaminases and ammonia level, as well as hypokalemia. On **imaging**, abdominal US shows presence of mild ascites.

Management:

1. Stabilize the patient (airway, breathing, circulation). Reverse potential triggers (eg, dehydration from gastroenteritis as in this patient).
2. Diagnostic paracentesis to rule out SBP.
3. Lactulose ± rifaximin; titrate to 3–4 bowel movements per day.

Complications:

- Permanent brain damage if severe.

HYF: The healthy liver metabolizes ammonia to urea, which is easily excreted. Decreased ammonia clearance due to liver dysfunction → ammonia accumulation → ammonia crosses blood-brain barrier and is converted to glutamine (osmolyte) → cerebral edema and neurotoxicity. Of note, ammonia levels do not consistently correlate with severity of HE in cirrhotic patients. Often triggered by stressors (eg, infection, dehydration, electrolyte abnormalities, GI bleed) or TIPS (blood bypasses liver).

HEPATORENAL SYNDROME (HRS)

A 55-year-old M with PMH of alcoholic cirrhosis presents with acute decompensated cirrhosis. On **exam**, he is jaundiced and has abdominal distension with fluid wave. **Labs** reveal elevated transaminases and creatinine 2× his baseline. Urine sodium is <10 mEq/L. Urine studies show biliary casts and no evidence of acute tubular necrosis. On **imaging**, abdominal US shows presence of severe ascites. Diagnostic and therapeutic paracentesis is done with 10 L of straw-colored fluid drained; fluid studies rule out SBP.

Management:

1. Trial volume repletion with IV fluids plus IV albumin. Rule out other causes of renal failure.
2. Consider octreotide (↓ splanchnic vasodilation) and midodrine (↑ BP). If ICU patient, consider telripressin or norepinephrine.
3. If refractory, consider dialysis.
4. Liver transplant can be curative.

Complications: Renal failure requiring dialysis.

HYF: Diagnosis of exclusion. Ascites is almost always present. HRS = pre-renal failure due to splanchnic vasodilation and decreased renal perfusion. Urine sodium is usually <10 mEq/L.

PORTAL VEIN THROMBOSIS

A 50-year-old M with PMH of alcoholic cirrhosis presents with hematochezia. On **exam**, he has splenomegaly, numerous spider angiomas, palmar erythema, and several ecchymoses on his extremities. **Labs** show mildly elevated AST and ALT and INR, as well as thrombocytopenia. Hgb is 8.0 (baseline 12). On **imaging**, abdominal US with Doppler shows small-volume ascites, cirrhotic liver morphology, and hyperechoic material within the portal vein that extends into the mesenteric and splenic veins.

Management:

1. Treat complications of portal hypertension (eg, GI bleed).
2. Once stabilized, consider anticoagulation on a case-by-case basis.
3. Screen for esophageal varices in patients with chronic PVTs. Prophylaxis for variceal bleed: EGD with band ligation and/or non-selective β-blockers (propranolol, nadolol).

Complications:

- Portal hypertension and its sequelae (eg, ascites, varices, GI bleeds).
- Portal cholangiopathy.
- Intestinal ischemia.

HYF: In cirrhotic patients, PVT is likely due to unbalanced hemostasis and slow portal flow. In contrast, PVT in patients with previously healthy livers is likely due to inherited or acquired prothrombotic states (eg, malignancy, inherited thrombophilias, IBD) or may be caused by trauma, severe primary peritonitis, or abdominal infections. With chronic PVTs, portal cavernomas (ie, cavernous transformation of the portal vein) develop due to formation of collateral blood vessels that bring blood around the area of obstruction. Patients with chronic PVT often form gastroesophageal varices due to portal hypertension; the most common presentation is GI bleeding. The decision to start anticoagulation is made on a case-by-case basis, as patients with chronic PVT are at risk for recurrent thrombosis, as well as variceal bleed.

2-8 Abdominal Pain

Chronic Upper
Ulcer, dyspepsia, reflux, gastroparesis, biliary colic, chronic pancreatitis, IBS/IBD, cancer (ie, stomach, pancreas, liver)

RUQ	Epigastric	LUQ
Biliary colic, cholecystitis, cholangitis, pancreatitis, hepatitis, Budd-Chiari, portal vein thrombosis, liver abscess	PUD, gastritis, GERD, esophagitis, pancreatitis, MI, pericarditis, ruptured AAA	Splenic infarct, splenic rupture, splenic abscess, gastritis, gastric ulcer, pancreatitis, subdiaphragmatic abscess
Right Lumbar Nephrolithiasis, pyelonephritis, perinephric abscess	**Pericumbilicus** Early appendicitis, gastroenteritis, bowel obstruction, IBS/IBD, ruptured AAA	**Left Lumbar** Nephrolithiasis, pyelonephritis, perinephric abscess
RLQ Appendicitis, salpingitis, inguinal hernia, ectopic pregnancy, nephrolithiasis, IBS/IBD, mesenteric adenitis, cecal volvulus	**Hypogastrium** Cystitis, acute urinary retention, IBS/IBD, ovarian cyst	**LLQ** Diverticulitis, salpingitis, ectopic pregnancy, nephrolithiasis, IBS/IBD, sigmoid volvulus

Diffuse
Gastroenteritis, mesenteric ischemia, SBO, IBS/IBD, peritonitis, diabetes, familial Mediterranean fever, metabolic disease, functional pain, psychiatric causes

Chronic Lower
IBS/IBD, diverticulitis, lactose intolerance, dysmenorrhea, endometriosis, hernia, cancer (eg, colon cancer, GU/GYN malignancies)

FIGURE 2.8

Differential diagnosis for abdominal pain based on area of pain. Abbreviations: AAA, abdominal aortic aneurysm; IBD, inflammatory bowel disease; IBS, irritable bowel syndrome; SBO, small bowl obstruction; MI, myocardial infarction; PUD, peptic ulcer disease; RUQ, right upper quadrant; RLQ, right lower quadrant; LUQ, left upper quadrant; LLQ, left lower quadrant.

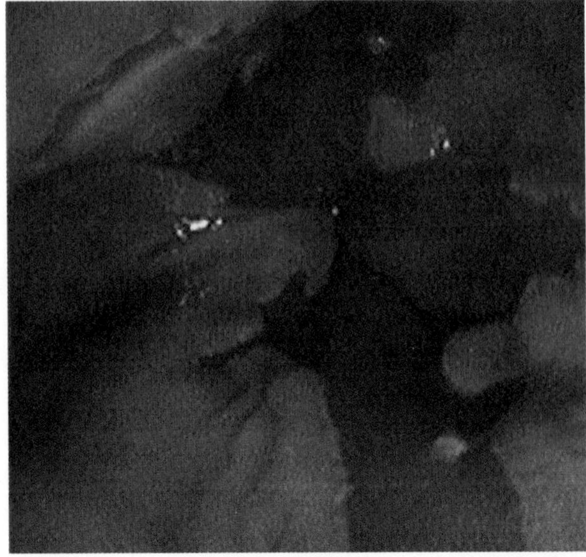
Barrett's esophagus.

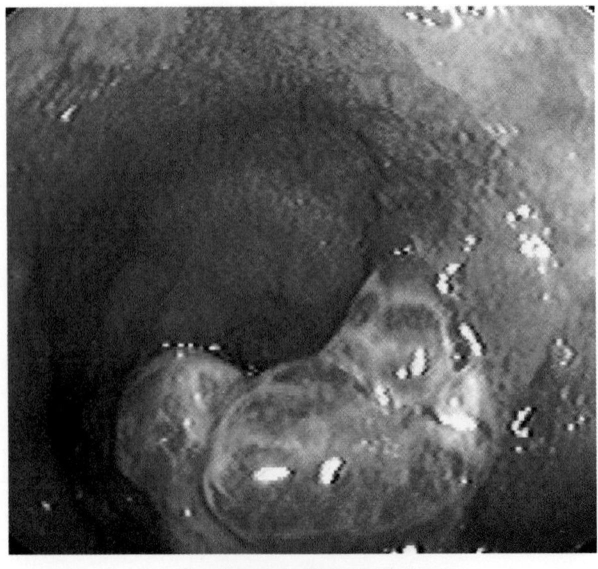
Esophageal adenocarcinoma with Barrett's esophagus.

2-8 Abdominal Pain

Abdominal pain is one of the most common presenting symptoms you will encounter as a clinician. The first step in diagnosing abdominal pain is to identify the location of the pain, which can sometimes help limit your differential diagnoses to those that cause pain in that quadrant of the abdomen. Of note, pain does not always localize precisely, so considering a broad differential is necessary no matter the location of the pain. Other parts of the history can narrow the differential. Time course of pain is crucial. Some disease processes present acutely within hours to days (eg, cholangitis, acute pancreatitis, small or large bowel obstruction), whereas others present subacutely or chronically over months to years (eg, inflammatory bowel disease, chronic mesenteric ischemia, peptic ulcer disease). Other important parts of the history include factors that alleviate or worsen the pain (eg, eating), pain quality and radiation, and any associated symptoms (nausea, vomiting, inability to pass stool and flatus, jaundice, fever, chills, weight loss, changes in bowel habits). Melena or hematochezia can be suggestive of an upper or lower GI bleed, respectively. Cardiac and pulmonary symptoms can be clues to diagnosing myocardial infarction or pneumonia presenting as abdominal pain. In women, sexual and gynecological histories are important to consider. Clarifying a history of alcohol consumption, as well as prescription and over-the-counter medications and supplements, can also be helpful. The physical exam is also key. Vital signs (eg, unexplained hypotension) and presence or absence of abdominal distension help narrow the differential. Peritoneal findings (rebound tenderness, guarding, rigidity) can suggest an intraabdominal catastrophe that requires emergent intervention (eg, bowel perforation, acute mesenteric ischemia).

Below, we discuss etiologies of abdominal pain based on their acuity of presentation: Acute or subacute/chronic.

Acute Abdominal Pain			
Diagnosis	**Clinical Presentation**	**Management**	**HYFs**
Cholelithiasis	A 45-year-old F with PMH of obesity, hyperlipidemia, and polycystic ovarian syndrome presents with recurrent RUQ pain. She reports post-prandial pain, especially with fatty foods. Her episodes always resolve. **Exam** is unremarkable. **Labs** show normal WBC, total bilirubin, ALP, and serum amylase. On **imaging**, RUQ ultrasound shows gallstones without any gallbladder wall thickening.	1. Supportive care: Pain management, diet (avoid trigger foods), rehydration. 2. Elective cholecystectomy if symptomatic. 3. Consider ursodeoxycholic acid in patients who cannot undergo cholecystectomy (dissolves gallstones).	Cholelithiasis refers to the presence of gallstones and can be asymptomatic or present with biliary colic, which is defined as self-resolving episodes of colicky pain in the RUQ that may be triggered by fatty foods. Composition of gallstones may include cholesterol, pigment (associated with cirrhosis, chronic hemolysis, biliary stasis), or mixed/brown (cholesterol + salt). Risk factors include obesity, female sex, middle age, and multiparity. Complications include chronic cholecystitis, as well as secondary infections (cholecystitis, cholangitis).
Cholecystitis	A 42-year-old F with PMH of obesity and hyperlipidemia presents with RUQ pain radiating to her right shoulder for the past 5 hours. She also reports fever, nausea, and vomiting. In the past, she has had similar RUQ pain after eating fatty foods that self-resolved, but this pain is constant and more severe. On **exam**, she has a fever and notable TTP in the RUQ, inspiratory arrest with palpation of the RUQ (positive Murphy's sign), and guarding. **Labs** show leukocytosis, elevated ALP, direct bilirubin, and ALP. On **imaging**, RUQ US shows presence of gallstones and a thickened gallbladder wall with pericholecystic fluid.	1. Supportive care (NPO, IV fluids, pain management). 2. IV antibiotics. 3. General surgery consult for non-emergent cholecystectomy within 72 hours. If not a surgical candidate, percutaneous drainage of gallbladder.	Cholecystitis can be calculous (gallstone impaction in the cystic duct) or acalculous (associated with gallbladder stasis, infection, and gallbladder hypoperfusion in critically ill patients who have been fasting or on total parenteral nutrition). In terms of imaging, RUQ US is 1st-line. If RUQ US is equivocal, obtain cholescintigraphy (HIDA scan); a lack of gallbladder visualization indicates obstruction. Risk factors are the same as cholelithiasis. Complications include gallbladder perforation and ascending cholangitis.

(Continued)

2-8 Abdominal Pain

Acute Abdominal Pain			
Diagnosis	**Clinical Presentation**	**Management**	**HYFs**
Cholangitis	A 62-year-old M with PMH of sickle cell disease presents with fever, chills, abdominal pain, and jaundice. On **exam**, he is febrile, hypotensive, and confused. He has tenderness to palpation in the RUQ, as well as jaundice. **Labs** show WBC 18, elevated AST/ALT, and total bilirubin of 8. On **imaging**, RUQ US shows biliary dilation and an impacted gallstone in the common bile duct.	Antibiotics and ERCP. If cause of cholangitis is gallstones, surgical cholecystectomy after resolution of cholangitis.	Charcot's triad (RUQ pain, fever, jaundice) is indicative of likely cholangitis. Reynolds' pentad includes Charcot's triad, plus altered mental status and hypotension. Sickle cell disease increases the risk of pigmented gallstones due to hemolysis and, as such, increases the risk of cholangitis.
Acute pancreatitis	A 22-year-old M college student presents with LUQ pain radiating to the back, associated with nausea and pain with PO intake. He notes increased alcohol consumption the past weekend. On **exam**, he is tender in the LUQ and hypotensive with dry mucous membranes. **Labs** show lipase of 450. On **imaging**, CT scan shows pancreatic edema and inflammation.	1. Supportive care: IV fluids, pain control, make NPO, and advance diet as tolerated. 2. For recurrent pancreatitis, consider obtaining RUQ US to evaluate for gallstone or pancreatic divisum anatomy, calcium level, triglyceride level, and IgG4 level based on clinical history. In young patients with recurrent pancreatitis without a clear etiology, consider sending a genetic work-up for hereditary pancreatitis.	Complications include pancreatic insufficiency, necrosis, or pseudocyst. Pancreatitis is diagnosed with 2/3 of the following: Abdominal pain, elevated lipase, CT findings of pancreatitis. The most common causes of acute pancreatitis are alcohol use and gallstones. If etiology is gallstones, consider cholecystectomy after resolution of pancreatitis. Etiologies of pancreatitis: **I GET SMASHED**: **I**diopathic, **G**allstones, **E**thanol, **T**umors/Trauma, **S**teroids, **M**umps, **A**utoimmune, **S**corpion sting, **H**ypercalcemia/triglyceridemia, **E**RCP, and **D**rugs.
Acute viral hepatitis	A 32-year-old M with no PMH presents with 4 days of nausea, vomiting, and RUQ abdominal discomfort. Today, he noted dark urine and yellowing of his eyes when he woke up. He recently returned from a coastal vacation where he ate a lot of seafood. Two friends have developed similar symptoms. He denies alcohol use. **Exam** reveals RUQ tenderness and scleral icterus. **Labs** show elevated AST and ALT of 1450 and 1300. Anti-HAV IgM is positive, while testing for HBV is negative.	Supportive care.	HAV is transmitted via fecal-oral route and is commonly transmitted via contaminated food, especially undercooked seafood. HBV is more commonly transmitted sexually, while HCV is more often transmitted via needles/blood-to-blood transmission. Vaccinations are available for HAV and HBV.
Ischemic colitis	A 74-year-old is in the ICU for septic shock complicated by hypotensive episodes and now has bright red blood per rectum. On **exam**, the abdomen is slightly tender to palpation in the upper quadrants. **Labs** are notable for stable hemoglobin. On **imaging**, CT shows colonic wall thickening at the hepatic and splenic flexure.	IV fluids, antibiotics, bowel rest.	Complications include bowel perforation, hemorrhage, infarction, septic shock. Ischemic colitis is usually due to decreased circulation and occurs in the watershed areas (splenic flexure, rectosigmoid junction).
Viral gastroenteritis	A 25-year-old M with no PMH presents with 2 days of watery diarrhea. He recently ate at a restaurant with several friends who also experienced similar symptoms. He has had 5–6 bowel movements per day and reports decreased appetite. On **exam**, he has poor skin turgor and increased capillary refill time. **Labs** show a mildly elevated Cr and mild hyponatremia and hypokalemia.	Supportive care: Encourage PO intake, IV fluids as needed.	Complications include prerenal AKI and electrolyte disturbances (hyponatremia, hypokalemia, hypomagnesemia, metabolic acidosis) due to dehydration and electrolyte loss in stool. Common viral etiologies include norovirus and rotavirus.

2-8 Abdominal Pain

Acute Abdominal Pain			
Diagnosis	**Clinical Presentation**	**Management**	**HYFs**
Acute mesenteric ischemia	A 75-year-old M with PMH of T2DM, extensive smoking history, hyperlipidemia, peripheral vascular disease, and STEMI 6 weeks ago s/p PCI presents with severe, acute periumbilical abdominal pain associated with nausea and vomiting. He reports 3 episodes of hematochezia since onset of pain. On **exam**, he has a fever of 39.0°C, BP 155/95, HR 120 and irregularly irregular, RR 18, and SpO_2 92% on room air. He is in significant distress due to pain. On abdominal exam, he has mild diffuse TTP and decreased bowel sounds. No rebound tenderness or rigidity. **Labs** are remarkable for leukocytosis, hemoconcentration, low bicarbonate, and elevated lactate. On **imaging**, abdominal XR is unrevealing. CT angiography confirms the diagnosis.	1. Stabilize patient. 2. Broad-spectrum IV antibiotics. 3. Anticoagulation. 4. Emergent surgical intervention: Visceral revascularization (embolectomy, thrombectomy, endarterectomy, or vascular bypass), based on specific lesion. Laparotomy and resection of necrotic bowel.	This patient likely developed atrial fibrillation and a mural thrombus after his recent MI that embolized to the mesenteric artery. Acute mesenteric ischemia is due to inadequate blood flow to the small intestine and can be caused by an acute thrombosis (peripheral arterial disease), cardioembolism (atrial fibrillation, valvular disease, infective endocarditis), or low blood-flow state (shock). Classically, patients present with severe abdominal pain out of proportion to their exam in the early stages. If untreated, bowel necrosis can occur, leading to development of focal abdominal tenderness, peritoneal signs (rebound tenderness), hematochezia, and sepsis with multi-organ failure. Labs usually show leukocytosis, elevated hemoglobin (hemoconcentration), and metabolic acidosis with high anion gap and lactate. Hyperphosphatemia and hyperkalemia are usually late signs and often associated with bowel infarction. CTA is preferred for diagnosis; if diagnosis is unclear, then opt for mesenteric angiography. Risk factors: Atherosclerosis, cardioembolic source, hypercoagulable disorders, recent AAA repair. Associated with high mortality and morbidity.
Ileus	A 42-year-old with PMH of hypertension presents with nausea and vomiting 2 days after a cholecystectomy. **Exam** reveals abdominal distention, tympanic percussion to abdomen, and sluggish bowel sounds. On **imaging**, CT shows small bowel distention without a transition point or obstruction.	Supportive care: Maintenance IV fluids, NPO, electrolyte repletion (K >4, Mg >2), encourage ambulation. Consider decompression with NG tube and/or rectal tube placement. Reverse possible causes (eg, nearby infection). Stop opioids. Consider prokinetic agents in some cases.	Ileus is common after surgery or intense illness and results in delayed transit of food through the small bowel. It will resolve over time with supportive care. Typically, patients will report no bowel movement or flatulence for days, as well as nausea and vomiting.
Splenic infarct	A 62-year-old with PMH of atrial fibrillation not on anticoagulation presents with LUQ pain, fever, nausea, and vomiting. **Exam** shows TTP in the LUQ. On **imaging**, CT A/P is concerning for splenic infarct. Subsequent TTE shows a left atrial thrombus.	Anticoagulation.	Complications include splenic abscess, infection or rupture. Splenic infarction can be caused by hypercoagulability, thromboembolisms, septic emboli (eg, endocarditis), and sickle cell disease. If septic emboli are suspected or splenic abscess develops, administer antibiotics.
Splenic rupture	An 18-year-old M high school football player with PMH of mononucleosis within the last 2 weeks presents with acute LUQ pain following a game in which he was tackled. **Exam** shows exquisite abdominal tenderness with guarding. **Labs** reveal a hemoglobin of 9 (baseline 13). On **imaging**, CT is concerning for splenic rupture and actively bleeding hematoma.	Supportive care to stabilize, followed by emergent splenectomy. After splenectomy, encapsulated vaccination series (pneumococcal, meningococcal, and *Haemophilus influenzae* [Hib]) is mandatory.	Mononucleosis is often seen in young adults and presents with fever, pharyngitis, and lymphadenopathy. Splenomegaly is often present, increasing the risk of splenic rupture if athletics are resumed too soon before full recovery. While splenic rupture can be observed in stable patients, surgery may be indicated if severe bleeding results.

(*Continued*)

2-8 Abdominal Pain

Diagnosis	Clinical Presentation	Management	HYFs
Acute Abdominal Pain			
Appendicitis	A 25-year-old M with no PMH presents with 2 days of abdominal pain that started around his umbilicus, but in the past hour now is located over the RLQ between the right anterior superior iliac spine and umbilicus, and is associated with fever and chills. On **exam**, patient has rebound tenderness at McBurney's point, as well as + Rovsing's, psoas, and obturator signs. **Labs** show a WBC of 12. On **imaging**, there is an enlarged, thickened appendix with surrounding fat stranding on CT scan.	Antibiotics, surgical consult for appendectomy.	Complications include appendiceal rupture, appendiceal abscess, and sepsis. McBurney's point: RLQ tenderness 1/3 distance from anterior superior iliac spine and umbilicus. Rovsing's sign: RLQ pain with palpation of LLQ. Psoas sign: RLQ pain with passive right hip extension. Obturator sign: RLQ pain with right hip flexion and internal rotation.
Diverticulitis	A 55-year-old with PMH of T2DM and hypertension presents with acute LLQ pain and fever. **Exam** shows fever and tenderness to palpation in the LLQ without rebound or guarding. **Labs** reveal WBC of 12.8. On **imaging**, CT A/P shows fat stranding around an enlarged diverticulum with contained abscess, suggestive of diverticulitis.	Antibiotics and fluids.	Complications include micro-/macro-perforation, abscess, and fistula formation. While colonoscopy is recommended to evaluate for colon cancer as a cause of diverticulitis, it should not be done acutely due to increased risk of perforation with acute infection/inflammation. Perform colonoscopy >6 weeks after an acute episode. While diverticulitis is associated with pain, it rarely causes bloody stools, as opposed to diverticulosis, which is not painful but is characterized by bloody stools.
Subacute/Chronic Abdominal Pain			
Gastroesophageal reflux disease (GERD)	A 52-year-old M with PMH of NSTEMI, OSA, smoking, alcohol use disorder, obesity, and chronic back pain presents with burning chest pain worse with lying down, cough, and waking with a sour taste at the back of his mouth. His symptoms worsen with spicy foods and caffeinated beverages and improve with antacids. **Exam** shows epigastric tenderness to palpation. **Labs** show negative troponin. EKG shows NSR without ST changes.	1. Empiric treatment with PPI. 2. Avoid NSAIDs, smoking/alcohol cessation, avoid large meals before bed, elevate head of bed. 3. EGD ± esophageal manometry with pH monitoring if no improvement on PPI. If symptoms correspond to reflux events or if hiatal hernia is present, consider surgical fundoplication.	GERD can present with cough, sore throat, hoarse voice, asthma, regurgitation, and/or globus sensation. If a patient has alarm symptoms such as dysphagia or weight loss, proceed with EGD. If the patient has GERD and ≥1 other risk factor for Barrett's esophagus (male, >50 years, white, hiatal hernia, smoking), consider screening EGD for Barrett's esophagus, as it increases risk of esophageal cancer. Other complications of GERD include reflux esophagitis and esophageal strictures.
Peptic ulcer disease, gastritis	A 36-year-old F with PMH of gastric bypass surgery and fibromyalgia presents with LUQ pain and acid reflux. For her chronic pain, she takes multiple ibuprofen a day. On **exam**, she has epigastric tenderness. EGD shows an ulcer at the previous anastomosis of her gastric bypass.	PPI, cessation of NSAIDs.	Complications include perforation and GI bleed. NSAIDs, *H. pylori* infection, and prior gastric bypass are all risk factors. All ulcers should be biopsied on EGD to rule out gastric cancer. If *H. pylori* is present, treatment consists of triple therapy with clarithromycin, amoxicillin, and a PPI; or quadruple therapy of metronidazole, tetracycline, bismuth, and PPI.

2-8 Abdominal Pain

Acute Abdominal Pain			
Diagnosis	**Clinical Presentation**	**Management**	**HYFs**
Zollinger-Ellison syndrome	A 35-year-old M with PMH of primary hyperparathyroidism presents with epigastric pain and diarrhea. On **exam**, he has mid-abdominal tenderness to palpation. After failed treatment with empiric PPI for GERD, he undergoes EGD that shows ulcerations in the distal duodenum and jejunum. PPI is stopped, and gastrin level measured after washout period is found to be 1500 pg/mL on **labs**.	1. PPI therapy. 2. Tumor localization with CT/MRI and somatostatin receptor-based imaging, followed by enucleation or surgical resection.	Complications include GI bleed or strictures from ulceration, as well as gastric and small bowel cancers secondary to ulceration. Patients with ZES should be screened for multiple endocrine neoplasia 1 and have parathyroid hormone levels, ionized calcium, and prolactin measured.
Chronic pancreatitis	A 62-year-old with PMH of recurrent acute pancreatitis presents with chronic abdominal pain, nausea, distention, and back pain with steatorrhea, polyuria, and polydipsia. **Exam** shows epigastric tenderness. On **imaging**, CT shows an atrophic pancreas with calcifications and a dilated main pancreatic duct. **Labs** show low pancreatic elastase, positive fecal fat, and A1C of 8.2%.	1. Analgesia: TCAs, celiac ganglion block, gabapentin. 2. Smoking and alcohol cessation. 3. For pancreatic insufficiency, insulin and exocrine pancreatic enzyme supplementation.	Recurrent episodes of acute pancreatitis can result in chronic pancreatitis. While alcohol and gallstones are common causes of acute and therefore chronic pancreatitis, IgG4/ANA, alpha-1-antitrypsin, and genetic testing for *CFTR, SPINK1,* and *PRSS1* can be considered based on history, as well as testing for hypertriglyceridemia. Screening for exocrine insufficiency (steatorrhea) and endocrine insufficiency resulting in diabetes is necessary. Other complications of chronic pancreatitis include pseudocysts and increased risk of pancreatic cancer.
Chronic mesenteric ischemia	A 78-year-old M with PMH of smoking, CAD s/p CABG and PCI presents with abdominal pain 1 hour after eating that lasts up to 2 hours and has resulted in avoidance of eating and weight loss. **Exam** shows slight abdominal tenderness to palpation throughout. **Labs** are unremarkable. On **imaging**, CTA shows calcifications of many vessels, as well as atherosclerosis resulting in stenosis of the celiac artery and superior mesenteric artery.	Surgical evaluation for stenting or surgical revascularization.	Chronic mesenteric ischemia results in "intestinal angina," or pain typically seen after eating. Patients often have risk factors for cardiovascular disease. Complications include bowel ischemia, necrosis, or perforation, as well as weight loss and malnutrition due to food aversion.
Inflammatory bowel disease	Crohn's disease: A 30-year-old with rheumatoid arthritis presents with cramping RLQ abdominal pain and frequent non-bloody diarrhea for 1 month associated with a 10-pound weight loss. **Exam** shows TTP in the RLQ. **Labs** show a new macrocytic anemia, low vitamin B_{12} level, and + FOBT. Colonoscopy reveals cobblestoning of the ileocolonic region with biopsy showing cryptitis with chronic inflammatory infitrates.	Prednisone is started for acute flare, with plans to start AZA/6-MP or other advanced therapy for maintenance once acute flare resolves.	Patients with IBD classically present with abdominal pain associated with diarrhea that may be bloody, weight loss, and extraintestinal manifestations such as rash, arthralgias, and eye irritation/redness. The patient in this vignette has Crohn's disease. Crohn's disease is associated with skip lesions and transmural inflammation and can occur anywhere along the GI tract. In contrast, ulcerative colitis is associated with continuous submucosal inflammation extending from the rectum.

(*Continued*)

2-8 Abdominal Pain

Acute Abdominal Pain			
Diagnosis	**Clinical Presentation**	**Management**	**HYFs**
Budd-Chiari syndrome	Patient with PMH of suggestive of hypercoagulable state (eg, SLE, antiphospholipid syndrome, multiple miscarriages) presents with RUQ. **Exam** reveals jaundice, ascites, TTP in the RUQ, and hepatomegaly. **Labs** show elevated transaminases. On **imaging**, Doppler shows abnormal flow patterns consistent with hepatic vein thrombosis.	1. Anticoagulation. 2. Thrombolysis ± TIPS 3. Investigate underlying risk factors/etiology.	Presents with the classic triad of abdominal pain, ascites, and liver enlargement. Complications include portal hypertension, liver failure, and cirrhosis. Hypercoagulability work-up should be done with a diagnosis of Budd-Chiari syndrome.
Small intestinal bacterial overgrowth (SIBO)	A 75-year-old F with PMH of poorly controlled T2DM complicated by gastroparesis and recent cellulitis s/p antibiotics presents with generalized abdominal pain with bloating, flatulence, and chronic watery diarrhea. **Exam** is unremarkable. On **imaging**, CT A/P is also unremarkable. Endoscopic and histopathologic examination of the small intestine and colon are unrevealing. **Labs** reveal macrocytic anemia, vitamin B_{12} deficiency, elevated folate level, and elevated fecal fat content. Carbohydrate breath test is positive. Jejunal aspirate culture reveals bacterial concentration of >1000 colony-forming units/mL.	Antibiotics (rifaximin, metronidazole, ciprofloxacin, tetracycline, amoxicillin-clavulanate, or neomycin). Replete vitamin and mineral deficiencies. If >4 episodes per year, consider antibiotic prophylaxis.	Bacterial overgrowth in the small intestine results when host defense mechanisms (gastric acid, bile, peristalsis, digestive enzymes, ileocecal valve, secretory IgA) fail. Associated with diabetes and scleroderma. Risk factors: Recent antibiotic therapy, chronic PPI use, elderly, intestinal dysmotility, pancreatic insufficiency, history of appendectomy. Complications include significant weight loss and malnutrition. Patients can present with macrocytic anemia; low thiamine, vitamin B_{12}, and niacin levels; high folate and vitamin K levels; and elevated fecal fat content.
Gastric cancer	A 75-year-old M with PMH of alcohol use disorder and extensive smoking history presents with persistent epigastric pain. He reports an unintentional weight loss of 20 lb in the past 3 months. On **exam**, he has epigastric TTP. EGD reveals a ulcer in the lesser curvature of the stomach. Biopsy reveals gastric adenocarcinoma.	Surgical resection, chemotherapy, and/or radiation depending on staging.	Gastric cancer may appear as an ulcer; all ulcers should be biopsied. Associated with Virchow node (metastasis to left supraclavicular node), Sister Mary Joseph nodule (periumbilical metastasis), and Krukenberg tumor (metastasis to the bilateral ovaries). Risk factors: *H. pylori*, nitrosamine exposure (preserved fish), tobacco, alcohol use, EBV. Gastric adenocarcinoma is the most common type of gastric cancer (>90% of cases) and is classified into 2 types: Intestinal-type (associated with *HER-2* mutation, nitrate ingestion, *H. pylori* infection) and diffuse-type (*linitis plastica*). Other gastric cancers include lymphoma, stromal (GIST, associated with *c-kit* mutation), and carcinoid tumor.
Colorectal cancer	A 65-year-old M with PMH of T2DM who has never had a colonoscopy presents with unintentional 15-pound weight loss, acute nausea/vomiting, and abdominal distention. On **exam**, he has RLQ tenderness, and his abdomen is distended with no stool in the rectal vault. A large volume of bilious fluid is aspirated on NG tube placement. **Labs** show iron deficiency anemia and + FOBT. On **imaging**, CT shows a transition point in the RLQ. Colonoscopy reveals a mass in the cecum.	Surgical resection, chemotherapy.	Hints for this diagnosis include unintentional weight loss, older age, family history, change in stool caliber, history of ulcerative colitis, and iron deficiency anemia in a male patient. Iron deficiency anemia in an individual age >45 without a recent normal colonoscopy is suspicious for colon cancer. Complications include bowel obstruction or perforation.

2-9 Melena

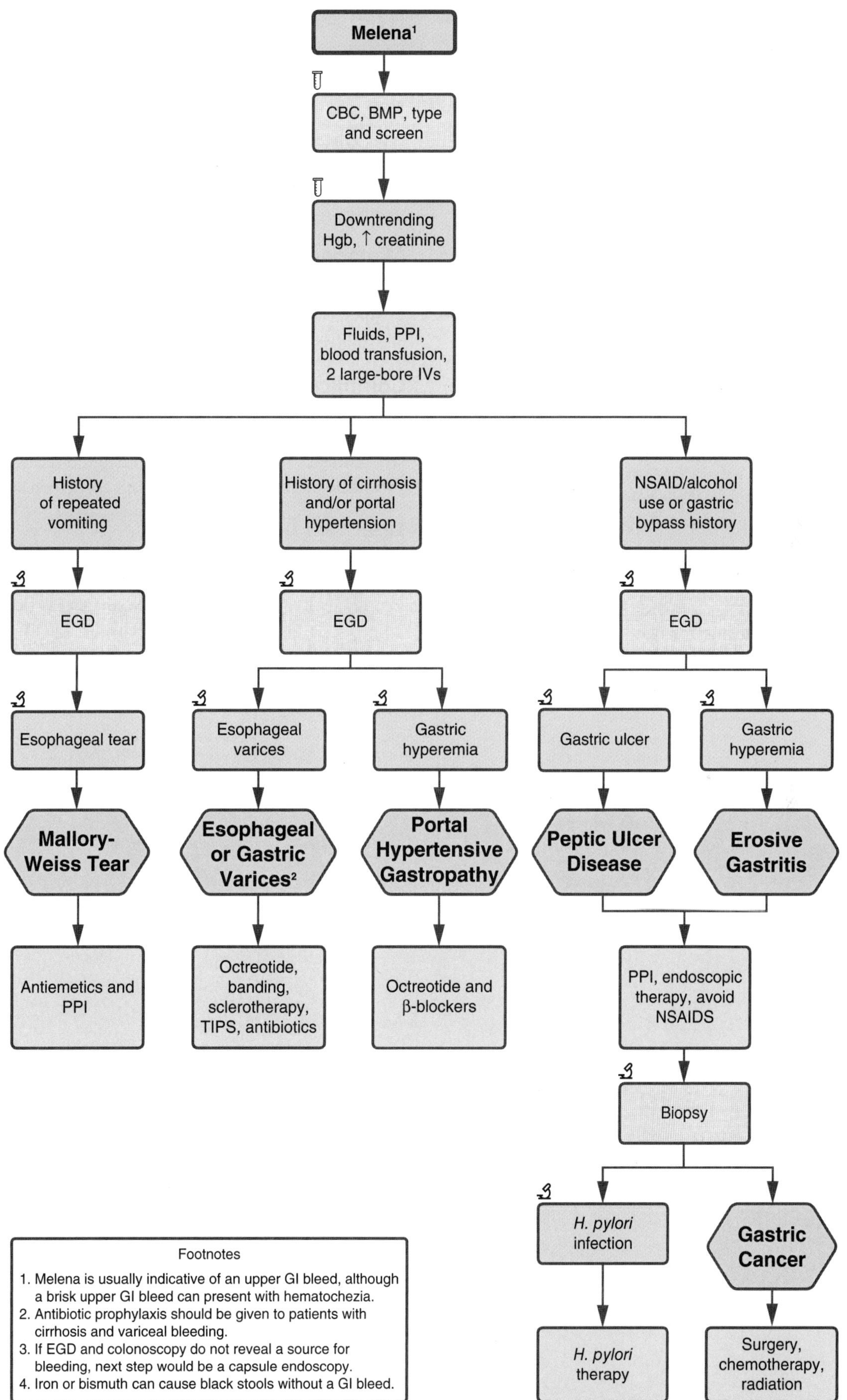

Melena[1]
CBC, BMP, type and screen
Downtrending Hgb, ↑ creatinine
Fluids, PPI, blood transfusion, 2 large-bore IVs
History of repeated vomiting
History of cirrhosis and/or portal hypertension
NSAID/alcohol use or gastric bypass history
EGD
EGD
EGD
Esophageal tear
Esophageal varices
Gastric hyperemia
Gastric ulcer
Gastric hyperemia
Mallory-Weiss Tear
Esophageal or Gastric Varices[2]
Portal Hypertensive Gastropathy
Peptic Ulcer Disease
Erosive Gastritis
Antiemetics and PPI
Octreotide, banding, sclerotherapy, TIPS, antibiotics
Octreotide and β-blockers
PPI, endoscopic therapy, avoid NSAIDS
Biopsy
H. pylori infection
Gastric Cancer
H. pylori therapy
Surgery, chemotherapy, radiation

Footnotes

1. Melena is usually indicative of an upper GI bleed, although a brisk upper GI bleed can present with hematochezia.
2. Antibiotic prophylaxis should be given to patients with cirrhosis and variceal bleeding.
3. If EGD and colonoscopy do not reveal a source for bleeding, next step would be a capsule endoscopy.
4. Iron or bismuth can cause black stools without a GI bleed.

FIGURE 2.9

2-9 Melena

PORTAL HYPERTENSIVE GASTROPATHY

A 35-year-old M with PMH of cirrhosis c/b portal hypertension presents with fatigue and melena. On **exam**, he appears pale. **Labs** indicate iron deficiency anemia. EGD shows a reticular "snake skin-like" pattern on pink mucosa in the stomach.

Management:

1. Nonselective β-blocker.
2. Iron repletion.
3. For acute bleeds or refractory bleeds, consider TIPS.

Complications: GI bleed.

HYF: If patients with cirrhosis and ascites have bleeding, also treat with antibiotic prophylaxis against SBP.

LARGE-VOLUME EPISTAXIS

A 22-year-old M presents with a large-volume nosebleed, after which he noted one dark, black, tarry bowel movement. **Exam** is benign. **Labs** show Hgb 14, platelets 250, INR 1.

Management:

1. Monitoring, typically no intervention required.
2. Intranasal packing.
3. Surgical ligation if treatment refractory or recurrent.

Complications: Blood loss anemia.

HYF: Swallowed blood, as from a large nosebleed, can present as melena.

EROSIVE GASTRITIS

A 55-year-old M with PMH of lung cancer is being treated for radiation pneumonitis in the ICU on high-dose steroids. He has an episode of melena. On **exam**, patient is intubated and sedated. **Labs** notable for Hgb 11, +FOBT. EGD shows diffuse gastric hyperemia.

Management:

1. PPI.
2. Biopsy to rule out *H. pylori*. If positive for *H. pylori*, treat with triple or quadruple therapies.

Complications: GI bleed.

HYF: Steroids and long ICU stay are factors associated with erosive gastritis. To avoid this, patients often receive prophylactic IV PPI while intubated in the ICU, especially if on steroids.

Peptic Ulcer Disease: See p. 406.

Gastric Cancer: See pp. 80, 407.

Esophageal Varices: See Gastroesophageal Varices, p. 74.

2-10 Hematochezia

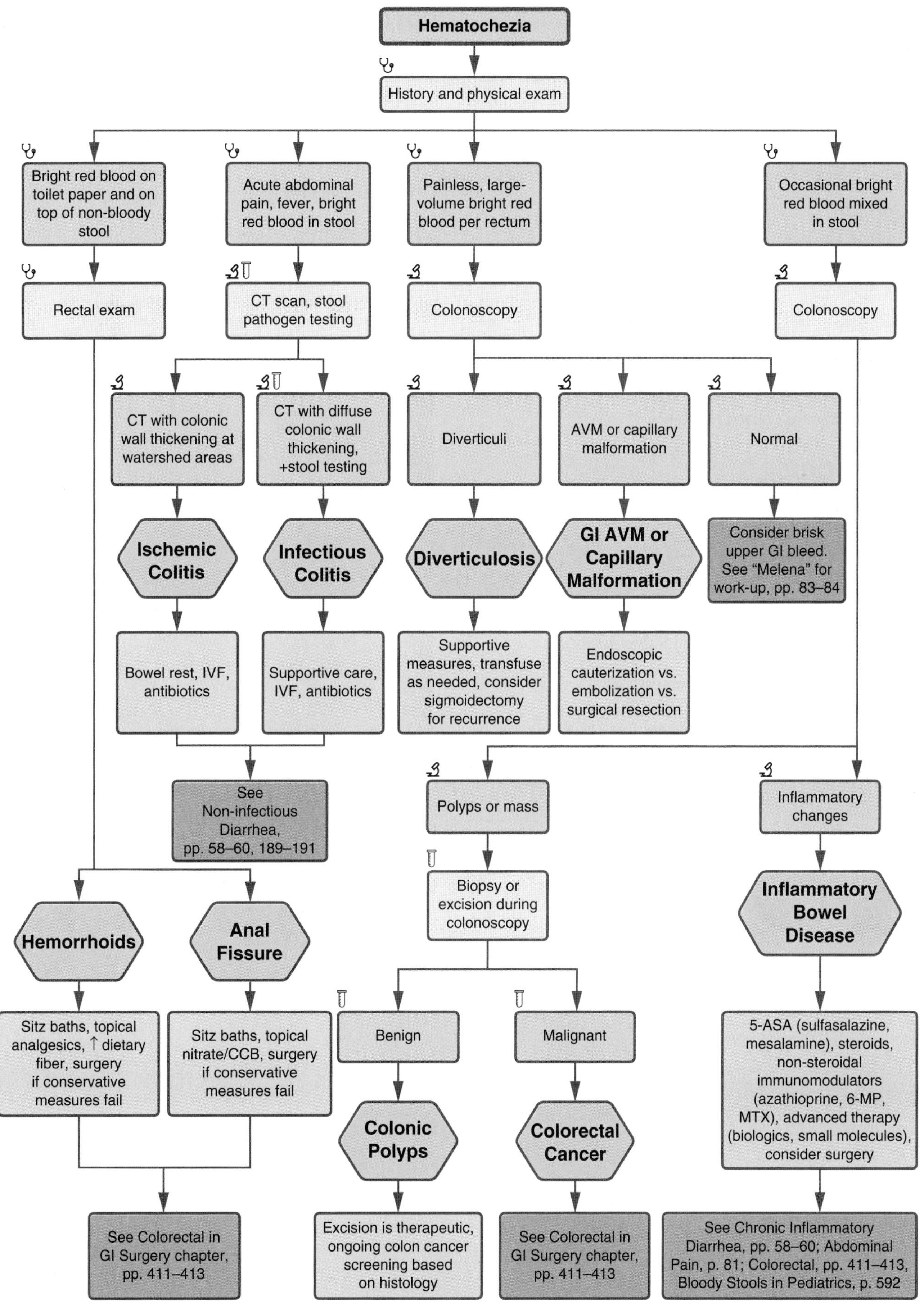
Hematochezia
History and physical exam
Bright red blood on toilet paper and on top of non-bloody stool
Acute abdominal pain, fever, bright red blood in stool
Painless, large-volume bright red blood per rectum
Occasional bright red blood mixed in stool
Rectal exam
CT scan, stool pathogen testing
Colonoscopy
Colonoscopy
CT with colonic wall thickening at watershed areas
CT with diffuse colonic wall thickening, +stool testing
Diverticuli
AVM or capillary malformation
Normal
Ischemic Colitis
Infectious Colitis
Diverticulosis
GI AVM or Capillary Malformation
Consider brisk upper GI bleed. See "Melena" for work-up, pp. 83–84
Bowel rest, IVF, antibiotics
Supportive care, IVF, antibiotics
Supportive measures, transfuse as needed, consider sigmoidectomy for recurrence
Endoscopic cauterization vs. embolization vs. surgical resection
See Non-infectious Diarrhea, pp. 58–60, 189–191
Polyps or mass
Inflammatory changes
Biopsy or excision during colonoscopy
Inflammatory Bowel Disease
Hemorrhoids
Anal Fissure
Benign
Malignant
Sitz baths, topical analgesics, ↑ dietary fiber, surgery if conservative measures fail
Sitz baths, topical nitrate/CCB, surgery if conservative measures fail
Colonic Polyps
Colorectal Cancer
5-ASA (sulfasalazine, mesalamine), steroids, non-steroidal immunomodulators (azathioprine, 6-MP, MTX), advanced therapy (biologics, small molecules), consider surgery
See Colorectal in GI Surgery chapter, pp. 411–413
Excision is therapeutic, ongoing colon cancer screening based on histology
See Colorectal in GI Surgery chapter, pp. 411–413
See Chronic Inflammatory Diarrhea, pp. 58–60; Abdominal Pain, p. 81; Colorectal, pp. 411–413, Bloody Stools in Pediatrics, p. 592

FIGURE 2.10

2-10 Hematochezia

DIVERTICULAR BLEED

A 62-year-old M with PMH of hypertension presents with painless bright red blood per rectum of large volume and resulting dizziness that have now resolved. On **exam**, he is tachycardic but otherwise appears well, with no tenderness to palpation of the abdomen. **Labs** reveal a Hgb 13 (baseline for patient). Colonoscopy shows many diverticula but no source of bleeding.

Management:

1. Monitoring. Most diverticular bleeds resolve spontaneously and are difficult to localize on colonoscopy, as bleeding has usually stopped by the time colonoscopy is done.

Complications: Blood loss anemia.

HYF: Caused by weakening of the vascular wall in a diverticulum with age. If diverticular bleeding continues to reoccur, consider surgical intervention (eg, bowel excision).

HEMORRHOIDS

A 38-year-old M with PMH of constipation presents with bright red blood on the toilet paper when he wipes. He is noted to have external hemorrhoids on rectal **exam**. **Labs** are notable for a normal Hgb of 14.

Management:

1. Sitz baths, increased fiber intake, lidocaine suppositories.

Complications: Thrombosis of hemorrhoid.

HYF: Hemorrhoids distal to the dentate line (external) can be painful, while internal hemorrhoids are not painful.

COLORECTAL CANCER

A 72-year-old M presents with worsening constipation, weight loss, and bright red blood per rectum mixed in stool. On **exam**, he appears cachectic. **Labs** reveal iron deficiency anemia. Colonoscopy shows a large left colonic mass.

Management:

1. Surgery, chemotherapy, immunotherapy, radiation.

Complications: Metastasis.

HYF: Iron deficiency anemia in an older individual should prompt a colonoscopy to look for colon cancer.

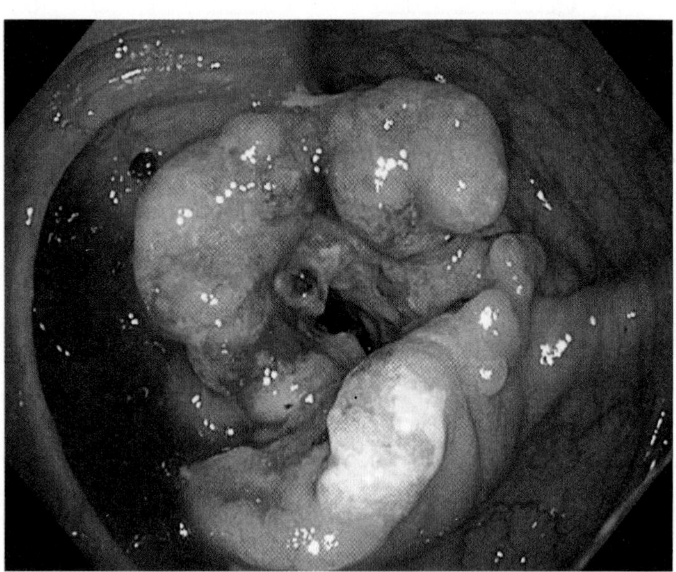

Colon adenocarcinoma on colonoscopy.

Inflammatory Bowel Disease: See pp. 58–60, 81, 411–413, 592.

Infectious Colitis: See pp. 59, 190–191.

Ischemic Colitis: See p. 59.

2-11 Vitamin and Mineral Deficiencies

Vitamin Deficiencies

The Vitamins			
Vitamin		Functions	Deficiency Disease
Lipid-soluble			
A	Retinol, β-carotene	Visual pigments in the retina; regulation of gene expression and cell differentiation (β-carotene is an antioxidant).	Night blindness, xerophthalmia; keratinization of skin.
D	Calciferol	Maintenance of calcium balance; enhances intestinal absorption of Ca^{2+} and mobilizes bone mineral; regulation of gene expression and cell differentiation.	Rickets = poor mineralization of bone in children; osteomalacia = bone demineralization in adults.
E	Tocopherols, tocotrienols	Antioxidant, especially in cell membranes; roles in cell signaling.	Extremely rare—serious neurologic dysfunction.
K	Phylloquinone: menaquinones	Coenzyme in formation of γ-carboxyglutamate in enzymes of blood clotting and bone matrix.	Impaired blood clotting, hemorrhagic disease.
Water-soluble			
B_1	Thiamine	Coenzyme in pyruvate and α-ketoglutarate dehydrogenases, and transketolase; regulates Cl^- channel in nerve conduction.	Peripheral nerve damage (beriberi) or central nervous system lesions (Wernicke-Korsakoff syndrome).
B_2	Riboflavin	Coenzyme in oxidation and reduction reactions (FAD and FMN); prosthetic group of flavoproteins.	Lesions of corner of mouth, lips, and tongue, seborrheic dermatitis.
Niacin	Nicotinic acid, nicotinamide	Coenzyme in oxidation and reduction reactions, functional part of NAD and NADP; role in intracellular calcium regulation and cell signaling.	Pellagra—photosensitive dermatitis, depressive psychosis.
B_6	Pyridoxine, pyridoxal, pyridoxamine	Coenzyme in transamination and decarboxylation of amino acids and glycogen phosphorylase; modulation of steroid hormone action.	Disorders of amino acid metabolism, convulsions.
	Folic acid	Coenzyme in transfer of one-carbon fragments.	Megaloblastic anemia.
B_{12}	Cobalamin	Coenzyme in transfer of one-carbon fragments and metabolism of folic acid.	Pernicious anemia = megaloblastic anemia with degeneration of the spinal cord.
	Pantothenic acid	Functional part of CoA and acyl carrier protein: fatty acid synthesis and metabolism.	Peripheral nerve damage (nutritional melalgia or "burning foot syndrome").
H	Biotin	Coenzyme in carboxylation reactions in gluconeogenesis and fatty acid synthesis; role in regulation of cell cycle.	Impaired fat and carbohydrate metabolism, dermatitis.
C	Ascorbic acid	Coenzyme in hydroxylation of proline and lysine in collagen synthesis; antioxidant; enhances absorption of iron.	Scurvy—impaired wound healing, loss of dental cement, subcutaneous hemorrhage.

Mineral Deficiencies

Mineral	Function	Disease(s)
Sodium (Na^+)	Involved in maintenance of fluid volume and osmotic pressure per the kidneys and associated hormones (eg, renin, aldosterone, antidiuretic hormone, atrial natriuretic peptide). Essential for generation and maintenance of electric or transport potential across membranes (eg, nerve conduction, muscle contraction, and membrane pumps).	Hyponatremia—Neurological symptoms secondary to cell swelling and electrolyte imbalance; potentially fatal. Hypernatremia—Deficit in free water in the body. Variable symptoms, including neurological, potentially fatal.
Potassium (K^+)	Usually the partner to sodium, essential for generation and maintenance of electric and transport potential across membranes (eg, nerve conduction, muscle contraction, and membrane pumps), as well as potassium-specific pumps.	Hypokalemia and hyperkalemia—Muscle and neurological symptoms; both may lead to fatal abnormal heart rhythm, especially hyperkalemia.
Chloride (Cl^-)	Involved in conjunction with sodium in maintenance of fluid volume and osmotic pressure per the kidney. Essential role in neurological functions (eg, glycine and GABA neurotransmitters) and acid–base balance via transport of bicarbonate.	Hypochloremia and hyperchloremia—Often secondary to vomiting and/or diarrhea; usually asymptomatic but may have respiratory symptoms.
Calcium (Ca^{2+})	Required for bone formation and remodeling; important cofactor for several enzymes and signal for signaling pathways (ie, diacylglycerol/IP_3), including blood clotting and muscle contraction; neurotransmitter for some neuron signals and plays a prominent role in maintaining a potential difference across membranes.	Hypocalcemia—neurological symptoms; may be followed by potentially fatal spasms of larynx and abnormal heart rhythm. Hypercalcemia—constipation (*groans*), psychotic episodes (*moans*), pain in *bones*, kidney *stones*, and depression (*psychiatric overtones*); abnormal heart rhythm can also develop.

(*Continued*)

2-11 Vitamin and Mineral Deficiencies

Mineral Deficiencies (Continued)

Mineral	Function	Disease(s)
Magnesium (Mg^{2+})	Magnesium stabilizes phosphate groups, including those in ATP; cofactor in several enzymatic processes.	Hypomagnesemia—muscle weakness, nerve problems/tremors, psychiatric episodes/epileptic fits; may lead to heart failure. Hypermagnesemia—weakness, breathing problems, and potentially fatal heart rhythms.
Phosphorous (P, usually found in the form of PO_4^{-3})	Essential structural and functional element for nucleic acids, bone/teeth, and phospholipid component of membranes; addition or removal of phosphate to/from a protein/enzyme serves as a key regulator of enzymes.	Hypophosphatemia—nerve, bone, red and white blood cells, membrane, and muscle functional problems. Hyperphosphatemia—interference with other minerals, promotes calcification of soft-tissue organs.
Iron (Fe^{2+} or Fe^{3+})	Essential cofactor in numerous enzymes and proteins (eg, heme); essential for oxidation processes or oxygen transport.	Iron deficiency (anemia). Iron excess (hemochromatosis).
Iodine (I_2)	Essential element for thyroid hormones; can act as antioxidant outside of thyroid, may play a role in the development of breast and/or stomach cancer, and affects immune system and salivary gland health.	Iodine deficiency (goiter; cretinism).
Zinc (Zn^{2+})	Cofactor in almost 100 enzymes, serving a multitude of roles in metabolism, transcription and translation, acid–base balance, immune function, and protein synthesis; part of nerve response of glutamate and essential for learning.	Zinc deficiency—initial signs may be seen in skin, hair, and nails (poor wound healing, alopecia); dysgeusia; hypogonadism. Zinc excess—can impair the absorption of other ions (eg, iron and copper); corrosive damage to soft tissues.
Manganese (Mn^{2+})	Essential cofactor for several types of enzymes involved in numerous biological functions as well as several specific types of peptides.	Manganese deficiency—possible association with inflammatory diseases, diabetes, and some neurological and psychiatric problems. Manganese excess (manganism)—progressive neurological/psychiatric symptoms.
Copper (Cu^{2+})	Cofactor in several enzymes involved in electron transport or oxidation–reduction reactions (eg, cytochrome *c* oxidase). Also, used for electron transport.	Copper deficiency—anemia symptoms, decreased metabolism, and psychiatric manifestations). Copper excess/Wilson's disease—neurological and psychological effects).
Sulfur (S, usually joined with H, O, and/or C)	As part of cysteine and methionine amino acids, plays an essential role in component of primary and tertiary protein structure via disulfide bond as well as role in sulphur-containing enzymes (eg, cytochrome c oxidase, coenzyme A (CoA); reduction of reactive species via glutathione.	NA
Cobalt (Co^{2+})	Component of cobalt-containing cofactors/enzymes, the most prominent of which is vitamin B_{12}.	Cobalt deficit—potentially fatal. Cobalt excess—pernicious anemia.
Nickel (Ni^{2+})	Important cofactor in some enzymes (eg, urease), especially those involved in reduction reactions.	Nickel deficiency—potential impact on involved enzymes, although not manifested as symptoms. Nickel excess—skin irritant and potential cancer-causing agent.
Chromium (Cr^{3+} and Cr^{6+})	Possible role in carbohydrate and/or lipid metabolism.	Chromium deficiency—extremely rare; effects controversial. Chromium excess—DNA damage; can act as a cancer-causing agent.
Fluoride (F^-)	Role in strengthening of teeth and bone and, as such, used for prevention of cavities and treatment of osteoporosis.	Fluoride deficiency—possible connection to weakened teeth and bones. Fluoride excess—neuromuscular and other symptoms that can result in death.
Selenium (Se)	Essential cofactor for certain antioxidant enzymes (eg, glutathione peroxidase), which remove reactive oxygen species; believed to be cofactor in thyroid hormone conversion of T_4 to T_3.	Selenium deficiency—destruction of heart or connective tissue; also affects thyroid hormone synthesis. Selenium excess (selenosis)—affects liver and lungs; potentially fatal.
Molybdenum (MoO_4^{2-})	Cofactor in several enzymes, including oxidizing enzymes (eg, xanthine oxidase).	Neurological symptoms may result; possible association with development of esophageal cancer.

3

Internal Medicine: Hematology-Oncology

3-1 Anemia

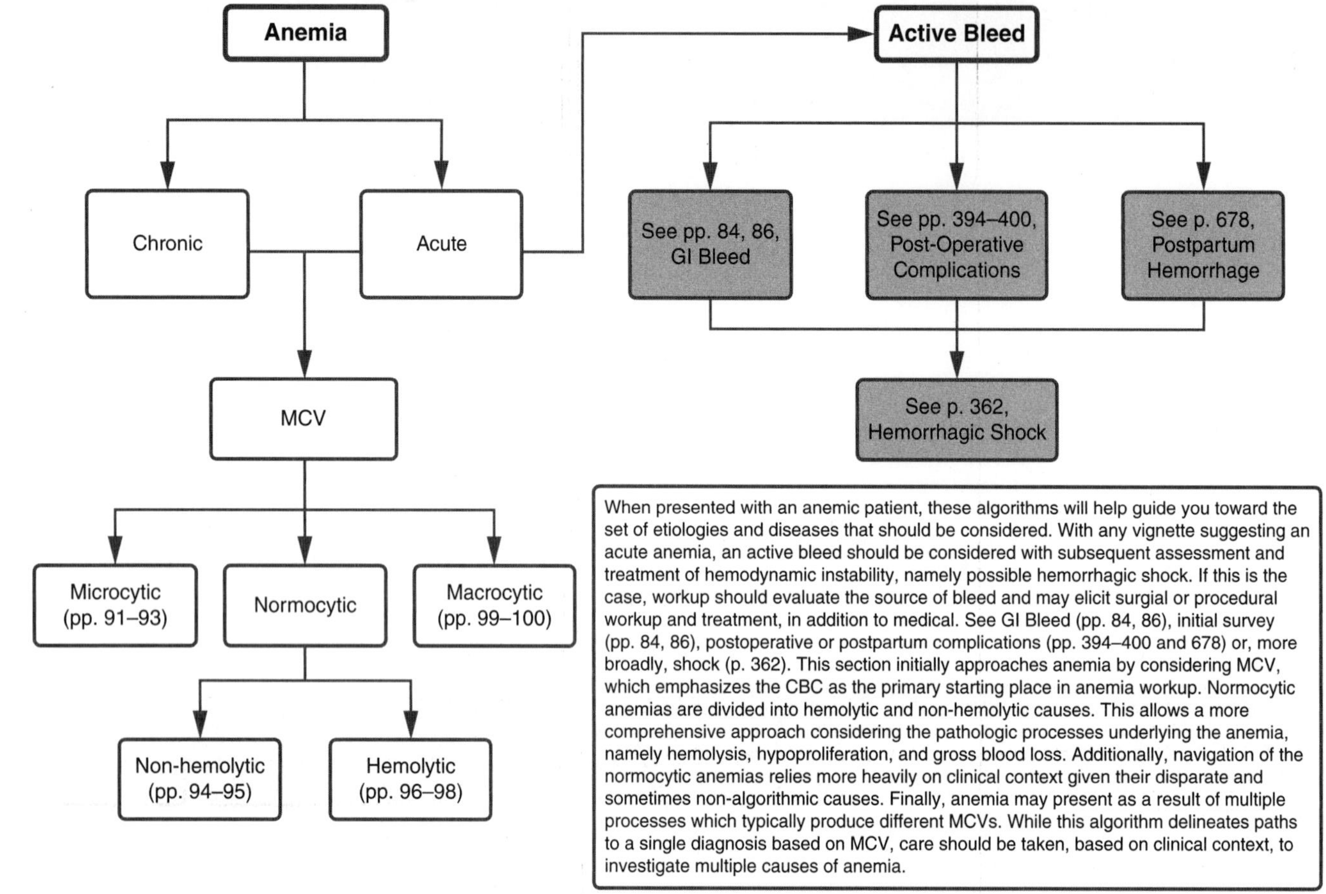
Anemia
Active Bleed
Chronic
Acute
See pp. 84, 86, GI Bleed
See pp. 394–400, Post-Operative Complications
See p. 678, Postpartum Hemorrhage
See p. 362, Hemorrhagic Shock
MCV
Microcytic (pp. 91–93)
Normocytic
Macrocytic (pp. 99–100)
Non-hemolytic (pp. 94–95)
Hemolytic (pp. 96–98)
When presented with an anemic patient, these algorithms will help guide you toward the set of etiologies and diseases that should be considered. With any vignette suggesting an acute anemia, an active bleed should be considered with subsequent assessment and treatment of hemodynamic instability, namely possible hemorrhagic shock. If this is the case, workup should evaluate the source of bleed and may elicit surgial or procedural workup and treatment, in addition to medical. See GI Bleed (pp. 84, 86), initial survey (pp. 84, 86), postoperative or postpartum complications (pp. 394–400 and 678) or, more broadly, shock (p. 362). This section initially approaches anemia by considering MCV, which emphasizes the CBC as the primary starting place in anemia workup. Normocytic anemias are divided into hemolytic and non-hemolytic causes. This allows a more comprehensive approach considering the pathologic processes underlying the anemia, namely hemolysis, hypoproliferation, and gross blood loss. Additionally, navigation of the normocytic anemias relies more heavily on clinical context given their disparate and sometimes non-algorithmic causes. Finally, anemia may present as a result of multiple processes which typically produce different MCVs. While this algorithm delineates paths to a single diagnosis based on MCV, care should be taken, based on clinical context, to investigate multiple causes of anemia.

FIGURE 3.1

3-2 Microcytic Anemia

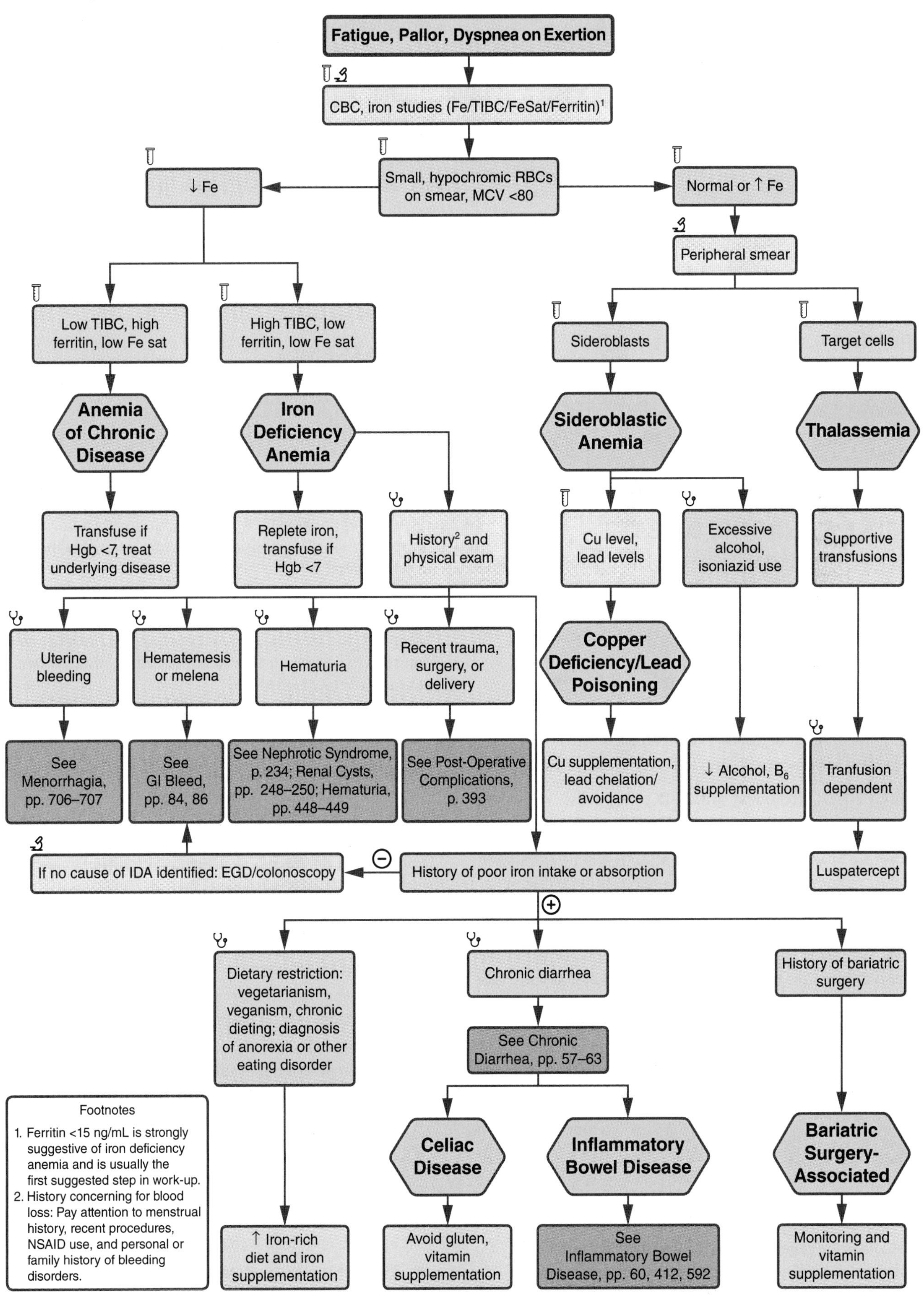
Fatigue, Pallor, Dyspnea on Exertion
CBC, iron studies (Fe/TIBC/FeSat/Ferritin)[1]
Small, hypochromic RBCs on smear, MCV <80
↓ Fe
Normal or ↑ Fe
Peripheral smear
Low TIBC, high ferritin, low Fe sat
High TIBC, low ferritin, low Fe sat
Sideroblasts
Target cells
Anemia of Chronic Disease
Iron Deficiency Anemia
Sideroblastic Anemia
Thalassemia
Transfuse if Hgb <7, treat underlying disease
Replete iron, transfuse if Hgb <7
History[2] and physical exam
Cu level, lead levels
Excessive alcohol, isoniazid use
Supportive transfusions
Uterine bleeding
Hematemesis or melena
Hematuria
Recent trauma, surgery, or delivery
Copper Deficiency/Lead Poisoning
See Menorrhagia, pp. 706–707
See GI Bleed, pp. 84, 86
See Nephrotic Syndrome, p. 234; Renal Cysts, pp. 248–250; Hematuria, pp. 448–449
See Post-Operative Complications, p. 393
Cu supplementation, lead chelation/ avoidance
↓ Alcohol, B_6 supplementation
Tranfusion dependent
If no cause of IDA identified: EGD/colonoscopy
⊖
History of poor iron intake or absorption
Luspatercept
⊕
Dietary restriction: vegetarianism, veganism, chronic dieting; diagnosis of anorexia or other eating disorder
Chronic diarrhea
History of bariatric surgery
See Chronic Diarrhea, pp. 57–63
Celiac Disease
Inflammatory Bowel Disease
Bariatric Surgery-Associated
↑ Iron-rich diet and iron supplementation
Avoid gluten, vitamin supplementation
See Inflammatory Bowel Disease, pp. 60, 412, 592
Monitoring and vitamin supplementation

Footnotes

1. Ferritin <15 ng/mL is strongly suggestive of iron deficiency anemia and is usually the first suggested step in work-up.
2. History concerning for blood loss: Pay attention to menstrual history, recent procedures, NSAID use, and personal or family history of bleeding disorders.

FIGURE 3.2

3-2 Microcytic Anemia

IRON DEFICIENCY ANEMIA (IDA)

A 71-year-old M with PMH of hypertension, coronary artery disease, and tobacco use is found to have Hgb 9 on yearly labs. He reports unintentional weight loss and occasional blood in the stool. On **exam:** Slightly pale conjunctiva are noted; otherwise, vitals and physical exam are within normal limits. **Labs/Imaging:** Hgb 9, MCV 76, low ferritin, low iron, high TIBC, elevated RDW. Colonoscopy reveals an intraluminal mass.

Management:

1. Blood transfusion as needed.
2. Start iron supplementation.
3. Treat underlying cause, if applicable (eg, malignancy, GI bleed).

Complications: Fatigue, dyspnea on exertion.

HYF: Can be caused by GI malabsorption (eg, prior gastric bypass surgery, inflammatory bowel disease). Refer adult men or post-menopausal women with IDA for diagnostic colonoscopy, as the underlying cause is colorectal cancer unless proven otherwise. IDA is associated with restless leg syndrome and pica. Antacids and proton pump inhibitors can decrease oral iron absorption.

ANEMIA OF CHRONIC DISEASE

A 75-year-old F with PMH of ESRD, lupus, and rheumatoid arthritis presents with persistent fatigue and dyspnea for the past 6 months. On **exam:** Slightly pale conjunctiva are noted; otherwise, vitals and physical exam are within normal limits. **Labs:** Hgb of 8.5, MCV of 76, ferritin high, iron low, TIBC low.

Management:

1. Blood transfusion as needed.
2. Treat underlying cause (lupus, rheumatoid arthritis).
3. If co-existing with anemia of chronic kidney disease, consider EPO.

Complications: Treatment with EPO can cause worsening hypertension.

HYF: Ferritin is an acute-phase reactant, so it will be elevated in inflammatory states (consistent with anemia of chronic disease).

SIDEROBLASTIC ANEMIA

A 40-year-old F with no significant PMH presents for persistent fatigue and dyspnea for the past 6 months. On **exam:** Slightly pale conjunctiva are noted; otherwise, vitals and physical exam are within normal limits. **Labs:** Hgb of 8.5, MCV of 76, ferritin high, normal/high iron, high saturation, sideroblasts on a blood smear. Low serum copper level and ceruloplasmin. Bone marrow aspirate shows normoblastic erythroid hyperplasia, poorly hemoglobinized cytoplasm in the RBC precursors, and telltale ring sideroblasts.

Management:

1. Blood transfusion as needed.
2. Stop potential offending agents (isoniazid, chloramphenicol, linezolid, alcohol).
3. If suspicious for genetic etiology, consider vitamin B6 supplementation. If acquired case, consider supplemental erythropoietin.
4. Replete copper with supplements.

Complications: Iron overload due to ineffective erythropoiesis and multiple transfusions (treat with iron chelation, serial phlebotomies), progression to acute leukemia.

HYF: Due to defective heme synthesis secondary to a genetic disorder or toxicity from various agents (eg, alcohol, lead, isoniazid). Patients with lead poisoning can present with malaise, gingival lead lines, and peripheral neuropathy with blood smear often showing basophilic stippling; treat with EDTA or dimercaptosuccinic acid (DMSA) if needed for lead chelation and add dimercaprol in children for severe lead poisoning. Lead chelation is indicated for levels >100 mcg/dL or >50 mcg/dL with significant signs or symotoms of lead toxicity. Mainstay of treatment is removing the exposure.

THALASSEMIA

A 22-year-old F undergoes routine evaluation for chronic anemia that was diagnosed 6 years ago. She mentions that her maternal aunt also has anemia. Her only medication is a combination oral contraceptive pill. On **exam:** Vitals and physical exam are within normal limits. **Labs:** Hgb of 6, MCV of 65, ferritin high, iron high, TIBC high. Blood smear shows microcytosis, nucleated erythrocytes, and target cells. Hemoglobin electrophoresis reveals a normal pattern of migration of hemoglobin A and normal levels of hemoglobin A2 and hemoglobin F.

Management:

1. Transfusions are guided more by symptoms since depending on severity (based on the mutations below), these patients have chronically low Hgb levels.
2. Supplement with folate and avoid iron supplementation if possible.

Complications: Iron overload from multiple transfusions.

HYF: Thalassemia arises from hemoglobin defects due to abnormal production of alpha- or beta-globin. East Asian, African, and Mediterranean ancestry is associated with a higher incidence of thalassemia. Diagnosis of thalassemia requires hemoglobin analysis and/or genetic testing; treatment depends on severity and type.

- α-thalassemia:
  - 1 α-gene mutation: α-thalassemia minima (silent carriers).
  - 2 α-gene mutations: α-thalassemia minor (reduced α-globin production → mild anemia).
  - 3 α-gene mutations: Hemoglobin H disease (minimal α-globin production leading to tetramer of β chains, chronic hemolytic anemia, and decreased lifespan).
  - 4 α-gene mutations: Hemoglobin Barts (tetramers of gamma chains. Hydrops fetalis and intrauterine demise occur unless in utero transfusions are administered.)
- β-thalassemia: Abnormal hemoglobin electrophoresis with an increase in hemoglobin A2.
  - 1 β-gene mutation: β-thalassemia minor (mild anemia).
  - 2 β-gene mutations: β-thalassemia major (severe symptomatic anemia diagnosed at an early age. Associated with growth retardation, developmental delays, and bony abnormalities).

3-2 Microcytic Anemia

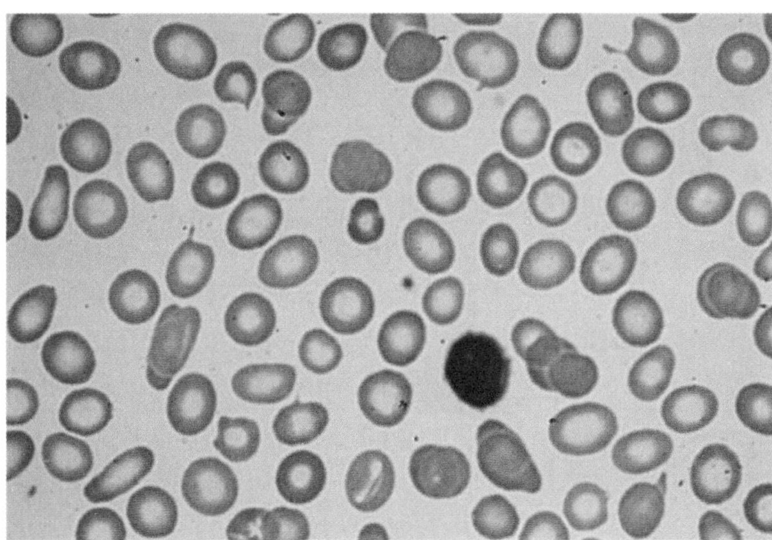

Hypochromic microcytic anemia.

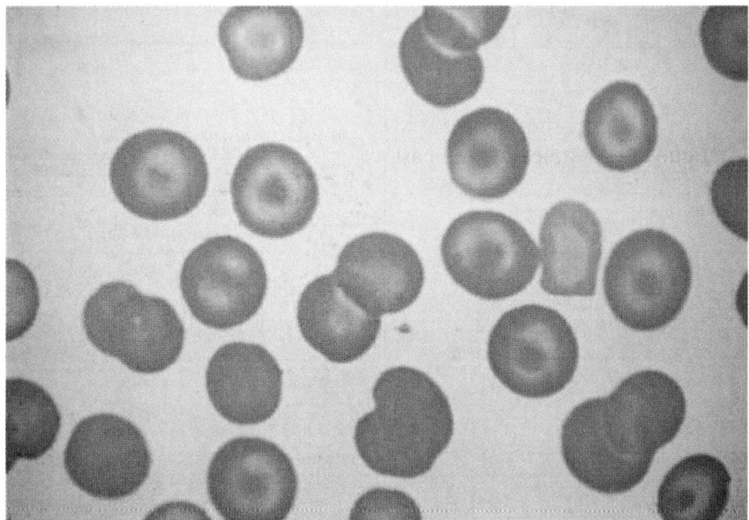

Target cells.

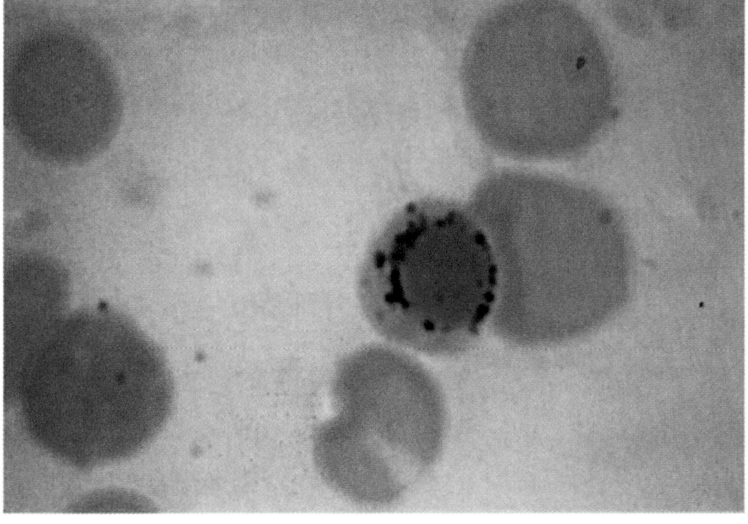

Ringed sideroblasts in bone marrow.

3-3 Normocytic Non-Hemolytic Anemia

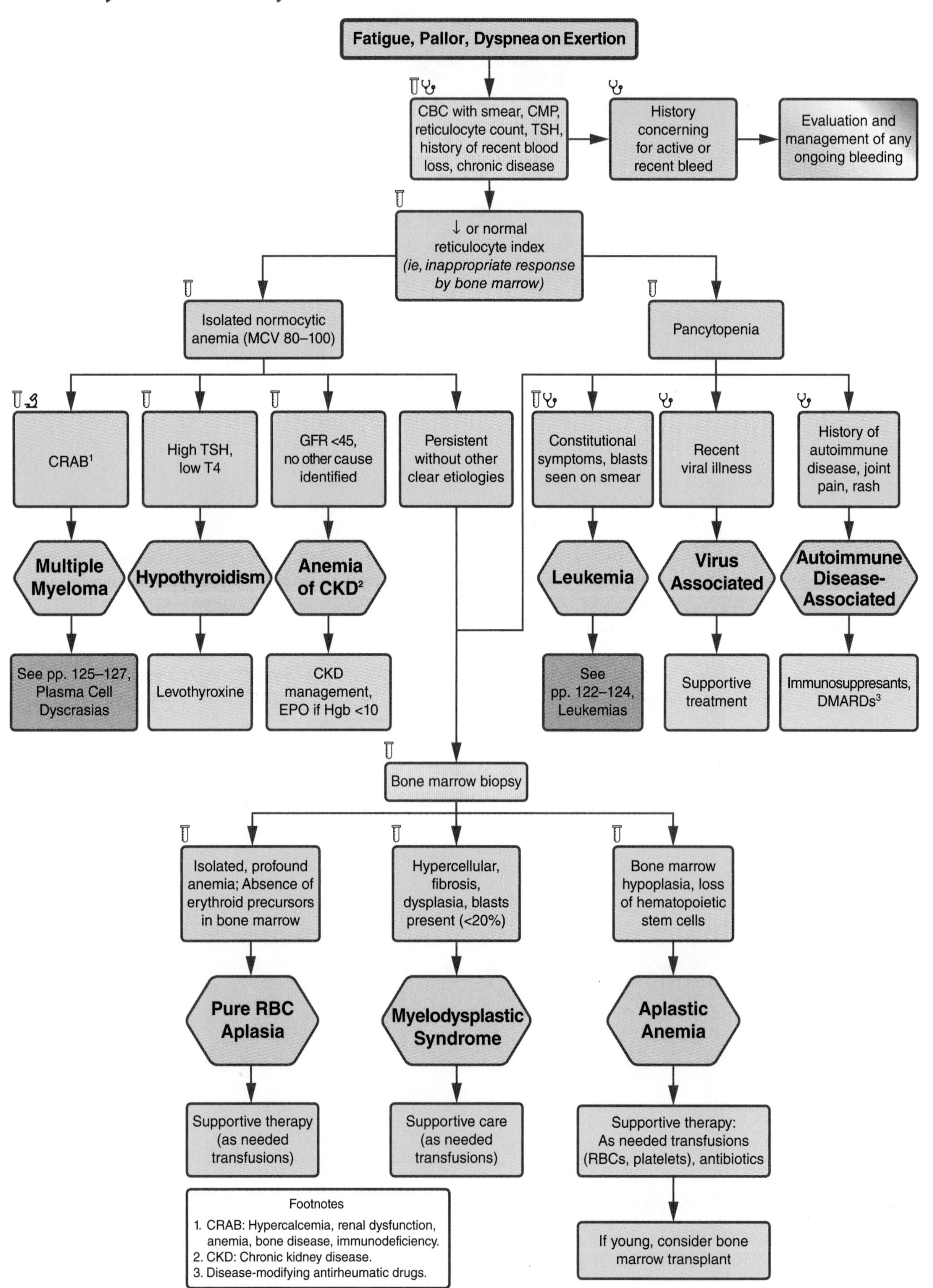

Fatigue, Pallor, Dyspnea on Exertion
CBC with smear, CMP, reticulocyte count, TSH, history of recent blood loss, chronic disease
History concerning for active or recent bleed
Evaluation and management of any ongoing bleeding
↓ or normal reticulocyte index (ie, inappropriate response by bone marrow)
Isolated normocytic anemia (MCV 80–100)
Pancytopenia
CRAB[1]
High TSH, low T4
GFR <45, no other cause identified
Persistent without other clear etiologies
Constitutional symptoms, blasts seen on smear
Recent viral illness
History of autoimmune disease, joint pain, rash
Multiple Myeloma
Hypothyroidism
Anemia of CKD[2]
Leukemia
Virus Associated
Autoimmune Disease-Associated
See pp. 125–127, Plasma Cell Dyscrasias
Levothyroxine
CKD management, EPO if Hgb <10
See pp. 122–124, Leukemias
Supportive treatment
Immunosuppresants, DMARDs[3]
Bone marrow biopsy
Isolated, profound anemia; Absence of erythroid precursors in bone marrow
Hypercellular, fibrosis, dysplasia, blasts present (<20%)
Bone marrow hypoplasia, loss of hematopoietic stem cells
Pure RBC Aplasia
Myelodysplastic Syndrome
Aplastic Anemia
Supportive therapy (as needed transfusions)
Supportive care (as needed transfusions)
Supportive therapy: As needed transfusions (RBCs, platelets), antibiotics
If young, consider bone marrow transplant
Footnotes
1. CRAB: Hypercalcemia, renal dysfunction, anemia, bone disease, immunodeficiency.
2. CKD: Chronic kidney disease.
3. Disease-modifying antirheumatic drugs.

FIGURE 3.3

3-3 Normocytic Non-Hemolytic Anemia

PURE RED BLOOD CELL APLASIA (PRCA)

A 32-year-old F with a PMH of sickle cell disease presents with dyspnea on exertion 1 week after a URI. On **exam:** Tachycardia, conjunctival pallor. **Labs:** Hgb of 4.5, MCV of 88, reticulocyte count severely reduced, marked reduction of all RBC precursors on bone marrow biopsy.

Management:

1. Blood transfusion for goal Hgb >7.
2. Treatment is specific to the suspected etiology:
   a. If persistent parvovirus infection, intravenous immunoglobulin.
   b. If drug-associated, discontinue medication and monitor with reticulocyte counts for 6 weeks.
   c. Appropriate therapy for hematologic malignancy.
   d. Immunosuppression if prolonged for 3–4 weeks.

Complications: Same as other anemias. Iron overload related to transfusions.

HYF: Anemia in PRCA occurs gradually, so patients may present with severe anemia as they have had time to compensate. Causes are diverse and include parvovirus B_{19}, medications, myeloproliferative neoplasms, and autoimmune disorders (eg, RA, SLE). Many cases are idiopathic. Associated drugs: EPO, immune checkpoint inhibitors, mycophenolate, and TMP-SMX. Diamond-Blackfan anemia presents with PRCA and congenital anomalies (eg, triphalangeal thumbs, cleft lip).

MYELODYSPLASTIC SYNDROME (MDS)

An 81-year-old M with no significant PMH presents for increasing fatigue. He has no other symptoms. On **exam:** Vital signs are normal, and the rest of the exam is unremarkable. **Labs:** Pancytopenia, MCV 98, blood smear with dysplastic cells (abnormal neutrophil segmentation, nucleated erythrocytes), normal folate and B_{12} levels, bone marrow biopsy with hypercellular marrow with dysplastic myeloid progenitor cells and lack of orderly maturation.

Management:

1. Treat anemia with transfusions and EPO.
2. Higher risk (based on Reviewed International Prognostic Scoring System): If medically fit and young, try intensive chemotherapy ± allogenic stem cell transplant.
3. If older and frail patients: Hypomethylating agents (azacytidine, decitabine) are better tolerated than intensive chemotherapy.
4. Lower Risk: Treatment includes transfusions, EPO, iron chelation, luspatercept, lenalidomide in 5q-, hypomethylating agents, immune modulators is allogeneic hematopoietic stem cell transplantation.

Complications: Same as other anemias. If other cell lines are involved, patients can have recurrent infections and easy bruising and bleeding. Risk of progression to acute myeloid leukemia.

HYF: On bone marrow biopsy, single or multilineage dysplasia and hypercellularity and blasts <20% point toward myelodysplastic syndrome. MDS can present as both isolated anemia (most commonly macrocytic but can be normocytic) or pancytopenia. Patients with MDS should be monitored for progression to AML.

APLASTIC ANEMIA

A 72-year-old M undergoing chemotherapy induction for AML presents with fatigue, SOB, and easy bruising. On **exam:** Tachycardia, pallor, petechiae. **Labs:** Marked pancytopenia, decreased reticulocyte count. Bone marrow biopsy is hypocellular without dysplasia or fibrosis.

Management:

1. Transfuse with RBCs and/or platelets. Monitor for iron overload, if patient requires multiple RBC transfusions.
2. If drug-associated, discontinue the offending medication.
3. If medically fit, young, and/or severe disease, consider hematopoietic stem cell transplant. If severe disease and unable to undergo bone marrow transplant, treat with immunosuppression (eg, cyclosporine, tacrolimus, antithymocyte globulin, eltrombopag).

Complications: Same as other anemias. Iron overload related to transfusions. Recurrent infections with opportunistic pathogens. Easy bruising and bleeding.

HYF: Drugs associated with aplastic anemia: "**C**an't **M**ake **N**ew **B**lood **C**ells **P**roperly": Carbamazepine, methimazole, NSAIDs, benzene, chloramphenicol, propylthiouracil. Associated with Fanconi syndrome (café au lait spots, short stature, radial/thumb hypoplasia).

Multiple Myeloma: See Plasma Cell Dyscrasias, pp. 125-127.

Hypothyroidism: See Endocrinology, pp. 136-138.

Leukemia: See pp. 122-124.

3-4 Normocytic Hemolytic Anemia

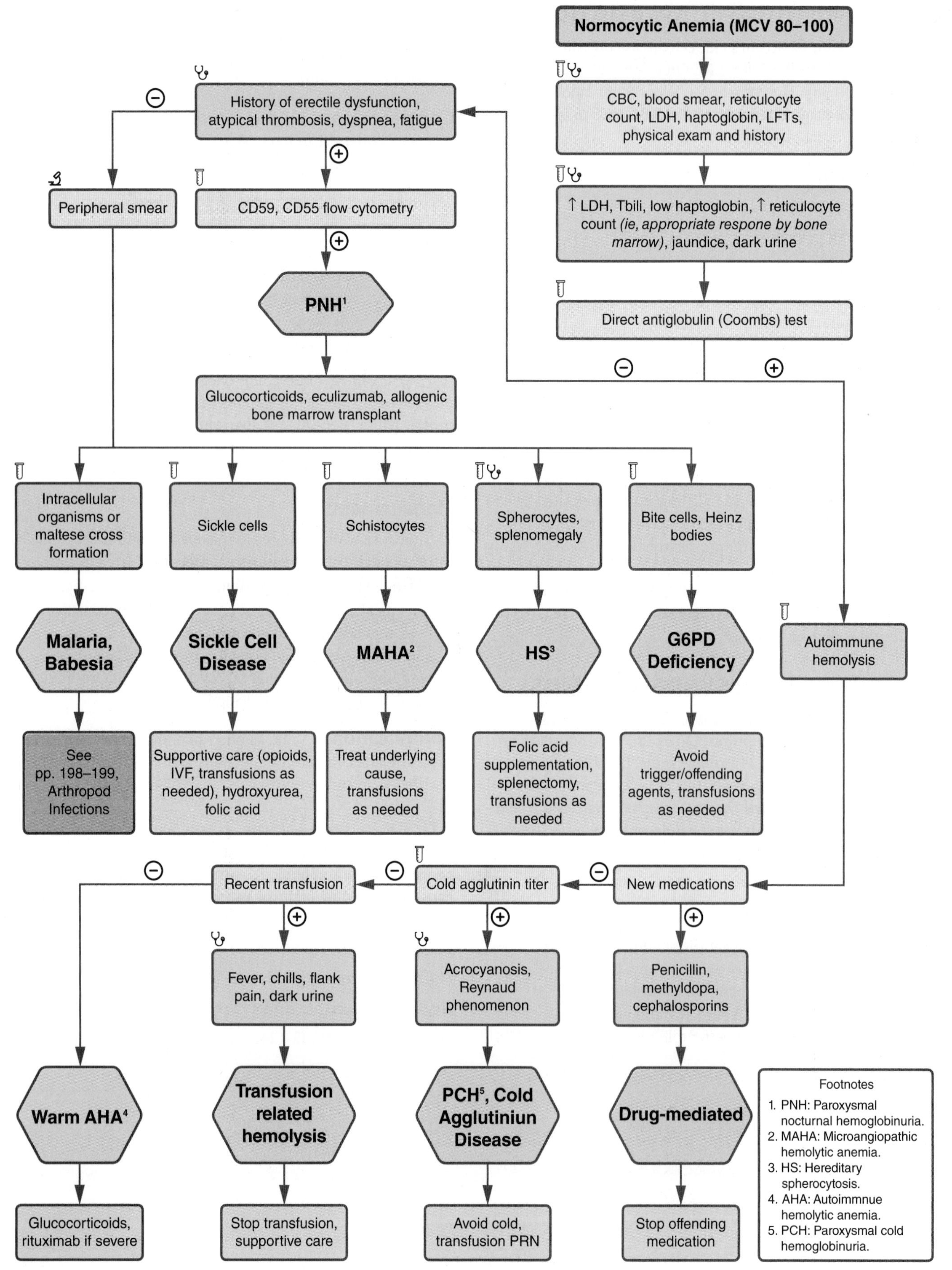
Normocytic Anemia (MCV 80–100)
CBC, blood smear, reticulocyte count, LDH, haptoglobin, LFTs, physical exam and history
↑ LDH, Tbili, low haptoglobin, ↑ reticulocyte count (ie, appropriate respone by bone marrow), jaundice, dark urine
Direct antiglobulin (Coombs) test
History of erectile dysfunction, atypical thrombosis, dyspnea, fatigue
Peripheral smear
CD59, CD55 flow cytometry
PNH[1]
Glucocorticoids, eculizumab, allogenic bone marrow transplant
Intracellular organisms or maltese cross formation
Sickle cells
Schistocytes
Spherocytes, splenomegaly
Bite cells, Heinz bodies
Malaria, Babesia
Sickle Cell Disease
MAHA[2]
HS[3]
G6PD Deficiency
Autoimmune hemolysis
See pp. 198–199, Arthropod Infections
Supportive care (opioids, IVF, transfusions as needed), hydroxyurea, folic acid
Treat underlying cause, transfusions as needed
Folic acid supplementation, splenectomy, transfusions as needed
Avoid trigger/offending agents, transfusions as needed
Recent transfusion
Cold agglutinin titer
New medications
Fever, chills, flank pain, dark urine
Acrocyanosis, Reynaud phenomenon
Penicillin, methyldopa, cephalosporins
Warm AHA[4]
Transfusion related hemolysis
PCH[5], Cold Agglutiniun Disease
Drug-mediated
Glucocorticoids, rituximab if severe
Stop transfusion, supportive care
Avoid cold, transfusion PRN
Stop offending medication
Footnotes
1. PNH: Paroxysmal nocturnal hemoglobinuria.
2. MAHA: Microangiopathic hemolytic anemia.
3. HS: Hereditary spherocytosis.
4. AHA: Autoimmnue hemolytic anemia.
5. PCH: Paroxysmal cold hemoglobinuria.

FIGURE 3.4

3-4 Normocytic Hemolytic Anemia

Etiologies of normocytic hemolytic anemia: MOM PASS me the GLUCOSE

- **Microangiopathic hemolytic anemia (TTP, HUS, DIC)**
- **Other: Malaria, hypersplenism**
- **Mechanical hemolysis**
- **Paroxysmal nocturnal hemoglobinuria**
- **Autoimmune anemia**
- **Sickle cell disease**
- **Spherocytosis**
- **GLUCOSE 6-phosphate dehydrogenase deficiency.**

PAROXYSMAL NOCTURNAL HEMOGLOBINURIA

A 24-year-old M with progressive fatigue and intermittent dark urine over several months is evaluated for exertional dyspnea, abdominal pain, and red urine. On **exam:** Pale, afebrile, BP 110/70, HR 112, SpO_2 98% on room air. Scattered petechiae are visible on the skin. Abdomen is non-distended and diffusely tender to palpation. Bowel sounds are normal. The remainder of the examination is normal. **Labs:** Hemoglobin 7.0, MCV 84, WBC 1300, platelets 30,000, elevated reticulocyte count and LDH, and low/undetectable haptoglobin. Urinalysis with 3+ blood and no RBCs on sediment. Absence of CD 55, CD 59 on RBCs by flow cytometry.

Management:

1. Steroids.
2. Eculizumab: Monoclonal antibody to C5 that inhibits activation of the terminal complement cascade.
3. Allogeneic bone marrow transplant is curative.

Complications: Thrombosis, bone marrow aplasia, episodic hemolysis. Aplasia can degenerate into leukemia.

HYF: PNH arises from intravascular hemolysis due to the lack of complement inhibitors CD59/CD55 on RBCs. Eculizumab is associated with *Neisseria* infections, so patients should receive meningococcal vaccination before use.

SICKLE CELL DISEASE

A 9-year-old F with PMH of mild anemia is evaluated for several hours of severe pain in her arms and legs. She has had 4 episodes of similar pain without precipitating factors that each resolved in 3–4 days. On **exam:** BP stable, HR 105, SpO_2 99% on room air, afebrile. Tenderness to palpation on arms and legs. No deformities or concerns for infections. **Labs:** Hgb 8, MCV 83, Hgb electrophoresis with >90% HbS and no HbA (hemoglobin SS—sickle cell disease).

Management:

1. Supportive care:
   a. Vaso-occlusive crises: Pain medication (opioids), IV fluids, and treat underlying trigger (eg, infections).
   b. Acute chest syndrome (clinical diagnosis: fever, tachypnea, hypoxia, cough, dyspnea, and CXR with new pulmonary infiltrate): Supplemental O_2, antibiotics, transfusions (either pRBCs or exchange transfusion).
2. Maintenance treatment: Hydroxyurea (increases hemoglobin F), folic acid.
3. Prophylactic pneumococcal vaccination and antibiotics due to functional asplenia.

Complications: Chronic hemolysis, vaso-occlusive disease with acute and chronic end-organ damage, nitric oxide depletion, immunocompromise from functional asplenia (autosplenectomy), pulmonary hypertension, stroke, recurrent cholelithiasis.

HYF: Autosomal recessive disorder due to mutation of adult hemoglobin (the β-chain has Glu replaced by Val → production of abnormal β globin chain → production of HbS instead of HbA. HbA2 and HbF are still produced into adulthood. Heterozygotes (HbAS) have the sickle cell trait, which offers protection against *Plasmodium falciparum*. Acute anemia in sickle cell patients commonly arises from aplastic crisis rather than hyperhemolysis and is usually triggered by infection (eg, parvovirus). For uncomplicated vaso-occlusive crises, avoid pRBC transfusions to treat chronic anemia, as they can predispose to iron overload and alloimmunization.

MICROANGIOPATHIC HEMOLYTIC ANEMIA (MAHA)

A 62-year-old F with PMH of mechanical aortic valve replacement is evaluated for mild anemia noted on routine labs. On **exam:** Vital signs within normal limits, no other abnormal findings. **Labs:** Hemoglobin 10, MCV 83, elevated total and indirect bilirubin, elevated LDH and reticulocyte count, undetectable haptoglobin, blood smear with schistocytes.

Management:

1. Blood transfusion as needed. Treat the underlying cause.

Complications: Hemorrhagic/hypovolemic shock if left untreated. Other complications related to anemia.

HYF: Intravascular hemolysis of RBCs due to fibrin deposition and platelet aggregation within damaged small vessels. Associated with DIC, HUS, TTP, SLE, mechanical valve malfunction, hypertensive emergency, and certain drugs.

G6PD DEFICIENCY

A 19-year-old M who recently started malaria prophylaxis prior to a trip to Africa presents with abdominal pain and dark urine. On **exam:** Jaundice, splenomegaly. **Labs/Imaging:** Hgb of 11.2, MCV of 85, bite cells and Heinz bodies on smear, G6PD assay abnormal.

Management:

1. Remove offending agent. Supportive care.

Complications: Periodical hemolysis in the presence of triggers (below).

(*Continued*)

3-4 Normocytic Hemolytic Anemia

HYF: X-linked recessive mutation in G6PD → inability to generate glutathione reductase → RBCs susceptible to hemolytic anemia with oxidative stress.

- "**Stress** makes me eat **bites** of **fava beans** with **Heinz** Ketchup" reinforces the smear findings of Heinz bodies and bite cells in those with G6PD deficiency, as well as the trigger of fava beans.
- Associated medications: "Hemolysis **IS D PAIN**" INH, sulfonamides, dapsone, primaquine (antimalarials), aspirin, ibuprofen, nitrofurantoin.
- Evaluation for G6PD deficiency should not be performed during an acute hemolytic episode because the older enzyme-deficient erythrocytes are preferentially destroyed during these episodes, which would lead to a false-negative result on testing. Wait 1–2 months after an acute episode before testing.

HEREDITARY SPHEROCYTOSIS

A 25-year-old M with recent URI presents with worsening exertional dyspnea. One week ago, he developed fever, sore throat, and cough. Those symptoms have resolved, but he has become more easily fatigued and short of breath. He had a cholecystectomy 2 years ago because of symptomatic cholelithiasis; at that time, he was noted to be anemic. On **exam:** Jaundiced, afebrile, BP 100/60, HR 120, RR 16, SpO_2 98% on room air. The spleen is palpable 3 cm below the left costal margin. **Labs:** Hgb 7, MCV 85, WBC 5000, platelets 230.000, elevated total and direct bilirubin. Blood smear with spherocytes. Negative Coombs tests. Eosin-5 maleimide flow cytometry and acidified glycerol lysis test confirm the diagnosis.

Management:

1. Splenectomy is curative.
2. Chronic folic acid replacement.

Complications: Complications related to anemia. Acute cholecystitis from pigmented gallstones.

HYF: Autosomal dominant defects in spectrin or ankyrin (RBC membrane proteins) lead to loss of RBC membrane surface area. This yield the spherical shape of RBCs characteristic of the disease and increases the chance of RBC destruction in the spleen.

PAROXYSMAL COLD HEMOGLOBINURIA (PCH)

A 10-year-old M presents with dark color urine, back pain, abdominal cramps, nausea, and vomiting while on a ski trip with his family. On **exam:** Vital signs stable, no other abnormal findings. **Labs:** Hgb 9, MCV 85, undetectable haptoglobin, elevated LDH, elevated total and indirect bilirubin, elevated reticulocyte count, blood smear with RBC couplets, and erythrophagocytosis. Coombs test is (+). Cold agglutinin titer confirms the diagnosis.

Management:

1. Avoid cold temperatures.
2. Rituximab (anti-CD20 antibody).

Complications: Sequelae of anemia.

HYF: Differentiate paroxysmal cold hemoglobinuria (IgG antibodies against the P antigen on RBC surface) from cold agglutinin disease (IgM antibodies against RBC surface). Cold agglutinin disease (but not paroxysmal cold hemoglobinuria) is associated with mycoplasma, EBV, lymphoproliferative disorders, and Waldenstrom's macroglobulinemia.

WARM AUTOIMMUNE HEMOLYTIC ANEMIA

A 29-year-old F who recently started penicillin for syphilis now presents with fatigue. On **exam:** Jaundice, splenomegaly. **Labs:** Hgb 11.2, MCV 85, elevated indirect bilirubin, (+) Coombs.

Management:

1. Glucocorticoids, IVIG, or rituximab.
2. For recurrent episodes, refer for splenectomy.

Complications: Sequelae of anemia. After a splenectomy, patients are at risk of sepsis with encapsulated bacteria and require pneumococcal, meningococcal, and *Haemophilus* vaccinations.

HYF: IgG-mediated AIHA is associated with SLE, chronic lymphocytic leukemia, lymphoma, and certain medications (**P Diddy Combs RAP**: **P**enicillin, methyl**d**opa, **c**ephalosporins, **r**ifampin, α-methyl**d**opa, **p**henytoin).

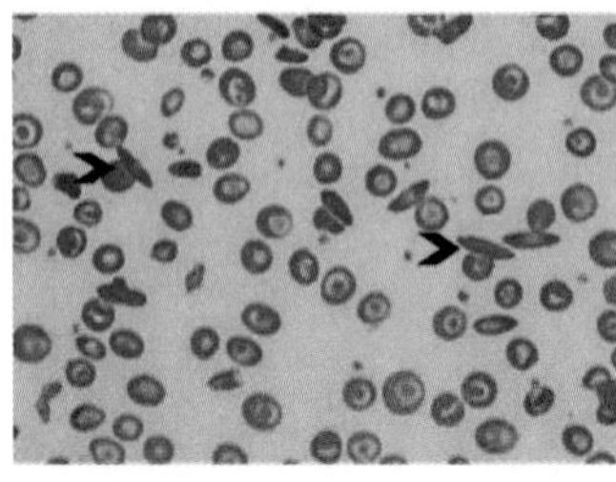
Sickled red blood cells.

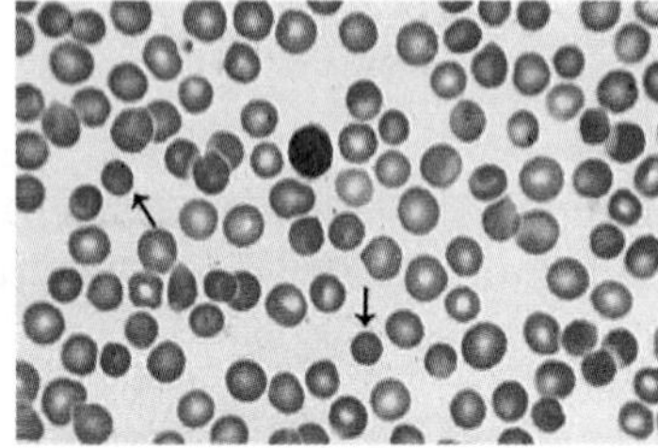
Spherocytes.

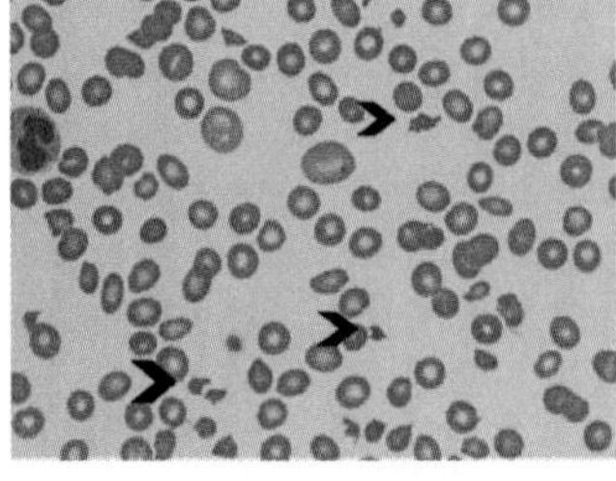
Schistocytes.

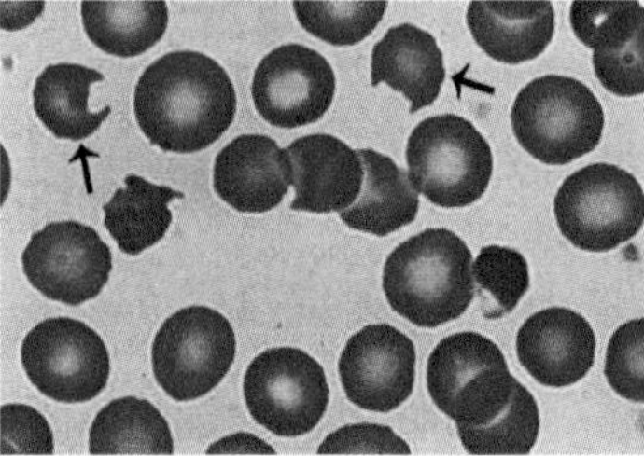
Bite cells.

3-5 Macrocytic Anemia

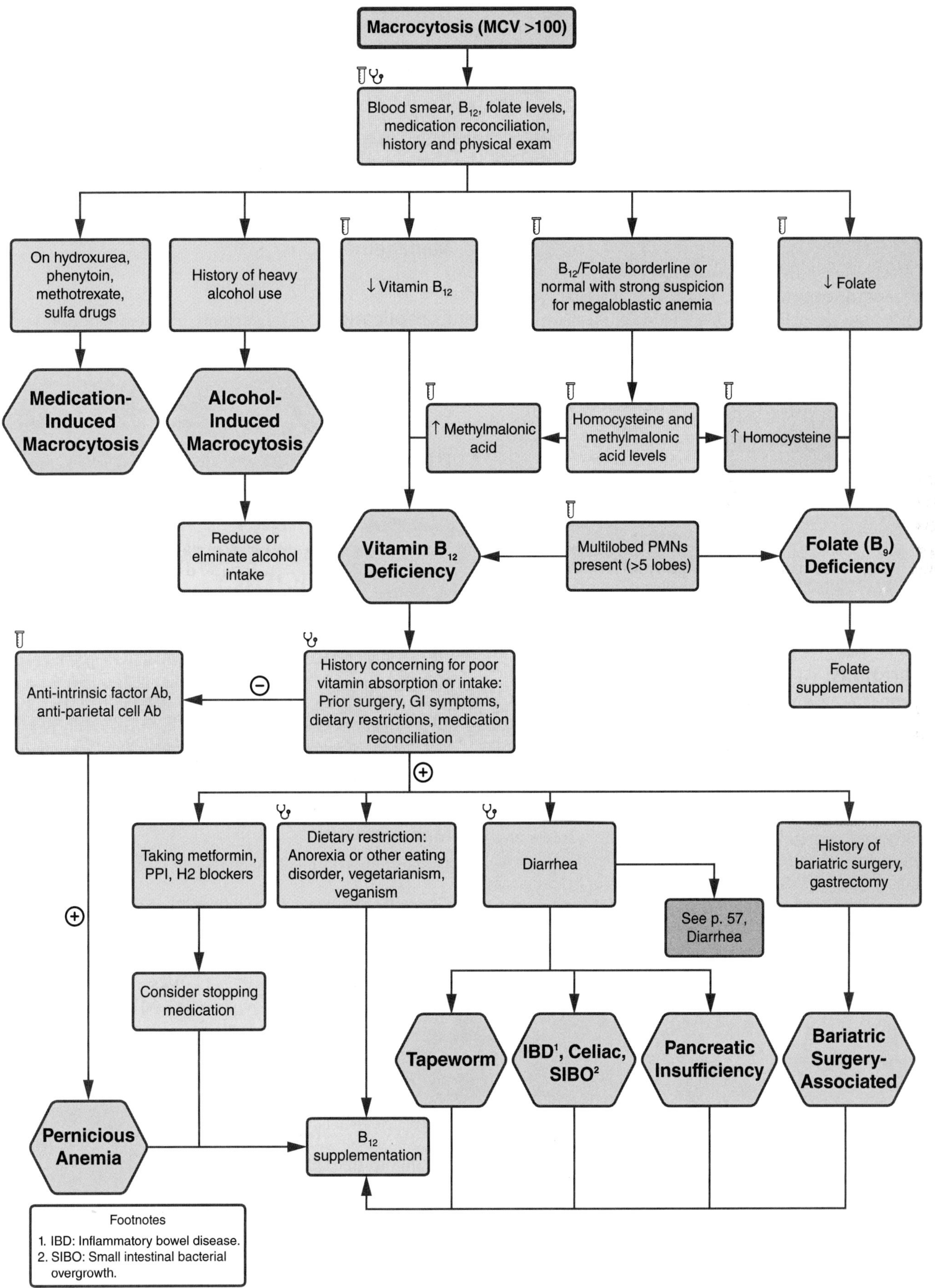

Macrocytosis (MCV >100)
Blood smear, B_{12}, folate levels, medication reconciliation, history and physical exam
On hydroxurea, phenytoin, methotrexate, sulfa drugs
History of heavy alcohol use
↓ Vitamin B_{12}
B_{12}/Folate borderline or normal with strong suspicion for megaloblastic anemia
↓ Folate
Medication-Induced Macrocytosis
Alcohol-Induced Macrocytosis
↑ Methylmalonic acid
Homocysteine and methylmalonic acid levels
↑ Homocysteine
Reduce or elminate alcohol intake
Vitamin B_{12} Deficiency
Multilobed PMNs present (>5 lobes)
Folate (B_9) Deficiency
Anti-intrinsic factor Ab, anti-parietal cell Ab
⊖
History concerning for poor vitamin absorption or intake: Prior surgery, GI symptoms, dietary restrictions, medication reconciliation
Folate supplementation
⊕
Taking metformin, PPI, H2 blockers
Dietary restriction: Anorexia or other eating disorder, vegetarianism, veganism
Diarrhea
History of bariatric surgery, gastrectomy
See p. 57, Diarrhea
⊕
Consider stopping medication
Tapeworm
IBD[1], Celiac, SIBO[2]
Pancreatic Insufficiency
Bariatric Surgery-Associated
Pernicious Anemia
B_{12} supplementation
Footnotes
1. IBD: Inflammatory bowel disease.
2. SIBO: Small intestinal bacterial overgrowth.

FIGURE 3.5

3-5 Macrocytic Anemia

ALCOHOL-INDUCED MACROCYTOSIS

A 52-year-old M with PMH of alcohol use disorder presents to the primary care clinic for routine follow-up. On **exam:** Vital signs are stable and exam is unremarkable. **Labs:** Hgb 15, MCV 102, normal B_{12}, normal folate.

Management:

1. Counsel on alcohol cessation.

Complications: Sequelae of anemia and alcohol use disorder.

HYF: Alcohol-induced macrocytosis occurs even in patients without liver disease who are folate and cobalamin replete. Abstinence from alcohol results in resolution of the macrocytosis within 2–4 months; return of the MCV to normal also confirms the diagnosis.

MEGALOBLASTIC ANEMIA DUE TO VITAMIN B_{12} DEFICIENCY

A 52-year-old F with PMH of gastric bypass surgery presents with 2 months of fatigue. On **exam:** Conjunctival pallor, glossitis. **Labs:** Hgb 10, MCV 106, multilobed PMNs on smear (>5 lobes), low B_{12} level, normal folate level.

Management:

1. Indefinite oral B_{12} supplementation, given persistently altered GI anatomy (gastric bypass). Consider IM repletion.

Complications: GI symptoms (diarrhea, appetite loss, glossitis), peripheral neuropathy, visual impairment, ataxia, loss of vibratory sense, loss of proprioception (subacute combined degeneration of the posterior and lateral columns of the spinal cord), dementia, hallucinations.

HYF: Methylmalonic acid and total homocysteine levels are helpful in differentiating cobalamin deficiency (both levels are elevated) from folate deficiency (elevated homocysteine level but normal methylmalonic acid level). High-risk populations for B_{12} deficiency include those with poor absorption due to history of gastric surgery (bypass, short bowel resection), IBD (especially Crohn's, given ileal involvement), poor intrinsic factor activation (pernicious anemia, PPI/H2 blocker use), and dietary restrictions.

- Megaloblastic anemia is the term for what occurs when cell division is impaired (nuclear abnormalities).
- Medications associated with megaloblastic anemia: hydroxyurea, phenytoin, methotrexate, sulfa drugs.
- B_{12} deficiency develops over 1–2 years given the significant physiologic stores within the body; folate deficiency can develop within weeks to months.
- B_{12} is only found in animal products or enriched plant products, so vegetarians and vegans are at higher risk.

PERNICIOUS ANEMIA

A 67-year-old F with PMH of Hashimoto thyroiditis and gastritis is evaluated for slowly worsening fatigue and exertional dyspnea of several months' duration. On **exam:** Afebrile, blood pressure 130/80, heart rate 100, SpO_2 98% on room air. The patient is pale, but the rest of the exam is within normal limits. **Labs:** Hgb of 6.4, MCV of 110, peripheral blood smear shows macrocytic erythrocytes and multi-lobed neutrophils. B_{12} is low at 150 pg/mL. Antibody against parietal cells is positive.

Management:

1. Oral or IM B_{12} supplementation.

Complications: GI symptoms (diarrhea, appetite loss, glossitis), peripheral neuropathy, visual impairment, ataxia, loss of vibratory sense, loss of proprioception (subacute combined degeneration of the posterior and lateral columns of the spinal cord), dementia, hallucinations.

HYF: Folate pernicious anemia is autoimmune gastritis against parietal cell or autoantibodies against intrinsic factor, which leads to B_{12} deficiency.

MEGALOBLASTIC ANEMIA DUE TO FOLATE DEFICIENCY

A 56-year-old M with PMH of alcohol use disorder is brought to the emergency department after being found lying unresponsive. He recently became homeless about 2 months ago. On **exam:** Vital signs are normal. The patient is disheveled, cachectic, and malodorous. He moans in response to painful stimuli and moves all extremities. He has poor dentition. Hepatomegaly is noted. **Labs:** Hgb 7.4, MCV 110, platelets 88000, WBC 7000, peripheral blood smear shows multi-lobed neutrophils. Folate is low, elevated homocysteine level, normal methylmalonic acid level.

Management:

1. Start folic acid supplementation.

Complications: GI symptoms (diarrhea, appetite loss), peripheral neuropathy, visual impairment, ataxia.

HYF:

- In folate deficiency, homocysteine level is elevated, but methylmalonic acid level is normal.
- Risk factors for folate deficiency: Malnutrition, malabsorption, chronic alcoholism, medications (methotrexate, trimethoprim), pregnancy, chronic hemolysis.
- Folate deficiency can develop within weeks to months.

*__Diamond-Blackfan anemia__ is a congenital erythroid aplasia resulting in macrocytosis. Presents with congenital malformations. Predisposes to MDS and AML.

3-6 Bleeding Disorders

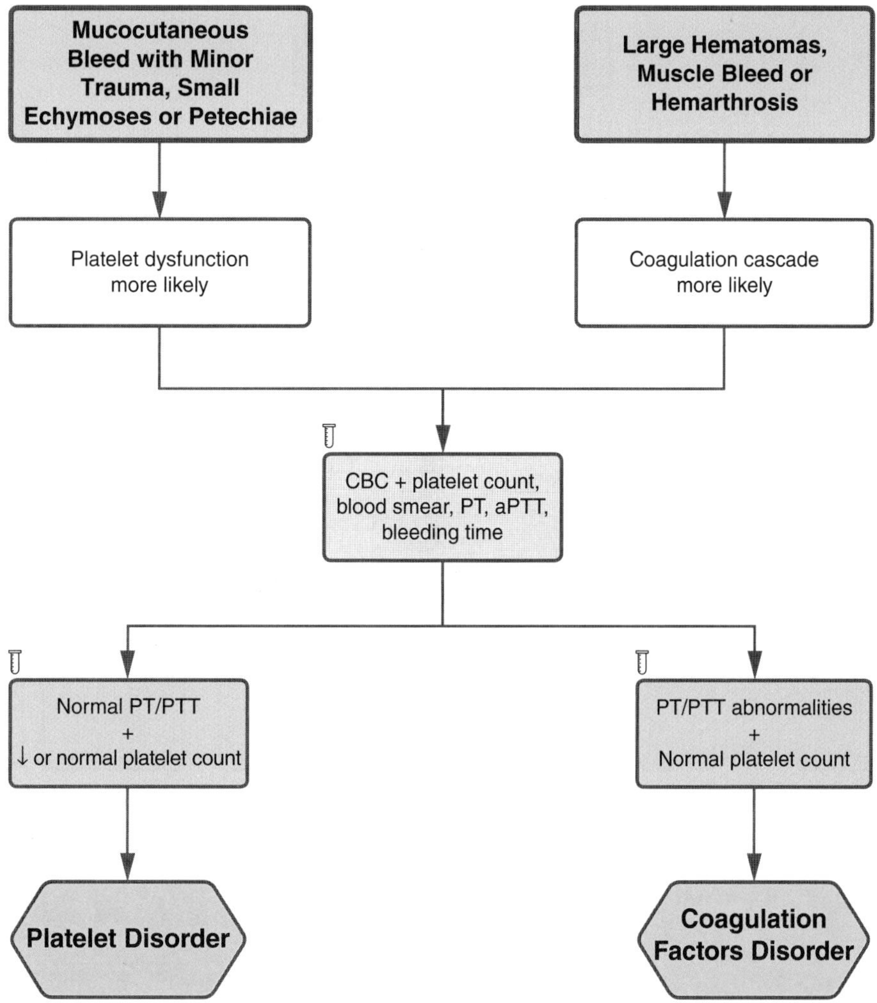
Mucocutaneous Bleed with Minor Trauma, Small Echymoses or Petechiae
Large Hematomas, Muscle Bleed or Hemarthrosis
Platelet dysfunction more likely
Coagulation cascade more likely
CBC + platelet count, blood smear, PT, aPTT, bleeding time
Normal PT/PTT + ↓ or normal platelet count
PT/PTT abnormalities + Normal platelet count
Platelet Disorder
Coagulation Factors Disorder

Bleeding disorders can be classified as disorders affecting platelets or disorders affecting coagulation factors, though certain disoders will affect both. When presented with a bleeding case, try to differentiate if it is a mucosal bleed versus a joint, deep muscle or tissue bleed. The former usually hints towards a defect of platelets and the latter toward a defect in the coagulation cascade. Additionally, keep in mind common medications that can affect both, like warfarin, direct oral anticoagulants, aspirin, and other antiplatelet agents.

FIGURE 3.6

3-7 Coagulation Factor Disorders

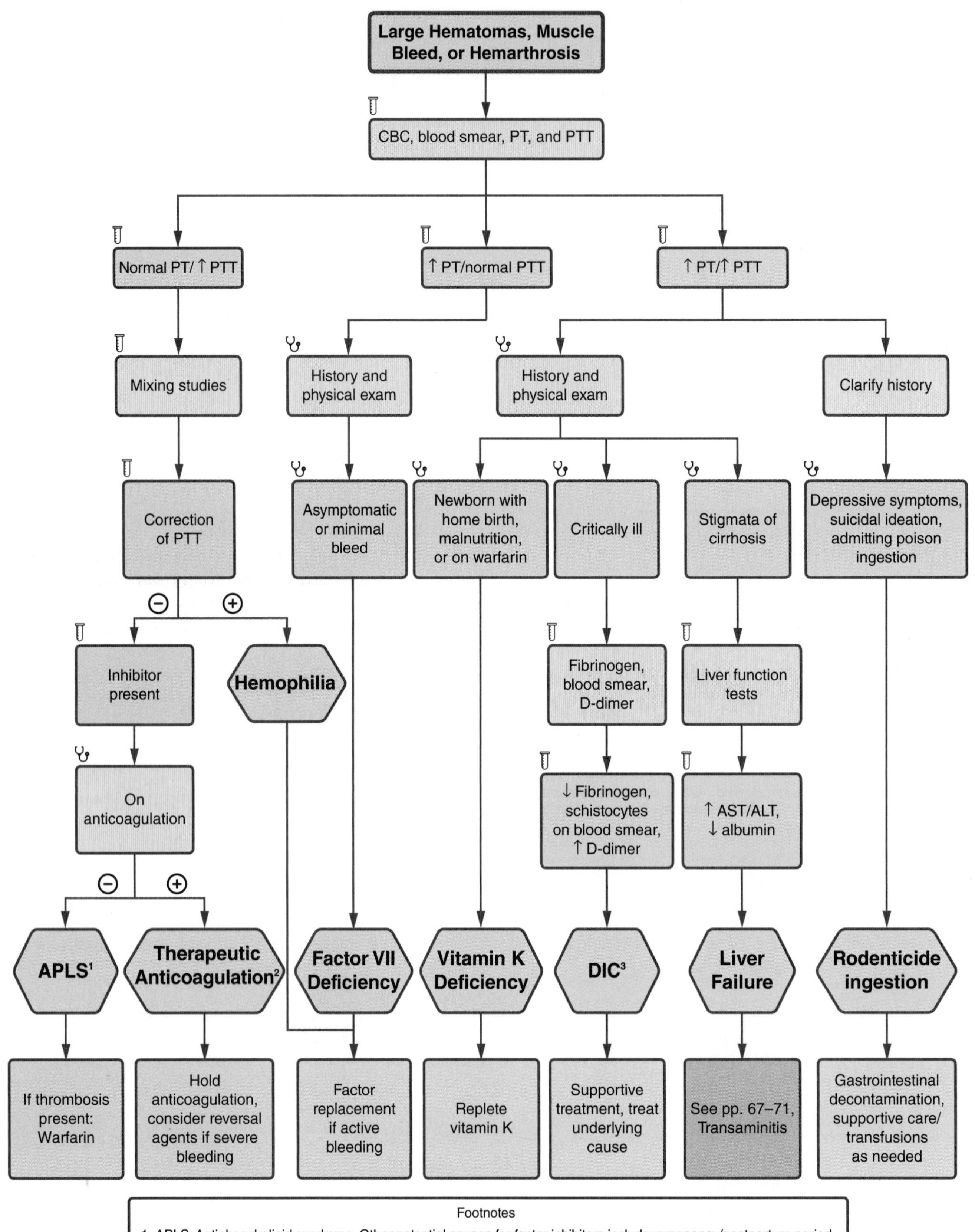
Large Hematomas, Muscle Bleed, or Hemarthrosis
CBC, blood smear, PT, and PTT
Normal PT/↑ PTT
↑ PT/normal PTT
↑ PT/↑ PTT
Mixing studies
History and physical exam
History and physical exam
Clarify history
Correction of PTT
Asymptomatic or minimal bleed
Newborn with home birth, malnutrition, or on warfarin
Critically ill
Stigmata of cirrhosis
Depressive symptoms, suicidal ideation, admitting poison ingestion
Inhibitor present
Hemophilia
Fibrinogen, blood smear, D-dimer
Liver function tests
On anticoagulation
↓ Fibrinogen, schistocytes on blood smear, ↑ D-dimer
↑ AST/ALT, ↓ albumin
APLS[1]
Therapeutic Anticoagulation[2]
Factor VII Deficiency
Vitamin K Deficiency
DIC[3]
Liver Failure
Rodenticide ingestion
If thrombosis present: Warfarin
Hold anticoagulation, consider reversal agents if severe bleeding
Factor replacement if active bleeding
Replete vitamin K
Supportive treatment, treat underlying cause
See pp. 67–71, Transaminitis
Gastrointestinal decontamination, supportive care/ transfusions as needed

Footnotes

1. APLS: Antiphospholipid syndrome. Other potential causes for factor inhibitors include: pregnancy/postpartum period, rheumatologic conditions (RA/SLE), malignancy, drugs (penicillin, sulfonamide, phenytoin). The most common factor inhibitor is usually factor VIII inhibitor.
2. Most commonly heparin and direct thrombin inhibitor anticoagulants (argatroban, dabigatran).
3. DIC: Diffuse intravascular coagulopathy.

FIGURE 3.7

3-7 Coagulation Factor Disorders

HEMOPHILIA

A 28-year-old M presents with acute-onset right knee pain, swelling, and redness. On **exam:** Right knee is edematous and erythematous with effusion present. **Labs/Imaging:** Knee US and arthrocentesis are (+) for hemarthrosis. Prolonged aPTT corrects in mixing studies. PT and CBC are normal. Assay of individual factors (VIII and IX) confirms the diagnosis.

Management:

1. For bleeding in hemophilia A and B: Virally inactivated factor concentrates.
2. For mild hemophilia A: Desmopressin, which stimulates the release of preformed factor VIII from endothelial cells.
3. Antifibrinolytic agents (eg, tranexamic acid) can help control bleeding from dental procedures.

Complications: Profound bleeding complications, hemorrhagic shock if not controlled, arthropathy from recurrent hemarthroses.

HYF: X-linked recessive disorder with deficiency of either factor VIII (hemophilia A) or factor IX (hemophilia B). Commonly presents with hemarthrosis, spontaneous deep muscle hematoma, or excessive bleeding after minimal trauma.

ANTIPHOSPHOLIPID SYNDROME (APLS)

A 36-year-old F presents with acute onset of right lower extremity pain and edema. She has a history of multiple pregnancy losses. She denies recent travel, surgery, or immobility and is not taking oral anti-contraceptives. On **exam:** Vitals are normal. Her right calf is notably swollen and erythematous. **Labs:**

- Start with coagulation times (PT/INR, aPTT): aPTT elevated, PT/INR usually normal.
- Lupus anticoagulant (3-step procedure):
  1. Screening: Either dilute Russell viper venom time (dRVVT) or an activated partial thromboplastin time (aPTT).
  2. Mixing patient plasma with normal plasma fails to correct the prolonged screening test.
  3. Addition of excess phospholipid shortens or corrects the prolonged coagulation test (demonstration of phospholipid dependence).
- Anti-cardiolipin antibodies.
- Anti-beta2-glycoprotein I antibodies.

Management:

1. Manage acute thrombosis depending on location and severity (anticoagulation vs. mechanical thrombectomy vs. catheter-directed thrombolysis).
2. Lifelong anticoagulation with warfarin.
3. Low-dose aspirin for patients with arterial thromboses.

Complications: Miscarriages, arterial and venous thrombotic events.

HYF: If testing is (+) for anticardiolipins, anti-beta2 glycoprotein, or lupus anticoagulant, repeat testing after >12 weeks to confirm persistence.

VITAMIN K DEFICIENCY

An 83-year-old F with PMH of alcohol use disorder and chronic pancreatitis is noted to have prolonged bleeding from venipuncture sites and new ecchymoses. She was admitted to the hospital 1 week ago for acute on chronic pancreatitis. She was recently treated for *Clostridioides difficile* diarrhea, and her oral intake has been poor. On **exam:** T 38 °C, BP 110/65 mmHg, HR 90/min, cachectic. **Labs:** PT is elevated, but aPTT is within normal limits. Hgb 10.2, WBC 8.0, platelets 130,000.

Management:

1. Vitamin K repletion.

Complications: Predisposition to significant bleeding. Patients on warfarin can become supratherapeutic.

HYF: Vitamin K is a fat-soluble vitamin. Deficiency is associated with GI malabsorption (eg, chronic pancreatitis).

DISSEMINATED INTRAVASCULAR COAGULATION (DIC)

A 46-year-old M admitted to the ICU is noted to have bleeding from venipuncture sites, hematuria, and increasing vasopressor requirements. He was admitted 1 week ago with septic shock secondary to endocarditis in the setting of IV drug use. On **exam:** T 37, BP 80/45 mmHg, HR 130/min, multiple bruises, active bleeding from venipuncture sites, bloody urine in Foley bag. **Labs:** Platelets 42,000, prolonged aPTT and PT, elevated INR, fibrinogen 70, and elevated D-dimer levels. Blood smear shows schistocytes and few platelets.

Management:

1. Supportive care: Platelet transfusions, cryoprecipitate, and fresh frozen plasma as needed.
2. Treat inciting cause (eg, septic shock).

Complications: Excessive bleeding, infarcts.

HYF: DIC causes profound bleeding and hypercoagulability simultaneously, as stressors cause activation of the clotting cascade → extensive clotting → depletion in clotting factors → abnormal bleeding.

LIVER FAILURE

A 52-year-old F with PMH of liver cirrhosis is hospitalized after severe hematemesis. On **exam:** BP 110/70, HR 106, and RR 22. She is jaundiced and has spider angiomata on the anterior chest. **Labs:** aPTT elevated, PT/INR elevated, hemoglobin 8.2, platelets 58,000.

Management:

1. If asymptomatic, no treatment required.
2. If active bleeding requiring blood product replacement, consider cryoprecipitate (increase fibrinogen levels) and platelet transfusions.
3. Consider vitamin K supplementation if INR is elevated.

(Continued)

3-7 Coagulation Factor Disorders

Complications: Hepatic encephalopathy, cirrhosis, ascites, hepatorenal syndrome, esophageal varices, hepatic malignancy.

HYF: Due to synthetic dysfunction of the liver. In severe cases, liver disease, DIC, and vitamin K deficiency can present with both PT and aPTT elevation. Distinguishing between liver disease and DIC can be clinically challenging; theoretically, factor VIII levels can differentiate the 2 diagnoses (ie, VIII is high in liver disease, low in DIC). Avoid using prothrombin complex concentrate (PCC) in managing the coagulopathy of liver disease, as it is associated with thrombotic complications. Prothrombin complex concentrate (Kcentra) contains the 4 Vitamin K-dependent factors (II, VII, IX, X) and is used for reversal of Vitamin K antagonists in bleeding or perioperatively. It can also be used off-label to reverse other anti-coagulants in the case of life-threatening bleeding or procedures.

Therapeutic Anticoagulation: See p. 113.

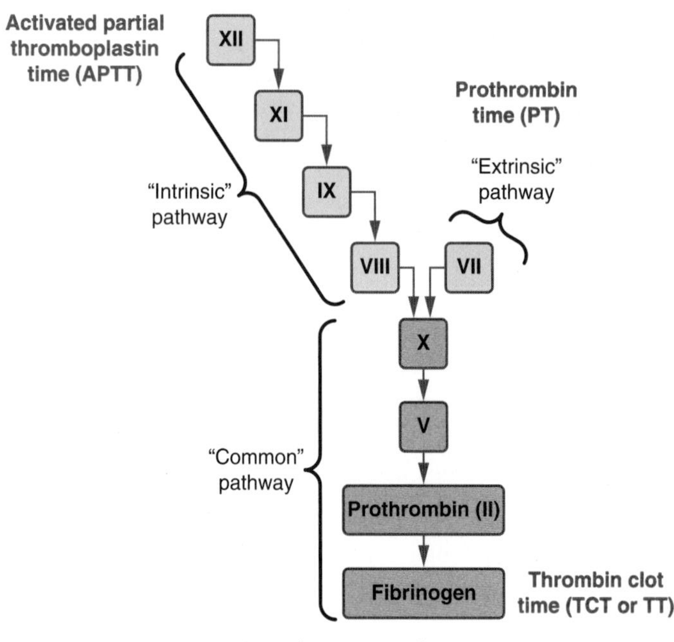
Activated partial thromboplastin time (APTT)
XII
XI
IX
VIII
VII
X
V
Prothrombin (II)
Fibrinogen
Prothrombin time (PT)
"Extrinsic" pathway
"Intrinsic" pathway
"Common" pathway
Thrombin clot time (TCT or TT)

Coagulation cascade.

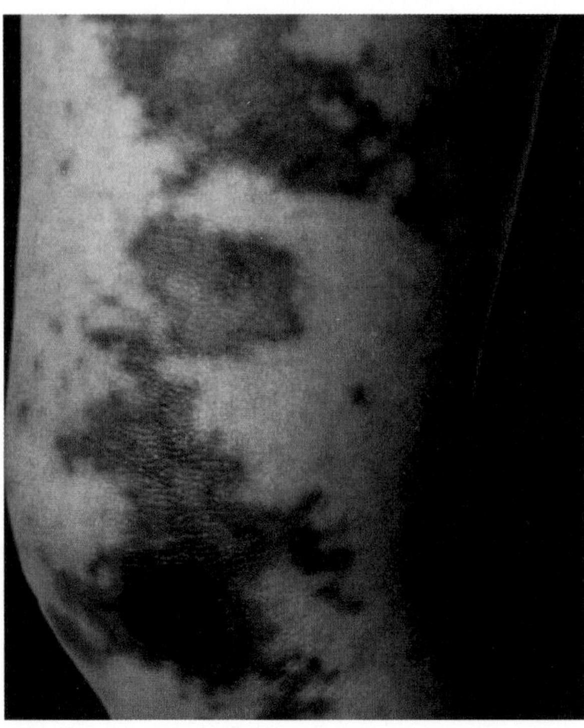

Purpuric lesions in DIC.

3-8 Platelet Disorders

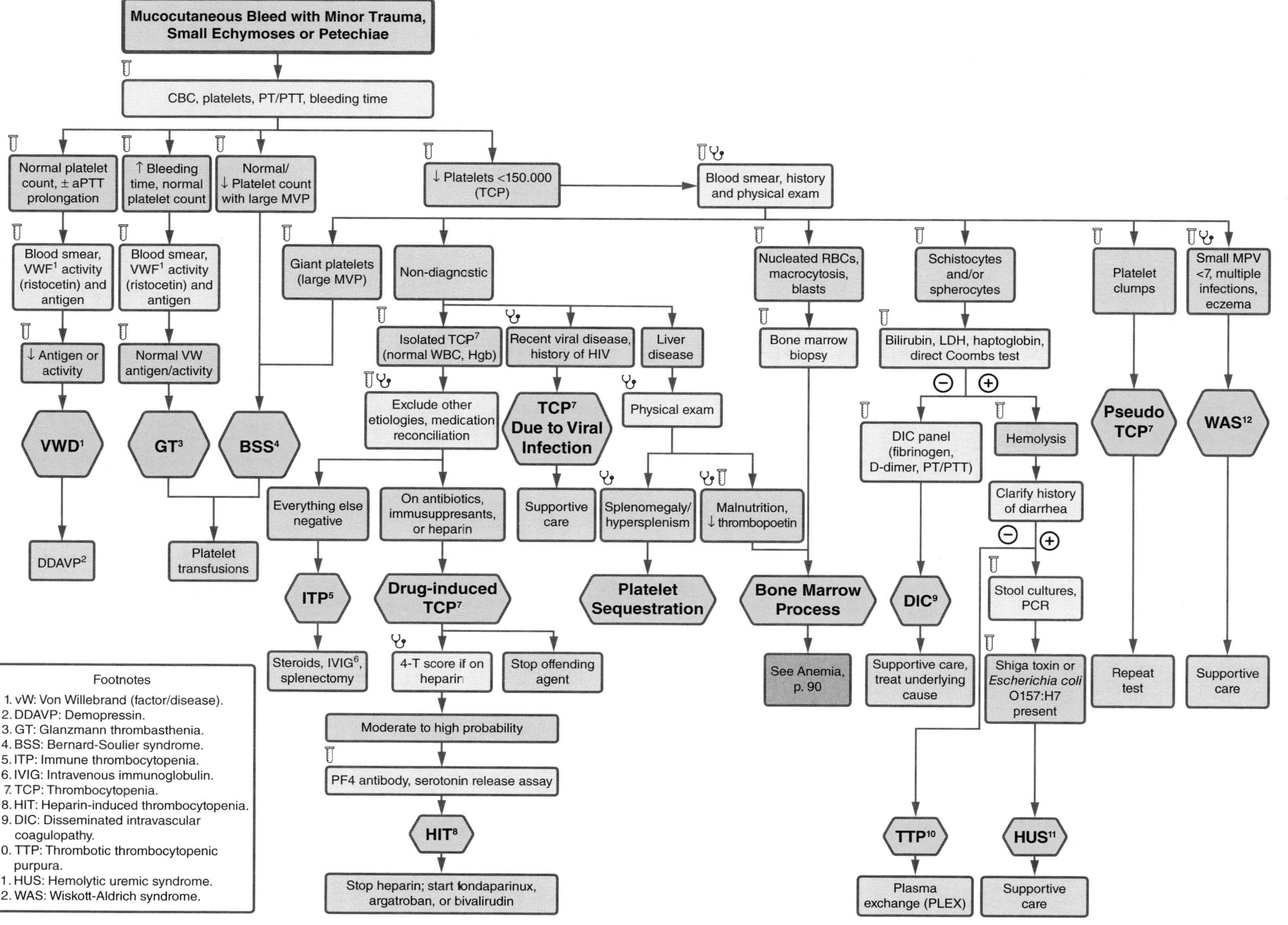

Mucocutaneous Bleed with Minor Trauma, Small Echymoses or Petechiae
CBC, platelets, PT/PTT, bleeding time
Normal platelet count, ± aPTT prolongation
↑ Bleeding time, normal platelet count
Normal/ ↓ Platelet count with large MVP
↓ Platelets <150.000 (TCP)
Blood smear, history and physical exam
Blood smear, VWF1 activity (ristocetin) and antigen
Blood smear, VWF1 activity (ristocetin) and antigen
Giant platelets (large MVP)
Non-diagnostic
Nucleated RBCs, macrocytosis, blasts
Schistocytes and/or spherocytes
Platelet clumps
Small MPV <7, multiple infections, eczema
↓ Antigen or activity
Normal VW antigen/activity
Isolated TCP7 (normal WBC, Hgb)
Recent viral disease, history of HIV
Liver disease
Bone marrow biopsy
Bilirubin, LDH, haptoglobin, direct Coombs test
VWD1
GT3
BSS4
Exclude other etiologies, medication reconciliation
TCP7 Due to Viral Infection
Physical exam
DIC panel (fibrinogen, D-dimer, PT/PTT)
Hemolysis
Pseudo TCP7
WAS12
Everything else negative
On antibiotics, immusuppresants, or heparin
Supportive care
Splenomegaly/ hypersplenism
Malnutrition, ↓ thrombopoetin
Clarify history of diarrhea
DDAVP2
Platelet transfusions
ITP5
Drug-induced TCP7
Platelet Sequestration
Bone Marrow Process
DIC9
Stool cultures, PCR
Steroids, IVIG6, splenectomy
4-T score if on heparin
Stop offending agent
See Anemia, p. 90
Supportive care, treat underlying cause
Shiga toxin or Escherichia coli O157:H7 present
Repeat test
Supportive care
Moderate to high probability
PF4 antibody, serotonin release assay
HIT8
TTP10
HUS11
Stop heparin; start fondaparinux, argatroban, or bivalirudin
Plasma exchange (PLEX)
Supportive care
Footnotes
1. vW: Von Willebrand (factor/disease).
2. DDAVP: Demopressin.
3. GT: Glanzmann thrombasthenia.
4. BSS: Bernard-Soulier syndrome.
5. ITP: Immune thrombocytopenia.
6. IVIG: Intravenous immunoglobulin.
7. TCP: Thrombocytopenia.
8. HIT: Heparin-induced thrombocytopenia.
9. DIC: Disseminated intravascular coagulopathy.
10. TTP: Thrombotic thrombocytopenic purpura.
11. HUS: Hemolytic uremic syndrome.
12. WAS: Wiskott-Aldrich syndrome.

FIGURE 3.8

3-8 Platelet Disorders

VON WILLENBRAND DISEASE (vWD)

A 26-year-old F is evaluated preoperatively for a scheduled elective meniscal surgery. Medical history is notable for heavy menstrual periods and bleeding with dental procedures. She does not take any medications. On **exam:** Vital signs and other findings are normal. **Labs:** Normal CBC, aPTT, and PT/INR. Platelet function analyzer-100 result is prolonged. There is a reduction in von Willebrand antigen (quantitative analysis) and/or reduced vWF ristocetin cofactor activity (depending on the type of vWD).

Management:

1. Desmopressin intravenously before a surgical procedure or intranasally as needed in the outpatient setting.
2. In type 2B (increased binding of high-molecular-weight fragments of vWF to platelet receptors) and 3 (severe factor deficiency), vWF concentrate is the preferred treatment.
3. Antifibrinolytic therapy (ie, tranexamic acid) is useful after surgical procedures to treat menorrhagia.

Complications: Excessive bleeding, anemia.

HYF: The most common hereditary bleeding disorder. It is due to an autosomal dominant defect or deficiency in vWF. vWF promotes platelet adhesion and functions as a protective carrier protein for factor VIII. When vWF is deficient, a secondary factor VIII deficiency results as well. vWF deficiency leads to mucocutaneous bleeding that mimics thrombocytopenia. Avoid NSAIDs and platelet function inhibitors, as they worsen bleeding.

GLANZMANN THROMBASTHENIA

A 34-year-old F presents to her PCP for regular follow-up. She complains of easy bleeding when she brushes her teeth. On **exam:** Vital signs within normal limits. No rashes, ecchymoses, hepatomegaly, splenomegaly, or lymphadenopathy are noted. **Labs:** CBC with Hgb 13, WBC 7000, platelets 150,000, PT/PTT within normal limits, blood smear with normal platelet morphology. If performed, platelet aggregometry is abnormal.

Management:

1. If bleeding, transfuse platelets (HLA-matched, leukocyte-depleted) or recombinant factor VIIa. Administer anti-fibrinolytics.

Complications: Excessive bleeding.

HYF: Glanzmann thrombasthenia is a bleeding disorder characterized by a defect in the platelet integrin αIIbβ3 (previously known as glycoprotein IIb/IIIa). It can be acquired or inherited. If inherited, it follows an autosomal recessive pattern. Avoid antiplatelet agents.

BERNARD-SOULIER SYNDROME

An 8-year-old M presents with leg pain and redness. He was playing soccer and was kicked on the affected extremity earlier in the day before the symptoms started. His parents also note that he bruises easily. On **exam:** There is a large hematoma on the affected area. **Labs:** Thrombocytopenia (usually not severe), giant platelets on blood smear.

Management:

1. Supportive care: HLA-matched platelets for transfusion as needed, ε-aminocaproic acid.

Complications: Excessive bleeding, anemia.

HYF: Autosomal recessive disorder of platelet adhesion due to low GpIb receptor for vWF on platelets, leading to impaired platelet adhesion. Avoid anti-platelet medications.

IMMUNE THROMBOCYTOPENIC PURPURA (ITP)

A 34-year-old F presents with a new rash on her lower extremities that appeared 3 days ago. She also reports easy bruising for the past week and bleeding when she brushes her teeth. On **exam:** Vital signs are within normal limits. Petechiae are noted on the lower extremities, and ecchymoses are present diffusely. No hepatomegaly, splenomegaly, or lymphadenopathy are noted. **Labs:** CBC with Hgb 13, WBC 7000, platelets 30,000.

Management:

1. If platelets >30,000 ± mild mucosal bleeding, observation.
2. If platelets <30,000 and mild bleeding, give glucocorticoids.
3. If severe bleeding or platelets <10,000, give glucocorticoids, IVIG, and platelet transfusion.
4. 2nd-line options if unresponsive to steroids: Thrombopoietin receptor agonist, splenectomy, rituximab.

Complications: Fatal hemorrhage.

HYF: ITP can occur on its own, be triggered by medications, or be associated with other disorders (eg, systemic lupus erythematosus, chronic lymphocytic leukemia, HIV, HCV, or *Helicobacter pylori* infection). Mediated by autoimmune B-cell directed production of antiplatelet antibodies.

HEPARIN-INDUCED THROMBOCYTOPENIA (HIT)

A 49-year-old F is evaluated in the hospital for swelling of her right leg. She was admitted 5 days ago with a deep venous thrombosis of the left leg and bilateral pulmonary emboli. Therapy with heparin was initiated on hospital day 1. On **exam:** T 38.1 °C (100.6 °F), BP 132/84 mmHg, HR 104/min, RR is 24/min, SpO_2 91% on room air. The right and left legs are swollen to mid-thigh. **Labs/Imaging:** Hemoglobin 12.8 g/dL (128 g/L), platelet count of 78,000 (platelet count 180,000 on admission). Doppler ultrasonography reveals new right femoral vein thrombosis. Platelet factor antibodies are positive (screening), and serotonin-release assay is positive (confirmatory).

Management:

1. Stop heparin products.
2. Start another anticoagulant: Argatroban, bivalirudin, danaparoid, fondaparinux, or a non–vitamin K antagonist oral anticoagulant (eg, rivaroxaban).
3. Continue anticoagulation for 3–6 months.
4. Avoid heparin products for life.

3-8 Platelet Disorders

HYF: Immune-mediated thrombocytopenia occurs 5–10 days after exposure to heparin. The mechanism involves antibodies produced against heparin—Platelet Factor 4 (PF4) complexes that activate platelets and cause further release of PF4 from the platelet alpha granules. Risk is higher with unfractionated heparin compared with low-molecular-weight heparin. Use 4-T score to categorize risk for HIT (level of thrombocytopenia, timing after exposure to heparin, thrombotic events, and other potential explanations for thrombocytopenia).

BONE MARROW PROCESS

An 89-year-old F presents with worsening fatigue, easy bruising, and bleeding gums with recent hospitalization for community-acquired pneumonia. On **exam:** BP 110/70, HR 100, SpO_2 93% on room air, pale conjunctiva, scattered petechiae in arms and legs. **Labs:** CBC shows pancytopenia. Blood smear with normocytic RBCs. Bone marrow shows profound hypocellularity.

Management: Treat underlying disorder.

1. Aplastic anemia: immunosuppression + bone marrow stimulants (ie, eltrombopag).
2. Megaloblastic anemia: Check B_{12} and folate; replete accordingly.
3. Myeloproliferative disorders, myelodysplastic syndrome, lymphoma, other malignancies: Varies based on low-risk or high-risk features and patient age. Usually supportive care (transfusions, bone marrow stimulants). For high risk or younger patients, consider bone marrow transplant.
4. Toxins: stop offending agent.

Complications: Fatal hemorrhage.

HYF: Disorders associated with bone marrow infiltration (myelofibrosis, metastatic tumors, granulomatous diseases) can decrease platelet production, as can nutritional deficiencies (vitamin B_{12} or folate).

DISSEMINATED INTRAVASCULAR COAGULATION (DIC)

A 38-year-old M with PMH of acute promyelocytic leukemia is being evaluated for persistent hematuria, oozing from different venipuncture sites, and now presence of melena. On **exam:** BP 100/60, HR 120, petechiae on lower extremities, oozing from venipuncture sites. **Labs:** Thrombocytopenia, anemia with hemoglobin of 5, prolonged PT/PTT, low fibrinogen, elevated D-dimer, schistocytes on blood smear, creatinine elevated with evidence of AKI.

Management:

1. Treat underlying cause (infection, trauma, cancer, etc.).
2. Supportive measures (transfusions, FFP, cryoprecipitate, hydration, vasopressors or ventilatory support, heparin for chronic thrombi).

Complications:

- Excessive bleeding, anemia.
- Thrombi can cause numerous infarcts.
- Death.

HYF: Disorder characterized by widespread abnormal coagulation due to neoplasm, trauma, sepsis, or obstetric complications. Characterized by initial coagulopathy due to extensive activation of the clotting cascade, then widespread clot formation, subsequent depletion of clotting factors, and abnormal bleeding due to clotting factor deficiencies.

THROMBOTIC THROMBOCYTOPENIC PURPURA (TTP)

A 40-year-old F is admitted to the hospital with an acute change in mental status and fever for the past 2 days. On **exam:** T 38.2 °C (100.7 °F), BP 108/70, HR 104, SPO_2 98% on room air. She is agitated and disoriented. Petechiae are noted on her shins. **Labs:** Low haptoglobin, anemia, thrombocytopenia, elevated LDH, and elevated creatine. Blood smear with schistocytes present. Negative Coombs test. ADAMST 13 low (<10%).

Management:

1. Therapeutic plasma exchange with FFP, corticosteroids (to decrease autoantibody production).
2. If recurrent, consider other immunosuppressors or splenectomy.

Complications: Chronic kidney disease (especially with quinine-induced TTP), permanent neurologic deficits, death.

HYF: Mediated by autoantibodies against ADAMTS13, leading to abnormally large vWF multimers that cause diffuse platelet aggregation and create platelet microthrombi. These occlude small blood vessels, leading to end-organ damage. RBCs are fragmented by contact with the microthrombi, causing hemolysis (microangiopathic hemolytic anemia). Platelet transfusion is contraindicated (worsens disease by feeding platelet consumption). Pentad of features: LMNOP—Low platelet count (thrombocytopenia), Microangiopathic hemolytic anemia, Neurologic changes, "Obsolete" renal function, Pyrexia.

HEMOLYTIC UREMIC SYNDROME (HUS)

An 8-year-old M presents with a 6-day course of abdominal cramping and bloody diarrhea. On **exam:** Afebrile, BP 98/60, HR 100, SpO_2 95% on room air. Abdomen is tender without guarding. **Labs:** Low/undetectable haptoglobin, anemia, thrombocytopenia, elevated LDH, and elevated creatine. Blood smear with schistocytes present. (–) Coombs test. Urinalysis with 3+ blood; 3+ protein; 0–2 erythrocytes/hpf; 0–2 leukocytes/hpf; several granular casts. Stool culture and PCR are (+) for Shiga toxin, free Shiga toxin, or O157:H7 antigen testing.

Management:

1. Supportive care: IV fluids, transfusions.

Complications: Acute renal failure (may require dialysis).

HYF: In children, HUS is usually preceded by O157:H7 *E. coli* hemorrhagic diarrhea (eg, eating contaminated meat). Atypical HUS is caused by Shiga toxin–producing *E. coli* (STEC) infection

(*Continued*)

3-8 Platelet Disorders

or as secondary HUS with a coexisting disease (eg, URI caused by *Streptococcus pneumoniae* or influenza). Characterized by microangiopathic hemolytic anemia, renal failure, thrombocytopenia without severe bleeding, and neurologic sequelae. Antibiotics do not alter the course of disease.

WISKOTT-ALDRICH SYNDROME (WAS)

A 3-year-old M is brought to the ED by his mother for a new rash. He has visited the hospital multiple times for upper respiratory infections over the past 2 years. On **exam:** Vital signs are stable. Petechiae on all 4 extremities and eczema are noted. **Labs:** Thrombocytopenia with platelets <70,000. Small platelets on peripheral blood smear. Diagnosis is confirmed with evidence of *WAS* gene mutation or absent WAS protein.

Management:

1. Supportive care: Prophylaxis with antibiotics/antivirals, platelet transfusions when bleeding (blood products should be irradiated and negative for CMV).

HYF: WAS is an X-linked disorder caused by mutations in the gene that encodes the Wiskott-Aldrich syndrome protein (WASP). The syndrome consists of susceptibility to infections (associated with adaptive and innate immunodeficiency), microthrombocytopenia, and eczema.

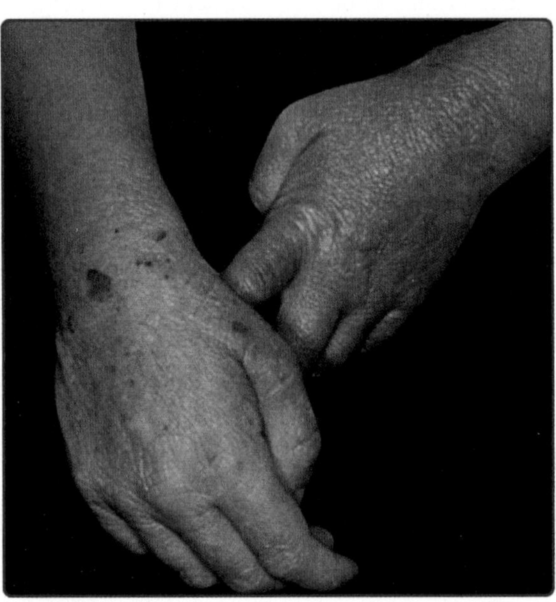

Atopic dermatitis in Wiskott-Aldrich syndrome.

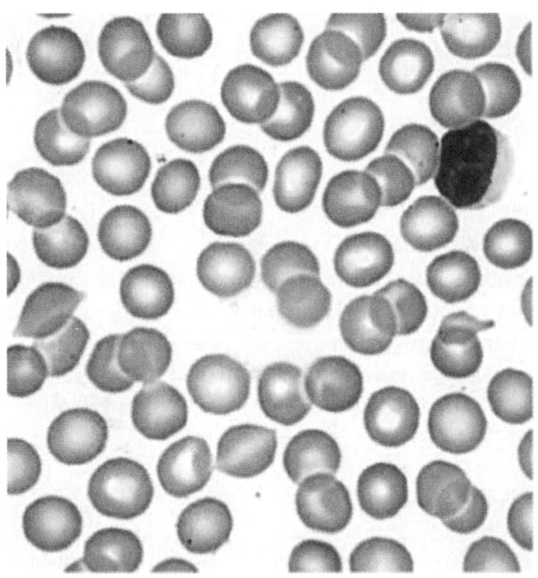

Thrombocytopenia.

3-9 Hypercoagulability

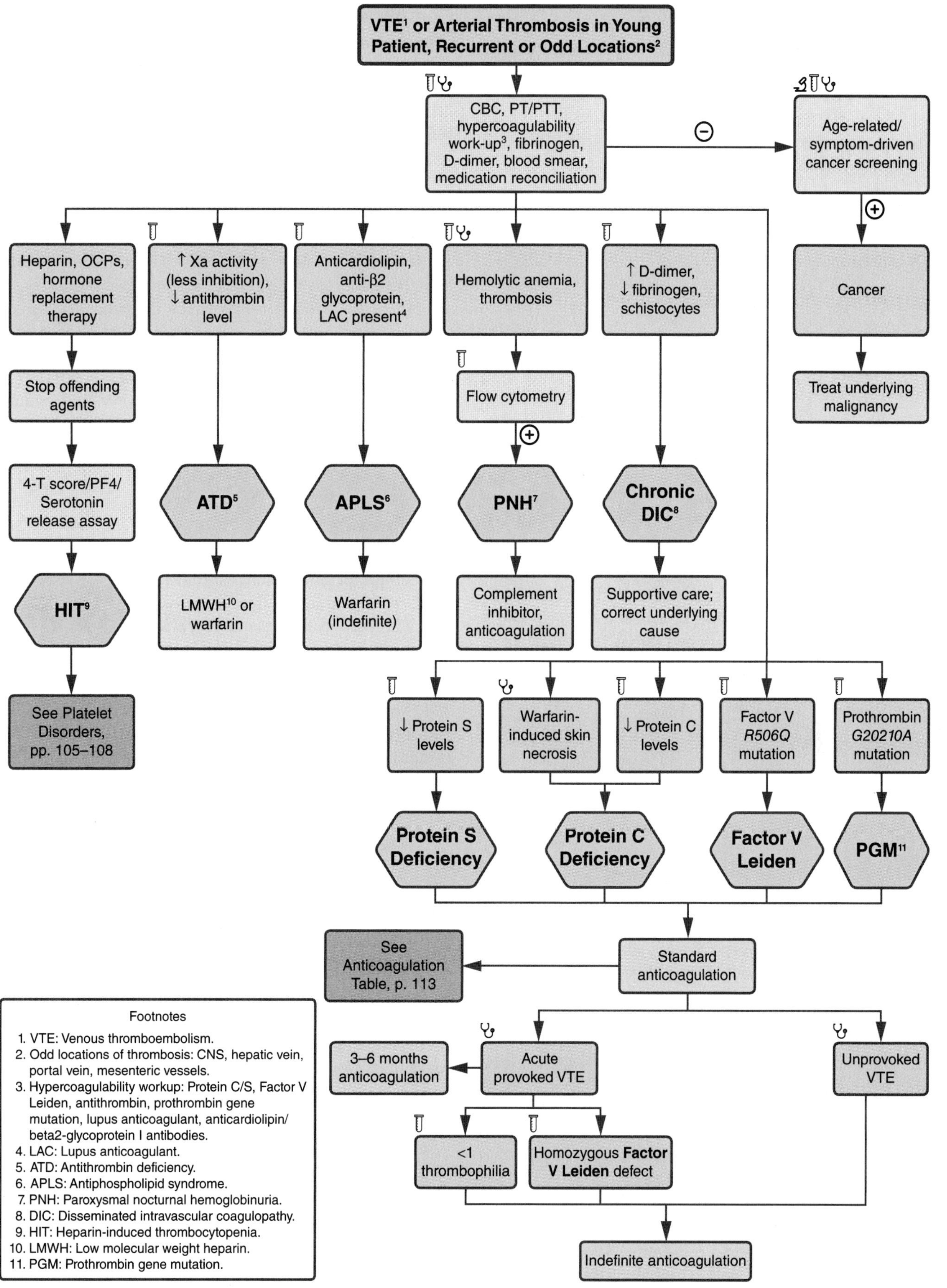

VTE[1] or Arterial Thrombosis in Young Patient, Recurrent or Odd Locations[2]
CBC, PT/PTT, hypercoagulability work-up[3], fibrinogen, D-dimer, blood smear, medication reconciliation
Age-related/ symptom-driven cancer screening
Cancer
Treat underlying malignancy
Heparin, OCPs, hormone replacement therapy
Stop offending agents
4-T score/PF4/ Serotonin release assay
HIT[9]
See Platelet Disorders, pp. 105–108
↑ Xa activity (less inhibition), ↓ antithrombin level
ATD[5]
LMWH[10] or warfarin
Anticardiolipin, anti-β2 glycoprotein, LAC present[4]
APLS[6]
Warfarin (indefinite)
Hemolytic anemia, thrombosis
Flow cytometry
PNH[7]
Complement inhibitor, anticoagulation
↑ D-dimer, ↓ fibrinogen, schistocytes
Chronic DIC[8]
Supportive care; correct underlying cause
↓ Protein S levels
Warfarin-induced skin necrosis
↓ Protein C levels
Factor V R506Q mutation
Prothrombin G20210A mutation
Protein S Deficiency
Protein C Deficiency
Factor V Leiden
PGM[11]
Standard anticoagulation
See Anticoagulation Table, p. 113
Acute provoked VTE
3–6 months anticoagulation
Unprovoked VTE
<1 thrombophilia
Homozygous Factor V Leiden defect
Indefinite anticoagulation
Footnotes
1. VTE: Venous thromboembolism.
2. Odd locations of thrombosis: CNS, hepatic vein, portal vein, mesenteric vessels.
3. Hypercoagulability workup: Protein C/S, Factor V Leiden, antithrombin, prothrombin gene mutation, lupus anticoagulant, anticardiolipin/ beta2-glycoprotein I antibodies.
4. LAC: Lupus anticoagulant.
5. ATD: Antithrombin deficiency.
6. APLS: Antiphospholipid syndrome.
7. PNH: Paroxysmal nocturnal hemoglobinuria.
8. DIC: Disseminated intravascular coagulopathy.
9. HIT: Heparin-induced thrombocytopenia.
10. LMWH: Low molecular weight heparin.
11. PGM: Prothrombin gene mutation.

FIGURE 3.9

3-9 Hypercoagulability

ANTITHROMBIN DEFICIENCY

A 27-year-old F is admitted to the hospital with pulmonary embolism. Her mother experienced a deep venous thrombosis 25 years ago. On **exam:** Tachycardic with heart rate ~110, SpO_2 89% on room air, BP stable. Remaining physical exam is normal. **Labs/Imaging:** CT angiogram of the chest shows evidence of PE. PTT remains normal despite heparin at appropriate doses.

Management:

1. Anticoagulation. Patients may require a non-heparin agent.
2. ATIII concentrate.

Complications: Thrombotic events, recurrent miscarriages.

HYF: Antithrombin III (ATIII) and proteins C and S serve as natural anticoagulants in the body. Mutations that lead to their loss of function contribute to a tendency to develop VTE. For patients in whom heparin is initiated and titration to a therapeutic range is difficult, consider ATIII deficiency because heparin requires ATIII to be effective. ATIII concentrate can be used to treat this condition.

PROTEIN S DEFICIENCY

A 7-year-old F is admitted to the hospital with portal vein thrombosis. On **exam:** Vital signs within normal limits. The abdomen is tender to palpation, but no guarding or rebound is noted. **Labs/Imaging:** CT abdomen and pelvis shows portal vein thrombosis. Hypercoagulability workup reveals protein S deficiency.

Management: Anticoagulation.

Complications: Thrombosis.

HYF: Protein S is a vitamin K–dependent factor synthesized by the liver; it circulates in a free form and is bound to a complement-binding protein.

PROTEIN C DEFICIENCY

A 28-year-old F presents with a painful rash on her bilateral lower extremities, which began 2 days ago. She was admitted to the hospital 5 days ago for diagnosis and treatment of pulmonary embolism with heparin and warfarin. She also has a family history of clotting disorders. On **exam:** Vital signs are normal. Non-blanchable macules and papules and areas of cutaneous necrosis in an angulated reticular pattern are seen on the lower legs. **Labs:** CBC and chemistry are within normal limits. INR is 3.8.

Management:

1. Treatment of acute VTE with direct oral anticoagulants, heparin, or warfarin.
2. If a patient develops warfarin-induced skin necrosis: Stop warfarin, treat with vitamin K and heparin, and consider fresh frozen plasma or protein C concentrate. Use alternative anticoagulation in these patients to prevent further episodes of warfarin-induced skin necrosis.

Complications: Calciphylaxis in the presence of warfarin. Otherwise, thrombotic events.

HYF: Protein C is a vitamin K–dependent protein that degrades activated factors V and VIII. Protein C deficiency predisposes to warfarin-induced skin necrosis, which is a rare complication of warfarin therapy. Do *not* test patients for protein C levels during acute VTE events or while receiving warfarin.

FACTOR V LEIDEN

A 45-year-old M presents with right lower extremity swelling and pain. He denies any recent travel, surgery, medications, or signs or symptoms concerning for malignancy. His father also had clotting issues at a young age. On **exam:** Exam is normal aside from erythema and tenderness to palpation in the right lower calf. **Labs/Imaging:** Lower extremity ultrasound shows acute DVT. Hypercoagulability work-up reveals a genetic factor V Leiden mutation.

Management: Anticoagulation (See Anticoagulation table, p. 113).

Complications: Venous thrombosis.

HYF: Factor V Leiden is resistant to cleavage by activated protein C, leading to predisposition of thrombus formation. Heterozygotes for the mutation have a fourfold to eightfold risk of developing a first VTE. Most patients remain asymptomatic.

PROTHROMBIN GENE MUTATION

A 40-year-old F presents with right lower extremity swelling and pain. He otherwise denies any recent travel, surgery, medications, or signs/symptoms concerning for malignancy. His father also had clotting problems at a young age. On **exam:** Vital signs within normal limits. **Labs/Imaging:** Lower extremity ultrasound with acute DVT. Hypercoagulability work-up shows a genetic prothrombin gene mutation.

Management: Anticoagulation (refer to the Anticoagulation table).

Complications: Thrombosis.

HYF: Prothrombin *G20210A* gene mutation causes increased production of prothrombin (Factor II), which leads to a twofold to fourfold risk for developing a first VTE.

- Not all patients with a DVT require a hypercoagulability work-up. Special factors to consider include:
  - Age <45 years, recurrent thromboses, thromboses in atypical locations (eg, mesenteric, cerebral, or hepatic beds), 1st-degree relative with DVT at a young age.
- Mnemonic for factors: S, C, (Factor) 5 P(ro)T(hrombin) A(nti) T(hrombin).
  - Sir Coagulable the 5th, ProTects A Turtle.

3-10 Acute Deep Vein Thrombosis

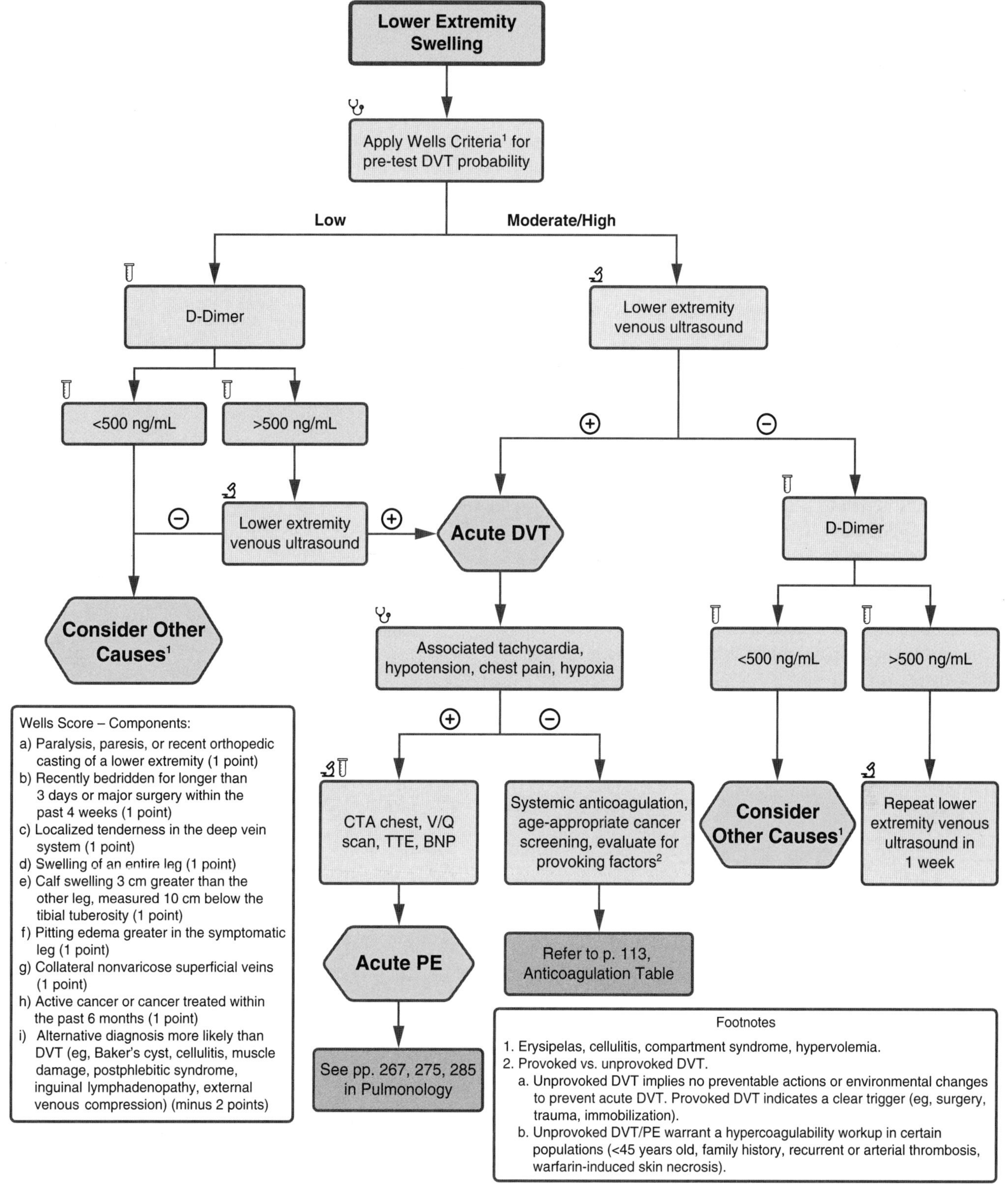
Lower Extremity Swelling
Apply Wells Criteria[1] for pre-test DVT probability
Low
Moderate/High
D-Dimer
Lower extremity venous ultrasound
<500 ng/mL
>500 ng/mL
Lower extremity venous ultrasound
Acute DVT
Consider Other Causes[1]
D-Dimer
Associated tachycardia, hypotension, chest pain, hypoxia
<500 ng/mL
>500 ng/mL
CTA chest, V/Q scan, TTE, BNP
Systemic anticoagulation, age-appropriate cancer screening, evaluate for provoking factors[2]
Consider Other Causes[1]
Repeat lower extremity venous ultrasound in 1 week
Acute PE
Refer to p. 113, Anticoagulation Table
See pp. 267, 275, 285 in Pulmonology

Wells Score – Components:

a) Paralysis, paresis, or recent orthopedic casting of a lower extremity (1 point)
b) Recently bedridden for longer than 3 days or major surgery within the past 4 weeks (1 point)
c) Localized tenderness in the deep vein system (1 point)
d) Swelling of an entire leg (1 point)
e) Calf swelling 3 cm greater than the other leg, measured 10 cm below the tibial tuberosity (1 point)
f) Pitting edema greater in the symptomatic leg (1 point)
g) Collateral nonvaricose superficial veins (1 point)
h) Active cancer or cancer treated within the past 6 months (1 point)
i) Alternative diagnosis more likely than DVT (eg, Baker's cyst, cellulitis, muscle damage, postphlebitic syndrome, inguinal lymphadenopathy, external venous compression) (minus 2 points)

Footnotes

1. Erysipelas, cellulitis, compartment syndrome, hypervolemia.
2. Provoked vs. unprovoked DVT.
   a. Unprovoked DVT implies no preventable actions or environmental changes to prevent acute DVT. Provoked DVT indicates a clear trigger (eg, surgery, trauma, immobilization).
   b. Unprovoked DVT/PE warrant a hypercoagulability workup in certain populations (<45 years old, family history, recurrent or arterial thrombosis, warfarin-induced skin necrosis).

FIGURE 3.10

3-10 Acute Deep Vein Thrombosis

ACUTE DVT (PROVOKED)

A 52-year-old F was recently discharged home from an elective right-hip total arthroplasty for severe osteoarthritis. Two weeks after discharge, she develops left-sided lower extremity swelling and pain with walking. On **exam:** Erythema and calf tenderness to palpation. **Labs/Imaging:** Venous doppler ultrasonography of her lower extremities reveals an acute thrombosis in her left popliteal and femoral veins.

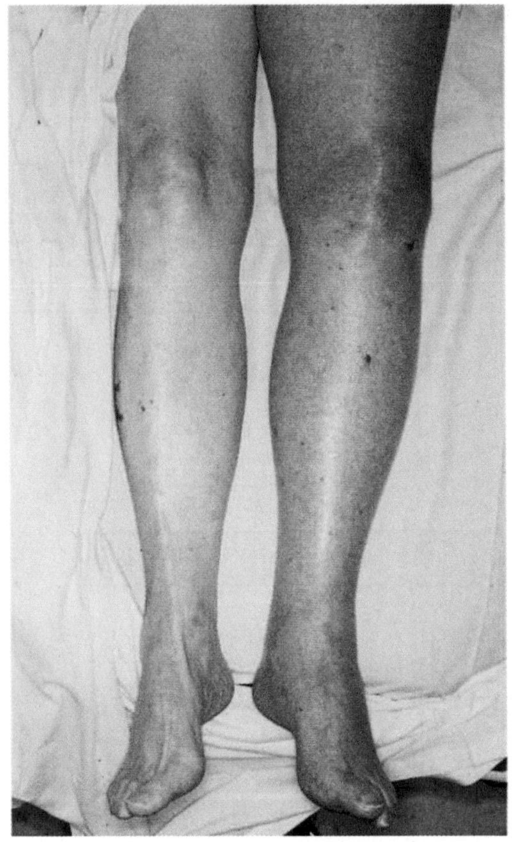

Acute DVT.

Management: Initiation of therapeutic anticoagulation. This is classified as a provoked DVT in the setting of her recent surgery and no hypercoagulability workup is warranted. Options for anticoagulation would most commonly include a direct oral anticoagulant (rivaroxaban/apixaban) or low molecular weight heparin (enoxaparin).

Complications: Pulmonary embolism, venous insufficiency.

HYF: Asymmetric leg swelling with associated warmth and tenderness is concerning for an acute DVT. Venous doppler ultrasound is the key diagnostic step to help differentiate from other causes of asymmetric leg swelling (cellulitis, erysipelas, compartment syndrome). Therapeutic anticoagulation should be completed for 3-6 months with hematology follow-up at that time. Hypercoagulability workup is usually reserved for repeat unprovoked venous thromboembolism (VTE), personal or family history of VTE before age 45, uncommon or arterial thrombi, or patients with a history of warfarin-induced skin necrosis.

3-11 Anticoagulation

Anticoagulation options	Mechanism	Complications	Indications	Contraindications	Reversal
Unfractionated heparin	Increases activity of antithrombin III → inhibits thrombin[1]	HIT, bleeding	For **acute** management (inpatient)	Hypersensitivity reaction or prior HIT	Protamine sulfate
Low molecular weight heparin (enoxaparin)	Increases activity of antithrombin III and inhibits Factor Xa	HIT, bleeding	For **acute or long-term** management. Preferred in pregnancy, malabsorption, or malignancy	Hypersensitivity reaction or prior HIT, renal impairment, prosthetic heart valves	Protamine sulfate
Warfarin	Inhibits Vit K epoxide reductase → inhibits Vit-K dependent FII, FVII, FIX, FX formation	Bleeding; clotting if not overlapped with heparin on initiation; drug interactions; dietary monitoring, skin necrosis	For **long-term** management only; preferred in renal insufficiency, APLS, or mechanical heart valves	Hypersensitivity, pregnancy, hemorrhagic tendencies, noncompliance	Vit K, PCC, FFP
Apixaban or Rivaroxaban	Direct FXa inhibitor	Bleeding, rivaroxaban must be taken with food for absorption	For **acute or long-term** management; typically first-line unless contraindicated	Hypersensitivity, pregnancy, renal impairment, mechanical heart valves, APLS, or recent GI/bariatric surgery	Andexanet alpha
Dabigatran	Direct thrombin inhibitor[2]	Bleeding, increased risk of thrombosis if prematurely discontinued	For **acute or long-term** management, preferred agent if HIT suspected	Hypersensitivity, APLS, vavular heart disease. Caution in renal impairment	Idarucizumab (only reverses dabigatran)
Fondaparinux	Antithrombin III-mediated selective inhibition of FXa	Bleeding	For **acute or long-term** management; not typically first-line	Hypersensitivity, severe renal dysfunction	PCC

APLS = antiphospholipid syndrome.
FFP = fresh frozen plasma.
HIT = heparin-induced thrombocytopenia.
PCC = prothrombin complex concentrate.
1. Unfractionated heparin (UFH), low molecular weight heparin (LMWH), and fondaparinux all bind to antithrombin III and act as indirect inhibitors of coagulation factors. While UFH causes inhibition of both thrombin and factor Xa, LMWH and fondaparinux inhibit only factor Xa.
2. Direct thrombin inhibitors come in both oral (dabigatran) and parenteral (argatroban, bivalirudin and desirudin) forms.

3-12 Eosinophilia, Neutropenia, Transplant

EOSINOPHILIA

Eosinophilia is defined as an absolute eosinophil count >500/μL (0.5–1.5 × 109/L). Allergies are the most common cause in the developed world, compared to parasitic infection in the developing world. Strongyloidiasis, which is endemic in the southeastern US, is another common cause. Eosinophilia may be the only manifestation of this disease, and affected patients can develop disseminated disease if glucocorticoids are mistakenly given to treat hypereosinophilic syndrome (HES).

- Etiologies for eosinophilia: CHINA.
  - C: Collagen vascular disease (eosinophilic granulomatosis with polyangiitis).
  - H: Helminth (parasitic worm) infection (Strongyloides).
  - I: Idiopathic hypereosinophilic syndrome.
  - N: Neoplasia (acute and chronic eosinophilic leukemia, CML, systemic macrocytosis).
  - A: Allergy, atopy, asthma.
- **Other etiologies:** Drug hypersensitivities, eg, DRESS syndrome, immunodeficiency syndromes like Hyper IgE syndrome and eosinophilic GI disorders.
- **Hypereosinophilic syndrome:** Sustained eosinophil count >1500/μL and associated with end-organ damage. Typically affects skin, lungs, heart, GI tract, and brain. It can be secondary or primary. Primary HES is a neoplastic disorder (part of myeloproliferative disorders) that can also be associated with other malignancies like AML, lymphoma, and solid tumors. Treatment consists of treating the underlying cause (if identified) and steroids if idiopathic.

NEUTROPENIA

Neutropenia is defined as absolute neutrophil count (ANC) <1500/μL [1–1.5 × 109/L]. It can be sub-classified as mild (1000–1500), moderate (500–1000), and severe (<500). Clinically significant infections usually don't occur if ANC >500. Isolated neutropenia can be inherited or acquired (eg, autoimmune conditions, immunodeficiencies, infections, medications, nutritional deficiencies, malignancy, idiopathic).

- Infections can either cause leukocytosis or neutropenia/leukopenia. Neutropenia can be seen with viral, bacterial, or rickettsial infections.
- Common offending medications: Chemotherapy, NSAIDs, anticonvulsants, cephalosporins, sulfa drugs, psychotropics (eg, clozapine).
- Autoimmune: Most commonly seen in systemic lupus erythematosus. Also part of the Felty syndrome triad (neutropenia, splenomegaly, and rheumatoid arthritis).

Treatment consists of treating the underlying cause and stopping offending agents. If thrombocytopenia or anemia is also present, perform bone marrow biopsy and aspirate for further evaluation. If profound and persistent neutropenia (eg, due to chemotherapy), consider granulocyte colony stimulators.

HYPERSENSITIVITY REACTIONS

Hypersensitivity reactions are allergen-induced immunologic responses, either via humoral or cellular mechanisms. There are 4 types of hypersensitivity reactions:

Types of Immunological (Hypersensitivity) Reactions

Type	Description	Examples
Type I	IgE-mediated. Activation of mast cells and basophils results in release of chemical mediators (histamine, leukotrienes, etc.)	Urticaria, angioedema, anaphylaxis
Type II	Cytotoxic reactions. IgG or IgM-mediated. Antibody binding to cells with subsequent binding of complement and cell rupture.	Blood cell dyscrasias (eg, hemolytic anemia, autoimmune thrombocytopenia)
Type III	Immune complex formation. Antigen-antibody immune complexes, usually with IgG or IgM. Deposition of immune complexes in skin, kidneys, joints, GI tract, etc.	Serum sickness, vasculitis
Type IV	Delayed cell-mediated hypersensitivity reactions. T-cell mediated. Can be further divided into subtypes based on T-lymphocyte subset and cytokine expression profiles.	Allergic contact dermatitis, SJS/TEN

ACID = Anaphylactic, Complement-mediated, Immune complex-mediated, Delayed.

- Work-up can include skin allergen testing and/or radioallergosorbent test (RAST) to determine specific allergen triggers.
- Treatment varies based on the type:
  - Type 1: antihistamines, leukotriene inhibitors, corticosteroids; consider desensitization.
  - Type 2: anti-inflammatories, immunosuppressive agents (eg, corticosteroids); consider plasmapheresis.
  - Type 3: anti-inflammatories.
  - Type 4: immunosuppressive agents (eg, corticosteroids).

HEMATOPOIETIC STEM CELL TRANSPLANT

Classified into 2 primary groups: autologous and allogeneic. Both are at risk for infections (short- and long-term) and delayed pulmonary toxicity.

- Autologous: "Auto – Self." This type of transplant uses the host's own stem cells. Typically used in multiple myeloma or relapsed aggressive lymphoma.
- Allogenic: "Allo – Different." This type of transplant uses a healthy donor's stem cells to replace the host's. Typically used in acute leukemia, aplastic anemia, and occasionally hemoglobinopathies. These patients are at risk for graft-vs.-host disease (GVHD). The donor and recipient are usually HLA- and ABO-matched, but rejection remains an issue. See Transplant Surgery, pp. 521-524 for discussion of graft rejection, immunosuppressive therapy, and infection prophylaxis after transplantation.

3-12 Eosinophilia, Neutropenia, Transplant

- A complication specific to allogeneic bone marrow transplantation is GVHD, in which donor T cells attack host tissues. It can be acute (typically <100 days post-transplant and associated with a triad of skin changes, GI upset and liver dysfunction) or chronic (typically >100 days post-transplant and more associated with skin/nail/MSK involvement and bronchiolitis obliterans, in addition to GI and liver manifestations). GVHD is thought to be due to minor histocompatibility antigens, and treatment consists of high-dose corticosteroids.
- The graft-vs.-leukemia effect is a variant of GVHD, in which leukemia patients who underwent allogeneic bone marrow transplant have lower relapse rates compared to those who received autologous transplants, likely due to recognition by donor T cells of cancer cells.

GRAFT VERSUS HOST DISEASE (GVHD)

A 72-year-old M with PMH of multiple myeloma who underwent an allogeneic bone marrow transplant about 3 weeks ago now presents with a new rash, diarrhea, and abdominal pain. On **exam:** A diffuse maculopapular erythematous rash is noted. The abdomen is tender to palpation, but the patient does not exhibit peritoneal signs. **Labs:** Elevated direct bilirubin, ± skin or liver biopsy confirming diagnosis.

Management:

1. Calcineurin inhibitors (prophylaxis).
2. Depending on severity, either only topical steroids or systemic steroids.
3. If resistant to steroids, other medications can be used, such as ruxolitinib, mycophenolate, etanercept.

Complications: Very high mortality.

HYF: Type IV hypersensitivity reaction secondary to the donor's T cells attacking recipient cells, causing end-organ dysfunction.

3-13 Transfusion Reactions

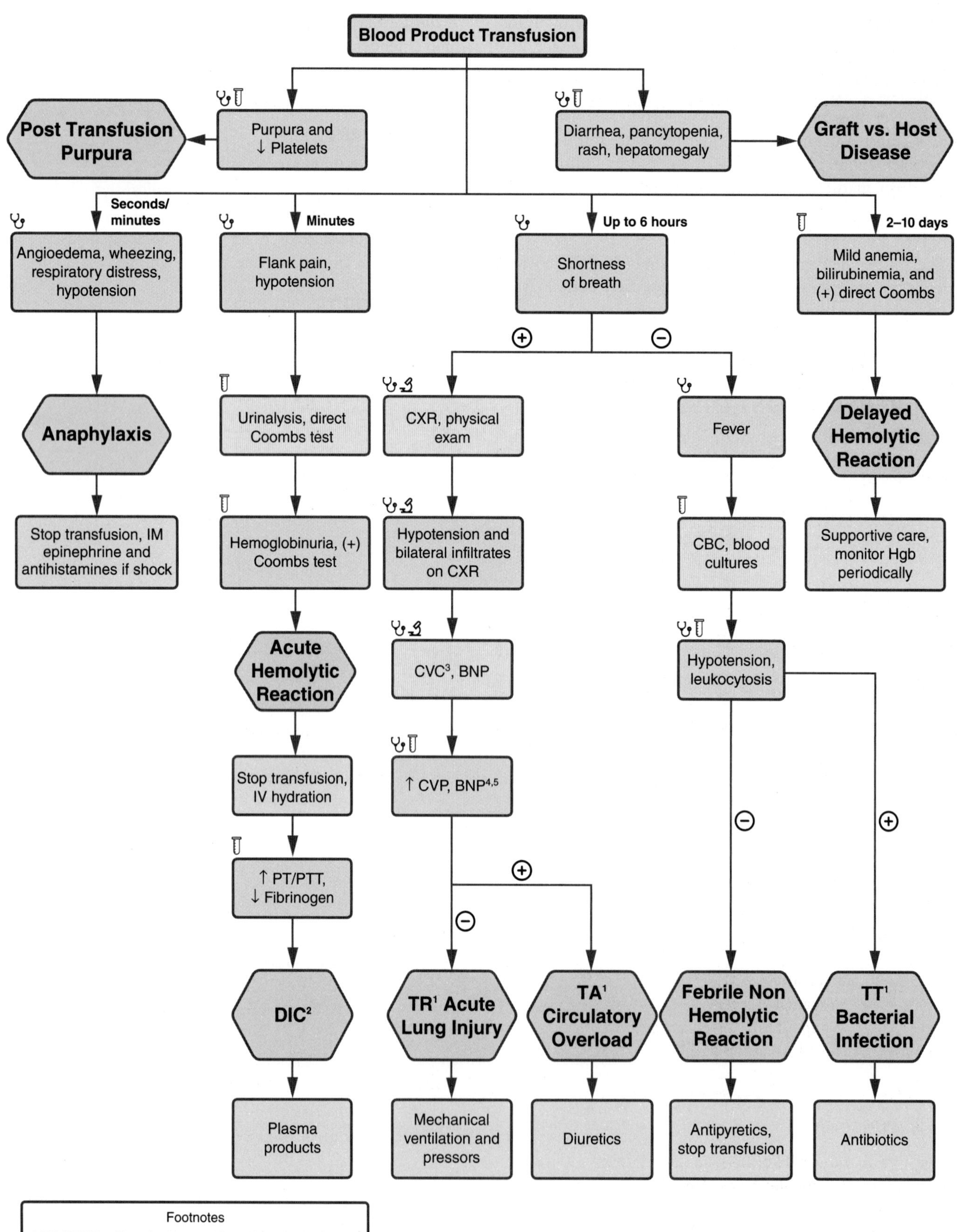
Blood Product Transfusion
Purpura and ↓ Platelets
Post Transfusion Purpura
Diarrhea, pancytopenia, rash, hepatomegaly
Graft vs. Host Disease
Seconds/ minutes
Angioedema, wheezing, respiratory distress, hypotension
Anaphylaxis
Stop transfusion, IM epinephrine and antihistamines if shock
Minutes
Flank pain, hypotension
Urinalysis, direct Coombs test
Hemoglobinuria, (+) Coombs test
Acute Hemolytic Reaction
Stop transfusion, IV hydration
↑ PT/PTT, ↓ Fibrinogen
DIC²
Plasma products
Up to 6 hours
Shortness of breath
CXR, physical exam
Hypotension and bilateral infiltrates on CXR
CVC³, BNP
↑ CVP, BNP⁴,⁵
TR¹ Acute Lung Injury
Mechanical ventilation and pressors
TA¹ Circulatory Overload
Diuretics
Fever
CBC, blood cultures
Hypotension, leukocytosis
Febrile Non Hemolytic Reaction
Antipyretics, stop transfusion
TT¹ Bacterial Infection
Antibiotics
2–10 days
Mild anemia, bilirubinemia, and (+) direct Coombs
Delayed Hemolytic Reaction
Supportive care, monitor Hgb periodically
Footnotes
1. TA/TT/TR = Transfusion associated/transmitted/related.
2. DIC = Disseminated intravascular coagulation.
3. CVC = Central venous catheter.
4. CVP = Central venous pressure.
5. BNP = Brain natriuretic peptide.

FIGURE 3.13

3-13 Transfusion Reactions

ANAPHYLAXIS

A 53-year-old M with PMH of IgA deficiency and diverticulosis presents with lower GI bleed and is found to have acute blood loss anemia. Several minutes after starting a blood transfusion, he becomes agitated. On **exam:** Fever, tachycardia, hypoxic, hypotension, wheezing on bilateral lung fields, and tongue swelling.

Management:

1. STOP transfusion.
2. Manage airway, breathing, circulation: Supplemental O_2 if needed, intubation to protect airway.
3. IM epinephrine, antihistamines, and ± vasopressors if persistent shock.

Complications: Shock leading to multi-organ failure, acute respiratory failure.

HYF: Type I hypersensitivity reaction that results from sudden systemic release of mediators such as histamine and tryptase by mast cells and basophils, typically in response to an IgE-mediated (or IgG-mediated) immune reaction. More common in IgA-deficient patients when they are exposed to an IgA-rich transfusion. IgA-deficient patients *must* receive blood products without IgA.

ACUTE HEMOLYTIC TRANSFUSION REACTION

A 52-year-old F with PMH of hemorrhoids presents with lower GI bleed and is found to have acute anemia. Minutes after transfusion was started, she develops flank pain. On **exam:** Fever, hypotension. **Labs:** Hemoglobinuria on UA, hemoglobinemia (plasma-free hemoglobin), elevated creatinine, positive direct antiglobulin test (Coombs), schistocytes on peripheral smear.

Management:

1. STOP transfusion.
2. Supportive care (eg, IV fluids).

Complications: Disseminated intravascular coagulopathy, acute kidney injury.

HYF: Type II hypersensitivity reaction due to preformed (acute) recipient antibodies against donor erythrocytes → intravascular hemolysis (ABO incompatibility) or extravascular hemolysis (host antibody reaction against foreign antigen on donor RBCs).

DELAYED HEMOLYTIC TRANSFUSION REACTION

A 63-year-old M with PMH of diverticulosis has been admitted to the hospital for a diverticular bleed. He has required transfusions of packed red blood cells but otherwise has been hemodynamically stable. He is complaining of worsening fatigue. On **exam:** Low-grade fever, jaundice, tachycardia to ~110s. **Labs:** Hemoglobin decreased from 12 to 7, positive direct antiglobulin (Coombs), schistocytes on peripheral smear, low haptoglobin, elevated lactate dehydrogenase, elevated total and indirect bilirubin, and elevated reticulocyte count.

Management:

1. STOP transfusion.
2. Supportive care (eg, IV fluids).
3. Consider steroids or other immunosuppressants if persistent.

Complications: Sequelae of anemia in the setting of brisk hemolysis, acute kidney injury.

HYF: Type II hypersensitivity reaction due to formed antibodies to non-ABO blood group antigens (so-called "minor" antigens) that develop in some individuals after a prior transfusion or pregnancy (sometimes years prior).

TRANSFUSION-ASSOCIATED CIRCULATORY OVERLOAD (TACO)

An 85-year-old F with PMH of aplastic anemia presents to the ED with fatigue. Her family also notes her to be paler than usual. On arrival, her hemoglobin was noted to be 4.0, and she was ordered a transfusion of 3 units of packed red blood cells. After the 1st unit of blood, she develops acute dyspnea and becomes more agitated. On **exam:** Tachypneic, tachycardic, SpO_2 86% on room air, bilateral crackles on lung exam, elevated jugular venous pressure. **Labs/Imaging:** Elevated BNP. CXR shows diffuse infiltrates consistent with pulmonary edema.

Management:

1. Manage ABCs (airway, breathing, circulation): Supplemental oxygen, mechanical ventilation if necessary.
2. Diuretics.

Complications: Acute respiratory failure.

HYF: Overt signs of volume overload (positive fluid balance, elevated central venous pressure, elevated B-type natriuretic peptide) are usually seen on exam. Risk factors: heart failure, nephrotic syndrome, liver failure.

TRANSFUSION-ASSOCIATED LUNG INJURY (TRALI)

A 35-year-old F with PMH of sickle cell disease presents to the ED with fatigue and diffuse pain. On arrival, hemoglobin was noted to be 4.0, and she was ordered a transfusion of 3 units of packed red blood cells. Around 6 hours after the transfusion, she develops acute dyspnea and becomes more agitated. On **exam:** Febrile, tachypneic, tachycardic, BP 85/50, SpO_2 84% on room air, bilateral crackles on lung exam. **Labs/Imaging:** CXR with diffuse infiltrates consistent with pulmonary edema.

Management:

1. Manage ABCs (airway, breathing, circulation): Supplemental O_2, mechanical ventilation if necessary, IV fluids to maintain BP, vasopressors as needed.
2. Consider corticosteroids.

(Continued)

3-13 Transfusion Reactions

Complications: Acute respiratory failure.

HYF: Non-cardiogenic pulmonary edema that occurs within 6 hours of transfusion. More likely to present with hypotension and fever due to donor anti-WBC antibodies that attack recipient pulmonary endothelial cells and neutrophils, as well as cytokine release that causes pulmonary vasodilation and further inflammatory pulmonary edema. Avoid diuretics during treatment, as they can worsen hypotension.

FEBRILE NON-HEMOLYTIC TRANSFUSION REACTION

An 85-year-old F with PMH of aplastic anemia presents for fatigue. Hemoglobin is noted to be 6.8, and she gets 1 unit of packed red blood cells. Around 4 hours after the transfusion, she develops a fever. On **exam:** T 39.0, chills, and rigors. **Labs:** Hemoglobin stable at 8, normal bilirubin, negative direct antiglobulin test (Coombs), no schistocytes on peripheral smear.

Management:

1. STOP transfusion.
2. Supportive care (eg, antipyretics).

Complications: Benign reaction that does not cause long-lasting sequelae.

HYF: Type II hypersensitivity reaction mediated by host antibodies to donor human leukocyte antigens (HLA) and WBCs, as well as accumulation of cytokines that occur during the storage of blood components and after transfusion.

TRANSFUSION-ASSOCIATED GRAFT VS. HOST DISEASE

A 68-year-old F with PMH of rheumatoid arthritis currently on methotrexate and a blood transfusion ~10 days ago presents with diffuse rash, subjective fever, and diarrhea. On **exam:** T 38.8, erythematous maculo-papular rash, hepatosplenomegaly, and diffuse abdominal tenderness. **Labs:** Pancytopenia, elevated LFTs.

Management: Hematopoietic stem cell transplantation.

Complications: Death.

HYF: Risk factors for transfusion-associated graft vs. host disease include chemotherapy for autoimmune disorders or malignancy, blood transfusions from 1st-degree relatives, and premature infants. Prevention involves γ irradiation of cellular blood components intended for at-risk recipients.

3-14 Lymphoma

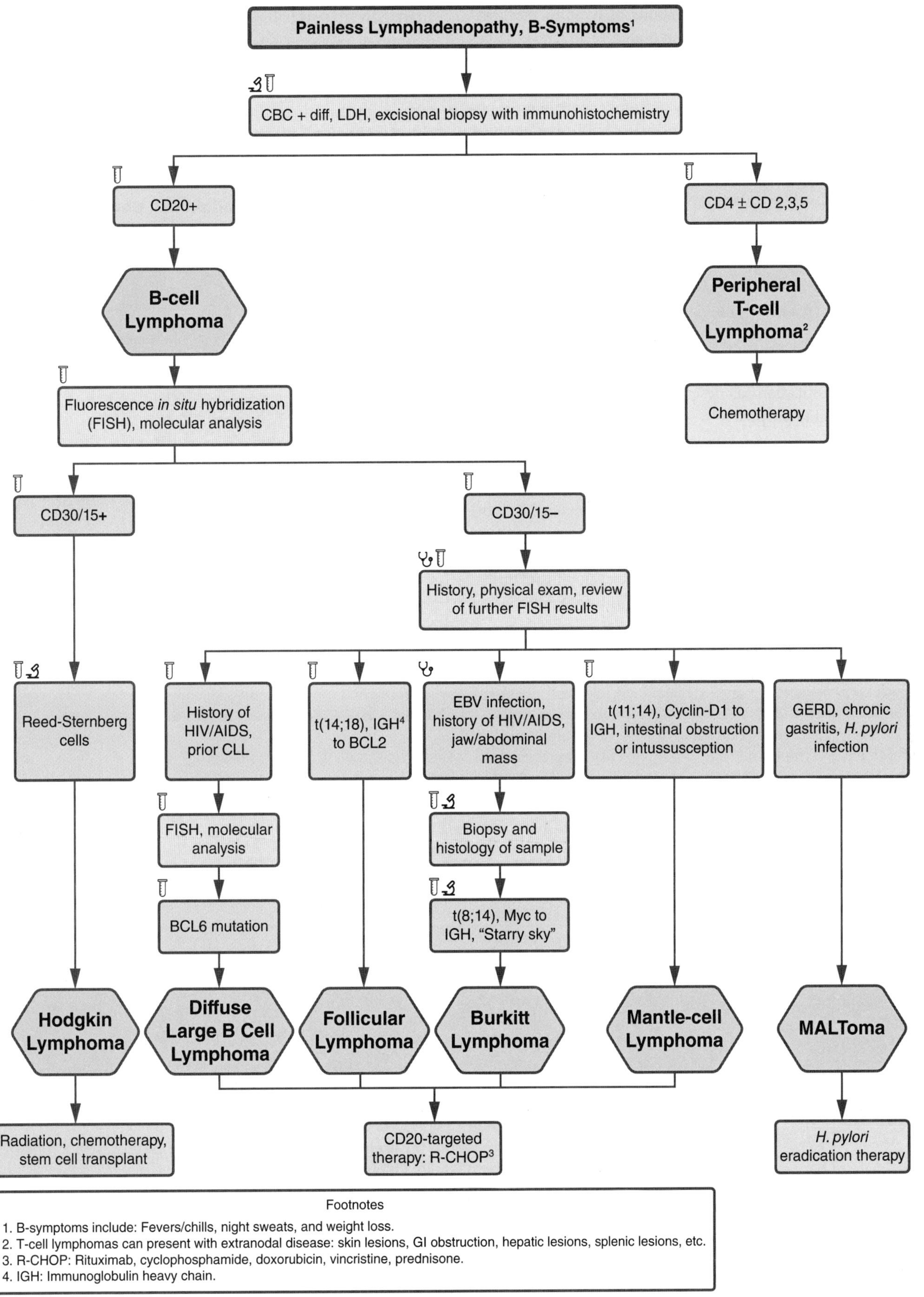
Painless Lymphadenopathy, B-Symptoms[1]
CBC + diff, LDH, excisional biopsy with immunohistochemistry
CD20+
B-cell Lymphoma
Fluorescence *in situ* hybridization (FISH), molecular analysis
CD30/15+
CD30/15–
History, physical exam, review of further FISH results
Reed-Sternberg cells
History of HIV/AIDS, prior CLL
FISH, molecular analysis
BCL6 mutation
t(14;18), IGH[4] to BCL2
EBV infection, history of HIV/AIDS, jaw/abdominal mass
Biopsy and histology of sample
t(8;14), Myc to IGH, "Starry sky"
t(11;14), Cyclin-D1 to IGH, intestinal obstruction or intussusception
GERD, chronic gastritis, *H. pylori* infection
Hodgkin Lymphoma
Diffuse Large B Cell Lymphoma
Follicular Lymphoma
Burkitt Lymphoma
Mantle-cell Lymphoma
MALToma
Radiation, chemotherapy, stem cell transplant
CD20-targeted therapy: R-CHOP[3]
H. pylori eradication therapy
CD4 ± CD 2,3,5
Peripheral T-cell Lymphoma[2]
Chemotherapy
Footnotes
1. B-symptoms include: Fevers/chills, night sweats, and weight loss.
2. T-cell lymphomas can present with extranodal disease: skin lesions, GI obstruction, hepatic lesions, splenic lesions, etc.
3. R-CHOP: Rituximab, cyclophosphamide, doxorubicin, vincristine, prednisone.
4. IGH: Immunoglobulin heavy chain.

FIGURE 3.14

3-14 Lymphoma

Lymphomas are malignant transformations of lymphocytes, primarily in the lymphoid tissue and lymph nodes. In advanced stages they can also involve the blood stream and/or non-lymphatic organs. Patients classically present with "B symptoms," including fevers, night sweats, and weight loss. Lymphomas are primarily categorized as Hodgkin (HL) vs. non-Hodgkin (NHL) lymphomas. NHL represents a diverse assortment of mature B- and T-cell neoplasms and is the most common hematopoietic neoplasm. HL is predominantly a B-cell neoplasm associated with EBV that classically presents above the diaphragm (eg, cervical lymphadenopathy).

LYMPHOMA

A 24-year-old M presents with intermittent fevers, night sweats, and an approximate 10-pound weight loss over the past 6 months. On **exam:** Cervical and axillary lymphadenopathy, palpable splenomegaly. **Labs:** WBC can be normal. Excisional biopsy FISH is important for classification (as described below), with bone marrow biopsy for staging purposes.

Management:

1. **Classic Hodgkin Lymphoma**
ABVD combination chemotherapy: (adriamycin, bleomycin, vinblastine, and dacarbazine) ± radiation therapy
2. **Non-Hodgkin Lymphoma**
R-CHOP chemoimmunotherapy: (rituximab, cyclophosphamide, doxorubicin, vincristine ie. oncovin, and prednisone) ± radiation therapy

Complications: Some lymphomas can be invasive to nearby structures and cause associated symptoms (eg, neuropathy due to nerve invasion, GI symptoms if obstruction/intussusception). Treatment of lymphomas can cause secondary toxicities from chemotherapy or radiation (cardiotoxicity from doxorubicin, pulmonary toxicity from bleomycin).

Characteristics of Non-Hodgkin vs. Hodgkin Lymphoma

	Hodgkin Lymphoma	Non-Hodgkin Lymphoma
Cells of origin	Reed-Sternberg cells (CD30+/CD15+ B cells)	Most commonly B cells, occasionally T cells
Patient population	Bimodal age distribution: Age 30 (primarily nodular sclerosing type) and age 60 (primarily lymphocyte-depleted type)	Peak incidence age 65–75 but can present in children
Risk factors	EBV	EBV, HIV, autoimmune disease, congenital immunodeficiencies

Non-Hodgkin Lymphomas

Type		High-Yield Facts
B-Cell Lymphomas	Diffuse large B-cell lymphoma	• Most common adult NHL. • Usually presents with a single fast-growing mass, rapidly progressive. • Labs show pancytopenia. • Associated with mutations in Bcl-2, Bcl-6.
	Burkitt lymphoma	• Endemic form presents as a jaw lesion in patients from Africa. Sporadic form presents as abdominal lesion in patients from Americas. • Associated with HIV and EBV. • Associated with t[8;14] (*MYC* oncogene overexpression). • "Starry sky" appearance on lymph node biopsy.
	Follicular lymphoma	• Mean age: 55 years. • Associated with t[14;18] *BCL2* gene overexpression.
	Mantle-cell lymphoma	• Classically presents in elderly men. • Rarest form of NHL. • CD5+, Cyclin-D1 overexpression. • Associated with t(11;14).
	Marginal zone lymphoma	• Associated with chronic inflammation. • Mucosa-associated lymphoid tissue (MALT) lymphoma is a type of marginal zone lymphoma secondary to *H. pylori*, HBV, HCV, or autoimmune disease. • In gastric MALT lymphoma, the likely source of inflammation is *H. pylori* gastritis. Therapy for *H. pylori* eradication is required for treatment.
T-Cell Lymphomas	Peripheral T-cell lymphoma	• CD3, CD2, and CD5 and almost always CD4. • Presents with extra-nodal lesions (skin, GI). • Associated with human T-lymphotropic virus (HTLV-I/II).
	Mycosis fungoides/Sezary syndrome	• Mycosis fungoides is a T-cell lymphoma that classically presents with cutaneous eczema-like lesions and pruritus. Skin biopsy shows "cerebriform" lymphoid cells. • Progression leads to Sezary syndrome, a T-cell leukemia with characteristic Sezary cells on blood smear.

3-14 Lymphoma

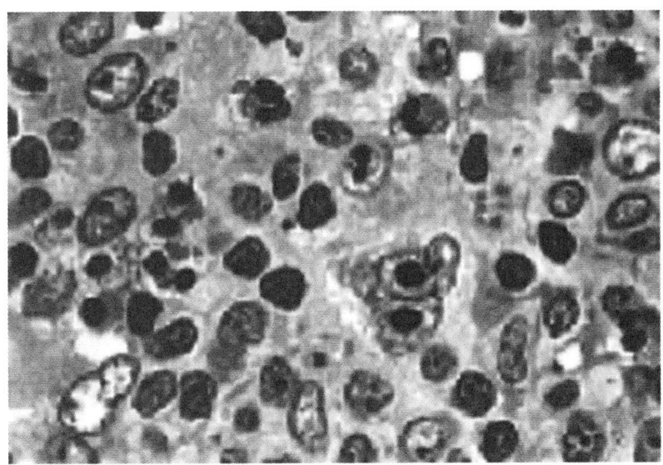

Reed-Sternberg cell.

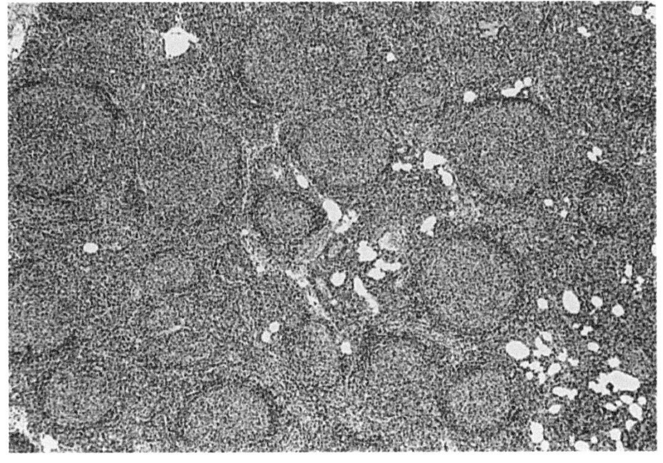

Follicular lymphoma.

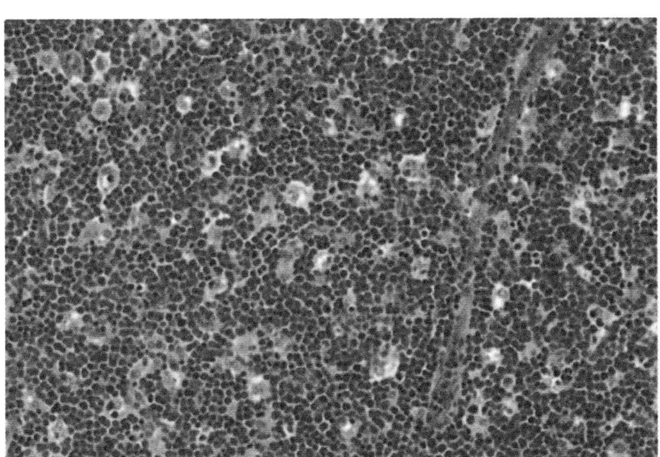

Burkitt lymphoma.

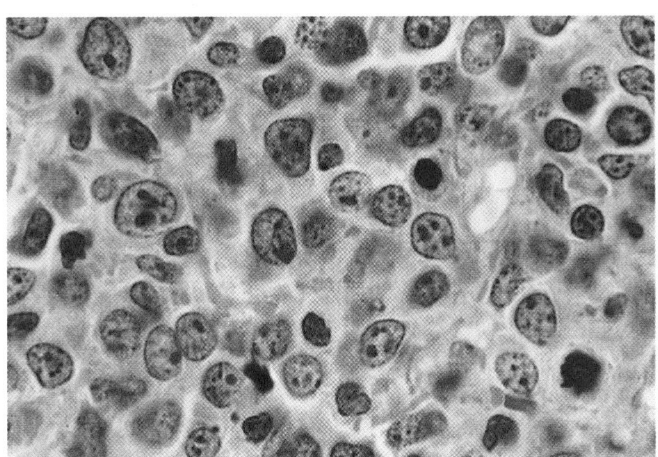

Diffuse large B-cell lymphoma.

3-15 Leukemia

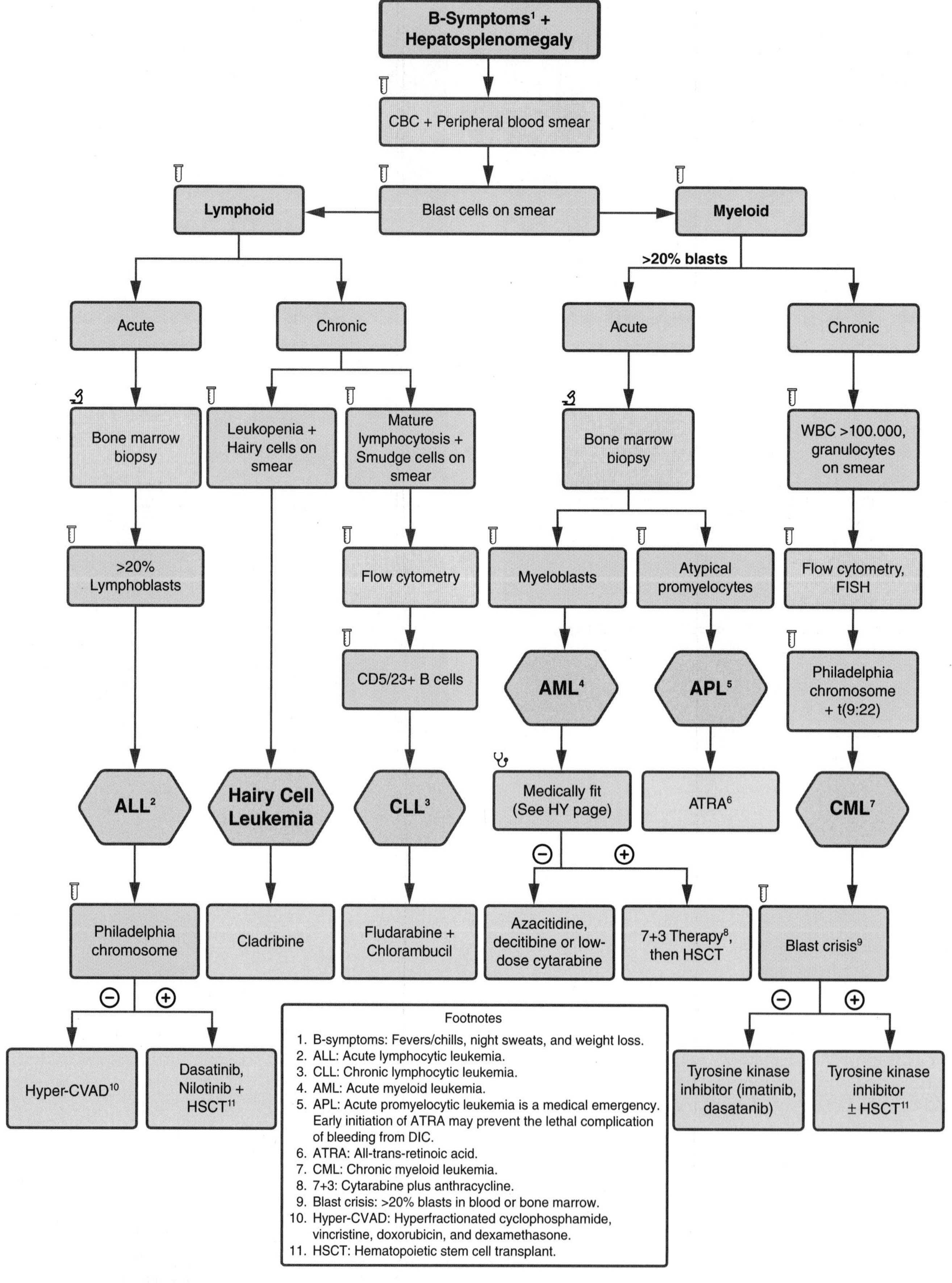

B-Symptoms[1] + Hepatosplenomegaly
CBC + Peripheral blood smear
Lymphoid
Blast cells on smear
Myeloid
>20% blasts
Acute
Chronic
Acute
Chronic
Bone marrow biopsy
Leukopenia + Hairy cells on smear
Mature lymphocytosis + Smudge cells on smear
Bone marrow biopsy
WBC >100.000, granulocytes on smear
>20% Lymphoblasts
Flow cytometry
Myeloblasts
Atypical promyelocytes
Flow cytometry, FISH
CD5/23+ B cells
AML[4]
APL[5]
Philadelphia chromosome + t(9:22)
ALL[2]
Hairy Cell Leukemia
CLL[3]
Medically fit (See HY page)
ATRA[6]
CML[7]
Philadelphia chromosome
Cladribine
Fludarabine + Chlorambucil
Azacitidine, decitibine or low-dose cytarabine
7+3 Therapy[8], then HSCT
Blast crisis[9]
Hyper-CVAD[10]
Dasatinib, Nilotinib + HSCT[11]
Tyrosine kinase inhibitor (imatinib, dasatanib)
Tyrosine kinase inhibitor ± HSCT[11]
Footnotes
1. B-symptoms: Fevers/chills, night sweats, and weight loss.
2. ALL: Acute lymphocytic leukemia.
3. CLL: Chronic lymphocytic leukemia.
4. AML: Acute myeloid leukemia.
5. APL: Acute promyelocytic leukemia is a medical emergency. Early initiation of ATRA may prevent the lethal complication of bleeding from DIC.
6. ATRA: All-trans-retinoic acid.
7. CML: Chronic myeloid leukemia.
8. 7+3: Cytarabine plus anthracycline.
9. Blast crisis: >20% blasts in blood or bone marrow.
10. Hyper-CVAD: Hyperfractionated cyclophosphamide, vincristine, doxorubicin, and dexamethasone.
11. HSCT: Hematopoietic stem cell transplant.

FIGURE 3.15

3-15 Leukemia

Leukemia results from malignant transformation of myeloid or lymphoid cells in the bloodstream and bone marrow. Acute myelogenous and lymphocytic leukemias usually involve early hematopoietic stem cells (ie, blasts), while chronic leukemias involve mature, well-differentiated cells. Many acute lymphoblastic leukemia subtypes are more common in children while CLL and hairy cell leukemia (HCL) are more common in older adults. In general, treatment involves chemotherapy and/or bone marrow transplant if patient is able. During treatment, the patient should undergo aggressive hydration and also start allopurinol or rasburicase with chemotherapy to prevent tumor lysis syndrome (renal insufficiency, hyperuricemia, hyperkalemia, hypocalcemia). Of note, rasburicase is contraindicated in G6PD deficiency.

ACUTE MYELOID LEUKEMIA

A 35-year-old M presents with fatigue, recurrent infections, and easy bruising. On **exam:** Hepatosplenomegaly, ecchymoses on extremities, bleeding gums, erythematous nodules on her back. **Labs:** CBC with Hgb 8.5, WBC 85,000, platelets 20,000. Peripheral blood smear shows myeloblasts with Auer rods (best initial test). Bone marrow biopsy and flow cytometry (most accurate test) shows 70% myeloblasts (best initial test). Myeloperoxidase (MPO) staining is (+). Bone marrow biopsy + flow cytometry (most accurate test) confirms the diagnosis.

Management: Medically fit patients are treated with 7+3 (cytarabine + daunorubicin) and allogeneic stem cell transplant. Otherwise for more fragile patients with worse functional status, consider azacytidine, anthracycline, decitabine, or low-dose cytarabine.

Complications: Frequent infections, hemorrhage.

HYF: Common chromosomal abnormalities: t(8;21), inv(16), t(16;16), t(9;11), t(6;9), inv(3). Associated with Down syndrome.

ACUTE LYMPHOBLASTIC LEUKEMIA (ALL)

A 5-year-old M with Down syndrome presents with easy bruising, purpura, and frequent infections. On **exam:** Cervical lymphadenopathy, hepatosplenomegaly, swollen/bleeding gums, and petechiae on extremities. **Labs:** CBC with Hgb 8.5, WBC 65,000, platelets 12,000. Peripheral blood smear shows lymphoblasts (best initial test). Bone marrow biopsy and flow cytometry (most accurate test) show 70% lymphoblasts positive for CD10/CD19/CD22/CD79a, and terminal deoxynucleotidyltranserase (TdT).

Management:

1. If (−) Philadelphia chromosome: hyper-CVAD (cyclophosphamide, vincristine sulfate, doxorubicin hydrochloride [Adriamycin], dexamethasone).
2. If Philadelphia chromosome (+): dasatinib or nilotinib + HSCT.

Complications:

- Lymphadenopathy and/or mediastinal mass can cause SVC syndrome.
- Leukostasis syndrome: Treat with hydroxyurea ± leukapheresis.

HYF: ALL is the most common childhood malignancy and usually presents in children aged 2–5 years. Associated with Down syndrome. Patients classically present with bone pain, frequent infections, bruising, purpura, and lymphadenopathy. Presence of the Philadelphia chromosome [t(9;22) in *BCR-ABL* genes] is associated with B-cell cancer and poor prognosis, while t(12;21) translocation confers a better prognosis. B-cell ALL is (+) for CD10, CD19, and CD20. T-cell ALL is (+) for CD2, CD3, CD4, CD5, and CD7.

ACUTE PROMYELOCYTIC LEUKEMIA (APL)

A 27-year-old F presents with symptoms of fatigue, petechiae, bleeding gums, and signs of DIC. On **exam:** Hepatosplenomegaly, skin pallor, purpura. **Labs:** CBC with smear shows myeloblasts with Auer rods (best initial test). Myeloperoxidase (MPO) staining is (+). Bone marrow biopsy and flow cytometry to classify leukemia type (most accurate test) confirms the diagnosis.

Management: All-trans-retinoic acid (ATRA) is highly effective in APL. To prevent tumor lysis syndrome, the patient should be aggressively hydrated and also start allopurinol with treatment.

Complications: DIC, pancytopenia.

HYF: APL is the FAB subtype M3 of AML with t(15;17) translocation, creating a *PML-RARA* fusion gene that prevents maturation of promyelocytes. Promyelocytes contain cytoplasmic granules that can cause DIC. Classically appear on blood smears as promyelocytes with reddish-blue or dark purple cytoplasmic granules and dumbbell-shaped nuclei. Treatment with ATRA promotes promyelocyte maturation. Treatment with ATRA can also cause differentiation syndrome due to maturation of a high burden of myelocytes consequently releasing cytokines: dyspnea, fever, peripheral edema, hypotension, weight gain, pleuro-pericardial effusion, acute renal failure, musculoskeletal pain, and hyperbilirubinemia.

CHRONIC MYELOID LEUKEMIA

A 50-year-old F presents with fever, fatigue, LUQ pain, and 10-pound weight loss in the past 3 months. On **exam:** Fever, splenomegaly, anemia, ecchymosis on extremities. **Labs:** CBC shows very high WBC count (neutrophils, eosinophils or basophils) >100,000/mm^3. Bone marrow biopsy shows granulocyte hyperplasia. PCR or FISH analysis shows the Philadelphia chromosome (t[9:22], *BCR-ABL* fusion protein) (most accurate test), which confirms the diagnosis.

Management:

1. Chronic: Treat with tyrosine kinase inhibitor (imatinib, dasatinib, nilotinib).
2. For blast crisis (>20% blasts on blood smear or bone marrow biopsy): Induction chemotherapy, followed by HSCT.

Complications: Hyperviscosity syndrome.

HYF: Characterized by the Philadelphia chromosome t(9:22), leading to *BCR-ABL* fusion protein. Tyrosine kinase inhibitors (imatinib) prevent autophosphorylation and inhibit downstream pathways leading to cell proliferation. It can be confused with a leukemoid reaction (↑ neutrophils and a left shift due to infection); leukocyte alkaline phosphatase (LAP) is low in CML and other hematologic malignancies but high in leukemoid reactions.

(Continued)

3-15 Leukemia

HAIRY CELL LEUKEMIA

A 52-year-old M presents with weakness, fatigue, easy bruising, recurrent infection, abdominal pain, early satiety, and approximately 15-pound weight loss in the past 3 months. On **exam:** Pancytopenia, bone marrow infiltrations, and splenomegaly. **Labs:** CBC with pancytopenia. Smear shows pathognomonic "hairy cells" that stain with tartrate-resistant acid phosphatase (TRAP) (best initial test). Flow cytometry (most accurate test) confirms the diagnosis.

Management:

1. Cladribine is the best initial treatment. Alternative treatment options: pentotastin, IFN-alpha, splenectomy.
2. If left untreated, most patients will develop progressive pancytopenia and splenomegaly, eventually requiring therapy.

Complications: Frequent infections, hemorrhage.

HYF: Most common in adult men. Classically presents with pancytopenia and splenomegaly; lymphadenopathy is rare. Bone marrow fibrosis can cause dry bone marrow aspiration.

CHRONIC LYMPHOCYTIC LEUKEMIA

A 65-year-old M presents with intermittent fevers, night sweats, malaise, and recurrent infections. On **exam:** Palpable lymphadenopathy, hepatosplenomegaly. **Labs:** CBC shows monoclonal lymphocytes (NK, T or B cells >5000/mm^3). Blood smear shows smudge cells (best initial test). Flow cytometry of bone marrow aspirate shows B cells (CD19+) that are CD5+ (most accurate test).

Management: Chemotherapy with chlorambucil or targeted therapy with ibrutinib once the patient becomes symptomatic (eg, severe lymphadenopathy, splenomegaly, thrombocytopenia, anemia, B symptoms).

Complications: Hypogammaglobulinemia, recurrent infections, autoimmune hemolytic anemia, Richter transformation into more aggressive disease (eg, diffuse large B-cell lymphoma, B symptoms).

HYF: Characterized by smudge cells on smear and CD5+, CD23+ cells.

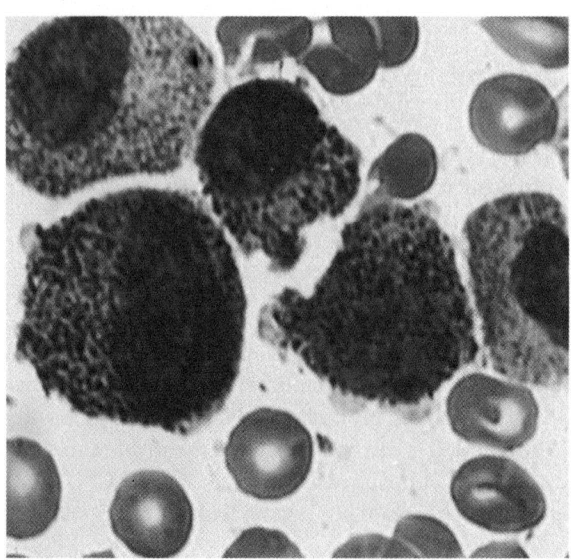

Hypergranular cells. Can occur in all AML subtypes.

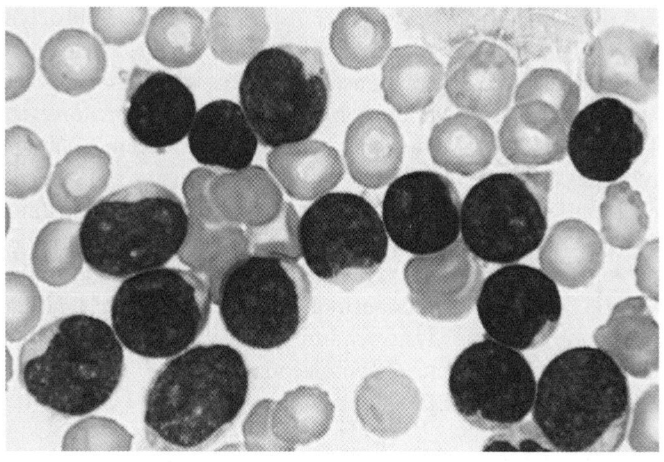

Acute lymphoblastic leukemia.

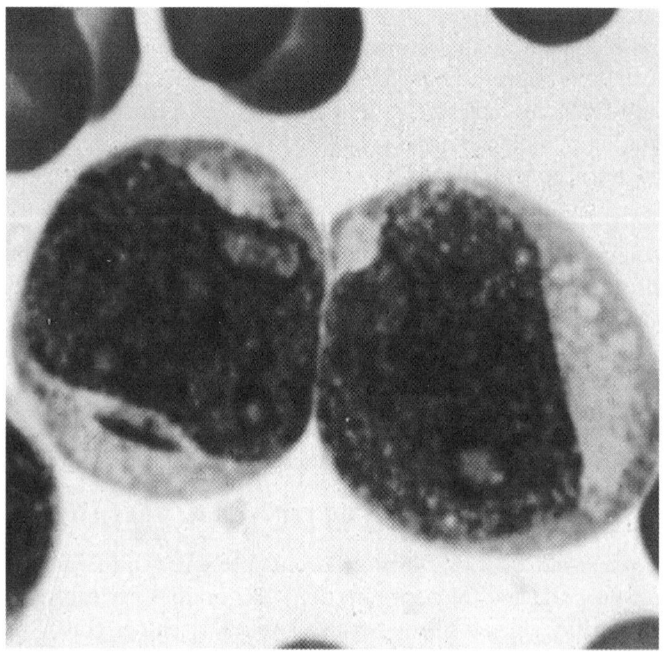

Acute promyelocytic leukemia.

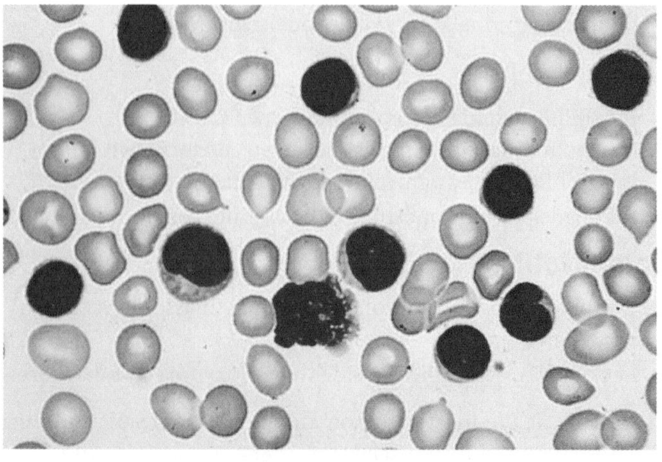

Smudge cells in chronic lymphocytic leukemia.

3-16 Plasma Cell Dyscrasias

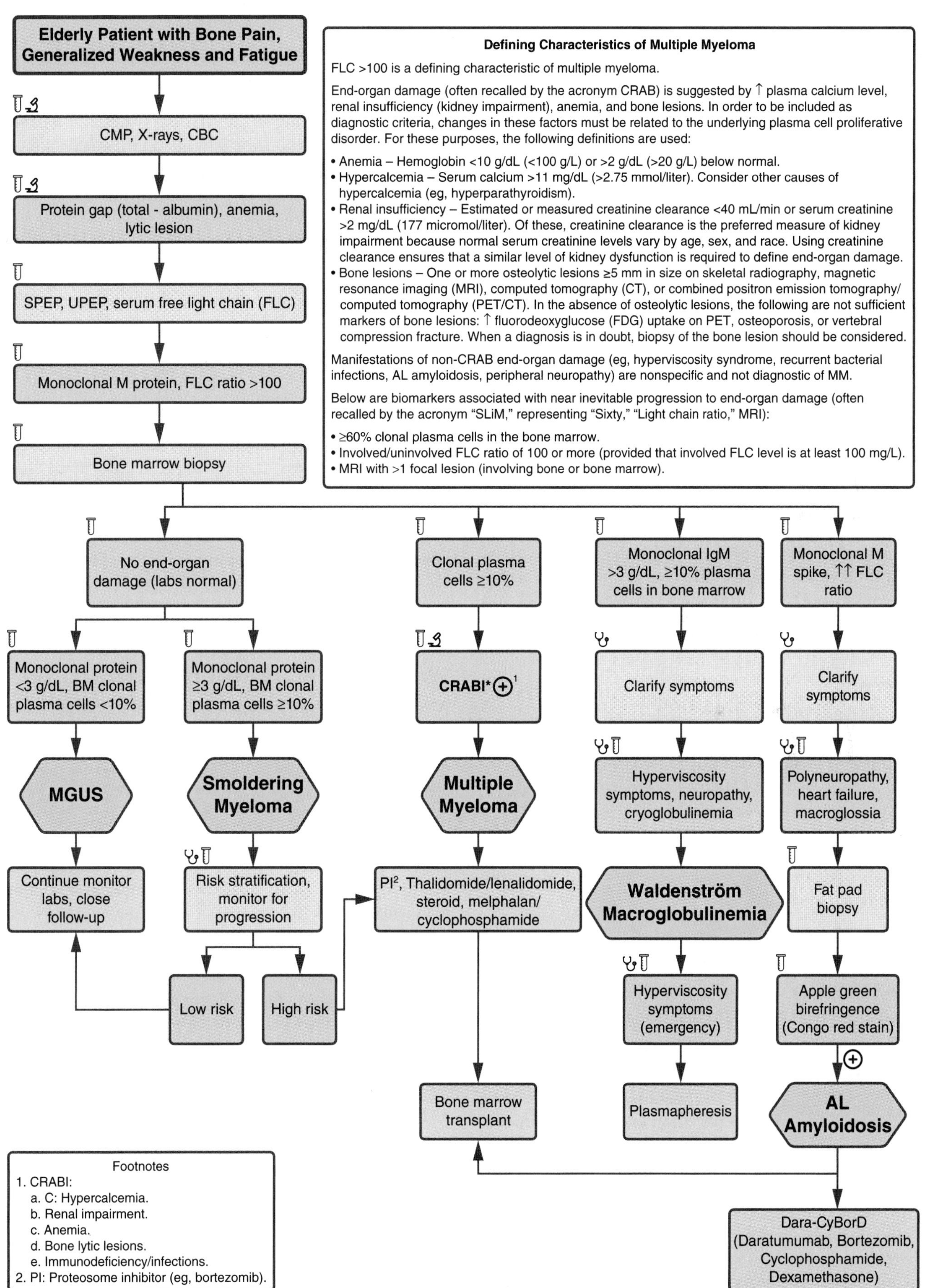

Elderly Patient with Bone Pain, Generalized Weakness and Fatigue
CMP, X-rays, CBC
Protein gap (total - albumin), anemia, lytic lesion
SPEP, UPEP, serum free light chain (FLC)
Monoclonal M protein, FLC ratio >100
Bone marrow biopsy
Defining Characteristics of Multiple Myeloma
FLC >100 is a defining characteristic of multiple myeloma.
End-organ damage (often recalled by the acronym CRAB) is suggested by ↑ plasma calcium level, renal insufficiency (kidney impairment), anemia, and bone lesions. In order to be included as diagnostic criteria, changes in these factors must be related to the underlying plasma cell proliferative disorder. For these purposes, the following definitions are used:
• Anemia – Hemoglobin <10 g/dL (<100 g/L) or >2 g/dL (>20 g/L) below normal.
• Hypercalcemia – Serum calcium >11 mg/dL (>2.75 mmol/liter). Consider other causes of hypercalcemia (eg, hyperparathyroidism).
• Renal insufficiency – Estimated or measured creatinine clearance <40 mL/min or serum creatinine >2 mg/dL (177 micromol/liter). Of these, creatinine clearance is the preferred measure of kidney impairment because normal serum creatinine levels vary by age, sex, and race. Using creatinine clearance ensures that a similar level of kidney dysfunction is required to define end-organ damage.
• Bone lesions – One or more osteolytic lesions ≥5 mm in size on skeletal radiography, magnetic resonance imaging (MRI), computed tomography (CT), or combined positron emission tomography/computed tomography (PET/CT). In the absence of osteolytic lesions, the following are not sufficient markers of bone lesions: ↑ fluorodeoxyglucose (FDG) uptake on PET, osteoporosis, or vertebral compression fracture. When a diagnosis is in doubt, biopsy of the bone lesion should be considered.
Manifestations of non-CRAB end-organ damage (eg, hyperviscosity syndrome, recurrent bacterial infections, AL amyloidosis, peripheral neuropathy) are nonspecific and not diagnostic of MM.
Below are biomarkers associated with near inevitable progression to end-organ damage (often recalled by the acronym "SLiM," representing "Sixty," "Light chain ratio," MRI):
• ≥60% clonal plasma cells in the bone marrow.
• Involved/uninvolved FLC ratio of 100 or more (provided that involved FLC level is at least 100 mg/L).
• MRI with >1 focal lesion (involving bone or bone marrow).
No end-organ damage (labs normal)
Clonal plasma cells ≥10%
Monoclonal IgM >3 g/dL, ≥10% plasma cells in bone marrow
Monoclonal M spike, ↑↑ FLC ratio
Monoclonal protein <3 g/dL, BM clonal plasma cells <10%
Monoclonal protein ≥3 g/dL, BM clonal plasma cells ≥10%
CRABI* ⊕1
Clarify symptoms
Clarify symptoms
MGUS
Smoldering Myeloma
Multiple Myeloma
Hyperviscosity symptoms, neuropathy, cryoglobulinemia
Polyneuropathy, heart failure, macroglossia
Continue monitor labs, close follow-up
Risk stratification, monitor for progression
PI2, Thalidomide/lenalidomide, steroid, melphalan/cyclophosphamide
Waldenström Macroglobulinemia
Fat pad biopsy
Low risk
High risk
Hyperviscosity symptoms (emergency)
Apple green birefringence (Congo red stain)
⊕
Bone marrow transplant
Plasmapheresis
AL Amyloidosis
Dara-CyBorD (Daratumumab, Bortezomib, Cyclophosphamide, Dexamethasone)

Footnotes
1. CRABI:
   a. C: Hypercalcemia.
   b. Renal impairment.
   c. Anemia.
   d. Bone lytic lesions.
   e. Immunodeficiency/infections.
2. PI: Proteosome inhibitor (eg, bortezomib).

FIGURE 3.16

3-16 Plasma Cell Dyscrasias

MONOCLONAL GAMMOPATHY OF UNDETERMINED SIGNIFICANCE (MGUS)

An 80-year-old M with no significant PMH is found to have abnormal annual labs and referred to hematology. On **exam:** Vital signs are stable. No abnormal findings. **Labs:** Elevated total protein gap (total protein – albumin), normal chemistry and CBC. Urine and serum electrophoresis and immunofixation show monoclonal spike <3 g/dL, and bone marrow biopsy shows <10% clonal plasma cells.

Management: Monitoring (repeat labs every 3–6 months).

Complications: Progression to multiple myeloma or AL amyloidosis, increased risk of osteoporosis and pathological fractures.

HYF: MGUS is defined as M protein level <3 g/dL, clonal plasma cells <10% of the bone marrow cellularity, and the absence of related signs and symptoms of end-organ damage. Patients with MGUS should be monitored for disease progression based on symptoms and blood work.

SMOLDERING MYELOMA

A 75-year-old M with no significant PMH is found to have abnormal annual labs and referred to hematology. On **exam:** Vital signs are stable. No abnormal findings. **Labs:** Elevated total protein gap, normal chemistry and CBC. Urine and serum electrophoresis and immunofixation show monoclonal spike ≥3 g/dL, and bone marrow biopsy shows 30% clonal plasma cells.

Management:

1. Risk stratification (bone marrow plasma cells >20%, monoclonal (M) protein >2 g/dL, OR involved/uninvolved free light chain (FLC) ratio >20).
   a. Low-intermediate risk: Observation and monitoring labs.
   b. High-risk: Lenalidomide or lenalidomide + dexamethasone.

Complications: Progression to multiple myeloma or AL amyloidosis (higher risk than MGUS), increased risk of osteoporosis and pathological fractures.

HYF: Smoldering myeloma is defined as a monoclonal (M) protein ≥3 g/dL and/or 10–60% bone marrow plasma cells but no end-organ damage. Patients with smoldering myeloma are at risk for progression to symptomatic multiple myeloma or AL amyloidosis.

MULTIPLE MYELOMA

A 74-year-old M without any PMH presents for new lower back pain. On **exam:** Tenderness to palpation on the spinal process of L2–L3, pale conjunctiva. **Labs/Imaging:** Hypercalcemia, normocytic anemia, elevated creatinine, elevated total protein gap (total protein – albumin). Lytic lesion on lumbar spine XRs. CBC with smear shows rouleaux formation. Urine and serum electrophoresis and immunofixation show monoclonal spike ≥3 g/dL and abnormal kappa/lambda ratio. Bone marrow biopsy confirms the diagnosis with a large population of monoclonal CD138+ plasma cells.

Management:

1. Risk stratification: If high-risk, patients should undergo induction (bortezomib, lenalidomide, low-dose dexamethasone) and auto-hematopoietic cell transplantation (HCT).
2. If not a candidate for HCT, give steroids (dexamethasone) + lenalidomide, bortezomib.

Complications:

- Renal failure, adult Fanconi syndrome (due to renal tubular damage).
- Hypercalcemia.
- Spinal cord compression.
- Recurrent infections.
- Amyloidosis.

HYF: Patients with multiple myeloma classically present with CRABi: HyperCalcemia, Renal injury, Anemia, Bone lytic lesions, Immunosuppression/Infections. Other multiple myeloma-defining characteristics include: ≥60% clonal plasma cells in the bone marrow, involved/uninvolved free light chain (FLC) ratio of 100 or more (provided that involved FLC level is at least 100 mg/L), and MRI with >1 focal lesion (involving bone or bone marrow). Multiple myeloma arises from abnormal clonal proliferation of plasma cells. This causes an excessive production of monoclonal immunoglobulins (usually IgA and IgG) or immunoglobulin fragments (light chains), also known as Bence-Jones proteins.

WALDENSTROM MACROGLOBULINEMIA

A 78-year-old M with no significant PMH is referred to hematology after he was found to have new-onset anemia. He reports a 2-month history of night sweats, fever, and weight loss. On **exam:** Vital signs are normal. Funduscopic examination is normal. No lymphadenopathy is present. Hepatosplenomegaly is noted. **Labs/Imaging:** Hgb 8.2, MCV 102, platelets 280.000, WBC 6500, reticulocyte count elevated. Calcium and creatinine are normal. Serum protein electrophoresis with immunofixation shows an IgM spike of 330 mg/dL (3.3 g/L). CT shows splenomegaly and prominent hilar lymph nodes.

Management:

1. If smoldering and asymptomatic, observation without therapy.
2. Rituximab ± chemotherapy (cyclophosphamide, bendamustine, and bortezomib, + glucocorticoids).
3. Ibrutinib (Bruton tyrosine kinase inhibitor).

Complications:

- Hyperviscosity syndrome is characterized by the symptoms and exam findings below. Treat with emergent plasmapheresis.
  - Central nervous system symptoms: Headache, altered mental status, change in vision and hearing, nystagmus, and ataxia.
  - Funduscopic: Dilated retinal veins, papilledema, and flame hemorrhages.
  - Mucosal bleeding: Related to platelet dysfunction, dysfibrinogenemia (prolonged thrombin time).

3-16 Plasma Cell Dyscrasia

HYF: Indolent B-cell lymphoma with clonal lymphoplasmacytic cells in the bone or lymph nodes that secrete clonal IgM in the blood.

AL AMYLOIDOSIS

An 82-year-old M is evaluated for bilateral lower extremity edema and lightheadedness for several months. On **exam:** T 37°C, BP 110/60 sitting and 83/50 standing, HR108. Tongue is enlarged. Elevated jugular venous pressure, crackles, S3 gallop, and decreased bilateral breath sounds are noted. Pitting edema is present. **Labs/Imaging:** Elevated creatinine, proteinuria >3 g/day. Serum protein electrophoresis shows an elevated IgG λ spike. Echocardiography shows increased thickening of the left ventricular wall and significant diastolic dysfunction. Left ventricular ejection fraction is preserved. Fat pad biopsy shows apple-green birefringence with Congo red staining.

Management:

1. Evaluate the patient for autologous HSCT (age, performance status and extent of organ involvement).
2. Patients ineligible for transplant: Melphalan- or bortezomib-based chemotherapy regimens.

Complications: Heart failure, renal failure, malabsorption.

HYF:

- Common signs and symptoms for light-chain amyloidosis:
  - Nephrotic syndromes.
  - Delayed gastric emptying, malabsorption.
  - Hepatomegaly.
  - Polyneuropathy.
  - Restrictive cardiomyopathy.
  - Bleeding disorders.
  - Macroglossia.
- To avoid invasive biopsy, fat pad or bone marrow biopsy is sometimes performed initially.
  - Patients with AL amyloidosis should undergo analysis for clonal plasma cell dyscrasias with serum and urine protein electrophoresis, serum FLC testing, and bone marrow biopsy.

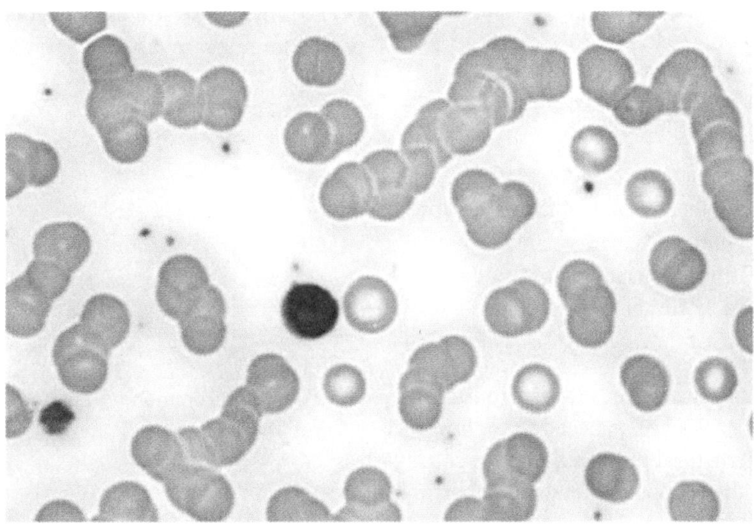

Rouleaux formation in multiple myeloma.

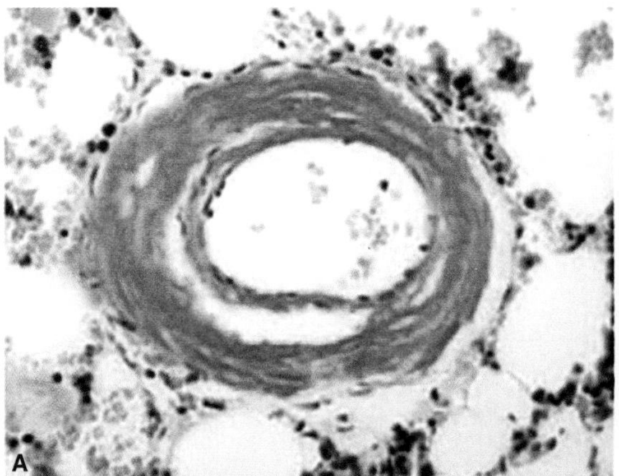
A

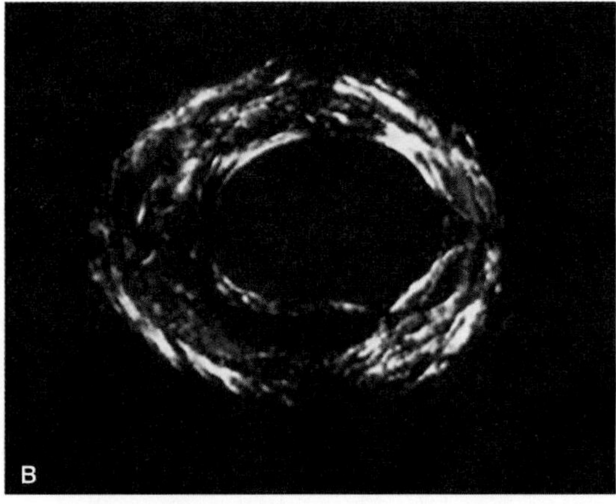
B

Apple-green birefringence with Congo red staining in AL amyloidosis.

3-17 Mediastinal Masses

Mediastinal masses can present with mass effect and/or systemic effects. Due to direct involvement or compression of normal mediastinal structures, mediastinal masses can cause a wide range of symptoms, including cough, stridor, hemoptysis, shortness of breath, pain, dysphagia, hoarseness, facial and/or upper extremity swelling due to vascular compression (eg, superior vena cava syndrome), hypotension due to tamponade physiology or cardiac compression, and Horner syndrome due to sympathetic chain involvement. Systemic symptoms such as fever, night sweats, and weight loss can be present in the case of lymphoma or may be due to a variety of paraneoplastic syndromes, such as myasthenia gravis with thymoma.

GERM CELL TUMORS

A 27-year-old F with no relevant PMH presents for routine follow-up with her PCP. She had a recent episode of upper respiratory infection which spontaneously resolved but in the ED got an CXR that showed a mediastinal mass. On **exam:** Normal physical exam with no lymphadenopathy or pulmonary findings. **Labs/Imaging:** CT chest with evidence of mediastinal mass, with calcifications, sebaceous material, and fatty tissue. Serologies including alpha-fetoprotein (AFP), beta-human chorionic gonadotropin (beta-hCG), and lactate dehydrogenase (LDH) are obtained. A biopsy establishes the diagnosis.

Management:

1. Mature teratoma: Resection.
2. Immature teratoma: Resection and chemo.
3. Seminomas: Cisplatin-based chemotherapy and radiation therapy.
4. Non-seminomas are aggressive tumors that are often metastatic at presentation. Treatment is usually multimodal: Chemotherapy initially, followed by surgery to resect any residual masses.

Complications: Tumors can metastasize into surrounding structures. Common sites of metastasis are adjacent bone, lungs, liver, and thoracic lymph nodes. Structural problems, such as compression syndromes that involve the bronchi or lungs or superior vena cava syndrome (SVCS), can also result.

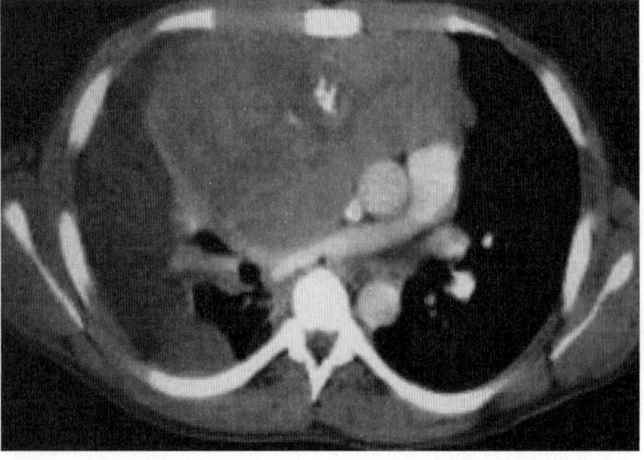

Mediastinal teratoma containing a tooth.

HYF: Seminomas have normal AFP. Nonseminomatous germ cell tumors have elevated AFP and/or bhCG. If mature teratoma, patients usually have a normal physical exam.

THYMOMA

A 52-year-old M with no relevant PMH presents with double vision and dysphagia. On **exam:** Bilateral ptosis, bulbar weakness, worse after repetitive movement. **Labs/Imaging:** CT chest with evidence of mediastinal mass. Labs reveal autoantibodies against acetylcholine receptors. Biopsy is consistent with thymoma.

Management:

1. Benign thymoma: Resection. If paraneoplastic (eg, myasthenia gravis), treat underlying disease prior to resection.
2. Thymic carcinoma: Resection if possible. If not a surgical candidate, then administer chemotherapy and radiation.

Complications: Structural problems, such as compression syndromes that involve the bronchi or lungs or superior vena cava syndrome (SVCS).

HYF: Thymomas are associated with paraneoplastic syndromes, most commonly myasthenia gravis.

Lymphoma: See pp. 119–121.

Mediastinal Masses	
Compartment	Etiology
Anterior (most common location) Terrible Ts: thymoma, teratoma/germ cell tumor, (terrible) lymphoma, and thyroid tissue	Enlarged or ectopic thyroid
	Germ cell tumors –Benign: **teratomas (most common GCT),** dermoid cysts –Malignant: seminomas, nonseminomatous germ cell tumors
	Lymphoma
	Thymus (most common) –Benign: thymoma –Malignant: thymic carcinoma
	Sarcomas (others)
Middle	Benign cyst (bronchogenic, enteric, pericardial)
	Esophageal tumors
	Lymphadenopathy (most common)
	Vascular masses
Posterior	Meningocele
	Neurogenic tumors (schwannomas, neurofibromas, neuroblastomas and ganglioneuroblastomas)
	Thoracic spine lesions

3-18 Commonly Tested Cancers

Commonly Tested Solid Cancers

	Diagnostic Tools	Treatment	Other Facts

Breast	• Screening with mammography biennially in the general population starting at age 50.
	• Ultrasound when clinically indeterminate lesion, cyst vs. solid, painful or varies with menstrual cycle. If age <30, start with US.
	• Fine needle aspiration with biopsy: Best initial test.
	• Core needle biopsy: can test for ER, PR, HER2.
	• Open biopsy (most accurate).
	• Sentinel lymph biopsy: Done during surgery/mastectomy.
	• CT/PET scan to determine extent of metastatic disease.
		1. Surgery:
		  • Lumpectomy + radiation
		  • Lumpectomy is contraindicated in metastatic/multifocal disease.
		2. Hormonal therapy: ER/PR positive patients should get tamoxifen, raloxifene, or aromatase inhibitors (eg, anastrozole).
		  • Aromatase inhibitors are preferred in post-menopausal women.
		  • Tamoxifen is preferred in pre-menopausal women.
		  • If HER2/neu+: Give trastuzumab.
		  • If triple (ER/PR/HER2)-negative: chemotherapy, immunotherapy
		Side effects:
		• Tamoxifen (selective estrogen modifier): endometrial cancer, blood clots.
		• Aromatase inhibitors: Osteoporosis.
		• Trastuzumab: Cardiotoxicity
			• Usually painless (early stages)
			• *BRCA1/2* mutation is associated with breast, ovarian, and pancreatic cancer.
			• Second most common cause of cancer death in women (behind lung cancer).
			• Classic features of cancer are a single, hard, immobile lesion with irregular borders.
			• Consider genetic testing/counseling for some patients and their families (Ashkenazi Jewish ancestry, male patients, triple-negative breast cancer).

Cervical	See Gynecology Chapter, p. 712		

Colon	Screening:
	• Endoscopy
	  ▪ Low-risk patients – Screen at age 45 and continue q10 years for colonoscopy, q5 years for flexible sigmoidoscopy.
	  ▪ 1st-degree relative with CRC – screen at age 40 or 10 years prior to their relative's age of presentation, whichever is earlier.
	• FIT (fecal immunochemical test): assesses for occult blood in the stool. Screen yearly. If positive, refer for diagnostic colonoscopy.
		• Surgical resection (most important in early stages) + adjuvant chemotherapy (locally invasive)
		• Metastatic: Multidisciplinary committee (± resection of metastasis and primary + adjuvant chemotherapy)
			• Risk factors: Hereditary syndromes (Lynch [AD mutation of DNA mismatch repair genes], familial adenomatous polyposis [AD mutation of *APC* tumor suppressor gene], *MYH*-associated polyposis, juvenile polyposis syndrome, Peutz-Jeghers syndrome), diets high in animal fat, inflammatory bowel disease cigarette smoking.
			• Associated conditions: *Streptococcus gallolyticus* bacteremia.

Lung	• Screen annually with low-dose CT in adults aged 50 to 80 years who have a 20 pack-year smoking history and currently smoke or have quit within the past 15 years	Surgery, except when: • Bilateral disease • Lymph node involvement • Malignant effusion • Heart, carina, aorta involvement If programmed death (PD) biomarker positive: Immunotherapy (pembrolizumab, nivolumab)	• Small cell carcinoma is unresectable in ~95% patients because it metastasizes quickly.
Ovarian	• No screening • Vignette: Middle-aged woman with increased abdominal girth, weight loss, and bloating • Best initial test: CT abdomen/pelvis • Most accurate: Biopsy	• Surgery (extensive and morbid) + chemotherapy. • CA-125 is used to monitor response to treatment.	• Risk factors: *BRCA1/2*, early menarche, family history, nulliparity, infertility, endometriosis, polycystic ovarian syndrome, Lynch syndrome. • Protective factors: Breastfeeding, oral contraceptive pills, chronic anovulation.
Prostate	• PSA correlates with volume of cancer. However, normal PSA does not exclude cancer. • Shared decision-making with patient regarding screening.	Prostatectomy: • More likely to cause erectile dysfunction and urinary incontinence Localized cancer: • Surgery = radiation = watchful waiting Hormonal therapy decreases size: flutamide, 17-hydroxylase inhibitor (abiraterone), GNRH agonist, ketoconazole, or orchiectomy.	• Presents with obstructive symptoms, similar to benign prostate hyperplasia. • Gleason: Grading system for aggressiveness/malignant potential. If high, refer for prostatectomy.

3-19 Oncologic Emergencies

Oncologic Emergencies

Oncologic Emergencies	Typical Causative Malignancies	Clinical Presentations	Pathophysiology	Complications	Relevant Labs/Imaging	Treatment
Hypercalcemia	Multiple myeloma, metastatic malignancies to bones (breast, renal, lung)	**Neurologic**: Depression, cognitive changes; **GI**: Constipation, nausea; **Renal**: Nephrolithiasis, nephrogenic DI	Tumor secretion of PTH-rP, osteolytic metastases, tumor secretion of 1,25-Vitamin D	Renal insufficiency, profound dehydration	**Calcium level typically >12**, CT-imaging with nephrolithiasis, **PTH and PTHrP levels, VitD levels,** TSH, SPEP and UPEP	**1st-line**: IV fluids. **2nd-line**: Zolendronic acid or pamidronate. **3rd-line:** Denosumab + calcitonin
Superior vena cava syndrome	Lung cancer (Pancoast tumor), lymphomas, thymic neoplasms, metastases	**Face or neck swelling, dyspnea**, chest pain, radiculopathy of right upper extremity, **cyanosis, plethora**	Extrinsic tumor compression of SVC or tumor invasion of SVC with subsequent CVP elevation	Hemodynamic compromise, renal insufficiency, cerebral edema, laryngeal edema	If lymphoma: anemia, thrombocytopenia, LDH, uric acid, etc. **Imaging:** CXR, venography, CT chest	Multimodal: **Secured airway + hemodynamic stability,** endovenous recanalization + stenting of SVC, radiation therapy, chemotherapy, glucocorticoids
Tumor lysis syndrome	Hematologic malignancies (NHL, ALL), rarely solid organ tumors	**Due to electrolyte abnormalities:** Nausea, vomiting, diarrhea, arrhythmias, tetany, muscle cramps	Rapid lysis of tumor cells and release of intracellular contents most commonly after chemotherapy initiation	Gout, seizures, heart failure, renal insufficiency, sudden cardiac death	Electrolytes: **Hyperkalemia, hyperphosphatemia, hyperuricemia,** hypocalcemia, elevated LDH	**Prevention:** IV fluids, allopurinol, febuxostat. **Treatment:** IV fluids, rasburicase, potassium and phosphate binders, dialysis if severe
Epidural spinal cord compression	Metastatic malignancies – prostate, lung, breast. Sarcomas and neuroblastomas in children	**Localized back pain,** radiculopathy, MSK weakness, numbness/tingling, **bladder/bowel dysfunction**	Arterial/venous tumor seeding → tumor invasion of epidural space → compression of thecal sac	Cauda equina syndrome, spinal cord infarction	**Imaging (MRI > CT)**–whole spine with/without contrast, diagnostic biopsy	**Supportive**: Pain control, glucocorticoids, bowel regimen + urinary foley. **Definitive**: Radiation therapy, spine stabilization and surgical resection, chemotherapy
Malignant effusions	Lung cancer, metastatic breast/ovarian, lymphomas	**Dyspnea**, cough, chest pain	Invasion into pleural space leading to decreased fluid absorption and increased fluid production	Respiratory failure. Poor prognostic sign overall	CXR/CT chest, **diagnostic thoracentesis** with **exudative fluid** studies (LDH, protein) and **cytology**	**Therapeutic thoracentesis,** chest tubes/catheters, **pleurodesis,** treat underlying malignancy
Increased intracranial pressure (ICP)	Primary brain malignancies (gliomas, primary CNS lymphomas), metastatic malignancies (lung, breast, melanoma)	Headache, nausea, **papilledema, CN VI palsy,** dilated pupil(s), **bradycardia, hypertension**	Given relatively fixed cranial vault volumes, malignant masses or obstructive hydrocephalus leads to increased ICP	Syncope, loss of consciousness, seizures, brain herniation	Brain MRI, ICP monitoring, transcranial Dopplers	**Head elevation, hyperventilation,** IV mannitol, isotonic saliness, BP control, sedation, **antiepileptic medications, glucocorticoids,** decompressive craniectomy

4

Internal Medicine: Endocrinology

4-1 Hypoglycemia

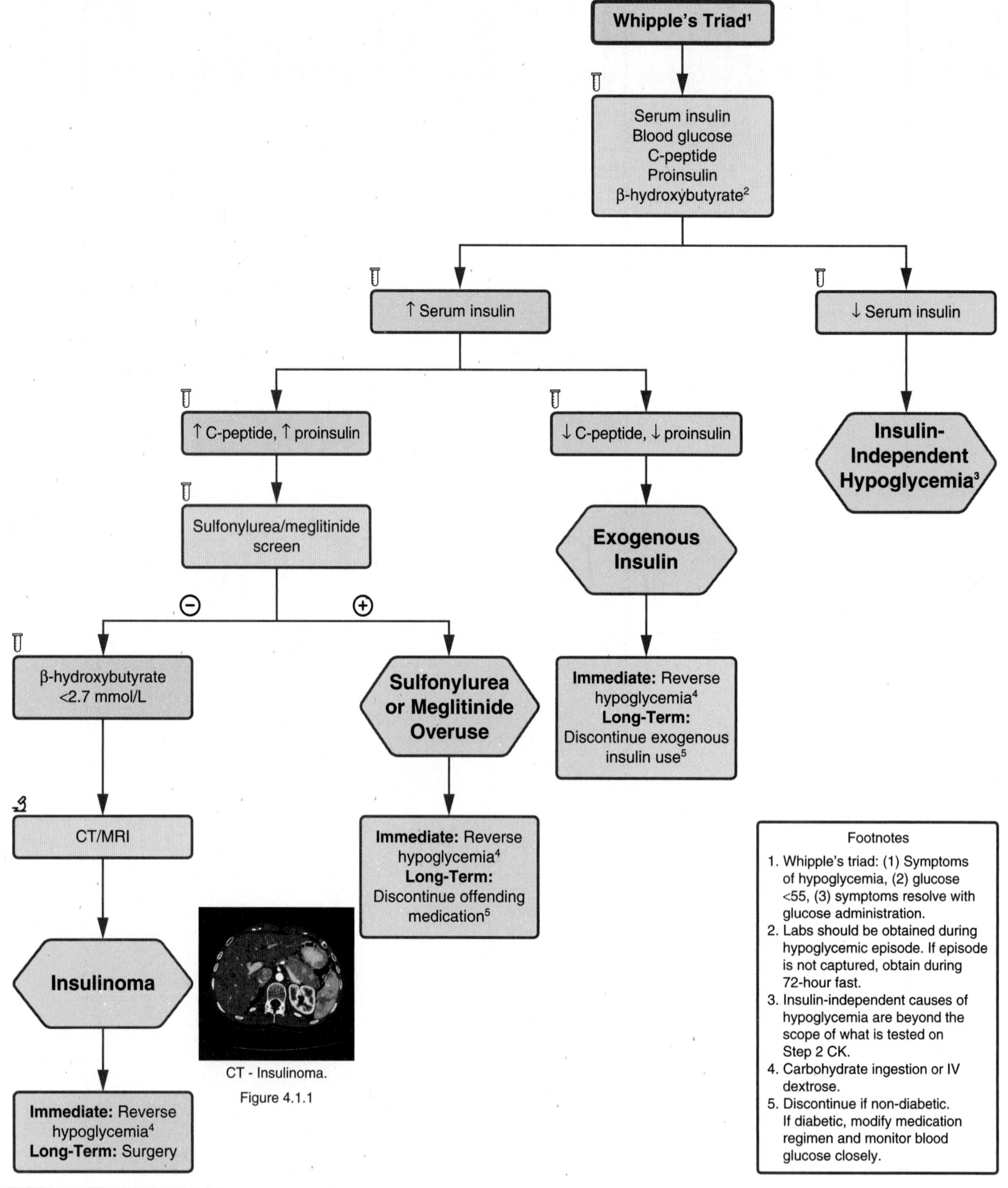
Whipple's Triad[1]
Serum insulin
Blood glucose
C-peptide
Proinsulin
β-hydroxybutyrate[2]
↑ Serum insulin
↓ Serum insulin
↑ C-peptide, ↑ proinsulin
↓ C-peptide, ↓ proinsulin
Insulin-Independent Hypoglycemia[3]
Sulfonylurea/meglitinide screen
Exogenous Insulin
⊖
⊕
β-hydroxybutyrate <2.7 mmol/L
Sulfonylurea or Meglitinide Overuse
Immediate: Reverse hypoglycemia[4] Long-Term: Discontinue exogenous insulin use[5]
CT/MRI
Immediate: Reverse hypoglycemia[4] Long-Term: Discontinue offending medication[5]
Insulinoma
Immediate: Reverse hypoglycemia[4] Long-Term: Surgery

CT - Insulinoma.

Figure 4.1.1

Footnotes

1. Whipple's triad: (1) Symptoms of hypoglycemia, (2) glucose <55, (3) symptoms resolve with glucose administration.
2. Labs should be obtained during hypoglycemic episode. If episode is not captured, obtain during 72-hour fast.
3. Insulin-independent causes of hypoglycemia are beyond the scope of what is tested on Step 2 CK.
4. Carbohydrate ingestion or IV dextrose.
5. Discontinue if non-diabetic. If diabetic, modify medication regimen and monitor blood glucose closely.

FIGURE 4.1

4-1 Hypoglycemia

HYPOGLYCEMIA IN PATIENTS WITHOUT DIABETES

Patients with low blood sugar require further evaluation if they demonstrate evidence of Whipple's triad:

1. Symptoms of hypoglycemia (tremors, fatigue, dizziness, diaphoresis, anxiety).
2. Low blood glucose levels <50.
3. Resolution of symptoms with glucose administration.

INSULINOMA

A 45-year-old M with a 7-month history of episodic shakiness and fatigue that resolves with eating. On **exam**, he may exhibit signs of hypoglycemia if he has not had a recent meal. Fasting **labs** show low blood glucose, elevated serum insulin, elevated proinsulin, elevated C-peptide, and β-hydroxybutyrate levels <2.7 mmol/L. On **imaging**, CT/MRI demonstrates a pancreatic mass.

Management:

1. Reverse hypoglycemia (carbohydrate ingestion or IV dextrose).
2. Resect tumor.

HYF: Associated with MEN 1. Beta cell tumor → increased insulin production → increased C-peptide and proinsulin levels.

INSULIN SECRETAGOGUE (SULFONYLUREA OR MEGLITINIDE) OVERUSE/ABUSE

A 31-year-old M who is otherwise healthy with family history of DM presents with tremors and dizziness. On **exam**, he may exhibit signs of hypoglycemia. Fasting **labs** show low blood glucose, elevated serum insulin, increased proinsulin, and increased C-peptide. Sulfonylurea level is high.

Management:

1. Reverse hypoglycemia (carbohydrate ingestion or IV dextrose).
2. Discontinue offending medication.

HYF: Sometimes seen in the context of factitious disorder ("factitious hypoglycemia"). In cases of large sulfonylurea overdose, give octreotide.

EXOGENOUS INSULIN USE

A 36-year-old F who is a health care professional presents with tremors, diaphoresis, and dizziness. On **exam**, she may exhibit signs of hypoglycemia. Fasting **labs** shows low blood glucose, elevated serum insulin, low proinsulin, and low C-peptide.

Management:

1. Reverse hypoglycemia (carbohydrate ingestion or IV dextrose).
2. Discontinue exogenous insulin.

HYF: Sometimes seen in the context of factitious disorder ("factitious hypoglycemia").

4-2 Hyperglycemia

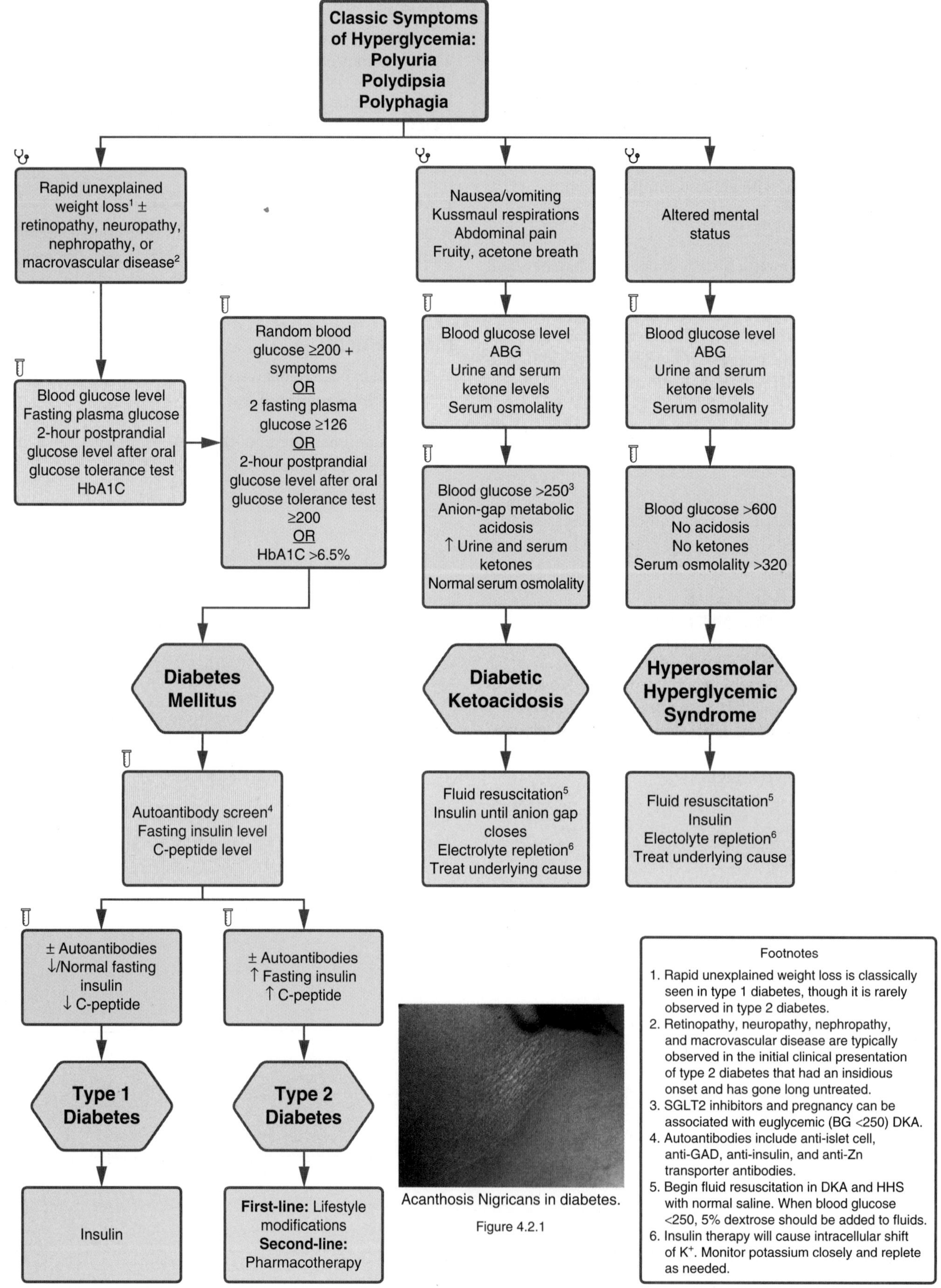

Classic Symptoms of Hyperglycemia: Polyuria Polydipsia Polyphagia
Rapid unexplained weight loss[1] ± retinopathy, neuropathy, nephropathy, or macrovascular disease[2]
Blood glucose level
Fasting plasma glucose
2-hour postprandial glucose level after oral glucose tolerance test
HbA1C
Random blood glucose ≥200 + symptoms
OR
2 fasting plasma glucose ≥126
OR
2-hour postprandial glucose level after oral glucose tolerance test ≥200
OR
HbA1C >6.5%
Diabetes Mellitus
Autoantibody screen[4]
Fasting insulin level
C-peptide level
± Autoantibodies
↓/Normal fasting insulin
↓ C-peptide
Type 1 Diabetes
Insulin
± Autoantibodies
↑ Fasting insulin
↑ C-peptide
Type 2 Diabetes
First-line: Lifestyle modifications
Second-line: Pharmacotherapy
Nausea/vomiting
Kussmaul respirations
Abdominal pain
Fruity, acetone breath
Blood glucose level
ABG
Urine and serum ketone levels
Serum osmolality
Blood glucose >250[3]
Anion-gap metabolic acidosis
↑ Urine and serum ketones
Normal serum osmolality
Diabetic Ketoacidosis
Fluid resuscitation[5]
Insulin until anion gap closes
Electrolyte repletion[6]
Treat underlying cause
Altered mental status
Blood glucose level
ABG
Urine and serum ketone levels
Serum osmolality
Blood glucose >600
No acidosis
No ketones
Serum osmolality >320
Hyperosmolar Hyperglycemic Syndrome
Fluid resuscitation[5]
Insulin
Electrolyte repletion[6]
Treat underlying cause

Acanthosis Nigricans in diabetes.

Figure 4.2.1

Footnotes

1. Rapid unexplained weight loss is classically seen in type 1 diabetes, though it is rarely observed in type 2 diabetes.
2. Retinopathy, neuropathy, nephropathy, and macrovascular disease are typically observed in the initial clinical presentation of type 2 diabetes that had an insidious onset and has gone long untreated.
3. SGLT2 inhibitors and pregnancy can be associated with euglycemic (BG <250) DKA.
4. Autoantibodies include anti-islet cell, anti-GAD, anti-insulin, and anti-Zn transporter antibodies.
5. Begin fluid resuscitation in DKA and HHS with normal saline. When blood glucose <250, 5% dextrose should be added to fluids.
6. Insulin therapy will cause intracellular shift of K^+. Monitor potassium closely and replete as needed.

FIGURE 4.2

4-2 Hyperglycemia

TYPE 1 DIABETES MELLITUS

A 6-year-old M presents with polydipsia, polyuria, polyphagia, and unexplained weight loss over 3 months. **Labs** may show elevated random blood glucose, elevated fasting glucose, elevated 2-hour postprandial glucose after glucose tolerance test, elevated Hb1AC, low/normal fasting insulin and C-peptide levels, and ± anti-islet cell, anti-GAD, anti-insulin, and/or anti-Zn transporter antibodies.

Management: Lifelong insulin.

Complications:

- **Diabetes complications: KNIVE** (Kidney, Neuromuscular, Infection, Vascular, Eyes)
- Acute: DKA.
- Chronic: Diabetic retinopathy, diabetic nephropathy, neuropathy, macrovascular disease (eg, cardiovascular, cerebrovascular, or peripheral vascular disease), infection.

HYF: Results from autoimmune destruction of pancreatic beta cells. Most commonly presents in children or young adults. Can present with ketoacidosis.

TYPE 2 DIABETES MELLITUS

A 45-year-old M with PMH of HLD presents with polydipsia, polyuria, and blurry vision. On **exam**, he shows acanthosis nigricans, retinal microaneurysms, and exudates. **Labs** may show elevated random blood glucose, elevated fasting glucose, elevated 2-hour postprandial glucose after glucose tolerance test, elevated Hb1AC, elevated fasting insulin and C-peptide levels, and ± anti-islet cell, anti-GAD, anti-insulin, and/or anti-Zn transporter antibodies.

Management:

1. First-line: Lifestyle modifications.
2. Second-line: Pharmacotherapy.

Complications:

- Acute: HHS, DKA.
- Chronic: Diabetic retinopathy, macrovascular disease (eg, cardiovascular, cerebrovascular, or peripheral vascular disease), microvascular disease (eg, retinopathy, nephropathy, erectile dysfunction), foot ulcers, infection (*Candida*), uric acid stones, chromium deficiency, neuropathic arthropathy (claw toe deformities).
  - Gastroparesis: Due to diabetic autonomic neuropathy. Diagnosis: nuclear gastric emptying study shows delayed transit into duodenum. Treatment: Small, frequent meals; metoclopromide (SE: extrapyramidal symptoms) or erythromycin (associated with tachyphylaxis).
  - Diabetic nephropathy: Initial hyperfiltration, then eGFR decreases with concomitant rise in Cr. Characterized by albuminuria that can progress to nephrotic syndrome. Use ACEi/ARB for renoprotection.
  - Symmetric distal sensorimotor neuropathy: Small nerve fiber injury = positive symptoms (eg, pain, paresthesia). Large nerve fiber injury = negative symptoms (numbness, diminished reflexes, loss of proprioception/vibration).
  - Intense glycemic control reduces microvascular endpoints but NOT macrovascular complications or mortality.

HYF: Caused by insulin resistance ± inadequate insulin secretion. Due to subtle onset, patients can present with chronic complications. New-onset diabetes mellitus can be a sign of pancreatic adenocarcinoma. Associated with carpal tunnel syndrome and necrotizing (malignant) otitis externa.

DIABETIC KETOACIDOSIS (DKA)

A 16-year-old F with PMH of type 1 DM presents with abdominal pain, nausea, and vomiting with recent non-compliance with her insulin regimen. On **exam**, she is lethargic, has Kussmaul respirations (deep rapid breathing), and fruity odor on breath. **Labs** show glucose >250 mg/dL, anion-gap metabolic acidosis, elevated serum β-hydroxybutyrate and acetoacetate, elevated ketones in urine, and normal serum osmolality.

Management: IV fluids, insulin until anion gap closes, electrolyte repletion as needed; treat underlying etiology.

Complications: Sepsis, ischemic processes; risk factor for mucormycosis.

HYF: Caused by hormonal imbalance (insulin deficiency with increased counter-regulatory hormones) that results in hyperglycemia and ketosis. More commonly seen in type 1 diabetics than type 2 diabetics. Can be triggered by non-compliance with insulin therapy, trauma, infection, or heavy alcohol use. Can be the initial presentation of type 1 diabetes.

Patients have a total body deficit of K^+ but may appear to have elevated K^+ due to extracellular shift ("paradoxical hyperkalemia"). Insulin therapy can cause an intracellular shift of K^+; therefore, K^+ needs to be monitored closely and repleted as needed.

HYPEROSMOLAR HYPERGLYCEMIC SYNDROME (HHS)

A 45-year-old F with PMH of T2DM presents with altered mental status. On **exam**, she shows lethargy, decreased skin turgor, dry oral mucosa, and low JVP. **Labs** show glucose >600 mg/dL and elevated serum osmolality without evidence of acidosis or ketosis.

Management: IV fluids, IV regular insulin, electrolyte repletion as needed; treat underlying etiology.

Complications: Rapid correction of hyperglycemia can lead to electrolyte abnormalities, cerebral edema.

HYF: Affects type 2 diabetics. Patients can present with focal neurologic deficits or altered mental status due to hyperglycemia-induced cerebral inflammation. Due to *relative* insulin deficiency with elevated counter regulatory hormones → hyperglycemic and hyperosmolar state. Though endogenous insulin can suppress ketogenesis, it cannot suppress hyperglycemia. Triggered by non-compliance with diabetes medications, glucocorticoids, trauma, infection, dietary indiscretion, or heavy alcohol use. As in DKA above, monitor for hypokalemia and replete potassium as needed.

4-3 Treatment for Type 2 Diabetes

First-Line: Lifestyle Modifications			
Dietary changes		Exercise	
Second-Line: Pharmacotherapy			
Drug Class	**Example Drug**	**Mechanism of Action**	**High-Yield Facts**
Biguanides	Metformin (first-line)	Enhances peripheral insulin sensitivity and inhibits gluconeogenesis in the liver	– SE: Weight loss, lactic acidosis, vitamin B_{12} deficiency, GI upset. – Should not be given to patients with renal failure, liver failure, or sepsis due to increased risk of lactic acidosis. – If anticipate IV iodine contrast exposure (nephrotoxic), temporarily discontinue metformin x48 hours to minimize risk of lactic acidosis – Weight neutral. Low hypoglycemia risk.
Sulfonylureas	Glipizide (short-acting), glyburide (long-acting)	Insulin secretagogue	– SE: Weight gain, hypoglycemia – For large overdose, give octreotide. Giving dextrose can cause transient hyperglycemia leading to even more insulin secretion.
Meglitinides (Sulfonylurea analogues)	Repaglinide, nateglinide	Insulin secretagogue	– SE: Weight gain, hypoglycemia (life-threatening). – Hypoglycemia risk increases with renal failure and ETOH use.
Thiazolidinediones	Pioglitazone	Activation of PPARγ to promote glucose utilization and reduce insulin resistance	– SE: Weight gain, increased risk of heart failure and bone loss, edema, bladder cancer. – Low hypoglycemia risk.
DDP-4 Inhibitors	Sitagliptin	Promotes insulin secretion and decreases glucagon secretion via inhibition of GLP-1 degradation	– SE: GI upset, early satiety, nasopharyngitis, URIs. – Low risk of hypoglycemia.
GLP-1 Receptor Agonists (Incretins)	Exenatide	Agonizes GLP-1 to delay food absorption, promote insulin secretion, and decrease glucagon secretion	– SE: GI upset, weight loss, pancreatitis (rare). – Low hypoglycemia risk.
SGLT-2 Inhibitors	Dapagliflozin	Reduces renal tubular glucose reabsorption by inhibiting SGLT-2	– SE: Vulvovaginal candidiasis, UTIs, hypotension (mild diuretic), weight loss, euglycemic ketoacidosis. – Low insulin:glucagon ratio → euglycemic diabetic ketoacidosis (blood glucose <250 mg/dL). Can be triggered by illness, exercise, alcohol, or abrupt decrease in concurrent insulin regimen. – Associated with decreased risk of heart failure. – Slow progression of albuminuria.
α-Glucosidase Inhibitors	Acarbose	Inhibits small intestinal carbohydrate absorption	– SE: GI upset, hypoglycemia.
Insulins	Insulin (long-acting, short-acting, combination preparations)	Stimulates peripheral glucose uptake	– SE: Hypoglycemia, weight gain, hypokalemia, pain and lipodystrophy at injection site.

4-4 Hypothyroidism

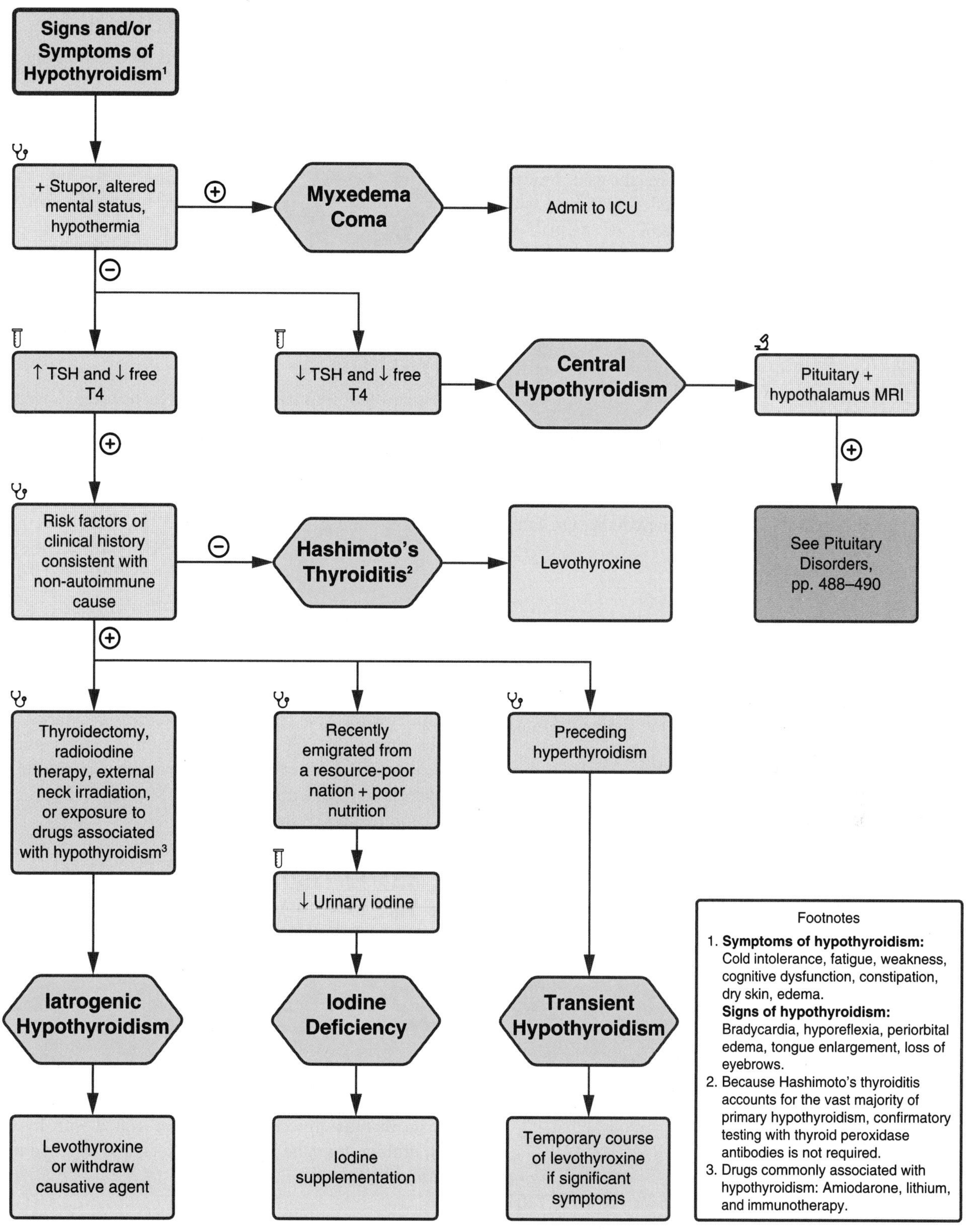
Signs and/or Symptoms of Hypothyroidism[1]
+ Stupor, altered mental status, hypothermia
Myxedema Coma
Admit to ICU
↑ TSH and ↓ free T4
↓ TSH and ↓ free T4
Central Hypothyroidism
Pituitary + hypothalamus MRI
Risk factors or clinical history consistent with non-autoimmune cause
Hashimoto's Thyroiditis[2]
Levothyroxine
See Pituitary Disorders, pp. 488–490
Thyroidectomy, radioiodine therapy, external neck irradiation, or exposure to drugs associated with hypothyroidism[3]
Recently emigrated from a resource-poor nation + poor nutrition
Preceding hyperthyroidism
↓ Urinary iodine
Iatrogenic Hypothyroidism
Iodine Deficiency
Transient Hypothyroidism
Levothyroxine or withdraw causative agent
Iodine supplementation
Temporary course of levothyroxine if significant symptoms

Footnotes

1. **Symptoms of hypothyroidism:** Cold intolerance, fatigue, weakness, cognitive dysfunction, constipation, dry skin, edema.
   Signs of hypothyroidism: Bradycardia, hyporeflexia, periorbital edema, tongue enlargement, loss of eyebrows.
2. Because Hashimoto's thyroiditis accounts for the vast majority of primary hypothyroidism, confirmatory testing with thyroid peroxidase antibodies is not required.
3. Drugs commonly associated with hypothyroidism: Amiodarone, lithium, and immunotherapy.

FIGURE 4.4

4-4 Hypothyroidism

Hypothyroidism is a state of low levels of free T3 and T4. Most cases are due to Hashimoto's thyroiditis, but there are a variety of other causes. Because thyroid hormone acts throughout the body, hypothyroidism has a wide variety of clinical manifestations, generally falling into two categories:

- Slowing of metabolic processes.
  - Fatigue, cold intolerance, constipation, weight gain, bradycardia, myopathy, delayed deep tendon reflex relaxation, hair loss, menstrual irregularities, hyperlipidemia, or anemia.
- Accumulation of glycosaminoglycans in interstitial spaces.
  - Coarse hair and skin, tongue enlargement, hoarseness, facial edema, or neuropathy.

Complications include myxedema coma, carpal tunnel syndrome, sleep apnea (due to macroglossisa), and decreased fertility (hyperprolectinemia).

MYXEDEMA COMA

A 40-year-old F with PMH of uncontrolled hypothyroidism is found down at home by her neighbor. On **exam**, she is obtunded, hypothermic, and bradycardic with non-pitting edema. On **labs**, she has a Na of 130.

Management:

1. Admit to ICU.
2. IV levothyroxine (T4) + T3.
3. IV hydrocortisone (if adrenal insufficiency is not ruled out).

Complications: Seizures (often due to hyponatremia), hypoventilation.

HYF: Medical emergency with high mortality rate. Do not wait to confirm diagnosis before starting treatment. Treat with glucocorticoids until adrenal insufficiency can be excluded.

CENTRAL HYPOTHYROIDISM

A 72-year-old M presents with signs and symptoms of hypothyroidism as well as polyuria and polydipsia. **Labs/imaging** show low TSH, low T4, Na of 150, and a pituitary mass on MRI.

Management:

1. Levothyroxine—titrate based on fT4 as TSH is not reliable (always low).
2. If pituitary tumor, surgical resection.

Complications: Pituitary apoplexy.

HYF: Central hypothyroidism is due to deficiency of TSH, TRH, or both. Causes include mass lesions, radiation, infections, infiltrative lesions, or infarction. There may be deficiency/excess of other pituitary hormones (eg, central diabetes insipidus as in the vignette, central hypogonadism).

SUBCLINICAL HYPOTHYROIDISM

A 33-year-old F with no PMH presents for a routine checkup. **Labs** show elevated TSH and normal T4.

Management: Treat with levothyroxine if TSH >10, planning for pregnancy, or symptomatic.

Complications: Progression to overt hypothyroidism.

HYF: Like hypothyroidism in general, most subclinical hypothyroidism is caused by Hashimoto's thyroiditis.

CHRONIC AUTOIMMUNE (HASHIMOTO'S) THYROIDITIS

A 40-year-old F with family history of lupus presents with signs and symptoms of hypothyroidism. **Exam** reveals diffuse goiter. **Labs** show elevated TSH, low T4, and anti-thyroid peroxidase antibodies.

Management: Levothyroxine.

Complications: Hashimoto's encephalopathy, increased risk of thyroid lymphoma, increased risk of myopathy with statins, hyponatremia.

HYF: Most patients with Hashimoto's have autoantibodies to thyroglobulin, thyroid peroxidase, or the thyroid sodium-iodide transporter. However, it is not necessary to routinely confirm the diagnosis with these tests. *Silent thyroiditis* is a variant of Hashimoto's thyroiditis characterized by painless goiter and transient hyperthyroidism (due to release of preformed hormone), followed by hypothyroidism with low TSH, (+)TPO antibody, and low radioactive iodine uptake. Self-resolves.

IATROGENIC HYPOTHYROIDISM

A 68-year-old F with PMH of atrial fibrillation treated with amiodarone presents with signs and symptoms of hypothyroidism.

Management: Levothyroxine OR withdraw causative agent (etiology-dependent).

HYF: Etiologies of iatrogenic hypothyroidism include history of thyroidectomy, radioiodine therapy, or external neck irradiation (eg, for Hodgkin's lymphoma). Drugs associated with hypothyroidism include amiodarone (also associated with hyperthyroidism), lithium, tyrosine kinase inhibitors, and checkpoint inhibitor immunotherapy.

IODINE DEFICIENCY

A 28-year-old M who recently emigrated from Haiti presents with symptoms of hypothyroidism. On **exam**, he has a goiter, with **labs** showing high TSH, low T4, and low urinary iodine levels.

4-4 Hypothyroidism

Management: Iodine supplementation.

Complications: Diffuse and nodular goiter.

HYF: Iodine is essential for thyroid hormone synthesis. Both insufficient and excessive iodine can result in thyroid disease. Iodine deficiency during pregnancy can cause congenital hypothyroidism in an infant.

TRANSIENT HYPOTHYROIDISM

A 47-year-old F with a history of URI 6 months ago followed by a painful thyroid gland and symptoms of hyperthyroidism now presents with symptoms of hypothyroidism and is found to have elevated TSH and low T4 on **labs**.

Management: Self-resolving. Treat with levothyroxine if symptomatic.

HYF: Transient hypothyroidism can follow many forms of thyroiditis, including postpartum (silent) thyroiditis or subacute thyroiditis (also called subacute granulomatous thyroiditis or de Quervain's thyroiditis, described in the vignette.)

*__Euthyroid sick syndrome/low T3 syndrome:__ An acutely sick patient is found to have low T3 due to decreased T4 → T3 conversion. Risk factors include severe illness (inflammatory cytokines) and certain medications (glucocorticoids). Thyroid function testing is unreliable in severe acute illness. Do not treat with levothyroxine; retest thyroid function once patient has returned to health.

4-5 Hyperthyroidism

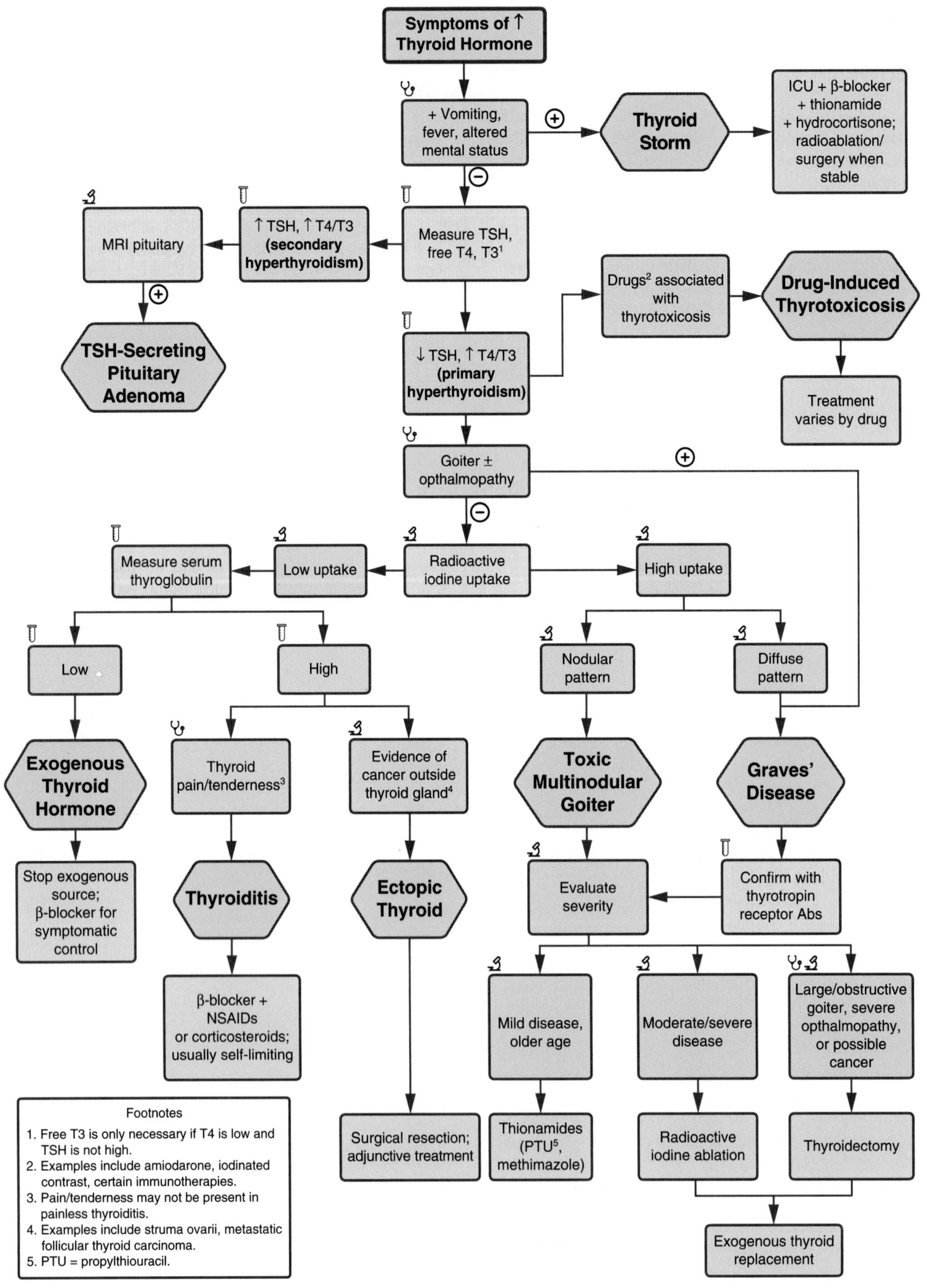

Symptoms of ↑ Thyroid Hormone
+ Vomiting, fever, altered mental status
Thyroid Storm
ICU + β-blocker + thionamide + hydrocortisone; radioablation/ surgery when stable
Measure TSH, free T4, T3[1]
↑ TSH, ↑ T4/T3 (secondary hyperthyroidism)
MRI pituitary
TSH-Secreting Pituitary Adenoma
↓ TSH, ↑ T4/T3 (primary hyperthyroidism)
Drugs[2] associated with thyrotoxicosis
Drug-Induced Thyrotoxicosis
Treatment varies by drug
Goiter ± opthalmopathy
Radioactive iodine uptake
Low uptake
Measure serum thyroglobulin
Low
Exogenous Thyroid Hormone
Stop exogenous source; β-blocker for symptomatic control
High
Thyroid pain/tenderness[3]
Thyroiditis
β-blocker + NSAIDs or corticosteroids; usually self-limiting
Evidence of cancer outside thyroid gland[4]
Ectopic Thyroid
Surgical resection; adjunctive treatment
High uptake
Nodular pattern
Toxic Multinodular Goiter
Diffuse pattern
Graves' Disease
Confirm with thyrotropin receptor Abs
Evaluate severity
Mild disease, older age
Thionamides (PTU[5], methimazole)
Moderate/severe disease
Radioactive iodine ablation
Large/obstructive goiter, severe opthalmopathy, or possible cancer
Thyroidectomy
Exogenous thyroid replacement
Footnotes
1. Free T3 is only necessary if T4 is low and TSH is not high.
2. Examples include amiodarone, iodinated contrast, certain immunotherapies.
3. Pain/tenderness may not be present in painless thyroiditis.
4. Examples include struma ovarii, metastatic follicular thyroid carcinoma.
5. PTU = propylthiouracil.

FIGURE 4.5

4-5 Hyperthyroidism

Common presenting symptoms of hyperthyroidism include heat intolerance, diaphoresis, muscle weakness/atrophy, anxiety, palpitations, weight loss, decreased appetite, lid lag, tremor, and hyperreflexia. Complications can include the following:

- Cardiovascular: HTN, arrhythmias (eg, Afib), high-output heart failure.
- Metabolic: Hypercalcemia, osteoporosis.
- Thyroid storm: Severe diaphoresis, vomiting, diarrhea, fever, altered mental status. Can be triggered by iodine load (eg, IV contrast) or stress (eg, infection, trauma). Treat with β-blockers (symptom control), thionamides (inhibit hormone synthesis), followed by iodine solution (inhibit hormone release) and glucocorticoids (inhibit conversion from T4 → T3).
- In the elderly, it can present atypically with depression, fatigue, malaise.

EXOGENOUS THYROID HORMONE

A 43-year-old M with PMH of obesity, hypothyroidism, and depression treated with levothyroxine presents with diaphoresis, tachycardia, and proximal muscle weakness. **Labs** show high T4, low TSH, and low serum thyroglobulin.

Management:

1. Stop exogenous source.
2. β-blockers (for symptom relief).

Complications: Thyroid storm.

HYF: Also known as "factitious hyperthyroidism." Can occur with over-prescription or accidental overdose.

TOXIC MULTINODULAR GOITER

A 72-year-old F presents with weight loss, palpitations, and diarrhea. On **exam**, she has diaphoresis, hyperreflexia, and tremor. **Labs/imaging** show high T4, low TSH, and high radioactive iodine uptake on scintigraphy with a nodular uptake pattern.

Management:

1. β-blockers (for symptoms relief).
2. Radioiodine ablation.
3. Thionamides (methimazole, propylthiouracil).
4. Thyroidectomy.

Complications: Thyroid storm.

HYF: Second most common cause of thyrotoxicosis. More common in areas without iodine fortification programs. May be called toxic adenoma if solitary nodule is present. Pathophysiology: Often results from iodine deficiency prompting increased TSH production and areas of thyroid hypertrophy, forming autonomous, hyperactive nodules.

GRAVES' DISEASE

A 32-year-old F with PMH of T1DM and SLE presents with weight loss, heat intolerance, and proximal muscle weakness. On **exam**, she has goiter and ophthalmopathy. **Labs** show high T4, low TSH, and thyrotropin receptor antibodies.

Management:

1. β-blockers (for symptom relief).
2. Thionamides (methimazole, propylthiouracil).
3. Radioiodine ablation (avoid if thyroid eye disease as it can get worse).
4. Thyroidectomy.

Complications:

- Thyroid storm, fetal hyperthyroidism.
- Thionamides cause agranulocytosis. Methimazole causes cholestasis and is a 1st-trimester teratogen. PPU causes liver failure and ANCA-associated vasculitis.
- Thyroidectomy is associated with risk of recurrent laryngeal nerve damage and hypoparathyroidism.

HYF: Most common cause of thyrotoxicosis. Exophthalmos (due to T-cell stimulation of orbital fibroblasts by thyrotropin receptor antibodies), pretibial myxedema, and thyroid bruits may also be distinguishing features on physical exam. Pathophysiology: Autoimmune thyroid-stimulating immunoglobulin binds to TSH receptors in thyroid and stimulates thyroid hormone production.

SUBACUTE (DE QUERVAIN'S) THYROIDITIS

A 33-year-old F with PMH of recent URI symptoms presents with fever. On **exam**, she has tender, enlarged thyroid. **Labs/imaging** show high T4, low TSH, high ESR/CRP, low radioactive iodine uptake on scintigraphy, and high serum thyroglobulin.

Management:

1. β-blockers (for symptom relief), NSAIDs (for pain).
2. Oral glucocorticoids.

Complications:

- Thyroid storm.
- Hypothyroid state 4–6 weeks after onset.

HYF: Many possible causes, including autoimmune (most common), infectious/subacute granulomatous, radiation-induced, drug-induced, and postpartum. Usually self-limiting. Pathophysiology: Transient, post-viral thyroid gland inflammation releases pre-formed thyroid hormone.

DRUG-INDUCED THYROTOXICOSIS

A 68-year-old F with PMH of atrial fibrillation treated with amiodarone presents with new palpitations, decreased appetite, and insomnia. On **exam**, she has tachycardia. **Labs** show elevated T4, low TSH, and elevated liver transaminases.

(Continued)

4-5 Hyperthyroidism

Management:

1. Stop offending agent.
2. Thionamides (methimazole, propylthiouracil) or oral glucocorticoids.
3. If refractory: Thyroidectomy.

Complications:

- Amiodarone: Hepatocellular injury, arrhythmias, neuropathy, pneumonitis, skin discoloration.
- Thyroid storm.

HYF: Amiodarone is the most common offending agent (amiodarone-induced thyrotoxicosis type 1: ↑ thyroid hormone synthesis with nodular thyroid disease or latent Graves' disease; amiodarone-induced thyrotoxicosis type 2: destructive thyroiditis causes release of pre-formed thyroid hormone). Other drugs associated with thyrotoxicosis include lithium, certain immunotherapies (IFN-alpha, IL-2, PD-1 inhibitors), and iodinated contrast.

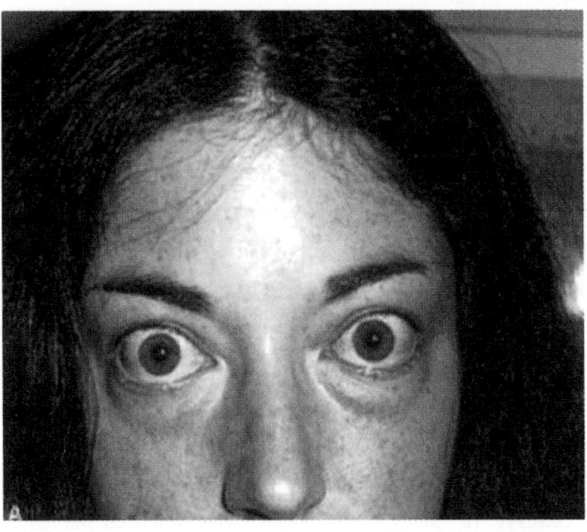

Thyroid eye disease in a patient with Graves' disease.

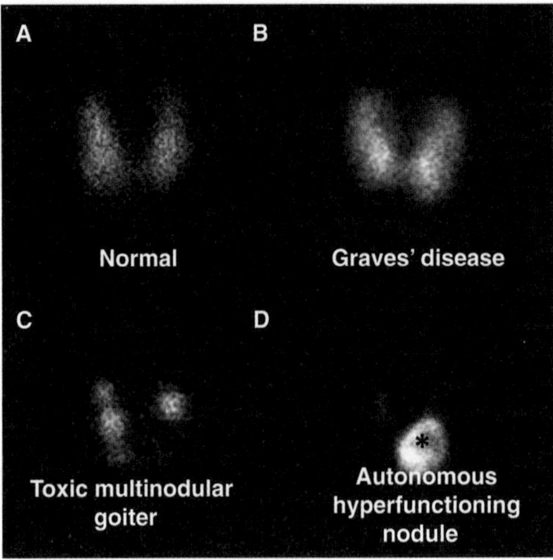
A
B
Normal
Graves' disease
C
D
Toxic multinodular goiter
*
Autonomous hyperfunctioning nodule

Radioactive iodine uptake test (RAIU) findings.

ECTOPIC THYROID

A 47-year-old F presents with fever, bloating, decreased appetite, and heat intolerance. She has a mass on bimanual exam. **Labs/imaging** show high T4, low TSH, and unilateral mass on pelvis US.

Management:

1. Struma ovarii: Surgical resection.
2. Metastatic follicular cancer: Radioactive iodine, radiation, surgery.

Complications: Thyroid storm, metastatic disease. Pathophysiology: Caused by either struma ovarii (ovarian teratoma) or metastatic follicular thyroid cancer.

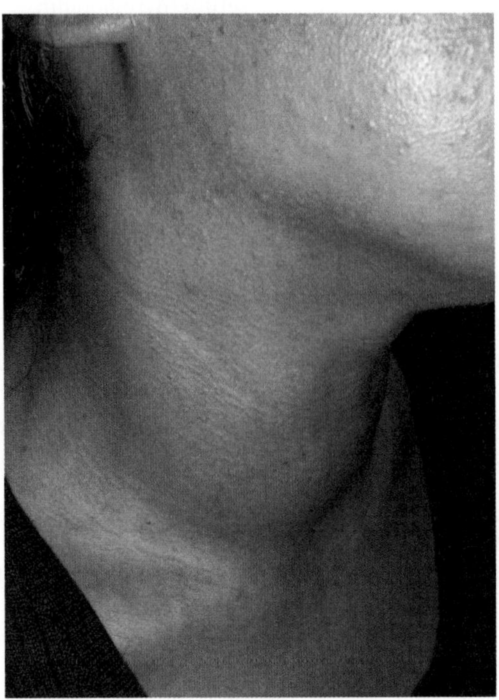

Goiter.

4-6 Thyroid Malignancies

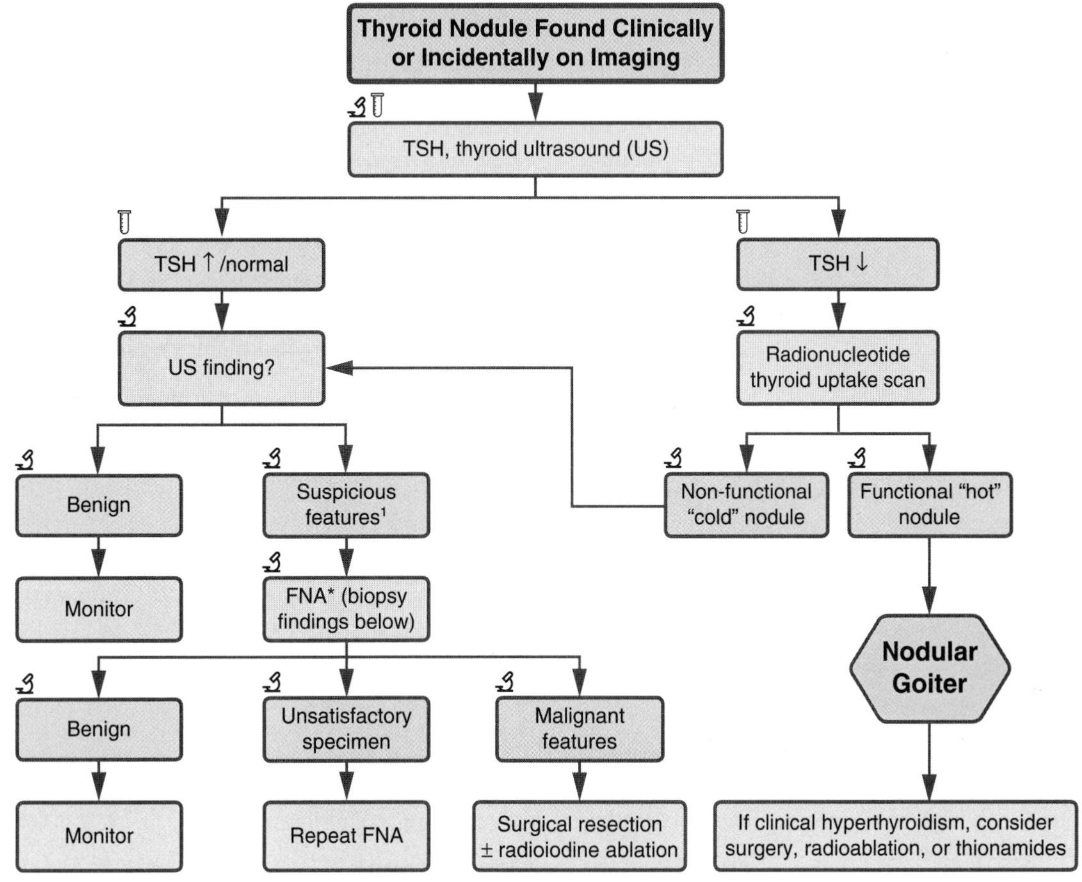
Thyroid Nodule Found Clinically or Incidentally on Imaging
TSH, thyroid ultrasound (US)
TSH ↑ /normal
TSH ↓
US finding?
Radionucleotide thyroid uptake scan
Benign
Suspicious features[1]
Non-functional "cold" nodule
Functional "hot" nodule
Monitor
FNA* (biopsy findings below)
Nodular Goiter
Benign
Unsatisfactory specimen
Malignant features
Monitor
Repeat FNA
Surgical resection ± radioiodine ablation
If clinical hyperthyroidism, consider surgery, radioablation, or thionamides

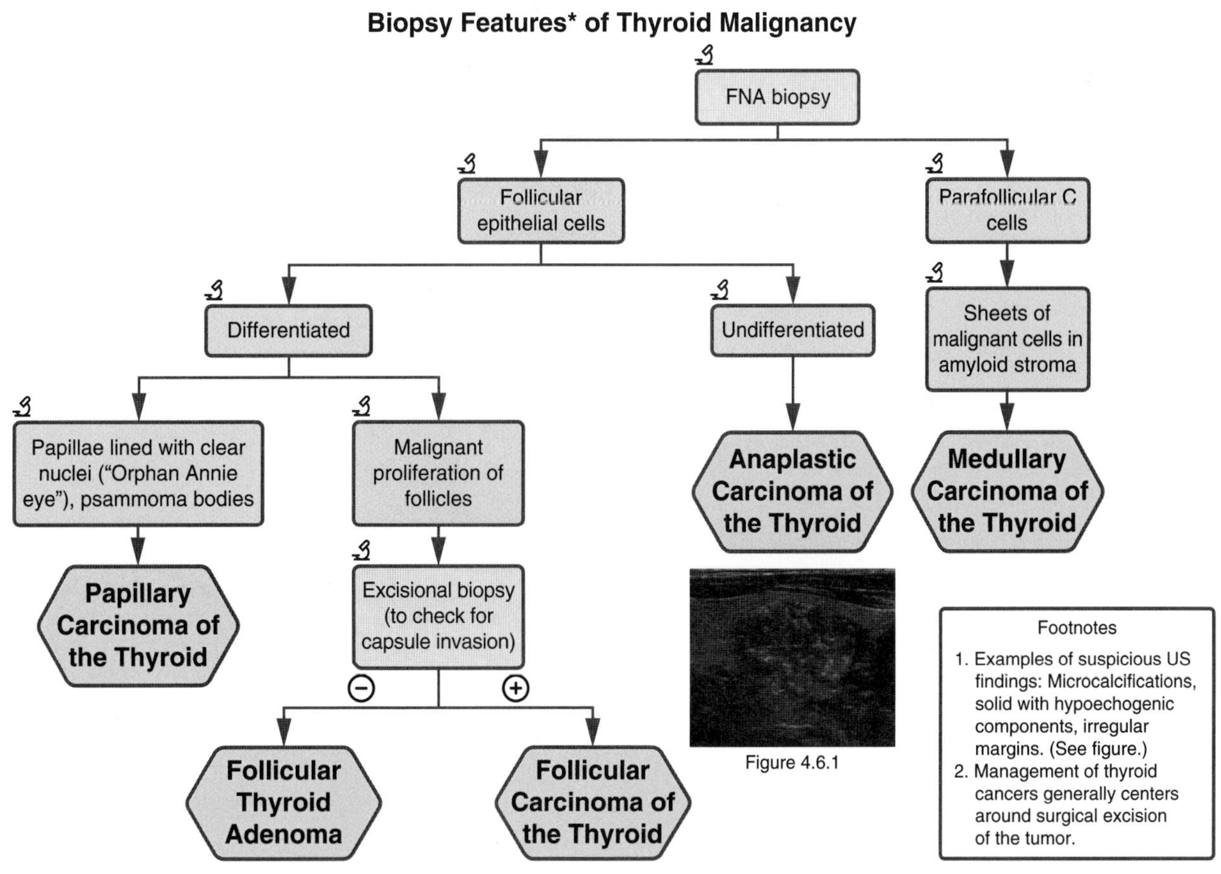
Biopsy Features* of Thyroid Malignancy
FNA biopsy
Follicular epithelial cells
Parafollicular C cells
Differentiated
Undifferentiated
Sheets of malignant cells in amyloid stroma
Papillae lined with clear nuclei ("Orphan Annie eye"), psammoma bodies
Malignant proliferation of follicles
Anaplastic Carcinoma of the Thyroid
Medullary Carcinoma of the Thyroid
Papillary Carcinoma of the Thyroid
Excisional biopsy (to check for capsule invasion)
⊖
⊕
Follicular Thyroid Adenoma
Follicular Carcinoma of the Thyroid

Figure 4.6.1

Footnotes

1. Examples of suspicious US findings: Microcalcifications, solid with hypoechogenic components, irregular margins. (See figure.)
2. Management of thyroid cancers generally centers around surgical excision of the tumor.

FIGURE 4.6

4-6 Thyroid Malignancies

PAPILLARY CARCINOMA

A patient with a PMH of leukemia treated with radiation presents with a small bump on the neck. On **exam**, the patient has a firm, fixed, non-tender nodule in the right thyroid lobe with cervical lymphadenopathy. **Labs/imaging** show elevated thyroglobulin, cold nodule on scintigraphy, and >2 cm hypoechogenic nodule with microcalcifications and irregular border on US.

Management:

1. Surgical resection with total thyroidectomy or unilateral lobectomy + lymph node dissection.
2. Radioiodine ablation.
3. Chemotherapy/radiotherapy.
4. Levothyroxine (if needed).

Complications: Metastasis, post-thyroidectomy hypothyroidism, SEs of radioactive iodine (sialadenitis, xerostomia, pulmonary fibrosis).

HYF:

- A major risk factor is ionizing radiation in childhood.
- Commonly associated mutations: *BRAF, RET*.
- Has an excellent prognosis: >95% 10-year survival rate.
- Metastasis through lymphatics causes cervical lymphadenopathy.
- TSH stimulates growth of occult residual tissue and metastatic disease. Individuals with high risk of recurrence need levothyroxine to suppress TSH secretion.
- In patients with total thyroidectomies, evaluate for cancer recurrence by measuring thyroglobulin levels after giving recombinant TSH or stopping levothyroxine (to increase thyroglobulin release from any residual cancer cells).
- PSaMmoma bodies (Papillary Carcinoma, Serous Cystadenoma, Meningioma) present in biopsy.

FOLLICULAR CARCINOMA

A patient presents with bone pain and a small bump on the neck with no lymphadenopathy. **Labs/imaging** show elevated thyroglobulin and microcalcifications of the nodule on US. Excisional biopsy shows extension of follicular cells beyond a fibrous capsule.

Management:

1. Surgical resection with total thyroidectomy or unilateral lobectomy.
2. Radioiodine therapy.
3. Chemotherapy/radiotherapy.
4. Levothyroxine (if needed).

Complications: Metastasis, post-thyroidectomy hypothyroidism.

HYF:

- Follicular carcinoma cannot be diagnosed on FNA alone! FNA only looks at cell morphology and does not analyze the capsule; diagnosis requires excisional biopsy to differentiate from follicular adenoma.
- Hematogenous metastasis (brain, lung, bone, liver).
- Give levothyroxine to patients with high risk of recurrence to suppress TSH secretion. Evaluate for cancer recurrence by measuring thyroglobulin levels.

ANAPLASTIC CARCINOMA

An elderly patient presents with progressive dysphagia and a bump on her anterior neck. Her history is notable for untreated papillary carcinoma of the thyroid. On **imaging**, US reveals a poorly demarcated solid mass with microcalcifications.

Management:

1. Surgery followed by chemotherapy and radiation.
2. Thyroid hormone replacement therapy to prevent hypothyroidism.
3. If unresectable, targeted therapy + chemoradiation.

Complications: Poor prognosis, locally invasive and rapidly enlarging. Can cause dyspnea, dysphagia. Post-thyroidectomy hypothyroidism.

HYF:

- Many patients with anaplastic thyroid cancer have a history of differentiated thyroid cancer. Commonly seen in elderly patients.

MEDULLARY CARCINOMA

A patient with PMH of severe HTN and severe pounding headaches presents with a small bump on the anterior neck. Physical **exam** reveals long arms and a tall stature. FNA biopsy is positive for calcitonin.

Management:

1. Surgical resection with total thyroidectomy.
   a. Thyroid hormone replacement therapy to prevent hypothyroidism.
   b. Calcitonin and CEA are useful biomarkers to measure post-surgery.

Complications: Metastasis, persistent hypercalcitoninemia, dyspnea, dysphagia, post-thyroidectomy hypothyroidism.

HYF:

- Neuroendocrine tumor of parafollicular C cells associated with MEN 2A and 2B (mutation in *RET* gene on chr. 10).
- Screen for pheochromocytoma prior to surgery to prevent hypertensive crisis during surgery; check urine VMA and metanephrine.

Nodular Goiter: See p. 141.

Clinical Features in Multiple Endocrine Neoplasia (MEN) Syndromes

MEN 1	MEN 2A	MEN 2B
Pituitary Adenoma		**Mucosal Neuromas & Marfanoid Habitus**
Parathyroid Hyperplasia	**Parathyroid Hyperplasia**	
	Medullary Thyroid Carcinoma	**Medullary Thyroid Carcinoma**
	Pheochromocytoma	**Pheochromocytoma**
Pancreatic Tumors		
MEN 1: 3 P's	**MEN 2A: 2 P's 1 M**	**MEN 2B: 2 M's 1 P**

4-7 Bone Mineral Disorders

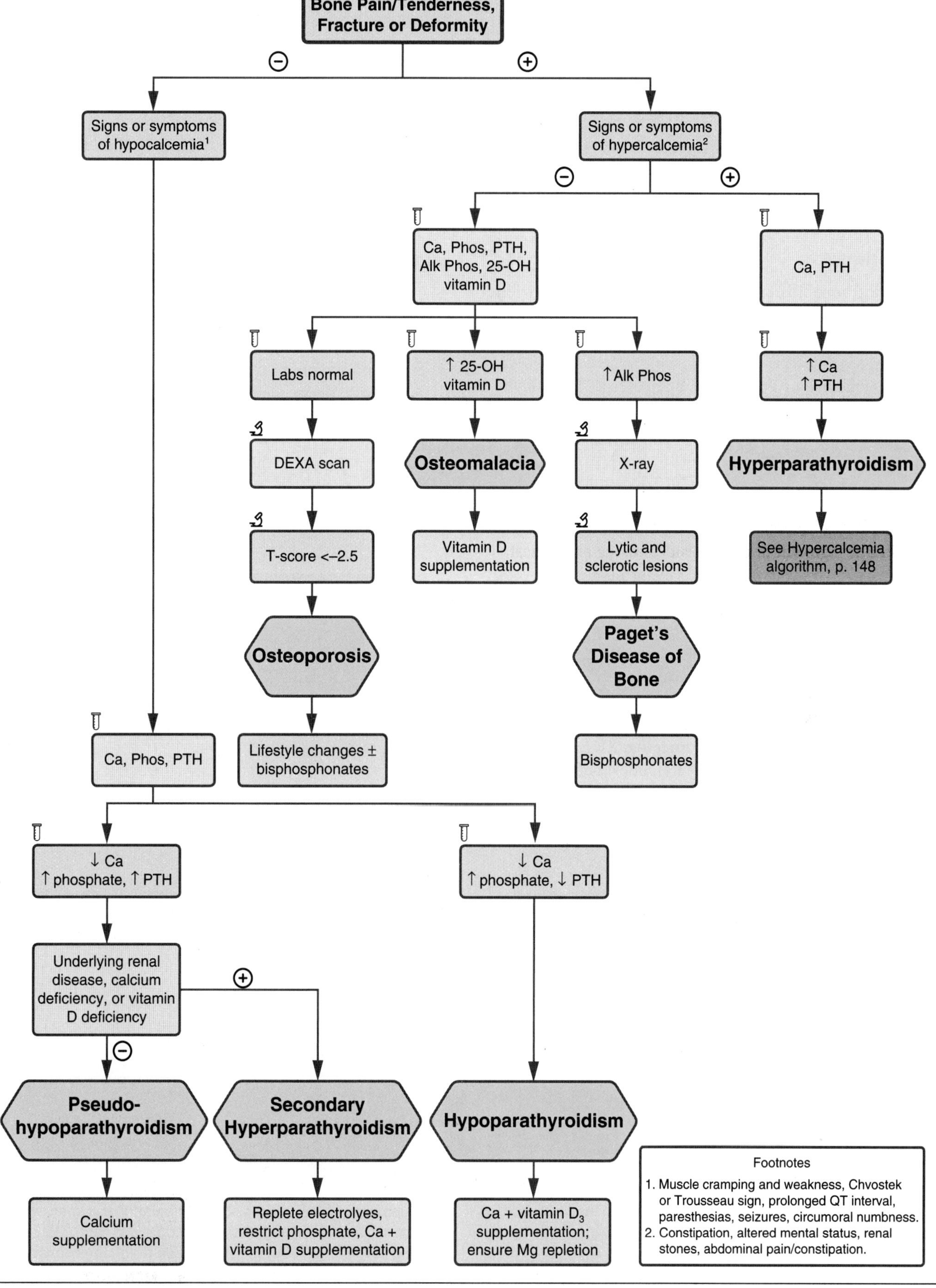
Bone Pain/Tenderness, Fracture or Deformity
⊖
⊕
Signs or symptoms of hypocalcemia[1]
Signs or symptoms of hypercalcemia[2]
⊖
⊕
Ca, Phos, PTH, Alk Phos, 25-OH vitamin D
Ca, PTH
Labs normal
↑ 25-OH vitamin D
↑ Alk Phos
↑ Ca ↑ PTH
DEXA scan
Osteomalacia
X-ray
Hyperparathyroidism
T-score <–2.5
Vitamin D supplementation
Lytic and sclerotic lesions
See Hypercalcemia algorithm, p. 148
Osteoporosis
Paget's Disease of Bone
Ca, Phos, PTH
Lifestyle changes ± bisphosphonates
Bisphosphonates
↓ Ca ↑ phosphate, ↑ PTH
↓ Ca ↑ phosphate, ↓ PTH
Underlying renal disease, calcium deficiency, or vitamin D deficiency
⊕
⊖
Pseudo-hypoparathyroidism
Secondary Hyperparathyroidism
Hypoparathyroidism
Calcium supplementation
Replete electrolyes, restrict phosphate, Ca + vitamin D supplementation
Ca + vitamin D_3 supplementation; ensure Mg repletion
Footnotes
1. Muscle cramping and weakness, Chvostek or Trousseau sign, prolonged QT interval, paresthesias, seizures, circumoral numbness.
2. Constipation, altered mental status, renal stones, abdominal pain/constipation.

FIGURE 4.7

4-7 Bone Mineral Disorders

OSTEOPOROSIS

A 72-year-old F with PMH of GERD and a 60-pack-year smoking history presents after a ground-level fall with severe hip pain. On **imaging**, X-ray shows a femoral neck fracture.

Management:

1. Lifestyle changes (weight-bearing exercise, smoking cessation) + calcium and vitamin D supplementation.
2. Bisphosphonates (inhibit osteoclasts).
3. Raloxifene (post-menopausal women).

Complications:

- Pathological bone fractures, especially at hip joint and in vertebral bodies.

HYF:

- Due to imbalance of the normal homeostasis: Breakdown > formation.
- RFs: Post-menopause (most significant), age, gender (F > M), smoking, ethnicity (white or Asian), ↓ BMI, hypothalamic amenorrhea, sedentary lifestyle, poor calcium and vitamin D intake, medications (steroids, PPI), rheumatoid arthritis.
- Screening DEXA scan for F > 65 (T-score < −2.5 means osteoporosis, T-score −1 to −2.5 means osteopenia).
- Raloxifene = selective estrogen receptor modulator. Associated with ↑ risk of VTE. Discontinue several weeks before any surgery with ↑ risk of VTE (eg, orthopedic surgery).

OSTEOMALACIA

A 65-year-old presents with generalized body pain, especially at the back and hips. On **exam**, the patient has a waddling gait. **Labs** show ↓ Ca and phosphate and ↑ PTH. On **imaging**, XR femur shows ↓ bone density with cortical thinning and pseudo-fractures.

Management: Supplement vitamin D.

Complications: Pathological bone fractures.

HYF:

- Inadequate calcium or phosphorus → ↓ mineralization of osteoid → weak bones.
- Vitamin D deficiency in children = rickets (growth plates present), in adults = osteomalacia.
- Causes: Vitamin D deficiency, malabsorption (celiac disease, gastric bypass), RTA type 2, CKD.
- Labs variable depending on etiology: ↓ Ca and phosphate if vitamin D deficiency, ↑ PTH (2° hyperparathyroidism), ↑ ALPs.

PAGET'S DISEASE OF BONE

A 65-year-old M presents with complaints of hearing loss and that his hats no longer fit. **Exam** shows frontal bossing and various cranial nerve deficits. **Labs** reveal ↑ ALP, P1NP, and c-telopeptide but normal calcium, phosphate, and PTH. On **imaging**, XR shows lytic + blastic lesions. Radionuclide bone scan shows focal ↑ uptake.

Management: Bisphosphonates (inhibit osteoclasts)—for every patient, even if ALP is normal.

Complications:

- Bone fracture.
- Osteosarcoma.
- Skull/cranial bones involved: Hearing loss, headache, cranial neuropathy, skull shape changes (frontal bossing).
- High-output heart failure.
- Spinal stenosis.

HYF:

- Osteoblast and osteoclast dysfunction→ ↑ bone turnover and abnormal remodeling → enlargement, fracture, bowing.
- Labs: ↑ ALP. Usually normal phos, Ca, PTH
- Signs and symptoms of Paget's disease of bone: PANICS (Pain, Arthralgia, Nerve compression/Neural deafness, Increased bone density, Cardiac failure, Skull involvement/Sclerotic vertebra.

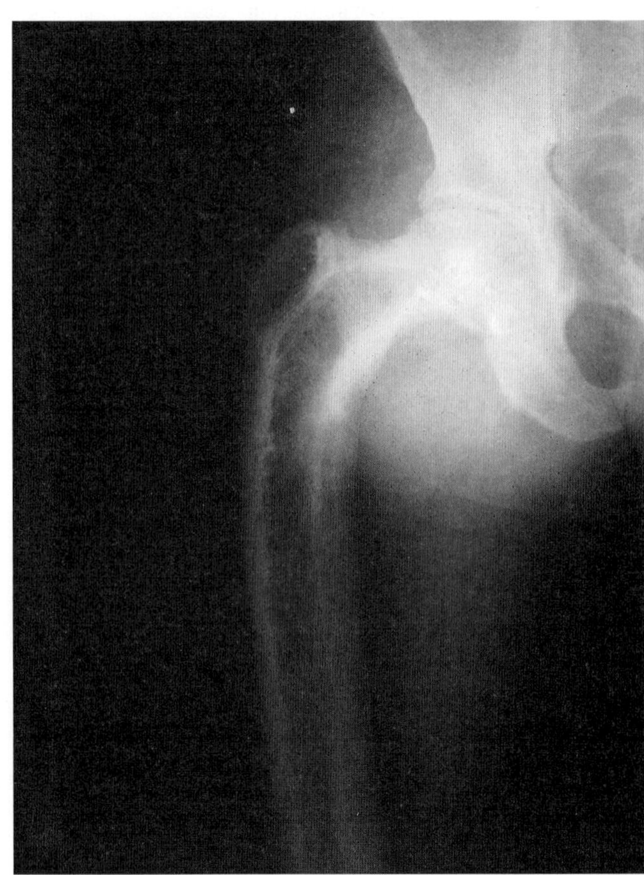

Right proximal femur and pelvis radiograph of a man with Paget's disease of bone involving both the femur and ilium. Note the lateral bowing of the femur with the stress fractures on the convex side of the femur.

4-7 Bone Mineral Disorders

HYPOPARATHYROIDISM

A 55-year-old with PMH of thyroid cancer presents a few weeks after thyroidectomy with muscle cramping and is found to have Chvostek and Trousseau signs on **exam**. **Labs** show ↓ PTH, ↑ phosphate, and ↓ calcium.

Management:

1. Supplement calcium (oral or IV) + vitamin D_3.
2. Recombinant PTH.

Complications: Hypocalcemia → tetany, seizure, arrhythmias (usually preceded by prolonged QT).

HYF:

- Labs: ↓ PTH, ↑ phosphate, ↓ Ca.
- Causes: Surgery (thyroidectomy) most common, genetic (DiGeorge's syndrome), autoimmune destruction, Wilson's disease, hemochromatosis, defective calcium-sensing receptor (*CaSR* gene).
- Hypomagnesemia can cause ↓PTH, leading to hypocalcemia. Replete magensium if low.

Pseudohypoparathyroidism: See p. 153.

SECONDARY HYPERPARATHYROIDISM

A 53-year-old M with PMH of autosomal dominant polycystic kidney disease on routine hemodialysis (eGFR 8 mL/min) is found to have hypocalcemia (8.9), phos (4.9), PTH (303.1), and vitamin D (16) on routine **labs**. On **imaging**, X-ray shows subperiosteal bone resorption, cysts, and osteopenia.

Management:

1. Calcium supplementation; treat hyperphosphatemia (dietary phosphate restriction, phosphate binders); correct vitamin D deficiency, lower PTH levels (calcimimetics, calcitriol, or synthetic vitamin D analogs).
2. If PTH levels are refractory to treatment without causing hyperphosphatemia or hypercalcemia or treatment is not tolerable (ie, nausea), subtotal (preferred, due to less risk of permanent hypoparathyroidism) or total parathyroidectomy with autograft may be considered.
3. If surgery, IV calcium immediately post-operatively, followed by vitamin D and OTC calcium supplementation.

Complications: Primary hyperparathyroidism symptoms (see p. 149). Refractory symptoms commonly include pruritus, anemia, fatigue, bone/joint pain (renal osteodystrophy), fractures, or calciphylaxis.

HYF:

- Pathophysiology: Secondary hyperplasia due to decreased Ca absorption and/or increased phosphate.
- Etiologies include chronic renal failure (hypovitaminosis D and hyperphosphatemia, decreased Ca), vitamin D deficiency, and low Ca intake.
- Renal osteodystrophy (high serum phos binds with Ca → tissue deposits → decreases serum Ca and 25-vitamin D → decreases intestinal Ca absorption → subperiosteal thinning of bones).
- Given expected hyperplasia, the role of localization studies is limited.

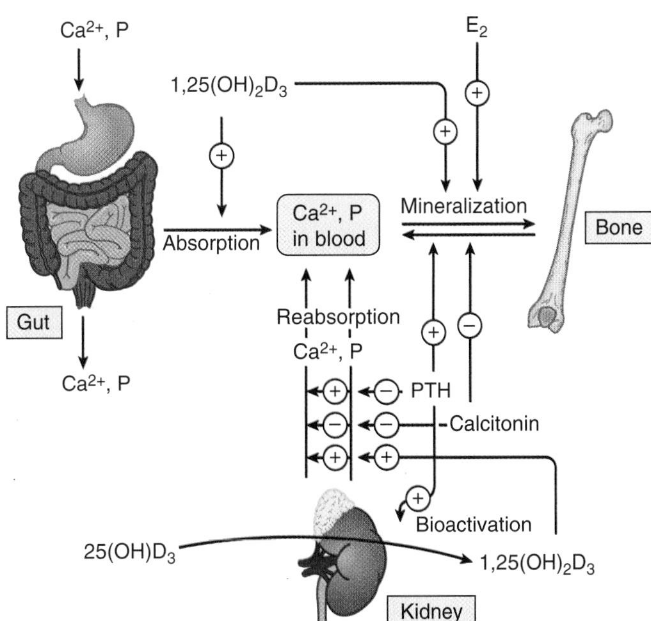

Ca^{2+}, P
E_2
$1,25(OH)_2D_3$
Mineralization
Absorption
Ca^{2+}, P in blood
Bone
Gut
Reabsorption
Ca^{2+}, P
Ca^{2+}, P
PTH
Calcitonin
Bioactivation
$25(OH)D_3$
$1,25(OH)_2D_3$
Kidney

Control of blood calcium and phosphate levels. Overview of the regulation of calcium (Ca^2) and phosphate (P) levels by the coordinated actions of active vitamin D [$1,25(OH)_2D_3$], parathyroid hormone (PTH), calcitonin, and estradiol (E_2).

4-8 Hypercalcemia

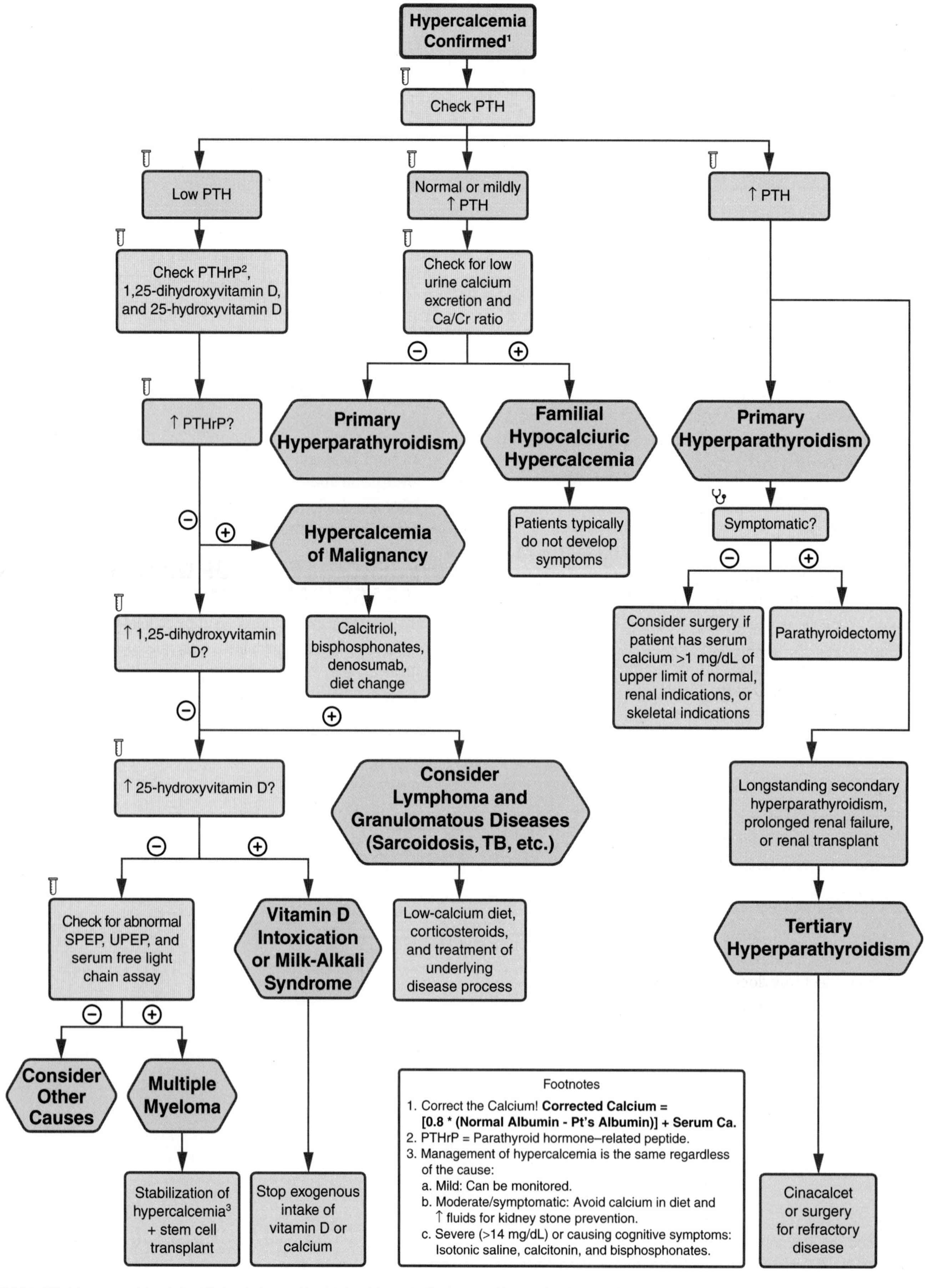

Hypercalcemia Confirmed[1]
Check PTH
Low PTH
Normal or mildly ↑ PTH
↑ PTH
Check PTHrP[2], 1,25-dihydroxyvitamin D, and 25-hydroxyvitamin D
Check for low urine calcium excretion and Ca/Cr ratio
↑ PTHrP?
Primary Hyperparathyroidism
Familial Hypocalciuric Hypercalcemia
Primary Hyperparathyroidism
Hypercalcemia of Malignancy
Patients typically do not develop symptoms
Symptomatic?
↑ 1,25-dihydroxyvitamin D?
Calcitriol, bisphosphonates, denosumab, diet change
Consider surgery if patient has serum calcium >1 mg/dL of upper limit of normal, renal indications, or skeletal indications
Parathyroidectomy
↑ 25-hydroxyvitamin D?
Consider Lymphoma and Granulomatous Diseases (Sarcoidosis, TB, etc.)
Longstanding secondary hyperparathyroidism, prolonged renal failure, or renal transplant
Check for abnormal SPEP, UPEP, and serum free light chain assay
Vitamin D Intoxication or Milk-Alkali Syndrome
Low-calcium diet, corticosteroids, and treatment of underlying disease process
Tertiary Hyperparathyroidism
Consider Other Causes
Multiple Myeloma
Stabilization of hypercalcemia[3] + stem cell transplant
Stop exogenous intake of vitamin D or calcium
Cinacalcet or surgery for refractory disease

Footnotes

1. Correct the Calcium! **Corrected Calcium = [0.8 * (Normal Albumin - Pt's Albumin)] + Serum Ca.**
2. PTHrP = Parathyroid hormone–related peptide.
3. Management of hypercalcemia is the same regardless of the cause:
   a. Mild: Can be monitored.
   b. Moderate/symptomatic: Avoid calcium in diet and ↑ fluids for kidney stone prevention.
   c. Severe (>14 mg/dL) or causing cognitive symptoms: Isotonic saline, calcitonin, and bisphosphonates.

FIGURE 4.8

4-8 Hypercalcemia

PRIMARY HYPERPARATHYROIDISM (HPTH)

A patient with PMH of nephrolithiasis and anxiety presents with fatigue, constipation, and diffuse body aches. **Exam** is unremarkable. **Labs** show hypercalcemia, hypophosphatemia, and significantly elevated PTH. 24-hour urinary calcium excretion is elevated. On **imaging**, US and Tc99m-sestamibi scan show a parathyroid adenoma.

Management:

1. Manage acute hypercalcemia: IV fluids, loop diuretics.
2. If symptomatic or at high risk of complications from hypercalcemia, ENT referral for parathyroidectomy.
   a. For those unable to get surgery, bisphosphonates and cinacalcet are options.
3. If asymptomatic, monitoring is recommended. Surgery is indicated in patients with signs of skeletal and renal damage.

Complications: Osteoporosis, nephrolithiasis, constipation, PUD, pseudogout, acute pancreatitis, hypertension, arrhythmias.

HYF: HPTH most commonly presents with nephrolithiasis, osteoporosis, constipation, and neuropsychiatric symptoms ("stones, bones, abdominal groans, psychiatric overtones"). PTH may be ↑ or inappropriately normal in the setting of hypercalcemia. Most commonly due to parathyroid adenoma but can be due to multi-gland parathyroid hyperplasia (eg, in CKD) or parathyroid carcinoma. Associated with MEN 1 and 2A. Hypocalcemia is a complication after parathyroidectomy; treat with calcium gluconate. Differentiate from secondary parahyperthyroidism (see p. 147), which is associated with hypocalcemia.

FAMILIAL HYPOCALCIURIC HYPERCALCEMIA (FHH)

A teenage patient presents for a well child visit and has no complaints. **Exam** is unremarkable, but **labs** reveal hypercalcemia, normal PTH, and low urine calcium excretion.

Management:

1. If there are no complications, no treatment is indicated.
2. If there are complications from hypercalcemia:
   a. Parathyroidectomy does not cure this disorder but can reduce risk of other sequelae of hypercalcemia.
   b. Screen family members to prevent unnecessary surgery.

Complications: Rare pancreatitis, chondrocalcinosis.

HYF: FHH is a benign autosomal dominant disorder caused by a mutation of the calcium-sensing receptor (*CaSR*).

HUMORAL HYPERCALCEMIA OF MALIGNANCY

An elderly patient with several months of worsening fatigue and unintentional weight loss presents with difficulty urinating. **Exam** reveals a focally enlarged prostate. **Labs** show hypercalcemia, low PTH, and elevated PSA and PTHrP.

Management:

1. Manage the primary malignancy.
2. Limit dietary calcium. Supplement with IV fluids as needed.
3. Bisphosphonates and denosumab are 1st-line therapy.

Complications: Usually presents with the common symptoms of hypercalcemia, alongside the symptoms associated with the primary malignancy.

Signs and Symptoms of Hypercalcemia:

- **Bones:** Bone pain, osteoporosis, osteitis fibrosa cystica
- **Stones:** Kidney stones
- **Abdominal Groans:** Constipation, pancreatitis, PUD
- **Psychiatric Overtones:** Lethargy, weakness, confusion

HYF: Humoral (PTHrP-mediated) hypercalcemia of malignancy is the most common cause of PTH-independent hypercalcemia. Associated with squamous ("sCa++mous") cell carcinoma (eg, lung, renal). Other causes of PTH-independent hypercalcemia in malignancy: Osteolytic bone metastases (evaluate with bone scan), ↑ 1,25-dihydroxyvitamin D production (eg, lymphoma), and ↑ IL-6 levels (eg, multiple myeloma).

HYPERCALCEMIA OF GRANULOMATOUS DISEASE (SARCOIDOSIS)

A young female presents with worsening dyspnea and cough. **Exam** is notable for elevated blood pressure and painful shin nodules. **Labs** show an elevated calcium and serum ACE. On **imaging**, CXR shows hilar lymphadenopathy with bilateral reticular opacities.

Management:

1. Glucocorticoids and management of underlying disease process.
2. Dietary calcium restriction; stop vitamin D supplementation.

Complications: Uncontrolled sarcoidosis can progress to involve other organ systems, but typically these episodes resolve spontaneously.

HYF: Any granulomatous syndrome can cause hypercalcemia-epithelioid histiocytes (macrophages) in granulomas to activate vitamin D. Steroids inhibit conversion to 1,25-dihydroxyvitamin D by activated macrophages but need 2–5 days to take effect.

TERTIARY HYPERPARATHYROIDISM

An elderly patient with PMH of type 2 diabetes and renal transplant presents with recurrent intermittent flank pain radiating to the groin. **Exam** is unremarkable. **Labs** show an elevated PTH, hypercalcemia, and hyperphosphatemia with a serum creatinine of 3.0.

Management:

1. Cinacalcet.
2. Consider parathyroidectomy for patients with refractory disease.

(Continued)

4-8 Hypercalcemia

Complications: Same as primary hyperparathyroidism and could lead to graft failure for transplant patients.

HYF: Chronic hypocalcemia due to untreated secondary hyperparathyroidism (eg, in CKD) causes parathyroid hyperplasia and autonomous PTH secretion → tertiary hyperparathyroidism.

MILK-ALKALI SYNDROME (MAS)/ VITAMIN D TOXICITY

A patient with osteoporosis and GERD who takes antacids and vitamins presents with kidney stones. **Exam** is unremarkable. **Labs** show hypercalcemia, hypophosphatemia, creatinine of 3.0 (baseline 1.0), metabolic alkalosis, and low PTH.

Management:

1. Stop exogenous intake of calcium, alkali (eg, calcium carbonate), and vitamin D.
2. Isotonic saline, then furosemide.

Complications: AKI, hypomagnesemia, complications of hypercalcemia

HYF: Hypercalcemia in MAS causes renal vasoconstriction and inhibition of Na-K-2Cl cotransporter → renal salt and water loss, ↑ bicarbonate reabsorption → AKI, metabolic alkalosis. Risk factors: CKD, thiazide diuretics, ACEi/ARBs, and NSAIDs.

MULTIPLE MYELOMA (MM)

A 65-year old patient with a PMH of multiple fractures and recurrent UTIs and pneumonia presents with worsening lower back pain, months of unintentional weight loss, neuropathy, and fatigue. **Exam** shows focal tenderness to palpation over his lower lumbar spine. **Labs** reveal hypercalcemia, anemia, elevated creatinine, elevated total serum protein, and a paraprotein gap. Peripheral blood smear shows stacks of RBCs in Rouleaux formation. SPEP shows an M-spike. UA shows proteinuria and granular casts. **Imaging** reveals multiple lytic lesions in the spine and other bones. Bone marrow biopsy reveals a large monoclonal plasma cell population.

Management:

1. Asymptomatic patients can be monitored; defer treatment until symptoms arise.
2. For symptomatic patients, stem cell transplant is the treatment of choice.
3. Supportive therapy:
   a. Bisphosphonates for bone pain.
   b. G-CSF and EPO for anemia.

Complications: Progression to renal failure, restrictive cardiomyopathy, and hypercalcemic crisis. MM can lead to secondary leukemia. Osteolytic spinal lesions can lead to spinal cord compression. Associated with cryoglobulinemia (type 1). Increased risk of infections (eg, UTIs) due to hypogammaglobulinemia and ineffective antibody production.

HYF: Multiple myeloma is a plasma cell dyscrasia that leads to large amounts of monoclonal IgG or IgA production. AKI is usually intrinsic due to ATN from obstruction of the tubules by casts consisting of Bence-Jones proteins (Ig light chains in urine). Nephrotic syndrome can result from damage of the monoclonal protein to the glomeruli.

4-8 Hypercalcemia

Disorders	Serum Calcium	Serum Phosphate	PTH	Urine Ca Excretion	PTHrP	1,25(OH)$_2$ Vitamin D	Manifestations
Primary hyperparathyroidism	↑	↓	↑	↑	N	↑	Kidney stones (hypercalciuria) Osteitis fibrosa cystica
Secondary hyperparathyroidism Chronic kidney disease Hypocalcemia Vitamin D deficiency	↓ or normal	↑ (if renal failure) or ↓ (other causes)	↑		N	↓	Renal osteodystrophy osteomalacia
Tertiary hyperparathyroidism	↑	↑	↑↑	↑	N	↓	Renal osteodystrophy
Familial hypocalciuric hypocalcemia	↑	↓	N	↓	N	↑	
Hypercalcemia of malignancy	↑	↓	↓	↑	↑/N	↑/N	
Granulomatous disease	↑	↑	↓	↑	N	↑↑↑	
Milk-alkali syndrome/vitamin D toxicity	↑	↑	↓	↑	N	↑	
Multiple myeloma	↑	↑	↓	↑	N	↓	

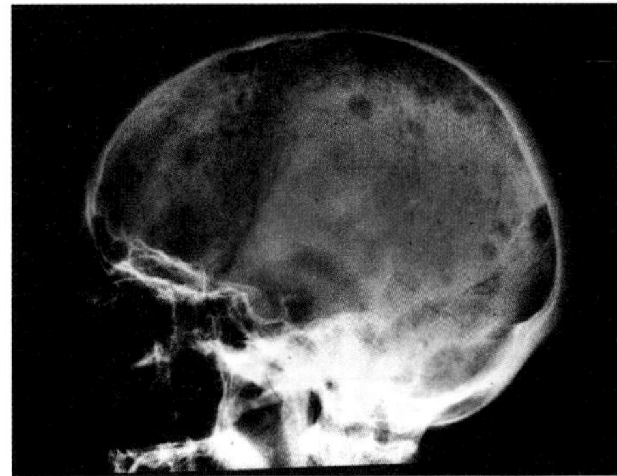

Lytic lesions in the skull of a patient with multiple myeloma.

4-9 Hypocalcemia

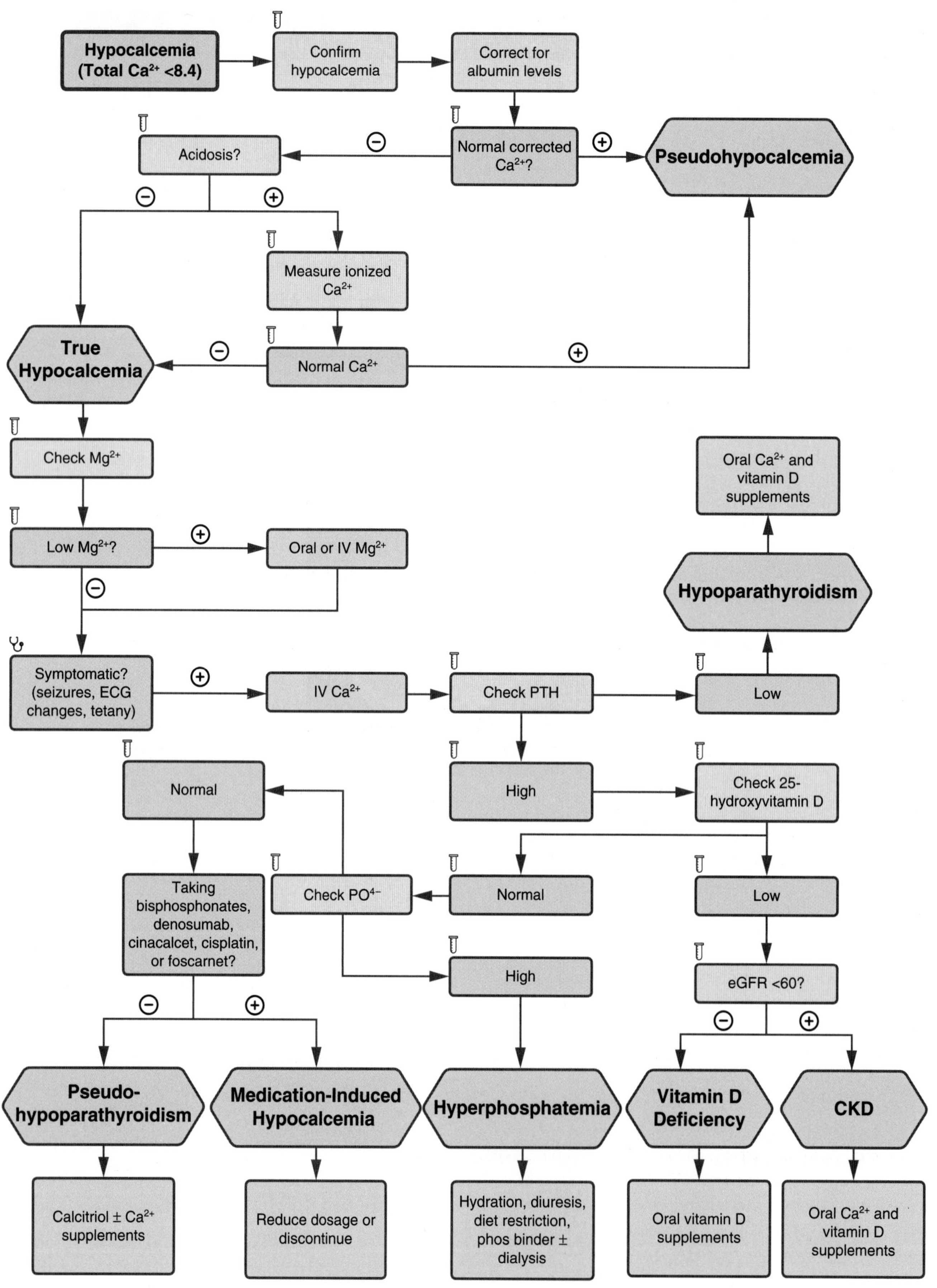

Hypocalcemia (Total Ca2+ <8.4)
Confirm hypocalcemia
Correct for albumin levels
Normal corrected Ca2+?
Pseudohypocalcemia
Acidosis?
Measure ionized Ca2+
Normal Ca2+
True Hypocalcemia
Check Mg2+
Low Mg2+?
Oral or IV Mg2+
Symptomatic? (seizures, ECG changes, tetany)
IV Ca2+
Check PTH
Low
Hypoparathyroidism
Oral Ca2+ and vitamin D supplements
High
Check 25-hydroxyvitamin D
Normal
Check PO4−
Normal
Taking bisphosphonates, denosumab, cinacalcet, cisplatin, or foscarnet?
High
Low
eGFR <60?
Pseudo-hypoparathyroidism
Medication-Induced Hypocalcemia
Hyperphosphatemia
Vitamin D Deficiency
CKD
Calcitriol ± Ca2+ supplements
Reduce dosage or discontinue
Hydration, diuresis, diet restriction, phos binder ± dialysis
Oral vitamin D supplements
Oral Ca2+ and vitamin D supplements

FIGURE 4.9

4-9 Hypocalcemia

PSEUDOHYPOCALCEMIA

A 32-year-old M with no PMH is admitted for minimal change disease. On exam, he has significant edema. Labs show total Ca 7.0 with albumin 1.5.

Management: Correct [Ca^{2+}] for hypoalbuminemia using Payne's formula: Corrected calcium (mg/dL) = measured total Ca (mg/dL) + 0.8 (4.0 – serum albumin [g/dL]), where 4.0 represents the average albumin level.

Complications: Inappropriate calcium repletion if hypoalbuminemia is not accounted for.

HYF: Serum calcium is mostly bound to albumin, so low serum albumin causes a reduction in measured calcium levels.

HYPOPARATHYROIDISM

A 55-year-old F with PMH of MEN2 is postoperative day 1 from a thyroidectomy, now reporting ipsilateral twitching of mouth upon tapping the right buccal region of the face (Chvostek sign) and carpal spasm after arterial occlusion by a BP cuff (Trousseau sign). Labs show a serum calcium level of 6.5 and PO_4^- of 6.0.

Management:

1. Acute setting: IV calcium repletion, vitamin D supplementation.
2. Long-term: Oral calcium and vitamin D supplements.

Complications: Seizures and arrhythmias if calcium is not properly repleted.

HYF: May be a transient or permanent symptom of neck surgery.

PSEUDOHYPOPARATHYROIDISM

A 21-year-old M with no PMH presents for a physical for a new job. Routine labs indicate serum calcium of 7.0 and PO_4^- of 6.0. Follow-up labs demonstrate a high PTH and normal vitamin D. The patient takes no dietary supplements or medications.

Management:

1. Oral Ca^{2+} and vitamin D supplements.
2. Aim to keep patient in low range of normal calcium.
3. Assess 24-hour urine [Ca^{2+}] to preclude renal calculi development.

Complications: Renal calculi and CKD if unmanaged.

HYF: Very rare (less than 1 per 100,000 individuals). Due to hereditary PTH resistance. PTH levels are increased but ineffective at target organs, leading to hypocalcemia and hyperphosphatemia. Associated with Albright's hereditary osteodystrophy (autosomal dominant, maternal imprinting): Shortened 4th/5th metatarsal or metacarpal bones, short stature, obesity, developmental delay.

MEDICATION-INDUCED HYPOCALCEMIA

A 75-year-old F with PMH of osteoporosis on risedronate and denosumab presents for follow-up. Patient has often forgotten to take her vitamin D and calcium supplements. Labs reveal a calcium of 7.2.

Management: Restart vitamin D and Ca^{2+} supplements.

Complications: Worsening of osteoporosis. Increased risk of long-bone fractures.

HYF: Bisphosphonates and denosumab inhibit osteoclasts, thus preventing bone resorption and release of calcium into systemic circulation. Other notable medications that can induce hypocalcemia are foscarnet, cisplatin, and cinacalcet.

HYPERPHOSPHATEMIA

A 66-year-old F with PMH of T2DM, HTN, HPL, CKD (GFR <30) presents at a nephrology outpatient clinic for CKD workup. Labs reveal a Ca of 6.7 and a PO_4^- of 6.0.

Management:

1. Dietary restriction, phosphate binders, sevelamer.
2. Peritoneal or hemodialysis.

Complications: Ectopic calcification and worsening of hypocalcemia.

HYF: Most commonly found in ESRD patients since their kidneys are unable to excrete phosphate. The phosphate binds with Ca to form complexes that are deposited throughout the body. If Ca * PO_4 >55, high risk of ectopic calcification and mortality.

VITAMIN D DEFICIENCY

A 56-year-old with no relevant PMH presents for routine follow-up. Labs show a Ca of 7.2. Further testing demonstrates an elevated PTH level and low vitamin D levels. Patient notably works night shifts in Boston.

Management: Vitamin D supplements.

Complications: Tiredness, muscle aches, depression, bone loss → rickets; 2° hyperparathyroidism.

HYF: Vitamin D increases intestinal absorption of calcium, magnesium, and phosphate. Vitamin D deficiency causes hypocalcemia → secondary hyperparathyroidism → phosphaturia and bone demineralization → rickets in children and osteomalacia in children and adults.

*In infants with hypocalcemia, consider DiGeorge syndrome.

4-10 Adrenal Insufficiency

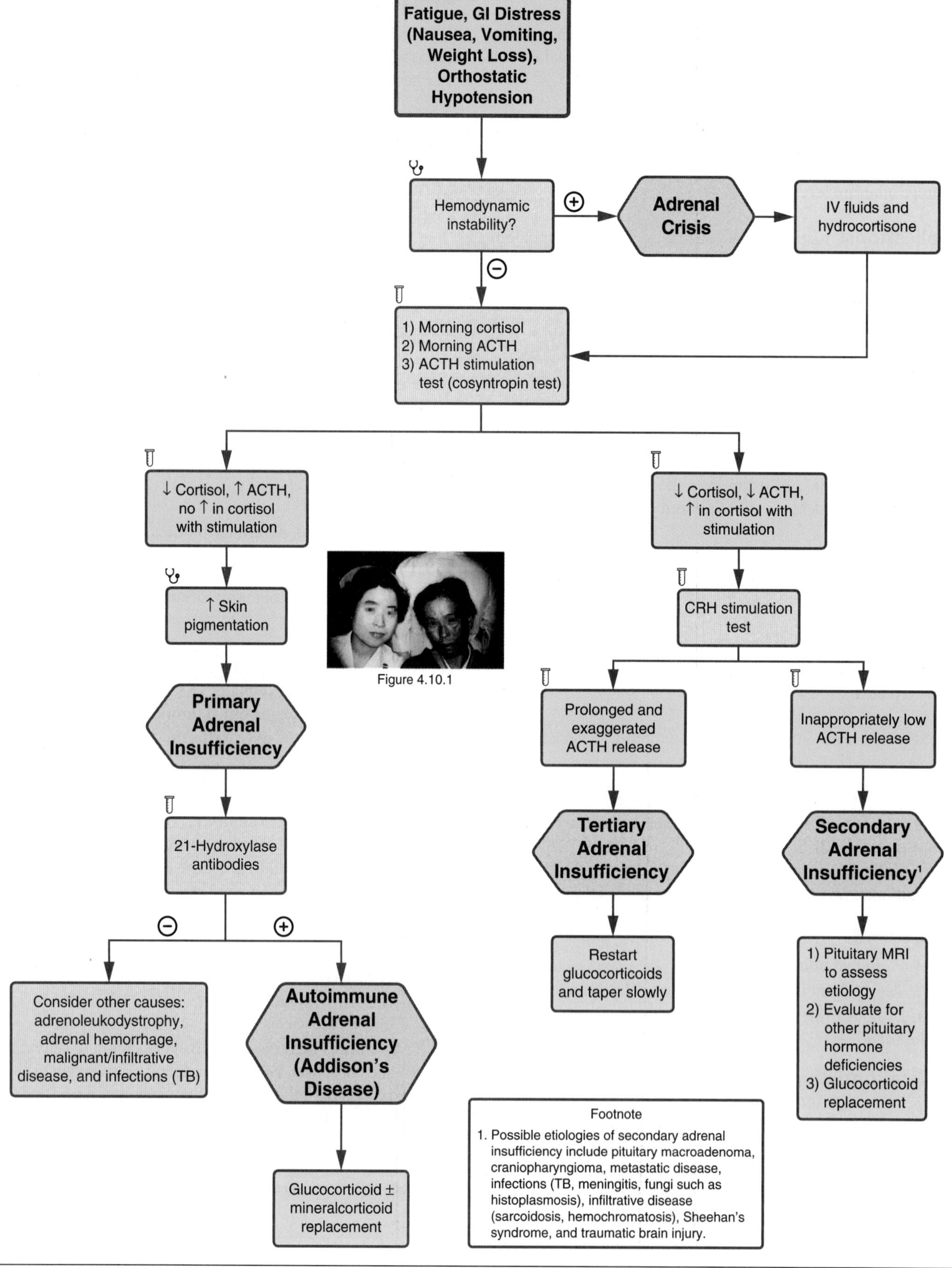
Fatigue, GI Distress (Nausea, Vomiting, Weight Loss), Orthostatic Hypotension
Hemodynamic instability?
Adrenal Crisis
IV fluids and hydrocortisone
1) Morning cortisol
2) Morning ACTH
3) ACTH stimulation test (cosyntropin test)
↓ Cortisol, ↑ ACTH, no ↑ in cortisol with stimulation
↑ Skin pigmentation
Primary Adrenal Insufficiency
21-Hydroxylase antibodies
Consider other causes: adrenoleukodystrophy, adrenal hemorrhage, malignant/infiltrative disease, and infections (TB)
Autoimmune Adrenal Insufficiency (Addison's Disease)
Glucocorticoid ± mineralcorticoid replacement
Figure 4.10.1
↓ Cortisol, ↓ ACTH, ↑ in cortisol with stimulation
CRH stimulation test
Prolonged and exaggerated ACTH release
Tertiary Adrenal Insufficiency
Restart glucocorticoids and taper slowly
Inappropriately low ACTH release
Secondary Adrenal Insufficiency[1]
1) Pituitary MRI to assess etiology
2) Evaluate for other pituitary hormone deficiencies
3) Glucocorticoid replacement
Footnote
1. Possible etiologies of secondary adrenal insufficiency include pituitary macroadenoma, craniopharyngioma, metastatic disease, infections (TB, meningitis, fungi such as histoplasmosis), infiltrative disease (sarcoidosis, hemochromatosis), Sheehan's syndrome, and traumatic brain injury.

FIGURE 4.10

4-10 Adrenal Insufficiency

PRIMARY ADRENAL INSUFFICIENCY (ADDISON'S DISEASE)

A 30-year-old F presents with chronic, progressive fatigue, chronic diarrhea, and 6 months of weight loss, and is now hypotensive after an appendectomy. On **exam**, she has hyperpigmentation. **Labs** shows hyponatremia, hyperkalemia, normal anion gap metabolic acidosis, ↓ 8 am cortisol, and ↑ ACTH. After receiving high-dose cosyntropin, basal cortisol remains low.

Management:

1. Hydrocortisone (glucocorticoid replacement) and fludrocortisone (mineralocorticoid replacement).
2. Androgen replacement.
3. ↑ Steroid dose in times of stress (eg, surgery).

Complications: Typically apparent during periods of stress (eg, surgery, trauma, infections).

- Shock, possibly without preceding hypotension.
- Seizure.
- Coma, death.
- Hyponatremia, hyperkalemia (not present in secondary AI).

HYF: Most common etiologies are autoimmune adrenalitis (in developed countries) and TB (in developing countries). Use presence of hyperpigmentation and hyperkalemia to distinguish from central AI.

ACUTE ADRENAL CRISIS (WATERHOUSE-FRIDERICHSEN SYNDROME)

A 15-year-old F with PMH of sickle cell disease presents with fever, abdominal pain, nausea, vomiting, and headache. On **exam**, she has severe hypotension, neck stiffness, and diffuse non-blanching petechial rash. **Labs** show ↓ cortisol, hypoglycemia, and hyponatremia, as well as acute anemia and thrombocytopenia.

Management:

1. Aggressive IV fluids to treat hypotension, manage hyponatremia, and treat hypoglycemia.
2. IV hydrocortisone (stress doses).
3. Treat underlying cause (antibiotics for meningococcemia).

Complications:

- Survivors may require chronic mineralocorticoid and glucocorticoid replacement.

HYF: Acute adrenal crisis is classically caused by bilateral adrenal hemorrhage from coagulopathy in *Neisseria* meningitis (Waterhouse-Friderichsen syndrome). Acute adrenal crisis can also be precipitated by abrupt withdrawal of chronic steroids or after surgical cure for Cushing's syndrome.

PROLACTINOMA

A 31-year-old F with PMH of irregular periods presents with headaches and reduced libido. On **exam**, she has bitemporal hemianopsia. **Labs/imaging** show ↑ prolactin, ↓ cortisol that remains low even after cosyntropin administration, ↓ ACTH, and >1 cm enhancing mass in the sella turcica on MRI with contrast.

Management:

1. Treat with dopamine agonist to inhibit prolactin production and reduce mass size over time (cabergoline is first-line; bromocriptine is preferred in pregnancy).
2. Monitor prolactin and mass size with MRI.
3. Consider transsphenoidal surgery if size, symptoms, and/or prolactin levels are unresponsive to high-dose dopamine agonists mostly needed in macroadenomas (>1 cm).

Complications:

- Visual impairment.
- Infertility.
- Osteoporosis.

HYF: Prolactinomas are the most common pituitary adenoma and may present with 2° adrenal insufficiency. Galactorrhea is seen in most premenopausal patients but usually not in postmenopausal patients. If concurrent central hypothyroidism, start hydrocortisone before levothyroxine as the increase in glucocorticoid metabolism induced by levothyroxine can precipitate adrenal crisis. Consider MEN1 syndrome in patients with pituitary adenoma, especially if early onset.

SHEEHAN'S SYNDROME

A 25-year-old F who is 6 weeks postpartum presents with fatigue, weakness, and inability to produce milk. She had an unremarkable pregnancy but suffered severe blood loss during delivery and required blood transfusions. She has not been able to produce milk. On **exam**, her BP is 88/64 and HR 85. On labs, she has low serum cortisol and plasma ACTH levels, as well as low TSH, LH, and FSH. On **imaging**, brain MRI reveals an empty sella turcica.

Management:

1. Hormone replacement therapy based on pattern of hormone deficiency (eg, hydrocortisone for glucocorticoid replacement, fludrocortisone for mineralocorticoid replacement, levothyroxine for thyroid hormone replacement).

Complications: Related to hormone deficiencies (eg, secondary adrenal insufficiency, hypothyroidism, hypogonadism).

HYF: Severe hemorrhage during childbirth leads to infarction and necrosis of the anterior pituitary gland. Damage to the pituitary can vary, affecting one to several or all pituitary hormones (panhypopituitarism). Sheehan's syndrome classically presents with failure to lactate postpartum (prolactin deficiency), hypotension (secondary adrenal insufficiency), and amenorrhea (hypogonadotropic hypogonadism).

(*Continued*)

4-10 Adrenal Insufficiency

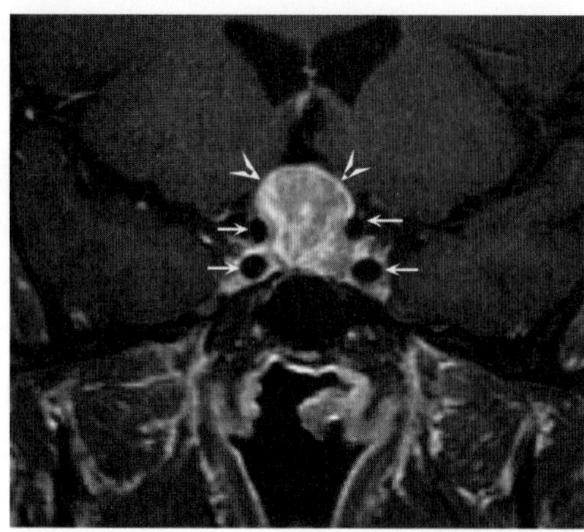

Pituitary adenoma. MRI shows a homogeneously enhancing mass (arrowheads) in the sella turcica and suprasellar region; the small arrows outline the carotid arteries.

GLUCOCORTICOID WITHDRAWAL (2°/3° ADRENAL INSUFFICIENCY)

A 56-year-old F with PMH of rheumatoid arthritis, who recently completed 4-week treatment of high-dose prednisone for recent flare, presents with fatigue, nausea, vomiting, and myalgia. On **exam**, she has Cushingoid features. **Labs** show ↓ cortisol that remains low even after cosyntropin administration, ↓ ACTH, normal aldosterone, and hypoglycemia.

Management:

1. Hydrocortisone (glucocorticoid replacement).
2. Slow taper of glucocorticoids.

Complications: Adrenal crisis (treatment: hydrocortisone or dexamethasone), death.

HYF: Most common cause of 2° adrenal insufficiency. Preserved mineralocorticoid function. Etomidate can precipitate acute adrenal crisis by inhibiting 11-beta-hydroxylase.

- ACTH stimulation test can fail due to the chronicity of the central AI leading to atrophic adrenal glands and suboptimal response to stimulation test.

4-11 Cushing's Syndrome

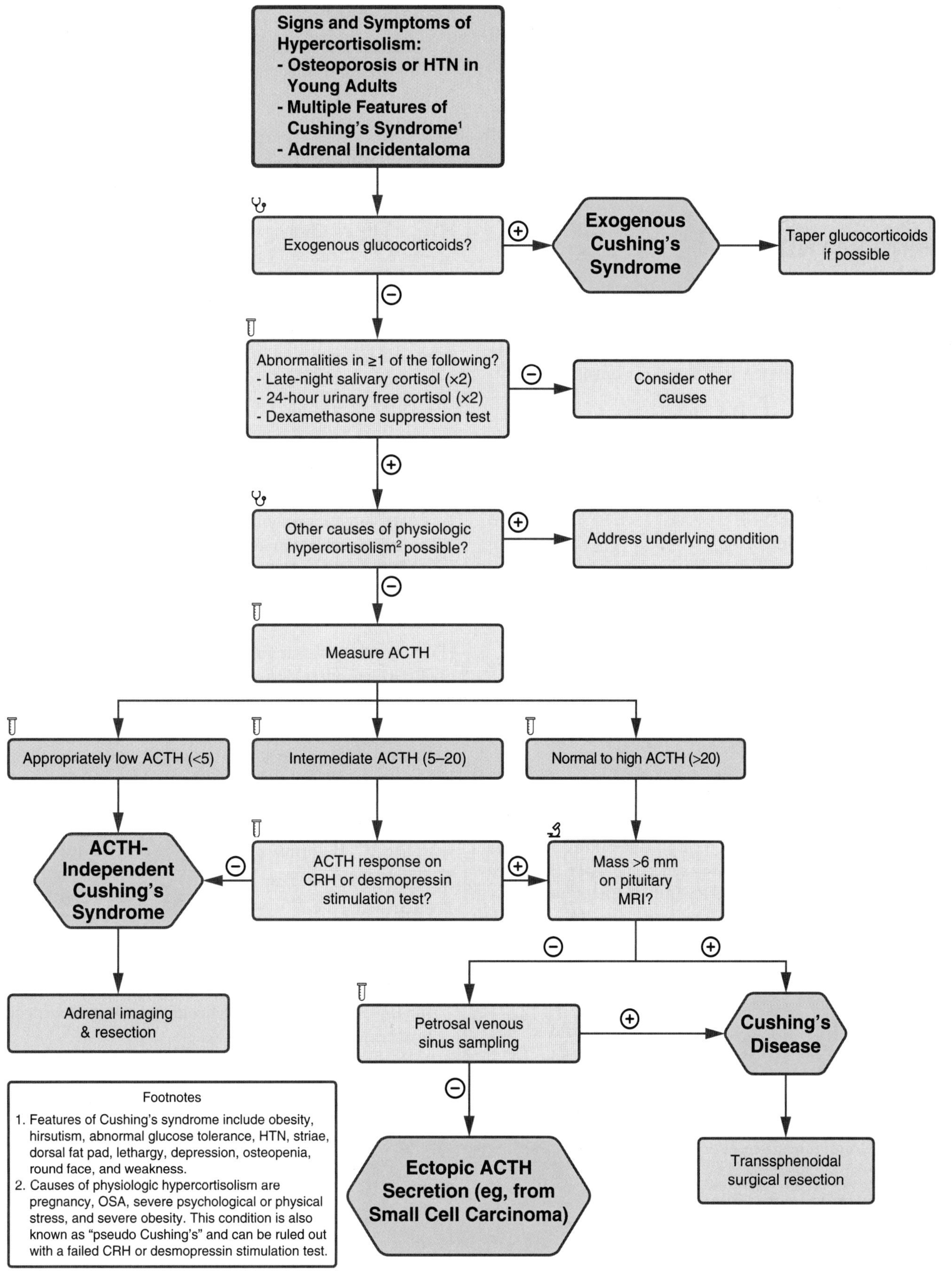
Signs and Symptoms of Hypercortisolism:
- Osteoporosis or HTN in Young Adults
- Multiple Features of Cushing's Syndrome[1]
- Adrenal Incidentaloma
Exogenous glucocorticoids?
Exogenous Cushing's Syndrome
Taper glucocorticoids if possible
Abnormalities in ≥1 of the following?
- Late-night salivary cortisol (×2)
- 24-hour urinary free cortisol (×2)
- Dexamethasone suppression test
Consider other causes
Other causes of physiologic hypercortisolism[2] possible?
Address underlying condition
Measure ACTH
Appropriately low ACTH (<5)
Intermediate ACTH (5–20)
Normal to high ACTH (>20)
ACTH-Independent Cushing's Syndrome
ACTH response on CRH or desmopressin stimulation test?
Mass >6 mm on pituitary MRI?
Adrenal imaging & resection
Petrosal venous sinus sampling
Cushing's Disease
Ectopic ACTH Secretion (eg, from Small Cell Carcinoma)
Transsphenoidal surgical resection
Footnotes
1. Features of Cushing's syndrome include obesity, hirsutism, abnormal glucose tolerance, HTN, striae, dorsal fat pad, lethargy, depression, osteopenia, round face, and weakness.
2. Causes of physiologic hypercortisolism are pregnancy, OSA, severe psychological or physical stress, and severe obesity. This condition is also known as "pseudo Cushing's" and can be ruled out with a failed CRH or desmopressin stimulation test.

FIGURE 4.11

4-11 Cushing's Syndrome

Cushing's syndrome represents a constellation of symptoms and signs resulting from chronic hypercortisolism. There are ACTH-independent (eg, adrenal adenoma) and ACTH-dependent causes (eg, ACTH-secreting pituitary tumor, ectopic ACTH secretion), with pituitary ACTH-dependent Cushing's syndrome referred to as Cushing's disease. All causes have similar clinical manifestations and complications, which are reviewed below. For cause-specific treatment recommendations and high-yield facts, refer to the individual sections.

CUSHING'S SYNDROME

A 50-year-old F with no PMH presents with oligomenorrhea, easy bruisability, weight gain most evident in the abdomen, proximal weakness, depression, and frequent colds. **Exam** shows hirsutism, abdominal striae, and new hypertension. **Labs** show new glucose intolerance. On **imaging**, DEXA scan shows osteopenia.

Treatment:

1. Until the underlying cause is addressed, treat manifestations like HTN and hyperglycemia as you would in any other patient.

Complications:

- Increased risk of infections.
- Sleep apnea.
- Glucocorticoid-induced myopathy.
- Fractures.

HYF: Though long-term exogenous glucocorticoid administration is associated with GI bleeding, cataracts, and leukocytosis, these are not common manifestations of endogenous Cushing's syndrome. ACTH-dependent Cushing's syndrome is associated with hyperpigmentation.

EXOGENOUS CUSHING'S SYNDROME

A 40-year-old F with PMH of SLE on chronic prednisone presents with signs and symptoms of Cushing's syndrome. **Labs** show elevated midnight salivary cortisol and low ACTH. Brain **imaging** is normal.

Treatment:

1. Taper glucocorticoids. Treat SLE with a steroid-sparing therapy.

Complications: Adrenal insufficiency if glucocorticoids are tapered too fast.

HYF: The most common cause of Cushing's syndrome is chronic use of exogenous glucocorticoids. Look for vignettes describing patients with autoimmune diseases on chronic steroids.

ACTH-INDEPENDENT CUSHING'S SYNDROME

A 45-year-old with no PMH presents with signs and symptoms of Cushing's syndrome. **Labs** show elevated midnight salivary cortisol and low ACTH. Adrenal **imaging** shows a left adrenal mass.

Management:

1. Unilateral adrenalectomy (adrenal adenoma) or bilateral adrenalectomy (bilateral adrenal hyperplasia).
2. Post-operative glucocorticoid therapy (ACTH and CRH have been suppressed).

Complications: High risk for post-op venous thromboembolism.

HYF: ~10% of Cushing's cases are due to benign adrenal adenomas. A small minority are due to bilateral adrenal hyperplasia or adrenal carcinomas.

ECTOPIC ACTH SECRETION

A 60-year-old with a 30-pack-year smoking history presents with signs and symptoms of Cushing's syndrome, as well as cough with hemoptysis. **Labs** show elevated 24-hour urinary cortisol and ACTH. After administration of high-dose dexamethasone, ACTH remains elevated. On **imaging**, CT chest shows a lung mass.

Treatment:

1. Tumor surgical excision and, if possible, chemotherapy.
2. For unresectable tumors, control hypercortisolism with enzyme inhibitors such as ketoconazole and metyrapone.

Complications: Complications related to primary tumors.

HYF: Neoplasms associated with ectopic ACTH secretion include small cell lung cancer, carcinoid tumors, and medullary thyroid cancer.

CUSHING'S DISEASE

A 30-year-old F presents with signs and symptoms of Cushing's syndrome, as well as headache and visual **exam** findings of bitemporal hemianopsia. **Labs** show hypokalemia and elevated midnight salivary cortisol and ACTH. After receiving high-dose dexamethasone, her ACTH normalizes. On **imaging,** MRI of the brain shows a pituitary mass.

Treatment:

1. Transsphenoidal pituitary surgery.
2. When surgery is delayed, contraindicated, or unsuccessful, use adrenal enzyme inhibitors ± bilateral adrenalectomy with subsequent lifelong glucocorticoid and mineralocorticoid replacement.

Complications:

- Hypopituitarism → infertility.
- Nelson's syndrome: Enlargement of ACTH-secreting pituitary adenoma and excess ACTH release after bilateral adrenalectomy.

HYF: Though pituitary ACTH-secreting tumors are somewhat resistant to negative feedback regulation, non-pituitary tumors are often *completely* resistant to regulation. Use the high-dose dexamethasone suppression test to distinguish between Cushing's disease and ectopic ACTH secretion. In response to high-dose dexamethasone, the pituitary will decrease secretion of ACTH, whereas an ectopic source will usually be unaffected.

4-11 Cushing's Syndrome

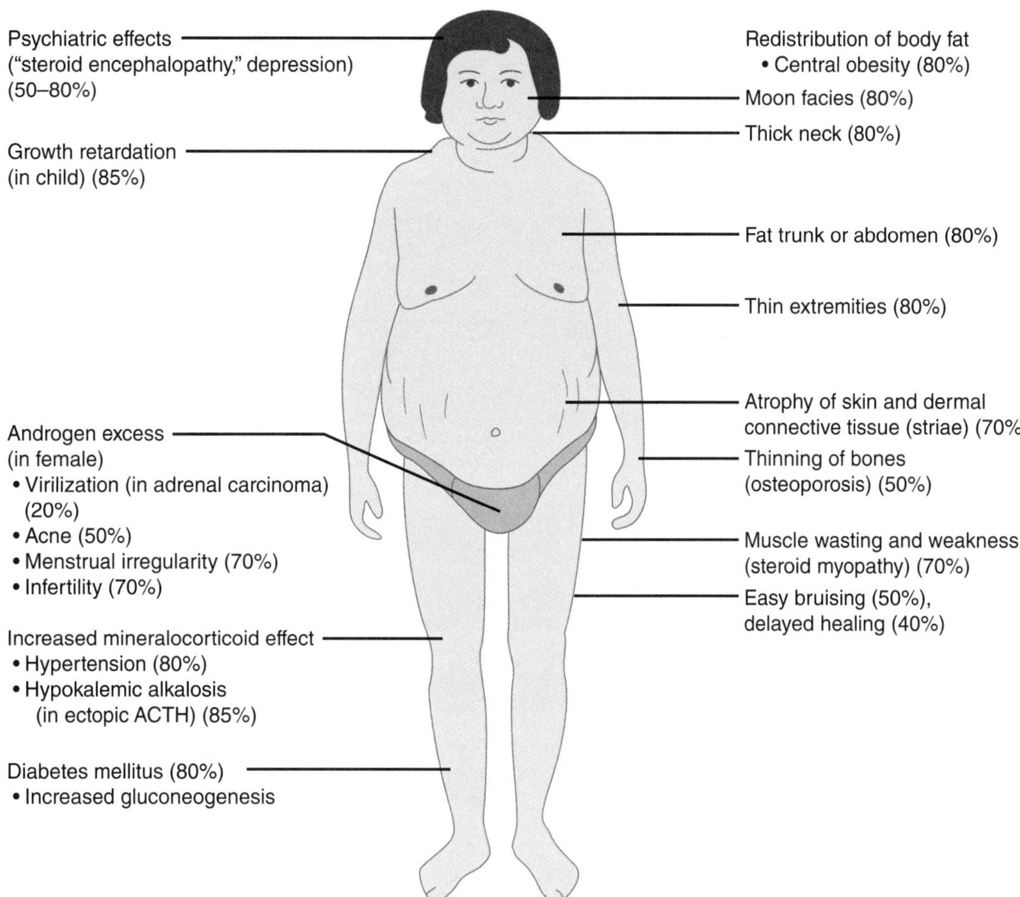
Psychiatric effects
("steroid encephalopathy," depression)
(50–80%)
Growth retardation
(in child) (85%)
Androgen excess
(in female)
• Virilization (in adrenal carcinoma)
(20%)
• Acne (50%)
• Menstrual irregularity (70%)
• Infertility (70%)
Increased mineralocorticoid effect
• Hypertension (80%)
• Hypokalemic alkalosis
(in ectopic ACTH) (85%)
Diabetes mellitus (80%)
• Increased gluconeogenesis
Redistribution of body fat
• Central obesity (80%)
Moon facies (80%)
Thick neck (80%)
Fat trunk or abdomen (80%)
Thin extremities (80%)
Atrophy of skin and dermal
connective tissue (striae) (70%)
Thinning of bones
(osteoporosis) (50%)
Muscle wasting and weakness
(steroid myopathy) (70%)
Easy bruising (50%),
delayed healing (40%)

Classic findings in Cushing's syndrome.

4-12 Etiologies of Secondary Hypertension

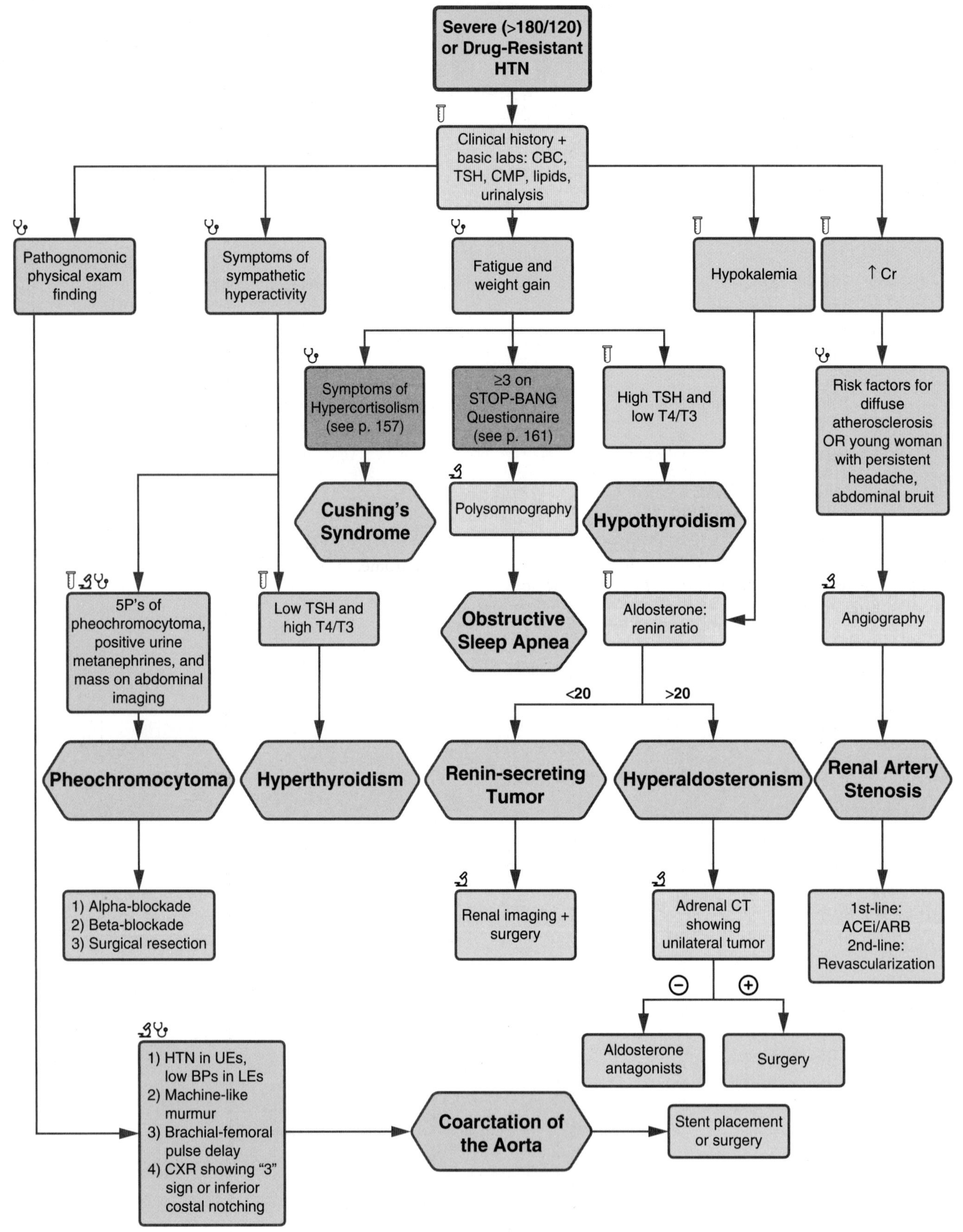
Severe (>180/120) or Drug-Resistant HTN
Clinical history + basic labs: CBC, TSH, CMP, lipids, urinalysis
Pathognomonic physical exam finding
Symptoms of sympathetic hyperactivity
Fatigue and weight gain
Hypokalemia
↑ Cr
Symptoms of Hypercortisolism (see p. 157)
≥3 on STOP-BANG Questionnaire (see p. 161)
High TSH and low T4/T3
Risk factors for diffuse atherosclerosis OR young woman with persistent headache, abdominal bruit
Cushing's Syndrome
Polysomnography
Hypothyroidism
5P's of pheochromocytoma, positive urine metanephrines, and mass on abdominal imaging
Low TSH and high T4/T3
Obstructive Sleep Apnea
Aldosterone: renin ratio
Angiography
<20
>20
Pheochromocytoma
Hyperthyroidism
Renin-secreting Tumor
Hyperaldosteronism
Renal Artery Stenosis
1) Alpha-blockade
2) Beta-blockade
3) Surgical resection
Renal imaging + surgery
Adrenal CT showing unilateral tumor
1st-line: ACEi/ARB
2nd-line: Revascularization
⊖
⊕
Aldosterone antagonists
Surgery
1) HTN in UEs, low BPs in LEs
2) Machine-like murmur
3) Brachial-femoral pulse delay
4) CXR showing "3" sign or inferior costal notching
Coarctation of the Aorta
Stent placement or surgery

FIGURE 4.12

4-12 Etiologies of Secondary Hypertension

PHEOCHROMOCYTOMA

A 56-year-old with PMH of HTN treated with lisinopril, HCTZ, and amlodipine presents with highly variable blood pressure readings and occasional headaches associated with palpitations and diaphoresis. **Exam** shows BP 170/100. **Labs** show hyperglycemia, but otherwise, CBC, creatinine, and TSH are normal. Plasma free metanephrines are elevated. 24-hour urine collection shows increased metanephrines, homovanillic acid, and vanillylmandelic acid. On **imaging**, CT shows a left adrenal mass.

Management:

1. Pre-operative alpha-blockade (phenoxybenzamine) followed by beta-blockade (metoprolol, propranolol).
2. Surgical resection of adrenal medullary tumor.

Complications:

- Catecholamine surge can be precipitated by anesthesia or surgery, leading to pheochromocytoma crisis (labile BP, fever, multi-organ failure). Beta-blockade before alpha-blockade will result in unopposed alpha stimulation, causing malignant HTN.
- Never biopsy an adrenal mass due to risk of adrenergic crisis.

HYF: Associated with MEN2, NF1, and VHL. An extra-adrenal catecholamine-secreting tumor that presents with similar signs and symptoms is referred to as a paraganglioma. Pheochromocytomas can cause hyperglycemia.

5P's of Pheochromocytoma:

1. Paroxysmal
2. Pain (headache)
3. Pressure (HTN)
4. Palpitations (tachycardia)
5. Perspiration

RENAL ARTERY STENOSIS

A 73-year-old M with PMH of DM2, HLD, 25-pack-year smoking history, peripheral artery disease, and CKD presents for resistant HTN despite being on multiple anti-hypertensives. **Exam** shows BP in the 160s/90s and a lateralizing systolic-diastolic abdominal bruit.

Management:

1. Confirm RAS with renal duplex Doppler ultrasound, CT angiography, or MR angiography.
2. BP control with multi-modal anti-hypertensives. First-line is ACEi/ARBs with careful monitoring.
3. Treatment of atherosclerotic disease (aspirin, statins, smoking cessation).
4. If refractory, revascularization (surgical or percutaneous angioplasty with stenting).

Complications:

- Malignant hypertension.
- Flash pulmonary edema.
- Heart failure.
- Renal failure after starting ACEi/ARB.
- Atrophy of the affected kidney.
- Secondary hyperaldosteronism.

HYF: Usually associated with atherosclerotic disease (eg, elderly patient with smoking history) or fibromuscular dysplasia. Fibromuscular dysplasia can present in a younger woman with 1) recurrent headache or stroke due to internal carotid artery stenosis, and 2) flank pain and secondary HTN due to renal artery stenosis. Exam can show an abdominal bruit (renal artery stenosis) or subauricular bruit (fibromuscular dysplasia). CTA/MRA and catheter-based angiography confirm the diagnosis. Treatment is ACEi/ARB, then percutaneous angioplasty or surgery for definitive management.

OBSTRUCTIVE SLEEP APNEA

A 54-year-old M with PMH of morbid obesity presents with daytime sleepiness. His wife states that he snores loudly in the nighttime. On **exam**, vitals show BP of 146/87. He has a thick neck and large abdomen. On **labs**, CBC and electrolytes are within normal limits.

Management:

1. Nocturnal polysomnography to confirm diagnosis.
2. BiPAP during sleep.
3. Important to differentiate from obesity hypoventilation syndrome.

Complications:

- Daytime somnolence.

HYF: Mnemonic to assess for risk factors for OSA:

STOP-BANG (**S**nore, **T**ired, **O**bserved apnea, High-blood **P**ressure, **B**MI >35, **A**ge >50, **N**eck circumference >40, **G**ender Male).
Scores >3 indicates high risk for OSA.

COARCTATION OF THE AORTA

A 26-year-old M with PMH of HTN presents with frequent headaches and fatigue. On **exam**, he has BP of 178/117. Repeat BP check on his other arm is 182/109. Femoral pulses are weak and delayed compared to brachial pulses. EKG shows evidence of LVH. **Labs** are normal. On **imaging**, CXR shows notching at the 4th, 5th, and 6th ribs and aortic indentation. Repeat BP on both ankles shows significantly decreased BP.

Management:

1. Echocardiography to confirm coarctation.
2. Surgery to fix the coarctation.

Complications:

- Hypertensive emergency of the upper extremities (ICH, intracranial hemorrhage).

HYF: Associated with Turner syndrome and Williams syndrome. Can also be acquired due to Takayasu's arteritis.

Cushing's Syndrome: See pp. 157–159.
Hypothyroidism: See pp. 137–139.
Hyperthyroidism: See pp. 140–142.

5
Internal Medicine: Infectious Diseases

5-1 Respiratory Tract Infections

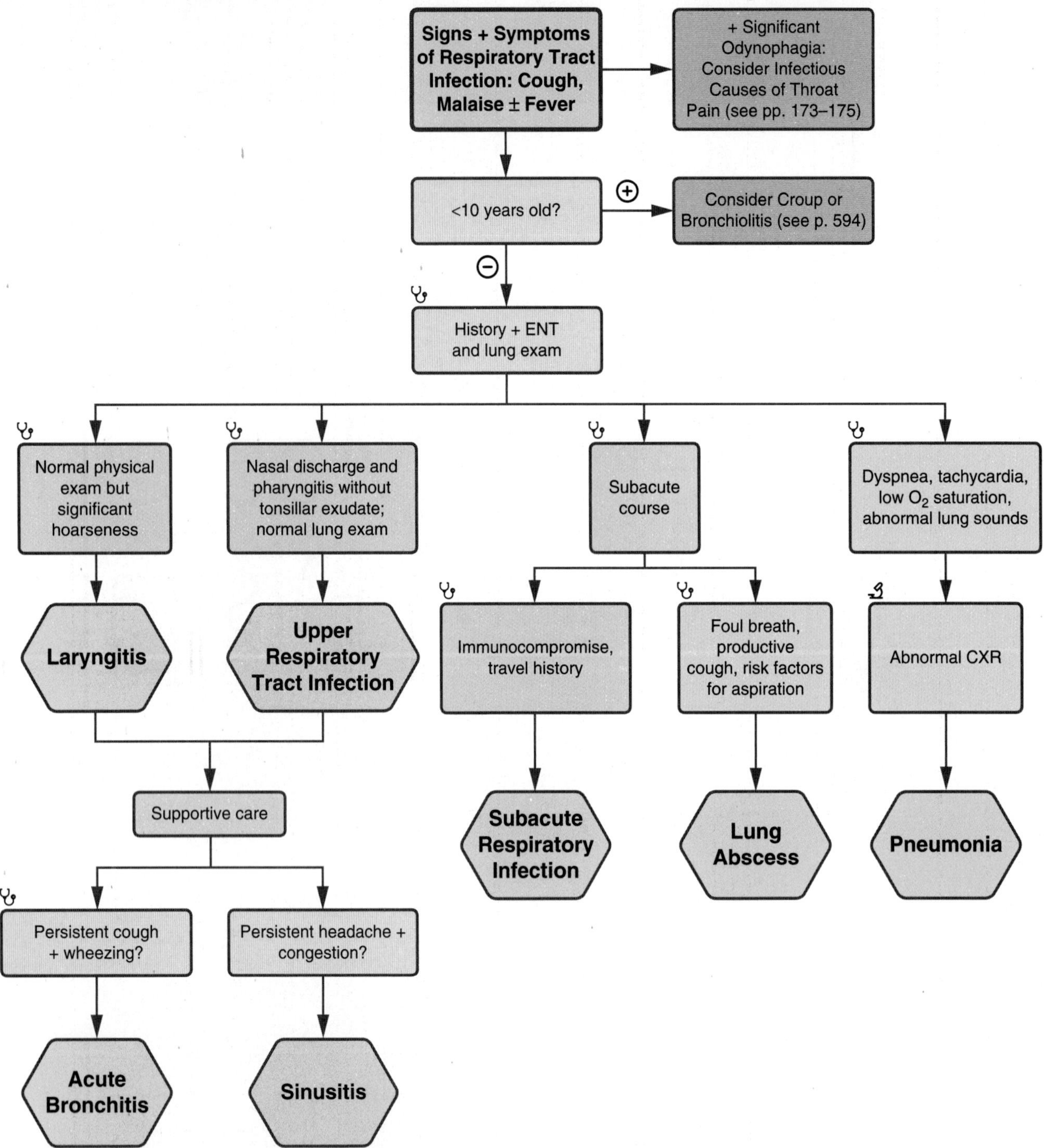
Signs + Symptoms of Respiratory Tract Infection: Cough, Malaise ± Fever
+ Significant Odynophagia: Consider Infectious Causes of Throat Pain (see pp. 173–175)
<10 years old?
Consider Croup or Bronchiolitis (see p. 594)
History + ENT and lung exam
Normal physical exam but significant hoarseness
Nasal discharge and pharyngitis without tonsillar exudate; normal lung exam
Subacute course
Dyspnea, tachycardia, low O2 saturation, abnormal lung sounds
Laryngitis
Upper Respiratory Tract Infection
Immunocompromise, travel history
Foul breath, productive cough, risk factors for aspiration
Abnormal CXR
Supportive care
Subacute Respiratory Infection
Lung Abscess
Pneumonia
Persistent cough + wheezing?
Persistent headache + congestion?
Acute Bronchitis
Sinusitis

The respiratory tract consists of the structures that air flows through on its way to the alveoli: The nose, nasal cavity, pharynx, larynx, trachea, bronchi, bronchioles, and finally, the alveoli themselves. These structures are divided into two parts, the upper respiratory tract and the lower respiratory tract (which begins with the trachea). Though infections affecting different parts of the respiratory tract can have overlapping clinical presentations, distinguishing upper respiratory tract infections and bronchitis from lower respiratory tract infections is critical for clinical decision making and antibiotic stewardship.

When a patient presents with symptoms of a respiratory tract infection, such as acute cough, fatigue, and fever, a physical exam is the most important step. Normal vital signs and lack of pulmonary findings or tonsillar exudate suggest an upper respiratory tract infection (common cold) that warrants only supportive therapy, while abnormal findings may require further laboratory testing and imaging. Significant hoarseness suggests involvement of the larynx, known as acute laryngitis. In patients with an acute onset but persistent cough lasting 1–3 weeks, consider acute bronchitis, which may be accompanied by mild dyspnea and wheezing on lung auscultation. Since most cases of bronchitis are caused by viruses, antibiotics are almost never warranted. In infants and children with respiratory distress, consider laryngotracheitis or bronchiolitis (see p. 594). Finally, in a patient with clinical suspicion for pneumonia (fever, dyspnea, pleuritic chest pain, tachypnea, abnormal breath sounds), you should obtain a chest radiograph. Lobar consolidations, interstitial infiltrates, or cavitations are consistent with pneumonia. In a patient with subacute respiratory symptoms, consider tuberculosis, endemic mycoses, lung abscess, and non-infectious etiologies such as lung cancer.

FIGURE 5.1

5-2 Pneumonia

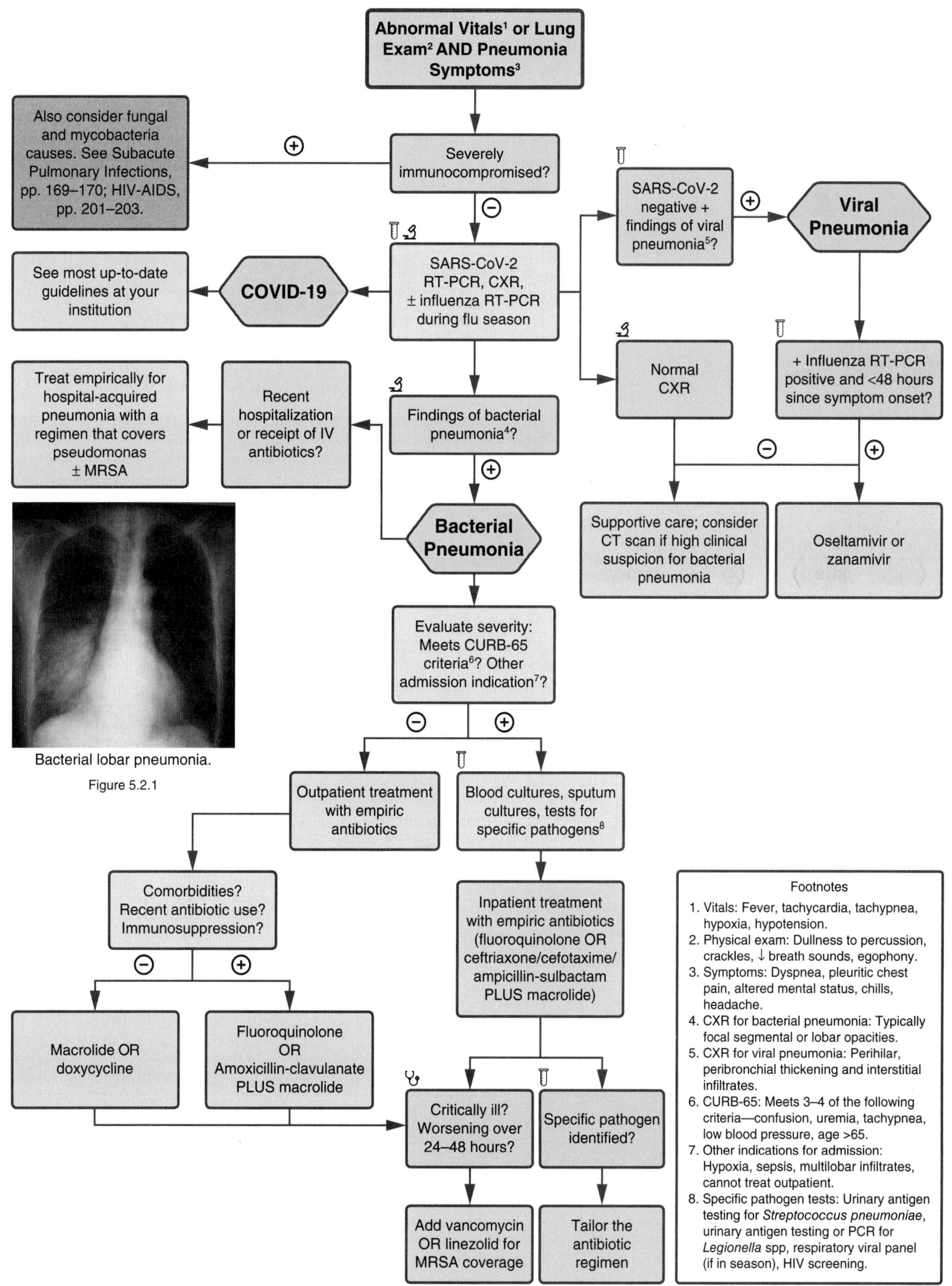
Abnormal Vitals[1] or Lung Exam[2] AND Pneumonia Symptoms[3]
Severely immunocompromised?
Also consider fungal and mycobacteria causes. See Subacute Pulmonary Infections, pp. 169–170; HIV-AIDS, pp. 201–203.
SARS-CoV-2 RT-PCR, CXR, ± influenza RT-PCR during flu season
COVID-19
See most up-to-date guidelines at your institution
SARS-CoV-2 negative + findings of viral pneumonia[5]?
Viral Pneumonia
Normal CXR
+ Influenza RT-PCR positive and <48 hours since symptom onset?
Supportive care; consider CT scan if high clinical suspicion for bacterial pneumonia
Oseltamivir or zanamivir
Findings of bacterial pneumonia[4]?
Recent hospitalization or receipt of IV antibiotics?
Treat empirically for hospital-acquired pneumonia with a regimen that covers pseudomonas ± MRSA
Bacterial Pneumonia
Bacterial lobar pneumonia.
Figure 5.2.1
Evaluate severity: Meets CURB-65 criteria[6]? Other admission indication[7]?
Outpatient treatment with empiric antibiotics
Blood cultures, sputum cultures, tests for specific pathogens[8]
Comorbidities? Recent antibiotic use? Immunosuppression?
Macrolide OR doxycycline
Fluoroquinolone OR Amoxicillin-clavulanate PLUS macrolide
Inpatient treatment with empiric antibiotics (fluoroquinolone OR ceftriaxone/cefotaxime/ ampicillin-sulbactam PLUS macrolide)
Critically ill? Worsening over 24–48 hours?
Specific pathogen identified?
Add vancomycin OR linezolid for MRSA coverage
Tailor the antibiotic regimen
Footnotes
1. Vitals: Fever, tachycardia, tachypnea, hypoxia, hypotension.
2. Physical exam: Dullness to percussion, crackles, ↓ breath sounds, egophony.
3. Symptoms: Dyspnea, pleuritic chest pain, altered mental status, chills, headache.
4. CXR for bacterial pneumonia: Typically focal segmental or lobar opacities.
5. CXR for viral pneumonia: Perihilar, peribronchial thickening and interstitial infiltrates.
6. CURB-65: Meets 3–4 of the following criteria—confusion, uremia, tachypnea, low blood pressure, age >65.
7. Other indications for admission: Hypoxia, sepsis, multilobar infiltrates, cannot treat outpatient.
8. Specific pathogen tests: Urinary antigen testing for Streptococcus pneumoniae, urinary antigen testing or PCR for Legionella spp, respiratory viral panel (if in season), HIV screening.

FIGURE 5.2

5-2 Pneumonia

PNEUMONIA

Pneumonia is an infection of the bronchoalveolar tree. Common symptoms include cough, fever, dyspnea, chills, headache, and pleuritic chest pain. Physical exam findings can include decreased breath sounds, rales, wheezing, egophony, dullness to percussion, and abnormal vitals (eg, hypoxia, hypotension). Note: Symptoms, especially fever, may be minimal in elderly or immunocompromised patients. Treatment is typically empiric, as the causative pathogen is rarely identified. Diagnosis is based on symptoms of acute respiratory infection, plus new consolidations on chest imaging; leukocytosis is common but not specific. In severe disease or high-risk patients, more specific testing for the causative pathogen may be pursued (eg, sputum culture with Gram stain or pathogen-specific tests), which we will discuss below.

Treatment:

- *Community-acquired pneumonia, low-risk*: Macrolide (eg, azithromycin) OR doxycycline.
- *Community-acquired pneumonia, high-risk:* Fluoroquinolone (eg, levofloxacin, moxifloxacin) OR β-lactam (amoxicillin-clavulanate, ceftriaxone) PLUS atypical coverage (azithromycin, doxycycline).
- *Hospital-acquired pneumonia*: Cefepime/ceftazidime/piperacillin-tazobactam OR carbapenem PLUS macrolide OR fluoroquinolone.

Complications:

- Acute respiratory distress syndrome.
- Sepsis.
- Pleural effusion, empyema, lung abscess.

BACTERIAL PNEUMONIA

Pathogen	Epidemiology/Risk Factors	Unique Clinical Features	Notes
Streptococcus pneumoniae	RFs: COPD, asplenia, EtOH/IVDU, immunocompromised. Higher risk of severe infection in children and age>65; pneumococcal vaccine is available for these patients.	Typically causes focal, lobar pneumonia. May be seen post-influenza. Can be detected with urine (or PCR) pneumococcal antigen tests, though rarely used.	Most common cause of community-acquired pneumonia. Covered by empiric β-lactam antibiotics.
Haemophilus influenzae	Most common in children. RFs: Similar to *S. pneumoniae* (above). Give Hib vaccination to higher-risk patients to prevent severe disease.	Also causes focal lobar pneumonia. Can be detected with cultures or PCR, though rarely used.	Type b ("Hib") is the most virulent subtype. Covered by empiric β-lactam antibiotics.
Staphylococcus aureus/MRSA	May be nosocomial. RFs similar to *S. pneumoniae* (above).	May present as classic community-acquired pneumonia or a more severe form (including cavitary lesions, hemoptysis, skin changes). May be seen post-influenza.	Can cause severe, necrotizing pneumonia. Expand empiric coverage to include vancomycin or linezolid if MRSA suspected, such as +MRSA nares swab.
Pseudomonas aeruginosa	RFs: Chronically ill, immunocompromised, cystic fibrosis, recent contact with healthcare system (often with ventilator tubing or other healthcare devices).	Sputum culture grows Gram-negative rods. Rapid in onset, commonly causes sepsis and can be severe/fatal.	Covered by carbapenems, piperacillin/tazobactam, cefepime, ceftazidime, ciprofloxacin, levofloxacin.
Enterobacteriacecae (Klebsiella, Escherichia coli, Serratia)	RFs: EtOH/IV drug use. *E. coli* is most common in neonates. *Klebsiella* and *Serratia marcescens* are nosocomial.	Gram-negative enteric rods. Commonly aspirated (vs. inspired), may be ventilator-associated. *Klebsiella pneumoniae* is associated with "currant jelly" sputum.	*Klebsiella pneumoniae* is associated with high antibiotic resistance.
Atypical bacteria:		More likely indolent in onset, less severe ("walking pneumonia").	
Mycoplasma pneumoniae	Epi: Younger adults, often sharing close quarters (eg, military, college students). Peaks fall/winter.	Causes URI and bronchitis more commonly than pneumonia. CXR shows diffuse interstitial infiltrates. Typically clinical diagnosis but may use PCR or serum cold agglutinins.	Covered by macrolides, doxycycline, fluoroquinolones.
Chlamydia pneumoniae	Epi: Younger adults, elderly.	No distinguishing symptoms apart from fever, cough, dyspnea. May identify with PCR.	Covered by empiric regimens; azithromycin is the best treatment.
Legionella pneumophila	RF: Contact with aerosolized water (eg, air conditioners, showers, fountains), COPD, DM.	Often presents with GI (diarrhea, nausea, vomiting,) or systemic (malaise, confusion) symptoms prior to pulmonary symptoms. Labs can show hyponatremia and elevated aminotransferases. Identify with urine antigen test or PCR.	Preferred treatment: Macrolides, fluoroquinolones.

5-2 Pneumonia

Aspiration pneumonia is a bacterial infection, most common in those with a mechanical/functional abnormality that impairs cough, swallowing, or airway protection. Often it has an indolent presentation with imaging showing infiltrates in gravity-dependent positions. Treat with or clindamycin ampicillin/sulbactam to cover anaerobes.

VIRAL PNEUMONIA

Pathogen	Epidemiology/Risk Factors	Unique Clinical Features	Notes
Influenza	Most common in December–March. RF: Not receiving yearly influenza vaccine (reduces infection risk by ~50%).	More rapid onset of high fever, myalgias, headache compared to bacterial pneumonia. Can detect with rapid NP swab, rapid molecular, or PCR tests.	Complications include secondary bacterial pneumonia (*S. pneumoniae, S. aureus*), COPD exacerbation, bronchitis. Treat with oseltamivir or zanamivir if within 48 hours of symptom onset.
SARS CoV-2	Transmitted mostly via respiratory droplets. Prevention includes 2 mRNA vaccines targeting surface spike proteins; 95% efficacy in preventing symptomatic disease.	80% of cases mild, 15% severe, 5% critical. Most common symptoms are cough, fever, fatigue, but may also present with myalgias, dyspnea, anosmia, GI symptoms. Labs may show elevated LDH/ferritin. Chest CT can show ground-glass opacities. Diagnosed with RT-PCR NP swab.	Complications include ARDS, septic shock, thrombosis, cardiac injury, persistent long-term systemic symptoms (fatigue, myalgias). Treatment includes remdesivir, low-dose dexamethasone, monoclonal antibodies.
Rhinovirus	Children are a major reservoir; typically causes pneumonia in elderly patients.	Often seen on NP/OP swabs in patients with community-acquired pneumonia.	A typical cause of the common cold. Most common virus isolated in pneumonia patients.
Other (RSV, parainfluenza, adenovirus, human metapneumovirus)	Older, immunocompromised adults. Adenovirus can cause "atypical pneumonia" in younger adults, associated with military	More commonly cause upper respiratory symptoms but may progress to pneumonia in vulnerable patients. Identify pathogens with a respiratory viral panel. Imaging findings are similar to other viral pneumonias (interstitial infiltrates, ground-glass opacities, bronchial wall thickening, peri-bronchial consolidation).	

Note: Viral pathogen is present in 44% of pneumonia patients; viral-bacterial coinfection is common.

5-3 Subacute Pulmonary Infections

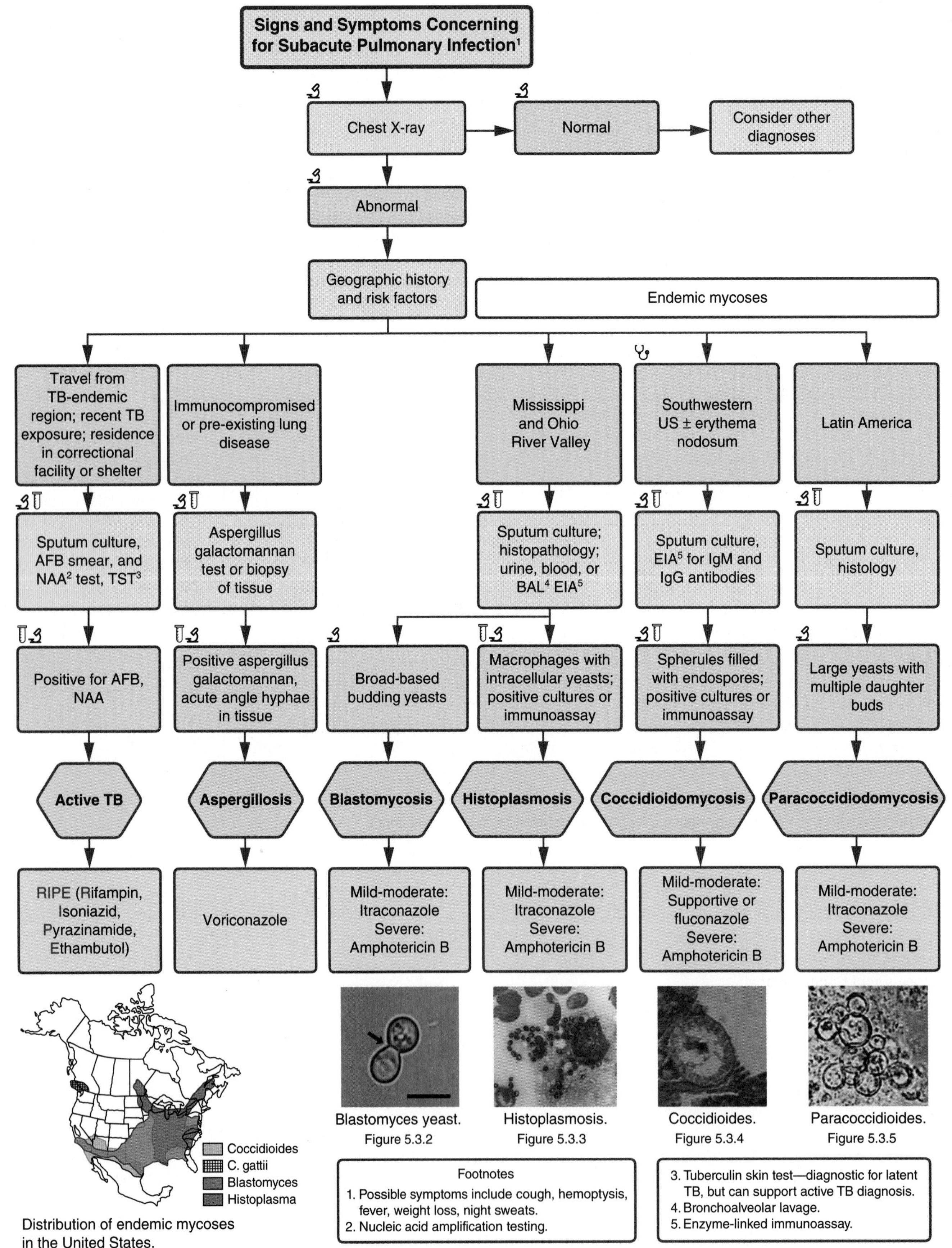
Signs and Symptoms Concerning for Subacute Pulmonary Infection[1]
Chest X-ray
Normal
Consider other diagnoses
Abnormal
Geographic history and risk factors
Endemic mycoses
Travel from TB-endemic region; recent TB exposure; residence in correctional facility or shelter
Immunocompromised or pre-existing lung disease
Mississippi and Ohio River Valley
Southwestern US ± erythema nodosum
Latin America
Sputum culture, AFB smear, and NAA[2] test, TST[3]
Aspergillus galactomannan test or biopsy of tissue
Sputum culture; histopathology; urine, blood, or BAL[4] EIA[5]
Sputum culture, EIA[5] for IgM and IgG antibodies
Sputum culture, histology
Positive for AFB, NAA
Positive aspergillus galactomannan, acute angle hyphae in tissue
Broad-based budding yeasts
Macrophages with intracellular yeasts; positive cultures or immunoassay
Spherules filled with endospores; positive cultures or immunoassay
Large yeasts with multiple daughter buds
Active TB
Aspergillosis
Blastomycosis
Histoplasmosis
Coccidioidomycosis
Paracoccidiodomycosis
RIPE (Rifampin, Isoniazid, Pyrazinamide, Ethambutol)
Voriconazole
Mild-moderate: Itraconazole Severe: Amphotericin B
Mild-moderate: Itraconazole Severe: Amphotericin B
Mild-moderate: Supportive or fluconazole Severe: Amphotericin B
Mild-moderate: Itraconazole Severe: Amphotericin B
Coccidioides
C. gattii
Blastomyces
Histoplasma

Distribution of endemic mycoses in the United States.
Figure 5.3.1

Blastomyces yeast.
Figure 5.3.2

Histoplasmosis.
Figure 5.3.3

Coccidioides.
Figure 5.3.4

Paracoccidioides.
Figure 5.3.5

Footnotes

1. Possible symptoms include cough, hemoptysis, fever, weight loss, night sweats.
2. Nucleic acid amplification testing.
3. Tuberculin skin test—diagnostic for latent TB, but can support active TB diagnosis.
4. Bronchoalveolar lavage.
5. Enzyme-linked immunoassay.

FIGURE 5.3

5-3 Subacute Pulmonary Infections

TUBERCULOSIS

A physician from southeast Asia presents with 5 weeks of productive cough, fevers, and weight loss. **Labs/Imaging:** CXR reveals a cavitary lesion in the right upper lobe. Sputum NAAT is (+) with AFB.

Management:

Active TB:	Latent TB:
2 months RIPE/4 months RI (6 months of total TB treatment) • Rifampin • Isoniazid • Pyrazinamide • Ethambutol	1. Isoniazid + Rifampin or Rifapentine for 3–4 months 2. Rifampin for 4 months 3. Isoniazid for 6–9 months

Complications: TB can spread to essentially any tissue in the body. Extrapulmonary manifestations include meningitis, Pott's disease, miliary TB, and constrictive pericarditis. Pulmonary cavitations increase risk for aspergillomas later.

HYF:

- Risk factors: Endemic countries, healthcare workers, communal living facilities, prisons, homelessness, IV drug use, and HIV.
- When active TB is suspected, get 3 sputum samples for culture (susceptibilities), smear (rapid diagnosis), and NAAT (rapid diagnosis).
- TST induration levels for latent TB diagnosis and treatment:
  - For those with no risk factors: 15 mm or more is positive.
  - Risk factors present: 10 mm or more is positive.
  - Immunocompromised: 5 mm or more is positive.
  - Of note, the BCG vaccine can affect this!
- Interferon gamma release assay (IGRA) can also be used.
- Drug side effects: INH causes neuropathy (prevented with vitamin B6 supplementation) and hepatotoxicity. Ethambutol can cause optic neuropathy.

INVASIVE ASPERGILLOSIS

An immunocompromised patient presents with a persistent cough, fever, and blood-tinged sputum. **Labs/Imaging:** CXR reveals a cavitary lesion in the upper lobes with negative AFB smear. Lung biopsy reveals acute-angle hyphae.

Management:

Medical	Surgical
Voriconazole, amphotericin B.	Debridement of necrotic tissue in some cases.

Complications: Disseminated infection can occur. Invasive aspergillosis has a high mortality rate in severely immunocompromised individuals.

HYF:

- The *Aspergillus* fungus can present as 3 clinical syndromes:
  - **Invasive aspergillosis:** In immunocompromised patients.
  - **Aspergilloma**: Non-invasive disease in which a fungus ball forms within a pre-existing lung lesion.
  - **Allergic bronchopulmonary aspergillosis:** Hypersensitivity reaction common in patients with cystic fibrosis or asthma.
- Morphology: Acute-angled hyphae.

BLASTOMYCOSIS

An avid hiker from Ohio presents with a nagging cough and warts on the cheek. **Labs/Imaging:** CXR reveals alveolar infiltrates without lymphadenopathy. Sputum culture reveals broad-based budding yeasts.

Management:

1. Mild to moderate: Itraconazole.
2. Severe: Amphotericin B.

Complications: Systemic infection, ARDS.

HYF:

- Found in moist soil and decaying plant matter in the central and eastern US (Ohio and the Mississippi River valley).
- Blastomycosis is most often asymptomatic.
- Morphology: Broad-based budding yeasts. **B for Broad.**

HISTOPLASMOSIS

A patient with PMH of HIV presents with 1 month of flu-like symptoms after spelunking in Mississippi caves. **Labs/Imaging:** CXR reveals patchy infiltrates with hilar lymphadenopathy. Sputum culture reveals intracellular yeasts.

Management:

1. Mild to moderate: Itraconazole.
2. Severe: Amphotericin B.

Complications: Systemic infection, ARDS.

HYF:

- Found in bird and bat droppings.
- Associated with GI symptoms and oral mucosal ulcers.
- Unlike blastomycosis, histoplasmosis often presents with hilar lymphadenopathy.
- Morphology: Macrophages with intracellular yeasts. "Histo likes to Hide."

COCCIDIOIDOMYCOSIS

A patient from California presents with months of fatigue, hemoptysis, and painful bumps on their shins. **Labs/Imaging:** CXR reveals a dense infiltrate in the left lower lobe with hilar lymphadenopathy. Sputum culture shows fungus.

(Continued)

5-3 Subacute Pulmonary Infections

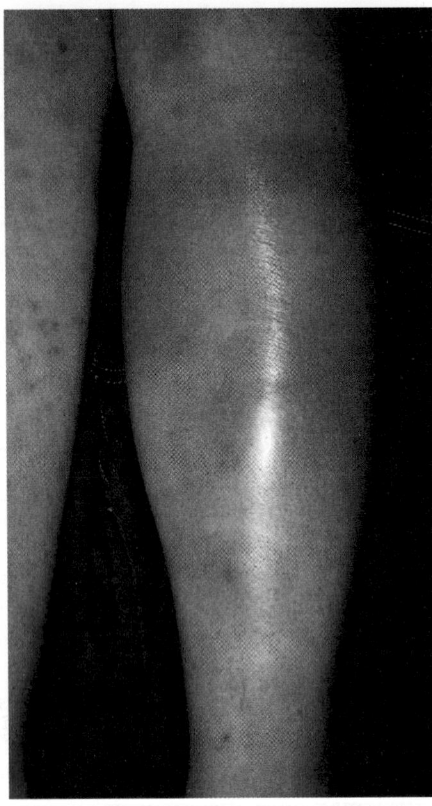

Erythema nodosum. Nodules on the legs are usually very tender.

Management:

1. Mild to moderate: Supportive measures or fluconazole.
2. Severe: Amphotericin B.

Complications: Dissemination → focal CNS findings.

HYF:

- Endemic to southwest US: California, Arizona, New Mexico.
- Skin lesions include erythema nodosum (painful lumps on shins) and erythema multiforme.
- Morphology: Spherules filled with endospores.

PARACOCCIDIOIDOMYCOSIS

A male traveler from Latin America presents with a month of fever and weight loss with diffuse lymphadenopathy. **Labs/Imaging:** CXR shows alveolar infiltrates without cavitation. Sputum microscopy reveals large yeasts with multiple attached daughter buds.

Management:

1. Mild to moderate: Itraconazole.
2. Severe: Amphotericin B.

Complications: Systemic infection, ARDS.

HYF:

- Risk factors: Contact with soil, travel from Latin America, male sex.
- Presents with warts, similar to blastomycosis.
- Morphology: Budding yeasts with multiple attached daughter buds (looks like a ship captain's wheel).

5-4 Tongue Lesions

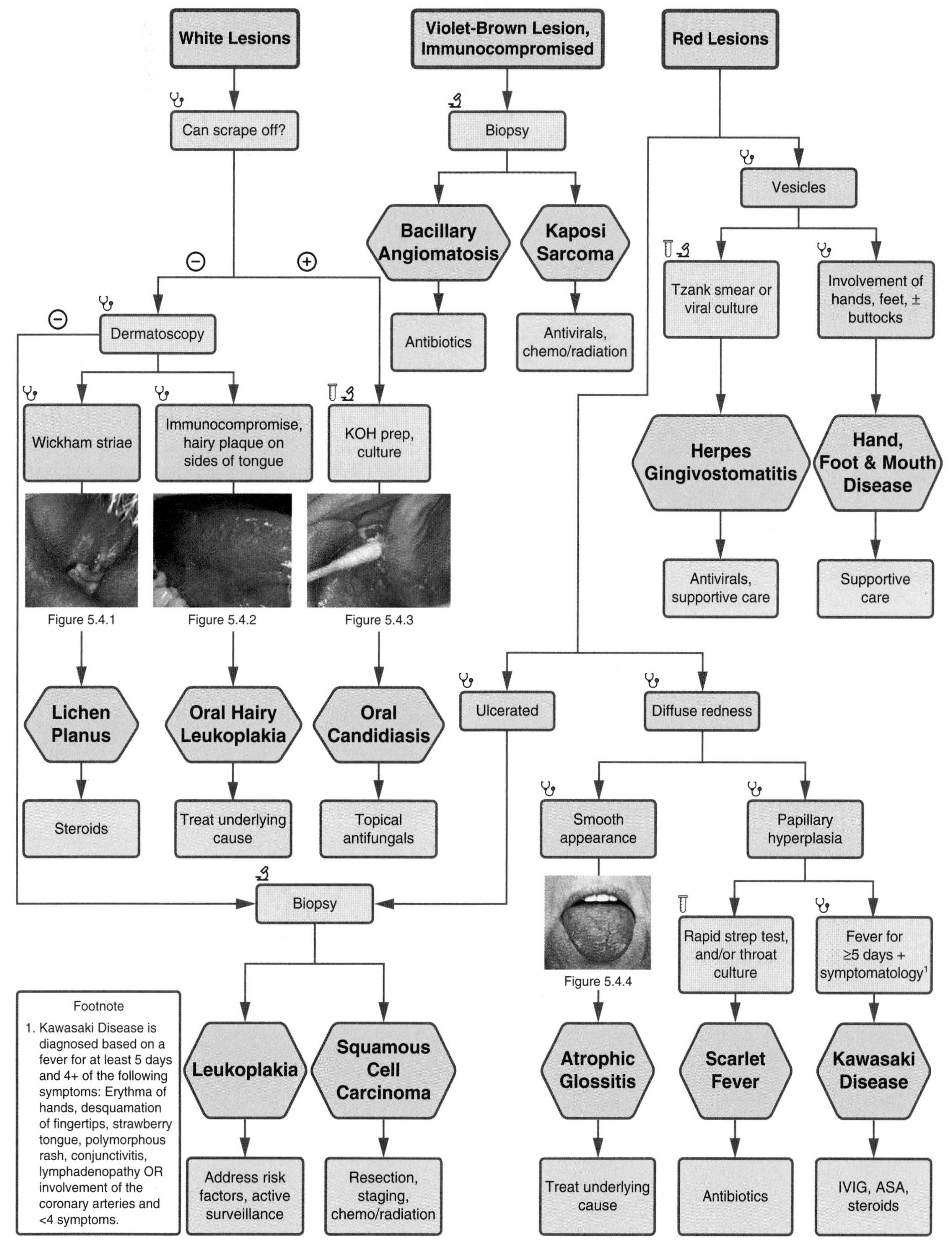
White Lesions
Can scrape off?
⊖
⊕
Dermatoscopy
⊖
Wickham striae
Immunocompromise, hairy plaque on sides of tongue
KOH prep, culture
Figure 5.4.1
Figure 5.4.2
Figure 5.4.3
Lichen Planus
Oral Hairy Leukoplakia
Oral Candidiasis
Steroids
Treat underlying cause
Topical antifungals
Biopsy
Leukoplakia
Squamous Cell Carcinoma
Address risk factors, active surveillance
Resection, staging, chemo/radiation
Violet-Brown Lesion, Immunocompromised
Biopsy
Bacillary Angiomatosis
Kaposi Sarcoma
Antibiotics
Antivirals, chemo/radiation
Red Lesions
Vesicles
Tzank smear or viral culture
Involvement of hands, feet, ± buttocks
Herpes Gingivostomatitis
Hand, Foot & Mouth Disease
Antivirals, supportive care
Supportive care
Ulcerated
Diffuse redness
Smooth appearance
Papillary hyperplasia
Figure 5.4.4
Rapid strep test, and/or throat culture
Fever for ≥5 days + symptomatology[1]
Atrophic Glossitis
Scarlet Fever
Kawasaki Disease
Treat underlying cause
Antibiotics
IVIG, ASA, steroids

Footnote

1. Kawasaki Disease is diagnosed based on a fever for at least 5 days and 4+ of the following symptoms: Erythma of hands, desquamation of fingertips, strawberry tongue, polymorphous rash, conjunctivitis, lymphadenopathy OR involvement of the coronary arteries and <4 symptoms.

FIGURE 5.4

5-4 Tongue Lesions

ORAL HAIRY LEUKOPLAKIA

A patient with PMH of HIV and EBV infection presents with painless corrugated white plaques ("hairy" or "feathered" appearance) on the lateral aspect of the tongue that cannot be scraped off.

Management:

1. If classic presentation, no biopsy is needed.
2. If lesion has unclear characteristics, then biopsy is indicated.
3. Treat underlying condition.

Complications: None – benign.

HYF: Caused by very high replication of EBV virus.

ORAL CANDIDIASIS

A patient with PMH of HIV and current tobacco use presents with loss of taste and pain while eating. **Exam** shows white plaques in the oral cavity that can be scraped off ("pseudomembranes") and red, inflamed mucosa. KOH prep shows budding yeasts and pseudohyphae.

Management:

1. Best initial test is KOH test.
2. Culture if needed.
3. Treat with topical nystatin or oral fluconazole.

Complications:

- Mucosal bleeding, pain.
- Mucosal translocation leading to candidemia.
- Disseminated organ infection (eg, endocarditis).

HYF: Populations at risk include newborns, immunosuppressed patients, those with inherited autoimmune disease (eg, *AIRE* gene mutation), uncontrolled diabetes, and inhaled corticosteroid use.

HERPES GINGIVOSTOMATITIS

A toddler presents with fever and difficulty eating. **Exam** shows erythematous gingiva, clusters of vesicles in oral cavity, and lymphadenopathy. **Labs** show reveals multinucleated giant cells and Cowdry A inclusion bodies on Tzanck smear.

Management:

1. Confirm diagnosis with viral culture or PCR.
2. Treatment with oral acyclovir.
3. Lesions typically resolve within 2 weeks.

Complications:

- Poor PO intake and dehydration.
- Herpetic keratitis through self-inoculation of the eye.
- Herpetic whitlow from thumb sucking in children or dentists in adults.

HYF: Herpes gingivostomatitis is most commonly caused by HSV-1 and is typically the initial presentation of an infection. Subsequent reactivation of the virus typically causes labial herpes. Labial herpes has tingling prodrome, more local symptoms, and primarily involves the vermilion borders of the lips. Tzanck smear, while traditionally used for initial testing, is now rarely used in common practice.

HAND, FOOT, AND MOUTH DISEASE

A child in daycare presents with fever and rash. **Exam** shows gray vesicles and ulcerations in the oropharynx, hands, and feet.

Management:

1. Supportive care.
2. Improves within 7–10 days.

Complications: Poor PO intake and dehydration.

HYF: Caused by the coxsackie A virus, which also causes herpangina. Primarily affects children ages 1–7 years old but also can infect adults. Highly contagious. Seasonal: Late summer and early fall.

Leukoplakia: See p. 353.

Squamous Cell Carcinoma: See p. 318.

Scarlet Fever: See pp. 584-585.

Kawasaki Disease: See pp. 330, 586.

Lichen Planus: See p. 339.

Bacillary Angiomatosis: See p. 203.

Kaposi's Sarcoma: See p. 203.

5-5 Throat Pain

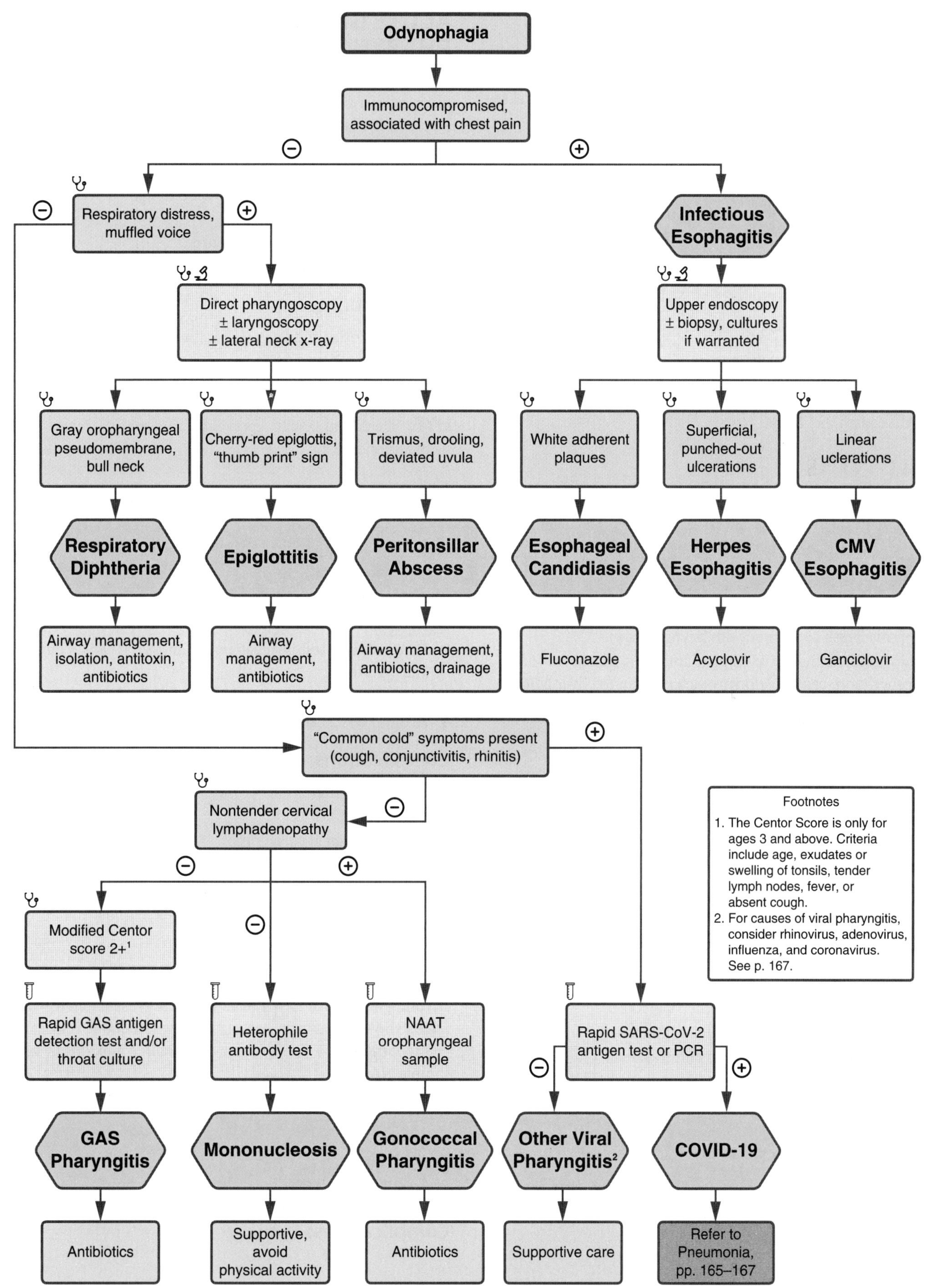
Odynophagia
Immunocompromised, associated with chest pain
Respiratory distress, muffled voice
Infectious Esophagitis
Direct pharyngoscopy ± laryngoscopy ± lateral neck x-ray
Upper endoscopy ± biopsy, cultures if warranted
Gray oropharyngeal pseudomembrane, bull neck
Cherry-red epiglottis, "thumb print" sign
Trismus, drooling, deviated uvula
White adherent plaques
Superficial, punched-out ulcerations
Linear uclerations
Respiratory Diphtheria
Epiglottitis
Peritonsillar Abscess
Esophageal Candidiasis
Herpes Esophagitis
CMV Esophagitis
Airway management, isolation, antitoxin, antibiotics
Airway management, antibiotics
Airway management, antibiotics, drainage
Fluconazole
Acyclovir
Ganciclovir
"Common cold" symptoms present (cough, conjunctivitis, rhinitis)
Nontender cervical lymphadenopathy
Modified Centor score 2+1
Rapid GAS antigen detection test and/or throat culture
Heterophile antibody test
NAAT oropharyngeal sample
Rapid SARS-CoV-2 antigen test or PCR
GAS Pharyngitis
Mononucleosis
Gonococcal Pharyngitis
Other Viral Pharyngitis2
COVID-19
Antibiotics
Supportive, avoid physical activity
Antibiotics
Supportive care
Refer to Pneumonia, pp. 165–167
Footnotes
1. The Centor Score is only for ages 3 and above. Criteria include age, exudates or swelling of tonsils, tender lymph nodes, fever, or absent cough.
2. For causes of viral pharyngitis, consider rhinovirus, adenovirus, influenza, and coronavirus. See p. 167.

FIGURE 5.5

5-5 Throat Pain

RESPIRATORY DIPHTHERIA

An unvaccinated adult with recent international travel presents with fever, fatigue, sore throat. **Exam** shows a gray pseudomembrane over the posterior pharynx, bulky lymphadenopathy, increased work of breathing, and stridor.

Management:

1. Airway management.
2. Droplet precautions.
3. Diphtheria antitoxin.
4. Cultures, IM penicillin G.

Complications:

- Myocarditis, arrhythmias.
- Polyneuropathy (primarily motor).

HYF: Antitoxin treatment is extremely important because the endotoxin causes the illness.

EPIGLOTTITIS

A child presents with high fever, sore throat, and drooling. **Exam** reveals a muffled voice and stridor, and the child is sitting in tripod position. On **imaging**, neck XR shows thumbprint sign.

Management:

1. If severe respiratory distress, give oxygen, endotracheal intubation (diagnosis is also confirmed with laryngoscopy).
2. Obtain cultures, then give empiric antibiotic treatment (often 3rd generation. cephalosporin + vancomycin to cover MRSA).
3. Consider steroids.

Complications: Airway obstruction.

HYF: Historically caused by *Haemophilus influenzae* type b, but, due to vaccination, *S. aureus* is now a leading cause.

PERITONSILLAR ABSCESS

A young adult presents with fever, severe sore throat, drooling, and dysphagia. **Exam** reveals "hot potato" voice, trismus, shifted uvula, fluctuant tonsil with exudates, and lymphadenopathy.

Management:

1. Airway management.
2. Empiric clindamycin or ampicillin-sulbactam.
3. I&D or needle aspiration, obtain cultures.

Complications:

- Spread to retropharyngeal space and mediastinum.
- Aspiration pneumonia.

HYF: Most common pathogen is *Streptococcus pyogenes*. If recurring, a tonsillectomy is indicated.

ACUTE GROUP A *STREPTOCOCCI* (GAS) PHARYNGITIS

A child presents with fever, sore throat, and no cough. **Exam** shows pharyngeal edema, tonsillar exudates, and tender cervical lymphadenopathy. **Labs** are positive for GAS on rapid test.

Management:

1. GAS rapid test if clinical suspicion in age <3 years, or Centor Score 2+ in ages 3+ years.
2. Can confirm with throat culture.
3. Treat with penicillin V or amoxicillin for 10 days.

Complications:

- Sinusitis, otitis media, peritonsillar abscess.
- Rheumatic fever.
- Poststreptococcal glomerulonephritis.

HYF: Treatment will prevent rheumatic fever but not glomerulonephritis.

MONONUCLEOSIS

An adolescent presents with sore throat and fatigue. **Exam** shows tonsillar exudates, tender lymphadenopathy, and splenomegaly.

Management:

1. Heterophile antibody test for EBV.
2. If heterophile test is negative, get anti-viral capsid antigen IgG and IgM tests.
3. Supportive care.
4. Avoid physical activity for 3 weeks.

Complications:

- Splenic rupture.
- Burkitt lymphoma.
- Nasopharyngeal carcinoma.

HYF: The majority of cases are caused by EBV. When caused by CMV, symptoms are often milder. Empiric treatment with penicillins causes maculopapular rash.

GONOCOCCAL PHARYNGITIS

A young adult with new sexual partners presents with sore throat. **Exam** shows pharyngeal exudates and nontender cervical lymphadenopathy. **Labs** are (+) for *Neisseria gonorrhoeae* on throat sample NAAT.

Management:

1. STI screening.
2. IM ceftriaxone.
3. Partner notification.

Complications: Dysphagia.

5-5 Throat Pain

HYF: Can be asymptomatic. If genitourinary chlamydia infection is not ruled out, then co-treat with azithromycin or doxycycline.

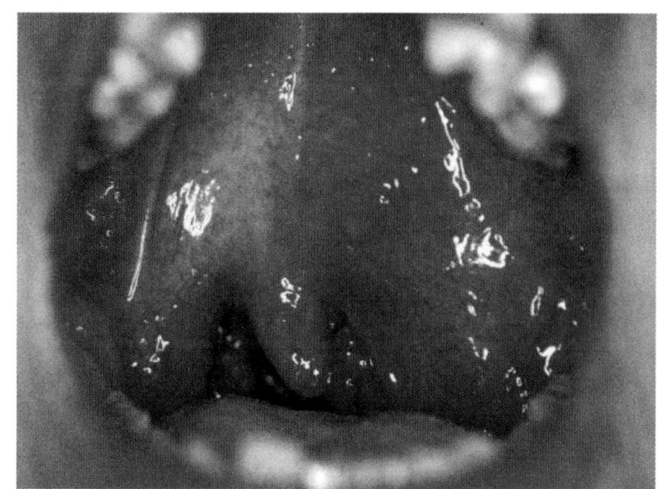

Peritonsillar abscess.

INFECTIOUS ESOPHAGITIS

An immunocompromised patient presents with dysphagia, retrosternal chest pain, and fever and is, found to have esophageal ulcers on endoscopy.

Management:

1. Supportive care, pain management.
2. Treatment per algorithm.
3. Treat underlying cause.

Complications:

- Dehydration.
- Erosions, strictures.
- Aspiration.

HYF: There are many etiologies for infectious esophagitis including *Candida* (most common), HSV, CMV, and other viral pathogens. Risk factors include immunocompromise, diabetes mellitus, and broad-spectrum antibiotic use. Diagnosis is usually made based on EGD with biopsy, along with cultures, serologies, and imaging as warranted.

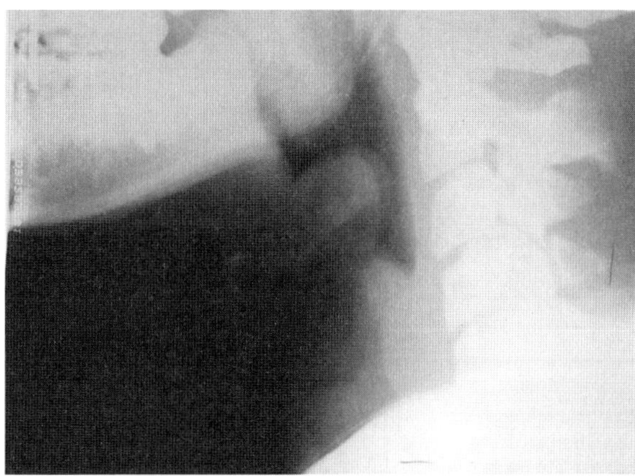

Thumbprint sign seen in epiglottitis.

5-6 Ear Pain

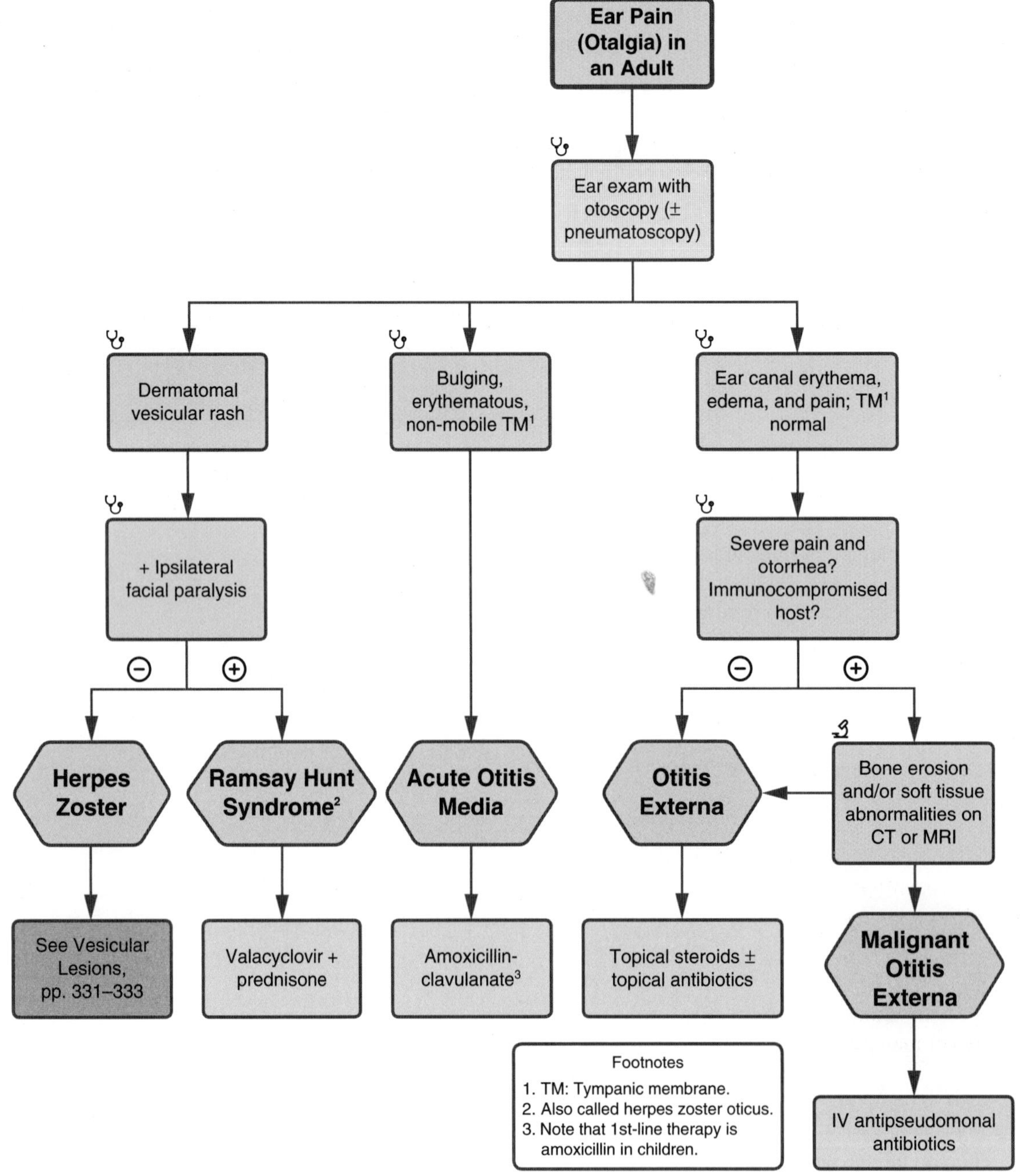
Ear Pain (Otalgia) in an Adult
Ear exam with otoscopy (± pneumatoscopy)
Dermatomal vesicular rash
Bulging, erythematous, non-mobile TM[1]
Ear canal erythema, edema, and pain; TM[1] normal
+ Ipsilateral facial paralysis
Severe pain and otorrhea? Immunocompromised host?
⊖
⊕
Herpes Zoster
Ramsay Hunt Syndrome[2]
Acute Otitis Media
Otitis Externa
Bone erosion and/or soft tissue abnormalities on CT or MRI
See Vesicular Lesions, pp. 331–333
Valacyclovir + prednisone
Amoxicillin-clavulanate[3]
Topical steroids ± topical antibiotics
Malignant Otitis Externa
IV antipseudomonal antibiotics
Footnotes
1. TM: Tympanic membrane.
2. Also called herpes zoster oticus.
3. Note that 1st-line therapy is amoxicillin in children.

FIGURE 5.6

5-6 Ear Pain

ACUTE OTITIS MEDIA

A 25-year-old F with PMH of seasonal allergies and recent URI presents with unilateral ear pain and hearing loss. Otoscopic **exam** shows a bulging, erythematous, and non-mobile tympanic membrane.

Management:

1. Empiric PO antibiotics (eg, amoxicillin-clavulanate).

Complications:

- TM rupture: Usually presents with sudden relief of pain with otorrhea.
- Mastoiditis: Infection/inflammation of mastoid bone; more common in children but highly morbid.
- Cholesteatomas.
- Chronic otitis media: May require tympanostomy tubes.
- CNS infection (eg, brain abscess, meningitis): More common in immunocompromised host.
- Labyrinthitis: Presents with nausea, vomiting, tinnitus, hearing loss, vertigo.
- Hearing loss.

HYF:

- Pathogens: *S. pneumoniae* and *H influenzae*, less commonly *Moraxella*, GAS, and *S. aureus*.
- Acute Otitis Media (AOM) = middle ear infection/inflammation (erythema, edema) with or without effusion. Otitis media with effusion (OME) = effusion without infection/inflammation.
- In children, AOM is usually managed without antibiotics unless <2 years old or recurrent/severe infection.

OTITIS EXTERNA

A 21-year-old competitive swimmer presents with unilateral ear pain and pruritus. **Exam** shows erythema and edema of the ear canal and pain with ear manipulation.

Management:

1. Clean ear canal (remove debris, cerumen, pus).
2. Topical therapy (ear drops usually consisting of steroid + acidifying agent ± antibiotics).

Complications:

- Malignant otitis externa.

HYF: Unlike AOM or malignant otitis externa, treatment is topical unless infection spreads beyond ear canal. Common pathogens: *Pseudomonas, Staphylococcus epidermidis*, and *S. aureus*.

MALIGNANT OTITIS EXTERNA

A 75-year-old M with PMH of T2DM presents with severe unilateral ear pain and discharge. **Exam** shows ear canal erythema, edema, and granulation tissue at the external auditory canal. **Labs** show elevated ESR and CRP.

Management:

1. IV antibiotics (eg, ciprofloxacin).

Complications:

- Osteomyelitis of skull base and temporomandibular joint.
- Cranial nerve deficits.
- CNS infection (eg, brain abscess, meningitis).

HYF: Pathogen: >95% *Pseudomonas*. Usually seen in elderly patients with diabetes mellitus.

Herpes Zoster: See pp. 332-333.

5-7 Sinusitis

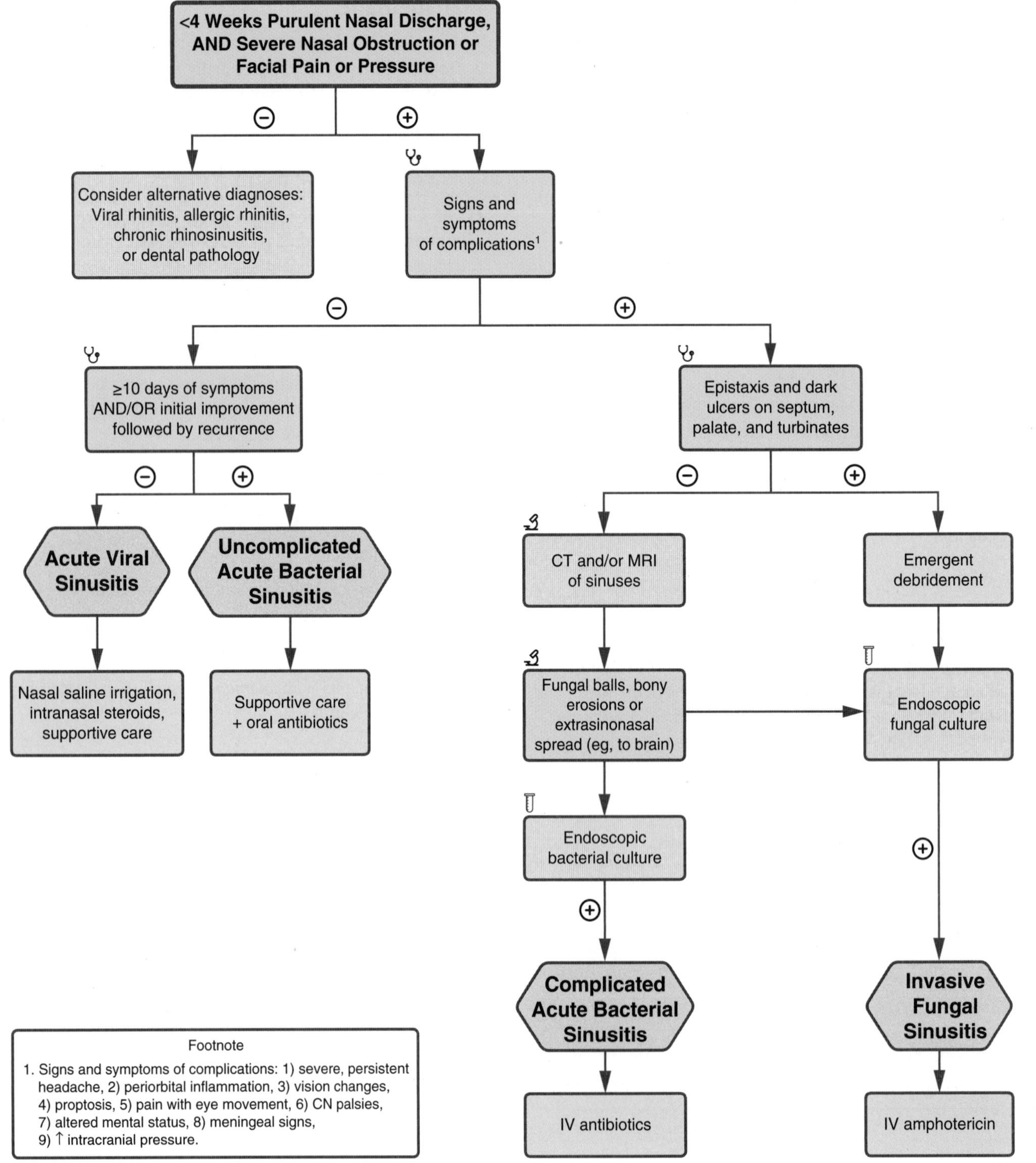
<4 Weeks Purulent Nasal Discharge, AND Severe Nasal Obstruction or Facial Pain or Pressure
Consider alternative diagnoses: Viral rhinitis, allergic rhinitis, chronic rhinosinusitis, or dental pathology
Signs and symptoms of complications[1]
≥10 days of symptoms AND/OR initial improvement followed by recurrence
Epistaxis and dark ulcers on septum, palate, and turbinates
Acute Viral Sinusitis
Uncomplicated Acute Bacterial Sinusitis
CT and/or MRI of sinuses
Emergent debridement
Nasal saline irrigation, intranasal steroids, supportive care
Supportive care + oral antibiotics
Fungal balls, bony erosions or extrasinonasal spread (eg, to brain)
Endoscopic fungal culture
Endoscopic bacterial culture
Complicated Acute Bacterial Sinusitis
Invasive Fungal Sinusitis
IV antibiotics
IV amphotericin
Footnote
1. Signs and symptoms of complications: 1) severe, persistent headache, 2) periorbital inflammation, 3) vision changes, 4) proptosis, 5) pain with eye movement, 6) CN palsies, 7) altered mental status, 8) meningeal signs, 9) ↑ intracranial pressure.

FIGURE 5.7

5-7 Sinusitis

ACUTE VIRAL RHINOSINUSITIS

A 36-year-old F with recent upper respiratory tract infection presents with 3 days of thick, white nasal discharge and worsening frontal pressure.

Management:

1. Supportive care: Nasal saline irrigation, oral analgesics, intranasal steroids, decongestants.
2. Monitor for unchanging or worsening symptoms.

Complications: Bacterial sinusitis.

HYF: May occur with acute otitis media or other symptoms of upper respiratory tract infections (sore throat, cough). Typically caused by rhinovirus, adenovirus, influenza virus, or parainfluenza virus.

ACUTE BACTERIAL RHINOSINUSITIS

A 38-year-old M with recent cold presents with 2 weeks of thick, white nasal discharge and pain with pressure below his eyes and in his forehead.

Management:

1. Rule out signs and symptoms indicating complicated infection (see flowchart).
2. If uncomplicated, observe for 3 days in children or 7 days in adults for improvement before treating with oral antibiotics.
3. If complicated, admit inpatient. Obtain CT or MRI of sinuses, consider endoscopic culture collection, and start IV antibiotics.

Complications:

- Preseptal cellulitis.
- Orbital cellulitis.
- Subperiosteal or orbital abscess.
- Cavernous sinus thrombosis.

HYF: Symptoms are usually stable or improve for 5–6 days and then worsen. Most commonly caused by *S. pneumoniae*, *H. influenzae*, and *Moraxella catarrhalis*.

ALLERGIC RHINOSINUSITIS

A 5-year-old F with PMH of eczema and seasonal allergies presents with sneezing, rhinorrhea, nasal obstruction, and nasal itching.

Management:

1. Allergen avoidance.
2. Glucocorticoid nasal spray.
3. Consider oral antihistamine.

Complications:

- Nasal polyps.
- Viral rhinosinusitis.
- Otitis media.

HYF: May present with transverse nasal crease and dark circles under the eyes (allergic shiners).

INVASIVE ASPERGILLUS SINUSITIS

A 56-year-old F with PMH of acute lymphocytic leukemia presents with fever, purulent nasal discharge, nosebleed, neck stiffness, and severe headache. **Exam** shows dark ulcers on the nasal septum. **Labs** show neutropenia. On **imaging**, MRI with contrast shows abnormal soft tissue filling of the ethmoidal air cell complex, nasal cavity, and maxillary sinus with sub-frontal intracranial extension and dural thickening.

Management:

1. If epistaxis and/or dark ulcers on septum, palate, and turbinates, emergent surgical debridement.
2. CT and/or MRI to evaluate extent of infection.
3. Fungal culture before IV amphotericin.

Complications:

- Abscesses (present as ring-enhancing lesions).
- Cortical or subcortical infarction.

HYF: Rapid onset and progression, typically in immunocompromised patients (hematologic malignancies, hematopoietic cell transplantation, chemotherapy-induced neutropenia, solid organ transplantation, advanced HIV infection, poorly controlled diabetes mellitus, and glucocorticoid therapy).

INVASIVE MUCORMYCOSIS SINUSITIS

A 30-year-old M with PMH of T2DM with A1c 10% presents with double vision, purulent nasal discharge, fever, and confusion. On **imaging**, CT with contrast shows bony erosions of the palate and orbit. Sinus endoscopic biopsy and culture confirm the diagnosis.

Management:

1. If epistaxis and/or dark ulcers on septum, palate, and turbinates, emergent surgical debridement.
2. CT and/or MRI to evaluate extent of infection.
3. Fungal culture before IV amphotericin.

Complications:

- Vascular invasion resulting in ischemic and/or hemorrhagic stroke.
- Orbital apex syndrome.
- Meningitis (rare).
- Brain abscess in chronic cases.
- Facial/nasal deformity.

HYF: Frequently progresses to orbital and brain involvement. More common in uncontrolled diabetes mellitus but also a complication in other immunocompromised conditions. Voriconazole is risk factor for developing mucormycosis in patients with hematologic cancer. Caused by *Rhizopus*. Can present with black eschar (not a feature in aspergillosis).

5-8 CNS Infection in an Immunocompetent Host

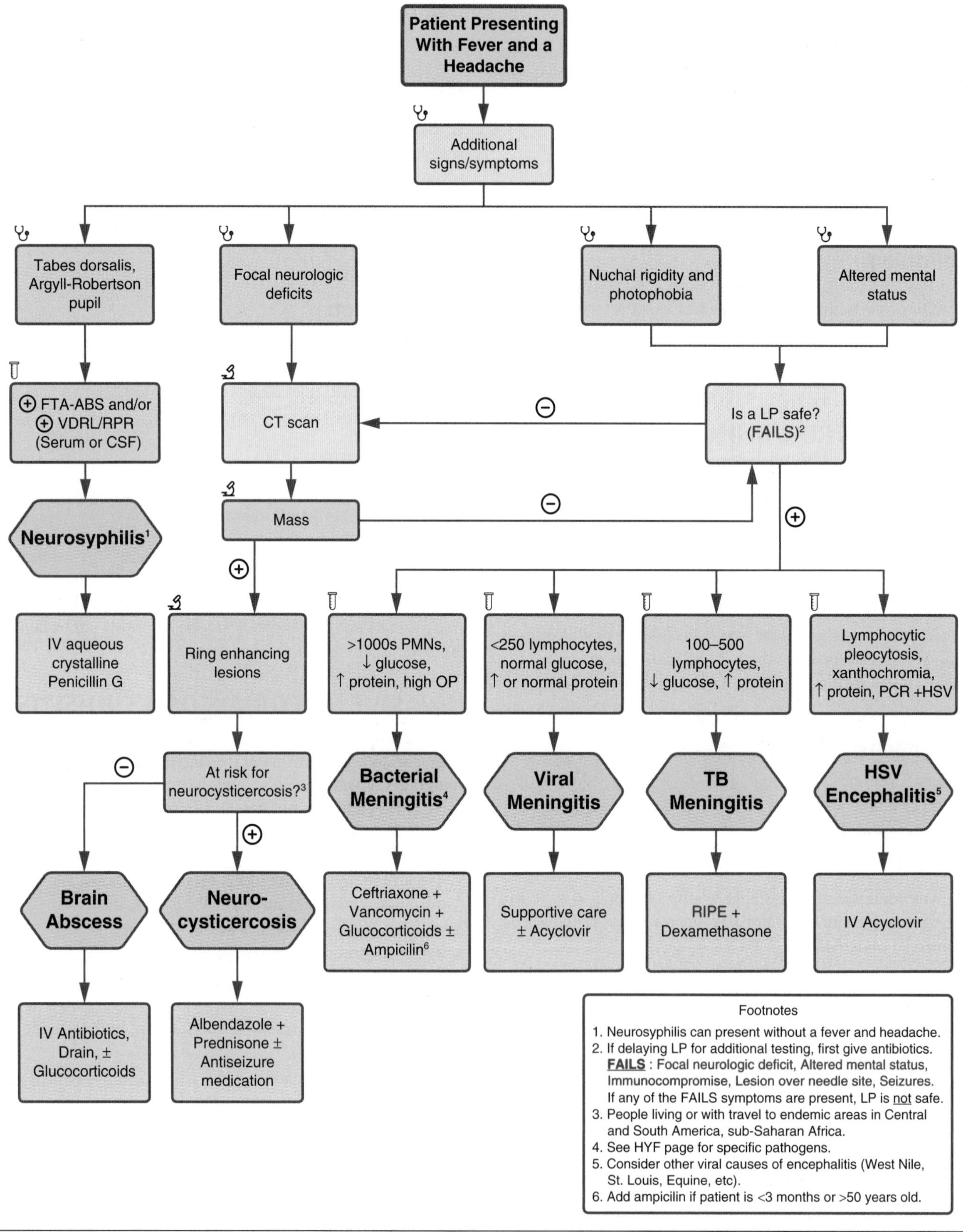
Patient Presenting With Fever and a Headache
Additional signs/symptoms
Tabes dorsalis, Argyll-Robertson pupil
Focal neurologic deficits
Nuchal rigidity and photophobia
Altered mental status
⊕ FTA-ABS and/or ⊕ VDRL/RPR (Serum or CSF)
CT scan
⊖
Is a LP safe? (FAILS)[2]
Neurosyphilis[1]
Mass
⊖
⊕
⊕
IV aqueous crystalline Penicillin G
Ring enhancing lesions
>1000s PMNs, ↓ glucose, ↑ protein, high OP
<250 lymphocytes, normal glucose, ↑ or normal protein
100–500 lymphocytes, ↓ glucose, ↑ protein
Lymphocytic pleocytosis, xanthochromia, ↑ protein, PCR +HSV
⊖
At risk for neurocysticercosis?[3]
Bacterial Meningitis[4]
Viral Meningitis
TB Meningitis
HSV Encephalitis[5]
⊕
Brain Abscess
Neuro-cysticercosis
Ceftriaxone + Vancomycin + Glucocorticoids ± Ampicilin[6]
Supportive care ± Acyclovir
RIPE + Dexamethasone
IV Acyclovir
IV Antibiotics, Drain, ± Glucocorticoids
Albendazole + Prednisone ± Antiseizure medication
Footnotes
1. Neurosyphilis can present without a fever and headache.
2. If delaying LP for additional testing, first give antibiotics. FAILS : Focal neurologic deficit, Altered mental status, Immunocompromise, Lesion over needle site, Seizures. If any of the FAILS symptoms are present, LP is not safe.
3. People living or with travel to endemic areas in Central and South America, sub-Saharan Africa.
4. See HYF page for specific pathogens.
5. Consider other viral causes of encephalitis (West Nile, St. Louis, Equine, etc).
6. Add ampicilin if patient is <3 months or >50 years old.

FIGURE 5.8

5-8 CNS Infection in an Immunocompetent Host

NEUROSYPHILIS

A 45-year-old M with PMH of gonorrhea and unprotected sexual intercourse presents with headache and difficulty ambulating. **Exam** shows small, irregular pupils that do not dilate to light, sensory ataxia, dysarthria, and decreased DTRs. **Labs** reveal (+) VDRL and FTA-ABS.

Management:

1. Consider LP for CSF testing regardless of known history of syphilis.
2. IV aqueous penicillin G for 10–14 days. If penicillin allergy, first undergo complete desensitization and then treat with penicillin.

Complications: Jarisch-Herxheimer reaction: Transient worsening in clinical condition (including worsening neurologic symptoms) after initiation of antibiotics due to dying *Treponema pallidum* (spirochete).

HYF: Neurosyphilis can happen at any stage of infection, early and late. Early neurosyphilis can present with meningitis. Late neurosyphilis can present with general paresis (affects cortex → memory loss, dysarthria, tremors, personality changes), tabes dorsalis (sensory ataxia, decreased DTRs, and pain), and Argyll-Robertson pupils. In late neurosyphilis, RPR may be non-reactive, but FTA-ABS will be reactive.

BRAIN ABSCESS

A 65-year-old M with PMH of endocarditis and IVDU presents with fever, headache. On **exam**, he has focal neurologic deficits and papilledema. **Labs** are notable for positive blood cultures. On **imaging**, CT head shows multiple ring-enhancing lesions.

Management:

1. Antibiotics.
2. Surgical drainage.
3. Glucocorticoids if significant mass effect.

Complications: Significant mass effect can cause herniation. Administer glucocorticoids if there is evidence of mass effect.

HYF: Brain abscesses can occur due to hematologic spread (via bacteremia) leading to multiple abscesses, direct spread (eg, untreated sinusitis, dental abscess) leading to 1 abscess, or direct inoculation (eg, head trauma, neurosurgery).

NEUROCYSTICERCOSIS

A 32-year-old M who immigrated from Central America 5 years ago presents with headache and new-onset seizures. On **exam**, he has papilledema. On **imaging**, CT head shows ring-enhancing lesions and multiple cysts.

Management:

1. Albendazole.
2. Prednisone to control inflammation and edema.
3. Anticonvulsant medications if seizures are present.
4. Consider intracranial hypertension and hydrocephalus management if present.

Complications:

- Intracranial hypertension (from the amount of cysts).
- Hydrocephalus (if cysts block CSF drainage).

HYF: Transmitted by *Taenia solium* (pork tapeworm) via fecal-oral human transmission, which is endemic in South and Central America, sub-Saharan Africa, and Asia. Symptoms appear after prolonged incubation (think of immigrants or farmers, not recent travelers). Imaging can have a "Swiss-cheese" appearance due to the number of lesions: cysts are new, whereas calcified lesions (often with central hyperdense foci) are old.

BACTERIAL MENINGITIS

A 30-year-old F presents with acute onset fever and headache. On **exam**, she has nuchal rigidity (positive Kernig and Brudzinski's sign) and photophobia. **Labs**: LP shows elevated opening pressure. CSF studies show WBCs >1000 of polymorphonuclear monocytes, glucose <40, protein >200, and (+) Gram stain.

Management:

1. Lumbar puncture with cell count, opening pressure, glucose, protein, and Gram stain.
2. Broad-spectrum antibiotics (ceftriaxone, vancomycin, ± ampicillin). Consider acyclovir while labs are pending.
3. Empiric steroids to prevent mass effect and herniation.
4. Once cultures speciate, narrow antibiotics.

Complications: Impaired mental status, seizures, sensorineural hearing loss, and focal neurologic deficits.

HYF: Diagnostics should not delay treatment! Give antibiotics before LP if you anticipate LP delay. Microbiological etiology for bacterial meningitis varies by age/underlying conditions and can impact presentation.

- <3 months old: Group B *Streptococci*, *E. coli*, *Listeria*.
- 3 months to 50 years: *Neisseria meningitidis* (#1 cause in teenagers. Presents with petechiae. Complications include Waterhouse-Friedrichsen syndrome. Post-exposure prophylaxis with rifampicin, or ciprofloxacin), *S. pneumoniae*, *H. influenzae*.
- >50 years: *S. pneumoniae*, *N. meningitidis*, *Listeria*.
- Recent neurosurgery (recent instrumentation): GNRs, MRSA, and coagulase negative *Staphylococcus*.
- If classic rashes are present, consider other, less common causes: Lyme (*Borrelia burgdorferi*), Rocky Mountain spotted fever (*Rickettsia rickettsii*).

If the following symptoms are present, obtain brain imaging to rule out a brain mass before performing a lumbar puncture to prevent herniation: "FAILS": Focal neurologic deficits, Altered mental status, Immunosuppression, Lesion, Seizures.

(Continued)

5-8 CNS Infection in an Immunocompetent Host

VIRAL MENINGITIS

A 10-year-old F presents with fever, headache, neck stiffness, and photophobia in July. **Exam** shows nuchal rigidity and a diffuse maculopapular exanthem. LP is performed. CSF **labs** show lymphocytes, normal protein and glucose, and no Gram staining.

Management:

1. LP with standard workup.
2. CSF PCR for viral pathogens.
3. If HSV is suspected (especially based on sexual history), consider acyclovir. Typically not needed for enterovirus.
4. If patient has risk factors for bacterial meningitis or is clinically unstable/deteriorating, start empiric antibiotics.

Complications: Typically none due to quick improvement.

HYF: Most common viral pathogens are enterovirus (especially in the summer/early fall) and HSV.

TB MENINGITIS

A 53-year-old M who works as a nurse presents with fever, headache, and vomiting. **Exam** shows nuchal rigidity and cranial nerve VI palsy. LP is performed. On **labs**, CSF studies show lymphocytes and low glucose. On **imaging**, CT head shows basal cistern meningeal enhancement and hydrocephalus.

Management:

1. LP with standard workup and acid-fast bacilli smear and culture.
2. Evaluate for systemic and pulmonary symptoms of TB.
3. Brain MRI and CT.
4. RIPE therapy [rifampin + isoniazid + pyrazinamide + ethionamide] therapy + dexamethasone.

Complications:

- Hydrocephalus: Closely monitor for clinical changes, consider serial LPs and/or surgical decompression.
- Hyponatremia.
- Long-term isoniazid requires Vitamin B_6 supplementation to prevent peripheral neuropathy.

HYF: Risk factors for TB include known/potential exposure to TB, travel to or residence in endemic area, and prior TB infection.

HSV ENCEPHALITIS

A 26-year-old M presents with acute onset fever, headache, altered mental status, and seizures. LP is performed. CSF **labs** show elevated lymphocytes, erythrocytes, and protein levels and normal glucose. CSF HSV PCR is positive. On **imaging**, CT head shows unilateral temporal lobe lesions with mass effect. EEG shows prominent intermittent high amplitude slow waves.

Management:

1. LP with standard workup and PCR for HSV.
2. IV acyclovir.

Complications: Early treatment with acyclovir is critical, as otherwise rates of mortality and morbidity are high.

HYF: HSV encephalitis has a predilection for the temporal lobes. CT head often reveals hypodense lesions in the temporal lobe but can be negative, so MRI is preferred. If symptoms point to encephalitis but PCR doesn't show HSV, consider other causes of encephalitis such as CMV, toxoplasmosis, West Nile virus, VZV, Lyme, RMSF, mycoplasma, and enterovirus.

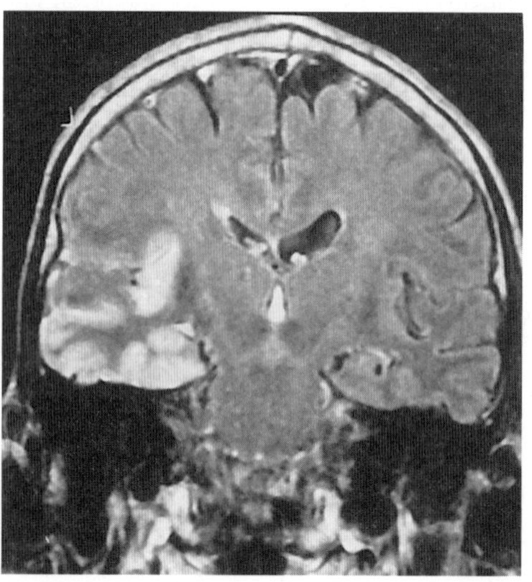

MRI/CT showing temporal lobe involvement in HSV encephalitis.

5-9 CNS Infection in an Immunocompromised Host

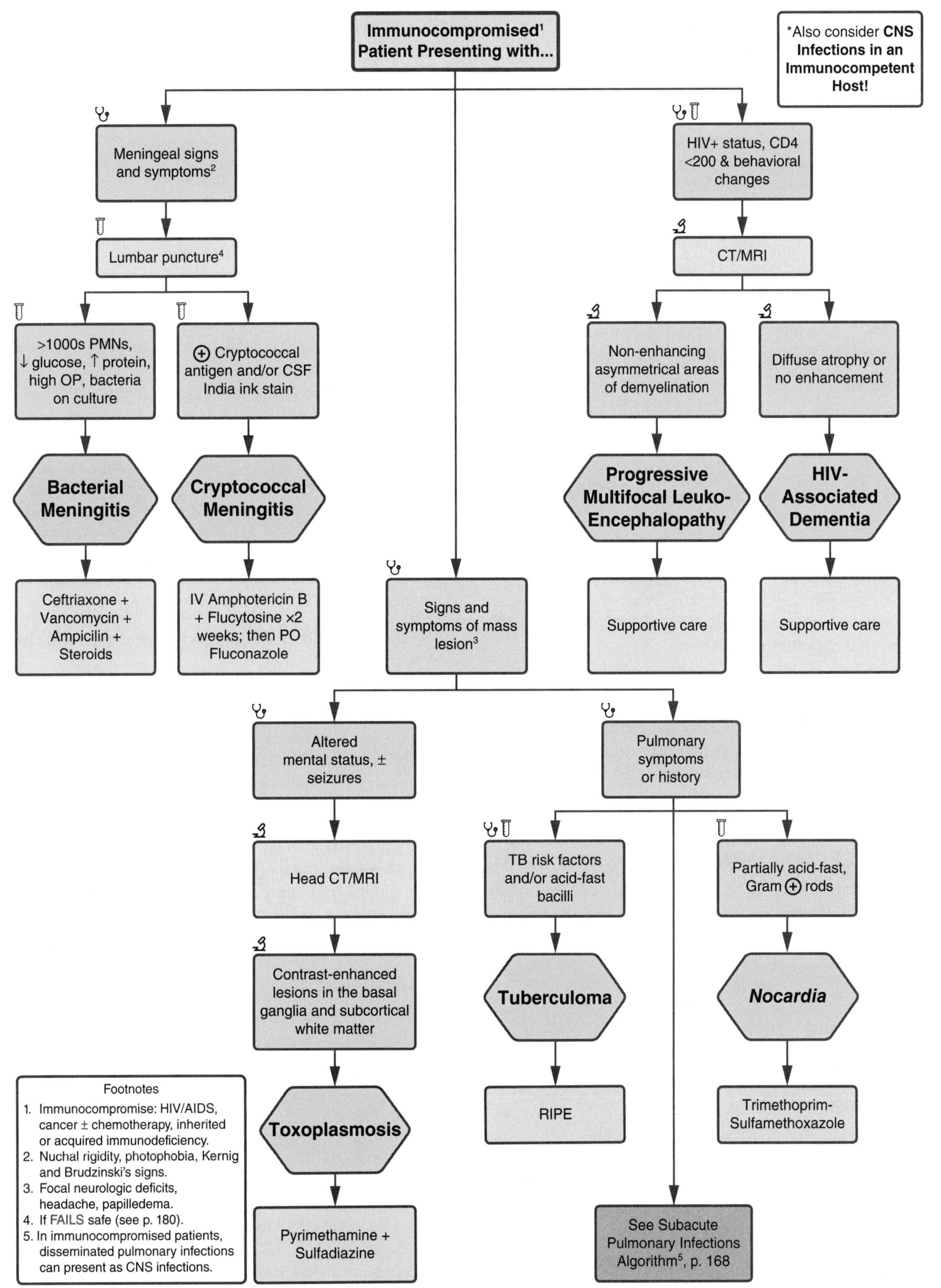

Immunocompromised[1] Patient Presenting with...
*Also consider CNS Infections in an Immunocompetent Host!
Meningeal signs and symptoms[2]
Lumbar puncture[4]
>1000s PMNs, ↓ glucose, ↑ protein, high OP, bacteria on culture
Bacterial Meningitis
Ceftriaxone + Vancomycin + Ampicilin + Steroids
⊕ Cryptococcal antigen and/or CSF India ink stain
Cryptococcal Meningitis
IV Amphotericin B + Flucytosine ×2 weeks; then PO Fluconazole
HIV+ status, CD4 <200 & behavioral changes
CT/MRI
Non-enhancing asymmetrical areas of demyelination
Progressive Multifocal Leuko-Encephalopathy
Supportive care
Diffuse atrophy or no enhancement
HIV-Associated Dementia
Supportive care
Signs and symptoms of mass lesion[3]
Altered mental status, ± seizures
Head CT/MRI
Contrast-enhanced lesions in the basal ganglia and subcortical white matter
Toxoplasmosis
Pyrimethamine + Sulfadiazine
Pulmonary symptoms or history
TB risk factors and/or acid-fast bacilli
Tuberculoma
RIPE
Partially acid-fast, Gram ⊕ rods
Nocardia
Trimethoprim-Sulfamethoxazole
See Subacute Pulmonary Infections Algorithm[5], p. 168
Footnotes
1. Immunocompromise: HIV/AIDS, cancer ± chemotherapy, inherited or acquired immunodeficiency.
2. Nuchal rigidity, photophobia, Kernig and Brudzinski's signs.
3. Focal neurologic deficits, headache, papilledema.
4. If FAILS safe (see p. 180).
5. In immunocompromised patients, disseminated pulmonary infections can present as CNS infections.

FIGURE 5.9

5-9 CNS Infection in an Immunocompromised Host

BACTERIAL MENINGITIS

See Bacterial Meningitis in CNS Infections in Immunocompetent hosts, pp. 181–182.

HYF: In immunocompromised hosts, consider *Listeria*, Gram-negative bacilli (including *Pseudomonas*), *Neisseria meningitidis* and *S. pneumoniae* as the most likely pathogens. In addition, also consider the same pathogens that affect immunocompetent hosts.

CRYPTOCOCCAL MENINGITIS

A 46-year-old M with PMH of HIV not on antiretroviral therapy (ART) presents with fever, headache, and impaired mentation. On **exam**, he has weak meningeal signs. LP is performed with very high opening pressure. CSF **labs** show monocytic predominance and + cryptococcal antigen testing.

Management:

1. LP with standard workup with fungal culture, CSF India ink stain and/or cryptococcal antigen testing (most sensitive).
2. IV Amphotericin B and Flucytosin for 2 weeks, followed by PO fluconazole (continue until CD4+ is >100 for ≥1 year).

Complications:

- High intracranial pressure (high opening pressure) might require serial LPs or VP shunt for management.
- Immune reconstitution inflammatory syndrome: Paradoxical worsening of symptoms after initiation of ART. Continue with ART and treat opportunistic infection.

HYF: *Cryptococcus neoformans* is the most common pathogen causing meningitis in patients with HIV/AIDS. Presentations of cryptococcal meningitis can vary from full meningeal symptoms to lack of concrete signs. Biopsy is characterized by "soap bubble lesions" and lack of inflammatory response. Exposure to pigeon droppings and soil is a risk factor.

PROGRESSIVE MULTIFOCAL LEUKOENCEPHALOPATHY

A 53-year-old F with PMH of HIV not on ART (last CD4 <200) presents with altered mental status. **Exam** shows dementia, hemianopia, and ataxia. On **imaging**, MRI brain shows non-enhancing multifocal demyelinating lesions.

Management:

1. CT or MRI to identify demyelinating lesions.
2. LP for routine studies and JC virus PCR.
3. Rule out other potential causes of reversible dementia.

Complications:

- Rapidly progressive with 50% mortality in months.

HYF: Caused by reactivation of latent JC virus (double stranded, circular, naked DNA virus). JC = Junky Cerebrum!

HIV-ASSOCIATED DEMENTIA

A 62-year-old M with PMH of HIV (CD4 count <200) presents with progressive cognitive deficits and apathy. On **imaging**, MRI brain shows diffuse atrophy.

Management:

1. Cognitive assessments.
2. Rule out reversible causes of dementia.
3. Initiating antiretroviral therapy has clear treatment and preventative benefits.

TOXOPLASMOSIS

A 62-year-old F with PMH of HIV/AIDS presents with subacute headache and confusion. On **exam**, she has right upper extremity paresthesias. On **imaging**, CT head shows 2 ring-enhancing lesions.

Management:

1. CT head or brain MRI (more sensitive) shows multiple isodense/hypodense ring-enhancing mass lesions, especially in the basal ganglia.
2. Serology, PCR, and tissue histology to identify *Toxoplasma*.
3. High-dose PO pyrimethamine + sulfadiazine (with leucovorin to prevent hematologic toxicity), then low-dose regimen until clinical and radiological improvement.
4. Prophylaxis with TMP-SMX or pyrimethamine + dapsone if CD4 <100 and (+) toxoplasmosis IgG.

Complications:

- Risk of congenital toxoplasmosis when affecting pregnant women (refer to TORCH infections on pp. 574-577).

HYF: Risk factors include eating undercooked meat and changing cat litter.

TUBERCULOMA

A 70-year-old F, previously incarcerated, with PMH of chronic cough presents with headache and slowly progressive hemiplegia. **Exam** shows mild papilledema. On **imaging**, CT head shows multiple discrete ring-enhancing brain lesions with surrounding edema.

Management:

1. Head CT/MRI to identify lesions.
2. Consider brain biopsy for acid-fast staining.
3. Consider workup for pulmonary and disseminated TB.
4. Treat with RIPE therapy.

Complications:

- Hydrocephalus and brainstem compression: Monitor size progression and consider surgical intervention.

NOCARDIA

An 89-year-old M with PMH of metastatic lung cancer s/p chemotherapy presents with headaches. On **exam**, he has worsened pain when lying down. On **imaging**, CT head shows brain abscess.

Management:

1. Consider tissue sampling for diagnosis if no pulmonary lesions are identified.
2. Treat with trimethoprim–sulfamethoxazole.

HYF: *Nocardia* is a weakly acid-fast, branching filamentous rod.

5-10 Endocarditis

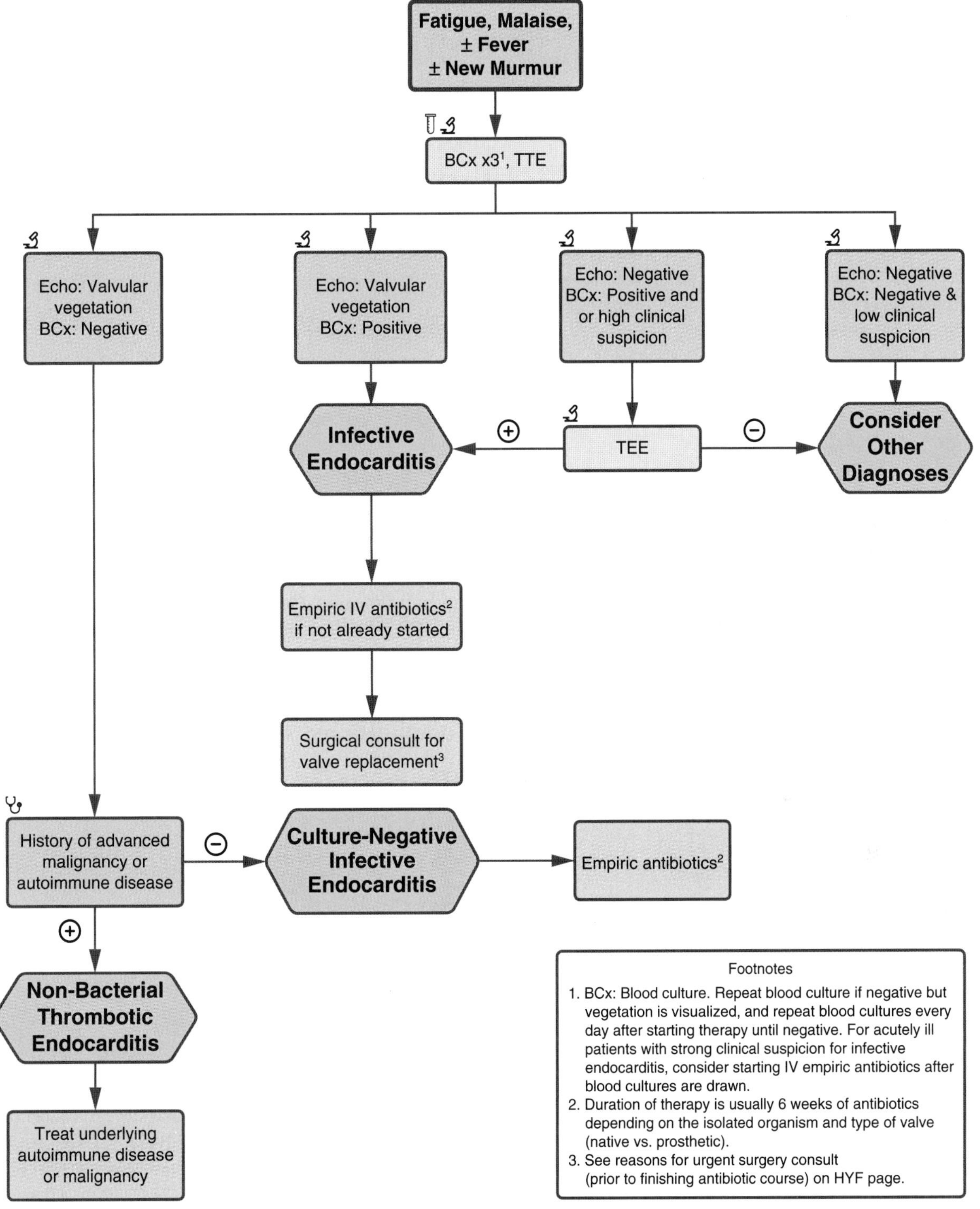
Fatigue, Malaise, ± Fever ± New Murmur
BCx x3[1], TTE
Echo: Valvular vegetation BCx: Negative
Echo: Valvular vegetation BCx: Positive
Echo: Negative BCx: Positive and or high clinical suspicion
Echo: Negative BCx: Negative & low clinical suspicion
Infective Endocarditis
TEE
Consider Other Diagnoses
Empiric IV antibiotics[2] if not already started
Surgical consult for valve replacement[3]
History of advanced malignancy or autoimmune disease
Culture-Negative Infective Endocarditis
Empiric antibiotics[2]
Non-Bacterial Thrombotic Endocarditis
Treat underlying autoimmune disease or malignancy
Footnotes
1. BCx: Blood culture. Repeat blood culture if negative but vegetation is visualized, and repeat blood cultures every day after starting therapy until negative. For acutely ill patients with strong clinical suspicion for infective endocarditis, consider starting IV empiric antibiotics after blood cultures are drawn.
2. Duration of therapy is usually 6 weeks of antibiotics depending on the isolated organism and type of valve (native vs. prosthetic).
3. See reasons for urgent surgery consult (prior to finishing antibiotic course) on HYF page.

FIGURE 5.10

5-10 Endocarditis

NATIVE VALVE ENDOCARDITIS (NVE)

A 30-year-old M with PMH of IVDU presents with 3 days of fever and anorexia. On **exam**, T is 38°C. On **labs**, WBC is 12000, and blood cultures grow *S. aureus*.

Management:

1. Empiric antibiotics are only necessary if there are acute signs or symptoms of endocarditis. Otherwise, wait for positive blood cultures.
2. If acute: Empiric IV vancomycin + IV cefepime, then narrow once cultures result for a total 6 weeks of antibiotic therapy.
3. All patients should get a surgical consult after antibiotics for consideration of valve repair/replacement.

Complications:

- Local infection → periannular abscess and conduction abnormalities (heart block).
- Emboli → systemic septic infarcts.
- Severe regurgitation → heart failure.
- Development of complications is consideration for surgery prior to completing antibiotics.

HYF:

- Most common bacterial causes:
  - *Staphylococcus aureus.*
  - Viridans group *streptococci.*
  - *Streptococcus gallolyticus (bovis).*
  - *Enterococcus* species.
  - HACEK organisms (*Haemophilus* species, *Aggregatibacter actinomycetemcomitans*, *Cardiobacterium hominis*, *Eikenella corrodens*, and *Kingella kingae*).
- Tricuspid valve > mitral valve = aortic valve.
  - Right-sided less likely to have murmur.
- TTE = 50% sensitive for IE; TEE >90% sensitive.
- Cutaneous exam findings: Petechiae, splinter hemorrhages in nail beds, Osler nodes (painful, pustular), Janeway lesions (non-painful).
- Presentation of endocarditis: FROM JANE (Fever, Roth spots, Osler nodes, Murmur, Janeway lesions, anemia, nail hemorrhage, emboli).
- Duke criteria for diagnosis: BE-FEVER
  - (Definite IE = 2 major OR 1 major + 3 minor).
  - Major criteria:
    - B: 2(+) blood cultures 12 hours apart with typical organism.
    - E: Echo very consistent.
  - Minor criteria:
    - F: Fever.
    - E: Immunologic evidence (eg, glomerulonephritis).
    - V: Vascular phenomena.
    - E: Microbial evidence (eg, BCx that don't meet major criteria).
    - R: Risk factors (IVDU, congenital valve disease).

PROSTHETIC VALVE ENDOCARDITIS

A 65-year-old M with PMH of aortic valve replacement presents with 5 weeks of night sweats, chills, and fatigue following a tooth extraction. On **exam**, he has a blowing diastolic murmur in the upper right sternal border. T is 37°C. On **labs**, WBC is 9000, and blood cultures grow *Enterococcus faecium*.

Management: 6 weeks of antibiotics.

Complications: All of the NVE complications + valvular dehiscence, which is an urgent surgical indication.

HYF:

- Most common causes:
  - *Staphylococcus aureus.*
  - Coagulase-negative staphylococci.
  - *Enterococcus* species.
- Antibiotic prophylaxis with amoxicillin is indicated prior to dental procedures for people with previous valve replacement.

CULTURE-NEGATIVE ENDOCARDITIS

A sheep farmer presents with a fever and is found to have a new murmur on **exam**. On **imaging**, a vegetation is seen on TTE and TEE. On **labs**, blood cultures ×3 have shown no growth for 7 days.

Management: Empiric antibiotics (IV vancomycin, ceftriaxone, and gentamicin).

Complications: Same as native valve endocarditis.

HYF:

- Most common causes (Under my umbr- "ella, ella, ella"):
  - *Coxiella burnetii.*
  - *Bartonella* species.
  - *Brucella* species.
  - Fungi (rare).
- HACEK organisms were traditionally culture-negative but are now routinely cultured using modern techniques.

NON-BACTERIAL THROMBOTIC ENDOCARDITIS

A 60-year-old F with PMH of metastatic breast cancer presents with new stroke and is found to have a valvular vegetation. On **exam**, she has no fever. On **labs**, she does not have leukocytosis. Blood cultures have been negative for 7 days.

Management: No antibiotics. Give heparin and treat underlying disease.

Complications: Sequelae of systemic emboli > heart failure.

HYF:

- Non-infectious. Associated with autoimmune disease or advanced malignancy.
- Also called Libman-Sacks or Marantic endocarditis.
- Both sides of the valve may be affected.

5-11 Cystitis

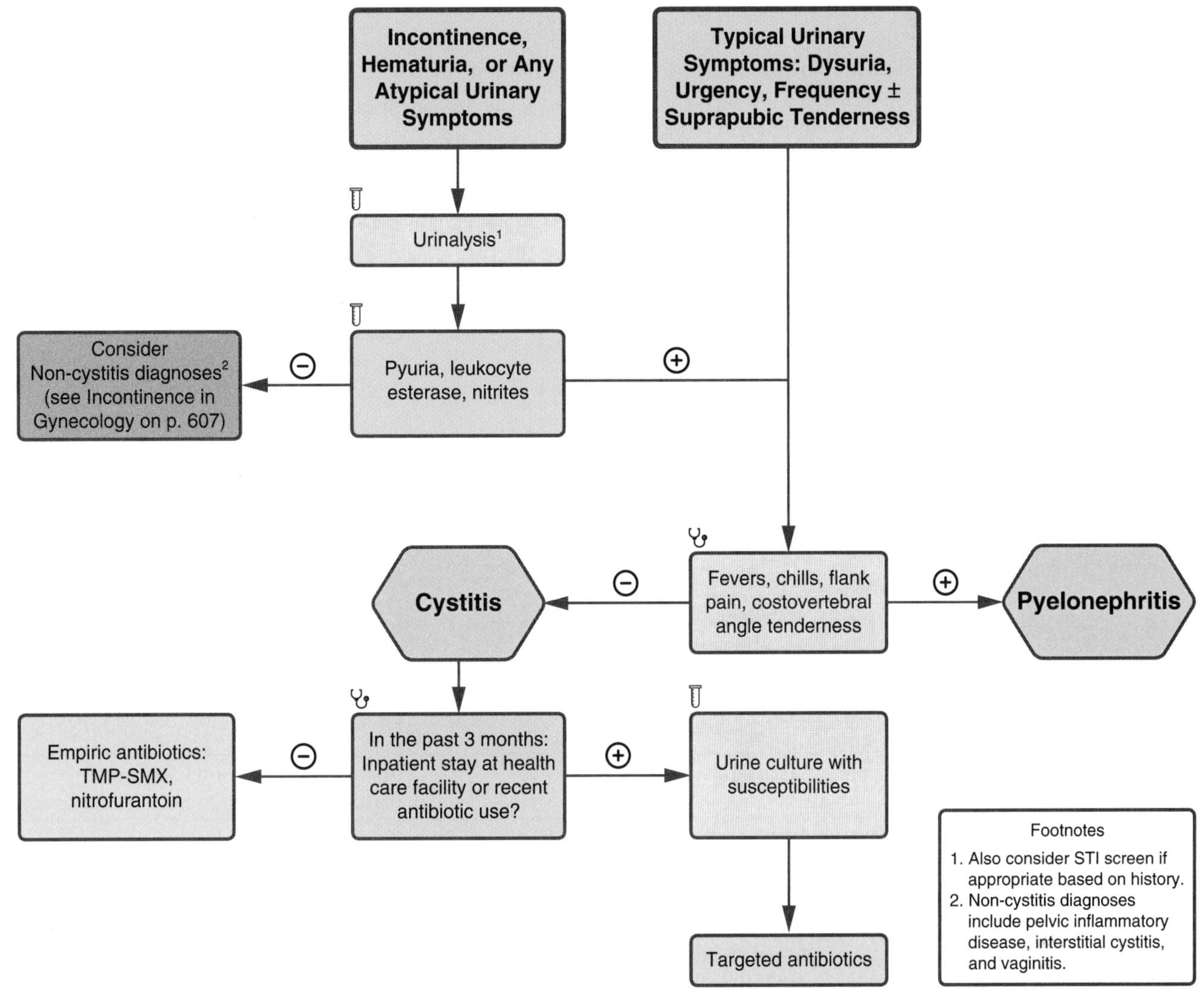
Incontinence, Hematuria, or Any Atypical Urinary Symptoms
Typical Urinary Symptoms: Dysuria, Urgency, Frequency ± Suprapubic Tenderness
Urinalysis[1]
Consider Non-cystitis diagnoses[2] (see Incontinence in Gynecology on p. 607)
Pyuria, leukocyte esterase, nitrites
Cystitis
Fevers, chills, flank pain, costovertebral angle tenderness
Pyelonephritis
Empiric antibiotics: TMP-SMX, nitrofurantoin
In the past 3 months: Inpatient stay at health care facility or recent antibiotic use?
Urine culture with susceptibilities
Targeted antibiotics
Footnotes
1. Also consider STI screen if appropriate based on history.
2. Non-cystitis diagnoses include pelvic inflammatory disease, interstitial cystitis, and vaginitis.

FIGURE 5.11

5-11 Cystitis

ACUTE SIMPLE CYSTITIS

A 45-year-old F with no PMH presents with burning with urination and increased urinary frequency. On **exam**, she has suprapubic tenderness to palpation. **Labs** show WBCs 20–50/hpf and (+) leukocyte esterase on UA.

Management:

1. TMP-SMX or nitrofurantoin.

Complications:

- Progression to pyelonephritis.
- If history of recent healthcare exposure, consider multi-drug resistant *E. coli* and perform urine cultures.

HYF:

- Common bacterial causes:
  - *E. coli* (most common).
  - *Klebsiella pneumoniae.*
  - *Proteus mirabilis.*
  - *S. saprophyticus* (in sexually active women).
  - If ESBL, consider carbapenem.
- UA is not required if symptoms clearly point toward cystitis.

Organism	Risk Factors	Treatment	HY Facts
E. coli	Most common UTI bacteria	If symptoms persist despite empiric treatment, consider culture and broadening antibiotics	Suspect MDR if recent healthcare or antibiotic exposure or if history of MDR
S. saprophyticus	Sexually active women	Susceptible to TMP-SMX or nitrofurantoin	
Enterococcus	Hospitalization, indwelling urinary catheter	Some strains are susceptible to nitrofurantoin May need vancomycin therapy. If VRE, then linezolid	
Proteus mirabilus	Prior history of *Proteus* infections	Susceptible to TMP-SMX	Urease causes urine alkalinization. Struvite stones are common (staghorn calculi)
Pseudomonas	Hospitalization Indwelling urinary catheter	Replace catheter if indwelling Susceptibility-driven treatment, though fosfomycin or ciprofloxacin are good 1st-line options	
Klebsiella pneumoniae		Susceptibility-driven treatment if resistant to TMP-SMX or nitrofurantoin	Can cause gas-forming UTIs Urease causes urine alkalinization Struvite stones common (staghorn calculi)
Enterobacter	Hospitalization	Susceptibility-driven treatment. Likely will require carbapenem.	

Pyelonephritis: See p. 245.

5-12 Acute Inflammatory Diarrhea

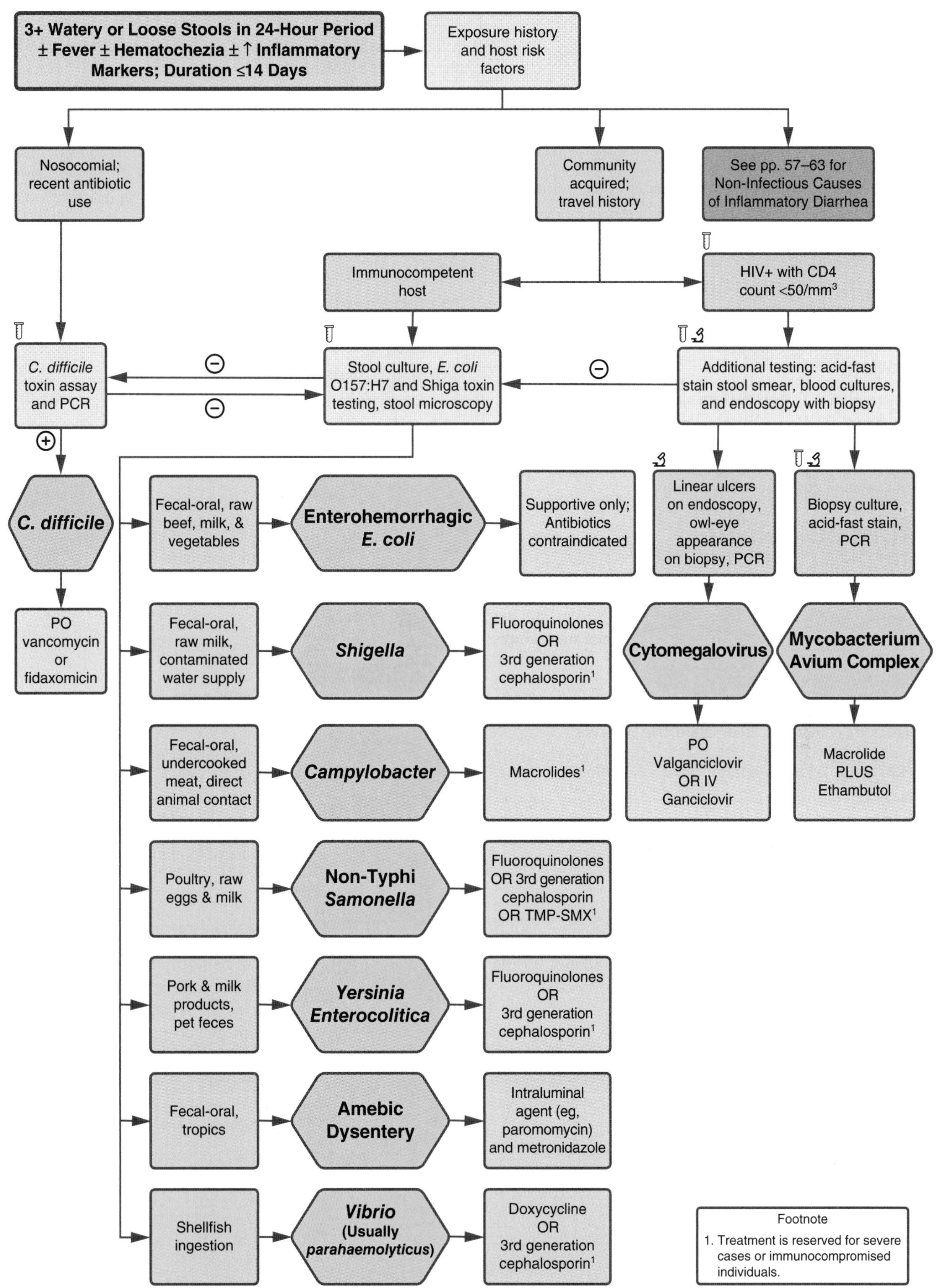

3+ Watery or Loose Stools in 24-Hour Period ± Fever ± Hematochezia ± ↑ Inflammatory Markers; Duration ≤14 Days
Exposure history and host risk factors
Nosocomial; recent antibiotic use
Community acquired; travel history
See pp. 57–63 for Non-Infectious Causes of Inflammatory Diarrhea
Immunocompetent host
HIV+ with CD4 count <50/mm3
C. difficile toxin assay and PCR
Stool culture, E. coli O157:H7 and Shiga toxin testing, stool microscopy
Additional testing: acid-fast stain stool smear, blood cultures, and endoscopy with biopsy
C. difficile
PO vancomycin or fidaxomicin
Fecal-oral, raw beef, milk, & vegetables
Enterohemorrhagic E. coli
Supportive only; Antibiotics contraindicated
Linear ulcers on endoscopy, owl-eye appearance on biopsy, PCR
Biopsy culture, acid-fast stain, PCR
Fecal-oral, raw milk, contaminated water supply
Shigella
Fluoroquinolones OR 3rd generation cephalosporin1
Cytomegalovirus
Mycobacterium Avium Complex
Fecal-oral, undercooked meat, direct animal contact
Campylobacter
Macrolides1
PO Valganciclovir OR IV Ganciclovir
Macrolide PLUS Ethambutol
Poultry, raw eggs & milk
Non-Typhi Samonella
Fluoroquinolones OR 3rd generation cephalosporin OR TMP-SMX1
Pork & milk products, pet feces
Yersinia Enterocolitica
Fluoroquinolones OR 3rd generation cephalosporin1
Fecal-oral, tropics
Amebic Dysentery
Intraluminal agent (eg, paromomycin) and metronidazole
Shellfish ingestion
Vibrio (Usually parahaemolyticus)
Doxycycline OR 3rd generation cephalosporin1
Footnote
1. Treatment is reserved for severe cases or immunocompromised individuals.

FIGURE 5.12

5-12 Acute Inflammatory Diarrhea

CLOSTRIDIOIDES DIFFICILE

A patient with an inpatient stay or antibiotic use in past 12 weeks OR on hospital day 3+ presents with new-onset watery diarrhea with trace mucus and blood. **Labs** are (+) for *C. difficile* toxins on stool analysis.

Management:

1. Endoscopy if diagnosis remains unclear after initial testing.
2. Antibiotic treatment is indicated in all symptomatic patients.
3. Initial episode: 1st-line is PO fidaxomicin or vancomycin; 2nd-line is metronidazole.
4. Recurrence: If initial episode was treated with vancomycin, then use fidaxomicin. Otherwise, give vancomycin followed by oral rifaximin. Consider fecal microbiota transplant.

Complications:

- Toxic megacolon with pseudomembranes.
- Paralytic ileus.

HYF: Only toxigenic strains cause infection; colonization with nontoxigenic strains does not require treatment.

ENTEROHEMORRHAGIC *ESCHERICHIA COLI*

A toddler with a history of eating undercooked beef burger presents with bloody diarrhea. On **exam**, he remains afebrile. He has decreased urine output, petechiae, and altered mental status. **Labs** are positive for O157:H7 on stool culture.

Management:

1. Antibiotics are contraindicated; supportive care only.

Complications: Most common cause of hemolytic uremic syndrome.

HYF: Produces shiga-like toxin (verotoxin).

SHIGELLA

A patient with recent travel to a low-resource setting presents with several days of high fever, tenesmus, and profuse mucoid-bloody diarrhea. **Labs** are positive for shiga toxin and non-motile Gram-negative rods on stool culture.

Management:

1. Severe cases: Fluoroquinolones or 3rd-generation cephalosporins.

Complications:

- Hemolytic uremic syndrome (2nd most common cause).
- Toxic megacolon.
- Febrile seizures in children.
- Reactive arthritis.

HYF: Also common among children, men who have sex with men, and skilled nursing facility residents. Invades M cells in Peyer's patches of the gastric mucosa.

CAMPYLOBACTER

A patient with recent consumption of undercooked meat OR direct contact with infected pet or livestock animal presents with high fever and bloody diarrhea. On **exam**, he has severe abdominal tenderness consistent with pseudo-appendicitis or colitis. On **labs**, stool testing shows curved, Gram-negative rods that replicate at 42°C.

Management:

1. Severe cases: Macrolides.

Complications:

- Guillain-Barre Syndrome.
- Reactive arthritis.

HYF: Most common cause of foodborne gastroenteritis in the US.

NON-TYPHOIDAL *SALMONELLA*

A patient with recent consumption of raw eggs, milk, and poultry OR contact with reptiles presents with mild fever, headaches, myalgias, severe vomiting, and watery-bloody diarrhea. On **labs**, stool testing shows motile Gram-negative rods.

Management:

1. Severe cases: Treat with fluoroquinolones, TMP-SMX, or cephalosporins depending on local sensitivities.

Complications:

- Reactive arthritis.
- Osteomyelitis, meningitis, myocarditis.

HYF: 2nd most common cause of foodborne gastroenteritis in the US.

YERSINIA ENTEROCOLITICA

An adult patient with PMH of hemochromatosis OR toddler with recent exposure to unpasteurized milk or dog feces presents with mild fever, vomiting, and diarrhea. On **exam**, the patient has abdominal tenderness consistent with pseudoappendicitis. On **labs**, stool testing shows growth of Gram-negative rod in cold environment.

Management:

1. Severe cases: Fluoroquinolones or 3rd-generation cephalosporins.

5-12 Acute Inflammatory Diarrhea

Complications:

- Reactive arthritis.
- Erythema nodosum.
- Toxic megacolon.

HYF: Can have prolonged course of many weeks.

VIBRIO PARAHAEMOLYTICUS

A patient with PMH of liver disease and/or hemochromatosis and recent consumption of shellfish presents with mild fever, bloody diarrhea, vomiting +/– bullous skin lesions. On **labs**, stool testing reveals growth of Gram-negative rods on a selective bile salt agar.

Management:

1. Antibiotic treatment is not indicated unless severe illness or co-occurring wound infection.
2. If severe illness or co-occurring wound infection, doxycycline OR 3rd-generation cephalosporin, surgical debridement.

Complications:

- Wound infection is more common with *V. vulnificus* but can occur with *V. parahaemolyticus* and can progress to septic shock and necrotizing fasciitis.

5-13 Acute Non-Inflammatory Diarrhea

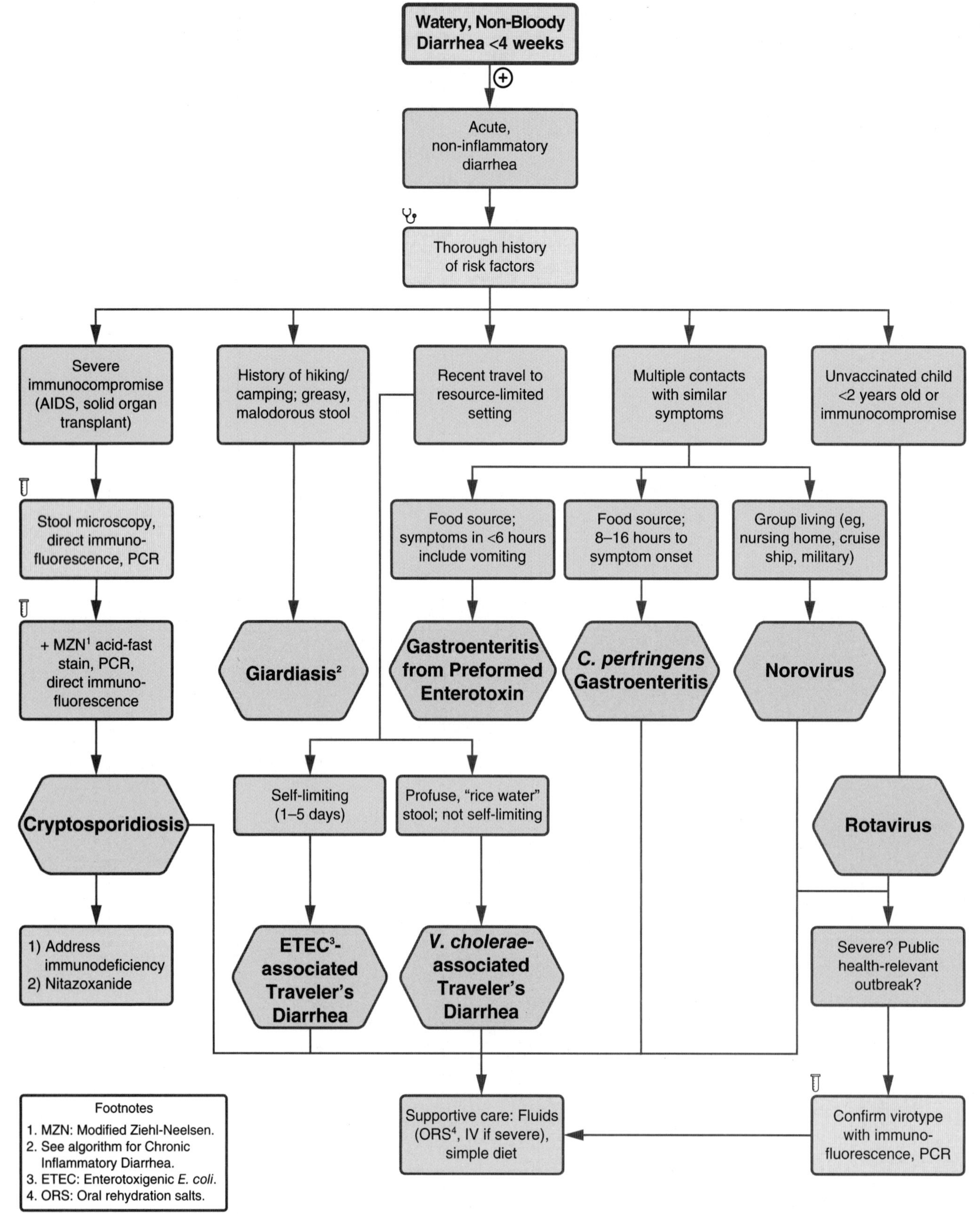
Watery, Non-Bloody Diarrhea <4 weeks
Acute, non-inflammatory diarrhea
Thorough history of risk factors
Severe immunocompromise (AIDS, solid organ transplant)
History of hiking/ camping; greasy, malodorous stool
Recent travel to resource-limited setting
Multiple contacts with similar symptoms
Unvaccinated child <2 years old or immunocompromise
Stool microscopy, direct immuno-fluorescence, PCR
+ MZN[1] acid-fast stain, PCR, direct immuno-fluorescence
Cryptosporidiosis
1) Address immunodeficiency
2) Nitazoxanide
Giardiasis[2]
Food source; symptoms in <6 hours include vomiting
Food source; 8–16 hours to symptom onset
Group living (eg, nursing home, cruise ship, military)
Gastroenteritis from Preformed Enterotoxin
C. perfringens Gastroenteritis
Norovirus
Rotavirus
Self-limiting (1–5 days)
Profuse, "rice water" stool; not self-limiting
ETEC[3]-associated Traveler's Diarrhea
V. cholerae-associated Traveler's Diarrhea
Severe? Public health-relevant outbreak?
Confirm virotype with immuno-fluorescence, PCR
Supportive care: Fluids (ORS[4], IV if severe), simple diet
Footnotes
1. MZN: Modified Ziehl-Neelsen.
2. See algorithm for Chronic Inflammatory Diarrhea.
3. ETEC: Enterotoxigenic E. coli.
4. ORS: Oral rehydration salts.

FIGURE 5.13

5-13 Acute Non-Inflammatory Diarrhea

GASTROENTERITIS FROM PREFORMED ENTEROTOXIN (*S. AUREUS, B. CEREUS*)

A 45-year-old F presents with vomiting and watery diarrhea 4 hours after eating with others who developed similar symptoms. **Exam** shows signs of dehydration. **Labs** show low stool osmotic gap (<50 mOsm/kg).

Management:

1. Supportive care.

Complications: None, typically self-resolves.

HYF: Symptoms appear <6 hours after exposure. *B. cereus* is associated with starchy food (eg, rice). *S. aureus* is associated with picnics and mayonnaise.

CLOSTRIDIUM PERFRINGENS GASTROENTERITIS

A 31-year-old M presents with watery diarrhea 12 hours after eating chicken at a new restaurant. **Exam** shows signs of dehydration. **Labs** show low stool osmotic gap (<50 mOsm/kg) and (+) stool culture for *C. perfringens*.

Management:

1. Supportive care.

Complications: None, typically self-resolves within 24–48 h.

HYF: 2nd most common cause of foodborne bacterial infection (after non-typhoidal *Salmonella*). Associated with improperly heated meats, poultry, and gravy, especially at restaurants.

NOROVIRUS

A 74-year-old F presents with diarrhea and vomiting 1 day after returning from vacation on a cruise ship where others had similar symptoms. **Exam** shows signs of dehydration. **Labs** show (+) RT-PCR and/or enzyme immunoassay for norovirus.

Management:

1. Supportive care.

Complications: None, typically self-resolves within 48–72 h.

HYF: Most common cause of gastroenteritis among all age groups. Symptom onset 24–48 hours after exposure. Outbreaks associated with restaurants, cruise ships, schools/daycares, and healthcare facilities.

CRYPTOSPORIDIOSIS (*CRYPTOSPORIDIUM PARVUM*)

A 52-year-old M with PMH of HIV/AIDS presents with 4 weeks of watery diarrhea, malaise, and ~10 lb weight loss. On **exam**, he has signs of dehydration. **Labs** show (+) *Cryptosporidium* on direct immunofluorescent antibody test and oocysts on modified Ziehl-Neelsen acid-fast stain.

Management:

If Immunocompetent:	If Immunocompromised:
1. Supportive care. 2. Nitazoxanide.	1. Address immunodeficiency (eg, start ART, stop immunosuppressive medication). 2. Nitazoxanide.

Complications:

- Biliary tract involvement.
- Persistent GI symptoms, arthralgias.

HYF: Spread by fecal-oral route. Resolves within 10–14 days in immunocompetent hosts but may persist indefinitely in immunocompromised hosts.

ROTAVIRUS

A 2-year-old M who attends daycare presents with watery diarrhea, vomiting, and fussiness for 12 hours. On **exam,** he has fever, signs of dehydration, and abdominal tenderness. **Labs** show no fecal leukocytes.

Management:

1. Supportive care.

Complications: None, self-resolves within 5–10 days.

HYF: Much more common in children than adults. Incubation period is 3–10 days. Rotavirus vaccine series (live attenuated) is administered orally at age 2–6 months.

ENTEROTOXIGENIC *E. COLI*-ASSOCIATED DIARRHEA

A 51-year-old M presents with watery diarrhea > vomiting 1 day after returning from travel to a resource-limited setting. **Exam** shows signs of dehydration. **Labs** show low stool osmotic gap (<50 mOsm/kg).

Management:

1. Supportive care.

Complications: None, typically self-resolves.

HYF: Due to enterotoxin formed in intestine. Symptoms appear >24 hours after exposure. Most common cause of "traveler's diarrhea."

V. CHOLERAE-ASSOCIATED DIARRHEA

A 24-year-old M presents with copious, watery diarrhea 2 days after returning from travel to a resource-limited setting. **Exam** shows signs of severe dehydration. **Labs** show low stool osmotic gap (<50 mOsm/kg).

Management:

1. IV fluids.

Complications: Severe dehydration, electrolyte abnormalities.

HYF: Copious "rice-water" stools begin >48 hours after exposure. Also associated with raw seafood consumption.

Giardiasis: Can present as inflammatory or non-inflammatory. See Chronic Inflammatory Diarrhea, pp. 58–60.

5-14 Roundworm and Tapeworm Infections

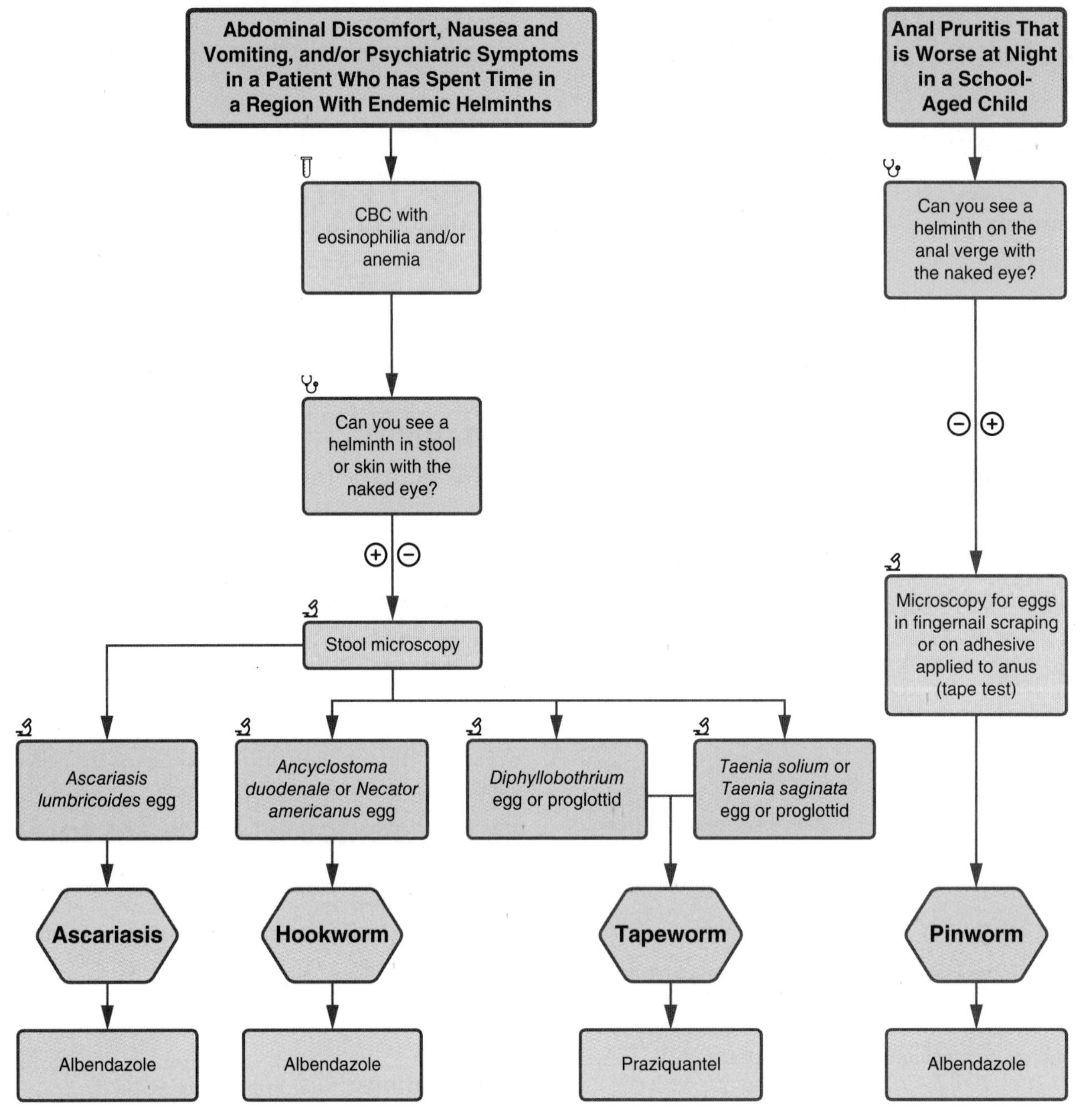
Abdominal Discomfort, Nausea and Vomiting, and/or Psychiatric Symptoms in a Patient Who has Spent Time in a Region With Endemic Helminths
CBC with eosinophilia and/or anemia
Can you see a helminth in stool or skin with the naked eye?
Stool microscopy
Ascariasis lumbricoides egg
Ancyclostoma duodenale or *Necator americanus* egg
Diphyllobothrium egg or proglottid
Taenia solium or *Taenia saginata* egg or proglottid
Ascariasis
Hookworm
Tapeworm
Albendazole
Albendazole
Praziquantel
Anal Pruritis That is Worse at Night in a School-Aged Child
Can you see a helminth on the anal verge with the naked eye?
Microscopy for eggs in fingernail scraping or on adhesive applied to anus (tape test)
Pinworm
Albendazole

FIGURE 5.14

5-14 Roundworm and Tapeworm Infections

ASCARIASIS (*ASCARIS LUMBRICOIDES*)

A 12-year-old M who recently emigrated from Laos presents with abdominal discomfort, nausea, vomiting, and diarrhea. The patient had a dry cough and wheeze 2 months ago that resolved. **Labs** show microcytic anemia and eosinophilia.

Management:

1. Albendazole (pyrantel pamoate if pregnant).

Complications:

- Obstruction of the small bowel or biliary tree.
- Malnutrition, growth retardation, and impaired cognitive development in children.

HYF: Transmitted via fecal-oral route. Larvae enter the bloodstream, migrate to the lungs, and mature to adults in the intestine. Approximately 1 billion people are infected, mostly in Asia.

HOOKWORM (*ANCYCLOSTOMA DUODENALE, NECATOR AMERICANUS*)

A previously healthy 25-year-old F presents with postprandial epigastric pain. She has been building septic tanks in rural Alabama and had an itchy rash between her toes, which has resolved. **Labs** show microcytic anemia and eosinophilia.

Management:

1. Treat with albendazole (pyrantel pamoate if pregnant).

Complications: Anemia, malnutrition, and growth retardation in children.

HYF: Hookworm larvae penetrate the bare feet of people walking in soil contaminated with feces. *A. duodenale* is endemic to the Mediterranean, the Middle East and Asia. *N. Americanus* is endemic to the Americas and Africa.

TAPEWORM (*TAENIA SAGINATA, TAENIA SOLIUM, DIPHYLLOBOTHRIUM LATUM*)

A 50-year-old Japanese fisherman presents with weakness and tingling in his extremities and loss of balance. He has 1–2 alcoholic drinks per month. On **exam**, ankle reflexes are absent bilaterally. Romberg sign is positive. **Labs** show macrocytic anemia.

Management:

1. Treat all species with praziquantel.

Complications:

- *D. latum* classically presents with vitamin B12 deficiency and megaloblastic anemia.
- *T. solium* autoinfection is associated with neurocysticercosis.
- All species can cause bowel obstruction.

HYF: *D. latum* is transmitted by eating raw fish and is endemic to Eastern Europe and Japan. It is the longest parasite that can infect humans (up to 10 meters!). *T. saginata* and *T. solium* are transmitted by eating undercooked beef and pork, respectively.

PINWORM (*ENTEROBIUS VERMICULARIS*)

A previously healthy 6-year-old girl complains that her anus is itchy, especially at night. **Exam** shows excoriations on the perianal skin. **Labs** are normal.

Management:

1. Diagnose by visualizing 8–13 mm mobile white worms on the anal verge or by microscopy of fingernail scrapings or tape applied to the anus (eggs are not present in stool).
2. Treat with albendazole (pyrantel pamoate if pregnant).

Complications:

- Abdominal pain, nausea, and vomiting.
- Eosinophilic enterocolitis.
- Extraintestinal migration: vulvovaginitis, salpingitis, cervicitis, peritoneal inflammation.

HYF: *E. vermicularis* is transmitted via fecal-oral route. Adult worms colonize the colon and lay eggs in the anal verge. It is the most common helminthic infection in the US and western Europe.

*__Trichinellosis__ is caused by parasitic roundworms of the genus *Trichinella*. It is acquired via ingestion of undercooked meat in developing countries (Mexico, Thailand). Patients present with a classic triad of myositis, periorbital edema, and eosinophilia. Treat with thiabendazole or mebendazole.

5-15 Zoonoses

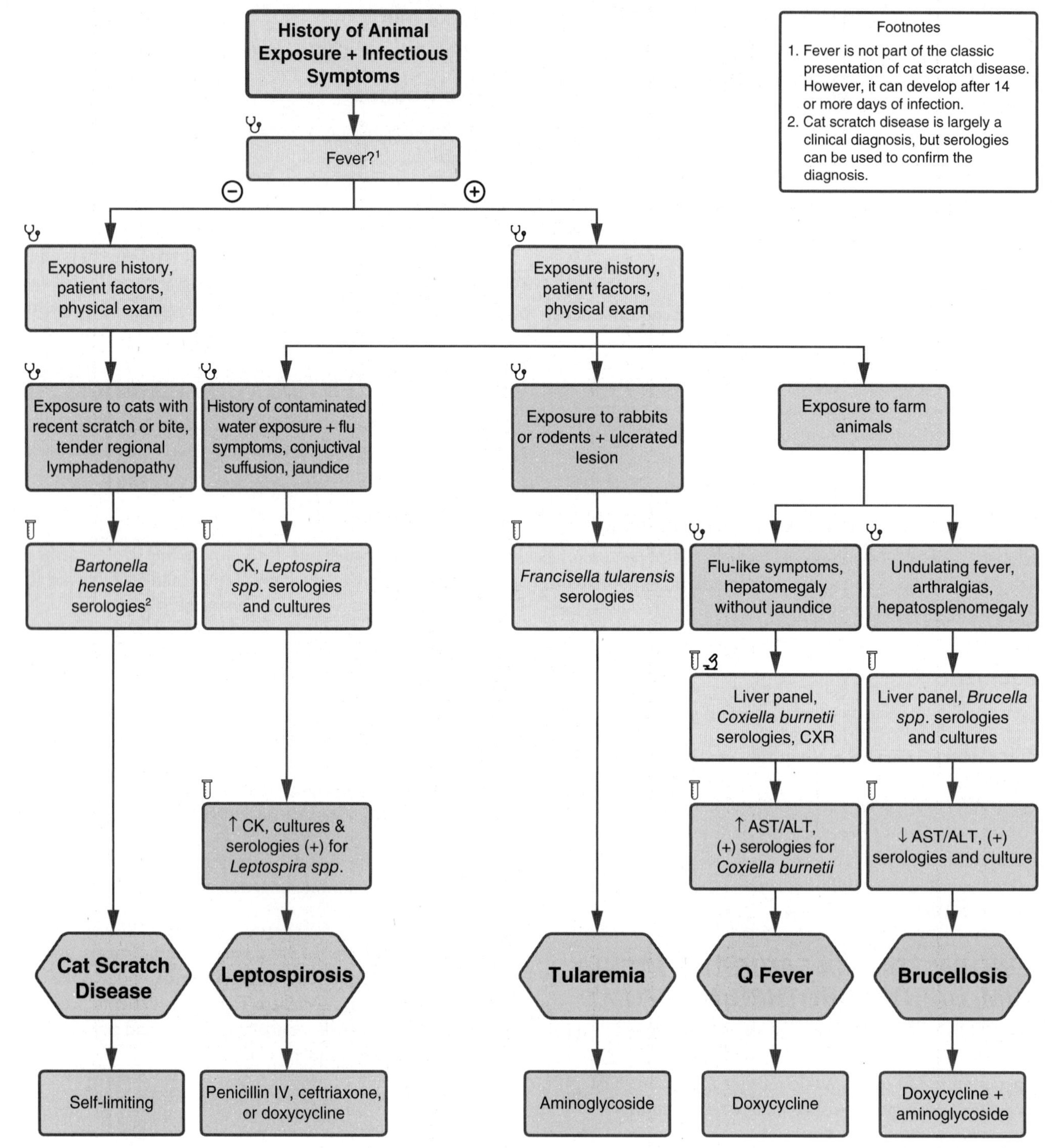
History of Animal Exposure + Infectious Symptoms
Fever?[1]
⊖
⊕
Exposure history, patient factors, physical exam
Exposure history, patient factors, physical exam
Exposure to cats with recent scratch or bite, tender regional lymphadenopathy
History of contaminated water exposure + flu symptoms, conjuctival suffusion, jaundice
Exposure to rabbits or rodents + ulcerated lesion
Exposure to farm animals
Bartonella henselae serologies[2]
CK, *Leptospira spp.* serologies and cultures
Francisella tularensis serologies
Flu-like symptoms, hepatomegaly without jaundice
Undulating fever, arthralgias, hepatosplenomegaly
Liver panel, *Coxiella burnetii* serologies, CXR
Liver panel, *Brucella spp.* serologies and cultures
↑ CK, cultures & serologies (+) for *Leptospira spp.*
↑ AST/ALT, (+) serologies for *Coxiella burnetii*
↓ AST/ALT, (+) serologies and culture
Cat Scratch Disease
Leptospirosis
Tularemia
Q Fever
Brucellosis
Self-limiting
Penicillin IV, ceftriaxone, or doxycycline
Aminoglycoside
Doxycycline
Doxycycline + aminoglycoside
Footnotes
1. Fever is not part of the classic presentation of cat scratch disease. However, it can develop after 14 or more days of infection.
2. Cat scratch disease is largely a clinical diagnosis, but serologies can be used to confirm the diagnosis.

FIGURE 5.15

5-15 Zoonoses

BRUCELLOSIS

A 45-year-old M farmer presents with 3 weeks of undulating fevers, arthralgias, night sweats, headache, and anorexia. On **exam**, he has hepatosplenomegaly and fever. **Labs** show elevated AST/ALT; positive cultures of the blood, CSF, urine, and bone marrow; and positive serologies.

Management: Doxycycline and aminoglycoside.

Complications: Spondylitis, endocarditis, neurobrucellosis, GU involvement.

HYF: **Causative Agent:** *Brucella spp.*; **Transmission:** Animal exposure (esp. farm), ingestion of contaminated animal products (eg, unpasteurized dairy products).

CAT SCRATCH DISEASE

A 35-year-old F with recent cat scratch injury now presents with nodular skin lesion at scratch site. On **exam**, she has tender regional lymphadenopathy ipsilateral to scratch site. **Labs** show (+) serologic tests (enzyme immunoassay or indirect fluorescence assay titers).

Management: Self-limiting, though azithromycin speeds recovery. If neuroretinitis or hepatosplenic disease, doxycycline/azithromycin + rifampin.

Complications: Disseminated infection (liver, spleen, eye, bone, or CNS).

HYF: **Causative Agent:** *Bartonella henselae*; **Transmission:** cat scratch or bite; **Other:** *B. henselae* can cause bacillary angiomatosis in HIV+ patients (presents with firm, red, friable, exophytic nodules).

LEPTOSPIROSIS

A 36-year-old F with recent travel to Puerto Rico presents with fever, myalgias, chills. On **exam**, she has conjunctival suffusion, fever, and jaundice. **Labs** show (+) blood and CSF cultures, positive serologic tests, and elevated CK.

Management: Mild disease: PO doxycycline; severe disease: IV penicillin, doxycycline, ceftriaxone, or cefotaxime + supportive care.

Complications: Weil's disease (severe form with hepatic and renal failure).

HYF: **Causative Agent:** *Leptospira spp.*; **Transmission:** Exposure to water or soil contaminated with animal urine; associated with swimming and water sports.

Q FEVER

A 38-year-old M farmer presents with high-grade fever, flu-like symptoms, and non-productive cough. On **exam**, he has fever and hepatomegaly without jaundice. **Labs** show AST/ALT elevation and (+) serologic tests (indirect immunofluorescence antibody titers). On **imaging**, CXR shows segmental opacification.

Management: Doxycycline, with the addition of hydoxychloroquine if end-organ involvement.

Complications: Endocarditis, vascular infection, bone and joint infection.

HYF: **Causative Agent:** *Coxiella burnetii*; **Transmission:** Inhalation of contaminated aerosols from or contact with fluids of laboring farm animals (eg, farmers, veterinarians).

TULAREMIA

A 27-year-old F farmer presents with fever and an ulcerated lesion on her left forearm. On **exam**, she has fever and regional lymphadenopathy. **Labs** show positive serologies.

Management: Streptomycin, gentamicin, or doxycycline.

Complications: Prolonged fever, sepsis, rhabdomyolysis, renal failure, hepatitis.

HYF: **Causative Agent:** *Francisella tularensis*; **Transmission:** Contact with infected animal (rabbits, rodents, prairie dogs, etc.), handling infected animal tissues, bites from ticks or flies.

5-16 Arthropod-Borne Diseases

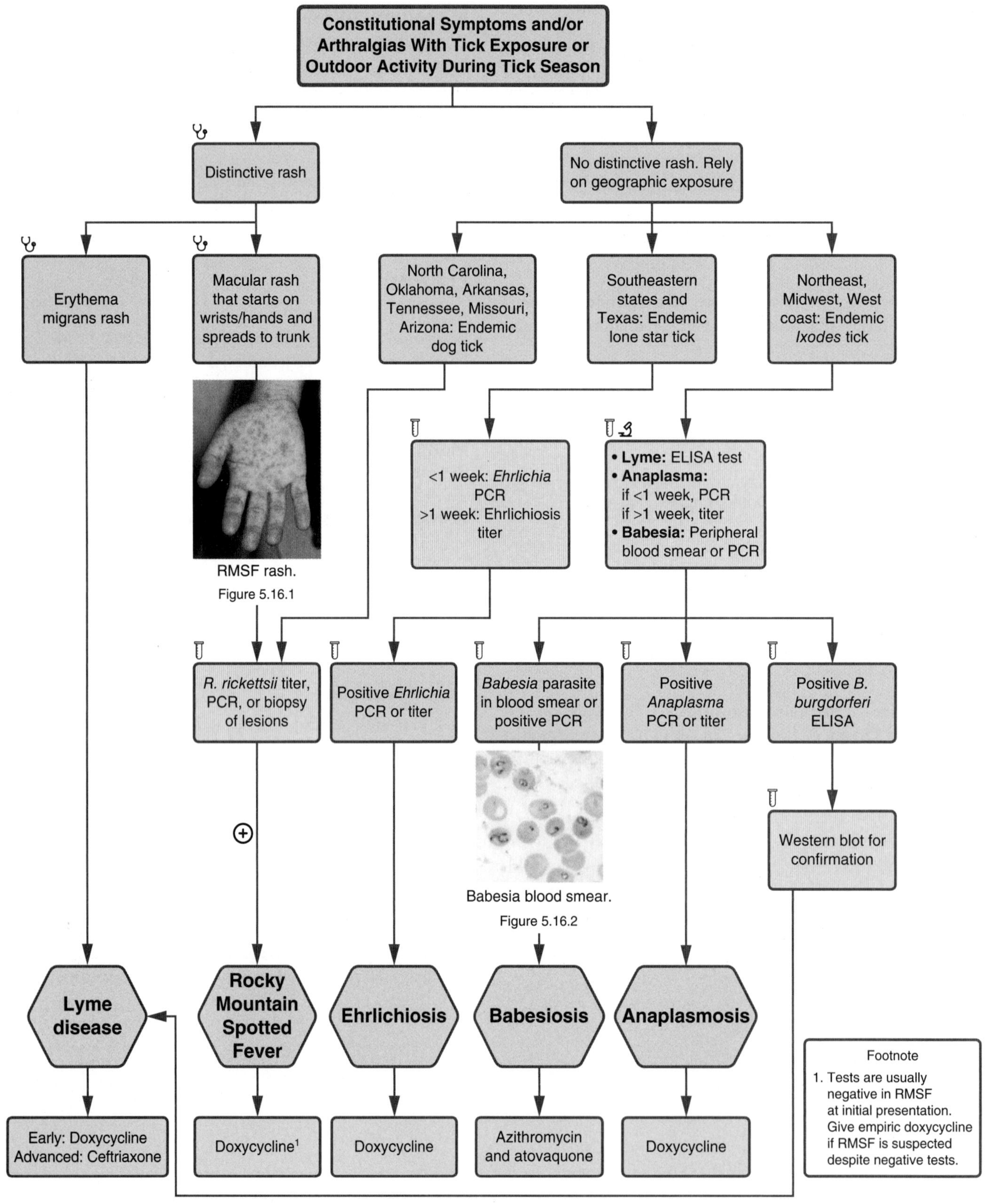

Constitutional Symptoms and/or Arthralgias With Tick Exposure or Outdoor Activity During Tick Season
Distinctive rash
No distinctive rash. Rely on geographic exposure
Erythema migrans rash
Macular rash that starts on wrists/hands and spreads to trunk
North Carolina, Oklahoma, Arkansas, Tennessee, Missouri, Arizona: Endemic dog tick
Southeastern states and Texas: Endemic lone star tick
Northeast, Midwest, West coast: Endemic *Ixodes* tick
RMSF rash.
Figure 5.16.1
<1 week: *Ehrlichia* PCR
>1 week: Ehrlichiosis titer
• **Lyme:** ELISA test
• **Anaplasma:** if <1 week, PCR if >1 week, titer
• **Babesia:** Peripheral blood smear or PCR
R. rickettsii titer, PCR, or biopsy of lesions
Positive *Ehrlichia* PCR or titer
Babesia parasite in blood smear or positive PCR
Positive *Anaplasma* PCR or titer
Positive *B. burgdorferi* ELISA
Western blot for confirmation
Babesia blood smear.
Figure 5.16.2
Lyme disease
Rocky Mountain Spotted Fever
Ehrlichiosis
Babesiosis
Anaplasmosis
Early: Doxycycline
Advanced: Ceftriaxone
Doxycycline[1]
Doxycycline
Azithromycin and atovaquone
Doxycycline
Footnote
1. Tests are usually negative in RMSF at initial presentation. Give empiric doxycycline if RMSF is suspected despite negative tests.

FIGURE 5.16

5-16 Arthropod-Borne Diseases

LYME DISEASE

A 12-year-old F with no PMH presents with fever and flu-like symptoms several days after returning from summer camp in Connecticut. On **exam**, she has a new target-shaped lesion on her arm.

Management:

1. If erythema migrans lesion is present, treat immediately with doxycycline.
2. If erythema migrans lesion is not present, confirm diagnosis with enzyme-linked immunoassay (ELISA) and Western blot test.
3. In advanced disease (eg, CNS involvement or arthritis), treat with ceftriaxone.

Complications:

- Early disseminated disease: Meningitis, Bell's palsy, radiculopathy, myocarditis, 3rd-degree AV block, migratory polyarthropathy.
- Late disease: Arthritis, encephalitis.

HYF: Caused by *Borrelia burgorferi,* a spirochete carried by *Ixodes scapularis* ticks, which are endemic to the Northeast, Midwest and West Coast of the US.

ROCKY MOUNTAIN SPOTTED FEVER

A 40-year-old F with no PMH presents with fever, headache, and rash 1 week after hiking with her dog in Missouri. On **exam**, she is febrile with a petechial rash on her wrists and ankles. **Labs** show thrombocytopenia.

Management:

1. Confirm diagnosis with titer, PCR, or biopsy of lesions.
2. Treat with doxycycline.

Complications: Altered mental status, disseminated intravascular coagulation (DIC).

HYF: Caused by *Rickettsia rickettsii,* a bacteria carried by American dog ticks in the central and southern US.

EHRLICHIOSIS

A 30-year-old F presents with altered mental status 1 week after clearing brush in Texas. On **exam**, she is febrile with nuchal rigidity. **Labs** show leukopenia, thrombocytopenia, and elevated ALT/AST. CSF sample shows elevated lymphocytes, elevated protein, and morulae in monocytes.

Management:

1. Diagnose with PCR or titer.
2. Treat with doxycycline.

Complications: Seizures, coma, renal and respiratory failure.

HYF: Caused by bacteria carried by the lone star tick, which is endemic to Texas and the southeastern US.

BABESIOSIS

A 65-year-old M with PMH of HTN presents with flu-like symptoms after returning from a hunting trip in northern of Michigan. On **exam**, he is febrile with jaundiced skin. **Labs** show hemolytic anemia.

Management:

1. Diagnose with PCR or peripheral blood smear.
2. Blood smear demonstrates ring-shaped or "Maltese cross" protozoa within RBCs.
3. Treat with azithromycin and atovaquone.

Complications: Intravascular hemolysis, anemia, jaundice.

HYF: Caused by protozoa carried by *Ixodes scapularis* tick, which has the same geographic distribution as Lyme disease and anaplasmosis.

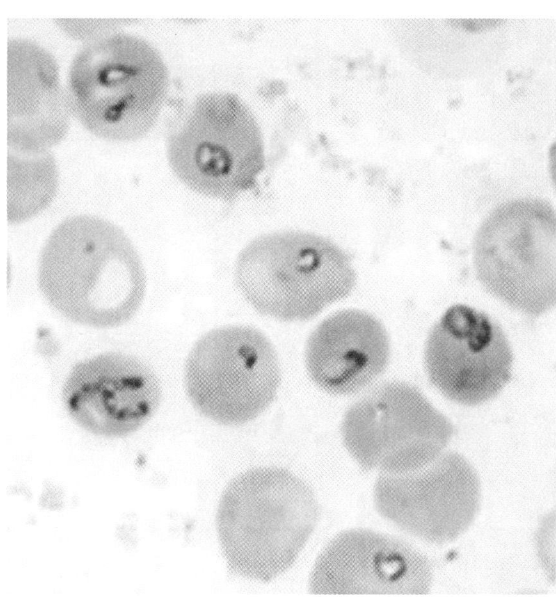

Babesia spp. parasitizes RBCs as shown in this blood film.

ANAPLASMOSIS

A 24-year-old M presents with flu-like illness 4 days after finding an engorged tick on his calf following a camping trip on the Oregon coast. On **exam**, he is febrile. **Labs** are notable for neutropenia.

Management:

1. Diagnose with PCR or titer.
2. Treat with doxycycline.

Complications:

- Seizure, coma, renal and respiratory failure.
- Opportunistic infections: HSV esophagitis, invasive aspergillosis, candidiasis.

HYF: Caused by bacteria carried by *Ixodes scapularis* tick. Same geographic distribution as Lyme and babesiosis. Blood smear shows morulae in granulocytes.

5-17 Fever in a Returning Traveler

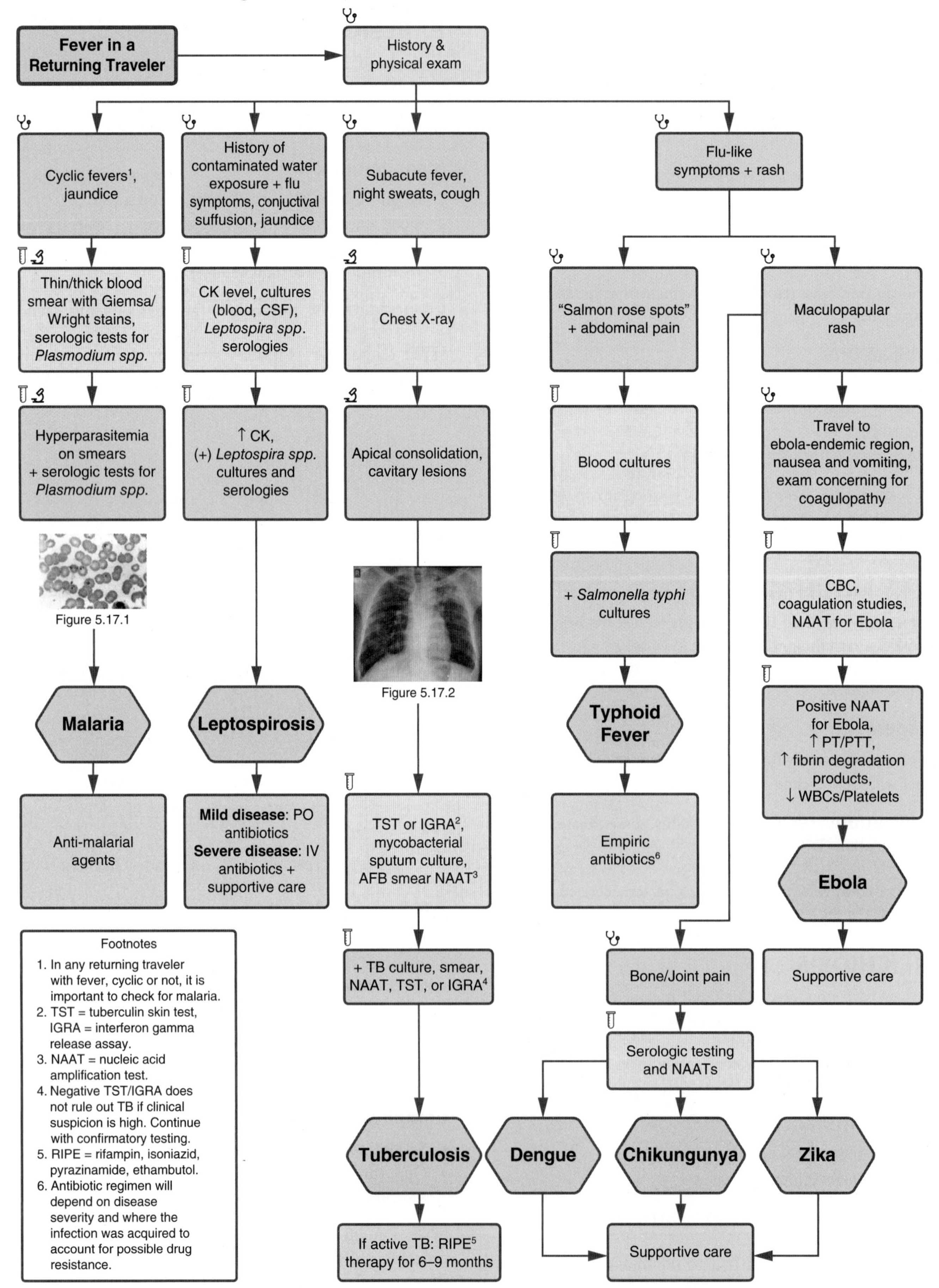
Fever in a Returning Traveler
History & physical exam
Cyclic fevers[1], jaundice
History of contaminated water exposure + flu symptoms, conjuctival suffusion, jaundice
Subacute fever, night sweats, cough
Flu-like symptoms + rash
Thin/thick blood smear with Giemsa/ Wright stains, serologic tests for Plasmodium spp.
CK level, cultures (blood, CSF), Leptospira spp. serologies
Chest X-ray
"Salmon rose spots" + abdominal pain
Maculopapular rash
Hyperparasitemia on smears + serologic tests for Plasmodium spp.
↑ CK, (+) Leptospira spp. cultures and serologies
Apical consolidation, cavitary lesions
Blood cultures
Travel to ebola-endemic region, nausea and vomiting, exam concerning for coagulopathy
Figure 5.17.1
Figure 5.17.2
+ Salmonella typhi cultures
CBC, coagulation studies, NAAT for Ebola
Malaria
Leptospirosis
Typhoid Fever
Positive NAAT for Ebola, ↑ PT/PTT, ↑ fibrin degradation products, ↓ WBCs/Platelets
Anti-malarial agents
Mild disease: PO antibiotics Severe disease: IV antibiotics + supportive care
TST or IGRA[2], mycobacterial sputum culture, AFB smear NAAT[3]
Empiric antibiotics[6]
Ebola
+ TB culture, smear, NAAT, TST, or IGRA[4]
Bone/Joint pain
Supportive care
Serologic testing and NAATs
Tuberculosis
Dengue
Chikungunya
Zika
If active TB: RIPE[5] therapy for 6–9 months
Supportive care
Footnotes
1. In any returning traveler with fever, cyclic or not, it is important to check for malaria.
2. TST = tuberculin skin test, IGRA = interferon gamma release assay.
3. NAAT = nucleic acid amplification test.
4. Negative TST/IGRA does not rule out TB if clinical suspicion is high. Continue with confirmatory testing.
5. RIPE = rifampin, isoniazid, pyrazinamide, ethambutol.
6. Antibiotic regimen will depend on disease severity and where the infection was acquired to account for possible drug resistance.

FIGURE 5.17

5-17 Fever in a Returning Traveler

TYPHOID FEVER

A 45-year-old M with recent travel to Asia presents with 1 week of high fever, new abdominal pain, and skin discoloration. On **exam**, he has a fever, salmon rose spots, and relative bradycardia. **Labs** show bacteremia with blood cultures positive for typhoidal *Salmonella*.

Management: Empiric antibiotic therapy (ceftriaxone, fluoroquinolones, etc.); narrow when susceptibilities are available.

Complications: Intestinal bleeding/perforation in week 3 if untreated, sepsis, death.

HYF: **Causative Agent:** Typhoidal *Salmonella* species (*S. typhi, S. paratyphi A*). **Transmission**: Fecal-oral via ingestion of contaminated food and water. Endemic to resource-limited nations with poor sanitation; travelers can get typhoid vaccine prior to travel.

DENGUE FEVER

A 32-year-old M with recent travel to Africa presents with fever, rash, myalgias, bone pain, and retro-orbital pain. On **exam**, he has a fever and morbilliform maculopapular rash with islands of skin with sparing of the palms and soles. **Labs** show thrombocytopenia, positive viral serologies, and nucleic acid amplification tests.

Manaagement: Supportive care (PRN fluids, blood products).

Complications: Severe thrombocytopenia, bleeding, shock; untreated disease can progress to dengue hemorrhagic fever.

HYF: Dengue virus is transmitted through the bite of the *Aedes* mosquito.

ZIKA

A 48-year-old F with recent travel to the Caribbean presents with fever, pruritic rash, arthralgias, myalgias, and headache. On **exam**, she has nonpurulent conjunctivitis and an erythematous maculopapular rash. **Labs** show positive viral serologic and nucleic acid amplification tests.

Management: Supportive care.

Complications: Guillain-Barre syndrome, microcephaly in congenital infection.

HYF: Zika virus is transmitted primarily through the bite of the *Aedes* mosquito, though it can also occur through maternal-fetal transmission, organ transplantation, blood product transfusion, and sex.

CHIKUNGUNYA

A 29-year-old F with recent travel to India presents with fever, rash, myalgias, symmetric polyarthralgias, and headache. On **exam**, she has a fever and generalized morbilliform maculopapular rash interrupted by areas of normal skin, peripheral edema, and cervical lymphadenopathy. **Labs** show positive viral serologic and nucleic acid amplification tests.

Management: Supportive care.

Complications: Chronic arthritis/arthralgias.

HYF: Chikungunya virus is transmitted through the bite of the *Aedes* mosquito.

EBOLA

A 38-year-old M veterinarian with recent work-related travel to West Africa presents with fever, vomiting, diarrhea, abdominal pain, and bloody stools. On **exam**, he has a fever, petechiae, ecchymoses, and diffuse maculopapular rash. **Labs** show thrombocytopenia, prolonged PT/PTT, elevated fibrin degradation products, and positive viral nucleic acid amplification tests.

Management: Supportive care.

Complications: Multiorgan failure and death; complications of treatment include sepsis, lung/renal injury, amd respiratory failure.

HYF: Ebola virus can be transmitted via person-to-person transmission through contact with infected body fluids or via infected animals.

MALARIA

A 42-year-old F traveler who returned from Africa 1 week ago who stopped prophylactic medications upon returning presents with with cyclic high-grade fevers, headaches, myalgias, abdominal pain, nausea, vomiting, and diaphoresis. On **exam**, she has fever, jaundice, and hepatosplenomegaly. **Labs** show hyperparasitemia ("ring" forms) on Giemsa/Wright stained thin/thick blood smears and positive serologic tests.

Management: If uncomplicated infection: chloroquine. If resistant: mefloquine, atovaquone-proguanil, artemisinins. Add atovaquone-proguanil if *Plasmodium vivax, P. ovale*, or unknown species.

Complications: Cerebral malaria, Gram-negative bacteremia, hemolytic anemia, renal and liver injury, hypoglycemia, lactic acidosis, pulmonary edema.

HYF: **Causative Agents:** *Plasmodium falciparum, P. vivax, P. ovale, P. malariae, P. knowlesi.* **Transmission:** Bite of infected female *Anopheles* mosquito in endemic areas. Other: Prevent by using mosquito repellants, bed nets, chemoprophylaxis (chloroquine; if resistant, use atovaquone-proguanil, mefloquine, doxycycline, or tafenoquine; start 2 weeks prior to travel, use through travel, end 4 weeks post-departure). Fever pattern varies depending on species involved. Hemoglobinopathies (eg, sickle cell disease) are protective.

5-18 HIV-AIDS

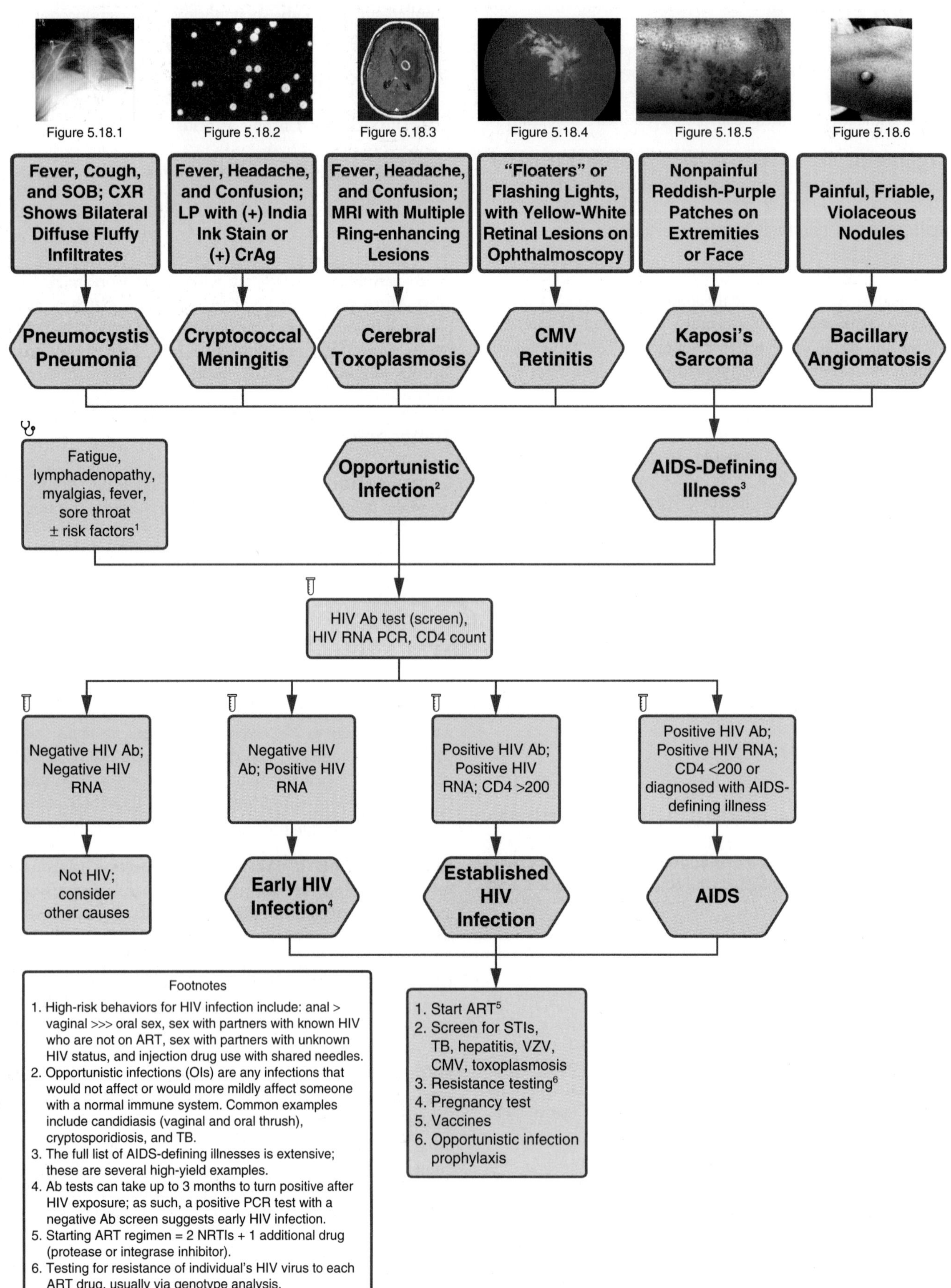

Figure 5.18.1
Figure 5.18.2
Figure 5.18.3
Figure 5.18.4
Figure 5.18.5
Figure 5.18.6
Fever, Cough, and SOB; CXR Shows Bilateral Diffuse Fluffy Infiltrates
Fever, Headache, and Confusion; LP with (+) India Ink Stain or (+) CrAg
Fever, Headache, and Confusion; MRI with Multiple Ring-enhancing Lesions
"Floaters" or Flashing Lights, with Yellow-White Retinal Lesions on Ophthalmoscopy
Nonpainful Reddish-Purple Patches on Extremities or Face
Painful, Friable, Violaceous Nodules
Pneumocystis Pneumonia
Cryptococcal Meningitis
Cerebral Toxoplasmosis
CMV Retinitis
Kaposi's Sarcoma
Bacillary Angiomatosis
Fatigue, lymphadenopathy, myalgias, fever, sore throat ± risk factors[1]
Opportunistic Infection[2]
AIDS-Defining Illness[3]
HIV Ab test (screen), HIV RNA PCR, CD4 count
Negative HIV Ab; Negative HIV RNA
Negative HIV Ab; Positive HIV RNA
Positive HIV Ab; Positive HIV RNA; CD4 >200
Positive HIV Ab; Positive HIV RNA; CD4 <200 or diagnosed with AIDS-defining illness
Not HIV; consider other causes
Early HIV Infection[4]
Established HIV Infection
AIDS
1. Start ART[5]
2. Screen for STIs, TB, hepatitis, VZV, CMV, toxoplasmosis
3. Resistance testing[6]
4. Pregnancy test
5. Vaccines
6. Opportunistic infection prophylaxis

Footnotes

1. High-risk behaviors for HIV infection include: anal > vaginal >>> oral sex, sex with partners with known HIV who are not on ART, sex with partners with unknown HIV status, and injection drug use with shared needles.
2. Opportunistic infections (OIs) are any infections that would not affect or would more mildly affect someone with a normal immune system. Common examples include candidiasis (vaginal and oral thrush), cryptosporidiosis, and TB.
3. The full list of AIDS-defining illnesses is extensive; these are several high-yield examples.
4. Ab tests can take up to 3 months to turn positive after HIV exposure; as such, a positive PCR test with a negative Ab screen suggests early HIV infection.
5. Starting ART regimen = 2 NRTIs + 1 additional drug (protease or integrase inhibitor).
6. Testing for resistance of individual's HIV virus to each ART drug, usually via genotype analysis.

FIGURE 5.18

5-18 HIV-AIDS

ACUTE HIV INFECTION

A patient presents with 3 days of fever, sore throat, myalgias, and non-tender enlarged cervical lymph nodes on **exam**. He had unprotected anal sex 2 weeks ago. On **labs**, HIV Ab test is negative, but HIV VL >100,000.

Management:

1. Start ART (NRTI x2 + PI/INSTI).
2. Screen for co-infections with other STIs.
3. Screen for diseases that progress more rapidly with a weakened immune system: TB, hepatitis, HPV (+ pap smear), toxoplasmosis, VZV, CMV.
4. Perform HIV genotype analysis to identify drug resistance.
5. Administer all age-indicated vaccines.
6. Start opportunistic infection prophylaxis if indicated (see below).

Complications: Opportunistic infections, progression to AIDS (usually ~8–10 years without ART).

HYF:

- Prototype ART drugs:
  - Nucleoside reverse transcriptase inhibitors (NRTIs): Emtricitabine, lamivudine, tenofovir.
  - Non-nucleoside reverse transcriptase inhibitors (NNRTIs): Efavirenz.
  - Protease inhibitors (PIs): Ritonavir-boosted darunavir.
  - Integrase strand transfer inhibitors (INSTIs): Dolutegravir.
- Opportunistic infection prophylaxis:
  - CD4 <200: PCP → TMP-SMX (Dapsone or atovaquone if allergy).
  - CD4 <100: Toxoplasmosis → same regimen as PCP.
  - CD4 <50: Disseminated MAC → azithromycin (not necessary if starting ART).
- In question stems, look for clues: Oropharyngeal candidiasis (thrush) often signifies HIV infection.
- AIDS = HIV+ with CD4 <200 OR AIDS-defining illness.

AIDS-DEFINING ILLNESSES

The aids-defining illnesses are pneumocystis, crytopcoccal meningitis, cerebral toxoplasmosis, cmv retinitis, kaposi's sarcoma, and bacillary angiomatosis. Acute HIV infection does not count.

PNEUMOCYSTIS JIROVECII PNEUMONIA

A 25-year-old M with PMH of IVDU presents with 2 weeks of fever, cough, and dyspnea. On **imaging**, CXR shows diffuse, bilateral, interstitial, and alveolar infiltrates.

Management: TMP-SMX, ART, + corticosteroids for moderate to severe disease.

CRYPTOCOCCAL MENINGITIS

A 40-year-old F with PMH of HIV not on ART presents with fever, headache, and altered mental status. CD4 <100. On **imaging**, brain MRI shows hydrocephalus.

Management: Anti-fungals (amphotericin B and flucytosine), LPs to reduce ICP, ART.

HYF: India ink staining of CSF shows encapsulated yeast (faster than testing for *Cryptococcus* antigen). Rarely presents with mass lesion on brain imaging.

CEREBRAL TOXOPLASMOSIS

A 30-year-old M with PMH of HIV not on ART presents with fever, headache, and altered mental status. CD4 <100. On **imaging** brain MRI shows multiple ring-enhancing lesions. On **labs**, serum is (+) for toxoplasma IgG.

Management: Sulfadiazine, pyrimethamine, and leucovorin or TMP-SMX.

CMV RETINITIS

A 40-year-old F sex worker presents with new "floaters" in 1 eye. On **exam**, fundoscopy shows yellow-white retinal lesions with associated hemorrhage.

Management: Anti-virals (valganciclovir) and ART.

Complications: Retinal detachment, blindness.

KAPOSI'S SARCOMA

A 50-year-old M with oral thrush presents with **exam** findings of non-painful elliptical reddish-purple patches on forearms.

Management: Start ART; chemoradiation therapy is rarely needed.

HYF: Vascular tumor caused by HHV-8.

BACILLARY ANGIOMATOSIS (*BARTONELLA HENSELAE*)

A 30-year-old F with PMH of HIV not on ART presents with several painful violaceous nodules on **exam** that bleed profusely with trauma. She has a cat.

Management: Doxycycline ×3 months; start ART.

6

Internal Medicine: Nephrology

6-1 Hyponatremia

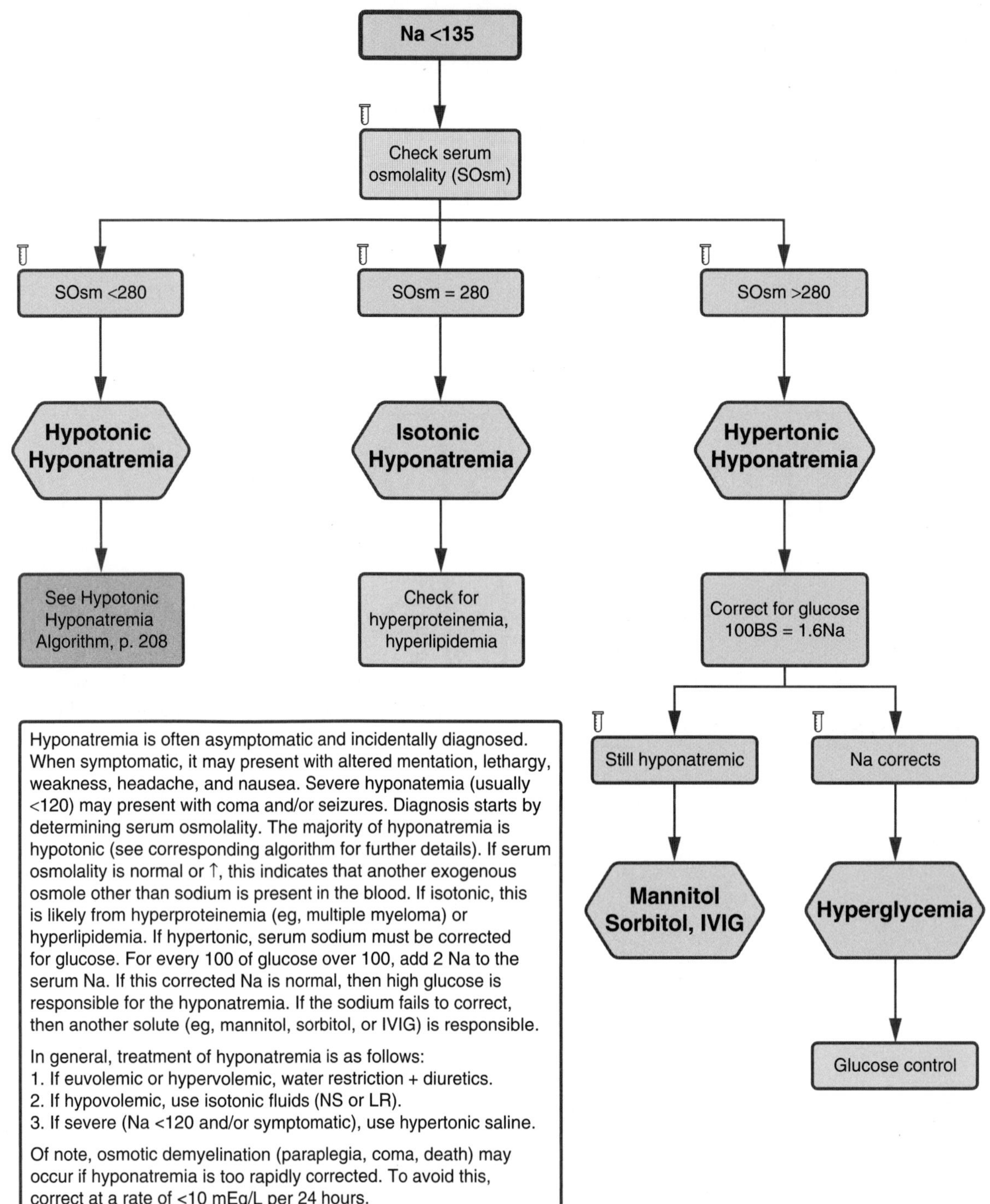
Na <135
Check serum osmolality (SOsm)
SOsm <280
SOsm = 280
SOsm >280
Hypotonic Hyponatremia
Isotonic Hyponatremia
Hypertonic Hyponatremia
See Hypotonic Hyponatremia Algorithm, p. 208
Check for hyperproteinemia, hyperlipidemia
Correct for glucose 100BS = 1.6Na
Still hyponatremic
Na corrects
Mannitol Sorbitol, IVIG
Hyperglycemia
Glucose control

Hyponatremia is often asymptomatic and incidentally diagnosed. When symptomatic, it may present with altered mentation, lethargy, weakness, headache, and nausea. Severe hyponatemia (usually <120) may present with coma and/or seizures. Diagnosis starts by determining serum osmolality. The majority of hyponatremia is hypotonic (see corresponding algorithm for further details). If serum osmolality is normal or ↑, this indicates that another exogenous osmole other than sodium is present in the blood. If isotonic, this is likely from hyperproteinemia (eg, multiple myeloma) or hyperlipidemia. If hypertonic, serum sodium must be corrected for glucose. For every 100 of glucose over 100, add 2 Na to the serum Na. If this corrected Na is normal, then high glucose is responsible for the hyponatremia. If the sodium fails to correct, then another solute (eg, mannitol, sorbitol, or IVIG) is responsible.

In general, treatment of hyponatremia is as follows:
1. If euvolemic or hypervolemic, water restriction + diuretics.
2. If hypovolemic, use isotonic fluids (NS or LR).
3. If severe (Na <120 and/or symptomatic), use hypertonic saline.

Of note, osmotic demyelination (paraplegia, coma, death) may occur if hyponatremia is too rapidly corrected. To avoid this, correct at a rate of <10 mEq/L per 24 hours.

FIGURE 6.1

6-1 Hyponatremia

ISOTONIC HYPONATREMIA (PSEUDOHYPONATREMIA)

A 50-year-old M with PMH of plasma cell dyscrasia (eg, multiple myeloma, Waldenström macroglobulinemia) or ↑↑ serum lipids/triglycerides is found to have hyponatremia. **Labs** show hyponatremia with normal serum osmolality (300).

Management:

1. Treat underlying condition.
2. If from blood dyscrasia, treat with chemotherapy, radiation therapy, biologic therapy, and/or hematopoietic stem cell transplant based on underlying disease.
3. If from hyperlipidemia, statin.

Complications: None.

HYF: Very rare. Due to lab error and/or in the technique used by lab equipment to measure serum Na, as some lab techniques measure the Na concentration in whole plasma. Remember to check serum osmolality. Pseudohyponatremia is most commonly due to accumulation of cholesterol components (eg, hyperlipidemia) but can also be due to abnormally high levels of proteins (eg, intravenous immunoglobulin therapy, myelodysplastic syndromes, immunoglobulin deposition diseases such as amyloidosis).

HYPERTONIC HYPONATREMIA: HYPERGLYCEMIA

A 60-year-old M with PMH of uncontrolled diabetes presents with hyperglycemia (eg, DKA, HHS). On **exam**, he has dry mucous membranes and ↓ skin turgor. **Labs** show ↑ serum osm (>300) and hyponatremia that corrects to normal for glucose.

Management:

1. Treat hyperglycemia with insulin.

Complications: Sequelae of underlying disorder.

HYF: To correct Na for hyperglycemia, add 2 Na for every 100 glucose over 100. So, if the serum glucose is 200, add 2 to the measured Na. If glucose is 450, add 7, and so on.

HYPERTONIC HYPONATREMIA: EXOGENOUS SOLUTES

A 45-year-old F with recent administration of mannitol, IVIG, or surgical irrigation with sorbitol is found to have hyponatremia on routine labs. **Labs** show ↑ serum osm (>300) and hyponatremia that fails to correct to normal for glucose.

Management:

1. Close monitoring.
2. If severe, dialysis.

HYF: To calculate correction for glucose, Na concentration ↓ by 2 for every 100 glucose above 100 (as noted previously). The hyponatremia in this instance is of the same mechanism that causes hyponatremia in the setting of hyperglycemia (ie, movement of fluid into the extracellular space because of the acutely increased extracellular osmolarity). In the case of mannitol administration, hypertonic hyponatremia typically only occurs in patients with impaired renal function, in whom the mannitol is retained.

Hypotonic Hyponatremia: See pp. 208–210.

6-2 Hypotonic Hyponatremia

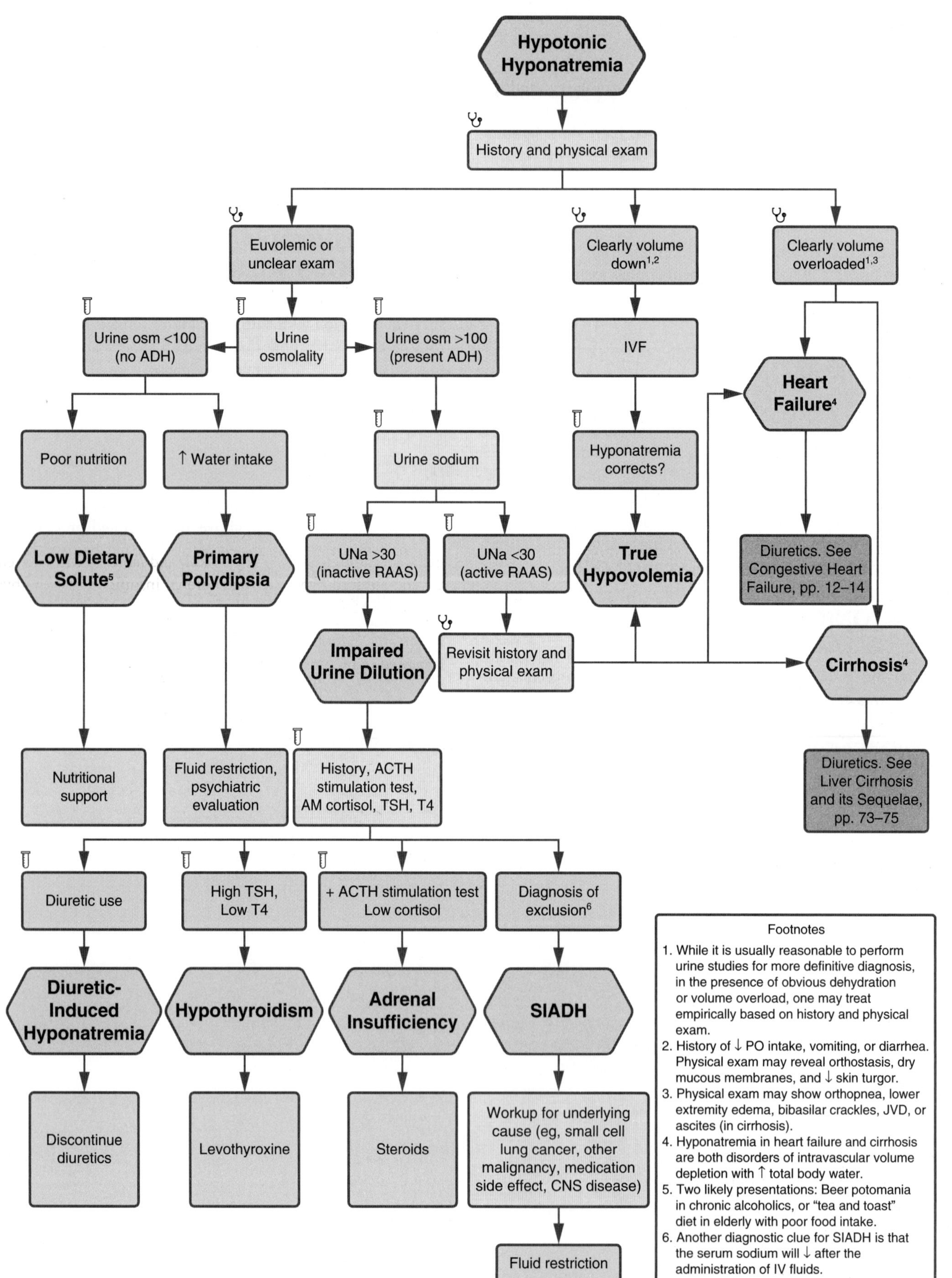
Hypotonic Hyponatremia
History and physical exam
Euvolemic or unclear exam
Clearly volume down[1,2]
Clearly volume overloaded[1,3]
Urine osm <100 (no ADH)
Urine osmolality
Urine osm >100 (present ADH)
IVF
Heart Failure[4]
Poor nutrition
↑ Water intake
Urine sodium
Hyponatremia corrects?
Low Dietary Solute[5]
Primary Polydipsia
UNa >30 (inactive RAAS)
UNa <30 (active RAAS)
True Hypovolemia
Diuretics. See Congestive Heart Failure, pp. 12–14
Impaired Urine Dilution
Revisit history and physical exam
Cirrhosis[4]
Nutritional support
Fluid restriction, psychiatric evaluation
History, ACTH stimulation test, AM cortisol, TSH, T4
Diuretics. See Liver Cirrhosis and its Sequelae, pp. 73–75
Diuretic use
High TSH, Low T4
+ ACTH stimulation test Low cortisol
Diagnosis of exclusion[6]
Diuretic-Induced Hyponatremia
Hypothyroidism
Adrenal Insufficiency
SIADH
Discontinue diuretics
Levothyroxine
Steroids
Workup for underlying cause (eg, small cell lung cancer, other malignancy, medication side effect, CNS disease)
Fluid restriction

Footnotes

1. While it is usually reasonable to perform urine studies for more definitive diagnosis, in the presence of obvious dehydration or volume overload, one may treat empirically based on history and physical exam.
2. History of ↓ PO intake, vomiting, or diarrhea. Physical exam may reveal orthostasis, dry mucous membranes, and ↓ skin turgor.
3. Physical exam may show orthopnea, lower extremity edema, bibasilar crackles, JVD, or ascites (in cirrhosis).
4. Hyponatremia in heart failure and cirrhosis are both disorders of intravascular volume depletion with ↑ total body water.
5. Two likely presentations: Beer potomania in chronic alcoholics, or "tea and toast" diet in elderly with poor food intake.
6. Another diagnostic clue for SIADH is that the serum sodium will ↓ after the administration of IV fluids.

FIGURE 6.2

6-2 Hypotonic Hyponatremia

PRIMARY (PSYCHOGENIC) POLYDIPSIA

A 45-year-old F with PMH of psychiatric disorder (eg, schizophrenia) presents with ↑ water consumption, complaint of dry mouth, and tonic-clonic seizure (if severe hyponatremia). On **exam**, she has moist mucous membranes and normal skin turgor. **Labs** show hyponatremia with urine osmolality <100.

Management:

1. Restrict water intake.
2. Psychiatric evaluation.

Complications: High risk of rapid correction; watch for osmotic demyelination syndrome.

HYF: Patients often present with polydipsia and polyuria and are found to have low-normal serum sodium levels. A water deprivation test will distinguish this diagnosis from nephrogenic and central DI, as free fluid restriction will cause increased urine osmolality and normalization of serum sodium because these patients have normal ability to concentrate urine.

TRUE HYPOVOLEMIA

A 30-year-old with no significant PMH presents with vomiting and diarrhea. On **exam**, the patient has dry mucous membranes and ↓ skin turgor. **Labs** show hyponatremia, urine osmolality >100, and urine Na <30.

Management:

1. IV fluids (NS or LR).
2. Correct underlying cause of losses.
3. Consider antiemetics or antidiarrheals.

Complications: Acute kidney injury.

HYF: When history and physical exam strongly indicate hypovolemia as the etiology (as in this case), you can empirically trial IV fluids. If hyponatremia persists despite IV fluids, obtain urine Na to assess for intrarenal losses. Urine Na <30 confirms that RAAS is active (ie, the kidney is concentrating well and not responsible for Na losses).

HEART FAILURE, CIRRHOSIS

A 75-year-old M with PMH of congestive heart failure or liver cirrhosis presents with SOB and dyspnea on exertion. On **exam**, he has JVD, pedal edema, and bibasilar lung crackles. **Labs** show hyponatremia.

Management:

1. Treat heart failure exacerbation/volume overload with loop diuretics (eg, furosemide, bumetanide) + water restriction.
2. If cirrhosis, treat exacerbation with spironolactone + furosemide.

Complications: Acute kidney injury (cardiorenal syndrome, hepatorenal syndrome).

HYF: Can trial empiric therapy when history and physical strongly suggest heart failure or cirrhosis as the etiology. Urine studies will show urine osmolality >100 and urine Na <30 because hyponatremia in heart failure and cirrhosis result from intravascular volume depletion with increased total body water. Treating fluid overload improves renal fluid dynamics and should correct hyponatremia.

DIURETIC-INDUCED HYPONATREMIA

A 55-year-old M with PMH of congestive heart failure with recent dose increase to his standing diuretics presents with weakness and dehydration. On **exam**, he has dry mucous membranes and ↓ skin turgor. **Labs** show hyponatremia, urine osmolality >100, and urine Na >30.

Management:

1. Hold diuretics. Gentle IV fluid resuscitation as needed.

Complications: Diuretic discontinuation may lead to exacerbation of underlying disease for which patient was taking diuretics (eg, heart failure).

HYF: Urine Na >30 indicates that RASS is not active and that losses are intrarenal. History, physical, and lab tests will differentiate diuretic-induced hyponatremia, adrenal insufficiency, hypothyroidism, and SIADH.

SYNDROME OF INAPPROPRIATE ANTIDIURETIC HORMONE SECRETION (SIADH)

A 54-year-old M with 50-pack-year smoking history is brought in by family for evaluation of altered mental status and is found to have serum sodium of 121. He notably has developed a cough with bloody sputum and had an unintentional weight loss of 20 lbs in the last 3 months. On **exam**, he is somnolent and appears euvolemic. Besides hyponatremia, **labs** show serum osmolality of 250, urine sodium 25, urine osmolality 120, and normal TSH and 8 am cortisol. On **imaging**, CT chest shows a spiculated mass in the right lung.

Management:

1. Fluid restriction.
2. If severe hyponatremia, administer hypertonic saline with frequent sodium monitoring. Ensure serum Na is not corrected by more than 8–10 mEq/L in 24 hours.
3. Loop diuretic and sodium tablets, as needed.
4. Consider ADH antagonists (conivaptan, tolvaptan, demeclocycline).

Complications: Osmotic demyelination syndrome if hyponatremia is corrected too quickly.

HYF: May be associated with paraneoplastic syndromes (small cell lung carcinoma, as in this patient's case), neurologic disease (brain tumor, traumatic brain injury), pulmonary disease (sarcoidosis, COPD, pneumonia), and medications (antipsychotics, antidepressants). Usually the following labs are seen: Serum osmolality

6-2 Hypotonic Hyponatremia

<280 mOsm/kg (hypotonic), urine osmolality >100 mOsm/kg, and urinary sodium level ≥20 mEq/L.

DECREASED SOLUTE INTAKE

A 75-year-old F with PMH of functional impairment and poor social support presents with fatigue, weight loss, and memory impairment. On **exam**, she has moist mucous membranes and normal skin turgor. **Labs** show hyponatremia with urine osmolality <100.

Management:

1. Increase solute intake via normal diet.
2. Assess social support.

Complications: High risk of rapid correction; watch for osmotic demyelination syndrome.

HYF: Classically occurs in an elderly patient with poor PO intake ("tea and toast" diet). May also occur in chronic alcoholics with decreased nutritional intake (beer potomania).

Hypothyroidism: See pp. 137-139.

Adrenal Insufficiency: See pp. 154-156.

6-3 Hypernatremia

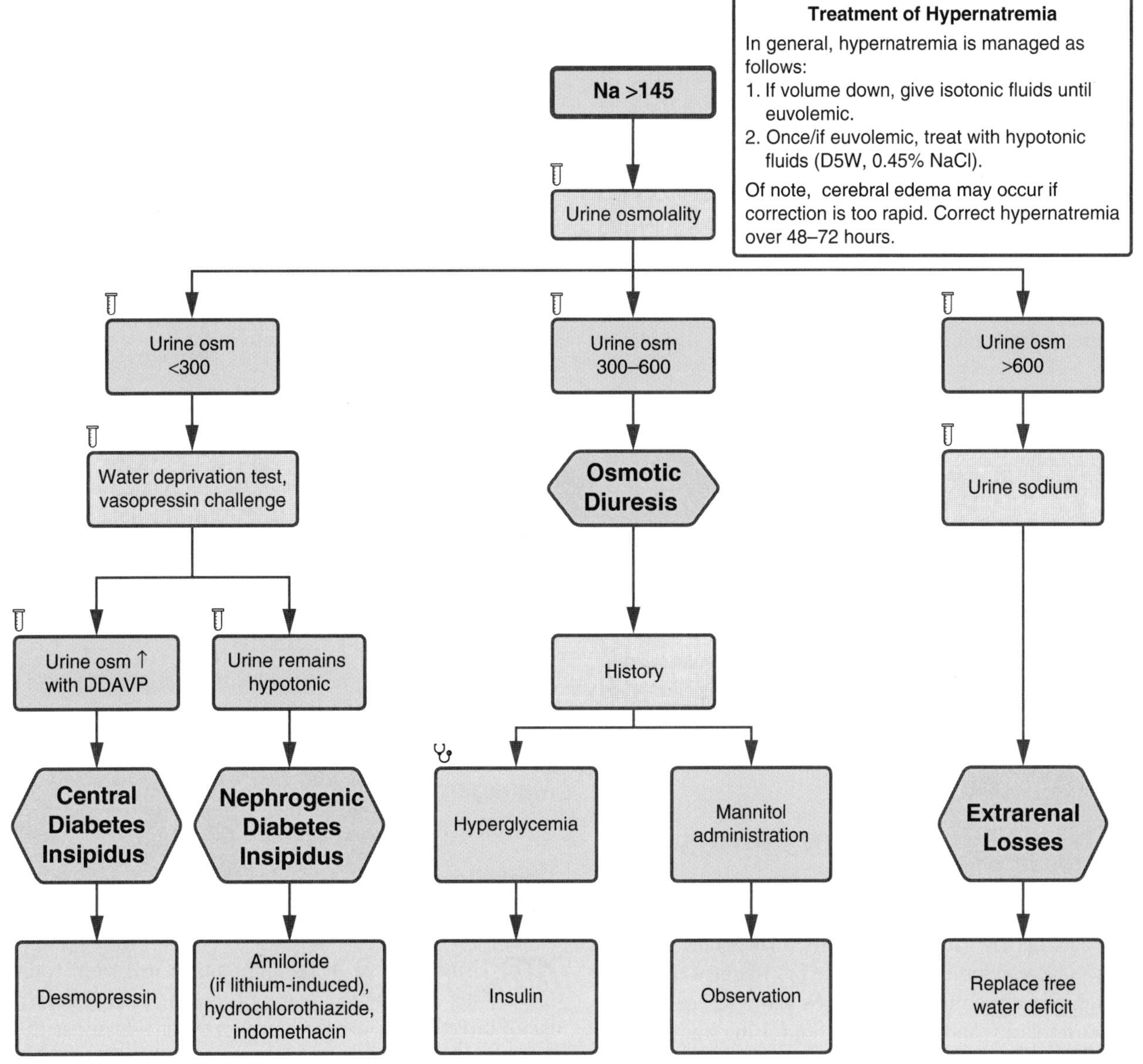
Treatment of Hypernatremia
In general, hypernatremia is managed as follows:
1. If volume down, give isotonic fluids until euvolemic.
2. Once/if euvolemic, treat with hypotonic fluids (D5W, 0.45% NaCl).
Of note, cerebral edema may occur if correction is too rapid. Correct hypernatremia over 48–72 hours.
Na >145
Urine osmolality
Urine osm <300
Urine osm 300–600
Urine osm >600
Water deprivation test, vasopressin challenge
Osmotic Diuresis
Urine sodium
Urine osm ↑ with DDAVP
Urine remains hypotonic
History
Central Diabetes Insipidus
Nephrogenic Diabetes Insipidus
Hyperglycemia
Mannitol administration
Extrarenal Losses
Desmopressin
Amiloride (if lithium-induced), hydrochlorothiazide, indomethacin
Insulin
Observation
Replace free water deficit

FIGURE 6.3

6-3 Hypernatremia

CENTRAL DIABETES INSIPIDUS

A 40-year-old M with PMH of traumatic brain injury during a car accident 4 weeks ago presents with polydipsia and polyuria. At the time of the accident, head imaging was normal. Since then, he reports constant thirst that is only relieved when he drinks large volumes of water. At one point, drinking water was not available, so he drank soap water. He reports frequent nocturia. **Exam** shows dry mucous membranes. **Labs** show serum sodium 160, ↑ serum osmolarity, and ↓ ADH. 24-hour urine studies show ↓ urine osmolality, ↓ urine sodium, and ↑ urine volume. Water deprivation test does not change urine osmolality or volume. Vasopressin challenge shows decreased urine volume and >50% ↑ in urine osmolality with DDVAP.

Management:

1. Start desmopressin.
2. Lifestyle modifications: low salt diet, hydration.

Complications: Sequelae of dehydration (eg, prerenal AKI), hypernatremia.

HYF: Central DI results from failure to produce ADH due to a pituitary tumor, pituitary injury (eg, history of traumatic brain injury), autoimmune disease, surgery, or ischemia (Sheehan syndrome). Desmopressin is an ADH analog that acts on the renal tubular cells to increase renal resorption of water and thus improve water retention.

NEPHROGENIC DIABETES INSIPIDUS

A 45-year-old M with PMH of bipolar disorder (recently started on lithium) and HTN presents with polydipsia and polyuria. Starting a month ago, he has had constant thirst that is only relieved when he drinks large volumes of water. He has frequent nocturia. **Exam** shows dry mucous membranes. **Labs** show serum sodium 160, ↑ serum osmolarity, and ↑ ADH. 24-hour urine studies show ↓ urine osmolality, ↓ urine sodium, and ↑ urine volume. Water deprivation test does not change urine osmolality or volume. Vasopressin challenge shows no change in urine volume or urine osmolality.

Management:

1. 1st-line: amiloride (if lithium-induced), hydrochlorothiazide, indomethacin.
2. Lifestyle modifications: low-salt diet, hydration.

Complications: Sequelae of dehydration (eg, prerenal AKI), hypernatremia, peripheral DI may be permanent if due to lithium toxicity.

HYF: Due to renal insensitivity or resistance to ADH. Etiologies include medication-induced (lithium, amphotericin, demeclocycline), electrolyte abnormalities (hypercalcemia, hypokalemia), and rarely genetic. Administration of DDAVP is used to distinguish between central and nephrogenic DI.

OSMOTIC DIURESIS

A 19-year-old M with PMH of type 1 diabetes mellitus presents with polyuria and dehydration. On **exam**, he has dry mucous membranes and ↓ skin turgor. **Labs** show hyperglycemia and urine osm 300–600.

Management:

1. If due to hyperglycemia, insulin.
2. If due to mannitol administration, dialysis.

Complications: Prerenal AKI from dehydration; seizures if hypernatremia is acute and profound.

HYF: Non-reabsorbed solutes (ie, mannitol, glucose, urea) are excreted in the urine, causing the urine to be hyperosmolar and hyponatremic compared to the serum. This "osmotic diuresis" results in hypernatremia. The serum Na concentration is variable. Mannitol and glucose typically cause hyponatremia first, with hypernatremia resulting after the rapid osmotic diuresis that may occur in patients with good renal function.

EXTRARENAL LOSSES

A 35-year-old F with no significant PMH presents with vomiting and diarrhea. On **exam**, she has dry mucous membranes and ↓ skin turgor. **Labs** show urine osm >600 and urine Na <25.

Management:

1. Replace free water deficit.

Complications: Prerenal AKI from dehydration; seizures if hypernatremia is acute and profound.

HYF: Urine Na <25 helps differentiate this from sodium overload. Water lost due to sweating is called "insensible loss," since it is not directly measured. Suspect extrarenal losses as the cause of hypernatremia when patients have a condition that predisposes to insensible losses (burns, emesis, diarrhea, sweating from fever) and limits oral intake (altered mental status, NPO). This is the most common cause of hypernatremia. The free water deficit is the volume of water replacement that is needed to correct hypernatremia and can be calculated as follows:

Free Water Deficit = (% Total Body Water) × Kg × [Na/(Ideal Na) – 1]

% Total Body Water:

- 60%: Children, adult males
- 50%: Adult females, elderly males
- 45%: Elderly females

SODIUM OVERLOAD

A 60-year-old F with recent administration of hypertonic saline for a traumatic brain injury now has hypernatremia. **Labs** show urine osm >600 and urine Na >25.

Management:

1. Replace free water deficit.

6-3 Hypernatremia

Complications: Seizures if hypernatremia is acute and profound.

HYF: Ingesting a large amount of salt (often accidental in children) can cause Na overload. Hypertonic saline or sodium bicarbonate administered to treat other disease processes can also cause Na overload as a complication. In the case of an acute Na overload (possibly secondary to an ingestion), rapidly treat hypernatremia with 2.5% dextrose in water (5% may cause hyperglycemia with the high volumes required). Urine Na of >25 helps to differentiate Na overload from extrarenal losses. Also note that Na overload tends to result in weight gain due to retention of water, whereas extrarenal losses result in weight loss.

6-4 Hypokalemia

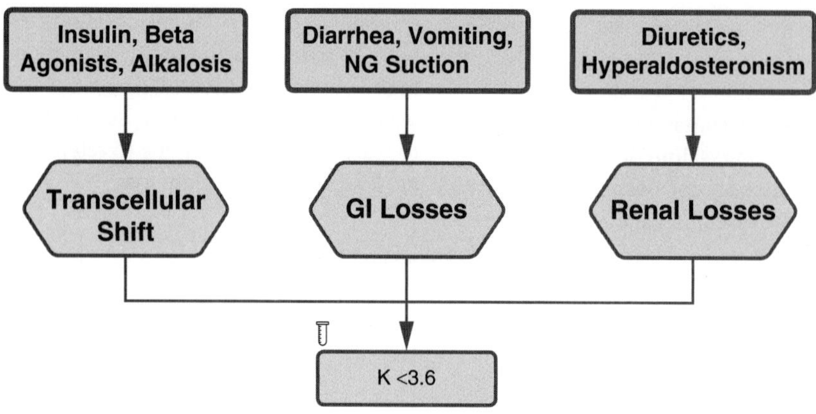
Insulin, Beta Agonists, Alkalosis
Diarrhea, Vomiting, NG Suction
Diuretics, Hyperaldosteronism
Transcellular Shift
GI Losses
Renal Losses
K <3.6

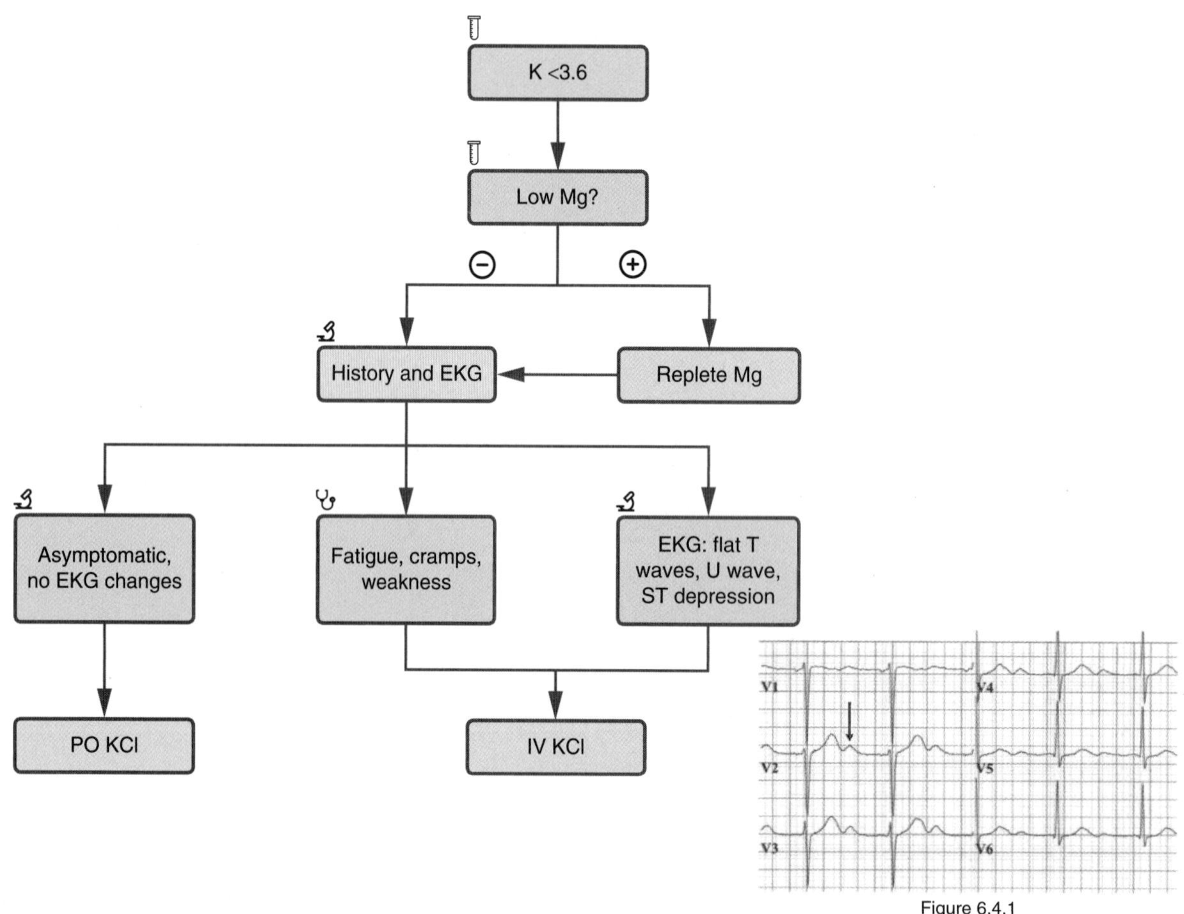
K <3.6
Low Mg?
History and EKG
Replete Mg
Asymptomatic, no EKG changes
Fatigue, cramps, weakness
EKG: flat T waves, U wave, ST depression
PO KCl
IV KCl
V1
V2
V3
V4
V5
V6

Figure 6.4.1

FIGURE 6.4

6-4 Hypokalemia

As with many things, treat hypokalemia acutely and then address the underlying cause. Hypomagnesemia can cause hypokalemia; if a patient is stable and asymptomatic, then it is reasonable to replete Mg before K. However, if a patient has symptoms or EKG changes, replete K and Mg at the same time. The method of potassium repletion is the same regardless of the etiology.

Management:

1. PO potassium repletion is always preferred.
2. If EKG changes or patient is unable to take PO: IV potassium.
3. Replete magnesium.

Complications: Severe hypokalemia may result in cardiac arrest.

HYF: Low magnesium may prevent successful repletion of K. Magnesium repletion should always be considered. EKG changes of hypokalemia: flat T waves, U waves, ST depression.

TRANSCELLULAR SHIFT

A 45-year-old M with PMH of DM1 presents with DKA. **Exam** reveals tachycardia, confusion, dry mucous membranes, and abdominal tenderness. **Labs** show glucose 560, anion gap 23, and K 3.8. Repeat labs show K 3.2 after insulin administration.

Management:

1. Treat emergent conditions (eg, give fluids for DKA).
2. Replete K.
3. Insulin (in the case of DKA or HHS).

HYF: In the case of DKA or hyperosmolar hyperglycemia, K must be >3.3 prior to starting insulin. The high doses of insulin required for these conditions will exacerbate the existing hypokalemia. Otherwise, be generally cautious with K repletion if a transcellular shift is suspected. The patient's total potassium stores may be normal, just shifted intracellularly. If the underlying condition resolves quickly, then you risk overcorrecting the K. Monitor K frequently during treatment.

GI LOSSES

A 60-year-old F with PMH of alcoholic cirrhosis presents with hepatic encephalopathy. **Exam** reveals altered mental status, asterixis, palmar erythema and caput medusae. She is treated with lactulose with improvement in mental status after several bowel movements. Subsequent **labs** show Mg 1.5 and K 3.0.

Management:

1. Replete K and Mg as noted above.

HYF: Patients who have emesis, diarrhea, or NG tube to suction can lose Mg and K. For cases in which the cause cannot be resolved, such as a patient with liver cirrhosis who needs to have 2-3 bowel movements per day to prevent onset of hepatic encephalopathy and a standing diuretic for ascites, then the patient may need long-term K supplementation and/or K-sparing diuretics.

RENAL LOSSES

A 75-year-old M with PMH of congestive heart failure presents with acute decompensated heart failure. **Exam** reveals elevated JVP, mild crackles on lung exam, and 3+ pitting edema to his thighs. Diuresis with furosemide is started. Subsequent **labs** show Mg 1.5 and K 3.3.

Management:

1. Replete Mg and K as noted above.

HYF: Patients on loop or thiazide diuretics are at risk of developing hypomagnesemia and/or hypokalemia due to renal losses. Hyperaldosteronism can also cause hypokalemia, as aldosterone causes renal excretion of K; suspect this diagnosis in a patient with refractory hypertension and hypokalemia.

6-5 Hyperkalemia: Etiologies

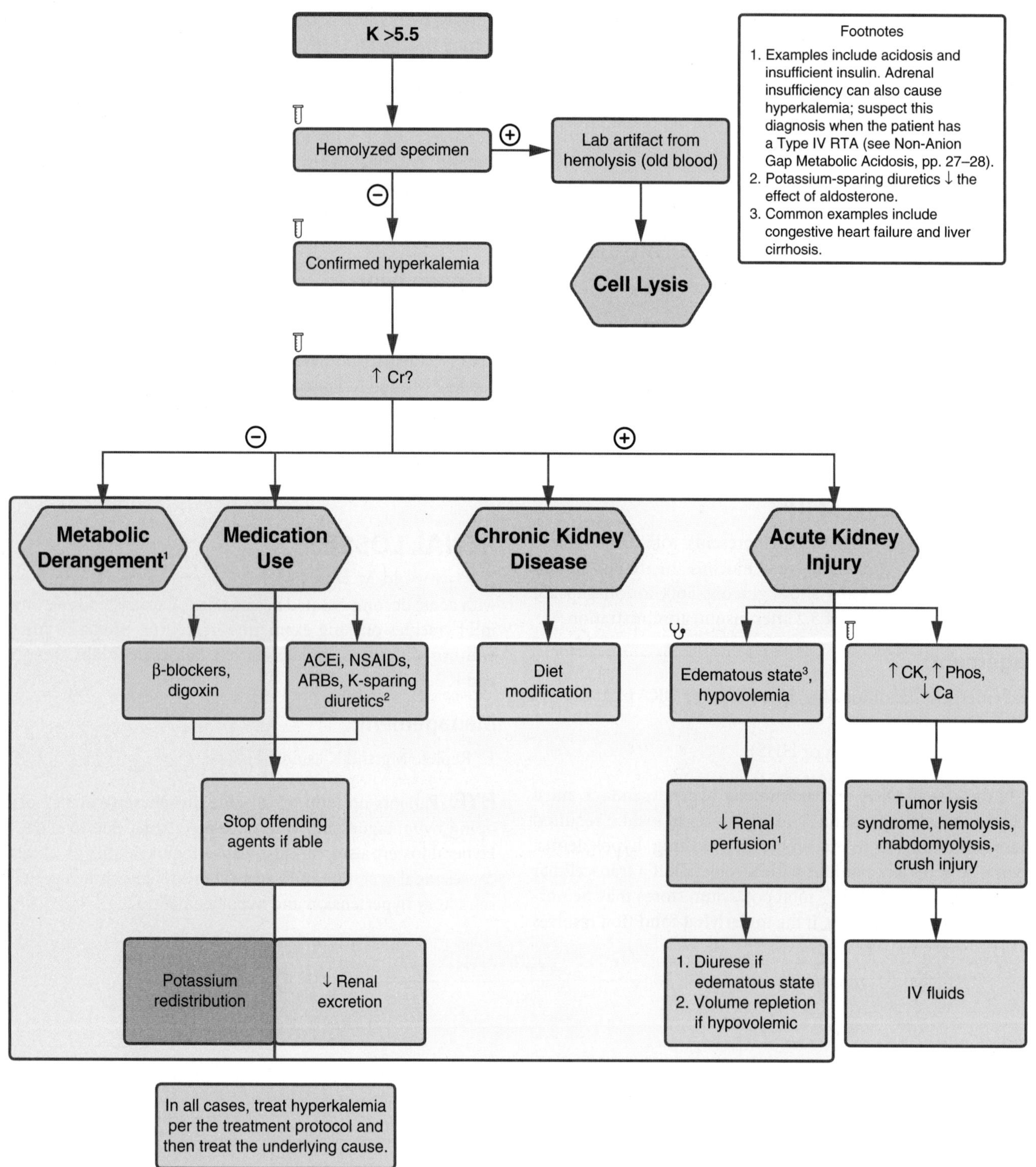
K >5.5
Hemolyzed specimen
Lab artifact from hemolysis (old blood)
Cell Lysis
Confirmed hyperkalemia
↑ Cr?
Metabolic Derangement[1]
Medication Use
Chronic Kidney Disease
Acute Kidney Injury
β-blockers, digoxin
ACEi, NSAIDs, ARBs, K-sparing diuretics[2]
Diet modification
Edematous state[3], hypovolemia
↑ CK, ↑ Phos, ↓ Ca
Stop offending agents if able
↓ Renal perfusion[1]
Tumor lysis syndrome, hemolysis, rhabdomyolysis, crush injury
Potassium redistribution
↓ Renal excretion
1. Diurese if edematous state
2. Volume repletion if hypovolemic
IV fluids
In all cases, treat hyperkalemia per the treatment protocol and then treat the underlying cause.
Footnotes
1. Examples include acidosis and insufficient insulin. Adrenal insufficiency can also cause hyperkalemia; suspect this diagnosis when the patient has a Type IV RTA (see Non-Anion Gap Metabolic Acidosis, pp. 27–28).
2. Potassium-sparing diuretics ↓ the effect of aldosterone.
3. Common examples include congestive heart failure and liver cirrhosis.

FIGURE 6.5a

6-5 Hyperkalemia: Management

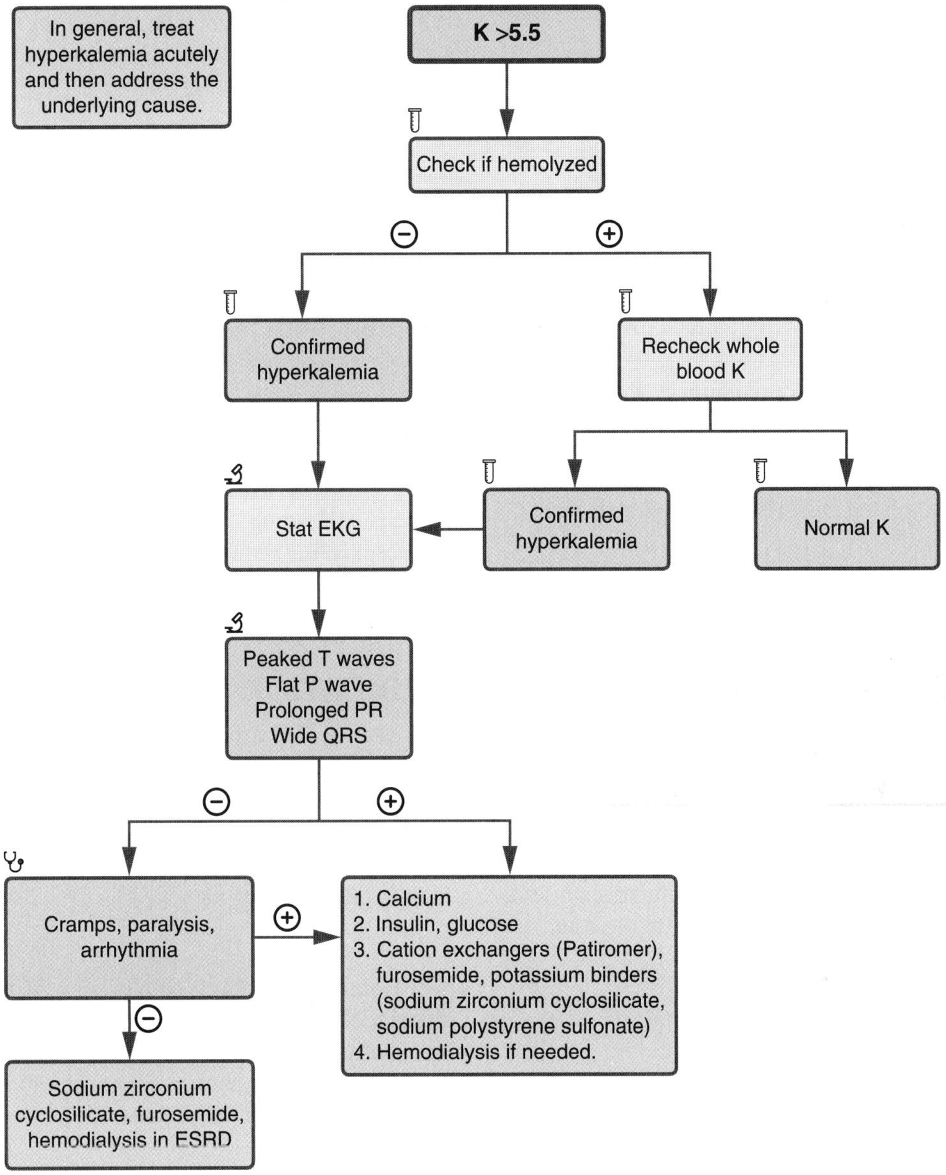

In general, treat hyperkalemia acutely and then address the underlying cause.

K >5.5

→ Check if hemolyzed

- ⊖ → Confirmed hyperkalemia → Stat EKG
- ⊕ → Recheck whole blood K
  - → Confirmed hyperkalemia → Stat EKG
  - → Normal K

Stat EKG → Peaked T waves / Flat P wave / Prolonged PR / Wide QRS

- ⊖ → Cramps, paralysis, arrhythmia
  - ⊕ → (treatment below)
  - ⊖ → Sodium zirconium cyclosilicate, furosemide, hemodialysis in ESRD
- ⊕ →
  1. Calcium
  2. Insulin, glucose
  3. Cation exchangers (Patiromer), furosemide, potassium binders (sodium zirconium cyclosilicate, sodium polystyrene sulfonate)
  4. Hemodialysis if needed.

FIGURE 6.5b

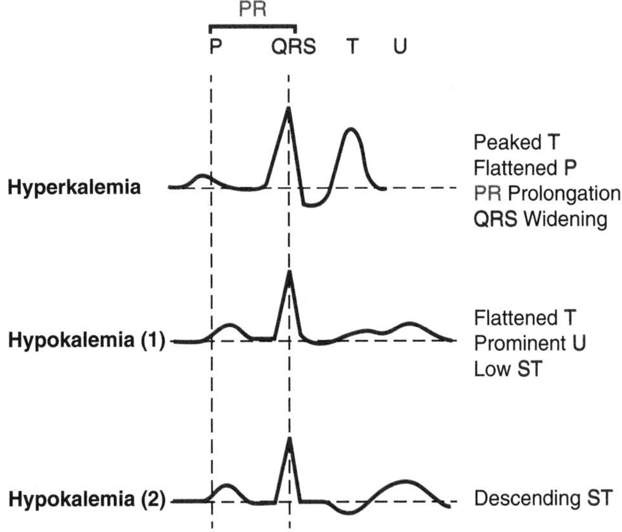
PR
P
QRS
T
U
Hyperkalemia
Peaked T
Flattened P
PR Prolongation
QRS Widening
Hypokalemia (1)
Flattened T
Prominent U
Low ST
Hypokalemia (2)
Descending ST

EKG changes in hyperkalemia and progressive changes in hypokalemia.

6-5 Hyperkalemia: Management

Management of Moderate Hyperkalemia:

1. Obtain EKG and confirm with repeat labs: 5.5 < K < 6.5 and no EKG changes.
2. Remove K from body with sodium zirconium cyclosilicate (feces) or loop diuretic (urine).

Management of Severe Hyperkalemia:

1. Obtain EKG and confirm with repeat labs: K >6.5 or EKG changes.
2. Stabilize myocardium with calcium gluconate.
3. Shift K into cells with insulin + glucose, ± albuterol. If low pH, give bicarbonate.
4. Remove K from body with sodium zirconium cyclosilicate (feces) or loop diuretic (urine).
5. If renal failure or refractory to above treatment: dialysis.

Complications: If untreated, high risk of cardiac arrhythmia.

HYF: Hyperkalemia may be a lab artifact from hemolysis of the blood sample. Mild cases can be treated slowly with a diuretic or sodium zirconium cyclosilicate. Severe hyperkalemia is an emergency and requires immediate decrease in serum K. Calcium gluconate decreases risk of arrhythmias, and temporizing measures (insulin, albuterol) shift K into cells while slower methods take effect (dialysis, diuretics, sodium zirconium cyclosilicate). EKG changes: peaked T wave, flat P wave, ↑ PR interval, wide QRS, BBB.

AKI

An 89-year-old M with PMH of Alzheimer's dementia presents with failure to thrive. On **exam**, he has temporal wasting, dry mucous membranes, and poor skin turgor. **Labs** show Na 148, Cr 1.5, and K 5.3.

Management:

1. Workup of AKI: UA, BMP, bladder scan.
2. EKG, IVFs, monitor electrolytes.

HYF: AKIs can decrease renal excretion of K. Mild hyperkalemia (as in this case) can be monitored if the patient is asymptomatic and without EKG changes. Hydrate and monitor BMP. Moderate-severe hyperkalemia can be treated as noted above. Common causes of AKI: dehydration, urinary retention, UTI, medications (diuretics), and edematous states (congestive heart failure, cirrhosis).

CKD

A 50-year-old M with PMH of DM2, HTN, and CKD presents for a routine visit. **Exam** is normal. **Labs** show Cr 1.8 and K 5.1, which are similar to previous values.

Management:

1. Consider nephrology referral for CKD.
2. Optimize management of comorbid diseases (HTN, DM2).
3. Counsel on low-K diet.

Complications:

- CKD can progress to ESRD.
- Acute renal injury superimposed on CKD can lead to severe hyperkalemia with subsequent arrhythmias.

HYF: Try to slow progression to ESRD by optimizing medical therapy. Treat diabetes and start the patient on an ACEi/ARB for HTN.

CELL LYSIS

A 30-year-old M with PMH of leukemia undergoing chemotherapy presents with palpitations, nausea, cramps. **Exam** is unremarkable. **Labs** show elevated uric acid, Cr 1.6, K 6.8, and phos 6. EKG reveals wide QRS, peaked T waves, and prolonged PR.

Management:

1. Treat severe hyperkalemia as noted above: temporizing measures + dialysis.
2. IV fluids (avoid lactated ringers since they contain K).

HYF: Cell lysis releases intracellular contents into the extracellular space, leading to acute electrolyte derangements. Cell lysis can occur in the setting of tumor lysis syndrome, rhabdomyolysis, crush injuries, or lab error (caused by improper handling of a blood sample).

MEDICATION USE

A 73-year-old M with PMH of HTN, chronic pain, and CHF on a β-blocker, ACEi, spironolactone, and naproxen presents for a routine visit. **Exam** is normal. **Labs** show Cr 1.2 and K 5.3.

Management:

1. Stop offending agents.
2. Low K diet.

HYF: Some medications (β-blockers, ACEi, K-sparing diuretics, digoxin, NSAIDs) can lead to hyperkalemia. Digoxin inhibits the Na/K antiporter. NSAIDs and ACEi decrease aldosterone secretion. K-sparing diuretics blunt response to aldosterone. Non-selective β-blockers inhibit cellular uptake of K.

METABOLIC DERANGEMENT

A 45-year-old M with PMH of DM1 presents with diabetic ketoacidosis. On **exam**, he has tachycardia, dry mucous membranes, and abdominal tenderness. **Labs** show glucose 560, anion gap 23, and K 5.3.

Management:

1. IV fluids.
2. Insulin gtt → insulin + dextrose.
3. K repletion once K starts to normalize while on insulin to avoid overcorrection.

HYF: Patients with DKA typically have normal or high K. Insulin deficiency results in an extracellular shift of K, which is subsequently excreted in the urine. The serum concentration of K remains high, but the patient's total body stores of K become low due to renal excretion. With insulin administration, serum K undergoes an intracellular shift, which can cause hypokalemia if not aggressively corrected. Metabolic acidosis can also cause an extracellular shift in K, leading to hyperkalemia; to reduce the acidity of the serum, cells will exchange a cytoplasmic K ion for a serum H ion.

6-6 Acid-Base Disorders

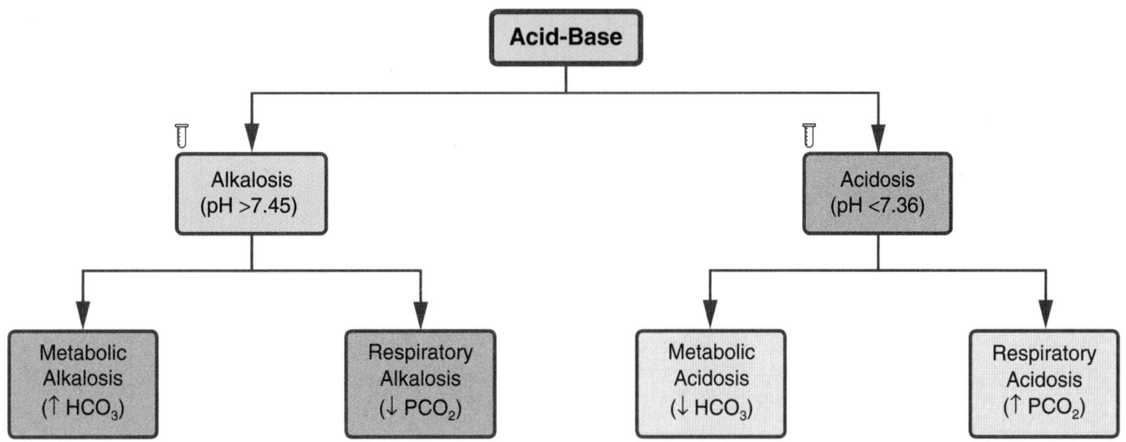
Acid-Base
Alkalosis (pH >7.45)
Acidosis (pH <7.36)
Metabolic Alkalosis ($\uparrow$ HCO_3)
Respiratory Alkalosis ($\downarrow$ PCO_2)
Metabolic Acidosis ($\downarrow$ HCO_3)
Respiratory Acidosis ($\uparrow$ PCO_2)

The major branch-point in acid-base disorders is whether the process is an acidosis or an alkalosis. As the names imply, an acidosis is a state in which there is an excess of acid or a lack of base. An alkalosis is the opposite: an excess of base or lack of acid. In any of these states, the primary issue may be due to abberations in production, clearance, or both. For example, a metabolic process that $\uparrow$ the production of acid may also coincide with a respiratory process that $\downarrow$ the clearance of acid. Acid-base problems can be complex, and we recommend having a systematic way of thinking through the clinical presentation. First, determine if the patient has an acidosis or alkalosis. Then determine if the primary driver is metabolic or respiratory. As noted above, there can be multiple processes occuring at the same time that add nuance and cloud the picture. However, this simple framework is a good place to start. The primary algorithms for each branch point will help guide you through the thought process to arrive at the final diagnosis.

FIGURE 6.6

6-7 Acidosis

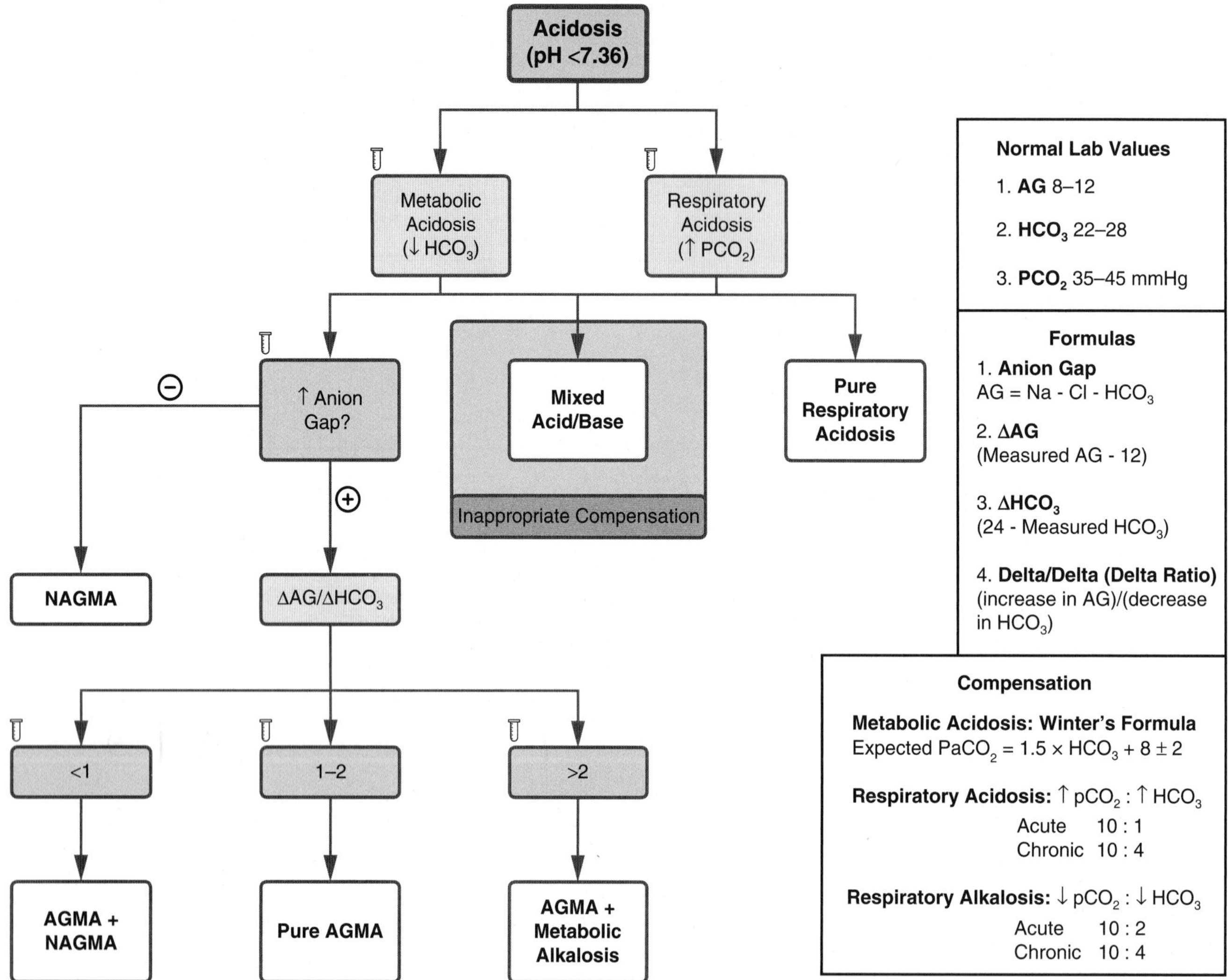
Acidosis
(pH <7.36)
Metabolic
Acidosis
(↓ HCO_3)
Respiratory
Acidosis
(↑ PCO_2)
↑ Anion
Gap?
Mixed
Acid/Base
Inappropriate Compensation
Pure
Respiratory
Acidosis
NAGMA
ΔAG/ΔHCO_3
<1
1–2
>2
AGMA +
NAGMA
Pure AGMA
AGMA +
Metabolic
Alkalosis
Normal Lab Values
1. AG 8–12
2. HCO_3 22–28
3. PCO_2 35–45 mmHg
Formulas
1. Anion Gap
AG = Na - Cl - HCO_3
2. ΔAG
(Measured AG - 12)
3. ΔHCO_3
(24 - Measured HCO_3)
4. Delta/Delta (Delta Ratio)
(increase in AG)/(decrease in HCO_3)
Compensation
Metabolic Acidosis: Winter's Formula
Expected $PaCO_2 = 1.5 \times HCO_3 + 8 \pm 2$
Respiratory Acidosis: ↑ pCO_2 : ↑ HCO_3
Acute 10 : 1
Chronic 10 : 4
Respiratory Alkalosis: ↓ pCO_2 : ↓ HCO_3
Acute 10 : 2
Chronic 10 : 4

Acidosis occurs when there is an excess of acid and/or a deficit of base. The first step is to determine the **primary** source of the derangement: Metabolic vs. Respiratory. Simply put, if there is not enough HCO_3, then it's primarily metabolic. If there is too much CO_2, then it's primarily respiratory. The body responds by producing more HCO_3 (metabolic compensation for primary respiratory acidosis) or by titrating CO_2 (respiratory compensation for primary metabolic acidosis). ↑ HCO_3 (metabolic compensation) takes time, so there is a difference in serum bicarbonate between the acute vs. chronic setting. CO_2 is rapidly titrated via the respiratory drive. If there is only one acid/base disorder, then the body will compensate in a predictable manner (see compensation box above). For example, in acute respiratory acidosis, HCO_3 will ↑ by 1 for every ↑ of 10 in CO_2. Similarly, the Winter's Formula can be used to check compensation for metabolic acidosis. If the HCO_3 and CO_2 do not properly compensate for one another, then there is a **secondary** process occuring, and you have a **Mixed Acid/Base Disorder**.

In metabolic acidosis, there are two final things to consider. The first is the **Anion Gap (AG)**, and the second is the **Delta/Delta (Delta ratio)**. Positive and negative charges in the blood equal. Na^+ comprises most of the positive charge, while Cl^- and HCO_3^- comprise most of the negative charge. The AG is the difference between the total Na^+ and the total Cl^- and HCO_3^-. Since we do not measure every ion in the blood, the measured AG is >0 (typically between 8 and 12). Some acidoses ↑ unmeasured anions. To keep the charges balanced, an ↑ in unmeasured anions causes a ↓ in measured anions (typically HCO_3). For example, an ↑ in lactate results in a roughly equal ↓ in HCO_3. Since HCO_3 ↓, the AG (Na - Cl - HCO_3) ↑. This is called an **Anion Gap Metabolic Acidosis (AGMA)**. Metabolic acidoses without an ↑ AG are called **Non-Anion Gap Metabolic Acidoses (NAGMA)**. Finally, there can be an ↑ AG without the expected change in HCO_3. Thus, we calculate the **Delta/Delta**, which is simply the ↑ in AG divided by the ↓ in HCO_3. Interpretation of the **Delta/Delta** is as follows: a) <0.4 is due to a pure NAGMA, b) 0.4–0.8 is generally due to a mixed NAGMA + AGMA or the patient has renal failure, c) 0.8–2 is usually due to a pure AGMA, and d) >2 is usually due to a mixed AGMA + pre-existing metabolic alkalosis (or compensated chronic respiratory acidosis).

FIGURE 6.7

6-8 Respiratory Acidosis

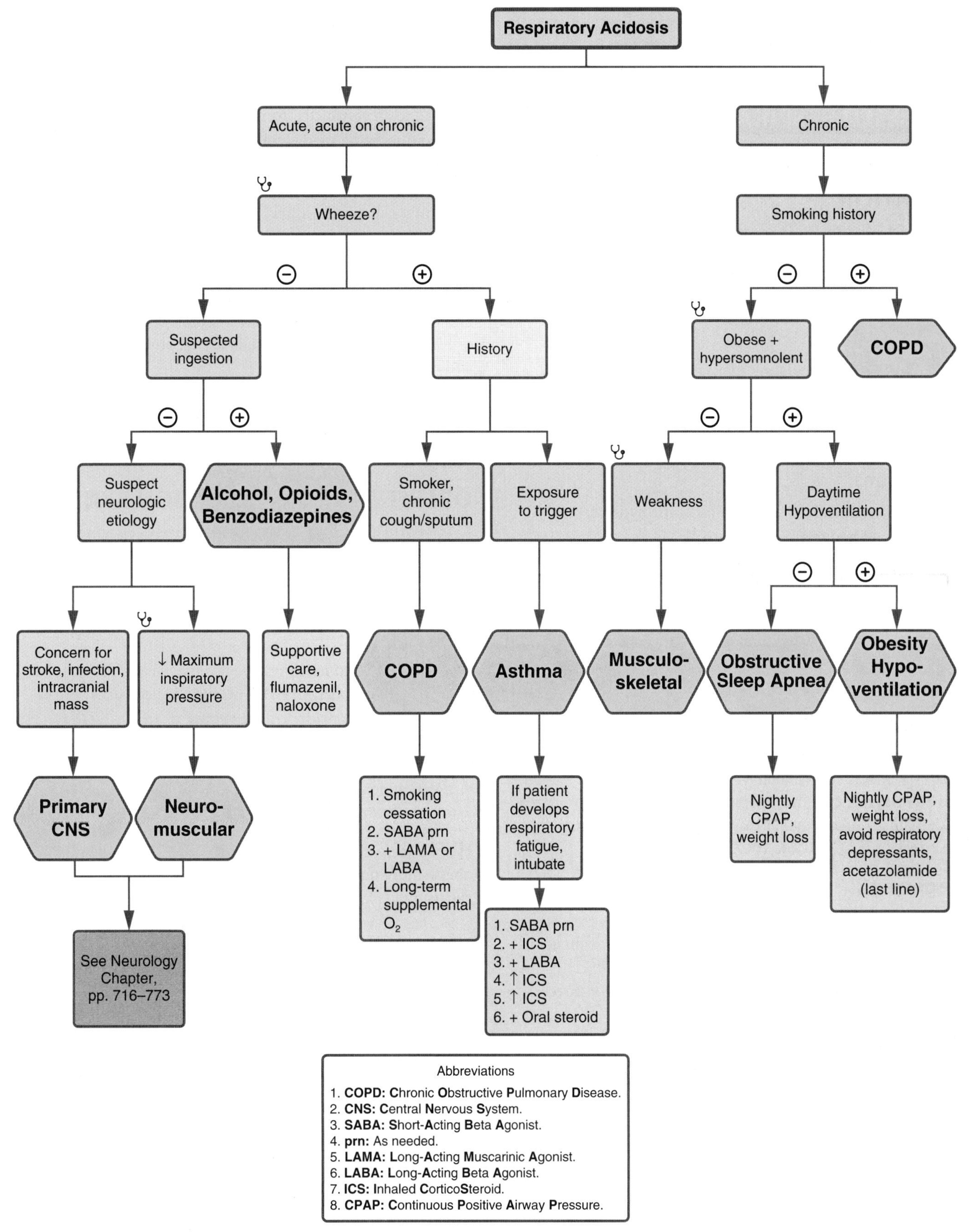
Respiratory Acidosis
Acute, acute on chronic
Chronic
Wheeze?
Smoking history
Suspected ingestion
History
Obese + hypersomnolent
COPD
Suspect neurologic etiology
Alcohol, Opioids, Benzodiazepines
Smoker, chronic cough/sputum
Exposure to trigger
Weakness
Daytime Hypoventilation
Concern for stroke, infection, intracranial mass
↓ Maximum inspiratory pressure
Supportive care, flumazenil, naloxone
COPD
Asthma
Musculo-skeletal
Obstructive Sleep Apnea
Obesity Hypo-ventilation
Primary CNS
Neuro-muscular
1. Smoking cessation
2. SABA prn
3. + LAMA or LABA
4. Long-term supplemental O_2
If patient develops respiratory fatigue, intubate
Nightly CPAP, weight loss
Nightly CPAP, weight loss, avoid respiratory depressants, acetazolamide (last line)
1. SABA prn
2. + ICS
3. + LABA
4. ↑ ICS
5. ↑ ICS
6. + Oral steroid
See Neurology Chapter, pp. 716–773
Abbreviations
1. COPD: Chronic Obstructive Pulmonary Disease.
2. CNS: Central Nervous System.
3. SABA: Short-Acting Beta Agonist.
4. prn: As needed.
5. LAMA: Long-Acting Muscarinic Agonist.
6. LABA: Long-Acting Beta Agonist.
7. ICS: Inhaled CorticoSteroid.
8. CPAP: Continuous Positive Airway Pressure.

FIGURE 6.8

6-8 Respiratory Acidosis

Below are quick overviews of how the following diagnoses present in the setting of respiratory acidosis. For more details, please see the primary algorithms and HYF pages for each of these diagnoses.

DECREASED RESPIRATORY DRIVE

RESPIRATORY ACIDOSIS DUE TO MEDICATION

A 55 year-old M with PMH of recent surgery prescribed opioids on discharge and HTN presents with progressive somnolence. On **exam**, he has bradypnea to 6 and pinpoint pupils. On **labs**, VBG has pH of 7.15 and CO_2 of 80. On **imaging**, CXR is normal.

Management:

1. Airway, breathing, circulation (consider BiPAP or intubation depending on mental status).
2. Intranasal naloxone for any patient with undifferentiated somnolence and pinpoint pupils.

Complications:

- Persistent altered mental status and chronic hypercarbia.
- Progression to hypoxia and PEA arrest.

HYF: pH <7.3 and pCO_2 >40 is consistent with respiratory acidosis. Minute ventilation = [tidal volume] × [respiratory rate]. Common culprit drugs include opioids, benzodiazepines, and alcohol.

RESPIRATORY ACIDOSIS DUE TO CENTRAL CAUSES (PRIMARY CNS)

An 89-year-old F with PMH of HTN and DM2 presents with left hemiparesis and is found to have extensive multifocal ischemic strokes on **imaging**. Over her hospital course, she develops increasing somnolence. On **exam**, her respiratory rate is 6. **Labs** are notable for arterial pH of 7.10 and $PaCO_2$ of 90.

Management:

1. Eliminate any sedating medications.
2. Consider non-invasive ventilation (eg, BiPAP) if within goals of care.
3. Consider neurologic rehabilitation if within goals of care.

Complications:

- Progression to chronic respiratory acidosis and chronic somnolence.
- Risk of decreased mental status and aspiration.

HYF: In acute stroke patients, reduced central respiratory drive → decreased total minute ventilation → respiratory acidosis.

NEUROMUSCULAR WEAKNESS

A 72-year-old M with no significant PMH presents with progressive dyspnea. On **exam**, he is noticeably tachypneic with shallow breaths and has fasciculations in his arms, legs, and tongue. **Labs** show an arterial pH of 7.22 and pCO_2 of 68 with impaired negative-inspiratory force testing. On **imaging**, CXR is clear.

Management:

1. Diagnostics with electromyogram (EMG).
2. Avoid sedating medications.
3. Utilize non-invasive ventilation such as BiPAP.
4. If progressive respiratory failure, consider intubation. If long-term mechanical ventilation is required, consider tracheostomy.

Complications: Respiratory failure, death.

HYF: Due to weakened respiratory muscles. Commonly tested etiologies include amyotrophic lateral sclerosis, Guillain-Barré syndrome, Duchenne's muscular dystrophy, myotonic dystrophy, and myasthenia gravis.

IMPAIRED VENTILATION DUE TO NON-PULMONARY CAUSES

OBESITY HYPOVENTILATION SYNDROME

A 44-year-old M with PMH of obstructive sleep apnea (OSA) and BMI of 55 presents with somnolence. **Exam** is normal. **Labs** show bicarbonate of 16, arterial pH of 7.18, $PaCO_2$ of 74, and an unremarkable urine drug screen. On **imaging**, CXR is clear.

Management:

1. Weight loss and non-invasive positive airway pressure: If concomitant OSA, CPAP. If no concomitant OSA, BiPAP.
2. If refractory, consider tracheostomy.

Complications:

- Sleep apnea and complications such as resistant hypertension, atrial fibrillation, and group 3 pulmonary hypertension.

HYF: Sleep disorder defined as alveolar hypoventilation in an obese individual while they are awake. This is a diagnosis of exclusion.

HYPOVENTILATION DUE TO MUSCULOSKELETAL CAUSES

A 68-year-old F with PMH of scoliosis presents with progressive dyspnea. **Exam** is notable for short stature and severe kyphosis. **Labs** show arterial pH of 7.20 and $PaCO_2$ of 72. On **imaging**, CXR shows diminished lung volumes.

Management:

1. Avoid sedating medications.
2. Postural support, spinal surgery for correction of kyphoscoliosis, and pulmonary rehab.

Complications: Chronic hypercarbic respiratory failure.

HYF: More often seen in post-menopausal, osteoporotic women.

6-8 Respiratory Acidosis

IMPAIRED PULMONARY VENTILATION

ACUTE COPD EXACERBATION

A 50-year-old F with PMH of 100-pack-year smoking history and emphysema presents with shortness of breath. On **exam**, he is somnolent; lung auscultation reveals rhonchi, wheezes, and a very prolonged expiratory phase. **Labs** show an arterial pH of 7.15, $PaCO_2$ of 85, and bicarbonate of 38. On **imaging**, CXR shows hyperinflated lungs that are clear.

Management:

1. Short-acting beta-agonists and antimuscarinics.
2. Prednisone.
3. Noninvasive ventilation with BiPAP.

Complications: Acute altered mental status and coma.

HYF: Patients with COPD may retain CO_2 at baseline; this is reflected in their VBG. **COPD treatment**: Corticosteroids, Oxygen, Prevention (pneumococcal and influenza vaccines, smoking cessation), BronchoDilators (β2-agonists, anticholinergics).

6-9 Anion Gap Metabolic Acidosis

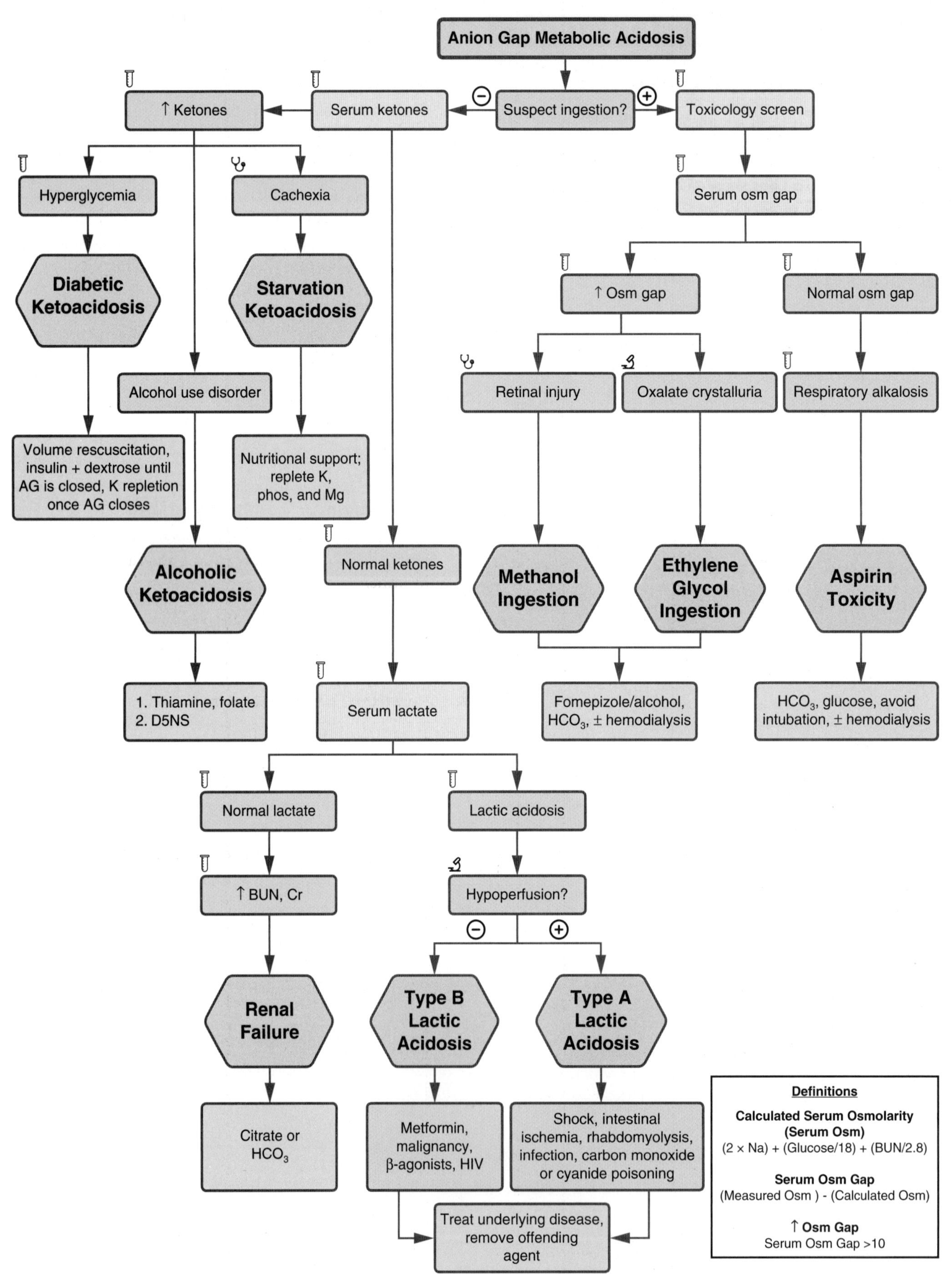

Anion Gap Metabolic Acidosis
Suspect ingestion?
Serum ketones
↑ Ketones
Toxicology screen
Hyperglycemia
Cachexia
Serum osm gap
Diabetic Ketoacidosis
Starvation Ketoacidosis
↑ Osm gap
Normal osm gap
Alcohol use disorder
Retinal injury
Oxalate crystalluria
Respiratory alkalosis
Volume rescuscitation, insulin + dextrose until AG is closed, K repletion once AG closes
Nutritional support; replete K, phos, and Mg
Alcoholic Ketoacidosis
Normal ketones
Methanol Ingestion
Ethylene Glycol Ingestion
Aspirin Toxicity
1. Thiamine, folate
2. D5NS
Serum lactate
Fomepizole/alcohol, HCO_3, ± hemodialysis
HCO_3, glucose, avoid intubation, ± hemodialysis
Normal lactate
Lactic acidosis
↑ BUN, Cr
Hypoperfusion?
Renal Failure
Type B Lactic Acidosis
Type A Lactic Acidosis
Citrate or HCO_3
Metformin, malignancy, β-agonists, HIV
Shock, intestinal ischemia, rhabdomyolysis, infection, carbon monoxide or cyanide poisoning
Treat underlying disease, remove offending agent
Definitions
Calculated Serum Osmolarity (Serum Osm)
(2 × Na) + (Glucose/18) + (BUN/2.8)
Serum Osm Gap
(Measured Osm) - (Calculated Osm)
↑ Osm Gap
Serum Osm Gap >10

FIGURE 6.9

6-9 Anion Gap Metabolic Acidosis

ETIOLOGIES OF AGMA

GOLDMARK (**G**lycols, **O**xoproline, **L**/**D**-Lactate, **M**ethanol, **A**spirin, **R**enal failure, **K**etoacidosis).

DIABETIC KETOACIDOSIS

A 24-year-old M with PMH of T1DM presents with nausea, vomiting, abdominal pain, and confusion. On **exam**, he has tachycardia and poor skin turgor. **Labs** show K 3.8, BG 500, elevated ketones, and AGMA.

Management:

1. IV fluids, insulin, dextrose.
2. K repletion (goal 4–5).

Complications: Arrhythmias, coma, hypoglycemia, hypokalemia.

HYF: Patients with DKA have a total body K deficit despite normal serum K; insulin will shift K into cells and possibly cause hypokalemia if K is not repleted aggressively.

STARVATION/ALCOHOLIC KETOACIDOSIS

A 45-year-old M with PMH of EtOH use disorder presents with nausea, vomiting, and abdominal pain after a recent EtOH binge. **Exam** shows tachycardia, hepatomegaly, and low BMI. **Labs** show AST > ALT elevation, AGMA, and undetectable EtOH level.

Management:

1. Alcoholic: Thiamine, then D5NS.
2. Starvation: Nutritional support; check Mg, K, Phos and replete electrolytes as needed for refeeding syndrome.

Complications:

- Wernicke encephalopathy in alcoholic patients if D5NS is given before thiamine.
- Refeeding syndrome: Abnormal electrolytes (hypoMg, hypoK, hypoPhos) → cardiac arrest.
- Altered mental status, cardiac arrhythmias.

HYF: Ketoacidosis occurs in low insulin scenarios. Serum EtOH may be undetectable at presentation and still contribute to development of AGMA. Serum EtOH, if present, may increase serum osm gap.

RENAL FAILURE

A 50-year-old M with PMH of CKD presents for a routine visit. On **exam**, he has lower extremity edema. **Labs** show bicarbonate 21, AGMA, Cr 4, and elevated phosphate.

Management:

1. Mild/moderate: sodium bicarbonate.
2. Severe (EKG changes, altered mental status): dialysis.

Complications: CKD progression, bone loss, increased mortality.

HYF: Acidosis in CKD is typically asymptomatic. Severe AGMA is likely if a patient has symptoms of uremia (eg, arrhythmias, fatigue, etc.).

LACTIC ACIDOSIS (LA)

A 76-year-old M with PMH of metastatic cancer presents with septic shock. On **exam**, he has fever, hypotension, tachypnea, and altered mental status. **Labs** show lactate 6, AGMA, and positive blood cultures.

Management:

1. Treat underlying cause (infection, shock, cancer).
2. $NaHCO_3$ for pH <7.1 (controversial).

Complications: Hemodynamic instability.

HYF: Type A lactic acidosis is due to cellular hypoxia. Type B is caused by disease/drugs. **D**-LA occurs in short-bowel syndrome after a carbohydrate-heavy meal.

GLYCOLS/METHANOL

A 4-year-old M with no PMH presents with suspected ingestion from the garage. On **exam**, he has bright liquid on his shirt and appears inebriated. **Labs** show AGMA and calcium oxalate crystals in the urine.

Management:

1. Manage ABCs, decontaminate the patient (remove clothing).
2. $NaHCO_3$.
3. Alcohol dehydrogenase inhibition: fomepizole, EtOH.
4. Dialysis if severe.

Complications:

- Methanol: blindness, death.
- Ethylene glycol: CKD, death.

HYF: Osm gap may not be present. Presence of calcium oxalate stones suggests ethylene glycol ingestion but is not sensitive or specific. Visual complaints → methanol (formic acid). Flank pain, hematuria, oliguria → ethylene glycol (metabolized to glycolic acid and oxalic acid).

ASPIRIN (SALICYLATE) TOXICITY

An 18-year-old F with PMH of depression presents with altered mental status, tinnitus, nausea, vomiting, and diarrhea. On **exam**, she has hyperpnea and tachycardia. **Labs** show pH 7.38, HCO_3 15, and PCO_2 24.

Management:

1. Do NOT intubate.
2. HCO_3 and IV fluids; dialysis if severe/pulmonary edema.

Complications: Pulmonary edema, altered mental status, arrhythmia.

HYF: Low pCO_2 and HCO_3 should make you suspect ASA toxicity. Pulmonary edema is an absolute indication for dialysis.

6-9 Anion Gap Metabolic Acidosis

ASA uncouples oxidative phosphorylation in mitochondria. Lack of hyperthermia does not rule out ASA toxicity.

5-OXOPROLINE

An 85-year-old F with PMH of chronic osteomyelitis presents with acidemia on routine checkup. She takes acetaminophen for chronic pain. On **exam**, she has cachexia. **Labs** show AGMA.

Management:

1. Stop acetaminophen.

HYF: 5-Oxoproline is an intermediate in the gamma-glutamyl cycle and is a rare cause of AGMA. Most commonly seen in elderly women who are chronically ill with malnutrition. Associated with acetaminophen use.

*Other causes of AGMA include uremia (uric acid), iron, isoniazid, and isopropyl alcohol.

6-10 Non-Anion Gap Metabolic Acidosis

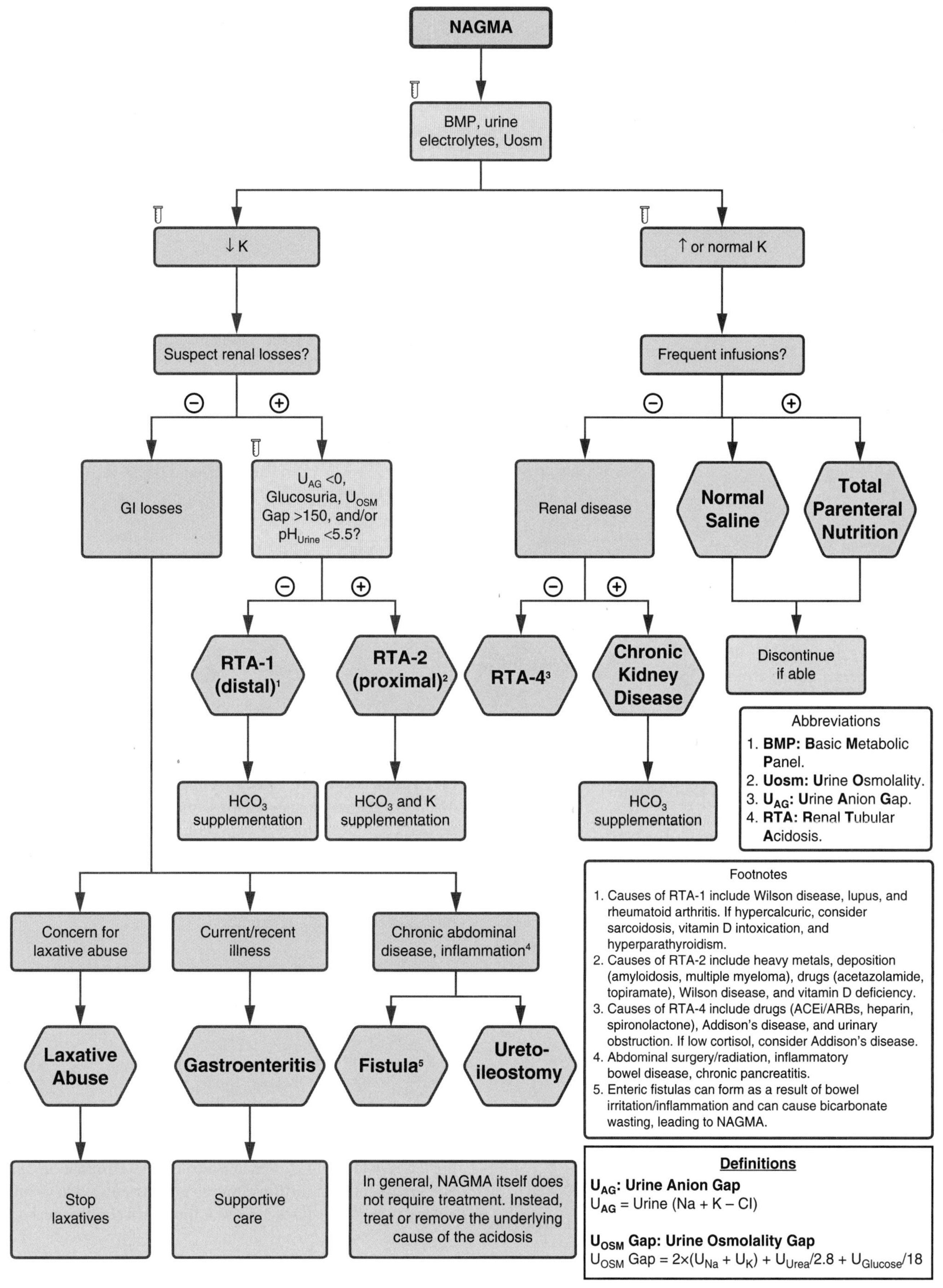
NAGMA
BMP, urine electrolytes, Uosm
↓ K
↑ or normal K
Suspect renal losses?
Frequent infusions?
⊖
⊕
GI losses
U_{AG} <0, Glucosuria, U_{OSM} Gap >150, and/or pH_{Urine} <5.5?
Renal disease
Normal Saline
Total Parenteral Nutrition
RTA-1 (distal)[1]
RTA-2 (proximal)[2]
RTA-4[3]
Chronic Kidney Disease
Discontinue if able
HCO_3 supplementation
HCO_3 and K supplementation
HCO_3 supplementation
Abbreviations
1. BMP: Basic Metabolic Panel.
2. Uosm: Urine Osmolality.
3. U_{AG}: Urine Anion Gap.
4. RTA: Renal Tubular Acidosis.
Concern for laxative abuse
Current/recent illness
Chronic abdominal disease, inflammation[4]
Laxative Abuse
Gastroenteritis
Fistula[5]
Ureto-ileostomy
Stop laxatives
Supportive care
In general, NAGMA itself does not require treatment. Instead, treat or remove the underlying cause of the acidosis
Footnotes
1. Causes of RTA-1 include Wilson disease, lupus, and rheumatoid arthritis. If hypercalcuric, consider sarcoidosis, vitamin D intoxication, and hyperparathyroidism.
2. Causes of RTA-2 include heavy metals, deposition (amyloidosis, multiple myeloma), drugs (acetazolamide, topiramate), Wilson disease, and vitamin D deficiency.
3. Causes of RTA-4 include drugs (ACEi/ARBs, heparin, spironolactone), Addison's disease, and urinary obstruction. If low cortisol, consider Addison's disease.
4. Abdominal surgery/radiation, inflammatory bowel disease, chronic pancreatitis.
5. Enteric fistulas can form as a result of bowel irritation/inflammation and can cause bicarbonate wasting, leading to NAGMA.
Definitions
U_{AG}: Urine Anion Gap
U_{AG} = Urine (Na + K – Cl)
U_{OSM} Gap: Urine Osmolality Gap
U_{OSM} Gap = 2×(U_{Na} + U_K) + U_{Urea}/2.8 + $U_{Glucose}$/18

FIGURE 6.10

6-10 Non-Anion Gap Metabolic Acidosis

Common Etiologies

Hyperalimentation	Hyperalimentation
Addison Disease	Acetazolamide
Renal Tubular Acidosis	Renal Tubular Acidosis
Diarrhea	Diarrhea/Diuretics
Acetazolamide	Uteroenterostomy
Spironolactone	Pancreatic fistula
Saline infusion	

TYPE 1 RTA

A 13-year-old M presents with abdominal pain and polyuria. On **exam**, he has short stature and abdominal tenderness. **Labs** show K 3.4, anion gap 8, UA with blood and urine pH 5.8. On **imaging**, renal US shows a large kidney stone.

Management:

1. Alkali therapy (bicarbonate).
2. If 2°, treat underlying disease and/or remove drug causing RTA.

Complications:

- Severe: osteoporosis, emesis, growth restriction in infants.
- Hypercalciuria → nephrolithiasis.

HYF: Due to deficiency in urine acidification, most commonly from defect in the proton pump in the alpha intercalated cells of the collecting duct → decreased H+ secretion in the urine → NAGMA. Patients often present with hypokalemia, urinary pH >5.5, and hypercalciuria. The most common cause is usually heritable and seen in children who present with nephrolithiasis and growth failure. Acquired RTA typically occurs in adulthood, is often asymptomatic, and found incidentally. Common causes of Type 1 RTA in adults: autoimmune (Sjögren, rheumatoid arthritis), various drugs (amphotericin B).

TYPE 2 (PROXIMAL) RTA

A 40-year-old M with PMH of epilepsy treated with valproic acid presents for routine check-up. **Exam** is normal. **Labs** show Na 137, Cl 108, HCO_3 20, K 2.9, phos 12.0, glucose 90, and UA with pH 5.2, 2+ glucose.

Management:

1. Treat underlying cause or remove offending agent.
2. Alkali therapy (bicarbonate or citrate).
3. May need K repletion or K-sparing diuretics.
4. Replete vitamin D and phos; ± K repletion, K-sparing diuretics.

HYF: Type 2 RTA is due to proximal tubule dysfunction leading to impaired reabsorption of bicarbonate and excess excretion in urine and creating a NAGMA. It can be isolated or part of Fanconi syndrome. Fanconi syndrome is accompanied by defects that also cause glucosuria, hypophosphatemia, and vitamin D deficiency. Common causes: anti-epileptics (valproic acid), carbonic anhydrase inhibitors, aminoglycosides, tenofovir, heavy metals, and multiple myeloma.

TYPE 4 RTA

A 65-year-old M with PMH of DM2, CKD, and HTN presents with routine check-up. **Labs** show AG 10, bicarb 17, K 5.3, and urine pH 5.1.

Management:

1. Treat underlying cause, stop offending agents.
2. Low K diet, diuretics.
3. Mineral/glucocorticoid supplementation if deficient.

HYF: Due to aldosterone resistance or insufficient aldosterone production (eg, renin deficiency). Can be primary (Addison's disease) or secondary to CKD, drugs (ACEi/ARB, NSAIDS, K-sparing diuretics, calcineurin inhibitors), or severe illness. Common diseases associated with CKD and type 4 RTA: diabetes, sickle cell disease, SLE.

GI LOSSES

A 25-year-old F nurse presents with fatigue, diarrhea. On **exam**, she has temporal wasting, BMI of 17, and poor skin turgor. She says she is concerned about being "fat." **Labs** show AG 10 and K 3.0.

Management:

1. Treat underlying cause, correct electrolyte abnormalities.

Complications: Hypokalemia, hypovolemia, fatigue.

HYF: Laxative abuse can cause metabolic alkalosis or acidosis. *Melanosis coli* is associated with senna abuse. Diarrhea and enteric fistulas (eg, due to surgery or inflammatory conditions) cause the loss of bicarbonate and other anions, leading to NAGMA. When urine comes in contact with GI mucosa (eg, enteric fistula, surgical ureteral diversion), there is increased Cl- absorption, which increases renal HCO_3 elimination.

INFUSIONS

A 25-year-old M is found to have NAGMA after receiving a large volume of normal saline infusion. **Labs** show AG 10 and low HCO_3.

Management:

1. Decrease normal saline infusion, switch fluids.

HYF: Large volumes of normal saline cause NAGMA by providing a heavy load of Cl-, which leads to renal elimination of HCO_3. Hyperalimentation (artificial supply of nutrients, such as total parenteral nutrition) causes NAGMA through a similar mechanism.

6-11 Metabolic Alkalosis

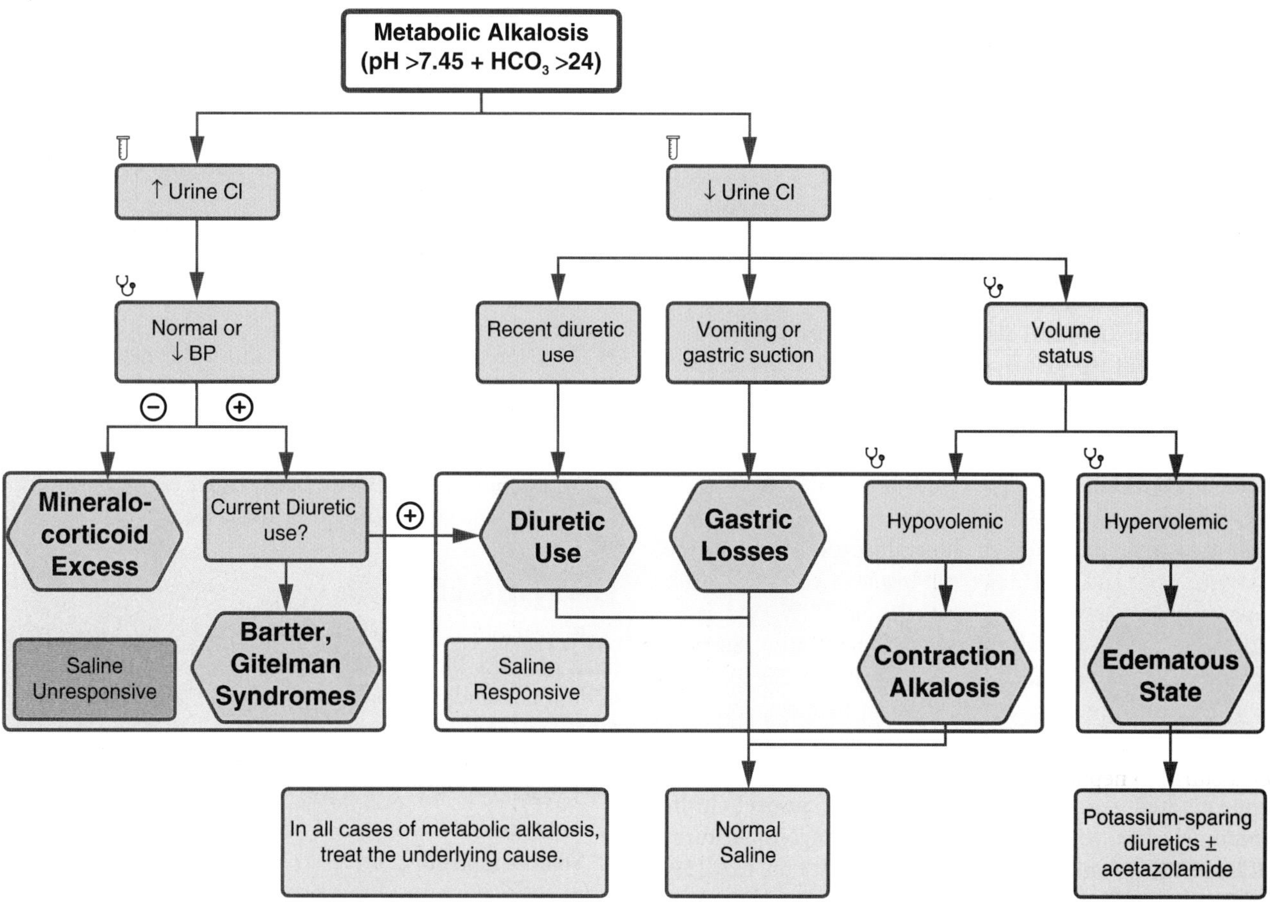

Metabolic Alkalosis
(pH >7.45 + HCO3 >24)
↑ Urine Cl
↓ Urine Cl
Normal or ↓ BP
Recent diuretic use
Vomiting or gastric suction
Volume status
Mineralo-corticoid Excess
Current Diuretic use?
Diuretic Use
Gastric Losses
Hypovolemic
Hypervolemic
Bartter, Gitelman Syndromes
Saline Unresponsive
Saline Responsive
Contraction Alkalosis
Edematous State
In all cases of metabolic alkalosis, treat the underlying cause.
Normal Saline
Potassium-sparing diuretics ± acetazolamide

Metabolic alkalosis is caused by impaired HCO_3 excretion, excess HCO_3 absorption, and/or ↑ H+ excretion. Hypovolemia, hypochloremia, hypokalemia, and mineralcorticoids all contribute to these processes. Since some clinical presentations may involve one or more of these processes simultaneously, we will discuss the pathophysiology first and then tie it all together.

HCO_3 excretion in the distal convoluted tubule depends upon Cl^-. When a patient's kidneys experience ↓ bloodflow, $NaHCO_3$ and Cl^- reabsorption ↑. With ↑ Cl^- reabsorption, less Cl^- reaches the distal tubules, limiting HCO_3 excretion. Thus, ↓ effective renal bloodflow ↑ HCO_3 reabsorption and ↓ excretion. In a true volume-depleted state, the intravascular volume ↓ while total HCO_3 remains stable. This results in a higher HCO_3 concentration and contraction alkalosis. As noted above, Cl^- is necessary for HCO_3 excretion in the distal tubules, but Cl^- is also tightly linked to volume status. Thus, hypochloremia is associated with alkalosis via two mechanisms.

Hypokalemia is another mechanism that can cause alkalosis. ↓ serum potassium concentration stimulates extracellular shift of potassium and intracellular shift of H+. Hypokalemia also ↑ renal reabsorption of HCO_3 by an unknown mechanism.

Aldosterone works in the kidneys to directly ↑ Na (and water) reabsorption, H excretion, and K excretion. The resultant K wasting causes hypokalemia, which leads to alkalosis by the mechanisms mentioned above. Volume retention also causes ↑ bloodflow to the kidneys. As a result, more total Na reaches the distal tubules, where it is reabsorbed with HCO_3. Thus, aldosterone directly (H+ excretion) and indirectly (↑ HCO_3 reabsorption, hypokalemia) causes metabolic alkalosis.

Loop and thiazide diuretics can cause hypovolemia and hypokalemia. Bartter and Gitelman syndromes are caused by mutations in nephron transport proteins. These mutations mimic the results of loop and thiazide diuretics, respectively.

Mineralocorticoid excess causes alkalosis via aldosterone. Gastric losses cause a ↓ in Cl^-, H+, and intravascular volume. Both contraction alkalosis and edematous states (cirrhosis, heart failure, nephrotic syndrome) cause alkalosis via ↓ effective intravascular volume. In the case of contraction alkalosis, this is secondary to ↓ total volume. In an edematous state, the total body fluid is ↑, but intravascular volume is ↓ due to third-spacing of fluid. The use of loop or thiazide diuretics may also contribute to alkalosis in edematous states.

Always treat the underlying disease. For saline-responsive etiologies, alkalosis resolves with normal saline as it provides both volume and Cl^-. Do not treat alkalosis with saline in non-responsive etiologies. Not only will patients not improve with volume, they can often worsen. In these cases, potassium-sparing diuretics (spironolactone, amiloride) ± acetazolamide may be used.

The etiology of metabolic alkalosis is typically obvious from the initial history, but urine Cl^- is a helpful way to group diagnoses on the differential and guide further investigation. Patients with metabolic alkalosis present with symptoms related to their underlying disease. Those who are volume depleted will have nausea, vomiting, fatigue, and/or dizziness. Patients with processes causing hypokalemia (mineralcorticoid excess, diuretics) can present with cramps and arrhythmias. Patients in an edematous state can present with orthopnea, encephalopathy, HTN, or various other symptoms, depending upon their underlying diagnosis.

FIGURE 6.11

6-11 Metabolic Alkalosis

MINERALOCORTICOID EXCESS

A 60-year-old M with PMH of OSA and drug-resistant HTN presents for a routine visit. On **exam**, he has BP 160/97 and is obese. **Labs** show K 3.6 and HCO_3 32.

Management:

1. Check plasma renin and aldosterone.
2. CT scan of adrenals.
3. ± adrenal vein sampling if CT not diagnostic.
4. Adrenalectomy in unilateral disease. Mineralocorticoid receptor antagonist (spironolactone, eplerenone) in bilateral disease.

Complications: Refractory HTN, increased cardiovascular risk, metabolic syndrome.

HYF: The two main examples of mineralocorticoid excess are hyperaldosteronism and Cushing's syndrome. Consider excess mineralocorticoids when you see hypokalemia, HTN, and metabolic alkalosis, though not all patients will have all 3. Suspect hyperaldosteronism in patients with severe HTN (>150/100) not controlled on 3 antihypertensives. To test for hyperaldosteronism, check plasma renin and plasma aldosterone. If renin is low and aldosterone is high → primary aldosteronism. If both renin and aldosterone are high → secondary aldosteronism. Suspect Cushing's syndrome when you see the classic "Cushingoid" features (eg, central obesity, abdominal striae, moon facies). See pp. 157–159, Cushing's Syndrome, for more information.

BARTTER AND GITELMAN SYNDROMES

A 25-year-old M with no PMH presents with chronic fatigue and cramps. On **exam**, he has BP 100/70. **Labs** show K 2.8 and HCO_3 28.

Management:

1. K, Na, Mg repletion.
2. K-sparing diuretics if repletion is ineffective.
3. Kidney transplant if progress to ESRD.

Complications: Electrolyte abnormalities, ESRD.

HYF: Bartter and Gitelman syndromes are salt-wasting tubulopathies. Bartter syndrome affects the thick ascending loop of Henle and mimics loop diuretics. Gitelman syndrome affects the DCT and mimics thiazide diuretics. These conditions are quite rare but should be considered in anyone who has hypokalemia, normo/hypotension, and metabolic alkalosis. When working these conditions up, rule out surreptitious etiologies: vomiting, diuretic abuse, and laxative abuse. Spot urine chloride will be persistently high over serial visits in Bartter and Gitelman syndromes.

DIURETIC USE, CONTRACTION ALKALOSIS

A 70-year-old M with PMH of newly diagnosed CHF, recently started on furosemide, presents for a routine visit. On **exam**, he has tachycardia and dry mucous membranes. **Labs** show K 3.1, HCO_3 29.

Management:

1. Stop diuretics (when able).
2. Volume repletion.

HYF: Diuretic use increases Na and water delivery to the distal tubule, resulting in increased hydrogen and K wasting → metabolic alkalosis. Diuresing a large volume also "contracts" the extracellular fluid around the relatively stable amount of HCO_3, causing a concomitant contraction alkalosis. Any cause of a large loss of HCO_3-poor fluid can cause contraction alkalosis.

GASTRIC LOSSES

A 30-year-old F with PMH of alcohol use disorder and pancreatitis presents with 1 week of nausea and vomiting. **Exam** reveals abdominal tenderness and dry mucous membranes. **Labs** show K 2.8, Cl 90, and HCO_3 30.

Management:

1. Antiemetics.
2. Volume repletion.

HYF: Metabolic alkalosis due to gastric losses is typically from vomiting. Emesis or NG suctioning removes acid from the body as well as volume, leading to a metabolic alkalosis with concomitant hypokalemia and hypochloridia. Diarrhea typically contains high HCO_3, except in some rare diseases, and thus doesn't typically cause metabolic alkalosis.

EDEMATOUS STATE

A 65-year-old M with PMH of liver cirrhosis presents with volume overload. On **exam**, he has ascites and 2+ pitting edema. **Labs** show Na 127, K 3.1, and HCO_3 28.

Management:

1. Do not give fluids.
2. K-sparing diuretic, replete K.

HYF: Alkalosis in edematous states (cirrhosis, CHF, nephrotic syndrome) is often exacerbated by diuretic use. However, even in the absence of diuretic use, there is an underlying physiologic cause: In an edematous state, there is decreased blood flow to the kidneys despite the overall volume-overloaded state, causing the kidneys to become sodium-avid and limiting their ability to excrete HCO_3. This results in a metabolic alkalosis.

6-12 Acute Kidney Injury

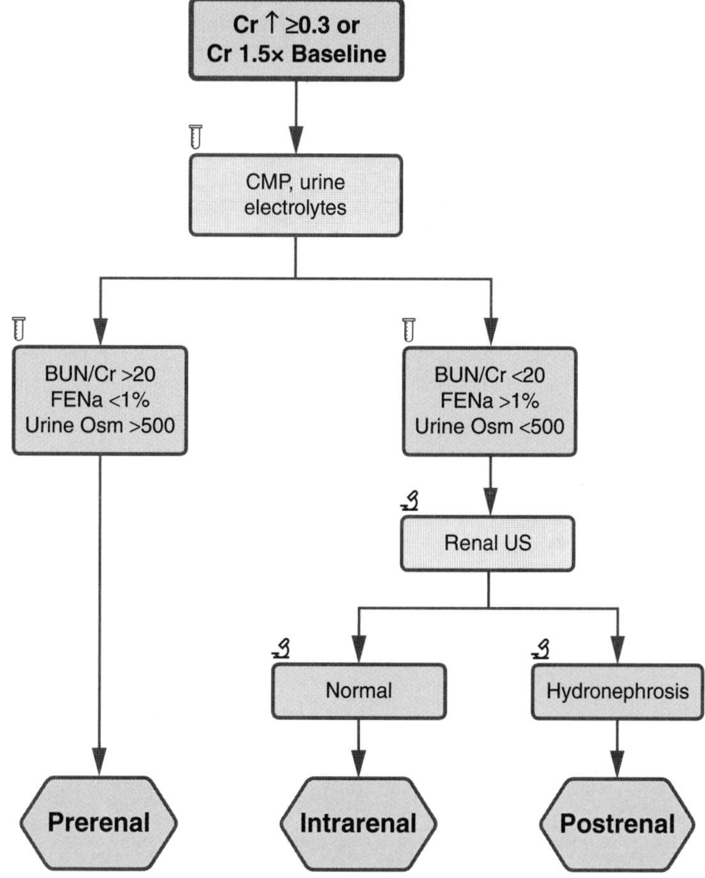
Cr ↑ ≥0.3 or
Cr 1.5× Baseline
CMP, urine electrolytes
BUN/Cr >20
FENa <1%
Urine Osm >500
BUN/Cr <20
FENa >1%
Urine Osm <500
Renal US
Normal
Hydronephrosis
Prerenal
Intrarenal
Postrenal

Acute kidney injury (AKI) is an acute and often reversible decline in kidney function. It is defined as 1) an ↑ in creatinine of 0.3 or greater, or 2) a creatinine greater than 1.5× baseline. There are 3 types of AKI: 1) Prerenal AKI, which occurs when there is a ↓ in blood flow to the kidneys due to conditions such as dehydration, severe bleeding, or heart failure, 2) Intrinsic AKI, which is characterized by direct damage to the kidneys, and 3) Post-renal AKI, which is due to obstruction of urine flow from the kidneys due to conditions such as nephrolithiasis, tumors, or an enlarged prostate gland in male patients.

The work-up for AKI typically involves a thorough medical history and physical exam to identify any underlying conditions that may predispose a patient to AKI (eg, recent gastroenteritis leading to dehydration, new medication that predisposes to nephrolithiasis, older male patient with benign prostatic hyperplasia). Laboratory tests may include measurement of electrolytes, BUN, creatinine, urine electrolytes, urinalysis, and urine output. Imaging studies, such as renal ultrasound or CT abdomen, may also be used to evaluate the urinary tract and identify any structural abnormalities. In some cases, renal biopsy may be indicated.

Treatment of AKI depends on the underlying etiology, severity, and associated conditions. AKIs are often associated with electrolyte abnormalities due to impaired kidney function (eg, hyperkalemia), which need to be considered when deciding on the course of treatment. In many cases, supportive care including IV fluids and close monitoring for resolution are sufficient. In other cases, dialysis or procedural interventions (eg, tumor resection, nephrostomy tube placement) may be required.

FIGURE 6.12

6-13 Prerenal Acute Kidney Injury

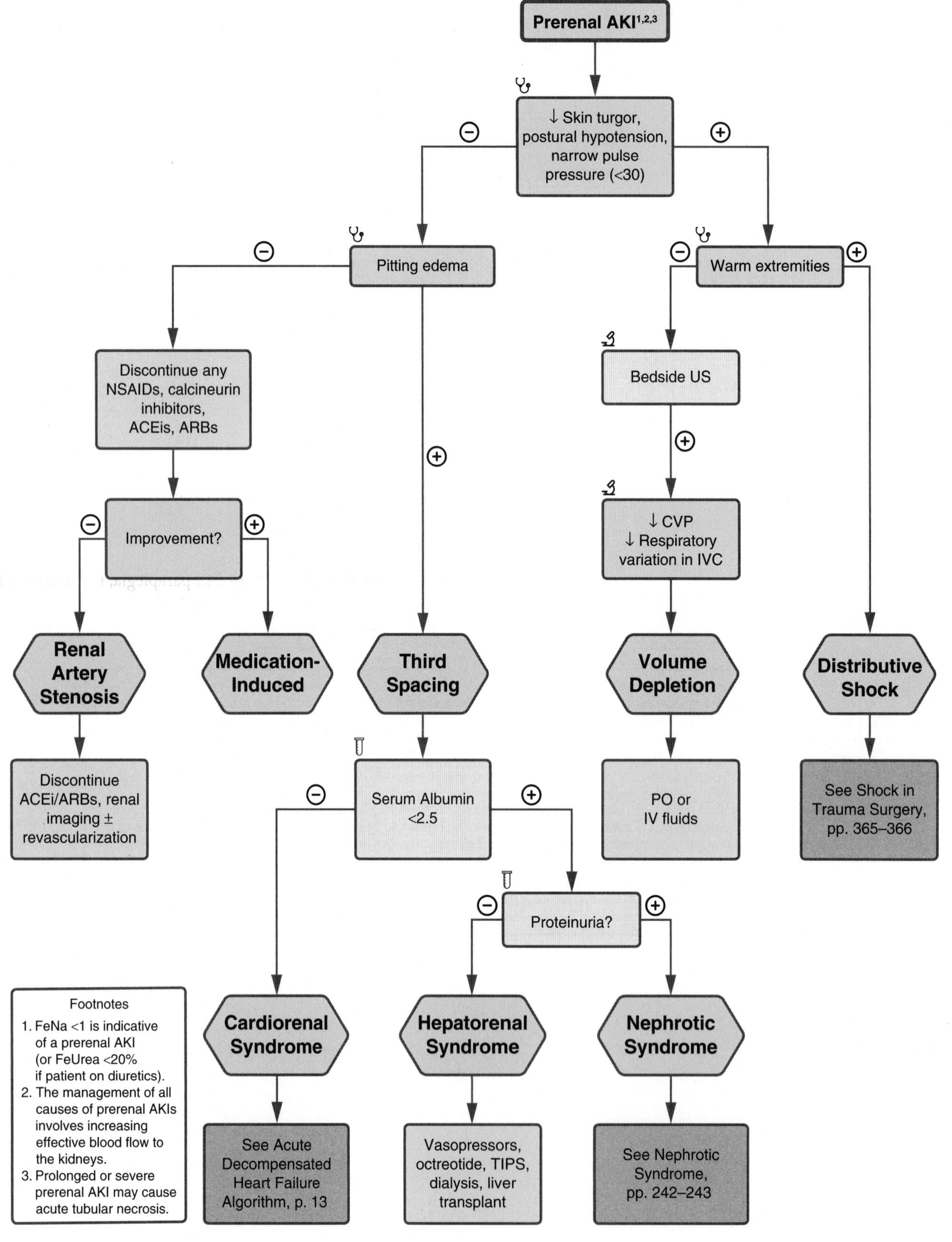

Prerenal AKI[1,2,3]
↓ Skin turgor, postural hypotension, narrow pulse pressure (<30)
Pitting edema
Warm extremities
Discontinue any NSAIDs, calcineurin inhibitors, ACEis, ARBs
Improvement?
Bedside US
↓ CVP
↓ Respiratory variation in IVC
Renal Artery Stenosis
Medication-Induced
Third Spacing
Volume Depletion
Distributive Shock
Discontinue ACEi/ARBs, renal imaging ± revascularization
Serum Albumin <2.5
PO or IV fluids
See Shock in Trauma Surgery, pp. 365–366
Proteinuria?
Cardiorenal Syndrome
Hepatorenal Syndrome
Nephrotic Syndrome
See Acute Decompensated Heart Failure Algorithm, p. 13
Vasopressors, octreotide, TIPS, dialysis, liver transplant
See Nephrotic Syndrome, pp. 242–243
Footnotes
1. FeNa <1 is indicative of a prerenal AKI (or FeUrea <20% if patient on diuretics).
2. The management of all causes of prerenal AKIs involves increasing effective blood flow to the kidneys.
3. Prolonged or severe prerenal AKI may cause acute tubular necrosis.

FIGURE 6.13

6-13 Prerenal Acute Kidney Injury

RENAL ARTERY STENOSIS

A 65-year-old M with PMH of vascular risk factors (smoking, diabetes, coronary artery disease, peripheral arterial disease) presents with medication-refractory hypertension and chronic kidney disease. **Exam** shows abdominal and carotid bruits. On **imaging**, doppler US confirms bilateral narrowing of the renal arteries. Urinalysis is negative on **labs**.

Management:

1. Discontinue ACEi, ARBs.
2. Renal arteriography, renal Doppler U/S, or ACE-I scintigraphy.
3. If stenosis <80%, observe. Otherwise revascularize (angioplasty).
4. Control hypertension with CCBs, not ACEi or ARBs.

Complications:

- ESRD requiring dialysis.
- Sequelae of HTN if it is not adequately controlled.

HYF: Also known as renovascular HTN. Most common cause of secondary HTN. Abdominal bruit sometimes noted on **exam**. Atherosclerosis is the leading factor in men age >45 and fibromuscular dysplasia in women age <50. Can be unilateral or bilateral. Severe refractory HTN or AKI after initiation of ACEi/ARB (not just the expected Cr bump) should raise suspicion for renovascular disease. Diagnose with duplex ultrasound.

MEDICATION-INDUCED

A 76-year-old M with PMH of HTN and DM2 admitted for CHF exacerbation s/p IV furosemide with excellent urine output, now has a Cr elevation 0.3 above baseline.

Management:

1. Decrease or discontinue IV furosemide.
2. Renal (or retroperitoneal) US to rule out obstruction.

Complications:

- Decrease in kidney function can be permanent.
- Increased risk of progression to CKD and mortality.

HYF: Common problem seen in hospitalized patients. Loop diuretics are the leading risk factor. Other medications that can induce prerenal AKI: NSAIDs, angiotensin-converting enzyme inhibitors, angiotensin receptor blockers, cyclosporine, tacrolimus. Differentiate between medication-induced prerenal AKI and medication-induced intrinsic AKI: Some medications cause injury to the kidney via inflammation or direct injury (eg, crystal formation, acute interstitial nephritis). In these instances, expect the UA to show evidence of this injury (ie, blood, WBCs, crystals). In contrast, drugs that reduce the effective perfusion of the kidneys and cause a prerenal AKI should result in a "bland" UA.

VOLUME DEPLETION

An 86-year-old F with PMH of Alzheimer's dementia and HTN is admitted for severe dehydration due to decreased PO intake. On **exam**, she has skin tenting with diminished turgor. **Labs** show Cr double that of baseline and contraction alkalosis.

Management:

1. IV fluids.
2. Address any electrolyte abnormalities.

Complications:

- Decrease in kidney function can be permanent.
- Increased risk of progression to CKD and mortality.

HYF: Patients can present with decreased PO intake, diarrhea (eg, viral gastroenteritis), or burns leading to insensible losses. Clinical signs/symptoms of decreased total volume include low skin turgor, hypernatremia, dry mucous membranes, contraction alkalosis, and hemoconcentration (an increase in concentration of WBCs, RBCs, and platelets). None of these are specific, but together they point to the diagnosis of decreased volume in conjunction with the history.

DISTRIBUTIVE SHOCK

A 44-year-old M with PMH of T12 paraplegia, recurrent UTIs, and decubitus ulcers presents with sepsis. On **exam**, he has hypotension, tachycardia, and tachypnea with extremities warm to touch, and **labs** show leukocytosis and Cr 1.5x that of baseline.

Management:

1. IV fluids and pressors as needed.
2. Blood cultures ×2.
3. IV antibiotics.

Complications: Acute tubular necrosis, end-stage renal disease if volume and hypotension not corrected.

HYF: Management of distributive shock involves 1) stabilizing the patient (eg, IV fluids, pressors), and 2) addressing the underlying cause (eg, broad-spectrum IV antibiotics for sepsis). Hypotension in the setting of distributive shock leads to renal hypoperfusion, which can lead to a pre-renal AKI or, if prolonged and/or severe, acute tubular necrosis.

CARDIORENAL SYNDROME

A 66-year-old F with PMH of CHF presents with acute decompensated heart failure. On **exam** she has an elevated JVP and pitting pedal edema, and **labs** show Cr 2× baseline.

Management:

1. Manage CHF exacerbation (ie, IV diuretics).

6-13 Prerenal Acute Kidney Injury

Complications:

- Respiratory failure due to pulmonary edema.
- ESRD.
- Liver failure.

HYF: Acute cardiac decompensation produces inappropriate RAAS activation and increased CVP. Decreased intravascular volume due to third-spacing and increased renal back-pressure decrease glomerular filtration, leading to AKI. Unlike many other pre-renal etiologies of AKI, treatment of cardiorenal syndrome involves diuresis; fluid repletion will only contribute to cardiorenal syndrome and worsen the AKI.

HEPATORENAL SYNDROME

A 45-year-old M with PMH of liver cirrhosis secondary to chronic HCV and EtOH use disorder presents with spontaneous bacterial peritonitis in the setting of decompensated cirrhosis with oliguria. On **exam**, he has jaundice and ascites, and **labs** show severe hyponatremia with Cr elevated 2.5× baseline.

Management:

1. IV norepinephrine or PO midodrine.
2. IV or PO octreotide, synthetic vasopressin analogues (eg, terlipressin).
3. IV albumin.
4. Consider dialysis if refractory to the above measures.
5. Definitive treatment is liver transplantation.

Complications: Development of HRS in decompensated cirrhosis is associated with poorer prognosis.

HYF: Cirrhosis produces splanchnic and systemic vasodilation via a neurohormonal cascade. Decrease in systemic hypoperfusion increases RAAS system activation, vasopressin, and catecholamine release, which in turn decrease renal perfusion and instigate AKI.

- Type 1 HRS (rapid): Cr >2.5× baseline in 2 weeks.
- Type 2 HRS: less severe AKI that is diuretic-resistant.

NEPHROTIC SYNDROME

A 43-year-old M with PMH of DM2 presents with nephrotic syndrome in the setting of membranous nephropathy. On **exam**, he has dependent edema, and **labs** show severe proteinuria (>300 mg/dL) and decreased serum albumin (<2.5).

Management:

1. See Nephrotic Syndrome, p. 242.

Complications:

- Respiratory distress due to pulmonary edema.
- Sepsis (particularly *Streptococcus pneumoniae*-induced).
- Pulmonary embolisms.
- Arterial or deep-vein thrombosis.

HYF: Nephrotic syndrome is due to an intrinsic process that can lead to extravascular fluid shifts and prerenal AKI. In children, the most common cause is MCD. In adults, the most common causes are MN or FSGS.

FIBROMUSCULAR DYSPLASIA

A 20-year-old F presents with new onset refractory hypertension and frequent headaches. **Exam** shows abdominal or carotid bruits. On **imaging**, doppler US reveals increased renal artery flow velocity.

Management

1. Treat hypertension.
2. Angioplasty is often the management of choice.

Complications: Stroke, TIA, CKD.

HYF: 90% of adults with fibromuscular dysplasia are women. The most common presentation is recurrent headaches. FMD is a cause of renovascular HTN. Subauricular or abdominal bruit may be auscultated. Internal carotid and renal arteries are most commonly affected. When FMD causes renal artery stenosis, the presenting sign may be AKI induced by ACEi/ARB.

6-14 Intrinsic Acute Kidney Injury

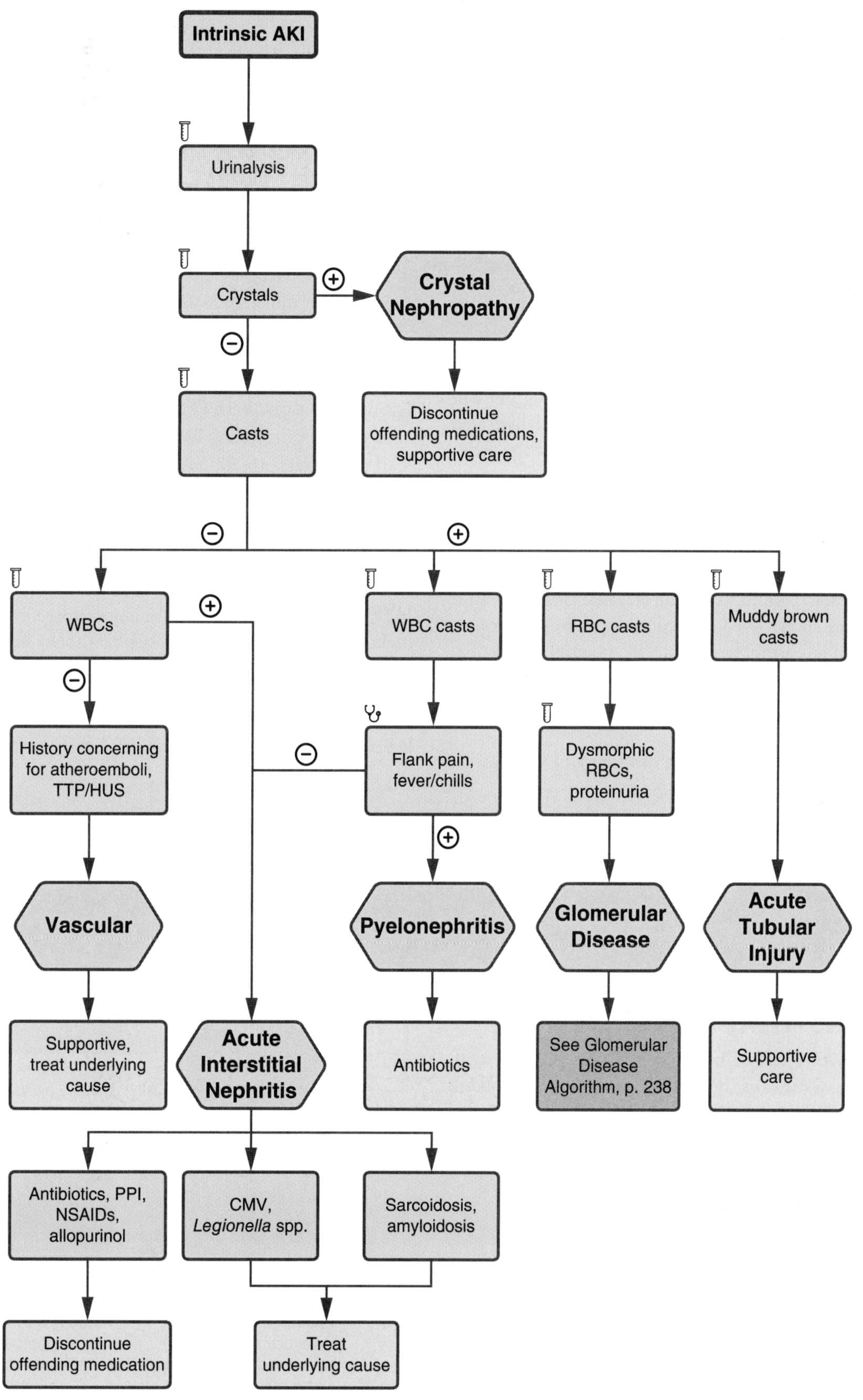
Intrinsic AKI
Urinalysis
Crystals
Crystal Nephropathy
Discontinue offending medications, supportive care
Casts
WBCs
WBC casts
RBC casts
Muddy brown casts
History concerning for atheroemboli, TTP/HUS
Flank pain, fever/chills
Dysmorphic RBCs, proteinuria
Vascular
Pyelonephritis
Glomerular Disease
Acute Tubular Injury
Supportive, treat underlying cause
Acute Interstitial Nephritis
Antibiotics
See Glomerular Disease Algorithm, p. 238
Supportive care
Antibiotics, PPI, NSAIDs, allopurinol
CMV, *Legionella* spp.
Sarcoidosis, amyloidosis
Discontinue offending medication
Treat underlying cause

FIGURE 6.14

6-14 Intrinsic Acute Kidney Injury

CRYSTAL NEPHROPATHY

A 45-year-old M with PMH of genital herpes with recent acyclovir use presents with elevated creatinine on routine labs. He is asymptomatic. **Exam** is normal. On **labs**, UA shows crystals.

Management:

1. Discontinue offending agent (acyclovir, methotrexate, sulfonamides, ethylene glycol).
2. Correct volume depletion with IV fluids.

Complications: Progression to ATN (± need for temporary dialysis), CKD.

HYF: Crystals, blood, and pyuria can be noted on UA. AKI typically occurs within 7 days of starting an offending drug but can occur at any time, especially when the patient becomes dehydrated or otherwise volume-depleted (eg, over diuresis, hemorrhage, emesis). CKD is a risk factor.

VASCULAR

A 65-year-old M with PMH of tobacco use disorder, T2DM, and coronary artery disease is found to have an elevated creatinine after coronary PCI. **Exam** shows livedo reticularis and a cyanotic toe. **Labs** show eosinophilia, eosinophiluria, and hypocomplementemia.

Management:

1. If from atheroemboli, supportive care.
2. If from TTP/HUS, correct underlying disorder and support with IV fluids.

Complications: Poor prognosis, often progresses to CKD or ESRD.

HYF: Vascular AKI can result from any cause of venous or arterial obstruction (eg, renal vein thrombosis, atheroemboli, scleroderma, renal crisis).

ACUTE INTERSTITIAL NEPHRITIS

A 45-year-old M with PMH of heavy NSAID use presents with elevated creatinine. On **exam**, he has no fever, chills, or flank tenderness. On **labs**, UA shows WBCs, >1% eosinophils, and rare WBC casts.

Management:

1. Allergic AIN: Discontinue offending medication (NSAID, allopurinol, sulfa, antibiotics, PPIs).
2. Infectious AIN: Treat underlying infection (CMV, *Leptospira*, EBV).
3. Infiltrative AIN: Treat sarcoid, sarcoidosis, amyloidosis.

Complications: Progression to CKD if untreated.

HYF: WBC casts are rare but indicative of interstitial inflammation. Typically occurs 7–10 days after exposure to the causative agent. Signs and symptoms include a rash, eosinophilia, WBC casts, pyuria, eosinophiluria, and fever. Acute interstitial nephritis may occur with certain diseases (eg, SLE) but is most commonly caused by medications.

ACUTE TUBULAR INJURY

A 45-year-old F being treated for septic shock in the ICU with episodes of hypotension is found to have decreased urine output and elevated creatinine. Her **exam** is consistent with hypovolemia. On **labs**, UA shows muddy brown casts.

Management:

1. Supportive care with IV fluids.
2. If from nephrotoxin, discontinue offending medication.
3. If from shock, treat underlying etiology (eg, IV antibiotics for sepsis).

Complications: Good prognosis with recovery usually within 3 weeks.

HYF: ATN can be the result of any extreme insult to the kidneys, including hypoperfusion (eg, septic shock) and toxins (medications [aminoglycosides, amphotericin B, sulfa drugs, acyclovir, calcineurin inhibitors, cisplatin], radiocontrast media, and heme-containing proteins [rhabdomyloysis, hemoglobinuria in hemolytic transfusion reactions]). Muddy brown casts are seen on UA.

Pyelonephritis: See pp. 244–245.

Glomerular Disease: See p. 238.

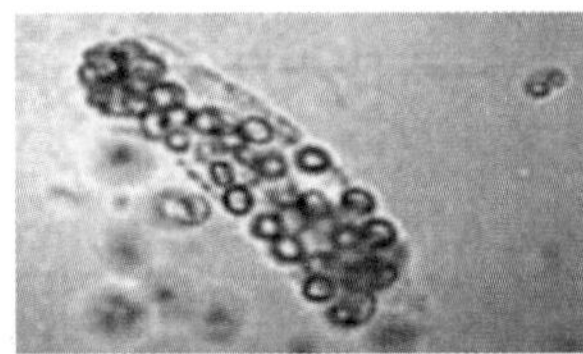
White blood cell casts suggest a diagnosis of acute interstitial nephritis (AIN) or acute pyelonephritis.

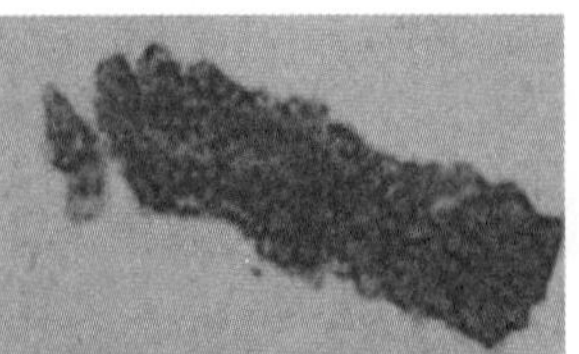
Red cell casts denote glomerular disease (eg, glomerulonephritis, small vessel vasculitis).

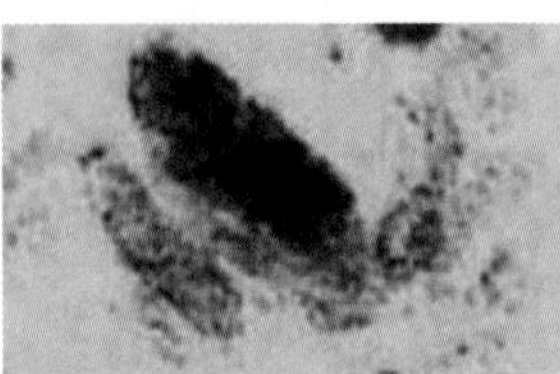
Muddy brown granular casts suggest acute tubular injury/necrosis (ATN) as the etiology of AKI.

6-15 Post-Renal Acute Kidney Injury

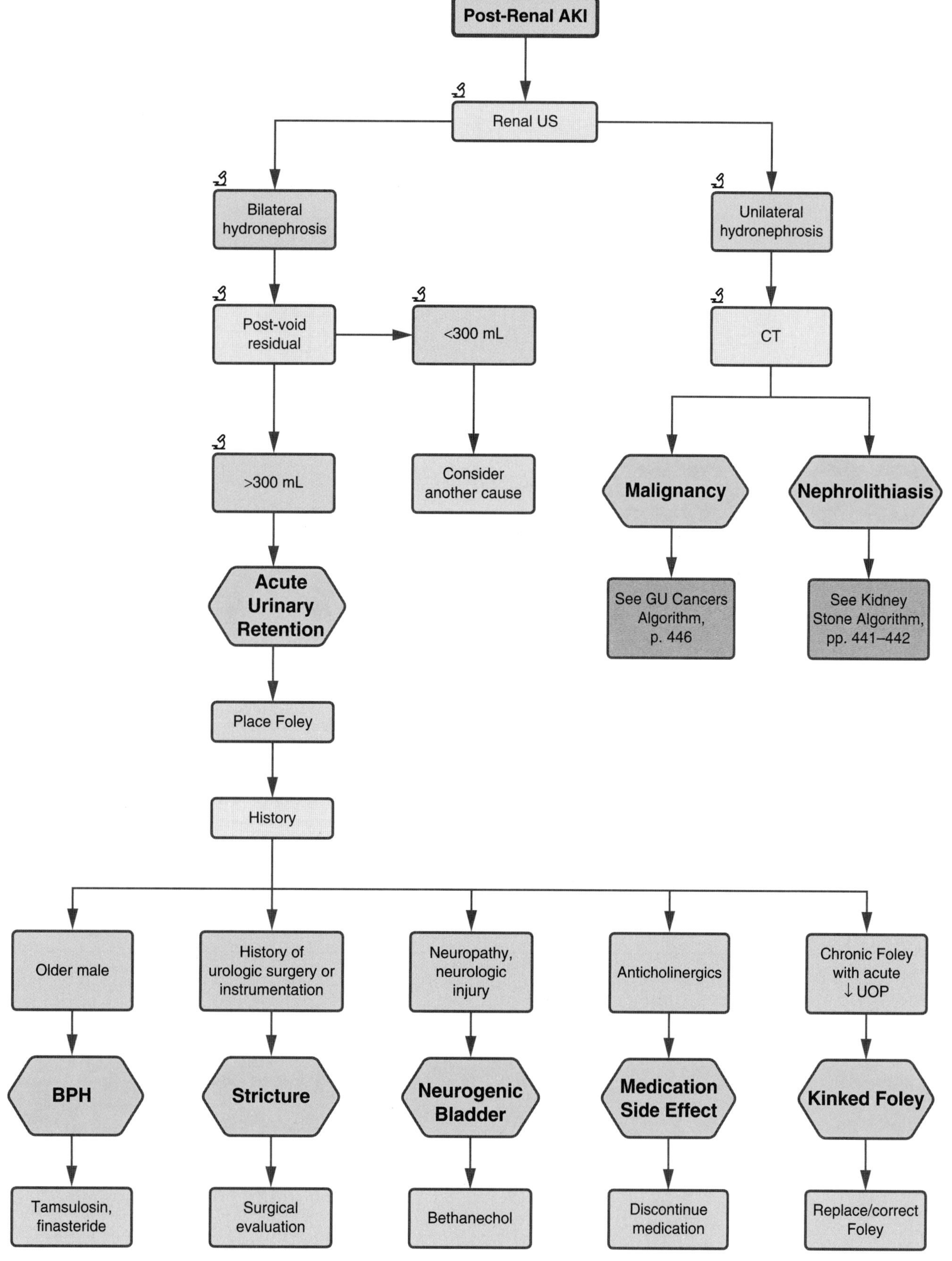
Post-Renal AKI
Renal US
Bilateral hydronephrosis
Unilateral hydronephrosis
Post-void residual
<300 mL
CT
>300 mL
Consider another cause
Malignancy
Nephrolithiasis
Acute Urinary Retention
See GU Cancers Algorithm, p. 446
See Kidney Stone Algorithm, pp. 441–442
Place Foley
History
Older male
History of urologic surgery or instrumentation
Neuropathy, neurologic injury
Anticholinergics
Chronic Foley with acute ↓ UOP
BPH
Stricture
Neurogenic Bladder
Medication Side Effect
Kinked Foley
Tamsulosin, finasteride
Surgical evaluation
Bethanechol
Discontinue medication
Replace/correct Foley

FIGURE 6.15

6-16 Glomerular Disease

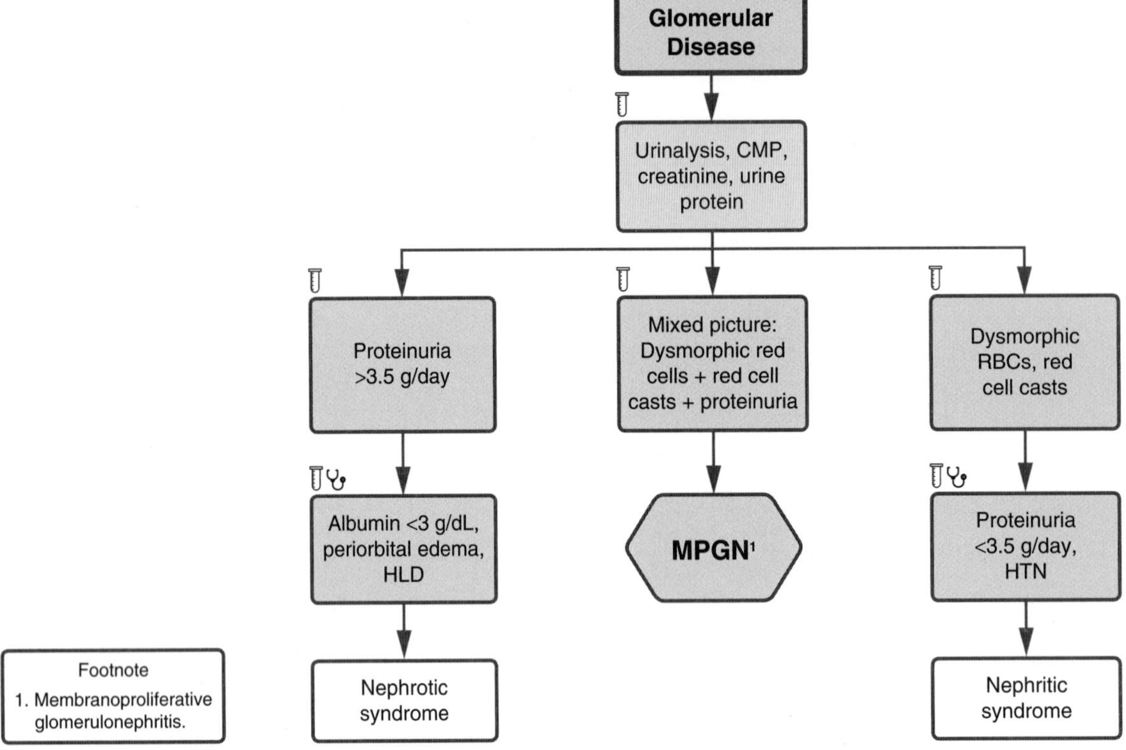
Glomerular Disease
Urinalysis, CMP, creatinine, urine protein
Proteinuria >3.5 g/day
Mixed picture: Dysmorphic red cells + red cell casts + proteinuria
Dysmorphic RBCs, red cell casts
Albumin <3 g/dL, periorbital edema, HLD
MPGN[1]
Proteinuria <3.5 g/day, HTN
Nephrotic syndrome
Nephritic syndrome

Footnote

1. Membranoproliferative glomerulonephritis.

Glomerular disease is a type of nephropathy that affects the glomeruli, which are tiny clusters of looping capillaries in the kidneys responsible for filtering toxins and excess fluid from the blood. Glomerular diseases can cause inflammation and damage to the glomeruli, which can lead to progressive kidney damage and the leakage of protein and red blood cells into the urine.

The glomerulus consists of several important components that, together, form the glomerular filtration barrier: 1) Capillary endothelium, which have small pores called fenestrations that are permeable to water and small solutes, 2) Glomerular basement membrane (GBM), which is comprised of a mesh of specialized proteins that prevent large molecules such as proteins from passing through, 3) Podocytes, which are specialized cells that wrap around the capillaries within the glomerulus. They have extensions called foot processes that interdigitate with each other to create the slit diaphragm, which helps regulate movement of fluid and solutes across the glomerular filtration barrier, and 4) Mesangial cells, which provide structural support, regulate blood flow through the glomerulus, and remove cellular debris and waste products from the glomerular filtration barrier. The proper function of these components is vital for maintaining normal kidney function and overall health.

Nephritic syndrome is characterized by inflammation of the glomeruli, which can result in hematuria, proteinuria, and hypertension. Patients with nephritic syndrome often present with rapid loss of renal function and dysmorphic RBCs in the urine.

Nephrotic syndrome is another type of glomerular disease that causes ↑ permeability of the glomerular filtration barrier, allowing large amounts of protein to leak into the urine. This can lead to symptoms such as proteinuria, hypoalbuminemia, edema, hypercholesterolemia, and blood clots.

Both nephritic syndrome and nephrotic syndromes can be caused by a variety of underlying conditions, including genetic disorders, autoimmune disorders, infections, and certain medications. In addition, there are certain diagnoses, such as membranoproliferative glomerulonephritis (MPGN), that can have components of both nephrotic and nephritic syndromes.

FIGURE 6.16

6-17 Nephritic Syndrome

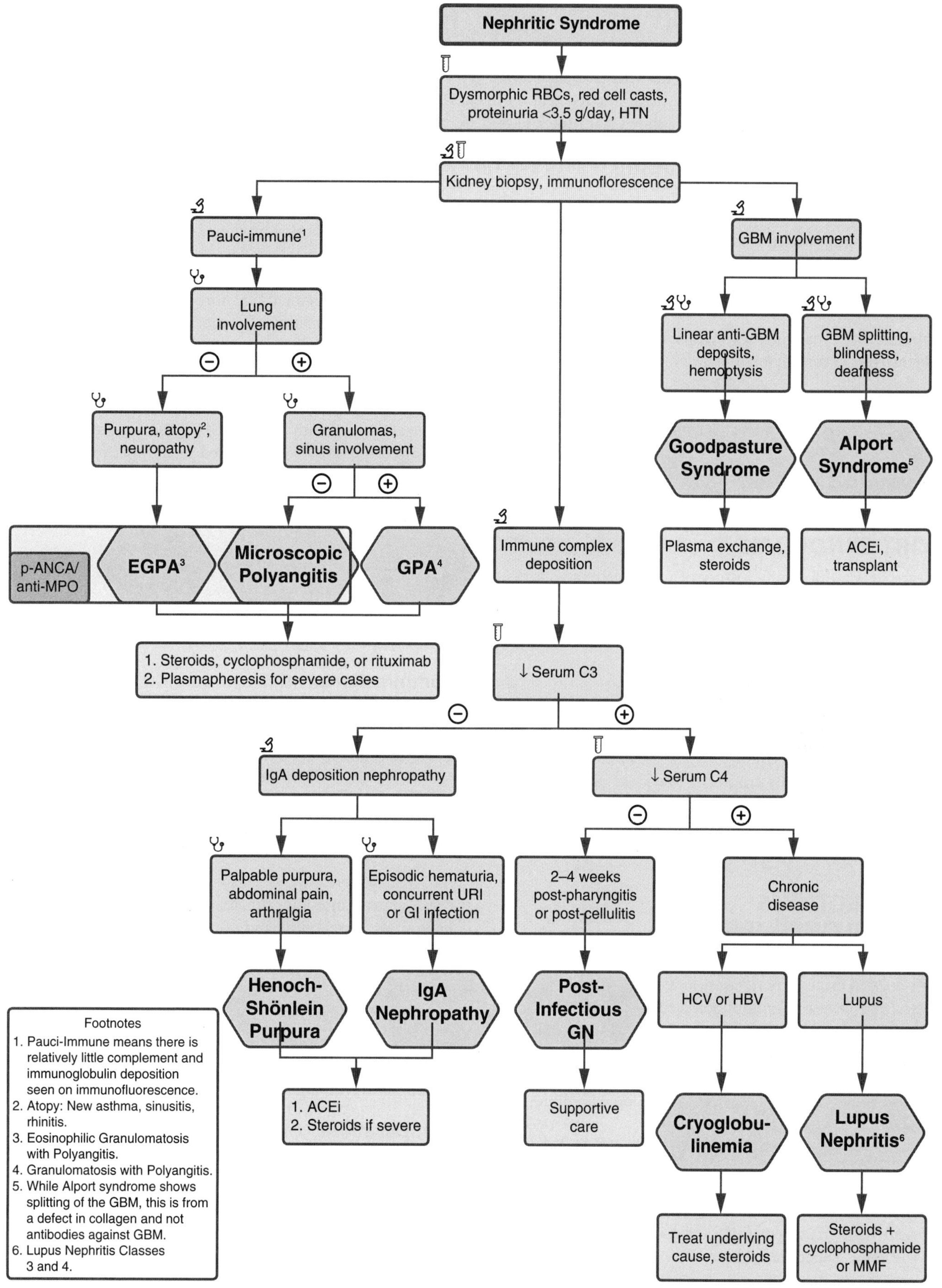

Nephritic Syndrome
Dysmorphic RBCs, red cell casts, proteinuria <3.5 g/day, HTN
Kidney biopsy, immunoflorescence
Pauci-immune[1]
Lung involvement
⊖
⊕
Purpura, atopy[2], neuropathy
Granulomas, sinus involvement
p-ANCA/ anti-MPO
EGPA[3]
Microscopic Polyangitis
GPA[4]
1. Steroids, cyclophosphamide, or rituximab
2. Plasmapheresis for severe cases
GBM involvement
Linear anti-GBM deposits, hemoptysis
GBM splitting, blindness, deafness
Goodpasture Syndrome
Alport Syndrome[5]
Plasma exchange, steroids
ACEi, transplant
Immune complex deposition
↓ Serum C3
IgA deposition nephropathy
↓ Serum C4
Palpable purpura, abdominal pain, arthralgia
Episodic hematuria, concurrent URI or GI infection
2–4 weeks post-pharyngitis or post-cellulitis
Chronic disease
Henoch-Shönlein Purpura
IgA Nephropathy
Post-Infectious GN
HCV or HBV
Lupus
1. ACEi
2. Steroids if severe
Supportive care
Cryoglobu-linemia
Lupus Nephritis[6]
Treat underlying cause, steroids
Steroids + cyclophosphamide or MMF
Footnotes
1. Pauci-Immune means there is relatively little complement and immunoglobulin deposition seen on immunofluorescence.
2. Atopy: New asthma, sinusitis, rhinitis.
3. Eosinophilic Granulomatosis with Polyangitis.
4. Granulomatosis with Polyangitis.
5. While Alport syndrome shows splitting of the GBM, this is from a defect in collagen and not antibodies against GBM.
6. Lupus Nephritis Classes 3 and 4.

FIGURE 6.17

6-17 Nephritic Syndrome

MEMBRANOPROLIFERATIVE GLOMERULONEPHRITIS

A 55-year-old M with PMH of HCV presents with gross hematuria and HTN. **Labs** show ↓ C3. UA reveals dysmorphic red cells with nephrotic-range proteinuria. Renal biopsy shows tram-track basement membrane with either sub-endothelial deposits (type I and III) or intramembranous dense deposits (type II).

Management:

1. Prednisone ± immunosuppression,
2. Treat underlying infection (eg, HBV, HCV).
3. Treat underlying autoimmune disease (lupus, rheumatoid arthritis).
4. Treat underlying malignancy (multiple myeloma, Waldenstrom, chronic lymphocytic leukemia).

Complications: May present as rapidly progressive (crescentic) glomerulonephritis.

HYF: Double-layered basement membrane (tram track), intramembranous dense deposits on biopsy.

ALPORT SYNDROME

A 15-year-old M with family history of male relatives with deafness, blindness, and kidney failure presents with gross hematuria following URI. On **labs**, UA shows numerous RBCs. Renal biopsy and electron microscopy reveal GBM splitting.

Management:

1. ACEi slows progression of renal disease.
2. Renal transplant once end-stage renal disease.

Complications: Usually progresses to end-stage renal disease.

HYF: X-linked recessive defect in formation of collagen-IV. Patients present with hematuria, hearing loss, and kidney disease.

POST-INFECTIOUS GLOMERULONEPHRITIS

A 9-year-old M with PMH of pharyngitis 2–3 weeks ago presents with tea-colored urine, hypertension, and edema. **Labs** show ↓ C3, ↑ ASO and anti-DNase. Immunofluorescence shows lumpy, bumpy appearance.

Management:

1. If symptomatic, treat edema and hypertension with diuretic.

Complications: Most patients make a full recovery. C3 normalizes within 8 weeks.

HYF: Post-strep GN occurs 10–21 days after infection. Patients will present with gross hematuria and have low C3, and a renal biopsy will show "subepithelial humps."

IgA NEPHROPATHY

A 20-year-old M presents with gross hematuria and concurrent URI. **Labs** show normal C3. Renal biopsy shows IgA deposits in immunofluorescence.

Management:

1. ACEi for hypertension/proteinuria.
2. If severe disease, glucocorticoids.

Complications: May progress to ESRD.

HYF: Occurs with an infection (typically within 5 days of an URI). Serum complements are normal. IgA deposits can be seen on biopsy. IgA nephropathy is the most common cause of glomerulonephritis in adults.

LUPUS NEPHRITIS

A 35-year-old M with PMH of SLE (discoid/malar rash, arthritis, oral ulcer) presents with elevated creatinine, proteinuria and/or hematuria. **Labs** show ↓ C3, C4. Renal biopsy shows mesangial proliferation and subendothelial, or subepithelial immune complex deposition.

Management:

1. Glucocorticoid + mycophenolate or cyclophosphamide.
2. ACEi for hypertension.
3. Treat lupus.

Complications: May progress to CKD.

HYF: May present as nephritic, nephrotic, or both. Occurs in half of SLE patients, though the severity varies widely. Serum C3 and C4 are low. Patients often also have low serum albumin due to urinary loss.

GRANULOMATOSIS WITH POLYANGIITIS

A 65-year-old presents with respiratory symptoms (cough ± hemoptysis), sinus symptoms (sinusitis, epistaxis), and gross hematuria. **Labs** show ↑ creatinine and (+) c-ANCA/anti-PR3. On **imaging**, CT shows cavitary lung lesions. Renal biopsy shows granulomatous inflammation.

Management:

1. High-dose steroids with rituximab, cyclophosphamide, or methotrexate.
2. For life-threatening cases, plasmapheresis.

Complications: Often presents as rapidly progressive (crescentic) glomerulonephritis.

HYF: GPA affects kidney + lung + sinus. Vasculitis that affects small- and medium-sized vessels. Upper respiratory tract is involved more frequently than lower. Serum complement levels are normal.

6-17 Nephritic Syndrome

MICROSCOPIC POLYANGIITIS

A 65-year-old presents with respiratory symptoms (cough ± hemoptysis), purpura on arms and legs, and gross hematuria. **Labs** reveal ↑ creatinine and (+) p-ANCA/anti-MPO. Biopsy does not show granulomatous inflammation.

Management:

1. High-dose steroids with rituximab, cyclophosphamide, or methotrexate.
2. For life-threatening cases, plasmapheresis.

Complications: Often presents as rapidly progressive (crescentic) glomerulonephritis.

HYF: MPA affects kidney + lung. No granulomas! "MPA has MPO(ANCA)." Vasculitis of the small vessels.

EOSINOPHILIC GRANULOMATOSIS WITH POLYANGIITIS

A 40-year-old F presents with purpura on arms and legs, neuropathy, and new atopy (asthma, sinusitis, rhinitis). **Labs** show ↑ eosinophils, ↑ IgE, and (+) p-ANCA.

Management:

1. High-dose steroids with rituximab, cyclophosphamide, or methotrexate.
2. For life-threatening cases, plasmapheresis.

Complications: Often presents as rapidly progressive (crescentic) glomerulonephritis.

HYF: EGPA affects kidney + lungs. Patients present with asthma, peripheral eosinophilia, and upper respiratory symptoms (rhinosinusitis).

GOODPASTURE SYNDROME

A 25-year-old M presents with hemoptysis, dyspnea, hematuria, and hypertension. On **imaging**, CXR shows pulmonary infiltrates. Renal biopsy shows linear anti-GBM deposits on immunofluorescence.

Management:

1. Plasmapheresis.
2. Pulsed steroids and cyclophosphamide.

Complications: Poor prognosis. May progress to ESRD.

HYF: Also known as anti-glomerular basement membrane disease. Patients typically have pulmonary symptoms (shortness of breath, cough, hemoptysis), and nephritic-range proteinuria. Fever and other systemic symptoms are not common. Biopsy shows linear IgG deposition along the glomerular basement membrane.

HENOCH-SCHONLEIN PURPURA (HSP)

A 5-year-old boy presents with palpable purpura, abdominal pain, arthralgias, and gross hematuria. **Labs** show normal C3. Renal biopsy shows IgA deposits in immunofluorescence.

Management:

1. ACEi for hypertension/proteinuria.
2. Severe disease: glucocorticoids.
3. Supportive therapy for all.

Complications: Excellent prognosis.

HYF: HSP is IgA with systemic sequelae (papular lower extremity rash, arthralgia, abdominal pain, and hematuria).

CRYOGLOBULINEMIA

A 50-year-old with PMH of chronic inflammation (HCV, HIV, or autoimmune disease) presents with purpura, arthralgia, and peripheral neuropathy. **Labs** show ↓ C3, (+) cryoglobulins, (+) rheumatoid factor, and urinalysis with nephritic (± nephrotic) syndrome.

Management:

1. Supportive treatment.
2. Acute: Glucocorticoids and rituximab.
3. Chronic: Treat underlying infection or autoimmune disease.

Complications:

- Risk of worsening chronic kidney disease.
- Increased risk of lymphoma.

HYF: Associated with a number of illnesses including HCV/HBV, HIV, and autoimmune disorders. The patient will have low complement levels. Vasculitis of the small vessels.

6-18 Nephrotic Syndrome

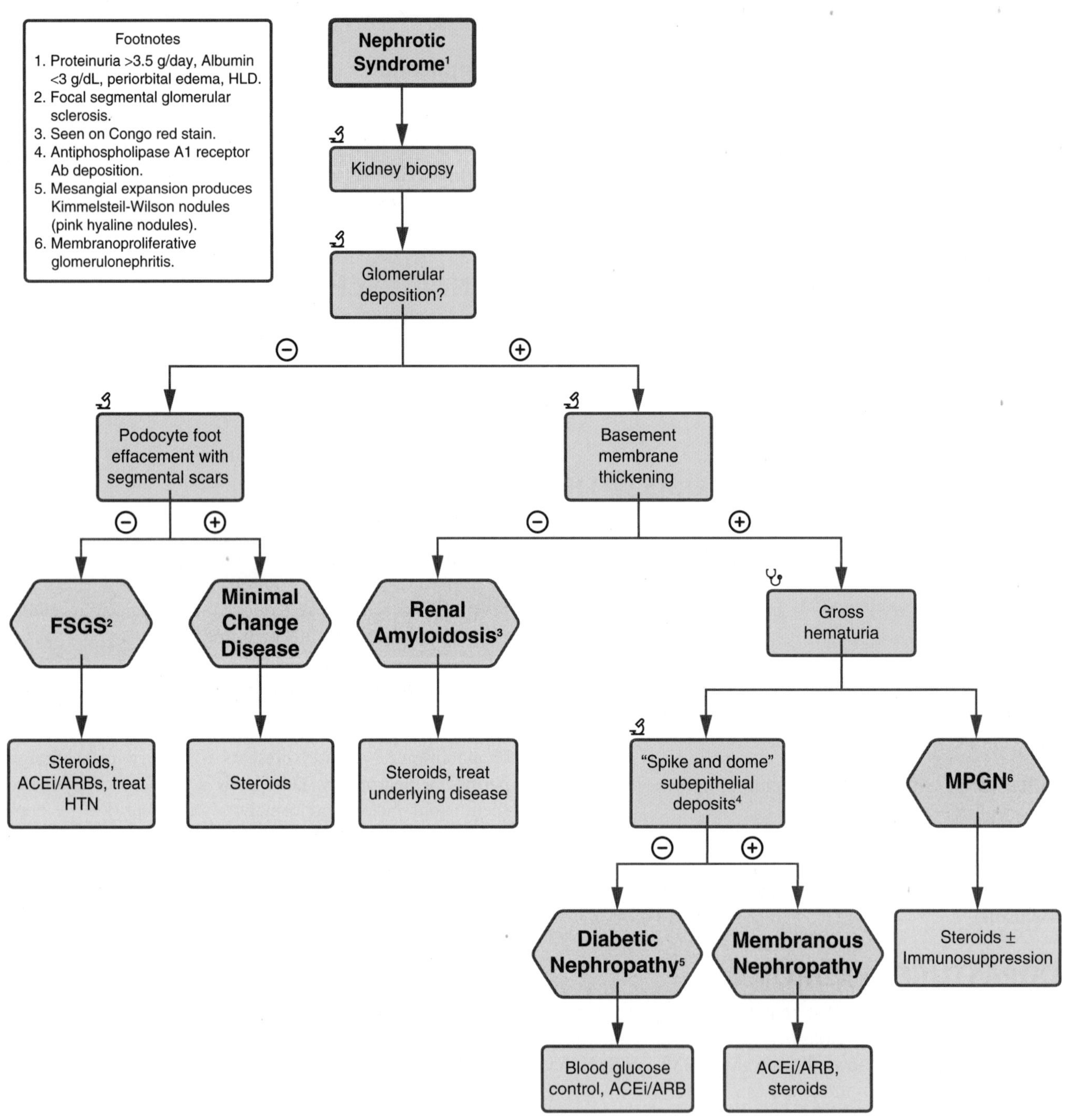
Footnotes
1. Proteinuria >3.5 g/day, Albumin <3 g/dL, periorbital edema, HLD.
2. Focal segmental glomerular sclerosis.
3. Seen on Congo red stain.
4. Antiphospholipase A1 receptor Ab deposition.
5. Mesangial expansion produces Kimmelsteil-Wilson nodules (pink hyaline nodules).
6. Membranoproliferative glomerulonephritis.
Nephrotic Syndrome[1]
Kidney biopsy
Glomerular deposition?
Podocyte foot effacement with segmental scars
Basement membrane thickening
FSGS[2]
Minimal Change Disease
Renal Amyloidosis[3]
Gross hematuria
Steroids, ACEi/ARBs, treat HTN
Steroids
Steroids, treat underlying disease
"Spike and dome" subepithelial deposits[4]
MPGN[6]
Diabetic Nephropathy[5]
Membranous Nephropathy
Steroids ± Immunosuppression
Blood glucose control, ACEi/ARB
ACEi/ARB, steroids

FIGURE 6.18

6-18 Nephrotic Syndrome

FOCAL SEGMENTAL GLOMERULOSCLEROSIS

A 35-year-old M with PMH of HIV, sickle cell disease, IV drug use, and obesity presents with **exam** findings of HTN and edema. On **labs,** UA shows protein >3.5 g/day. Renal biopsy shows focal segmental sclerosis in capillary tufts.

Management:

1. Prednisone, immunosuppressive therapy.
2. ACEi/ARBs for proteinuria and hypertension.

Complications: Poor prognosis, often progresses to ESRD.

HYF: Often idiopathic but can be associated with IVDU (heroin), HIV, obesity, and sickle cell disease. Most common cause of nephrotic syndrome in adults. Associated with *ApoL1* mutation.

RENAL AMYLOIDOSIS

A 65-year-old M with PMH of multiple myeloma and sarcoidosis presents with ↑ creatinine and proteinuria. Renal biopsy shows nodular glomerulosclerosis, amyloid fibrils, and apple-green birefringence with Congo red stain.

Management:

1. Prednisone, melphalan.
2. Treat underlying cause (eg, bone marrow transplant for multiple myeloma, biologic agents for autoimmune disease).

Complications: May progress to ESRD.

HYF: Associated with plasma cell dyscrasias, autoimmune disease (rheumatoid arthritis, sarcoidosis), and infections (TB). May present with other symptoms of systemic amyloidosis like restrictive cardiomyopathy, hepatosplenomegaly, and cerebral amyloidosis.

MEMBRANOUS NEPHROPATHY

A 45 -year-old M with PMH of HBV/HCV and hepatocellular carcinoma presents with severe generalized edema. **Labs** are consistent with nephrotic syndrome and positive for anti-phospholipase A2 (PLA2R) antibodies. Renal biopsy shows thick GBM with C3/IgG subepithelial deposits.

Management:

1. ACEi/ARB.
2. Prednisone and immunosuppression for severe disease.

Complications: Highest rate of thrombosis of all nephrotic syndromes.

HYF: Associated with autoimmune diseases (SLE), solid tumor malignancies, infections (HBV, malaria), NSAIDs, and gold toxicity. Renal biopsy shows "spike and hole" appearance of immune complex deposits.

DIABETIC NEPHROPATHY

A 55-year-old M with PMH of uncontrolled diabetes complicated by diabetic retinopathy and neuropathy presents with incidental albuminuria on screening. Renal biopsy shows thickened GBM, mesangial expansion, and Kimmelstiel-Wilson nodules.

Management:

1. ACEi/ARB.
2. Tight glucose control.

Complications: If untreated, may progress to ESRD.

HYF: Only severe cases present as true nephrotic syndrome. Diabetic nephropathy has two forms: diffuse hyalinization vs. nodular glomerulosclerosis with Kimmelstiel-Wilson lesions. Albuminuria tracks disease severity.

MINIMAL CHANGE DISEASE

A 2-year-old boy with PMH of recent URI presents with sudden onset generalized edema. On **labs,** UA shows nephrotic-range proteinuria. Renal biopsy reveals effacement of foot processes on electron microscopy.

Management:

1. Steroids.

Complications: Excellent response to steroids with favorable prognosis.

HYF: Usually occurs in children but may also occur in adults around age 40. Most common cause of nephrotic syndrome in children. Associated with NSAID use and lymphomas.

*[*]**Lupus nephritis** is a nephritis that can present with a nephrotic syndrome. Patients can present with hematuria, proteinuria, HTN, or edema. Labs classically show low serum C3 and C4. Renal biopsy shows mesangial expansion and subendothelial or subepithelial immune complex deposition. Treat with ACE/ARB, as well as prednisone and other immunosuppressants.*

6-19 Dysuria in Men

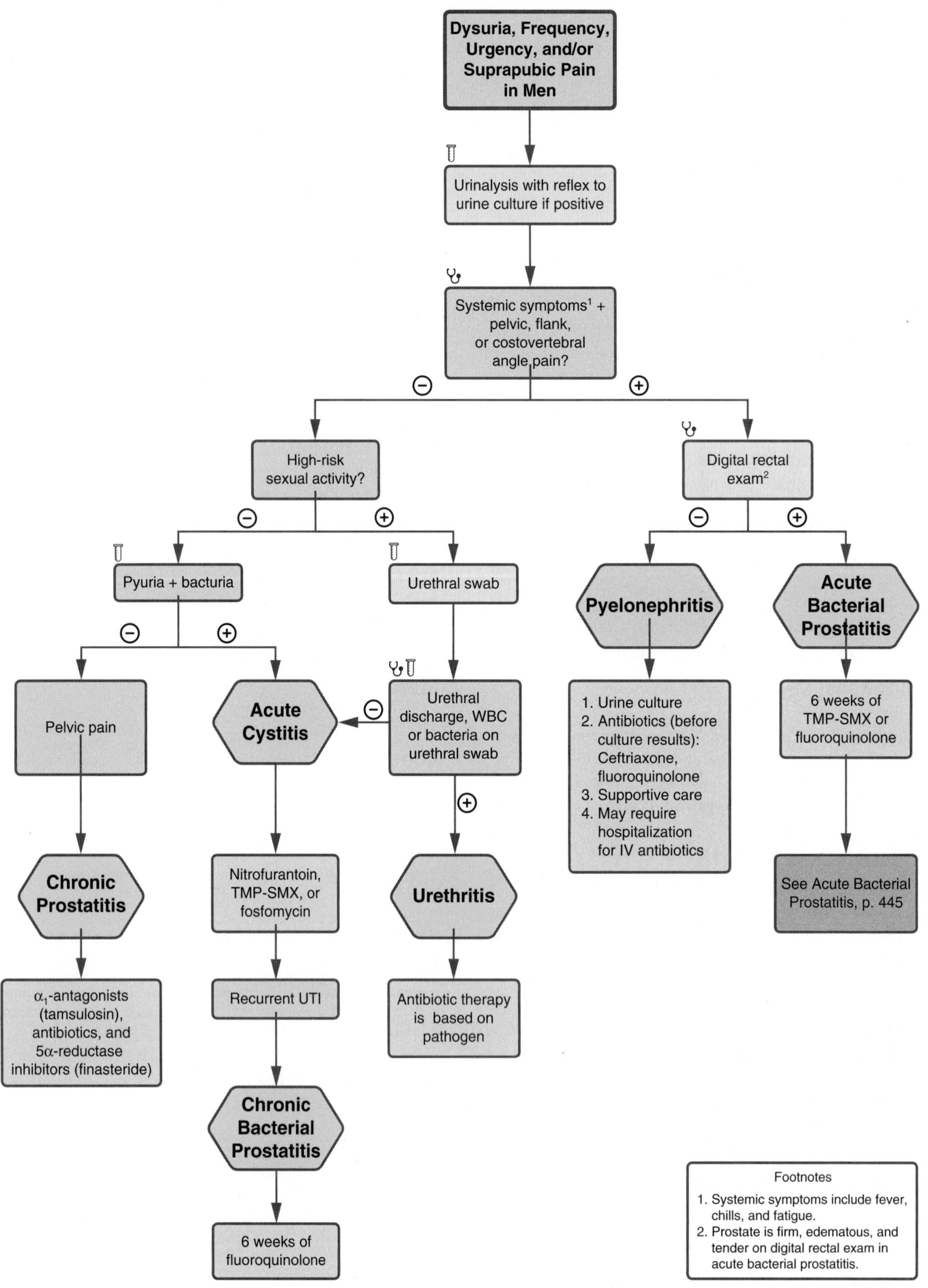

Dysuria, Frequency, Urgency, and/or Suprapubic Pain in Men
Urinalysis with reflex to urine culture if positive
Systemic symptoms[1] + pelvic, flank, or costovertebral angle pain?
High-risk sexual activity?
Digital rectal exam[2]
Pyuria + bacturia
Urethral swab
Pyelonephritis
Acute Bacterial Prostatitis
Pelvic pain
Acute Cystitis
Urethral discharge, WBC or bacteria on urethral swab
1. Urine culture
2. Antibiotics (before culture results): Ceftriaxone, fluoroquinolone
3. Supportive care
4. May require hospitalization for IV antibiotics
6 weeks of TMP-SMX or fluoroquinolone
Chronic Prostatitis
Nitrofurantoin, TMP-SMX, or fosfomycin
Urethritis
See Acute Bacterial Prostatitis, p. 445
α1-antagonists (tamsulosin), antibiotics, and 5α-reductase inhibitors (finasteride)
Recurrent UTI
Antibiotic therapy is based on pathogen
Chronic Bacterial Prostatitis
6 weeks of fluoroquinolone
Footnotes
1. Systemic symptoms include fever, chills, and fatigue.
2. Prostate is firm, edematous, and tender on digital rectal exam in acute bacterial prostatitis.

FIGURE 6.19

6-19 Dysuria in Men

CHRONIC PROSTATITIS/CHRONIC PELVIC PAIN SYNDROME

A middle-aged M presents with pelvic/perineal pain, pain with ejaculation, and dysuria. Digital rectal **exam** shows a tender prostate. On **labs**, urinalysis does not have leukocyte esterase, white blood cells, or bacteria.

Management:

1. α_1-antagonist (eg, tamulosin, terazosin) ± 5α-reductase inhibitor (eg, finasteride, dutasteride).

Complications: Chronic pain.

HYF: The most common presenting symptom is pelvic or perineal pain; there is no fever or other signs/symptoms of infection. Do not confuse this with chronic bacterial prostatitis, which has urinary symptoms in addition to pain, is associated with an abnormal UA, and is treated with antibiotics.

ACUTE CYSTITIS

A 65-year-old M presents with frequency, urgency, and dysuria. On **exam**, he is afebrile and has suprapubic tenderness. **Labs** show UA with pyuria and bacteriuria. Urine culture is pending.

Management:

1. UA with urine culture.
2. Nitrofurantoin or trimethoprim-sulfamethoxazole × 7 days or fosfomycin once.
3. Targeted antibiotics based on culture results.

Complications: Pyelonephritis, sepsis if untreated.

HYF: If recurrent UTIs, assess for obstruction, BPH, or prostatitis. In high-risk individuals (HIV, poorly controlled DM) or those with systemic signs/symptoms, initiate workup for complicated UTI (see Pyelonephritis below). See also Cystitis in Infectious Disease, p. 188.

PYELONEPHRITIS

A middle-aged man presents with fever, chills, nausea/vomiting, UTI symptoms (dysuria, urinary frequency and urgency), and flank pain. He has CVA and suprapubic tenderness on **exam**. On **labs**, urinalysis shows (+) leukocyte esterase, WBCs, and bacteria. Urine culture is pending.

Management:

1. Hydration.
2. If stable: outpatient fluoroquinolone.
3. If septic or unstable: admit for IV antibiotics.
   a. If risk factors for drug resistant bacteria: piperacillin-tazobactam.
   b. If no risk factors: ceftriaxone.
4. Narrow/broaden based on urine cultures.

Complications: Renal abscess, sepsis.

HYF: A complicated UTI is one that is associated with systemic signs/symptoms, occurs in a high-risk patient (immunocompromised, pregnant), is refractory to antibiotics, or is the result of an obstruction. This designation includes pyelonephritis. Imaging may be helpful to assess for obstruction (ie, CT abdomen or renal US can reveal hydronephrosis) or renal abscess (CT preferred). The yield of a UA and urine culture may be decreased if antibiotics are given prior to urine collection; urine collection should ideally occur before antibiotic administration if clinically able.

URETHRITIS

A 25-year-old M presents with dysuria for the past 5 days. He has had multiple sexual partners recently. On **exam**, there is purulent discharge at the urethral meatus. On **labs**, UA of first-void urine shows (+) leukocyte esterase. A urethral swab is obtained. Gram stain reveals ≥2 WBC/hpf and gram-negative diplococci are visualized within WBCs. Nucleic acid amplification tests identify *N. gonorrhoeae* and *C. trachomatis*.

Management:

1. 1st-line for gonococcal urethritis: IM Ceftriaxone and PO azithromycin. Of note, this combination covers both *N. gonorrhoeae* urethritis and non-gonococcal urethritis due to *C. trachomatis*.
2. 1st-line for non-gonococcal urethritis: PO doxycycline or azithromycin. Of note, azithromycin also covers *M. genitalium*.

Complications: Gonococcal urethritis: acute epididymitis, prostatitis, pharyngitis, conjunctivitis, disseminated gonococcal infection. Non-gonococcal urethritis: acute epididymitis, reactive arthritis (triad of urethritis, conjunctivitis, and arthritis).

HYF: Infectious urethritis is most commonly seen in young, sexually active men and usually caused by a sexually transmitted pathogen (*Neisseria gonorrhoeae* and *Chlamydia trachomatis*, less commonly *Mycoplasma genitalium*). Co-infection with *N. gonorrhoeae* and *C. trachomatis* is common, so presumptive therapy for both (ie, IM ceftriaxone for gonorrhea and PO azithromycin for chlamydia) is recommended if Gram-stain reveals gonococci but test results for chlamydia are not available at the time of treatment. Coinfection with other sexually transmitted pathogens are common, so consider screening for HIV and syphilis.

CHRONIC BACTERIAL PROSTATITIS

A middle-aged man presents with recurrent UTIs and bacteriuria. On **labs**, urinalysis shows (+) leukocyte esterase, WBCs, and bacteria. Digital rectal **exam** reveals mild prostate tenderness.

Management:

1. Fluoroquinolone for 6 weeks.

Complications: Bacteremia and sepsis. Prostate abscess. Progression from acute to chronic bacterial prostatitis. Chronic pelvic pain.

HYF: Chronic bacterial prostatitis has a subtler and more chronic presentation than acute bacterial prostatitis. Patients with acute bacterial prostatitis may need to be hospitalized if septic or have severe comorbidities. Suspect chronic bacterial prostatitis if a patient presents with multiple episodes of simple cystitis with the same strain of bacteria. Chronic bacterial prostatitis is typically a clinical diagnosis but can be confirmed by testing prostatic fluid for bacteria; if higher than in urine, then diagnosis is confirmed. Do not confuse this diagosis with chronic prostatitis/chronic pelvic pain syndrome, which is characterized by unremarkable urinalysis.

6-20 Dysuria in Women

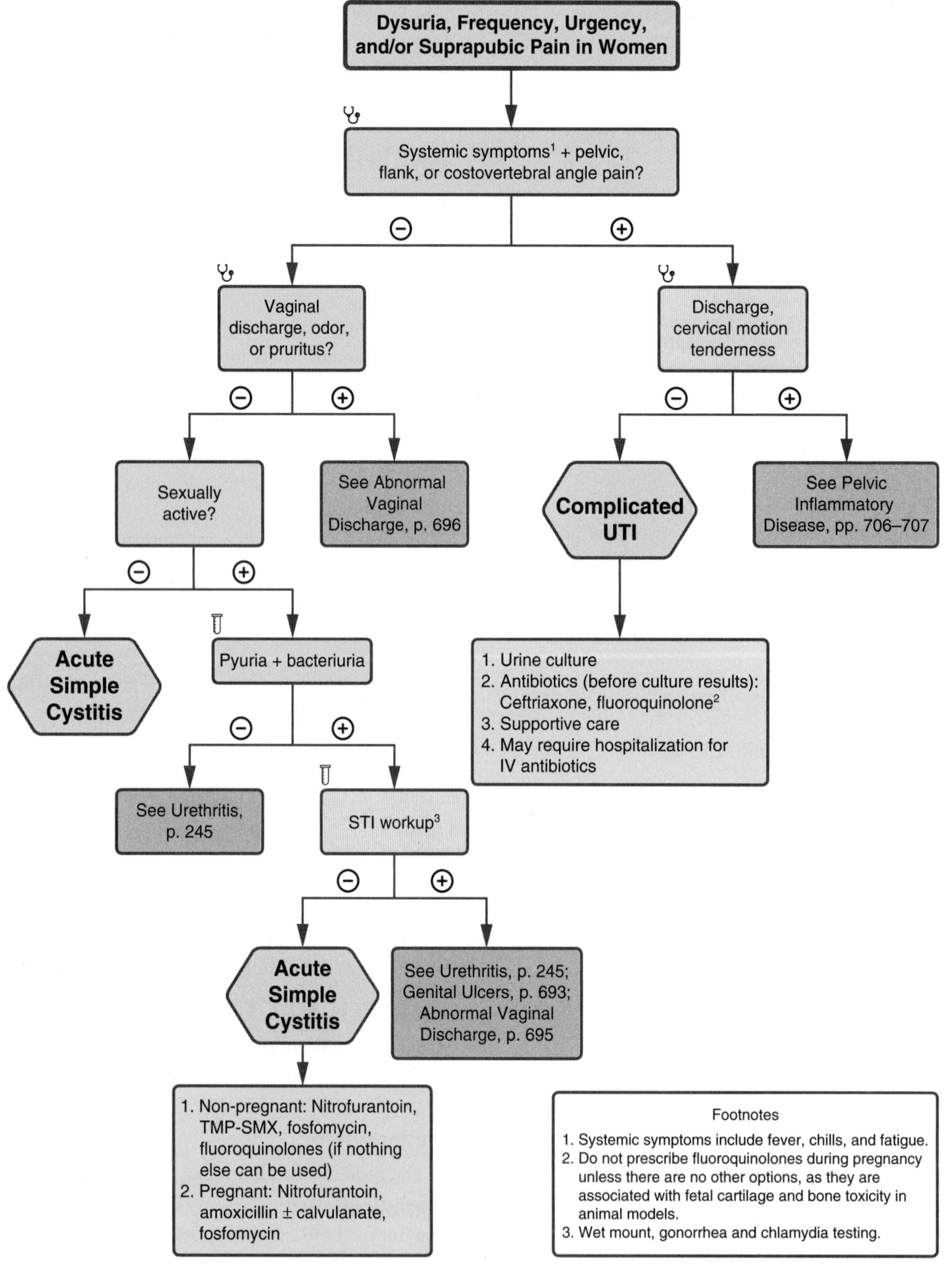
Dysuria, Frequency, Urgency, and/or Suprapubic Pain in Women
Systemic symptoms[1] + pelvic, flank, or costovertebral angle pain?
Vaginal discharge, odor, or pruritus?
Discharge, cervical motion tenderness
Sexually active?
See Abnormal Vaginal Discharge, p. 696
Complicated UTI
See Pelvic Inflammatory Disease, pp. 706–707
Acute Simple Cystitis
Pyuria + bacteriuria
1. Urine culture
2. Antibiotics (before culture results): Ceftriaxone, fluoroquinolone[2]
3. Supportive care
4. May require hospitalization for IV antibiotics
See Urethritis, p. 245
STI workup[3]
Acute Simple Cystitis
See Urethritis, p. 245; Genital Ulcers, p. 693; Abnormal Vaginal Discharge, p. 695
1. Non-pregnant: Nitrofurantoin, TMP-SMX, fosfomycin, fluoroquinolones (if nothing else can be used)
2. Pregnant: Nitrofurantoin, amoxicillin ± calvulanate, fosfomycin
Footnotes
1. Systemic symptoms include fever, chills, and fatigue.
2. Do not prescribe fluoroquinolones during pregnancy unless there are no other options, as they are associated with fetal cartilage and bone toxicity in animal models.
3. Wet mount, gonorrhea and chlamydia testing.

FIGURE 6.20

6-20 Dysuria in Women

ACUTE SIMPLE CYSTITIS

A 25-year-old F presents with dysuria and urinary frequency. On exam, she is afebrile and has suprapubic tenderness to palpation. On labs, UA shows pyuria and bacteriuria.

Management:

1. Urine culture with susceptibilities.
2. Empiric antibiotics: 1st-line is nitrofurantoin, fosfomycin, or trimethoprim/sulfamethoxazole. 2nd-line is ciprofloxacin.
3. Tailor antibiotics to urine culture and susceptibility results.

Complications: Pyelonephritis, urosepsis.

HYF: Most common pathogen is *Escherichia coli.* Women are more susceptible to UTI because they have shorter urethras than men. Only treat asymptomatic bacteriuria if the patient is pregnant (due to increased susceptibility to pyelonephritis, which can harm mother and fetus) or undergoing urologic procedures (because instrumentation in the urinary tract can introduce bacteria into bloodstream and cause bacteremia and sepsis). See also acute cystitis in Infectious Disease and Dysuria (male, pp. 188 and 245).

Complicated UTI: See pyelonephritis on p. 245.

6-21 Renal Cysts

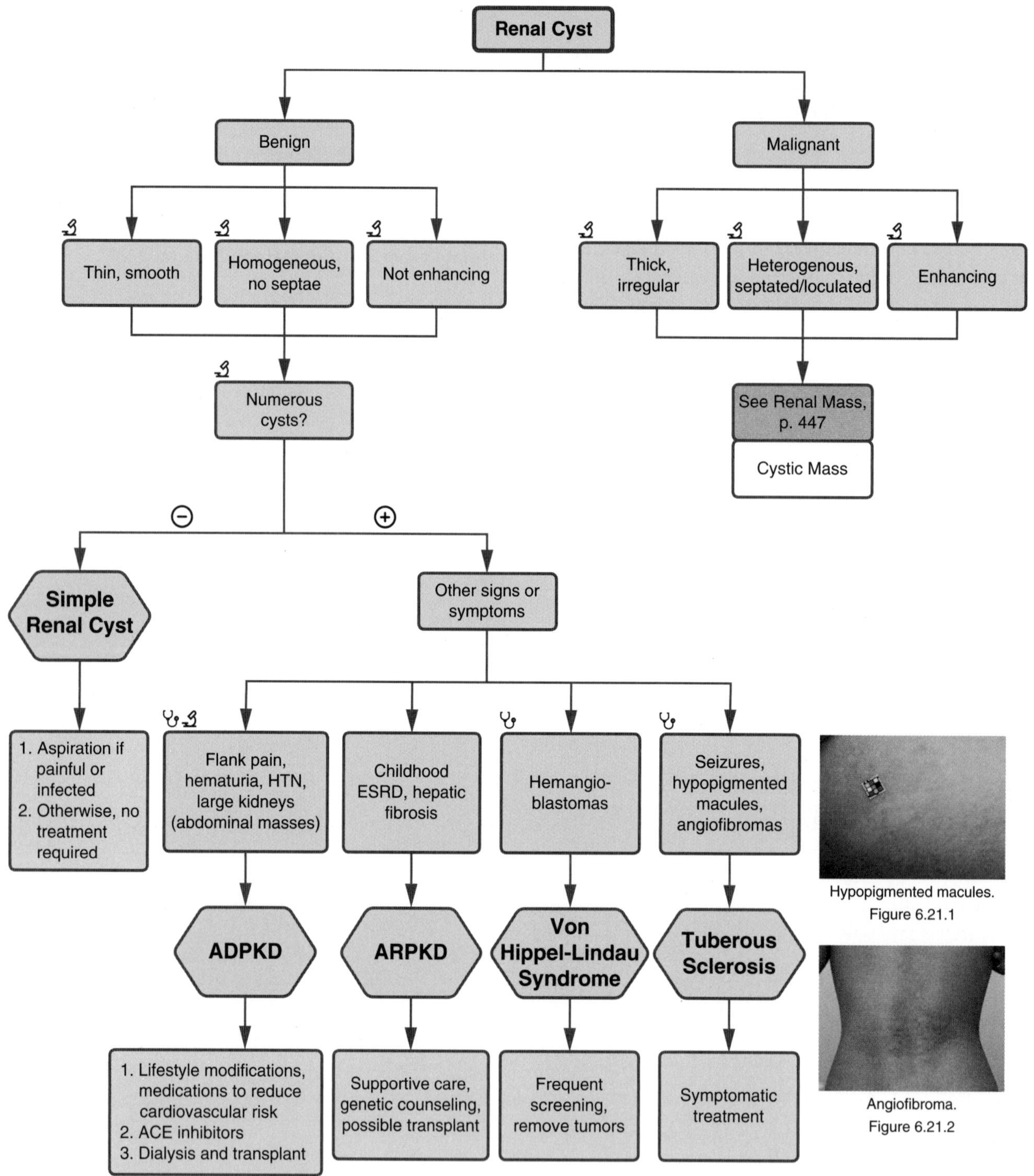
Renal Cyst
Benign
Malignant
Thin, smooth
Homogeneous, no septae
Not enhancing
Thick, irregular
Heterogenous, septated/loculated
Enhancing
Numerous cysts?
See Renal Mass, p. 447
Cystic Mass
Simple Renal Cyst
Other signs or symptoms
1. Aspiration if painful or infected
2. Otherwise, no treatment required
Flank pain, hematuria, HTN, large kidneys (abdominal masses)
Childhood ESRD, hepatic fibrosis
Hemangio-blastomas
Seizures, hypopigmented macules, angiofibromas
ADPKD
ARPKD
Von Hippel-Lindau Syndrome
Tuberous Sclerosis
1. Lifestyle modifications, medications to reduce cardiovascular risk
2. ACE inhibitors
3. Dialysis and transplant
Supportive care, genetic counseling, possible transplant
Frequent screening, remove tumors
Symptomatic treatment

Hypopigmented macules.
Figure 6.21.1

Angiofibroma.
Figure 6.21.2

FIGURE 6.21

6-21 Renal Cysts

SIMPLE RENAL CYSTS

A 55-year-old M with PMH of HTN is noted to have an incidental cyst noted on **imaging**. He has no symptoms. On US, it is round, anechoic, and without calcifications. **Exam** and **labs** are normal.

Management:

1. No treatment or monitoring required.

Complications: Pain, infection (typically seeded from other source), rupture, bleeding.

HYF: Simple renal cysts are typically asymptomatic and found incidentally on imaging. They are benign and do not alter renal function. Benign features on US: smooth, anechoic, no septations, no calcifications. Incidence of renal cysts increases with age. Cysts are associated with hypertension.

AUTOSOMAL DOMINANT POLYCYSTIC KIDNEY DISEASE (ADPKD)

A 47-year-old M with PMH of HTN presents with hematuria. On **exam**, he is noted to have hypertension with BP 155/83, as well as bilateral flank masses. **Labs** show Cr 1.8 and UA with hematuria and proteinuria. On **imaging**, CT abdomen reveals multiple large cysts on bilateral kidneys and the liver.

Management:

1. ACEi/ARB for HTN and/or proteinuria.
2. Increase fluid intake, low Na diet.
3. Consider tolvaptan.
4. Dialysis or transplant for ESRD.

Complications:

- Progression to ESRD.
- Cyst rupture/hemorrhage.
- Extra-renal cysts.
- Associated with intracranial berry aneurysms → rupture can lead to subarachnoid hemorrhage.

HYF: Patients often present with hypertension, hematuria, proteinuria, and/or flank pain (from cyst rupture, UTI, or nephrolithiasis). Caused by mutations in *PKD1* (chr. 16) and *PKD2* (chr. 4). Most common cause of death for patients with ADPKD is cardiac (eg, myocardial infarction). ADPKD is also associated with intracranial cerebral aneurysms, mitral valve prolapse, diverticulosis, nephrolithiasis, extra-renal cysts (pancreas, liver), and UTIs.

AUTOSOMAL RECESSIVE POLYCYSTIC KIDNEY DISEASE (ARPKD)

An infant presents for routine newborn exam. On **exam**, he has hypertension, abdominal distension, and bilateral palpable flank masses. On **imaging**, ultrasound reveals hepatomegaly, intrahepatic ductal dilation, and large echogenic kidneys with poor corticomedullary differentiation.

Management:

1. Supportive care.
2. If intrauterine diagnosis, serial ultrasounds to monitor amniotic fluid level.
3. Treat HTN with ACEi/ARBs, hyponatremia with fluid restriction, and respiratory distress with mechanical ventilation.
4. Dialysis or transplant for ESRD.
5. Genetic counseling.

Complications:

- ESRD, HTN, hyponatremia.
- Portal HTN, cholangitis.

HYF: Presents in infants and children with renal failure, liver fibrosis, and portal hypertension. Caused by mutation in *PKHD1* on chromosome 6. Associated with oligohydramnios leading to Potter's sequence and pulmonary hypoplasia.

VON HIPPEL-LINDAU SYNDROME (RENAL CELL CARCINOMA)

A 26-year-old F with PMH of retinal hemangioblastoma presents with flank pain and hematuria. Her family history is notable for several maternal relatives with pancreatic and brain cancers. On **exam**, there is a palpable right flank mass. **Labs** are significant for elevated Cr and UA positive for RBCs. On **imaging**, CT abdomen demonstrates a right-sided renal mass with sites of necrosis and calcifications.

Management:

1. Chemotherapy ± radiation ± surgical resection of tumors depending on tissue of origin and cancer staging.
2. Frequent surveillance imaging.
3. Genetic counseling.

Complications: Depends on origin of cancers (eg, vision loss with retinal hemangioblastoma, jaundice with pancreatic mass, renal failure with renal cell carcinoma).

HYF: VHL is autosomal dominant and caused by a mutation in the *VHL* gene (chr. 3). Associated with CNS and retinal hemangioblastomas, clear cell renal cell carcinomas, pheochromocytomas, and both benign and malignant pancreatic tumors. Patients require frequent surveillance imaging from a young age to detect new tumors. RCC is associated with paraneoplastic syndromes (ectopic EPO, PTHrP, renin).

TUBEROUS SCLEROSIS

A 5-year-old F presents after having spells of "tensing and jerking" behavior concerning for seizures. **Exam** reveals elliptic hypopigmented macules and facial angiofibromas. On **imaging**, routine EEG demonstrates epileptiform abnormalities. MRI demonstrates cortical glioneuronal hamartomas (cortical tubers), as well as a renal angiomyolipoma and multiple small renal cysts.

6-21 Renal Cysts

Management:

1. Treat individual manifestations: epilepsy (antiepileptic drugs), brain tumors (surgery or mTOR inhibitors), renal angiomyolipoma (surgical excision).
2. Frequent surveillance imaging.
3. Genetic counseling.

Complications: Seizures, heart failure (severe cardiac rhabdomyoma), pulmonary fibrosis, pneumothorax, kidney disease.

HYF: Tuberous sclerosis is autosomal dominant and caused by a mutation in the *TSC1* (hamartin on chr. 9) or *TSC2* (tuberin on chr. 16) genes. Characterized by growth of hamartomas in various organs. Common manifestations include epilepsy, cognitive/behavioral disorders, and cardiac rhabdomyoma. Characteristic lesions include ash leaf spots, shagreen patches, and facial angiofibromas.

7

Internal Medicine: Pulmonology

7-1 Dyspnea

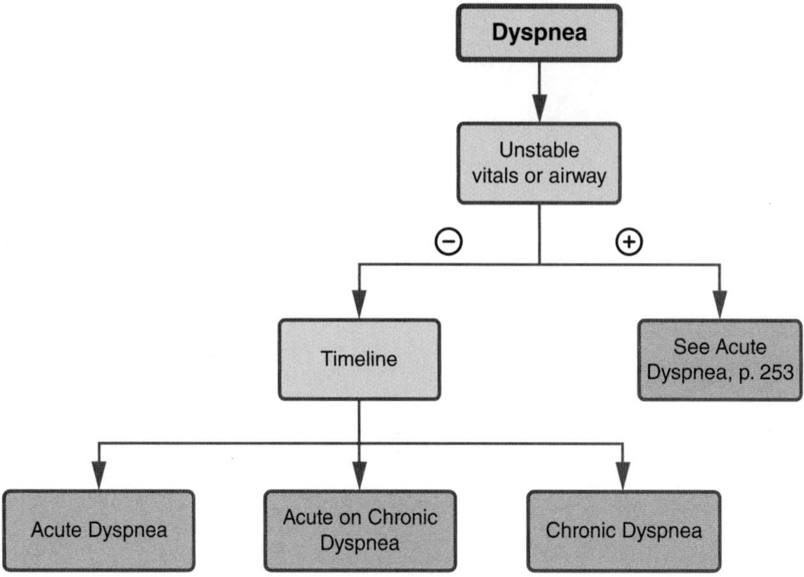
Dyspnea
Unstable vitals or airway
⊖
⊕
Timeline
See Acute Dyspnea, p. 253
Acute Dyspnea
Acute on Chronic Dyspnea
Chronic Dyspnea

Dyspnea may be one of the most daunting clinical presentations in medicine. Its etiologies range from benign to immediately life-threatening, and it can be related to essentially any organ system in the body. Such a broad differential requires a systematic way of approaching this chief complaint. This algorithm attempts to walk you through a practical way to think about dyspnea. As with most chief complaints, the first question to be answered is, "How sick is this patient?" **Secure the ABCs first and foremost**. Tension pneumothorax, tamponade, airway edema, and similar conditions should always be considered given their potential to quickly kill the patient. Once you have determined that the patient is stable, the next step is to determine the time period over which the dyspnea developed.

Broadly, we think of dyspnea occuring over a relatively short period of time (acute or acute on chronic) or slowly worsening over an extended period of time. It can be helpful to **think in order from acute to chronic** because, in general, acute presentations tend to be more likely to be immediately dangerous to the patient. For example, a pulmonary embolism is more likely to be lethal in the short term if not caught, even though it is not necessarily fatal in the long run with proper treatment. Compare this to a slowly worsening anemia caused by a malignancy. The anemia is not likely to be immediately fatal, even if the cancer is incurable.

In the acute setting, consider etiologies that can develop rapidly. A severe infection, toxic ingestions, and coronary etiologies should be at the top of the differential. However, keep in mind that the "acute" presentation may in fact be the initial presentation of more chronic processes, such as heart failure. Next, consider chronic diseases that can worsen acutely. The classic examples of these would include asthma and COPD exacerbations. Finally, consider chronic processes. Think of this category as a collection of diagnoses that can progressively worsen over time. For example, dyspnea that has been insidiously deteriorating could be the initial presentation of a variety of interstital lung diseases.

Finally, it is always reasonable to use a mnemonic to ensure you are not forgetting a potential etiology. One popular mnemonic is **VINDICATE Me:** **V**ascular, **I**nfectious/Intoxication, **N**eoplastic, **D**egenerative, **I**atrogenic, **C**ongenital, **A**utoimmune, **T**raumatic, **E**ndocrine, **Me**tabolic.

FIGURE 7.1

7-2 Acute Dyspnea

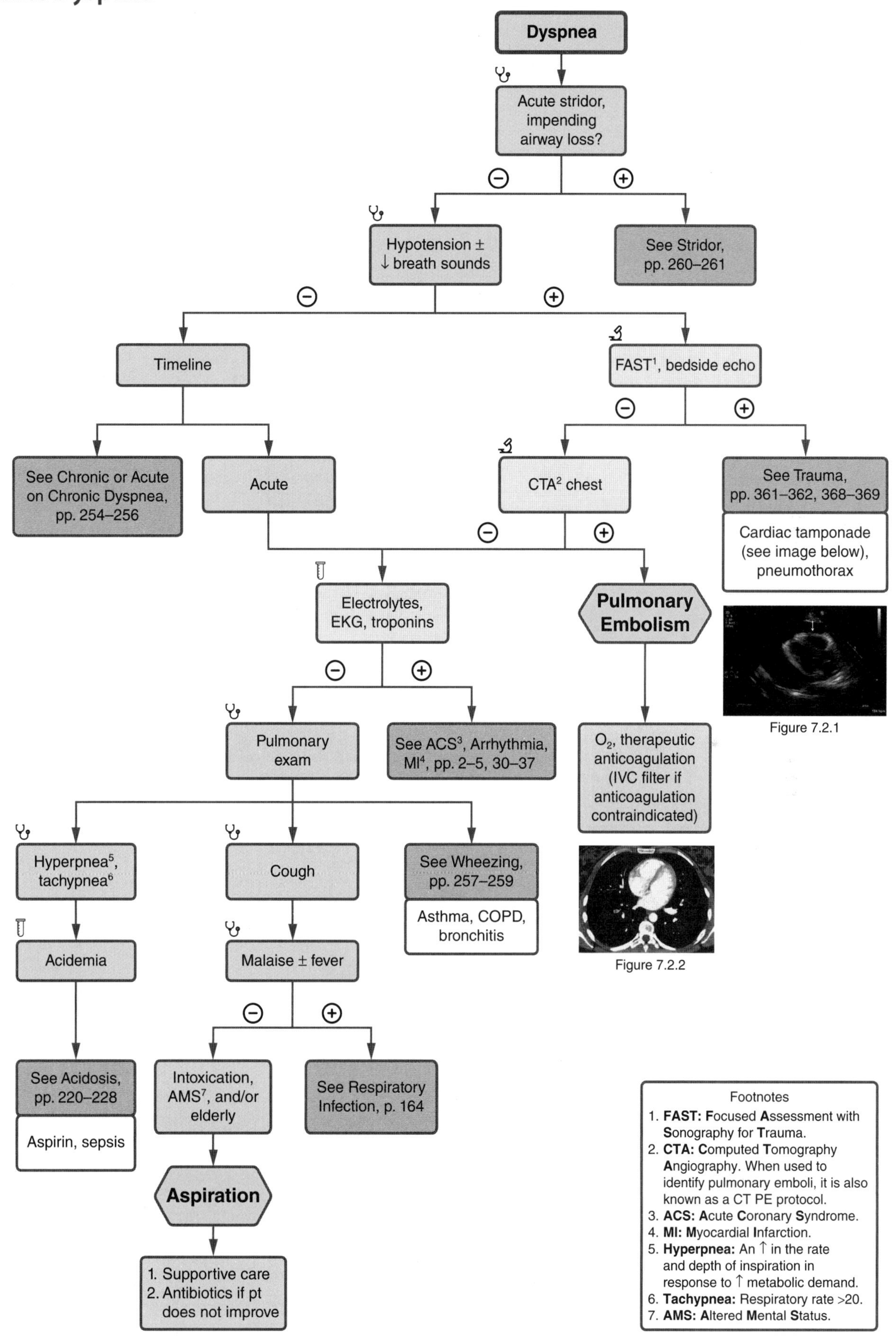

Dyspnea
Acute stridor, impending airway loss?
Hypotension ± ↓ breath sounds
See Stridor, pp. 260–261
Timeline
FAST[1], bedside echo
See Chronic or Acute on Chronic Dyspnea, pp. 254–256
Acute
CTA[2] chest
See Trauma, pp. 361–362, 368–369
Cardiac tamponade (see image below), pneumothorax
Electrolytes, EKG, troponins
Pulmonary Embolism
Pulmonary exam
See ACS[3], Arrhythmia, MI[4], pp. 2–5, 30–37
O2, therapeutic anticoagulation (IVC filter if anticoagulation contraindicated)
Hyperpnea[5], tachypnea[6]
Cough
See Wheezing, pp. 257–259
Asthma, COPD, bronchitis
Acidemia
Malaise ± fever
See Acidosis, pp. 220–228
Aspirin, sepsis
Intoxication, AMS[7], and/or elderly
See Respiratory Infection, p. 164
Aspiration
1. Supportive care
2. Antibiotics if pt does not improve
Figure 7.2.1
Figure 7.2.2
Footnotes
1. FAST: Focused Assessment with Sonography for Trauma.
2. CTA: Computed Tomography Angiography. When used to identify pulmonary emboli, it is also known as a CT PE protocol.
3. ACS: Acute Coronary Syndrome.
4. MI: Myocardial Infarction.
5. Hyperpnea: An ↑ in the rate and depth of inspiration in response to ↑ metabolic demand.
6. Tachypnea: Respiratory rate >20.
7. AMS: Altered Mental Status.

FIGURE 7.2

7-3 Acute-on-Chronic Dyspnea

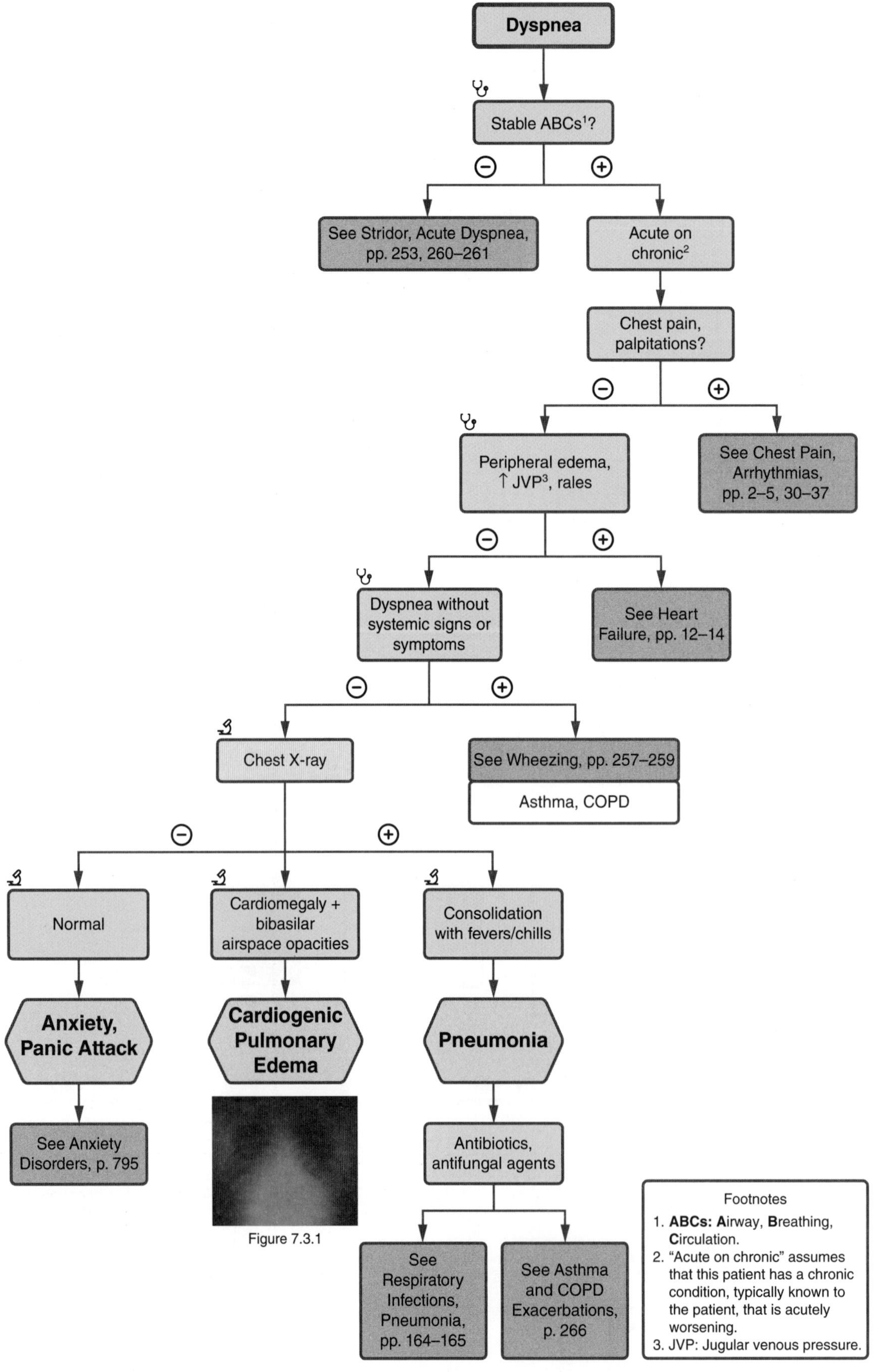
Dyspnea
Stable ABCs[1]?
⊖
⊕
See Stridor, Acute Dyspnea, pp. 253, 260–261
Acute on chronic[2]
Chest pain, palpitations?
⊖
⊕
Peripheral edema, ↑ JVP[3], rales
See Chest Pain, Arrhythmias, pp. 2–5, 30–37
⊖
⊕
Dyspnea without systemic signs or symptoms
See Heart Failure, pp. 12–14
⊖
⊕
Chest X-ray
See Wheezing, pp. 257–259
Asthma, COPD
⊖
⊕
Normal
Cardiomegaly + bibasilar airspace opacities
Consolidation with fevers/chills
Anxiety, Panic Attack
Cardiogenic Pulmonary Edema
Pneumonia
See Anxiety Disorders, p. 795
Figure 7.3.1
Antibiotics, antifungal agents
See Respiratory Infections, Pneumonia, pp. 164–165
See Asthma and COPD Exacerbations, p. 266
Footnotes
1. ABCs: Airway, Breathing, Circulation.
2. "Acute on chronic" assumes that this patient has a chronic condition, typically known to the patient, that is acutely worsening.
3. JVP: Jugular venous pressure.

FIGURE 7.3

7-4 Chronic Dyspnea

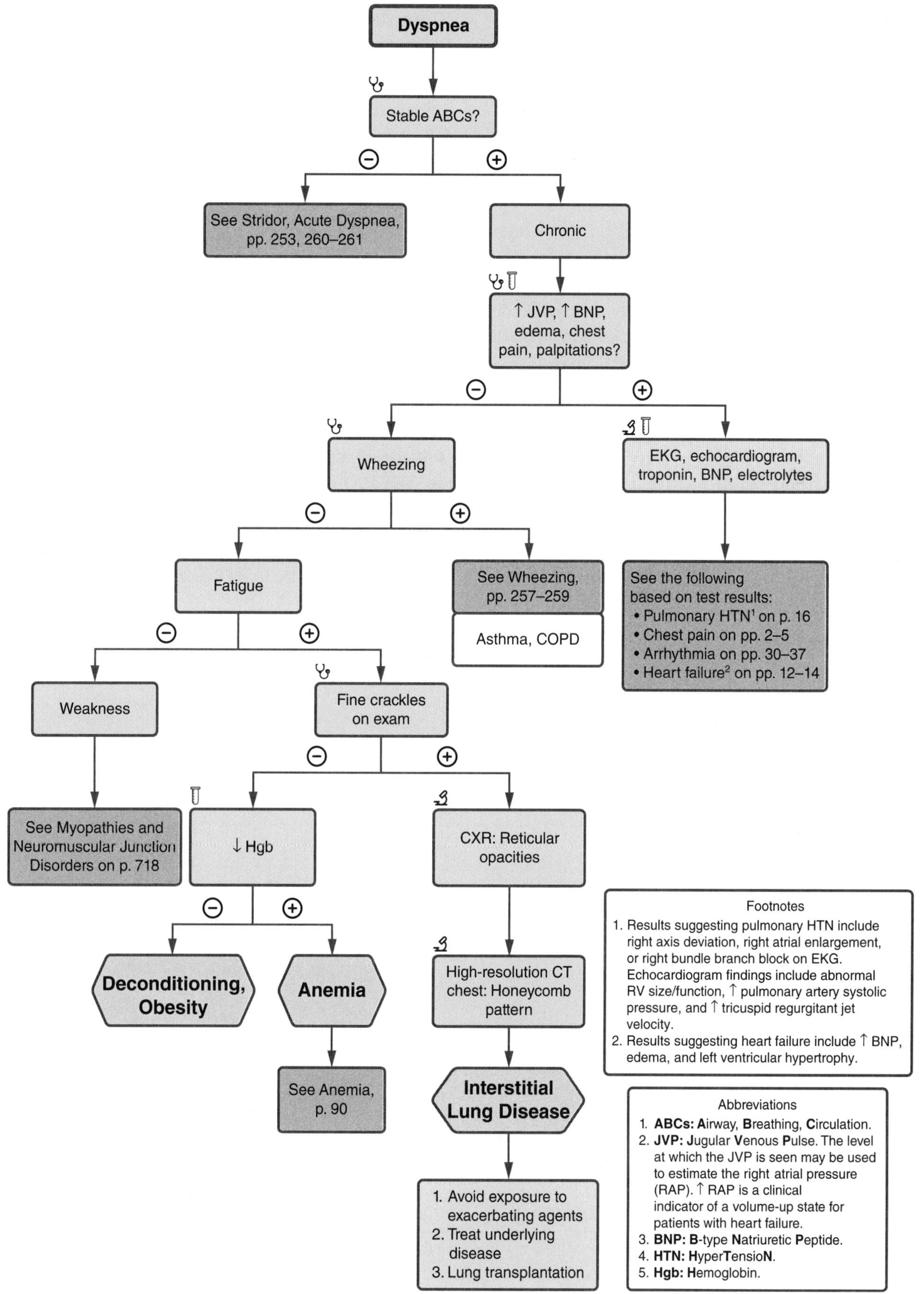
Dyspnea
Stable ABCs?
See Stridor, Acute Dyspnea, pp. 253, 260–261
Chronic
↑ JVP, ↑ BNP, edema, chest pain, palpitations?
Wheezing
EKG, echocardiogram, troponin, BNP, electrolytes
Fatigue
See Wheezing, pp. 257–259
Asthma, COPD
See the following based on test results:
• Pulmonary HTN[1] on p. 16
• Chest pain on pp. 2–5
• Arrhythmia on pp. 30–37
• Heart failure[2] on pp. 12–14
Weakness
Fine crackles on exam
See Myopathies and Neuromuscular Junction Disorders on p. 718
↓ Hgb
CXR: Reticular opacities
Deconditioning, Obesity
Anemia
High-resolution CT chest: Honeycomb pattern
See Anemia, p. 90
Interstitial Lung Disease
1. Avoid exposure to exacerbating agents
2. Treat underlying disease
3. Lung transplantation
Footnotes
1. Results suggesting pulmonary HTN include right axis deviation, right atrial enlargement, or right bundle branch block on EKG. Echocardiogram findings include abnormal RV size/function, ↑ pulmonary artery systolic pressure, and ↑ tricuspid regurgitant jet velocity.
2. Results suggesting heart failure include ↑ BNP, edema, and left ventricular hypertrophy.
Abbreviations
1. ABCs: Airway, Breathing, Circulation.
2. JVP: Jugular Venous Pulse. The level at which the JVP is seen may be used to estimate the right atrial pressure (RAP). ↑ RAP is a clinical indicator of a volume-up state for patients with heart failure.
3. BNP: B-type Natriuretic Peptide.
4. HTN: HyperTensioN.
5. Hgb: Hemoglobin.

FIGURE 7.4

7-4 Chronic Dyspnea

DECONDITIONING, OBESITY

A sedentary 75-year-old M with PMH of T2DM and morbid obesity presents with chronic dyspnea. He denies chest pain, diaphoresis, nausea, or vomiting. On **exam**, the patient is morbidly obese and becomes out of breath adjusting his position on the exam table. Cardiovascular workup (EKG, troponin, BNP) is negative. **Labs** and **imaging** are normal.

Management

1. Lifestyle changes
2. Optimize treatment of any existing comorbidities

HYF: Obesity and deconditioning are one of the most common causes of dyspnea; however, more acute causes must first be ruled out. Patients who have suffered recent major medical events (stroke, trauma, extended hospitalization) are at risk of becoming deconditioned. Elderly patients and those with limited mobility are also at a high risk.

ASPIRATION (PNEUMONITIS)

An 80-year-old M with PMH of stroke presents with mild dyspnea and cough after eating. On **exam**, he is afebrile, HR 80, RR 15, SpO_2 92% on room air. He has crackles in the right lung base. **Labs** are normal. On **imaging**, CXR demonstrates an opacity in the right lower lobe.

Management:

1. Oropharyngeal suctioning.
2. Supportive care.
3. Antibiotics if respiratory function does not improve.

Complications: Progression to bacterial pneumonia or acute respiratory distress syndrome (ARDS).

HYF: Aspiration pneumonitis occurs when gastric contents are inhaled. This typically occurs in patients with altered mental status (drugs, toxins, infection, etc.) or with impaired ability to swallow. Low-grade fever can be present, even in the absence of infection. There is no need for prophylactic antibiotics or steroids in most patients.

Anemia: See in Hematology/Oncology, p. 90.

Cardiogenic Pulmonary Edema: See heart failure in Cardiology, pp. 12–14. See Acute Cough and Shunt in Pulmonology, pp. 263–264, 274–276.

Interstitial Lung Disease: See V/Q Mismatch, Chronic Cough, and PFTs in Pulmonology, pp. 265–267, 271–273, 277–280.

Pulmonary Embolism: See Wheeze, Acute Cough, Hemoptysis, and V/Q mismatch in Pulmonology, pp. 257–259, 265–267, 274–276, 281–282.

Anxiety, Panic Attack: See Psychiatry, pp. 794–795.

Pneumonia: See Infectious Diseases, pp. 165–167.

7-5 Wheezing

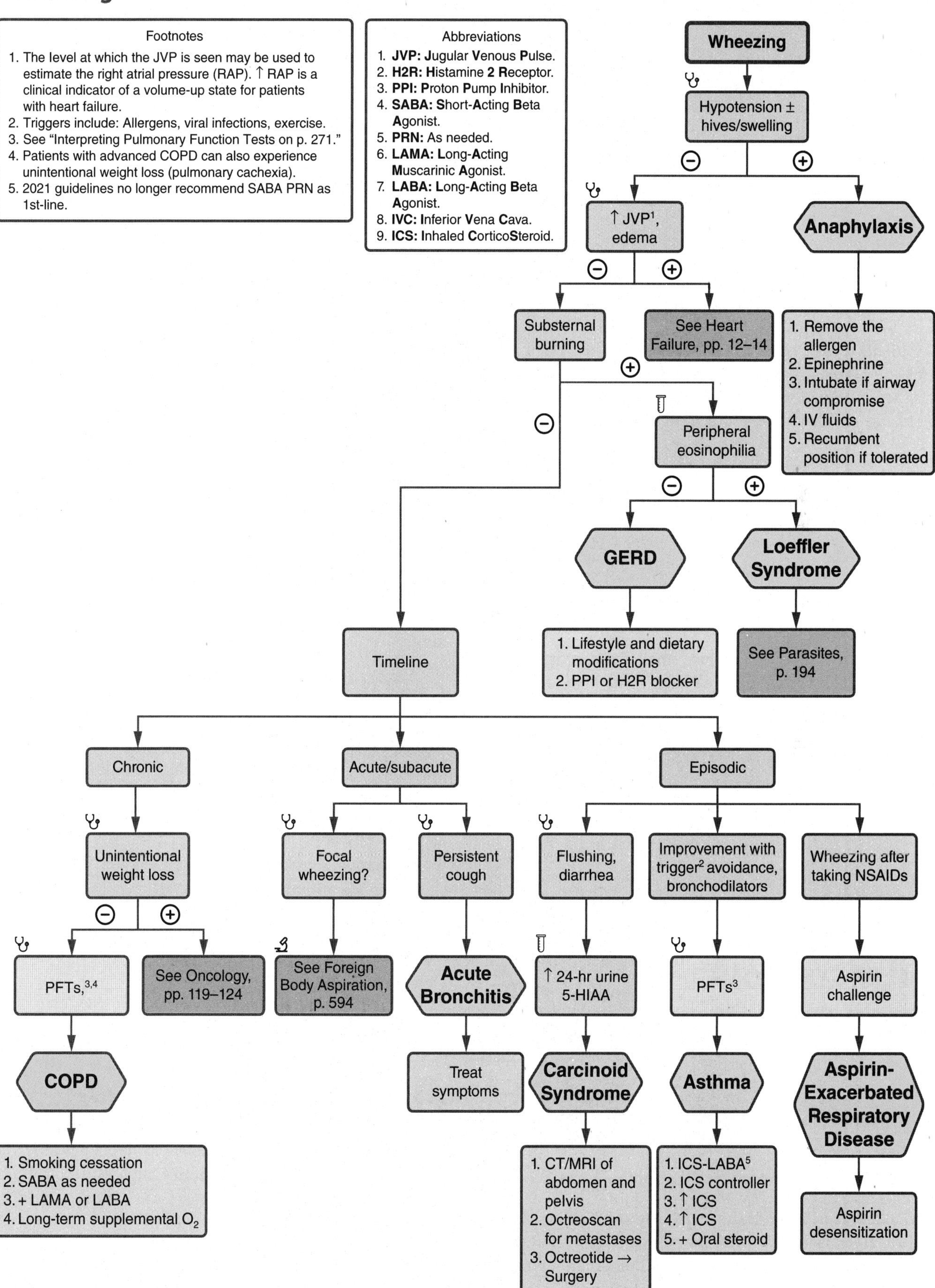
Footnotes
1. The level at which the JVP is seen may be used to estimate the right atrial pressure (RAP). ↑ RAP is a clinical indicator of a volume-up state for patients with heart failure.
2. Triggers include: Allergens, viral infections, exercise.
3. See "Interpreting Pulmonary Function Tests on p. 271."
4. Patients with advanced COPD can also experience unintentional weight loss (pulmonary cachexia).
5. 2021 guidelines no longer recommend SABA PRN as 1st-line.
Abbreviations
1. JVP: Jugular Venous Pulse.
2. H2R: Histamine 2 Receptor.
3. PPI: Proton Pump Inhibitor.
4. SABA: Short-Acting Beta Agonist.
5. PRN: As needed.
6. LAMA: Long-Acting Muscarinic Agonist.
7. LABA: Long-Acting Beta Agonist.
8. IVC: Inferior Vena Cava.
9. ICS: Inhaled CorticoSteroid.
Wheezing
Hypotension ± hives/swelling
↑ JVP[1], edema
Anaphylaxis
Substernal burning
See Heart Failure, pp. 12–14
1. Remove the allergen
2. Epinephrine
3. Intubate if airway compromise
4. IV fluids
5. Recumbent position if tolerated
Peripheral eosinophilia
GERD
Loeffler Syndrome
Timeline
1. Lifestyle and dietary modifications
2. PPI or H2R blocker
See Parasites, p. 194
Chronic
Acute/subacute
Episodic
Unintentional weight loss
Focal wheezing?
Persistent cough
Flushing, diarrhea
Improvement with trigger[2] avoidance, bronchodilators
Wheezing after taking NSAIDs
PFTs,[3,4]
See Oncology, pp. 119–124
See Foreign Body Aspiration, p. 594
Acute Bronchitis
↑ 24-hr urine 5-HIAA
PFTs[3]
Aspirin challenge
COPD
Treat symptoms
Carcinoid Syndrome
Asthma
Aspirin-Exacerbated Respiratory Disease
1. Smoking cessation
2. SABA as needed
3. + LAMA or LABA
4. Long-term supplemental O2
1. CT/MRI of abdomen and pelvis
2. Octreoscan for metastases
3. Octreotide → Surgery
1. ICS-LABA[5]
2. ICS controller
3. ↑ ICS
4. ↑ ICS
5. + Oral steroid
Aspirin desensitization

FIGURE 7.5

7-5 Wheezing

ANAPHYLAXIS

A 60-year-old F with PMH of IgA deficiency presents with dyspnea after a blood transfusion. On **exam**, she has wheezing, hypotension, vomiting, and urticaria.

Management:

1. Stop transfusion or medication infusion.
2. Give IM epinephrine.
3. IV fluids, steroids, antihistamines.
4. Intubate if airway compromise.

Complications: Shock, airway constriction, death.

HYF: Patients usually have prior exposure to the allergen to form IgE antibodies (type 1 hypersensitivity). Common triggers: Food, insect stings, medications. Signs of airway compromise include stridor, hoarse/muffled voice, oropharyngeal swelling.

GASTROESOPHAGEAL REFLUX DISEASE (GERD)

A 45-year-old M with PMH of obesity presents with cough, morning hoarseness, and postprandial substernal burning. **Exam** and **labs** are normal.

Management:

1. Lifestyle modifications (weight loss, small meals; avoid smoking, chocolate, coffee, and alcohol) if <2x/week.
2. PPIs, H2-receptor blockers.
3. EGD if refractory, longstanding, or "alarm" symptoms (eg, weight loss, black/tarry stool, dysphagia).

Complications:

- Strictures, Barrett's esophagus, erosive esophagitis, cancer.
- Upper GI bleeding.

HYF: Associated with pregnancy, smoking, obesity, alcohol, and hiatal hernias.

LOEFFLER SYNDROME

A 30-year-old M recent immigrant presents with cough, dyspnea, and fever. On **exam**, he has lung crackles and wheezing. **Labs** show eosinophilia. On **imaging**, CT chest shows migratory pulmonary nodules.

Management:

1. Symptomatic treatment.
2. Stool O&P in 2 months, then treat with anti-helminthic.

HYF: Can be caused by multiple parasites, including *Ascaris* (treat with albendazole or pyrantel pamoate if pregnant) and *Strongyloides* (treat with ivermectin). Pulmonary phase is self-limited. Helminth eggs do not show in stool until later in the disease course.

CHRONIC OBSTRUCTIVE PULMONARY DISEASE (COPD)

A 65-year-old M smoker presents with dyspnea, chronic cough, and sputum production. On **exam**, he has wheezing, prolonged expiration, and distant heart sounds. **Labs** show hypercapnia. On **imaging**, CXR reveals hyperinflated lungs. PFTs show ↓ FVC, ↓ FEV1, and ↓ FEV1/FVC.

Management:

1. Annual flu shot. Pneumococcal vaccines: Polysaccharide (PPSV23) + conjugate (PCV13, if age ≥65). Smoking cessation.
2. SABA as needed → add scheduled LAMA if more symptomatic.
3. Long-term O_2 if hypoxemic (goal SpO_2 90–93%).

Complications:

- Pulmonary infections, COPD exacerbations.
- Pulmonary hypertension, cor pulmonale.
- Hypercarbia.
- Frequent hospitalizations and steroids.

HYF: Chronic bronchitis is characterized by a productive cough >3 months/year for 2 consecutive years. Emphysema is a pathologic diagnosis marked by destruction and dilation of structures distal to terminal bronchioles. Smoking causes centrilobular destruction. α-1 antitrypsin deficiency causes panlobular destruction and liver disease.

CARCINOID SYNDROME

A 64-year-old F with recent unintentional weight loss presents with periodic facial flushing and profuse watery diarrhea. **Exam** shows multiple small blanching skin macules and diffuse wheezes. **Labs** show elevated urinary 5-hydroxyindoleacetic acid (5-HIAA).

Management:

1. Localize the tumor with CT/MRI abdomen.
2. Octreotide prior to surgical removal.

Complications: Severe tricuspid regurgitation causing right heart failure.

HYF: Tumor commonly originates in the ileum or appendix. Patients only become symptomatic with metastasis to the liver due to first-pass hepatic metabolism.

ASTHMA (EXERCISE-INDUCED)

A 20-year-old F presents with wheezing, cough, and dyspnea with exercise. On **exam**, she has lichenoid plaques in a flexural distribution. PFTs show ↓ FEV1/FVC with 15% improvement with albuterol.

Management:

1. Avoid triggers.
2. Chronic: 2021 guidelines recommend beginning with ICS-LABA inhaler PRN. Previous recommendation was albuterol inhaler PRN.
3. Oral montelukast and leukotriene antagonists are add-on therapies. Control allergies.

7-5 Wheezing

Complications: Asthma exacerbation (see Acute Cough on pp. 274–276 for management.)

HYF: Exercise-induced asthma is a variant characterized by onset of dyspnea or cough after 10 minutes of exercise that usually resolves 1 hour after exercise; treatment includes prophylactic use of SABA 10 minutes before exercise and, if refractory, use of ICS. Patients with asthma are at higher risk for any pulmonary infections (influenza, bacterial pneumonia). If PFTs are normal, perform methacholine challenge for diagnosis. Normalizing pH, $PaCO_2$, and ↓ PaO_2 are signs of respiratory fatigue → imminent respiratory collapse.

ASPIRIN-EXACERBATED RESPIRATORY DISEASE

A 27-year-old F with PMH of chronic sinusitis, asthma, and nasal polyps presents with progressive dyspnea after taking naproxen for an ankle sprain. **Exam** is notable for bilateral nasal gray mucoid masses.

Management:

1. Avoid NSAIDs and ASA.
2. Inhaled corticosteroids for asthma, antileukotrienes (eg, montelukast, zileuton).
3. Consider nasal polyp resection.
4. If patient would benefit from taking long-term aspirin (eg, history of coronary artery disease or stroke), consider aspirin desensitization.

Complications:

- Severe bronchospasm.
- Need for ASA desensitization if ASA is required for another disease (eg, CAD).

HYF: Characterized by chronic sinusitis, recurrent nasal polyps, asthma symptoms, and acute upper and lower respiratory tract symptoms exacerbated by ASA or NSAID use. Pseudoallergic reaction (not IgE-mediated) due to COX inhibition, leading to leukotriene overproduction and airway constriction.

7-6 Stridor

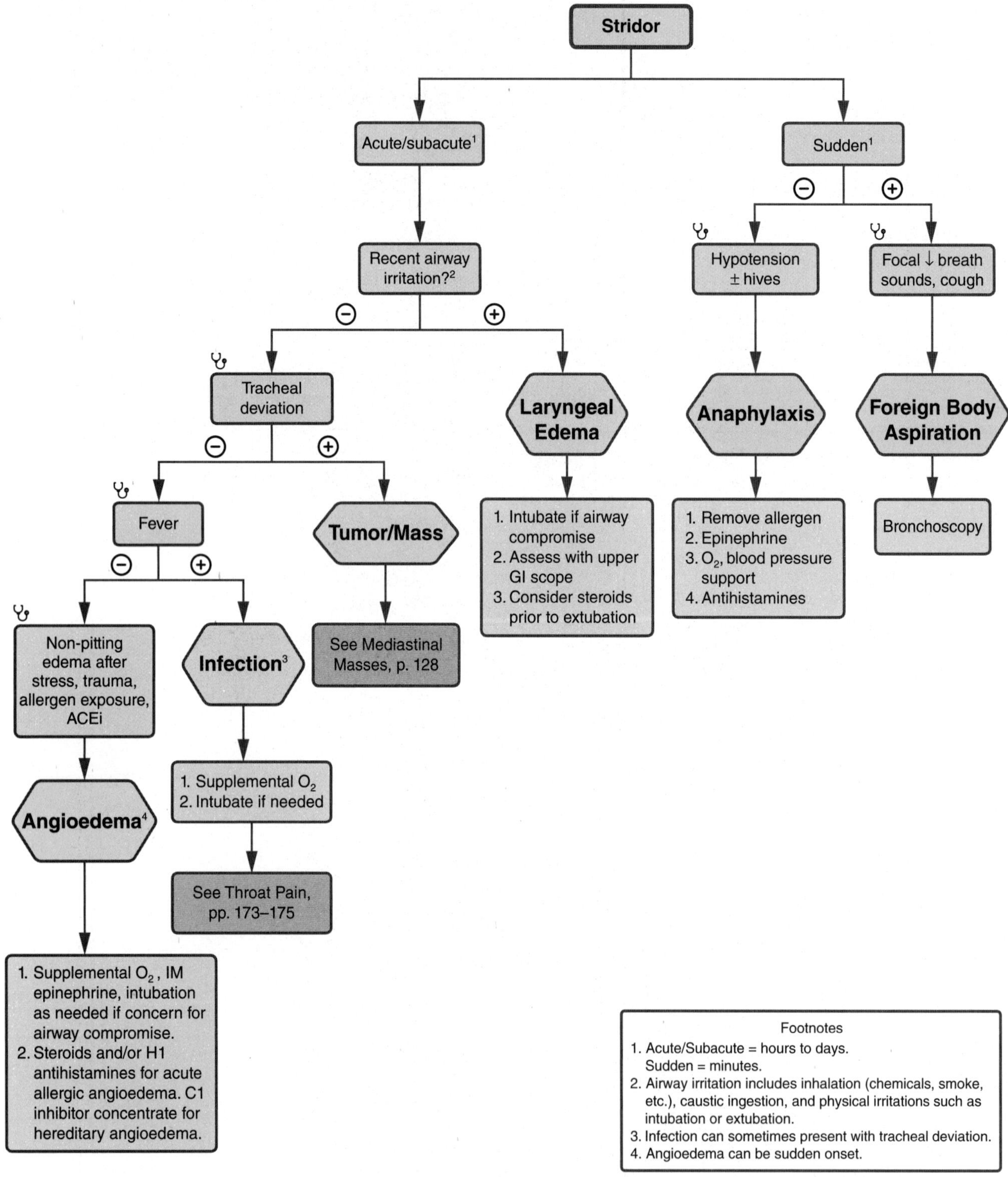
Stridor
Acute/subacute[1]
Sudden[1]
Recent airway irritation?[2]
Hypotension ± hives
Focal ↓ breath sounds, cough
Tracheal deviation
Laryngeal Edema
Anaphylaxis
Foreign Body Aspiration
Fever
Tumor/Mass
1. Intubate if airway compromise
2. Assess with upper GI scope
3. Consider steroids prior to extubation
1. Remove allergen
2. Epinephrine
3. O_2, blood pressure support
4. Antihistamines
Bronchoscopy
Non-pitting edema after stress, trauma, allergen exposure, ACEi
Infection[3]
See Mediastinal Masses, p. 128
1. Supplemental O_2
2. Intubate if needed
Angioedema[4]
See Throat Pain, pp. 173–175
1. Supplemental O_2, IM epinephrine, intubation as needed if concern for airway compromise.
2. Steroids and/or H1 antihistamines for acute allergic angioedema. C1 inhibitor concentrate for hereditary angioedema.
Footnotes
1. Acute/Subacute = hours to days. Sudden = minutes.
2. Airway irritation includes inhalation (chemicals, smoke, etc.), caustic ingestion, and physical irritations such as intubation or extubation.
3. Infection can sometimes present with tracheal deviation.
4. Angioedema can be sudden onset.

FIGURE 7.6

7-6 Stridor

LARYNGEAL EDEMA

A 75-year-old M was rescued from a house fire. Exam shows singed beard and mustache, facial burns, stridor, moderate accessory muscle use, and drooling.

Management:

1. Decontaminate by removing any clothing and copiously irrigate.
2. Intubate if signs of airway decompensation.
3. Give steroids prior to extubation if high risk.

Complications:

- May perforate intestines and need surgery.
- Airway or GI stricture.

HYF: Common triggers include intubation and other mechanical trauma, smoke and heat trauma, and alkalizing agents such as harsh cleaners or chemicals. For ingestions, do not give charcoal or induce vomiting due to risk of friable esophagus and oropharynx; assess extent of injury with upper GI endoscopy.

ANGIOEDEMA

A 57-year-old F with PMH of HTN on lisinopril presents with tongue swelling without redness, rash, or itchiness. On exam, she is found to have severe respiratory distress with tripoding and accessory muscle use, stridor, raspy voice, and enlarged tongue and lips.

Management:

1. IM epinephrine. Supplemental O_2 and emergent intubation if concern for impending airway compromise. Remove the offending agent.
2. If acute allergic angioedema, steroids and/or H1 antihistamines (eg, cetirizine).
3. If C1 inhibitor deficiency (hereditary angioedema), C1 inhibitor concentrate, kallikrein inhibitor (ecallantide), bradykinin-B2-receptor antagonist (icatibant), or fresh frozen plasma (FFP).

Complications: Airway compromise → acute respiratory failure and cardiac arrest.

HYF: Most commonly due to ACEi and can occur at any time during use. Other triggers include NSAIDS, ASA, and blood transfusions. Can also be due to C1 esterase inhibitor deficiency (hereditary angioedema), which causes higher bradykinin levels leading to an increase in smooth muscle relaxation in the walls of blood vessels and resultant edema in the extremities, GI tract, and, in severe cases, the larynx.

Anaphylaxis: See pp. 117, 258.

Foreign Body Aspiration: See p. 594.

7-7 Hypoxemia

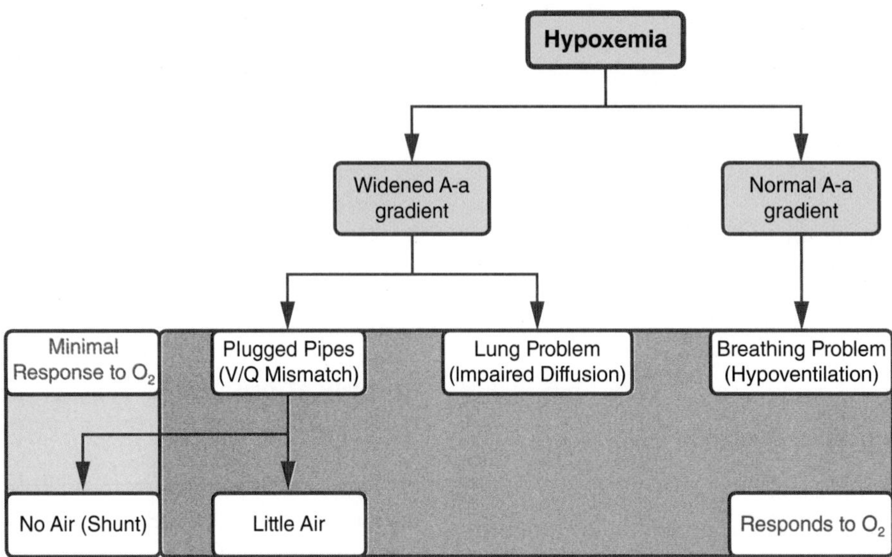
Hypoxemia
Widened A-a gradient
Normal A-a gradient
Minimal Response to O_2
Plugged Pipes (V/Q Mismatch)
Lung Problem (Impaired Diffusion)
Breathing Problem (Hypoventilation)
No Air (Shunt)
Little Air
Responds to O_2

Hypoxemia is a condition where there is an abnormally low level of oxygen in the arterial blood, leading to inadequate oxygen delivery to the organs. It is typically defined as an arterial oxygen tension (PaO_2) below 60 mmHg or an arterial oxygen saturation (SaO_2) below 90%. It can be caused by a variety of factors, including a low inspired oxygen concentration, impaired ventilation, reduced perfusion, or diffusion impairment.

When a patient is hypoxemic, the **alveolar-arterial gradient (A-a gradient)** helps us pinpoint the cause. The A-a gradient evaluates the efficiency of gas exchange in the lungs by measuring the difference in the partial pressure of oxygen between the alveoli **(PAO_2)** and the arteries **(PAO_2)**. Under normal conditions, gas exchange in the lungs is efficient, so there is a small A-a gradient. In healthy patients, the A-a gradient increases slightly with age but generally remains between 5–10 mmHg. Hypoxemia with a **normal A-a gradient** may be due to factors such as decreased inspired oxygen concentration (eg, high altitude) or hypoventilation (eg, obesity hypoventilation syndrome, central nervous system depression). Hypoxemia with an **increased A-a gradient** may indicate impaired gas exchange in the lungs, which can occur due to a variety of conditions that affect perfusion or ventilation and cause a **ventilation-perfusion (V/Q) mismatch**. Additionally, **diffusion impairment**, as seen in interstitial lung disease, can also cause an elevated A-a gradient.

Ventilation refers to the movement of air in and out of the lungs via the respiratory tract. **Alveolar ventilation (V)** is the volume of inspired air that reaches the alveoli. Gas exchange of oxygen and carbon dioxide occurs via diffusion across the blood-air barrier, following pressure gradients. The volume of ventilated air that does not take part in gas exchange is known as the physiologic dead space, which is comprised of anatomic dead space (eg, nostrils, trachea, bronchioles) and alveolar dead space (ie, total volume of alveoli – mostly in the lung apices – that do not participate in gas exchange because they are ventilated but not perfused). **Perfusion (Q)** is the pulmonary blood flow (ie, cardiac output) that reaches the capillaries surrounding the alveoli. While upright, Q is highest in the lung base due to the effects of gravity; while supine, Q is approximately equal throughout the lung. V and Q are closely regulated to optimize gas exchange. The V/Q ratio depends on the location but is generally higher at the apex of the lungs than at the base. The ideal V/Q ratio is 1. The average V/Q in a healthy patient is 0.8.

There are two types of **V/Q mismatch. Shunt** (V/Q = 0) occurs when there is sufficient perfusion but inadequate ventilation (eg, airway obstruction in pneumonia or ARDS). PaO_2 cannot be improved by supplemental oxygen. **Dead space ventilation** ($V/Q \rightarrow \infty$) occurs when there is sufficient ventilation but inadequate blood flow to the alveoli (eg, blood flow obstruction in pulmonary embolism). PaO_2 can be improved by supplemental oxygen. In the following pages, we will discuss etiologies of V/Q mismatch.

Footnotes

A-a Gradient = $PAO_2 - PaO_2$.
PAO_2 = Partial pressure of alveolar oxygen = $(FiO_2) \times (P_{atm} - P_{H2O}) - (PaCO_2/0.8)$.
FiO_2 = Fraction of inspired O_2, 0.21 in room air.
P_{atm} = Atmospheric pressure, 760 mmHg.
P_{H2O} = Vapor pressure of water, 47 mmHg.
$PaCO_2$ = Partial pressure of arterial CO_2 from arterial blood gas.
At sea-level, $PAO_2 = (FiO_2) \times (713) - (PaCO_2/0.8)$.
Normal A-a gradient estimate = (Age/4) + 4.

FIGURE 7.7

7-8 V/Q Mismatch: Shunt

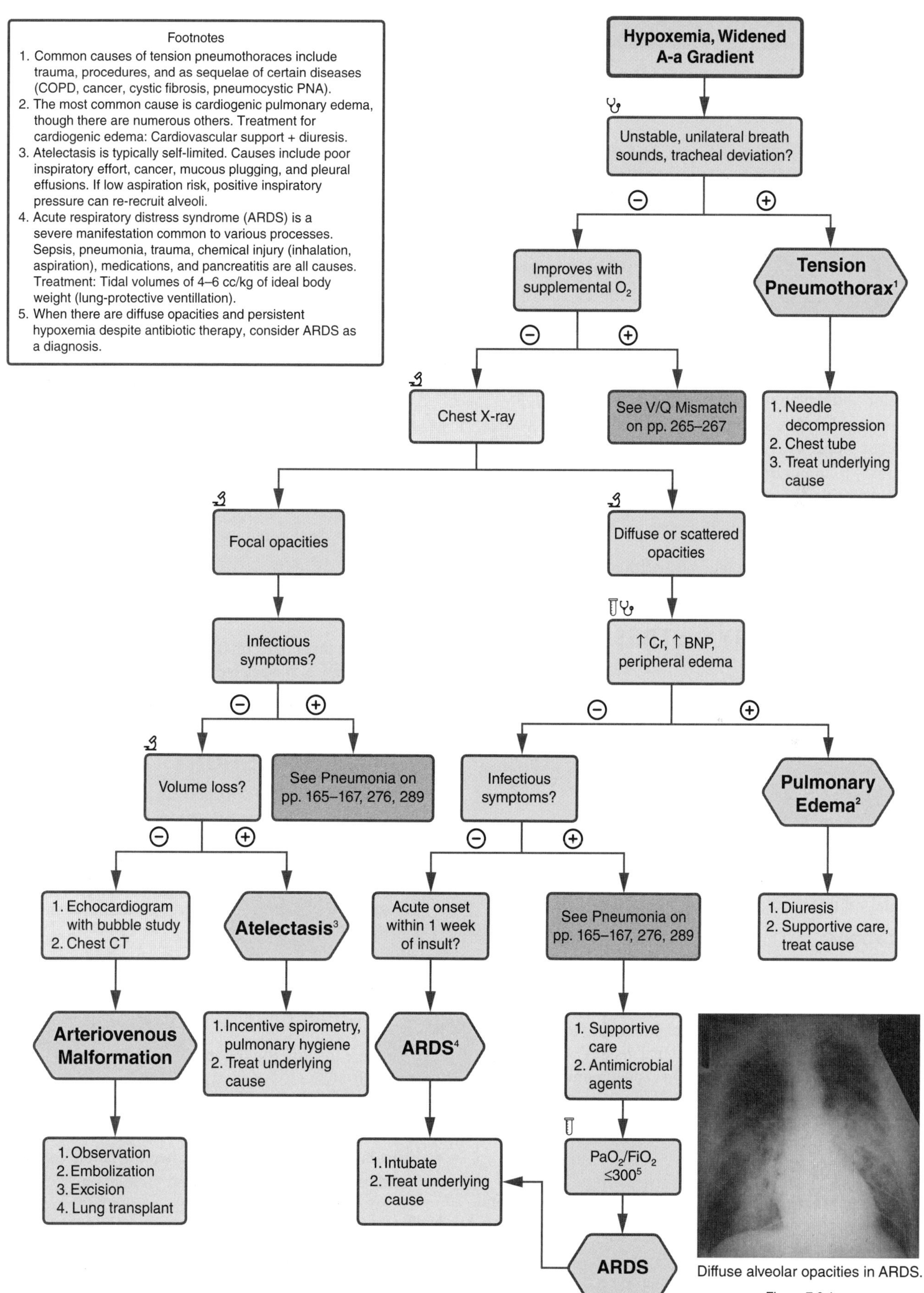
Footnotes
1. Common causes of tension pneumothoraces include trauma, procedures, and as sequelae of certain diseases (COPD, cancer, cystic fibrosis, pneumocystic PNA).
2. The most common cause is cardiogenic pulmonary edema, though there are numerous others. Treatment for cardiogenic edema: Cardiovascular support + diuresis.
3. Atelectasis is typically self-limited. Causes include poor inspiratory effort, cancer, mucous plugging, and pleural effusions. If low aspiration risk, positive inspiratory pressure can re-recruit alveoli.
4. Acute respiratory distress syndrome (ARDS) is a severe manifestation common to various processes. Sepsis, pneumonia, trauma, chemical injury (inhalation, aspiration), medications, and pancreatitis are all causes. Treatment: Tidal volumes of 4–6 cc/kg of ideal body weight (lung-protective ventillation).
5. When there are diffuse opacities and persistent hypoxemia despite antibiotic therapy, consider ARDS as a diagnosis.
Hypoxemia, Widened A-a Gradient
Unstable, unilateral breath sounds, tracheal deviation?
Improves with supplemental O_2
Tension Pneumothorax[1]
1. Needle decompression 2. Chest tube 3. Treat underlying cause
Chest X-ray
See V/Q Mismatch on pp. 265–267
Focal opacities
Diffuse or scattered opacities
Infectious symptoms?
↑ Cr, ↑ BNP, peripheral edema
Volume loss?
See Pneumonia on pp. 165–167, 276, 289
Infectious symptoms?
Pulmonary Edema[2]
1. Echocardiogram with bubble study 2. Chest CT
Atelectasis[3]
Acute onset within 1 week of insult?
See Pneumonia on pp. 165–167, 276, 289
1. Diuresis 2. Supportive care, treat cause
Arteriovenous Malformation
1. Incentive spirometry, pulmonary hygiene 2. Treat underlying cause
ARDS[4]
1. Supportive care 2. Antimicrobial agents
1. Observation 2. Embolization 3. Excision 4. Lung transplant
1. Intubate 2. Treat underlying cause
$PaO_2/FiO_2 \leq 300$[5]
ARDS
Diffuse alveolar opacities in ARDS.

Figure 7.8.1

FIGURE 7.8

7-8 V/Q Mismatch: Shunt

LUNG ABNORMALITY

TENSION PNEUMOTHORAX

See Pneumothorax in "Chest Trauma" in the General Surgery section on pp. 367–369.

ATELECTASIS

A 57-year-old M with PMH of ALS complicated by respiratory muscle weakness presents with acute hypoxemia to 79%. On **exam**, he is not responsive to maximal supplemental oxygen and has absent lung sounds on the left. On **imaging**, CXR shows complete opacification of left lung with tracheal deviation to the left. Bronchoscopy shows mucous impaction of the left mainstem.

Management:

1. Prevention with pulmonary hygiene, aspiration precautions.
2. Non-invasive therapies such as hypertonic saline or mucolytics for mucous plugging.
3. If secondary to tumor or foreign body, definitive management is direct removal of obstruction with bronchoscopy.

Complications: Pneumonia, PEA arrest from hypoxemia.

HYF: Causes include mucous plug obstruction, foreign body, or large unilateral pleural effusion.

ACUTE RESPIRATORY DISTRESS SYNDROME (ARDS)

A 48-year-old F presents with several days of fever and productive cough. On **imaging**, initial CXR shows R-sided lobar consolidation. Subsequently, she develops progressive profound hypoxemia to 72%, refractory to maximal non-invasive O_2. Repeat CXR shows bilateral diffuse alveolar opacities.

Management:

1. Treat the underlying cause (pneumonia, pancreatitis, etc.).
2. Frequently requires intubation for refractory hypoxemia.
3. Low-tidal volume ventilation at 6 mL/kg of ideal body weight.

Complications:

- Prolonged ventilation and ICU course.
- Death from hypoxemia, multi-system organ failure.

HYF: ARDS is defined as acute, bilateral pulmonary infiltrates, not entirely attributable to a cardiac cause, that require supplemental oxygen. Etiologies include direct lung injury (pneumonia, aspiration, inhalation, transfusion-related), systemic illness (sepsis, pancreatitis, DIC), or medications (amiodarone, blood transfusion reactions).

PULMONARY EDEMA

A 75-year-old M with PMH of DM2, ESRD on hemodialysis, and HFpEF presents after missing 3 sessions of dialysis with dyspnea, swelling in his legs, and hypoxemia to 76% refractory to supplemental O_2. On **exam**, he has diffuse wet crackles on auscultation and 2+ pitting edema to the knees bilaterally. On **imaging**, CXR shows bilateral alveolar opacities in a bat-wing pattern.

Management:

1. Diuretic therapy in patients that make urine.
2. Dialysis for volume overload in this patient with ESRD.

See Acute Cough on pp. 275–276 for further information on Pulmonary Edema.

BLOOD-FLOW ABNORMALITY

ARTERIOVENOUS MALFORMATION (AVM)

A 34-year-old M with PMH of recurrent epistaxis presents with a minor lobar pneumonia. He has a family history of hereditary hemorrhagic telangiectasias (HHT). On **exam**, he is tachypneic with SpO_2 of 83%. On **imaging**, chest CT angiography shows a large pulmonary AVM.

Management:

1. Embolization with interventional radiology.

Complications:

- Occult hypoxemia out of proportion to lung parenchyma pathology.
- Massive pulmonary hemorrhage.
- Paradoxical VTE clot transit and systemic embolization.

HYF: Can be diagnosed on TTE with bubble study and delayed bubble appearance. Associated with hereditary vascular disorders (eg, HHT).

INTRACARDIAC SHUNT

A. A 45-year-old F with PMH of recurrent DVTs and paradoxical ischemic CVAs presents with minor pneumonia. On **exam**, she has acute hypoxemia to 85% and a fixed split.
B. A 75-year-old M with PMH of recent MI 1 week ago s/p PCI to the LAD experiences acute hypoxemia. **Exam** is notable for hypotension, SpO_2 of 82% on room air, and a harsh holosystolic murmur heard best at the LLSB.

Management:

1. Echocardiography with bubble study to determine cause of shunt.
2. Procedure to close the shunt (endovascular or cardiac surgery).

Complications:

- Heart failure, cardiogenic shock, hemodynamic collapse.
- Paradoxical emboli to the systemic circulation.

HYF: Diagnosed with early reappearance of bubbles on echocardiogram bubble study. Causes: Congenital malformations (ASD, VSD) and acquired septal rupture after MI.

7-9 V/Q Mismatch: Other Causes

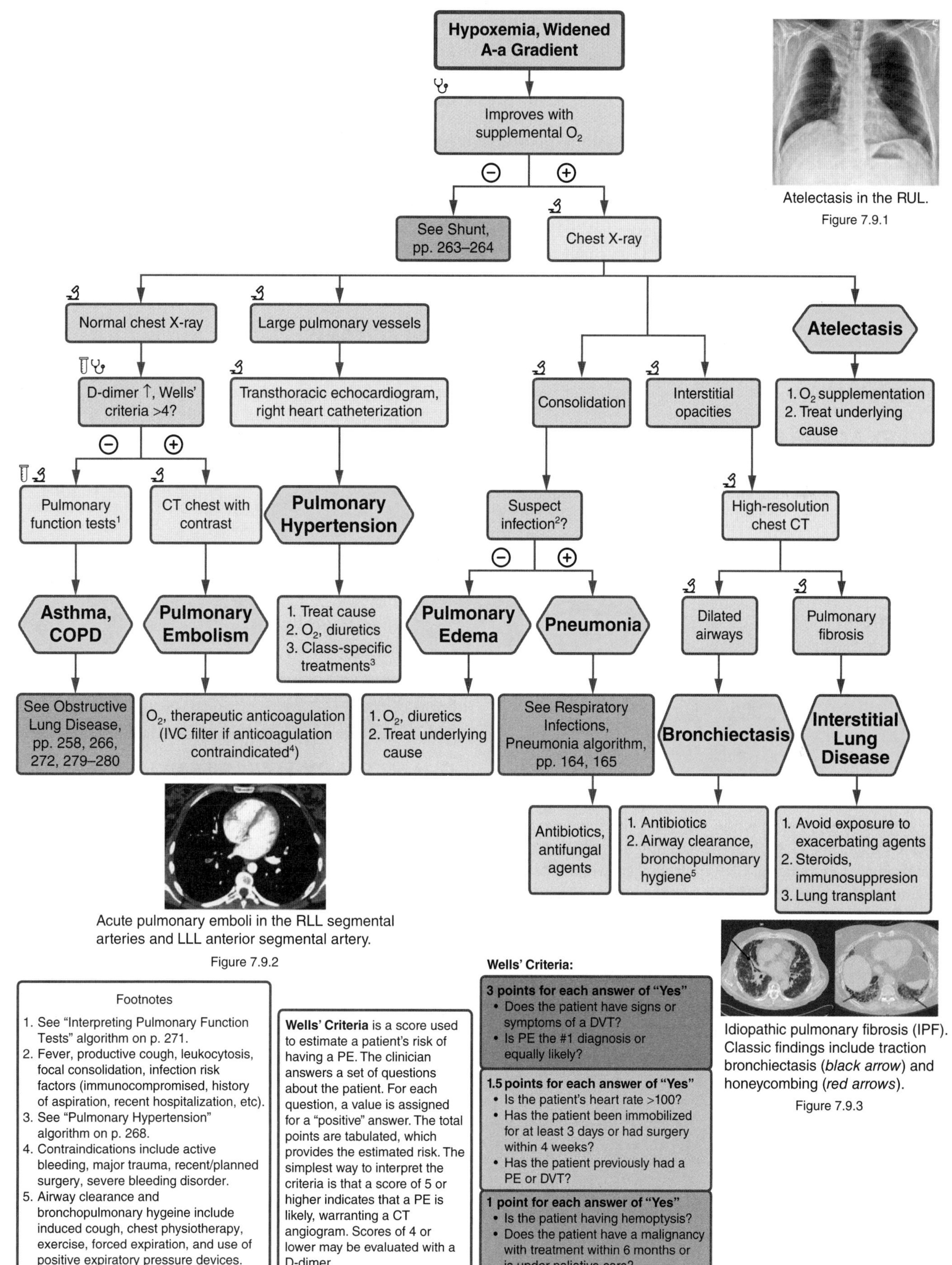

Hypoxemia, Widened A-a Gradient
Improves with supplemental O_2
⊖
⊕
See Shunt, pp. 263–264
Chest X-ray
Normal chest X-ray
Large pulmonary vessels
Atelectasis
D-dimer ↑, Wells' criteria >4?
Transthoracic echocardiogram, right heart catheterization
Consolidation
Interstitial opacities
1. O_2 supplementation
2. Treat underlying cause
⊖
⊕
Pulmonary function tests[1]
CT chest with contrast
Pulmonary Hypertension
Suspect infection[2]?
High-resolution chest CT
⊖
⊕
Asthma, COPD
Pulmonary Embolism
1. Treat cause
2. O_2, diuretics
3. Class-specific treatments[3]
Pulmonary Edema
Pneumonia
Dilated airways
Pulmonary fibrosis
See Obstructive Lung Disease, pp. 258, 266, 272, 279–280
O_2, therapeutic anticoagulation (IVC filter if anticoagulation contraindicated[4])
1. O_2, diuretics
2. Treat underlying cause
See Respiratory Infections, Pneumonia algorithm, pp. 164, 165
Bronchiectasis
Interstitial Lung Disease
Antibiotics, antifungal agents
1. Antibiotics
2. Airway clearance, bronchopulmonary hygiene[5]
1. Avoid exposure to exacerbating agents
2. Steroids, immunosuppresion
3. Lung transplant
Atelectasis in the RUL.
Figure 7.9.1
Acute pulmonary emboli in the RLL segmental arteries and LLL anterior segmental artery.
Figure 7.9.2
Idiopathic pulmonary fibrosis (IPF). Classic findings include traction bronchiectasis (black arrow) and honeycombing (red arrows).
Figure 7.9.3
Footnotes
1. See "Interpreting Pulmonary Function Tests" algorithm on p. 271.
2. Fever, productive cough, leukocytosis, focal consolidation, infection risk factors (immunocompromised, history of aspiration, recent hospitalization, etc).
3. See "Pulmonary Hypertension" algorithm on p. 268.
4. Contraindications include active bleeding, major trauma, recent/planned surgery, severe bleeding disorder.
5. Airway clearance and bronchopulmonary hygeine include induced cough, chest physiotherapy, exercise, forced expiration, and use of positive expiratory pressure devices.
Wells' Criteria is a score used to estimate a patient's risk of having a PE. The clinician answers a set of questions about the patient. For each question, a value is assigned for a "positive" answer. The total points are tabulated, which provides the estimated risk. The simplest way to interpret the criteria is that a score of 5 or higher indicates that a PE is likely, warranting a CT angiogram. Scores of 4 or lower may be evaluated with a D-dimer.
Wells' Criteria:
3 points for each answer of "Yes"
• Does the patient have signs or symptoms of a DVT?
• Is PE the #1 diagnosis or equally likely?
1.5 points for each answer of "Yes"
• Is the patient's heart rate >100?
• Has the patient been immobilized for at least 3 days or had surgery within 4 weeks?
• Has the patient previously had a PE or DVT?
1 point for each answer of "Yes"
• Is the patient having hemoptysis?
• Does the patient have a malignancy with treatment within 6 months or is under paliative care?

FIGURE 7.9

7-9 V/Q Mismatch: Other Causes

AIRWAY DISEASE: DECREASED VENTILATION

ASTHMA EXACERBATION

A 33-year-old F with PMH of severe persistent asthma presents with severe dyspnea after missing inhaler doses and an allergen exposure. On exam, she is found to be hypoxemic with SaO_2 85%, which corrects with 5 L O_2. She is in severe respiratory distress with tripoding and small air movement and diffuse wheezes on lung auscultation. On labs, ABG on room air shows pH 7.37, PaO_2 60, and $PaCO_2$ 40.

Management:

1. Severe asthma management: IV steroids, nebulized albuterol, Mg.

See Wheezing and Acute Cough on pp. 258–259 and 275–276 for further information.

COPD EXACERBATION

A 75-year-old M with PMH of COPD presents with acute cough productive of scant sputum and progressive dyspnea, and he is found to be hypoxemic to 83% SaO_2 requiring 7 L to correct to 94% SaO_2. Exam shows diffuse coarse rhonchi. On imaging, CXR shows hyperinflation. On labs, ABG on RA shows pH 7.35, PaO_2 66, and $PaCO_2$ 55.

Management:

1. COPD exacerbation management: Systemic steroids, azithromycin, albuterol-ipratropium inhalers.

See Wheezing and Acute Cough on pp. 258–259 and 275–276 for further information.

BRONCHIECTASIS

A 26-year-old M with PMH of cystic fibrosis presents with increasing cough and sputum production. On exam, he is hypoxemic to 87% on RA requiring 3 L O_2, afebrile, and lung auscultation reveals diffuse rhonchi. On imaging, CXR shows finger-in-glove pattern.

See Hemoptysis on pp. 281–282 for further information.

ALVEOLAR FILLING (WATER, PUS, OR ATELECTASIS): DECREASED VENTILATION AT THE CAPILLARY MEMBRANE

PULMONARY EDEMA

A 66-year-old M with PMH of ischemic HFrEF (EF 20%) presents with 15 lb weight gain, leg edema, orthopnea, and progressive dyspnea. On exam, he is found to be hypoxemic to 85% requiring 3 L oxygen with warm, well-perfused extremities and bilateral wet crackles in his lower lung fields. On imaging, CXR shows bilateral basilar-predominant fluffy opacities and engorged vasculature. On labs, ABG on RA shows pH 7.38, PaO_2 62, and $PaCO_2$ 42.

Management:

1. Acute CHF management: If perfusing and no concern for cardiogenic shock, give IV loop diuretics like furosemide.

See Heart Failure on p. 12 for further information.

PNEUMONIA

A 77-year-old F with PMH of HTN presents with 1 week of cough, fevers, and chills. On exam, she is found to be febrile and requires 5 L O_2 to maintain SaO_2 >92%. On imaging, CXR shows RLL dense opacity. On labs, ABG on RA with SaO_2 82% shows pH 7.37, PaO_2 60, and $PaCO_2$ 40.

See Pneumonia on pp. 166–167 for further information.

ATELECTASIS

A 67-year-old M with PMH of morbid obesity underwent a hip replacement yesterday. This morning, he is hypoxemic to 85% on RA requiring 3 LO_2 and afebrile. Lung exam reveals diminished breath sounds throughout and trace crackles at the bilateral bases. On imaging, CXR shows diminished lung volumes without infiltrates.

Management:

1. Mobilization out of bed to a chair.
2. Pulmonary hygiene with maneuvers such as incentive spirometry.

See Shunt on p. 264 for further information.

DESTRUCTION OF CAPILLARY BED: DECREASED PERFUSION

PULMONARY HYPERTENSION

A 36-year-old F with PMH of HIV and prior methamphetamine use presents with chronic progressive dyspnea on exertion and lower extremity edema. On exam, she is found to be hypoxemic to 85% on RA requiring 4 L O_2 with elevated JVP to 12 cm H_2O. On imaging, CXR shows an enlarged right atrium and right ventricle. TTE shows a dilated RV with estimated pulmonary artery pressure of 50 mmHg.

Management:

1. Right heart catheterization to confirm pulmonary artery pressures and cardiac output.
2. O_2 supplementation as needed to maintain SaO_2 >95%.
3. Disease-specific therapy as below.
4. Manage secondary CHF symptoms with loop diuretics.

Complications: Cardiogenic shock.

HYF: Pulmonary hypertension.

7-9 V/Q Mismatch: Other Causes

Pulmonary Hypertension

	Causes	Treatment
Group 1: Pulmonary arterial hypertension (PAH)	Idiopathic Drugs (methamphetamine) HIV Connective tissue disease (eg, scleroderma) Portopulmonary hypertension	Vasodilators: PDE-5 inhibitors (sildenafil) Prostacyclin analogues (epoprostenol, treprostinil) Endothelin-receptor antagonists (bosentan, macitentan)
Group 2: Left heart failure	Left heart failure (systolic or diastolic) Left-sided valve disease	Guideline-directed medical therapy for congestive heart failure (see Heart Failure on p. 12)
Group 3: Lung disease	Severe lung disease, both obstructive (COPD) and restrictive (ILD)	Treat the underlying lung disease
Group 4: Chronic thromboembolic pulmonary hypertension (CTEPH)	Chronic PEs	Anticoagulation
Group 5: Miscellaneous	All others (eg, sarcoidosis, schistosomiasis)	Treat the underlying disease

INTERSTITIAL LUNG DISEASE (ILD)

A 55-year-old F with PMH of Crohn's disease presents with progressive dyspnea. On **exam**, she is found to be hypoxemic to 85% on room air requiring 4 L, with lung auscultation notable for shallow breaths, inspiratory squeaks, and fine dry crackles. On **imaging**, CT chest shows fibrosis of lung parenchyma. PFTS show ↓ TLC, ↓ FVC, ↓ FEV1, ↓ DLCO, and normal FEV1/FVC ratio.

Management:

1. Supplemental O_2 as needed.
2. Avoid triggers (eg, environmental irritants, medications).
3. Some forms may respond to steroids or anti-inflammatory biologic therapies.
4. Lung transplant for end-stage disease.

Complications:

- Progressive acute respiratory failure.
- Pulmonary hypertension and right heart failure.

HYF: Causes include the following

- Idiopathic (idiopathic pulmonary fibrosis, crypogenic organizing pneumonia, acute interstitial pneumonia).
- Pneumoconiosis (environmental exposures like silicosis).
- Connective tissue and autoimmune disorders (rheumatoid arthritis, scleroderma, anti-synthetase syndrome).
- Medications (amiodarone, bleomycin).
- Chest radiation (eg, prior radiation therapy for cancer).

PULMONARY EMBOLISM (PE)

An 85-year-old F with PMH of breast cancer presents with dyspnea and pleuritic chest pain. On **exam**, she has tachycardia, hypoxemia, and a swollen left calf. **Labs** show elevated D-dimer. On **imaging**, CTA chest shows an acute PE.

Management:

1. If hemodynamically unstable: Thrombolysis vs. thrombectomy.
2. Anticoagulation vs. IVC filter.
3. Supplemental O_2 as needed.

Complications:

- Pulmonary hypertension, pulmonary infarction.
- Acute right heart failure, death.

HYF: Obtain V/Q scan if CT with contrast is contraindicated. CXR is often normal. Acute anticoagulation: LMWH, UFH, direct Xa inhibitor, fondaparinux. Chronic anticoagulation: LMWH, warfarin, DOACs. Avoid direct Xa inhibitors in cancer and renal failure. In pregnancy, avoid warfarin and use LMWH. Wells' criteria >4 means that PE is likely.

Mnemonic for Wells' criteria: **SHIT PMH.**
Signs and symptoms of DVT: 3 points.
History of DVT: 1.5 points.
Immobilization (>2 days): 1.5 points.
Tachycardia (HR >100): 1.5 points.
Post-op (recent surgery): 1.5 points.
Malignancy: 1 point.
Hemoptysis: 1 point.

See Acute Cough and Hemoptysis on pp. 275–276 and 281–282 for further information.

7-10 Pulmonary Hypertension

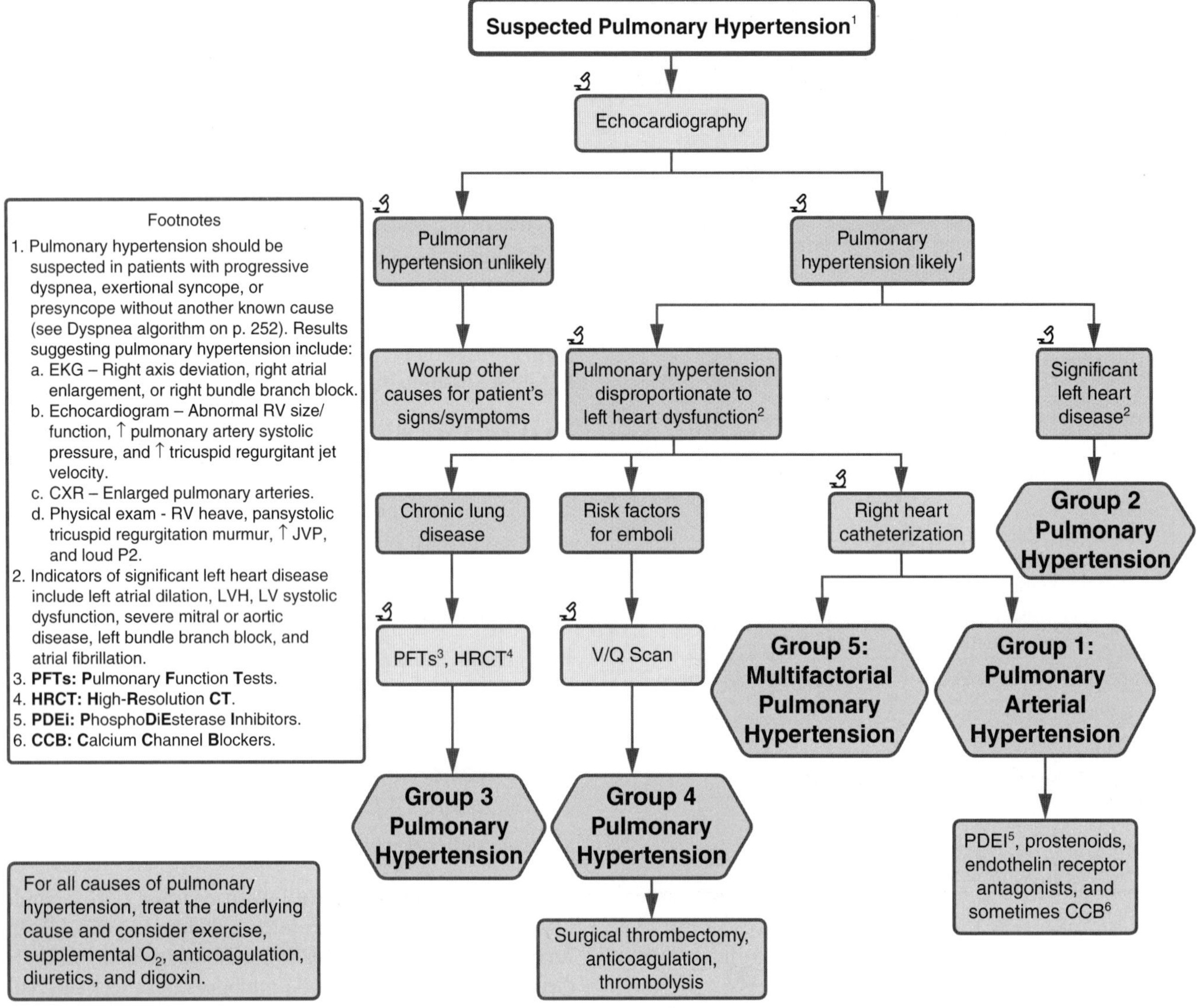
Suspected Pulmonary Hypertension[1]
Echocardiography
Pulmonary hypertension unlikely
Pulmonary hypertension likely[1]
Workup other causes for patient's signs/symptoms
Pulmonary hypertension disproportionate to left heart dysfunction[2]
Significant left heart disease[2]
Chronic lung disease
Risk factors for emboli
Right heart catheterization
Group 2 Pulmonary Hypertension
PFTs[3], HRCT[4]
V/Q Scan
Group 5: Multifactorial Pulmonary Hypertension
Group 1: Pulmonary Arterial Hypertension
Group 3 Pulmonary Hypertension
Group 4 Pulmonary Hypertension
PDEI[5], prostenoids, endothelin receptor antagonists, and sometimes CCB[6]
Surgical thrombectomy, anticoagulation, thrombolysis

Footnotes

1. Pulmonary hypertension should be suspected in patients with progressive dyspnea, exertional syncope, or presyncope without another known cause (see Dyspnea algorithm on p. 252). Results suggesting pulmonary hypertension include:
   a. EKG – Right axis deviation, right atrial enlargement, or right bundle branch block.
   b. Echocardiogram – Abnormal RV size/function, ↑ pulmonary artery systolic pressure, and ↑ tricuspid regurgitant jet velocity.
   c. CXR – Enlarged pulmonary arteries.
   d. Physical exam - RV heave, pansystolic tricuspid regurgitation murmur, ↑ JVP, and loud P2.
2. Indicators of significant left heart disease include left atrial dilation, LVH, LV systolic dysfunction, severe mitral or aortic disease, left bundle branch block, and atrial fibrillation.
3. **PFTs: P**ulmonary **F**unction **T**ests.
4. **HRCT: H**igh-**R**esolution **CT**.
5. **PDEi: P**hospho**D**i**E**sterase **I**nhibitors.
6. **CCB: C**alcium **C**hannel **B**lockers.

For all causes of pulmonary hypertension, treat the underlying cause and consider exercise, supplemental O_2, anticoagulation, diuretics, and digoxin.

Pulmonary hypertension (PH) presents clinically with non-specific symptoms. These include syncope, dyspnea on exertion, fatigue, and symptoms related to any underlying illness that resulted in PH. These underlying disease processes cover a wide spectrum of conditions and are divided into 5 groups, which we will discuss below. PH should be suspected when a patient has a condition known to lead to PH or when there are signs, symptoms, or test results concerning for PH (see footnotes).

The first step in evaluating a patient for PH is an echocardiogram. This is a non-invasive test that can potentially provide strong evidence in favor of, or against, a diagnosis of PH. If clinical suspicion for PH is low and the echocardiogram does not favor PH, then other causes for the patient's symptoms should be considered. However, if PH is likely, then the next step is to identify the underlying cause.

The most common etiology of PH is left heart disease (LHD), or group 2. If the echocardiogram demonstrates LHD significant enough to explain the patient's degree of PH, then the diagnosis is made. However, if LHD is absent or not severe enough to cause PH, then other causes must be investigated. If patients have hypoxemia or known chronic lung disease (CLD), then consider PH caused by CLD, or group 3. If CLD is suspected, workup includes high-resolution chest CT and pulmonary function tests. In patients with known risk factors for vascular occlusion (eg, clotting disorders, malignancy), then they should undergo a V/Q scan to evaluate for chronic thromboembolic PH, or CTEPH, which is the most common diagnosis in group 4 (pulmonary artery obstruction).

Finally, groups 1 and 5 are diagnoses of exclusion. If all other testing has not revealed the cause, then the patient should undergo right heart catheterization (RHC). In the absence of other explanations, demonstration of an ↑ pulmonary artery pressure as well as ↑ pulmonary vascular resistance is diagnostic of group 1 (pulmonary arterial hypertension). Disease processes that lead to group 1 PH include HIV, connective tissue disorders (scleroderma, lupus, rheumatoid arthritis), and portal hypertension. Non-invasive workup with labs and imaging (eg, rheumatologic serologies, RUQ US) to determine the presence of these diseases is done prior to RHC, but a RHC is required to definitively diagnose pulmonary arterial hypertension. Group 5 PH is multifactorial in nature and includes patients who do not fit neatly into any of the other four categories.

Regardless of the etiology for PH, management steps may include exercise, supplemental O_2, anticoagulation, diuretics, and digoxin. For group 1, phosphodiesterase inhibitors, prostenoids, endothelin receptor antagonists, and sometimes calcium channel blockers can be considered. Group 4 patients should be evaluated for surgical thrombectomy with anticoagulation or, alternatively, thrombolysis in poor surgical candidates. In all groups, treat the underlying disease when possible.

FIGURE 7.10

7-10 Pulmonary Hypertension

The mainstay of management for pulmonary hypertension (PH) is to treat the underlying cause, if known. A potential complication of all causes of PH is progression to right-sided heart failure. Right heart catheterization (RHC) is the gold standard for diagnosis. RHC can measure the pressure in the right side of the heart, the resistance of the pulmonary vasculature, and the pulmonary capillary wedge pressure (PCWP). Estimated right atrial pressure (RAP) >35 mmHg is indicative of PH, though it is not specific to any particular cause. The PCWP reflects the pressure in the left side of the heart and, when elevated (>15 mmHg), is indicative of left heart disease.

GROUP 1 PH (PULMONARY ARTERIAL HYPERTENSION)

A 40-year-old F with PMH of scleroderma presents with progressive dyspnea and fatigue. On **exam**, she has clear lung fields and loud P2. On **imaging**, TTE shows estimated RAP 50 mmHg. PFTs without restrictive pattern. PCWP <15 mmHg on RHC.

Management:

1. Rule out other causes of symptoms: Pulmonary (PFTs, imaging), cardiac (TTE, RHC), other (history of systemic diseases, drugs, etc.).
2. Endothelin receptor agonists, prostacyclin analogs, and phosphodiesterase inhibitors.
3. If refractory to the above treatments, consider IV prostanoid and lung transplant.

HYF: Group 1 PH is increased pressure in the pulmonary vasculature that occurs as a primary disease process (PAH) and is not due to left heart disease, pulmonary disease, or other systemic causes (group 5 PH). About 50% of cases are idiopathic. Some PAH cases are inherited (eg, *BMPR2* gene mutation).

GROUP 2 PH (LEFT HEART DISEASE)

A 65-year-old M with PMH of CHF presents with progressive dyspnea, fatigue, and lower extremity edema. **Labs** show elevated Cr and BNP consistent with acute decompensated heart failure. On **exam**, he has lower extremity edema, elevated JVP, and parasternal heave. On **imaging**, CXR shows cardiomegaly and pulmonary edema. EKG without acute ischemia. TTE shows est. RAP of 40 mmHg.

Management:

1. Optimize guideline-directed medical therapy for heart failure (diuretics, SGLT2, BB, ACEi/ARB, etc.).

HYF: Group 2 is due to left heart disease and the most common cause of PH. No indication for PH-specific medications (PDE-5); treat the underlying left heart disease.

GROUP 3 PH (LUNG DISEASE)

A 65-year-old M with PMH of tobacco use disorder presents with progressive dyspnea and fatigue. On **exam**, he has hypoxemia and fine crackles in the lungs. On **imaging**, high-resolution CT is consistent with interstitial lung disease, TTE demonstrates est. RAP 42 mmHg, and PFTs show a restrictive pattern.

Management:

1. Treatment of underlying lung disease.
2. Treprostinil (prostacyclin agonist).
3. If medication fails → consider lung transplant.

HYF: Due to chronic lung disease and hypoxemia. Causes of group 3 PH include COPD, restrictive lung diseases, pulmonary developmental disorders, and hypoxemia without structural lung disease. Workup begins with TTE. If the patient has risk factors for lung disease, obtain PFTs with possible subsequent high-resolution CT. PAH-directed drugs are used in group 3 PH with limited efficacy.

GROUP 4 PH (CTEPH)

A 60-year-old M with PMH of prior PE presents with progressive dyspnea and fatigue. On **exam**, he has lower extremity edema and elevated JVP. On **imaging**, TTE demonstrates normal left heart function, est. RAP 60 mmHg.

Management:

1. TTE to rule out left heart disease.
2. V/Q scan. If V/Q scan is indeterminate, consider pulmonary angiography.
3. Anticoagulation (IVC filter if high-bleed risk).
4. Refer to a CTEPH center.
5. Evaluate for pulmonary thromboendarterectomy (curative).

HYF: Once CTEPH is confirmed, all patients require anticoagulation indefinitely. All patients must be evaluated for clot removal via pulmonary thromboendarterectomy, as it is curative.

GROUP 5 PH (MULTIFACTORIAL MECHANISMS)

A 60-year-old M with PMH of CKD, sarcoidosis, and sickle cell disease presents with progressive dyspnea and fatigue. On **exam**, he has a loud P2. On **imaging**, TTE shows est. RAP 40 mmHg and normal LV function, V/Q scan without occlusive disease, and PFTs without restrictive disease. RHC reveals PCWP <15 mmHg and elevated pulmonary arterial pressures.

HYF: Group 5 is a diagnosis of exclusion. If a patient has PH that does not fit into groups 1–4, then they likely have group 5. There are a number of diseases that can cause PH via multifactorial mechanisms: renal disease, hematologic disorders (sickle cell disease), sarcoidosis, neurofibromatosis, glycogen storage diseases, and some congenital heart conditions.

7-11 Approach to Pulmonary Function Tests

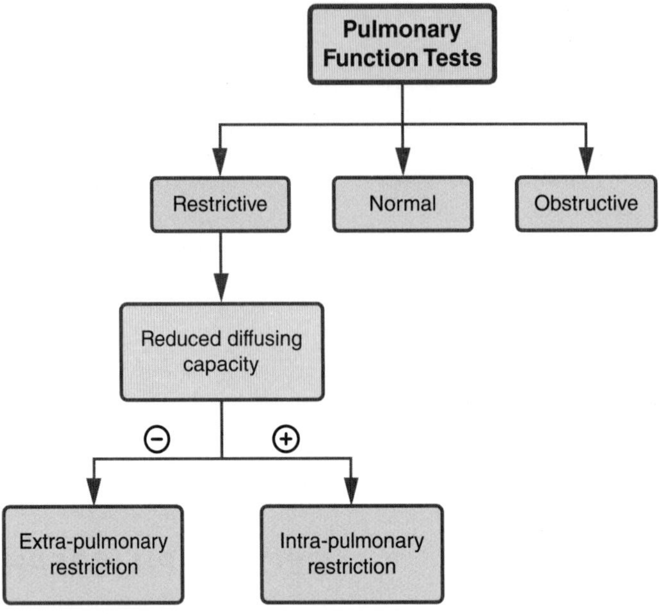
Pulmonary Function Tests
Restrictive
Normal
Obstructive
Reduced diffusing capacity
⊖
⊕
Extra-pulmonary restriction
Intra-pulmonary restriction

Pulmonary function tests (PFTs) measure the flow and volume of gas that a patient inhales and exhales. The patient is first instructed to breathe normally. The air breathed in and out for a breath cycle is called the tidal volume (TV). When undergoing PFTs, the patient will then be asked to inhale as much as they can. At their maximum, the volume of air in their lungs is called the total lung volume (TLV). The patient then exhales as much as they can. It is impossible to expel all air out of the lungs, and the remaining air is called the residual volume (RV). The total amount of air that the patient can move, from maximum inhalation to maximum exhalation, is called the vital capacity (VC) or forced vital capacity (FVC). This can be thought of as the TLC minus the RV. When the patient exhales as much as they can, the amount expelled in 1 second is called the forced expiratory capacity in 1 second (FEV1). One of the measures noted in PFTs is the ratio between FEV1 and FVC.

Inspiration is an active process and expiration a passive one. The diaphragm pulls the lungs open, creating lower pressure that pulls outside air in. The alveoli are elastic, and the more they expand, the more they resist further expansion—think of how rubber bands are more difficult to stretch the further they are pulled. Eventually, the respiratory muscles are unable to overcome the elasticity of the alveoli and the chest wall. This is the point of maximal inspiration. Expiration is driven by the elastic recoil of alveoli and the thoracic cavity.

Some patients have a disease that restricts expansion. This can be due to stiffness (pulmonary fibrosis), mass (obesity), or pathologic weakness (neuromuscular disorders). Since the alveoli and thorax are not fully stretched, they do not recoil as forcefully. Thus, the FEV1 is reduced. However, restrictive disease reduces all lung volumes proportionally. Hence, FEV1/FVC is normal, even though FEV1 is lower. The restrictive pattern is therefore normal FEV1/FVC (>70% predicted) with reduced TLC or FVC (<80% predicted).

Other patients have a process that obstructs air expulsion. This can be due to the reduction in alveolar elasticity (elastin destruction in emphysema) or to physical airway obstruction (bronchoconstriction in asthma). Whatever the cause, patients with an obstructive process have impaired expiration, which leads to air trapping (↑ RV and TLV). Inhalation is unaffected, so TV is normal. The obstructed expiration means that FEV1 is reduced (<70% predicted), and exhalation takes longer. Significant improvement of this obstruction with bronchodilators is diagnostic of asthma.

The final aspect of PFTs looks at the ability of the lungs to exchange the gas that makes it to the alveoli. This is done by having the patient inhale a known concentration of carbon monoxide (CO) and then exhale. Since Hgb has a higher affinity for CO than for O_2 and the concentration of CO in the blood is assumed to be zero, the absorption of CO never reaches steady state and is limited only by the amount of Hgb and the ability of CO to diffuse into the capillaries. Since the concentration of inhaled CO is known, the amount of CO absorbed can be calculated from the concentration of CO exhaled. This results in the patient's calculated diffusion capacity of CO (DLCO). Disease processes that ↓ the amount of Hgb in the lungs (anemia directly, and pulmonary embolus indirectly by limiting blood flow) or impair diffusion of CO across capillary membranes will ↓ the DLCO.

So, a patient with emphysema would have FEV1 <70% (obstructive) and ↓ DLCO since the alveoli and capillaries are destroyed (thus less diffusion). A patient with chronic bronchitis would have obstructive disease, but since their disease doesn't involve the alveoli, the DLCO would be normal. An asthmatic would have obstruction and normal or high DLCO (alveoli are intact → normal DLCO, but there can be an element of relatively ↑ blood flow → ↑ DLCO). A patient with pulmonary fibrosis would have stiff lungs, resulting in ↓ FEV1, ↓ FVC, and normal FEV1/FVC. Since there is fibrosis of the alveoli and capillaries, diffusion would be limited, and they would have ↓ DLCO. Finally, a patient with neuromuscular weakness would have a restrictive pattern with normal diffusion.

FIGURE 7.11

7-12 Pulmonary Function Tests

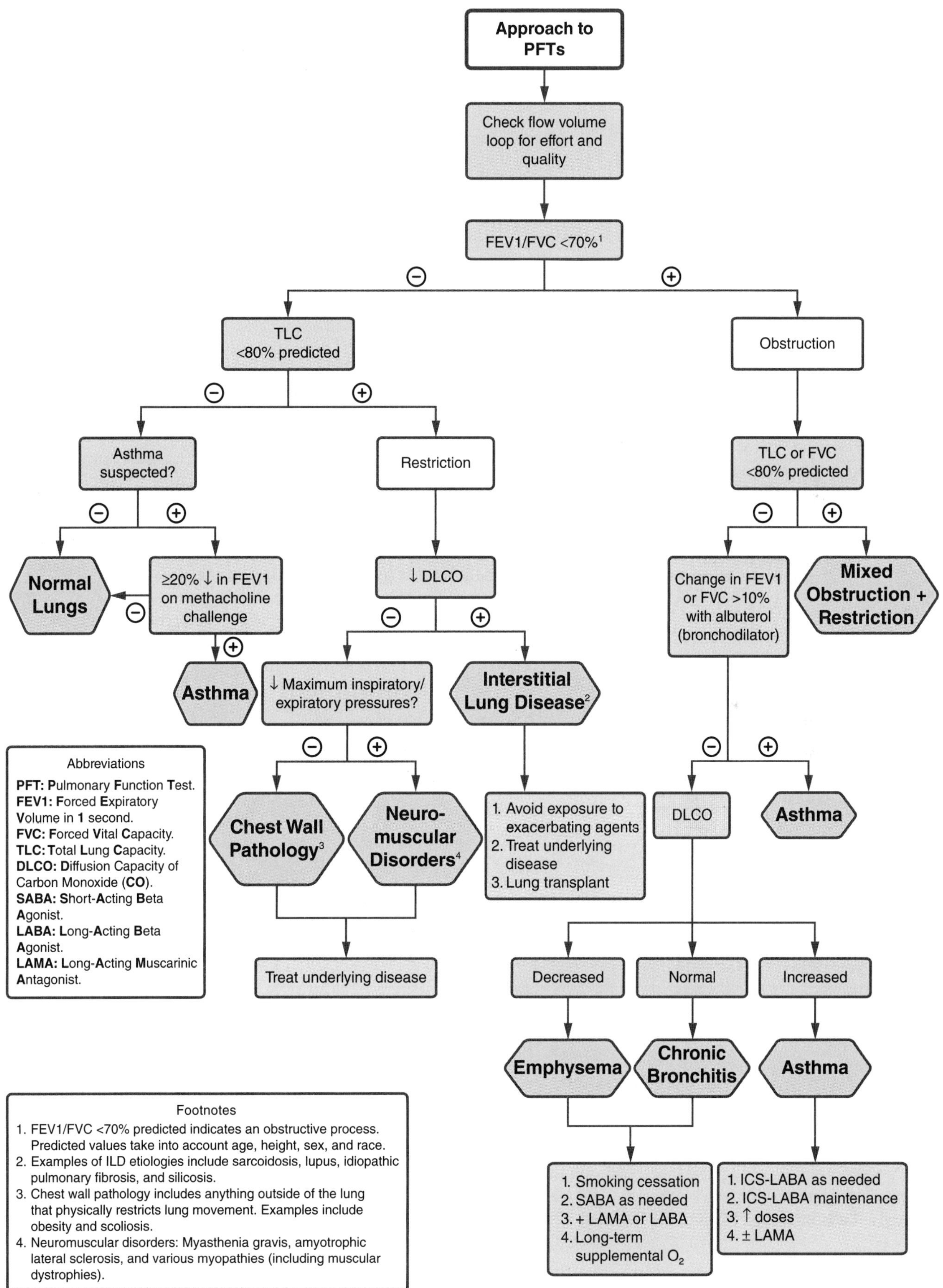
Approach to PFTs
Check flow volume loop for effort and quality
FEV1/FVC <70%[1]
⊖
⊕
TLC <80% predicted
Obstruction
⊖
⊕
Asthma suspected?
Restriction
TLC or FVC <80% predicted
⊖
⊕
Normal Lungs
≥20% ↓ in FEV1 on methacholine challenge
↓ DLCO
Change in FEV1 or FVC >10% with albuterol (bronchodilator)
Mixed Obstruction + Restriction
Asthma
↓ Maximum inspiratory/ expiratory pressures?
Interstitial Lung Disease[2]
Chest Wall Pathology[3]
Neuro-muscular Disorders[4]
1. Avoid exposure to exacerbating agents
2. Treat underlying disease
3. Lung transplant
DLCO
Asthma
Treat underlying disease
Decreased
Normal
Increased
Emphysema
Chronic Bronchitis
Asthma
1. Smoking cessation
2. SABA as needed
3. + LAMA or LABA
4. Long-term supplemental O_2
1. ICS-LABA as needed
2. ICS-LABA maintenance
3. ↑ doses
4. ± LAMA
Abbreviations
PFT: Pulmonary Function Test.
FEV1: Forced Expiratory Volume in 1 second.
FVC: Forced Vital Capacity.
TLC: Total Lung Capacity.
DLCO: Diffusion Capacity of Carbon Monoxide (CO).
SABA: Short-Acting Beta Agonist.
LABA: Long-Acting Beta Agonist.
LAMA: Long-Acting Muscarinic Antagonist.
Footnotes
1. FEV1/FVC <70% predicted indicates an obstructive process. Predicted values take into account age, height, sex, and race.
2. Examples of ILD etiologies include sarcoidosis, lupus, idiopathic pulmonary fibrosis, and silicosis.
3. Chest wall pathology includes anything outside of the lung that physically restricts lung movement. Examples include obesity and scoliosis.
4. Neuromuscular disorders: Myasthenia gravis, amyotrophic lateral sclerosis, and various myopathies (including muscular dystrophies).

FIGURE 7.12

7-12 Pulmonary Function Tests

ASTHMA

A 19-year-old F presents with nocturnal cough and episodic wheezing and chest tightness after exercise. **Exam** is unremarkable. PFTs show FEV1/FVC 0.60, TLC 85%. After albuterol, FEV1 increases 15%.

Management:

1. Avoid triggers.
2. Stepwise approach: ICS-LABA PRN → CS-LABA BID scheduled → dose escalation of ICS-LABA → add LAMA or phenotypic targets. See the Table on p. 278 for more information.
3. IV steroids, Mg, and albuterol nebulizers for severe exacerbation.

Complications: Respiratory failure during severe attack.

HYF: Asthma is a type I (IgE-mediated) hypersensitivity reaction. Aspirin, exercise, allergens, and respiratory pathogens are common causes of exacerbations. Pulsus paradoxus (decrease in SBP >10 mmHg with inspiration) can be seen in severe attacks. Hyperventilation during an asthma attack decreases $PaCO_2$, causing a respiratory alkalosis. Normal blood gas during an acute attack is a sign of respiratory fatigue and impending respiratory failure. PFTs may be normal when not in acute exacerbation; in this case, exaggerated bronchoconstriction with a methacholine challenge can help diagnose asthma.

INTERSTITIAL LUNG DISEASE (ILD)

A 70-year-old M carpenter with PMH of tobacco use disorder presents with months of dry cough and progressive dyspnea. On **exam**, he has fine inspiratory crackles, digital clubbing, no edema, no JVD, and SpO_2 87% on room air. **Labs** show normal BNP and negative, rheumatologic panel (ANA, RF, CCP). On **imaging**, CXR shows a reticular pattern. Chest CT demonstrates reticular opacities and honeycombing. PFTs show a restrictive pattern with ↑ FEV1/FVC, ↓ FVC, ↓ FEV1, ↓ TLC, ↓ FVC, ↓ DLCO. TTE is normal. Tissue biopsy confirms the diagnosis.

Management:

1. Rule out rheumatologic or cardiac etiologies.
2. Remove potential environmental triggers.
3. Treat underlying disease, if applicable.
4. O_2 supplementation if needed. Influenza and pneumococcal vaccination.
5. Further management varies by ILD subtype (see below).

Complications: Aspiration, right heart failure.

HYF: ILD can be caused by many exposures and conditions: Systemic or connective tissue diseases (including sarcoidosis, vasculitis, scleroderma, rheumatoid arthritis, amyloidosis), environmental exposures (mold, birds, dust particles, hypersensitivity pneumonitis, pneumoconioses as described below), and medications (amiodarone, methotrexate, nitrofurantoin, bleomycin). Treatment for idiopathic pulmonary fibrosis (IPF) includes antifibrotics (pirfenidone) and tyrosine kinase inhibitors (nintedanib). ILD due to exposure or underlying disease may respond to steroids or biologics (rituximab). Treat cryptogenic organizing pneumonia (COP) with prednisone. Treatment for acute interstitial pneumonia (AIP) is supportive care; high-dose steroids can be trialed, but it is not typically steroid-responsive.

Pneumoconioses

Disorder	Risk Factors	Objective Findings	Complications
Silicosis	Mine worker with silica or glass, sandblasting, ceramics	Upper zone predominant nodular infiltrates ± calcifications, hilar adenopathy	Massive fibrosis, emphysema, risk for TB
Asbestosis	Jobs involving insulation, demolition, construction or shipbuilding decades prior to presentation	Calcified linear pleural plaques, ferruginous bodies in alveolar septae	Increased risk for lung cancer (especially in smokers), particularly bronchogenic carcinoma; mesothelioma
Anthracosis (Coal Dust)	Coal Miners	Upper zone nodular infiltrates	Massive fibrosis, emphysema
Berylliosis	Nuclear or aerospace field worker, ceramics worker	Diffuse opacities, hilar adenopathy, noncaseating granulomas	Respiratory impairment, may require long-term corticosteroids

COPD (EMPHYSEMA AND CHRONIC BRONCHITIS)

A 65-year-old M with 50-pack-year smoking history presents to the office with progressive dyspnea and cough. On **exam**, he has prolonged expiration, expiratory wheezes, and decreased breath sounds. **Labs/imaging**: NT-proBNP normal, CXR with hyperinflation and diaphragm flattening, EKG with poor R-wave progression and low voltages, and PFTs with obstructive pattern.

Management:

1. Smoking cessation.
2. Albuterol as needed.
3. Long-acting muscarinic antagonist and/or beta agonist.
4. Long-term supplemental O_2.

7-12 Pulmonary Function Tests

5. Steroids ± azithromycin for exacerbations.
6. Vaccines: Influenza, Pneumococcal, and, COVID.
7. Lung cancer screening (age 55–80 + 30 pack-year smoking history + active user or quit (<15 years ago).

Complications: COPD exacerbations, cor pulmonale.

HYF: Two subtypes of COPD with significant overlap in pathology and presentation: Chronic bronchitis and emphysema. Chronic bronchitis is defined by productive cough for ≥ 3 months/year for 2 consecutive years (and other causes ruled out). These patients are described as "blue bloaters" because they tend to be overweight and are hypercarbic/hypoxemic early in their disease course (hence "blue"). Emphysema is defined by distal airway destruction and dilation. Patients with emphysema are described as "pink puffers." They appear more cachectic and develop hypoxemia/hypercarbia later in their disease course (so they stay "pink"). COPD exacerbation is a clinical diagnosis that includes worsening cough, sputum production, and/or dyspnea.

Neuromuscular Disorders: See p. 718.

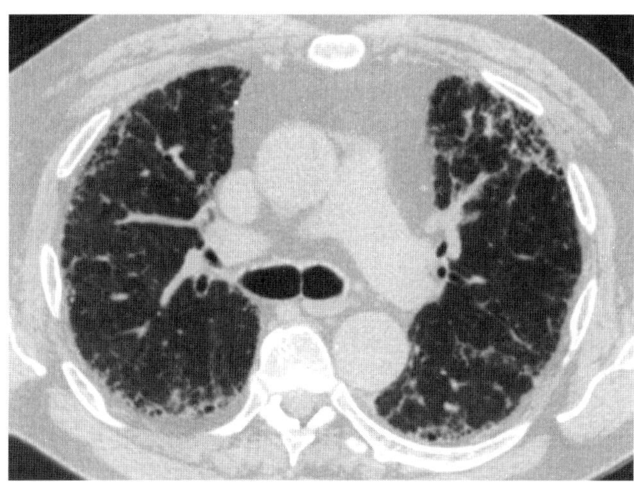

A

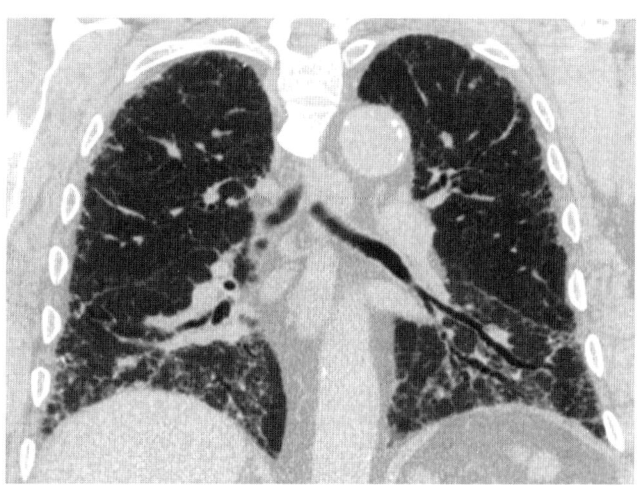

B

(**A**) Axial and (**B**) coronal CT images of interstitial pulmonary fibrosis, depicting symmetric, basilar- and peripheral-predominant reticular opacities, traction bronchiectasis, and honeycombing.

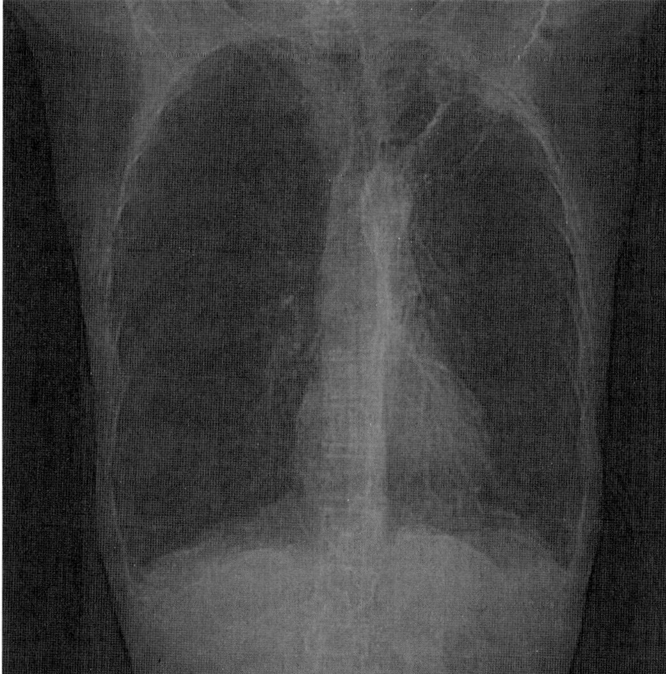

Lung hyperinflation with flattened hemidiaphragms and increased bronchovascular markings seen in COPD.

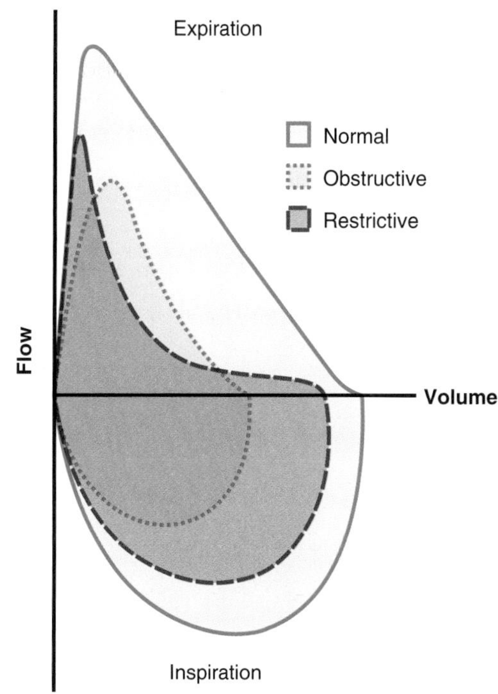
Expiration
Normal
Obstructive
Restrictive
Flow
Volume
Inspiration

PFT flow volume loops.

7-13 Acute Cough

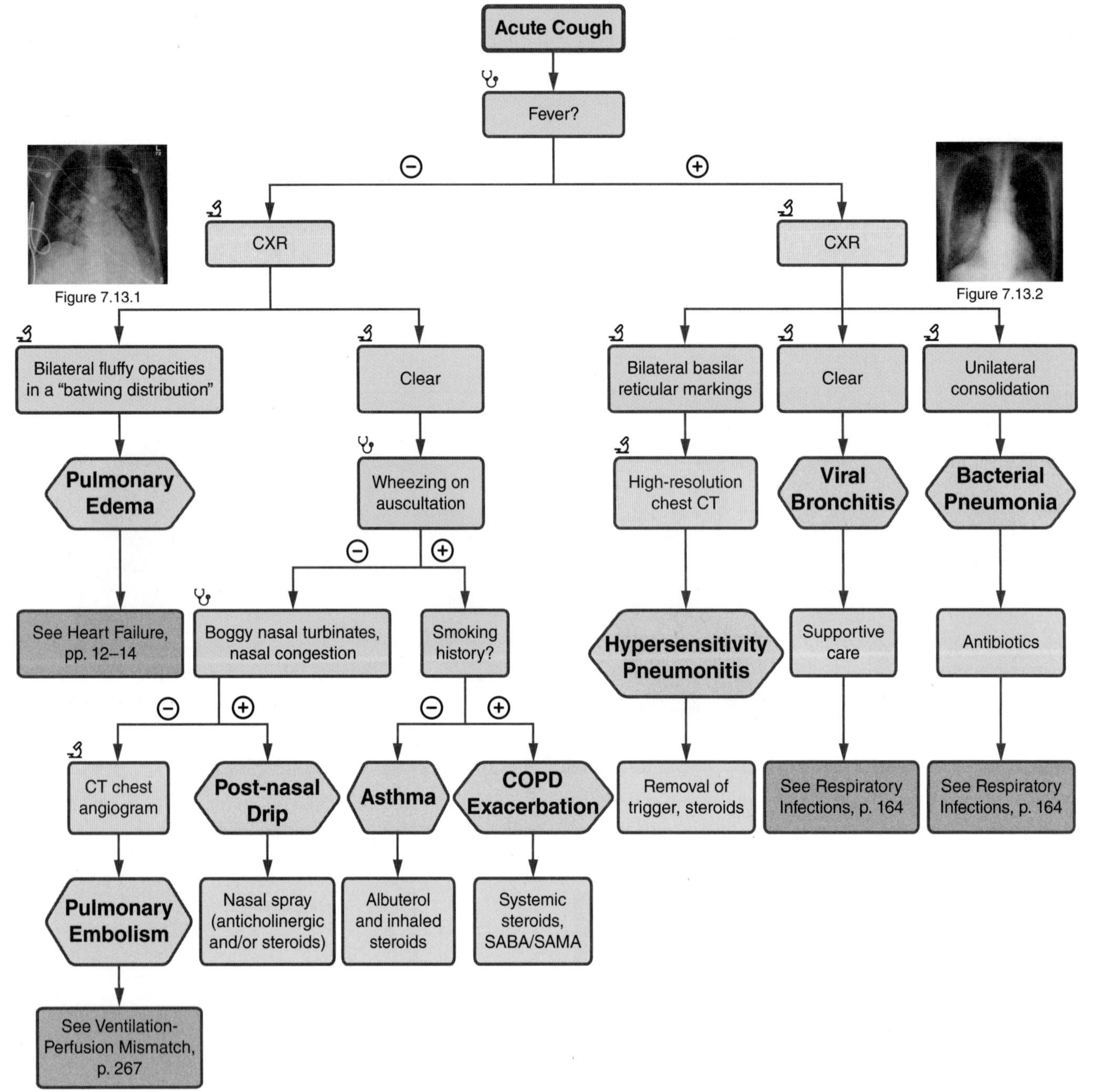
Acute Cough
Fever?
⊖
⊕
CXR
CXR
Figure 7.13.1
Figure 7.13.2
Bilateral fluffy opacities in a "batwing distribution"
Clear
Bilateral basilar reticular markings
Clear
Unilateral consolidation
Pulmonary Edema
Wheezing on auscultation
High-resolution chest CT
Viral Bronchitis
Bacterial Pneumonia
See Heart Failure, pp. 12–14
Boggy nasal turbinates, nasal congestion
Smoking history?
Hypersensitivity Pneumonitis
Supportive care
Antibiotics
CT chest angiogram
Post-nasal Drip
Asthma
COPD Exacerbation
Removal of trigger, steroids
See Respiratory Infections, p. 164
See Respiratory Infections, p. 164
Pulmonary Embolism
Nasal spray (anticholinergic and/or steroids)
Albuterol and inhaled steroids
Systemic steroids, SABA/SAMA
See Ventilation-Perfusion Mismatch, p. 267

FIGURE 7.13

7-13 Acute Cough

PULMONARY EDEMA

A 60-year-old F with PMH of STEMI s/p PCI and HTN presents with 2 weeks of leg swelling, orthopnea, and cough. Exam shows elevated JVP, bibasilar crackles, and symmetric 2+ pitting edema up to both knees. Labs show hyponatremia and elevated BNP. On imaging, CXR reveals increased vascular congestion bilaterally.

Management:

1. Diuresis with loop diuretics (eg, furosemide).
2. Correct the trigger for decompensated heart failure (eg, arrhythmia, diet indiscretion, infection).

Complications: Acute hypoxemia requiring noninvasive ventilation.

HYF: Pulmonary edema is secondary to a primary process (eg, heart failure as in this patient, mitral stenosis/regurgitation, malignant HTN). Stabilize the patient, if applicable, and treat the underlying etiology.

PULMONARY EMBOLISM

A 43-year-old F with PMH of obesity, tobacco use disorder, PCOS on oral contraceptive pills, and recently diagnosed breast cancer presents after a long car trip with unilateral calf swelling, pleuritic chest pain (worse on inspiration), and cough productive of scant hemoptysis. Exam shows sinus tachycardia. Labs reveal elevated D-dimer and leukocytosis. On imaging, CTA chest shows large bilateral PEs.

Management:

1. Anticoagulation with heparin drip.
2. If hemodynamically unstable, thrombectomy or tPA.

Complications:

- Obstructive shock and death.
- Lung infarction.
- Pulmonary hypertension and right heart failure.

HYF: Risk stratify using Wells' criteria (score >4 means that PE is likely). In patients with high probability of PE, give anticoagulation before confirmatory testing. Thrombolysis or thrombectomy is indicated in cases of massive PE (saddle PE) causing right heart failure and hemodynamic instability; patients would present with hypotension, pulmonary edema, and JVD, with point-of-care TTE showing signs of right heart strain.

See Ventilation-Perfusion Mismatch, p. 267 for further information.

POST-NASAL DRIP (UPPER AIRWAY COUGH SYNDROME)

A 38-year-old F with PMH of seasonal allergies and recent URI presents with a cough that is worse at night. Exam shows boggy nasal mucosa and cobblestoning of posterior oropharynx.

Management:

1. Intranasal steroid sprays.
2. Antihistamines (eg, cetirizine, loratadine) to treat allergies.

Complications:

- Sore throat.
- Halitosis.
- Ear infections (due to blocked eustachian tubes).

HYF: Refer to Chronic Cough on p. 278.

ASTHMA

A 14-year-old M with PMH of eczema and seasonal allergies presents with nonproductive cough and dyspnea. Exam shows diffuse bilateral expiratory wheezes and prolonged expiratory phase.

Management:

1. Short-acting albuterol inhalers for rescue.
2. If stable, inhaled steroids as maintenance. If significant dyspnea or progressive symptoms, systemic steroids.

Complications: Frequent hospitalizations and sequelae of steroid use.

HYF: Normal blood gasses, rather than the expected respiratory alkalosis due to tachypnea, are a sign of fatigue and impending respiratory failure. Diagnose asthma with PFTs showing ↓ FEV1/FVC ratio that improves with bronchodilators. On PFTs, the pre-bronchodilator exam will be normal (for patients with well-controlled asthma) or demonstrate obstruction, while the post-bronchodilator exam will show an improvement in obstruction. If the pre-bronchodilator exam is normal and clinical suspicion is high for asthma, then a methacholine challenge test may be performed. A baseline FEV1 is obtained and the patient then inhales methacholine; a FEV1 decrease of ≥20% supports a diagnosis of asthma.

COPD Exacerbation: See p. 266.

(Continued)

7-13 Acute Cough

HYPERSENSITIVITY PNEUMONITIS

A 53-year-old F zookeeper presents with several weeks of cough, fevers, and myalgias. **Exam** shows trace dry crackles on auscultation. **Labs** show eosinophilia. On **imaging**, CT chest shows reticular markings.

Management:

1. Avoidance of the trigger.
2. Systemic steroids.

Complications: Chronic lung disease, upper lobe fibrosis

HYF: Repeat exposure to irritants causes alveolar thickening and granulomatous inflammation. Acutely, patients may have cough, dyspnea, fever, and malaise, all of which arise within 6 hours of antigen exposure. Common irritant antigens include mold and bird droppings. Chronic exposure can lead to pulmonary fibrosis. The best treatment is antigen avoidance.

VIRAL BRONCHITIS

A 37-year-old M presents with harsh nonproductive cough and concurrent nasal congestion. **Exam** and **imaging** are unremarkable.

Management:

1. No antibiotics indicated.
2. Supportive care with antitussives.

Complications: Bacterial superinfection.

HYF: Common viral pathogens include rhinovirus, adenovirus, influenza, parainfluenza, RSV.

BACTERIAL PNEUMONIA

A 65-year-old M with PMH of DM2 and COPD presents with productive cough, fevers. **Exam** shows right base crackles and dullness on percussion. **Labs** show leukocytosis. On **imaging**, CXR shows lobar consolidation.

Management:

1. Antibiotics (refer to ID section on p. 166).

Complications: Empyema, sepsis.

HYF: Healthy young patients: *S. pneumoniae, M. pneumoniae, C. pneumoniae, H. influenzae,* viral. Elderly with comorbidities: *S. pneumoniae,* aerobic GNRs (*E. coli, Klebsiella*), *S. aureus, Legionella,* viruses.

7-14 Chronic Cough

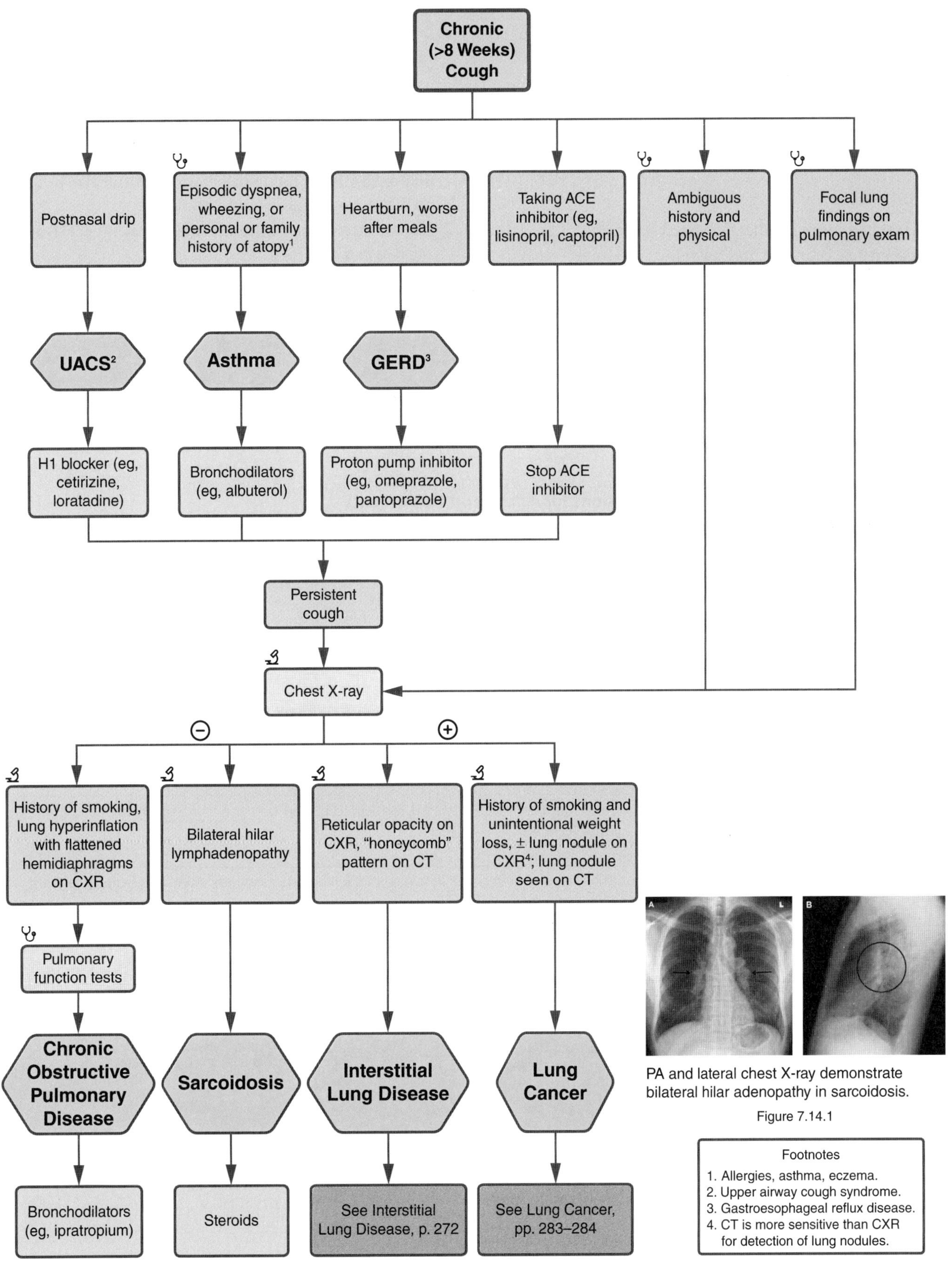
Chronic (>8 Weeks) Cough
Postnasal drip
Episodic dyspnea, wheezing, or personal or family history of atopy[1]
Heartburn, worse after meals
Taking ACE inhibitor (eg, lisinopril, captopril)
Ambiguous history and physical
Focal lung findings on pulmonary exam
UACS[2]
Asthma
GERD[3]
H1 blocker (eg, cetirizine, loratadine)
Bronchodilators (eg, albuterol)
Proton pump inhibitor (eg, omeprazole, pantoprazole)
Stop ACE inhibitor
Persistent cough
Chest X-ray
⊖
⊕
History of smoking, lung hyperinflation with flattened hemidiaphragms on CXR
Bilateral hilar lymphadenopathy
Reticular opacity on CXR, "honeycomb" pattern on CT
History of smoking and unintentional weight loss, ± lung nodule on CXR[4]; lung nodule seen on CT
Pulmonary function tests
Chronic Obstructive Pulmonary Disease
Sarcoidosis
Interstitial Lung Disease
Lung Cancer
Bronchodilators (eg, ipratropium)
Steroids
See Interstitial Lung Disease, p. 272
See Lung Cancer, pp. 283–284
A
L
B

PA and lateral chest X-ray demonstrate bilateral hilar adenopathy in sarcoidosis.

Figure 7.14.1

Footnotes

1. Allergies, asthma, eczema.
2. Upper airway cough syndrome.
3. Gastroesophageal reflux disease.
4. CT is more sensitive than CXR for detection of lung nodules.

FIGURE 7.14

7-14 Chronic Cough

UPPER AIRWAY COUGH SYNDROME (POST-NASAL DRIP)

A 24-year-old F with PMH of seasonal allergies presents with a chronic nonproductive cough that is worse at night. On exam, she has normal vitals and lung auscultation, boggy nasal turbinates, and cobblestoning on her posterior pharynx.

Management:

1. Intranasal steroids (eg, fluticasone nasal spray).
2. H1 blockers (eg, cetirizine, loratidine).

Complications:

- Sore throat.
- Halitosis.
- Ear infections (due to blocked eustachian tubes).

HYF: Also known as upper airway cough syndrome. Characteristic history is nocturnal worsening.

ASTHMA (COUGH VARIANT)

A 26-year-old M with PMH of eczema presents with chronic cough worse with exertion, seasonal changes, and cat exposures. On exam, he has diffuse expiratory wheezes on lung auscultation.

Management:

1. ICS-LABA PRN, though albuterol PRN can also be used as the first step for cough-variant asthma.
2. Treat concomitant environmental allergies (eg, H1-blockers such as cetrizine).
3. Inhaled corticosteroids.

Complications: Asthma exacerbation leading to respiratory failure.

HYF: See treatment options below. Refer to "Wheezing" or "Pulmonary Function Tests" on pp. 257–259, 270–273 for additional information.

Initial Asthma Treatment: Recommended Options for Adults and Adolescents

Presenting Symptoms	Preferred Initial Treatment
All patients.	SABA-only treatment (without ICS) is not recommended.
Infrequent asthma symptoms (eg, less than twice a month).	• As-needed low-dose ICS-formoterol. Other options include taking ICS whenever SABA is taken, in combination or separate inhalers.
Asthma symptoms or need for reliever twice a month or more.	• Low-dose ICS with as needed SABA, *or* • As needed low-dose ICS-formoterol. Other options include LTRA (less effective than ICS) or ICS whenever SABA is taken either in combination or separate inhalers. Consider likely adherence with controller if reliever is SABA.
Troublesome asthma symptoms most days; or waking due to asthma ≥1 time per week, especially if any risk factors exist.	• Low-dose ICS-LABA as maintenance and reliever therapy with ICS-formoterol, or as conventional maintenance treatment with as-needed SABA, *or* • Medium-dose ICS with as-needed SABA.
Initial asthma presentation is with severely uncontrolled asthma or with an acute exacerbation.	• Short course of OCS *and* start regular controller treatment with high-dose ICS or medium-dose ICS-LABA.

ICS, inhaled corticosteroids; LABA, long-acting β_2-agonist; LTRA, leukotriene-receptor antagonist; OCS: oral corticosteroids; SABA: short-acting β_2-agonist.

GERD: See, p. 80.

COPD: See p. 258, 266, 272, 279–280.

7-14 Chronic Cough

Pharmacologic Therapy for COPD

	Principal Action	Benefits	Indication	Adverse Effects
Bronchodilators				
β_2-Agonists. Short-acting β-agonists (SABAs; albuterol, levalbuterol). Long-acting β-agonists (LABAs; formoterol, salmeterol).	Promote smooth muscle relaxation by stimulating β_2-adrenergic receptors and increasing cyclic adenosine monophosphate (AMP).	SABAs: Improve FEV1 and symptoms. LABAs: Improve FEV1 and lung volumes, dyspnea, and health status; reduce exacerbations and number of hospitalizations.	SABAs: First-line initial therapy for mild intermittent symptoms as needed. LABAs: For patients with persistent symptoms at a dose of 1 or 2 puffs BID.	Resting tachycardia, cardiac rhythm disturbances, tremor, sleep disturbances, hypokalemia.
Anticholinergics. Short-acting antimuscarinics (SAMAs; ipratropium, oxitropium). Long-acting antimuscarinics (LAMAs; tiotropium, umeclidinium).	Promote smooth muscle relaxation by blocking muscarinic receptors.	SAMAs: Small benefits in lung function, health status, and requirement for oral steroids. LAMAs: Improve symptoms and health status, decrease exacerbations and hospitalizations.	Short-acting: Can be used for symptoms as needed, less rapid onset than β_2-agonists but effect lasts longer. Long-acting: first-line therapy for patients with persistent symptoms at a dose of 1 puff daily.	Dry mouth, bitter or metallic taste. Closed-angle glaucoma using solutions with a facemask.
Methylxanthines (theophylline).	Promote smooth muscle relaxation by acting as a nonspecific phosphodiesterase inhibitor that increases intracellular cyclic AMP.	Less effective than long-acting bronchodilators, improved FEV1 and symptoms when added to salmeterol.	Third-line agent for patients with persistent symptoms.	Toxicity is dose-related, clearance declines with age, atrial and ventricular arrhythmias, grand mal convulsions, headaches, insomnia, nausea, heartburn, significant interactions with medications including warfarin and digoxin.
Anti-inflammatory Agents				
Inhaled corticosteroids (ICS).	Reduce inflammation.	Possible slower decline in FEV1.	For patients with stage III–IV COPD or for those with repeated exacerbations, blood eosinophil counts may predict the effect of ICS.	Increased likelihood of oral candidiasis, hoarseness, bruising, and pneumonia, possibly associated with decreased bone mineral density.
PDE4 inhibitors (roflumilast).	Reduce inflammation through inhibition of the breakdown of intracellular AMP.	Improves lung function and reduces exacerbations.	For patients with stage III or IV COPD and history of exacerbations.	Cannot give with theophylline, nausea, anorexia, abdominal pain, diarrhea, sleep disturbances, headache.
Antibiotics.	Antimicrobial agents.	For COPD exacerbations, reduces risk of treatment failure and death.	Not generally recommended for use in chronic COPD management. May consider azithromycin (250 mg 3 times a week) in patients who have optimized other therapies with frequent hospitalizations. Use for COPD exacerbations.	Increased incidence of bacterial resistance, tinnitus, and hearing impairment.
Mucolytic agents. (erdosteine, carbocysteine, and *N*-acetyl cysteine).	Decrease sputum viscosity and adhesiveness to facilitate expectoration.	Reduces exacerbations in select populations.		
Oral glucocorticoids.	Reduce inflammation.	Use for COPD exacerbations to increase the time to subsequent exacerbations, decrease rate of treatment failure, shorten hospital stays, and improve hypoxemia and FEV1.	Avoid for chronic COPD management. Use for COPD exacerbations.	Hypertension, hyperglycemia, osteoporosis, myopathy, delirium.

COPD, chronic obstructive pulmonary disease; FEV1, forced expiratory volume in 1 second.

7-14 Chronic Cough

Management of COPD Based on Clinical Severity

Symptom Severity	Non-pharmacologic	Medications (first choice)
Few symptoms and 0–1 exacerbations per year, and/or mild impairment.	Smoking cessation, physical activity, vaccinations.[1]	Short-acting bronchodilator as needed: β_2-agonist (albuterol) OR anticholinergics (ipratropium).
More symptoms and 0–1 exacerbations per year, and/or mild impairment.	Smoking cessation, physical activity, vaccinations, pulmonary rehabilitation.	Long-acting bronchodilator: Anticholinergics (tiotropium) OR β_2-agonist (salmeterol).
Few symptoms and ≥2 exacerbations per year, and/or severe impairment.	Smoking cessation, physical activity, vaccinations, pulmonary rehabilitation.	Inhaled corticosteroid (prednisone) AND long-acting bronchodilator OR combination long-acting β_2-agonist and anticholinergic.
More symptoms and ≥2 exacerbations per year, and/or severe impairment.	Smoking cessation, physical activity, vaccinations, pulmonary rehabilitation.	Long-term oxygen therapy (15–20 hours daily) as appropriate.[2]

1. Vaccinations: <65 years of age: PPSV 23 alone; ≥65 years of age: PCV 13 + PPSV 23; all ages: Influenza annually.
2. Of note, supplemental O_2 can worsen hypercapnia. Titrate O_2 to goal SpO_2 90–93%.

SARCOIDOSIS

A 26-year-old F with PMH of uveitis and erythema nodosum presents with chronic nonproductive cough, night sweats, and weight loss. **Exam** shows tender subcutaneous nodules along the extensor surface of her legs. On **imaging**, CXR shows bilateral bulky hilar lymphadenopathy.

Management:

1. Immunosuppression with steroids (1st-line).
2. Transition to steroid-sparing agents (methotrexate, TNF-α inhibitors such as infliximab and adalimumab, anti-CD20 agents such as rituximab).

Complications:

- Restrictive lung disease.
- Multisystem involvement: Cardiomyopathy and cardiac conduction abnormalities, uveitis, arthritis, polyneuropathies, 7th cranial nerve palsy (often mistaken for Bell's palsy), skin (erythema nodosum, lupus pernia).

HYF: Clinical and radiologic evidence can suggest sarcoidosis, but diagnosis requires biopsy, often transbronchial. Pathologic hallmark is noncaseating granulomas. Can be associated with hypercalcemia due to excess 1–25-OH vitamin D from granulomas. Chest imaging demonstrates bilateral hilar adenopathy. Presentation can be subacute (a few months) with non-specific symptoms: Malaise, cough, fever, and rash. More common in younger adults, especially African-American women. Löfgren's syndrome is a specific acute clinical presentation that consists of erythema nodosum, hilar adenopathy, migratory polyarthralgias, and fever.

INTERSTITIAL LUNG DISEASE

A 54-year-old F with PMH of rheumatoid arthritis presents with chronic cough and dyspnea. On **exam**, she has shallow inspirations, and lung auscultation is notable for bilateral fine dry crackles. On **imaging**, CXR shows diffuse interstitial and reticular markings.

Management:

1. High-resolution CT is best next step (evaluate for honeycombing, lobular septal thickening).
2. PFTs will show restrictive pattern and decreased DLCO.
3. Treat underlying autoimmune disease (steroids, immunosuppression).

Complications:

- Recurrent flares, high mortality.
- Chronic progressive respiratory failure.
- Pulmonary hypertension.

HYF: Usually due to underlying rheumatologic or autoimmune conditions: SLE, rheumatoid arthritis, systemic sclerosis, sarcoidosis. See "Interstitial Lung Disease" in the PFTs section on p. 272.

LUNG CANCER (POST-OBSTRUCTIVE PNEUMONIA)

An 82-year-old M with PMH of recurrent right middle lobe PNA, weight loss, and 80-pack-year smoking history presents with chronic cough and scant hemoptysis. On **exam**, he is tachypneic and frequently coughs. On **imaging**, CXR shows atelectasis of RML, and CT chest shows a spiculated 2-cm nodule obstructing the RML bronchus.

Management:

1. Antibiotics for post-obstructive pneumonia.
2. Diagnose lung cancer with biopsy (endobronchial or CT-guided).
3. Treatment depends on the type of cancer.

Complications:

- Post-obstructive pneumonia can lead to empyema, lung abscess, and fistula formation.
- Hypercalcemia if squamous cell cancer (via PTHrP).
  - Pancoast syndrome or SVC syndrome due to mechanical compression.
- Paraneoplastic syndromes (esp. with small cell lung cancer): SIADH, hypercortisolism, encephalomyelitis, cerebellar degeneration, Lambert-Eaton myasthenic syndrome (LEMS).

HYF: Post-obstructive pneumonia can be a complication of lung cancer, particularly in advanced stages, and may be the first clinical manifestation of malignancy. Suspect underlying lung cancer in a patient with risk factors (eg, extensive smoking history) who presents with recurrent pneumonia in the same location. Screen for lung cancer with yearly low-dose CT for age 55–80, >30-pack-year history, and smoking within 15 years.

7-15 Hemoptysis

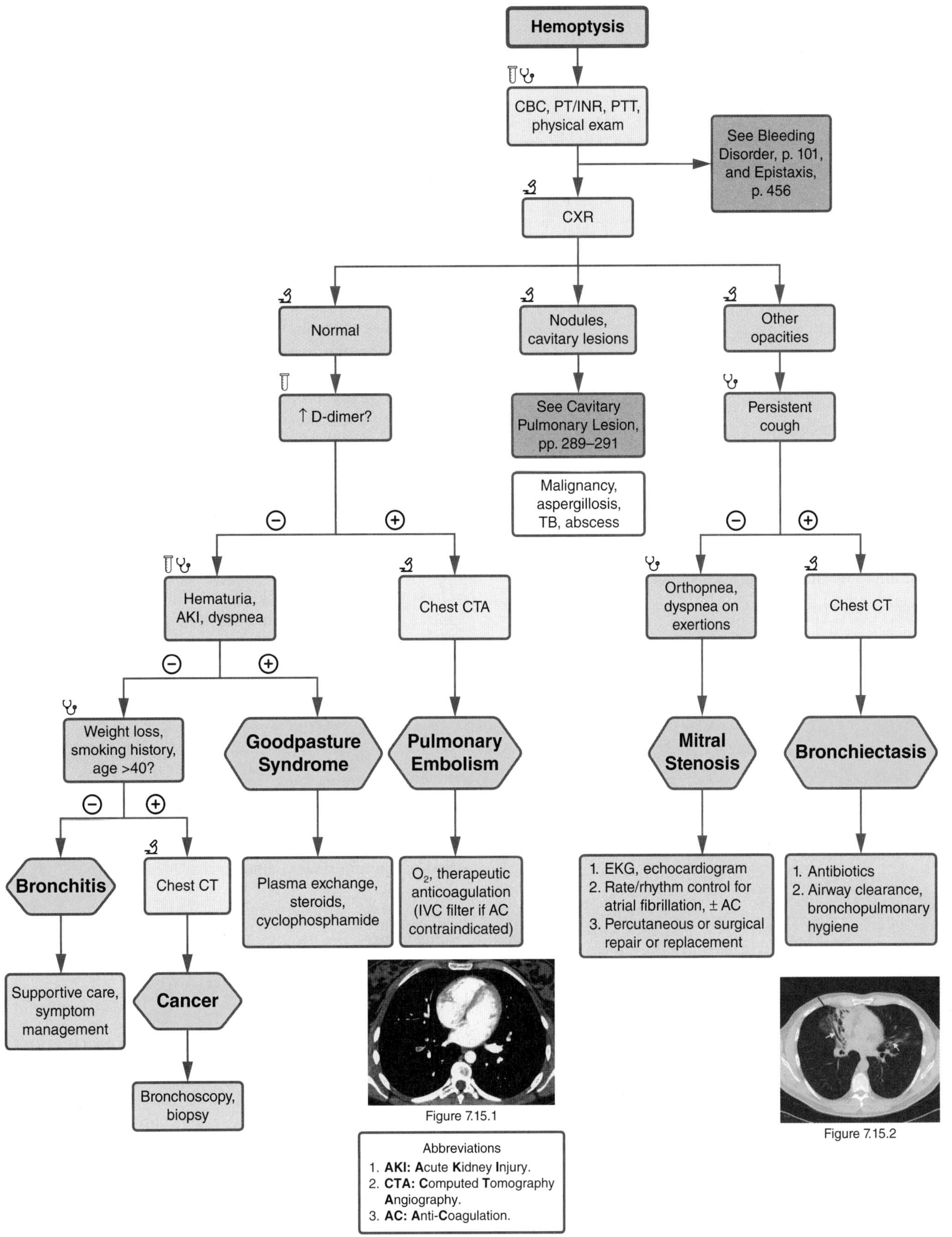
Hemoptysis
CBC, PT/INR, PTT, physical exam
See Bleeding Disorder, p. 101, and Epistaxis, p. 456
CXR
Normal
Nodules, cavitary lesions
Other opacities
↑ D-dimer?
See Cavitary Pulmonary Lesion, pp. 289–291
Malignancy, aspergillosis, TB, abscess
Persistent cough
Hematuria, AKI, dyspnea
Chest CTA
Orthopnea, dyspnea on exertions
Chest CT
Weight loss, smoking history, age >40?
Goodpasture Syndrome
Pulmonary Embolism
Mitral Stenosis
Bronchiectasis
Bronchitis
Chest CT
Plasma exchange, steroids, cyclophosphamide
O_2, therapeutic anticoagulation (IVC filter if AC contraindicated)
1. EKG, echocardiogram
2. Rate/rhythm control for atrial fibrillation, ± AC
3. Percutaneous or surgical repair or replacement
1. Antibiotics
2. Airway clearance, bronchopulmonary hygiene
Supportive care, symptom management
Cancer
Bronchoscopy, biopsy
Figure 7.15.1
Figure 7.15.2
Abbreviations
1. AKI: Acute Kidney Injury.
2. CTA: Computed Tomography Angiography.
3. AC: Anti-Coagulation.

FIGURE 7.15

7-15 Hemoptysis

BRONCHITIS

A. A 27-year-old M presents with rhinorrhea and a harsh cough with scant bloody sputum without fevers or chills. Exam is normal.

B. A 76-year-old M smoker with HTN and PAD presents with chronic morning cough productive of scant bloody sputum without weight loss or night sweats. On exam, lung auscultation reveals diffuse coarse rhonchi without crackles.

Management:

1. Symptomatic management with expectorants (guaifenesin).
2. Smoking cessation.
3. If chronic bronchitis, refer to COPD on pp. 258, 266, 272, 279–280 for further information.

Complications:

- Acute: Self-limiting.
- Chronic: Supplemental O_2 if resting SaO_2 is ≤88%.

HYF: Chronic bronchitis is defined as productive cough for >3 months per year for 2 consecutive years. Bronchitis can be chronic associated with COPD and smoking or acute and associated with a viral infection. Acute on chronic symptoms are usually from a viral etiology.

BRONCHIECTASIS

A. A 22-year-old M with PMH of chronic pulmonary infections and exocrine pancreatic insufficiency presents with chronic cough, scant hemoptysis, and recurrent bouts of productive purulent sputum. Exam reveals diffuse rales. On imaging, CT chest shows dilated bronchial cysts. PFTs show ↓ FEV1/FVC ratio on PFTs.

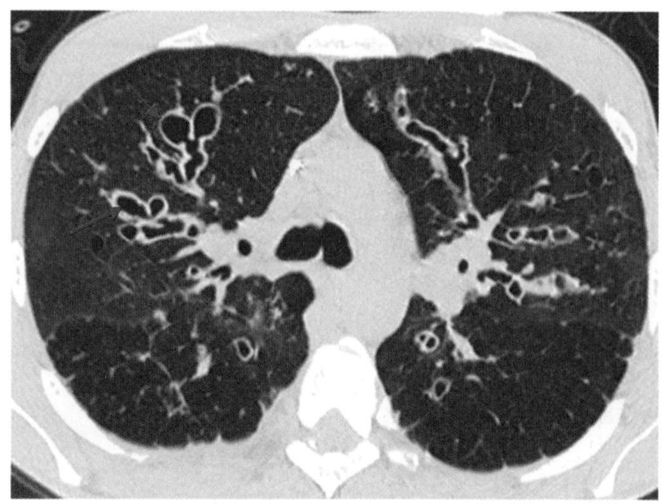

CT scan of diffuse, cystic bronchiectasis (red arrows).

B. A 44-year-old M with PMH of Crohn's disease presents with progressive dyspnea and periodic bouts of sputum production and scant hemoptysis. On imaging, CXR shows finger-tracing.

Management:

1. Treat the underlying inflammatory condition.
2. Pulmonary hygiene with chest physiotherapy.
3. Antibiotics for acute exacerbations and purulent sputum.
4. Definitive therapy is lobectomy or lung transplant.

Complications: Chronic respiratory infections, pulmonary fibrosis.

HYF: Most common with history of lung infections, cystic fibrosis (CF), immunodeficiency, localized airway obstruction, autoimmune disease, or inflammatory bowel disease. CXR can show tram lines and dilated bronchi with peribronchial inflammation ("finger-tracing"). CT chest can show dilated balloon cysts with debris (lower lobe predominant).

GOODPASTURE SYNDROME

A 24-year-old M with PMH of asthma presents with malaise, hematuria, progressive leg and facial swelling, and hemoptysis. Exam shows a blood pressure of 164/95 and periorbital edema. On labs, UA shows 3+ blood with RBC casts. On imaging, CXR shows pulmonary infiltrates. Renal biopsy shows linear deposits on immunofluorescence.

Management:

1. Plasma exchange therapy and pulse dose steroids.

Complications: Acute hypoxemic respiratory failure, ESRD.

HYF: Also known as anti-glomerular basement membrane (anti-GBM) disease. Peak incidence in males aged 20. Anti-glomerular basement membrane disease with antibasement membrane antibodies. Sputum shows hemosiderin-laden macrophages.

Lung Cancer: See pp. 280, 284, 290.

Pulmonary Embolism: See pp. 16, 267, 275, 285.

Mitral Stenosis: See Valvular diseases, pp. 42–43.

Tuberculosis: See Infectious Diseases Section on TB, p. 169.

7-16 Pulmonary Nodules

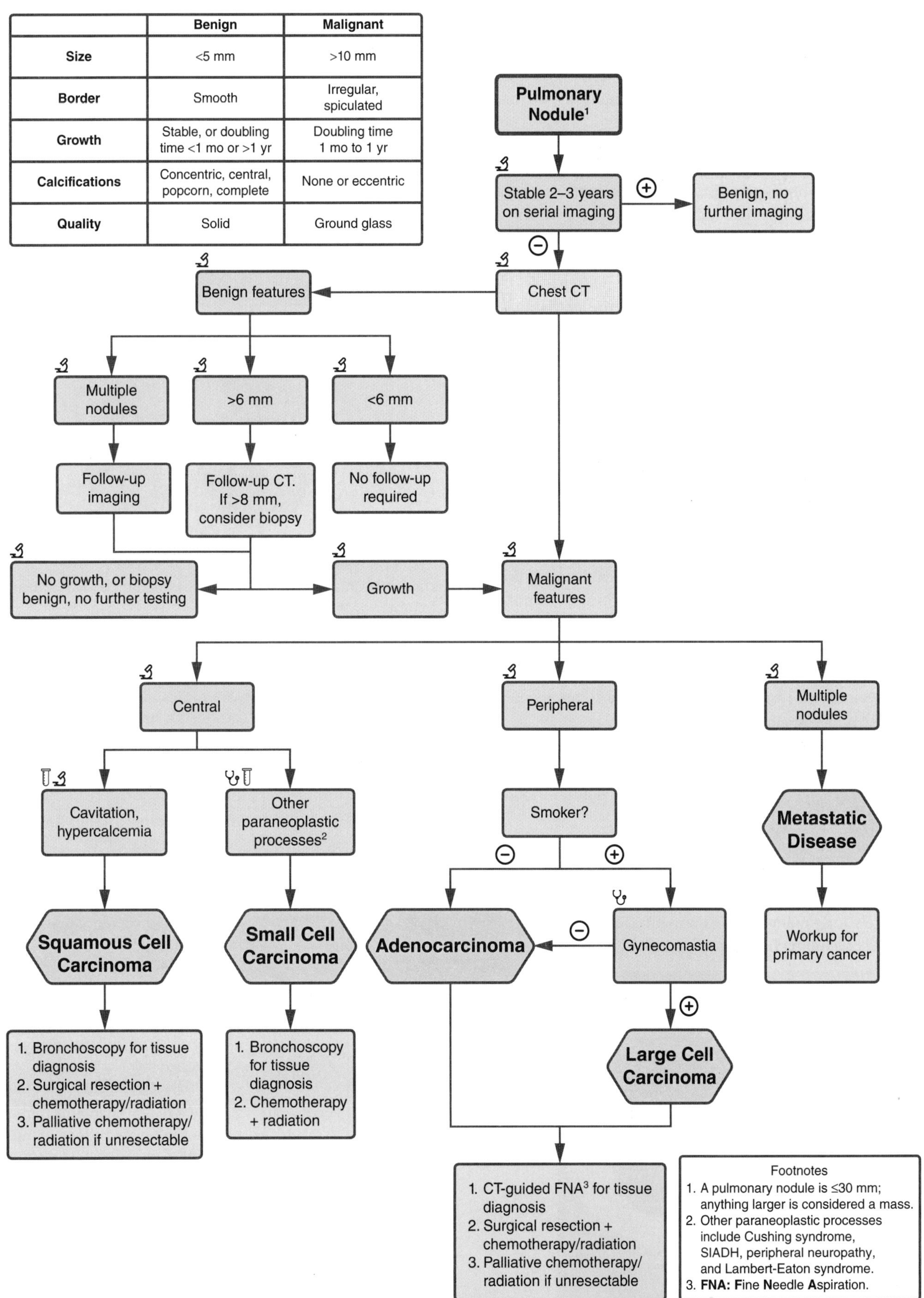

	Benign	Malignant
Size	<5 mm	>10 mm
Border	Smooth	Irregular, spiculated
Growth	Stable, or doubling time <1 mo or >1 yr	Doubling time 1 mo to 1 yr
Calcifications	Concentric, central, popcorn, complete	None or eccentric
Quality	Solid	Ground glass

Pulmonary Nodule[1]
Stable 2–3 years on serial imaging
Benign, no further imaging
Chest CT
Benign features
Multiple nodules
>6 mm
<6 mm
Follow-up imaging
Follow-up CT. If >8 mm, consider biopsy
No follow-up required
No growth, or biopsy benign, no further testing
Growth
Malignant features
Central
Peripheral
Multiple nodules
Cavitation, hypercalcemia
Other paraneoplastic processes[2]
Smoker?
Metastatic Disease
Squamous Cell Carcinoma
Small Cell Carcinoma
Adenocarcinoma
Gynecomastia
Workup for primary cancer
Large Cell Carcinoma
1. Bronchoscopy for tissue diagnosis
2. Surgical resection + chemotherapy/radiation
3. Palliative chemotherapy/ radiation if unresectable
1. Bronchoscopy for tissue diagnosis
2. Chemotherapy + radiation
1. CT-guided FNA[3] for tissue diagnosis
2. Surgical resection + chemotherapy/radiation
3. Palliative chemotherapy/ radiation if unresectable
Footnotes
1. A pulmonary nodule is ≤30 mm; anything larger is considered a mass.
2. Other paraneoplastic processes include Cushing syndrome, SIADH, peripheral neuropathy, and Lambert-Eaton syndrome.
3. FNA: Fine Needle Aspiration.

FIGURE 7.16

7-16 Pulmonary Nodules

LUNG CANCER

A. A 66-year-old M with PMH of severe COPD presents with worsening cough with bloody sputum and weight loss. **Exam** is unremarkable. **Labs** show Na of 120. On **imaging**, CT chest shows a central lung mass.

B. A 74-year-old M Navy veteran with PMH of recurrent LLL pneumonia presents with progressive hemoptysis, weight loss, constipation, and bone pain. **Exam** shows diminished breath sounds over the RML area. **Labs** show Ca level of 13. On **imaging**, CT chest shows an obstructing mass with necrosis and cavitation.

C. A 70-year-old F with PMH of Hodgkin lymphoma s/p chemotherapy and radiation presents with progressive right chest pain, hemoptysis, and weight loss. **Exam** shows finger clubbing. On **imaging**, CT chest shows a peripheral lung mass.

Management:

1. Best imaging test: CT chest.
2. Tissue diagnosis: Bronchoscopy + biopsy for central lesions; CT-guided percutaneous biopsy for peripheral lesions.
3. Treatment depends on the type of cancer.

Complications:

- From mass effect:
  - Pancoast syndrome: Shoulder pain, Horner syndrome (miosis, ptosis, anhidrosis), C8-T1 involvement → intrinsic hand muscle weakness.
  - SVC syndrome: Face and neck swelling, dyspnea, cerebral edema.
  - Hoarse voice from recurrent laryngeal nerve compression.
  - Post-obstructive pneumonia.
- Paraneoplastic syndromes (see table).
- Metastasis to brain, liver, bone, and adrenal glands.
- Malignant pericardial effusion: Sinus tachycardia, pulsus paradoxus.
- Post-obstructive pneumonia.

HYF: Lung cancer risk factors include tobacco use, environmental exposures (eg, asbestos, which is common in ship and heavy metal industries), and prior chest radiation (eg, prior cancer treatment). The most likely lung malignancy to present as a cavitary lesion is squamous cell carcinoma (usually necrotic).

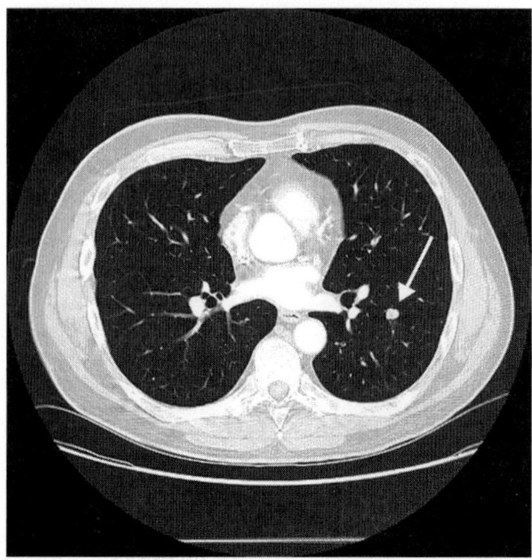

Biopsy-proven lung adenocarcinoma on CT chest.

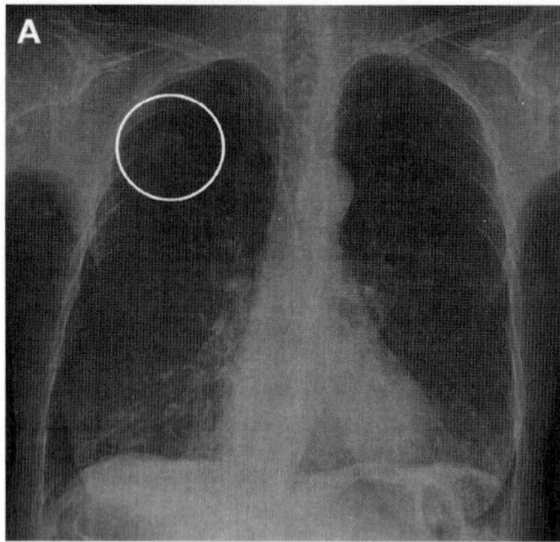
A

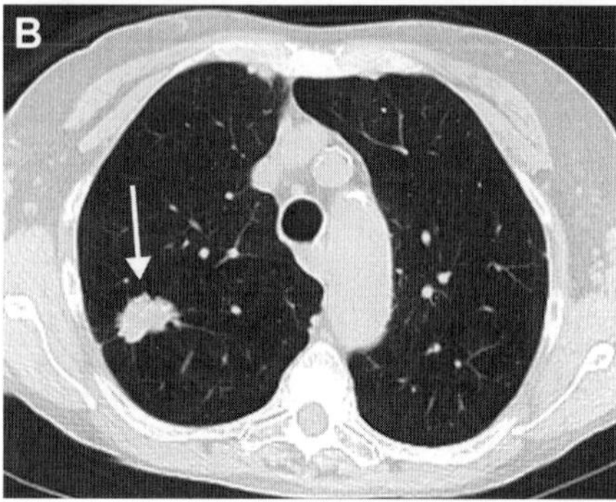
B

Biopsy-proven small cell carcinoma of the lung on (A) CXR, and (B) CT chest.

Types of Lung Cancer and Their Characteristics

Type	Location	
Adenocarcinoma	Peripheral	• In non-smokers • + Hypertrophic pulmonary osteoarthropathy (finger clubbing) • Tx: Resection if able, chemo + radiation • Paraneoplastic: Migratory thrombophlebitis, nonbacterial verrucous endocarditis
Squamous cell carcinoma	Central	• + Smokers • Paraneoplastic: Hypercalcemia via PTHrP • Tx: Same as adenocarcinoma
Small cell carcinoma	Central	• + Smokers • Paraneoplastic (many due to neuroendocrine tumor origin): ▪ SIADH ▪ Cushing (+ ACTH release) ▪ Lambert-Eaton myasthenic syndrome ▪ Myasthenia gravis ▪ Tx: Unresectable. Chemo + radiation
Large cell carcinoma	Peripheral	• Undifferentiated anaplastic tumor with pleomorphic giant cells on pathology • Tx: Surgical resection. Less responsive to chemotherapy. Poor prognosis • Paraneoplastic: β-HCG (gynecomastia)
Bronchial carcinoid tumor	---	• Symptoms usually caused by mass effect, rare metastases. Good prognosis • Histology shows nests of neuroendocrine cells • Paraneoplastic: Carcinoid syndrome due to 5-HT secretion

7-17 Pulmonary Vascular Diseases

ACUTE PULMONARY EMBOLISM

A 77-year-old F with PMH of osteoporosis develops sharp chest pain worse on deep inhalation during POD #3 from open reduction internal fixation of a right femoral shaft fracture. On **exam**, the patient is tachycardic and tachypneic. EKG indicates a large S wave in lead I, a Q wave in lead III, and an inverted T wave in lead III ("S1Q3T3" pattern).

Management:

1. Use Wells' criteria to determine pretest probability of PE.
2. Obtain CT PE protocol if intermediate or high pretest probability.
3. Treat based on risk stratification once diagnosed:
   a. Low risk: DOACs.
   b. Intermediate risk (submassive) and high risk (massive): Unfractionated heparin, systemic thrombolytic, catheter-directed therapy, surgical embolectomy, mechanical support if cardiogenic shock.

Complications: Pulmonary infarcts, RV dysfunction, death.

HYF: Start anticoagulation as soon as PE diagnosis suspected. See Ventilation-Perfusion Mismatch on p. 267 for further information.

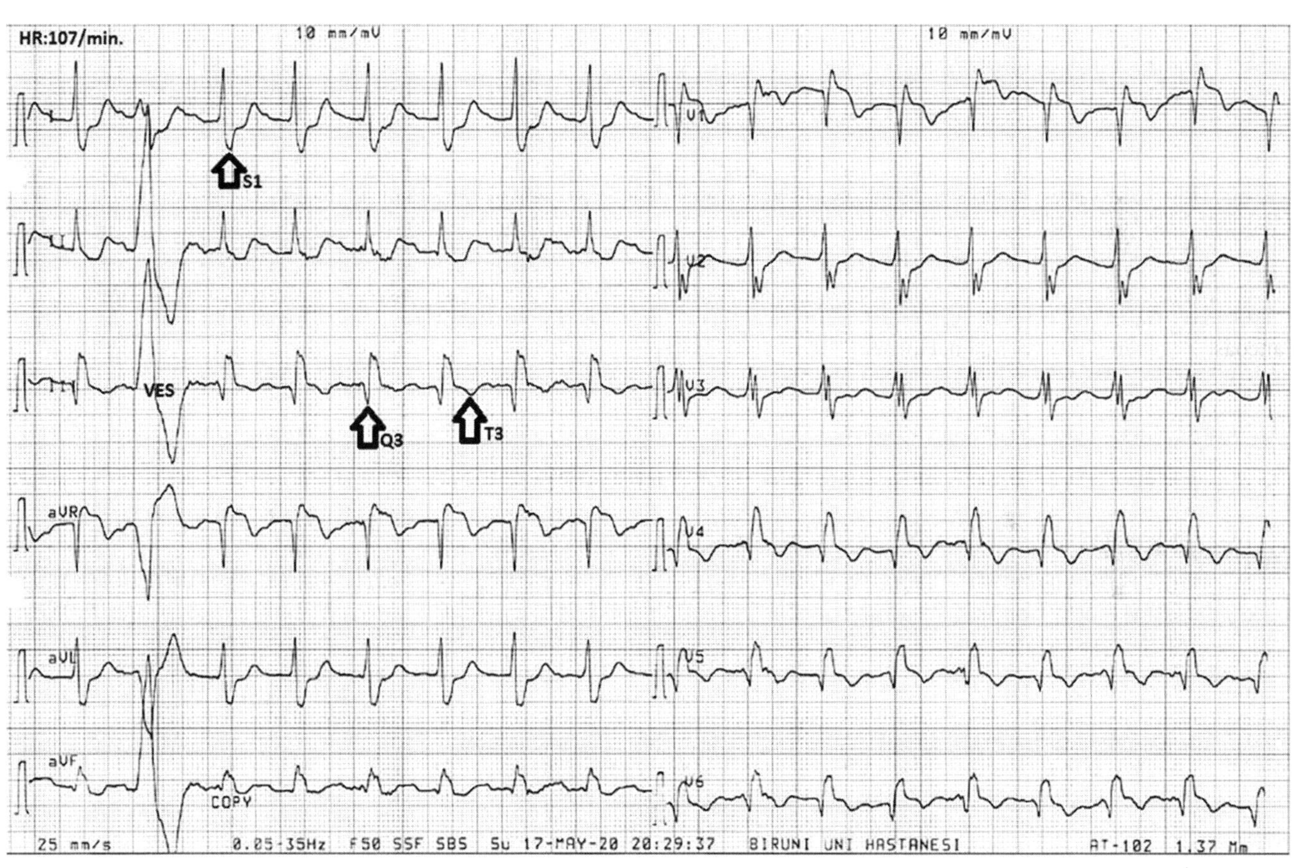
HR:107/min.
10 mm/mV
10 mm/mV
S1
VES
Q3
T3
aVR
aVL
aVF
V1
V2
V3
V4
V5
V6
COPY
25 mm/s
0.05-35Hz F50 SSF SBS Su 17-MAY-20 20:29:37 BIRUNI UNI HASTANESI
AT-102 1.37 Mm

"S1Q3T3" pattern in a patient with pulmonary embolism.

CHRONIC THROMBOEMBOLIC PULMONARY HYPERTENSION (CTEPH)

A 62-year-old M with PMH of resolved acute pulmonary embolism 5 months ago develops progressive SOB and exercise intolerance. **Exam** reveals normal neck veins. However, flow murmurs can be appreciated over lung fields. EKG is unremarkable. On **imaging**, cardiac Doppler US is notable for pulmonary hypertension.

Management:

1. Immediate anticoagulation if suspected.
2. Imaging: V/Q scan > CT pulmonary angiography with contrast due to higher sensitivity. If V/Q scan is positive, then obtain CT pulmonary angiography for further evaluation.
3. Right heart catheterization to confirm.
4. If surgical candidate: Pulmonary endarterectomy or pulmonary balloon angioplasty.
5. If not surgical candidate: Medical management of pulmonary hypertension.

Complications: Right heart failure that eventually leads to death.

HYF: Late complication of acute PE. Pulmonary HTN from unresolved PE causes RV failure.

7-17 Pulmonary Vascular Diseases

PULMONARY ARTERIOVENOUS MALFORMATIONS

A 43-year-old M with PMH of hereditary hemorrhagic telangiectasia develops progressive dyspnea, platypnea, and hemoptysis. On **exam**, SpO_2 is persistently low, and orthodeoxia is present and does not significantly improve with external oxygen delivery devices, such as high-flow nasal cannula or BiPAP. On **imaging**, CT reveals pulmonary AVMs.

Management:

1. Non-contrast CT or transthoracic contrast echocardiography (echocardiogram with bubble study) to confirm right-to-left shunts.
2. Embolotherapy (coil AVMs).

Complications: Stroke, cerebral abscess, hemoptysis, or death.

HYF: Platypnea is a classic presenting symptom, and orthodeoxia is a classic sign of pulmonary AVMs.

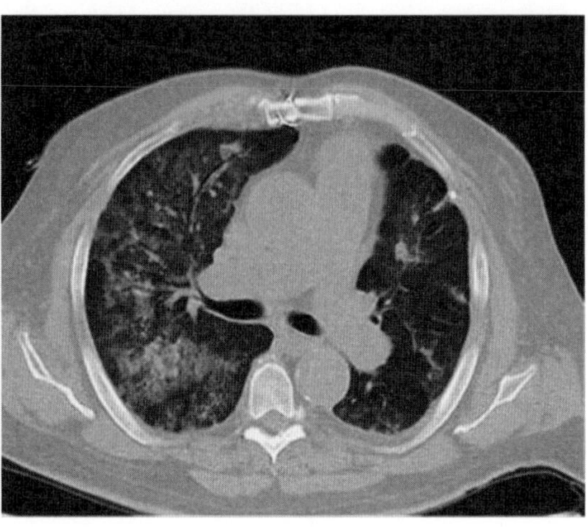

CT showing bilateral ground-glass infiltrates due to alveolar hemorrhage, which can occur in granulomatosis with polyangiitis, microscopic polyangiitis, or eosinophilic granulomatosis with polyangiitis.

PULMONARY VASCULITIS

A 68-year-old M with PMH of HTN and T2DM complains of progressive dyspnea with frequent coughing and occasional hemoptysis. On **imaging**, CXR reveals bilateral hazy opacities. CT demonstrates ground-glass opacities.

Management:

1. Respiratory support.
2. ANCA assay.
3. Bronchoscopy to confirm diffuse alveolar hemorrhage.
4. Glucocorticoids, immunosuppression.

Complications: DVT, ESRD, stroke.

HYF: Granulomatosis with polyangiitis (GPA) is c-ANCA (+), whereas microscopic polyangiitis (MPA) is p-ANCA (+). See Rheumatologic Serologies and Petechiae on pp. 298–302.

Pulmonary Hypertension (PH): See p. 16.

7-18 Pleural Disease

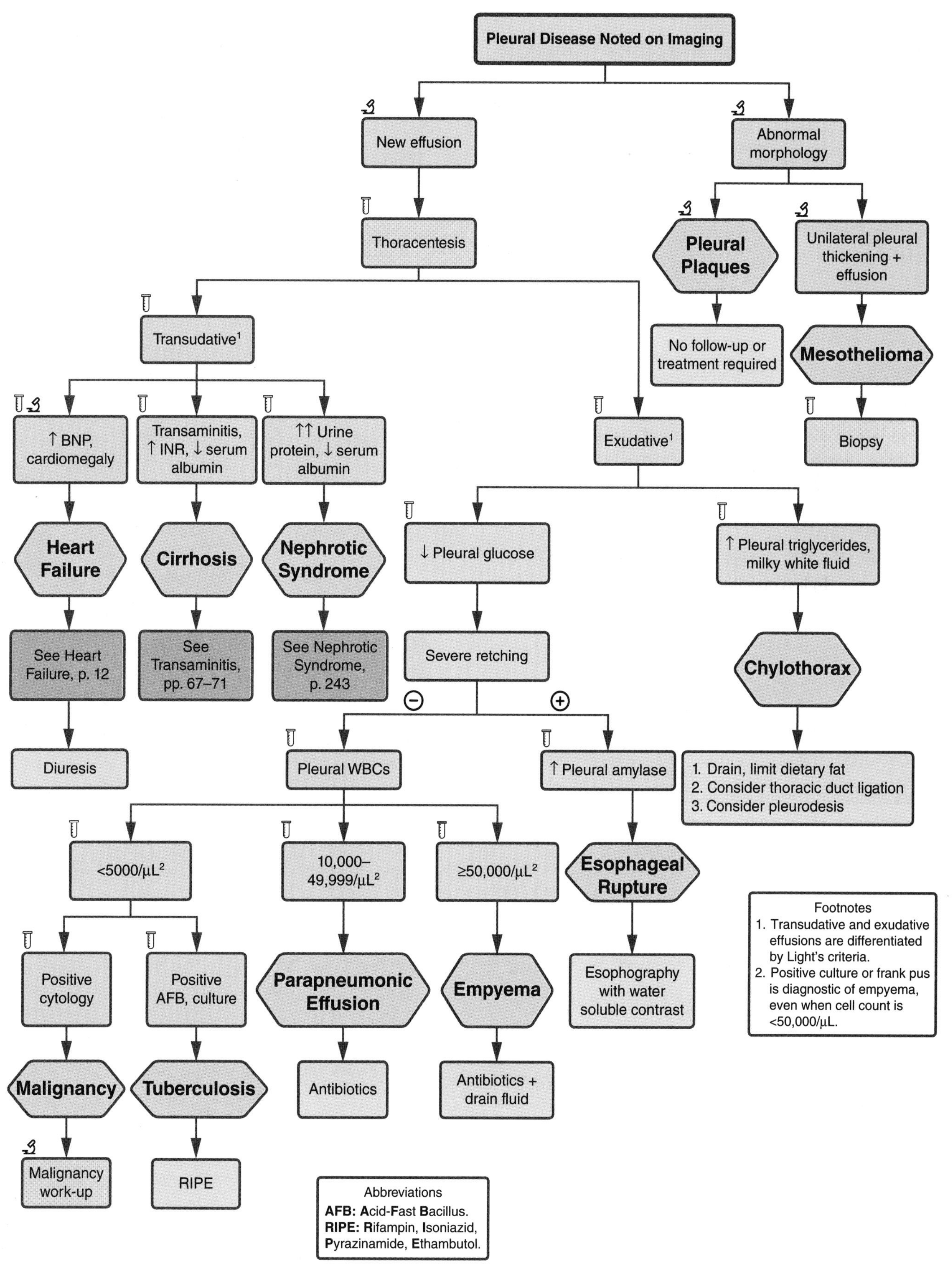
Pleural Disease Noted on Imaging
New effusion
Abnormal morphology
Thoracentesis
Pleural Plaques
Unilateral pleural thickening + effusion
Transudative1
No follow-up or treatment required
Mesothelioma
↑ BNP, cardiomegaly
Transaminitis, ↑ INR, ↓ serum albumin
↑↑ Urine protein, ↓ serum albumin
Exudative1
Biopsy
Heart Failure
Cirrhosis
Nephrotic Syndrome
↓ Pleural glucose
↑ Pleural triglycerides, milky white fluid
See Heart Failure, p. 12
See Transaminitis, pp. 67–71
See Nephrotic Syndrome, p. 243
Severe retching
Chylothorax
−
+
Diuresis
Pleural WBCs
↑ Pleural amylase
1. Drain, limit dietary fat
2. Consider thoracic duct ligation
3. Consider pleurodesis
<5000/μL2
10,000–49,999/μL2
≥50,000/μL2
Esophageal Rupture
Footnotes
1. Transudative and exudative effusions are differentiated by Light's criteria.
2. Positive culture or frank pus is diagnostic of empyema, even when cell count is <50,000/μL.
Positive cytology
Positive AFB, culture
Parapneumonic Effusion
Empyema
Esophography with water soluble contrast
Malignancy
Tuberculosis
Antibiotics
Antibiotics + drain fluid
Malignancy work-up
RIPE
Abbreviations
AFB: Acid-Fast Bacillus.
RIPE: Rifampin, Isoniazid, Pyrazinamide, Ethambutol.

FIGURE 7.18

7-18 Pleural Disease

Light's Criteria for Pleural Effusions

	Transudative	Exudative
Protein (pleural/serum)	≤0.5	>0.5
LDH (pleural/serum)	≤0.6	>0.6
LDH (pleural)	≤2/3 upper limit of normal serum	>2/3 upper limit of normal serum

PLEURAL PLAQUES

A 60-year-old M who worked in a shipyard presents for routine check-up. **Exam** and **labs** are unremarkable. On **imaging**, CXR shows scattered calcified plaques throughout the pleura.

Management:

1. No follow-up or treatment required.

HYF: Pleural plaques are the most common pathology related to asbestos exposure. They are asymptomatic and typically found incidentally on radiograph or CT. They are benign and do not require treatment or follow-up.

MESOTHELIOMA

A 70-year-old M with PMH of asbestos exposure presents with dyspnea, night sweats, and chest pain. **Exam** has palpable chest wall masses, unilateral decreased breath sounds, and dullness to percussion. On **imaging**, chest CT demonstrates a unilateral pleural effusion with a pleural mass.

Management:

1. Resection, radiation, chemotherapy ± immunotherapy.

Complications: Metastatic spread.

HYF: Mesothelioma is a rare cancer, though it is the most common primary tumor of the pleura. A history of asbestos exposure is found in 70% of cases. Pleural malignant mesothelioma is the most common manifestation, but peritoneal mesothelioma is another potential site. Patients who develop this malignancy typically have a long exposure history (10–20 years) with an extended latency period (20–30 years since exposure) before developing symptoms. Death is usually caused by respiratory failure due to local spread. Mesothelioma has a poor prognosis.

CHYLOTHORAX

A 60-year-old M with recent cardiothoracic surgery presents with dyspnea. On **exam**, he has dullness to percussion over the right lung field. On **imaging**, CXR shows a right pleural effusion. **Labs** show serum protein 7 and LDH 200. A thoracentesis is performed with pleural fluid studies that show lymphocyte predominance on cell count, protein 4, LDH 80, and triglycerides 150.

Management:

1. Pleurodesis.
2. Limit dietary fat.
3. Consider thoracic duct ligation.

HYF: Patients often have a unilateral pleural effusion, most often on the right. Causes of chylothorax can be thought of as traumatic vs. non traumatic. The most common traumatic causes are cardiothoracic surgeries. Non-traumatic causes are typically due to malignancy.

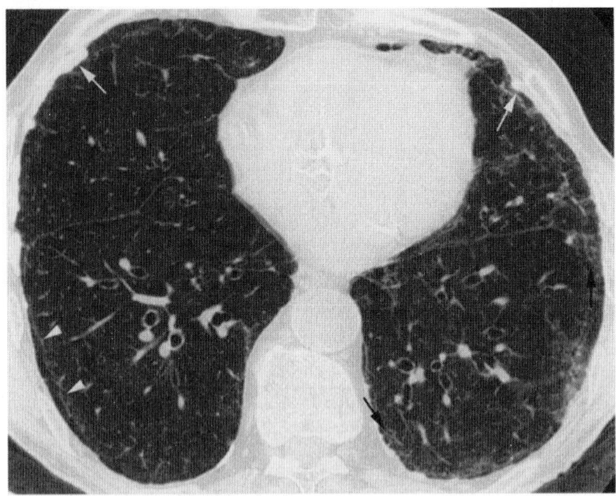

Asbestosis. Note the calcified pleural plaques (*white arrows*) and bilateral, subpleural reticulation (*black arrows*) representing fibrotic lung disease.

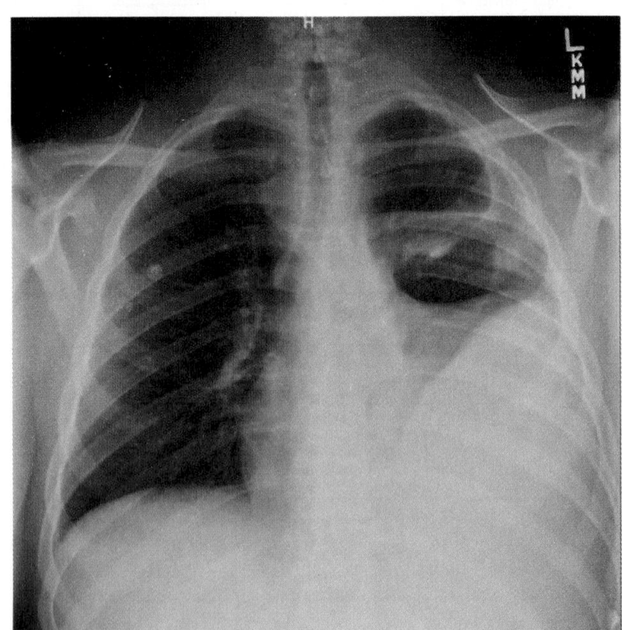

Pleural effusion in the context of mesothelioma.

Malignancy: See Pulmonary Nodules, p. 284.

Tuberculosis: See Cavitary Pulmonary Lesions, p. 291.

Parapneumonic Effusion, Empyema: See Pneumonia, pp. 164–165, 276, 290.

Esophageal Rupture: See General Surgery, p. 403.

Heart Failure: See Cardiology, pp. 12–14.

Cirrhosis: See Gastroenterology, pp. 72–75.

Nephrotic Syndrome: See Nephrology, p. 243.

7-19 Cavitary Pulmonary Lesion

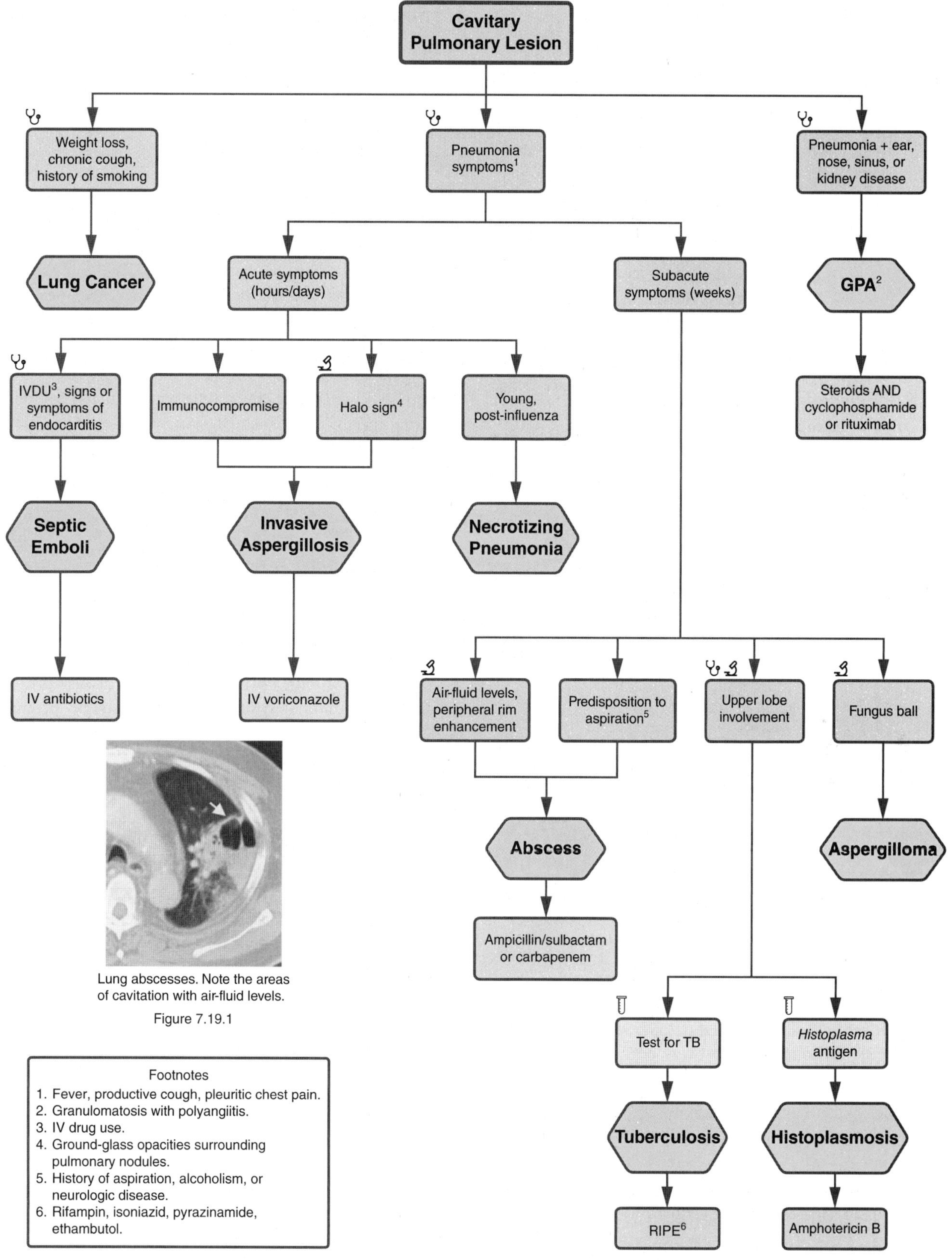

Cavitary Pulmonary Lesion
Weight loss, chronic cough, history of smoking
Pneumonia symptoms[1]
Pneumonia + ear, nose, sinus, or kidney disease
Lung Cancer
Acute symptoms (hours/days)
Subacute symptoms (weeks)
GPA[2]
IVDU[3], signs or symptoms of endocarditis
Immunocompromise
Halo sign[4]
Young, post-influenza
Steroids AND cyclophosphamide or rituximab
Septic Emboli
Invasive Aspergillosis
Necrotizing Pneumonia
IV antibiotics
IV voriconazole
Air-fluid levels, peripheral rim enhancement
Predisposition to aspiration[5]
Upper lobe involvement
Fungus ball
Abscess
Aspergilloma
Ampicillin/sulbactam or carbapenem
Test for TB
Histoplasma antigen
Tuberculosis
Histoplasmosis
RIPE[6]
Amphotericin B

Lung abscesses. Note the areas of cavitation with air-fluid levels.

Figure 7.19.1

Footnotes

1. Fever, productive cough, pleuritic chest pain.
2. Granulomatosis with polyangiitis.
3. IV drug use.
4. Ground-glass opacities surrounding pulmonary nodules.
5. History of aspiration, alcoholism, or neurologic disease.
6. Rifampin, isoniazid, pyrazinamide, ethambutol.

FIGURE 7.19

7-19 Cavitary Pulmonary Lesion

LUNG CANCER

A 60-year-old M smoker presents with chronic cough, hemoptysis, and unintentional weight loss. **Labs** show hyponatremia. On **imaging**, chest CT reveals a cavitary lesion in the RUL.

Management:

1. Biopsy to confirm diagnosis.

Complications:

- Metastases to liver, brain, and bone.
- SVC syndrome: Face and neck swelling, dyspnea, cerebral edema.
- Pancoast syndrome: Shoulder pain, Horner syndrome, C8-T1 involvement → intrinsic hand muscle weakness.
- Malignant pericardial effusion: Sinus tachycardia, pulsus paradoxus.
- Paraneoplastic syndromes.
- Post-obstructive pneumonia.

HYF: The most likely lung malignancy to present as a cavitary lesion is squamous cell carcinoma (usually necrotic). Labs may suggest a paraneoplastic syndrome (eg, PTHrP-mediated hypercalcemia, hyponatremia due to SIADH).

GRANULOMATOSIS WITH POLYANGIITIS

A 65-year-old M with PMH of CKD and recent unintentional weight loss presents with fever, malaise, arthralgia, and hemoptysis.

Management:

1. Measure ANCA + tissue biopsy.
2. Steroids + (cyclophosphamide OR rituximab).

Complications:

- Hearing loss.
- Nasal septal perforation.
- Diffuse pulmonary hemorrhage.

HYF: Associated with a "saddle nose" deformity.

SEPTIC EMBOLI

A 25-year-old F with PMH of IV drug use is being treated for endocarditis and now has new pleuritic chest pain, dyspnea, and cough. **Labs/imaging:** Blood cultures have been persistently positive. Chest CT shows bilateral cavitation at the lung peripheries.

Management:

1. IV antibiotics.

HYF: Septic emboli are treated with antibiotics, not anticoagulation. Also associated with indwelling catheters.

INVASIVE ASPERGILLOSIS

A 50-year-old M with PMH of rheumatoid arthritis on chronic prednisone presents with fever, pleuritic chest pain, and hemoptysis. On **imaging**, chest CT shows cavitary lung nodules that are surrounded by ground-glass opacities.

Management:

1. Bronchoalveolar lavage to obtain fungal stain and cultures. Serum galactomannan assay is specific, but if negative, lung biopsy should be performed to confirm the diagnosis.
2. Voriconazole or echinocandin (eg, caspofungin).

Complications: Massive hemoptysis.

HYF: CT can show "halo sign" due to alveolar hemorrhage. Immunodeficiency + acute hemoptysis + halo sign = invasive aspergillosis. Do not confuse with chronic pulmonary aspergillosis (aspergilloma), a chronic disease for which a major risk factor is lung damage (not necessarily immunosuppression).

NECROTIZING PNEUMONIA

A 20-year-old F with PMH of recent viral upper respiratory infection presents with severe pneumonia symptoms and hemoptysis. On **imaging**, chest CT shows unilateral cavitary lesions in the lungs.

Management:

1. Vancomycin or linezolid.
2. Sputum culture and narrow antibiotics when able.

Complications: Hemoptysis, abscess, empyema.

HYF: Commonly due to community-acquired MRSA.

ABSCESS

A 75-year-old M with PMH of Parkinson's disease presents with subacute pneumonia symptoms and a cough productive of foul-smelling sputum.

Management:

1. Ampicillin/sulbactam or a carbapenem (clindamycin reserved for penicillin allergies).

Complications: Rupture into pleural space → empyema.

HYF: Associated with aspiration risk factors (eg, alcohol, neurologic dysfunction). If sputum is described as foul-smelling or putrid, think lung abscess.

ASPERGILLOMA

A patient with PMH of TB presents with chronic weight loss, productive cough, and hemoptysis. On **imaging**, chest CT reveals lung cavities with fungus balls.

Management:

1. Itraconazole or voriconazole.
2. Surgery to resect the fungus ball.

Complications:

- Pulmonary fibrosis.
- Hemorrhage, sometimes fatal.

7-19 Cavitary Pulmonary Lesion

HYF: Patients classically have history of TB or allergic bronchopulmonary aspergillosis. Do not confuse with invasive aspergillosis, an acute and severe disease for which immunosuppression (not lung damage) is a major risk factor.

TUBERCULOSIS

A previously incarcerated patient presents with subacute cough, weight loss, and night sweats. On **imaging**, chest X-ray shows apical opacities and right hilar lymphadenopathy.

Management:

1. RIPE: Rifampin + isoniazid + pyrazinamide + ethambutol.

Complications:

- Hemoptysis.
- Bronchiectasis.
- Chronic pulmonary aspergillosis.

HYF: Clues pointing to TB include immigration from endemic areas (such as Mexico, South America, Asia, and Eastern Europe), history of immunodeficiency or substance use, or living in a correctional facility or homeless shelter (crowded areas). Classic therapy is RIPE, 4 for 2 and 2 for 4: Rifampin, isoniazid, pyrazinamide, and ethambutol for 2 months, followed by rifampin and isoniazid for 4 months. Reactivation TB classically affects the upper lung lobes.

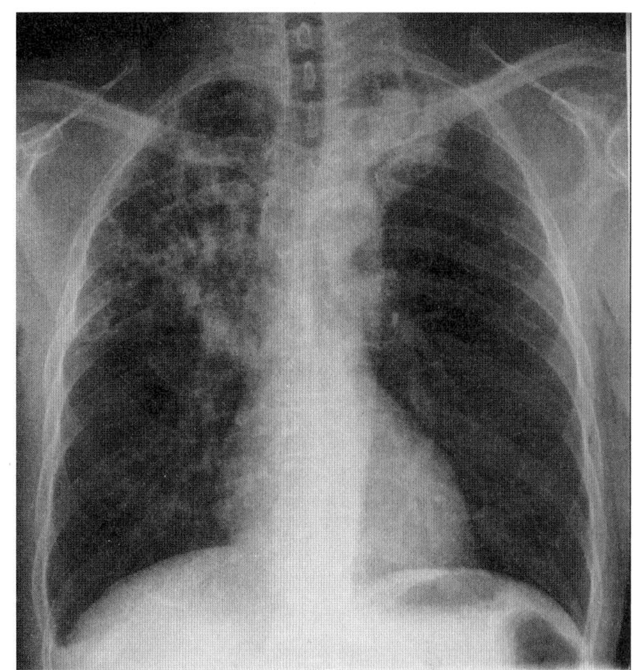

Reactivation TB with patchy airspace opacities in the right upper lung.

Histoplasmosis: See p. 169.

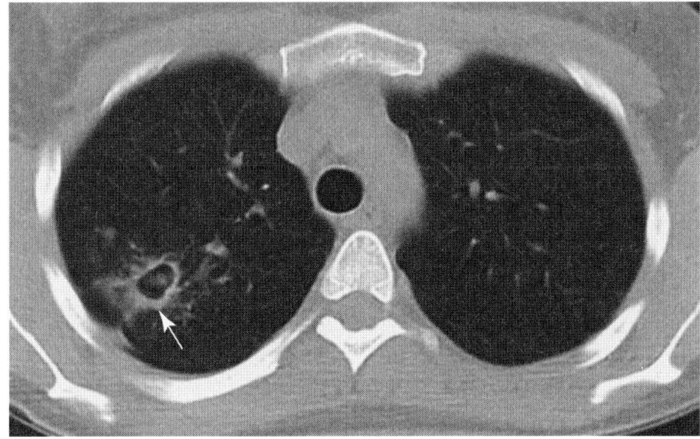

Aspergilloma.

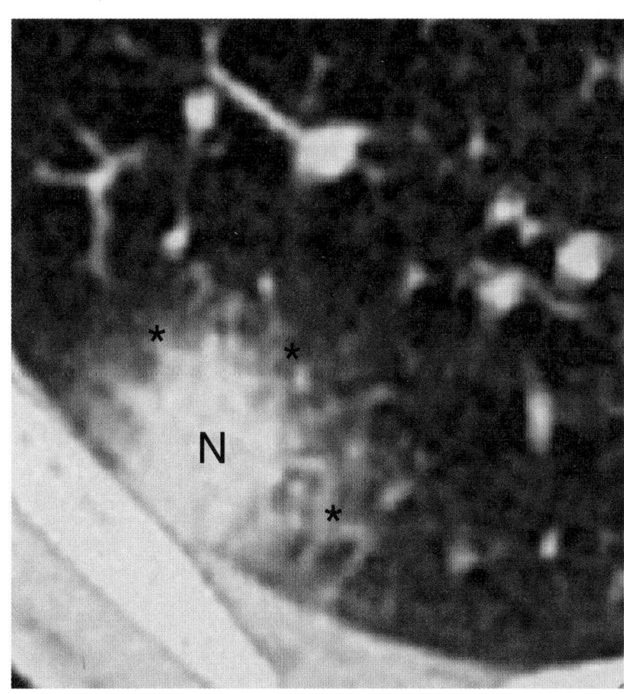
*
*
N
*

"Halo" sign in angioinvasive aspergillosis.

8

Internal Medicine: Rheumatology

8-1 Polyarticular Joint Pain

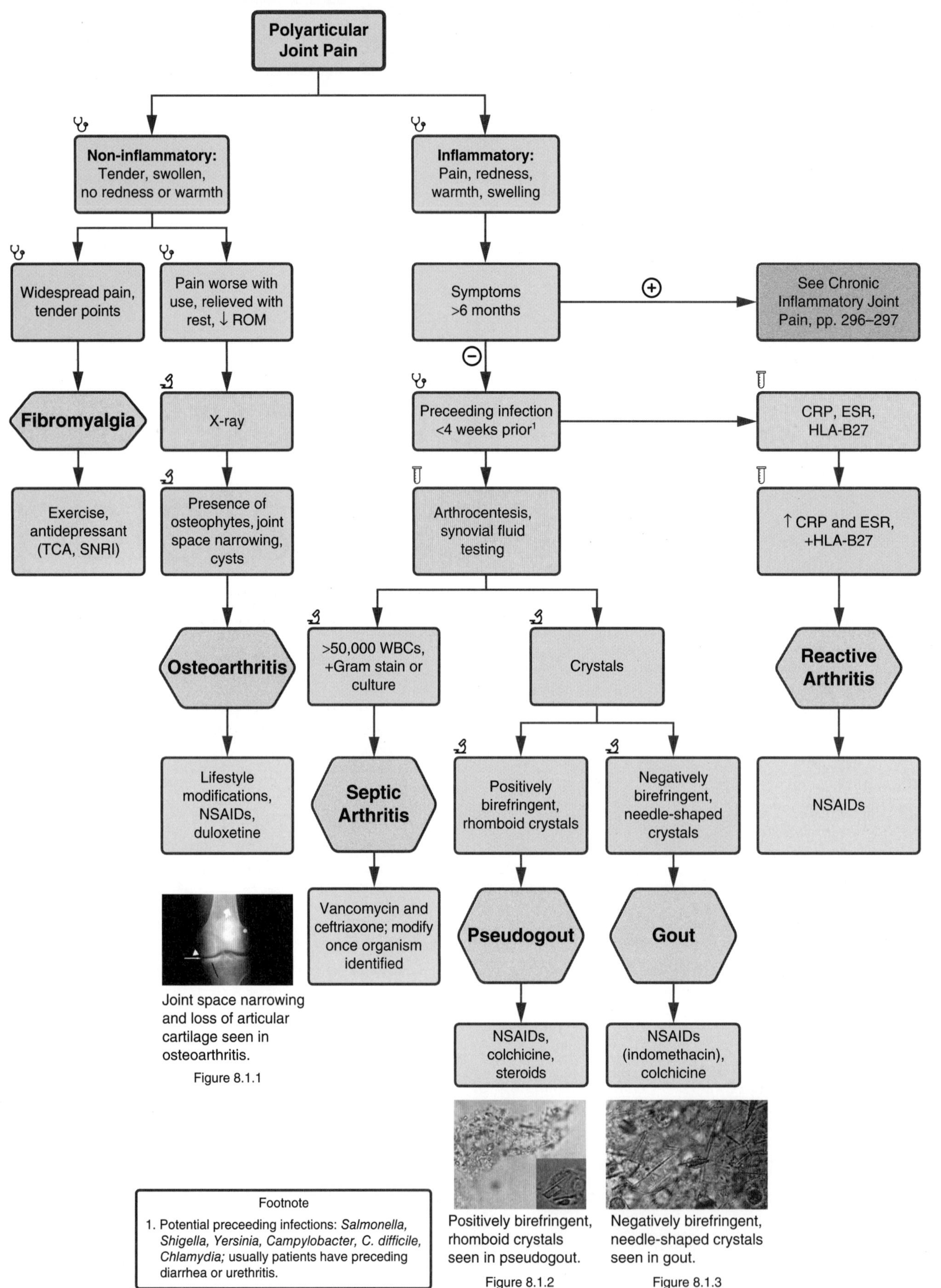
Polyarticular Joint Pain
Non-inflammatory: Tender, swollen, no redness or warmth
Inflammatory: Pain, redness, warmth, swelling
Widespread pain, tender points
Pain worse with use, relieved with rest, ↓ ROM
Symptoms >6 months
See Chronic Inflammatory Joint Pain, pp. 296–297
Fibromyalgia
X-ray
Preceeding infection <4 weeks prior[1]
CRP, ESR, HLA-B27
Exercise, antidepressant (TCA, SNRI)
Presence of osteophytes, joint space narrowing, cysts
Arthrocentesis, synovial fluid testing
↑ CRP and ESR, +HLA-B27
Osteoarthritis
>50,000 WBCs, +Gram stain or culture
Crystals
Reactive Arthritis
Lifestyle modifications, NSAIDs, duloxetine
Septic Arthritis
Positively birefringent, rhomboid crystals
Negatively birefringent, needle-shaped crystals
NSAIDs
Vancomycin and ceftriaxone; modify once organism identified
Pseudogout
Gout
NSAIDs, colchicine, steroids
NSAIDs (indomethacin), colchicine

Joint space narrowing and loss of articular cartilage seen in osteoarthritis.

Figure 8.1.1

Positively birefringent, rhomboid crystals seen in pseudogout.

Figure 8.1.2

Negatively birefringent, needle-shaped crystals seen in gout.

Figure 8.1.3

Footnote

1. Potential preceeding infections: *Salmonella, Shigella, Yersinia, Campylobacter, C. difficile, Chlamydia;* usually patients have preceding diarrhea or urethritis.

FIGURE 8.1

8-1 Polyarticular Joint Pain

FIBROMYALGIA

A 33-year-old F with PMH of depression presents with 4 months of fatigue, headaches, diffuse aching, and stiffness. On **exam**, she has tenderness to palpation at the lower back, neck, and shoulders with 5/5 strength. **Labs** are within normal limits.

Management:

1. Conservative measures: Patient education, good sleep hygiene, low-impact aerobic exercise.
2. Tricyclic antidepressants (eg, amitriptyline), SNRIs (eg, duloxetine), SSRIs (eg, fluoxetine), or pregabalin.
3. Cognitive-behavioral therapy (CBT).

Complications:

- Decreased functionality.
- Health-related depression and anxiety.

HYF: Occurs most frequently in women aged 20–55. Patients may require a combination of CBT and pharmacologic therapies. TCAs inhibit re-uptake of norepinephrine and serotonin (similar to SNRIs) but also cause many SEs due to interactions with other receptors: M1 (anticholinergic symptoms such as constipation), alpha-adrenergic (orthostatic hypotension), and histamine (somnolence).

OSTEOARTHRITIS (OA)

A 72-year-old M with PMH of T2DM and obesity presents with pain and stiffness in knees. On **exam**, he has ↓ range of motion (ROM) and crepitus. On **imaging**, knee X-ray shows osteophytes and a narrowed joint space.

Management:

1. Lifestyle modifications are mainstay of treatment: Weight management, exercise, braces, assistive device use.
2. Mild OA: Topical non-steroidal anti-inflammatory drugs (NSAIDs).
3. Moderate to severe OA: Oral NSAIDs or duloxetine.
4. Severe hip/knee OA: Joint replacement surgery.

Complications:

- Bone and joint deformities, pain.
- Popliteal (Baker) cyst.
- Functional/lifestyle impairment.

HYF: Commonly affects the DIP (Heberden nodes), PIP (Bouchard nodes), hip, and knee joints. Patients have <30 minutes of morning stiffness that improves with rest.

SEPTIC ARTHRITIS

A 60-year-old F with PMH of T2DM presents with acute-onset severe right knee pain and fever. The **exam** shows an erythematous, warm, tender knee with ↓ passive ROM. Joint drainage is performed via needle aspiration. On **labs**, synovial fluid shows 100,000 WBCs/μL with neutrophil predominance and Gram-positive cocci in clusters. Blood cultures and synovial fluid cultures are pending.

Management:

1. Empiric IV antibiotics based on initial Gram stain of synovial fluid: For Gram-positive cocci, empiric treatment with IV vancomycin. For Gram-negative bacilli, treatment is guided by risk for *Pseudomonas* infection (immunocompromised, IV drug use). If no risk factors for *Pseudomonas*, give a 3rd-generation cephalosporin (IV ceftriaxone or cefotaxime); if the patient has risk factors for *Pseudomonas*, give IV cefepime and/or ceftazidime.
2. Modify antibiotic treatment after receiving culture results.
3. Joint drainage for source control: Needle aspiration, arthroscopic drainage, or arthrotomy (open surgical drainage) based on clinical scenario.

Complications:

- Joint damage, osteomyelitis.
- Bacteremia, sepsis.

HYF: Most commonly due to *S. aureus* or streptococci. If prosthetic joint, think *S. epidermidis*.

CRYSTALLINE ARTHRITIS (GOUT AND PSEUDOGOUT)

A 65-year-old M with PMH of T2DM, hypertension, and hyperlipidemia presents with severe pain in the big toe. On **exam**, the toe is red, swollen, and warm. Aspiration of the MTP joint shows negatively birefringent, needle-shaped crystals and ↑ WBCs (consistent with gout) or positively birefringent, rhomboid crystals and ↑ WBCs (consistent with pseudogout).

Management:

1. Gout:
   a. Acute attack: NSAIDs (indomethacin), colchicine, steroids if NSAIDs are contraindicated.
   b. Maintenance therapy: Lifestyle modifications (weight loss, diet changes), xanthine oxidase inhibitors, uricosuric agents.
2. Pseudogout: NSAIDs, colchicine, glucocorticoids.

Complications:

- Gout: Flares, tophi, pain, joint damage, kidney stones or damage.
- Pseudogout: Pain, joint damage.

HYF: Gout most commonly affects the big toe first (podagra). and can be precipitated by protein-rich food or alcohol binges, use of diuretics, or volume depletion. Pseudogout most commonly affects the knees and is caused by calcium pyrophosphate dihydrate (CPPD) crystal deposition; look for chondrocalcinosis on imaging.

8-2 Chronic Inflammatory Polyarticular Joint Pain

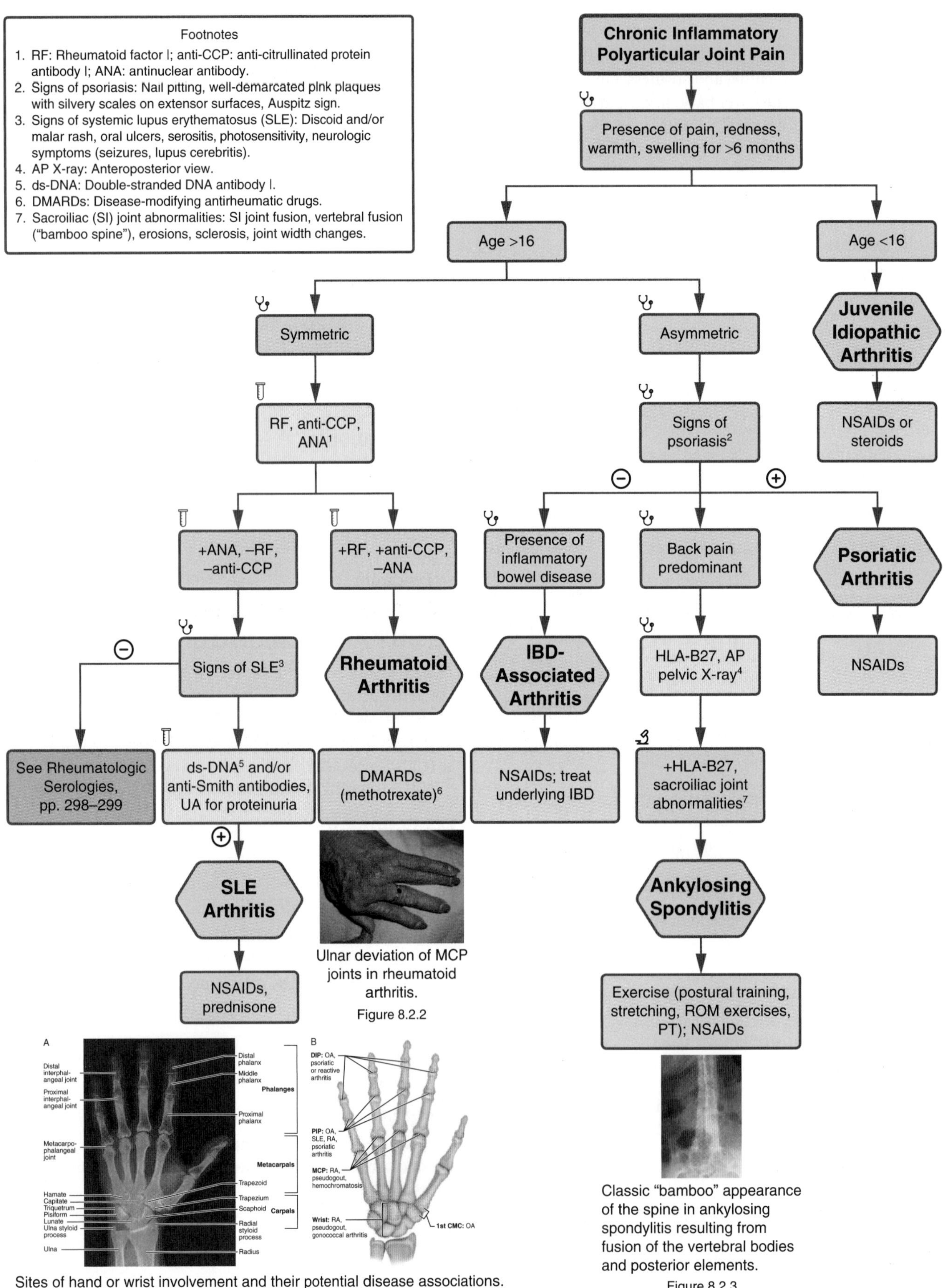
Footnotes
1. RF: Rheumatoid factor I; anti-CCP: anti-citrullinated protein antibody I; ANA: antinuclear antibody.
2. Signs of psoriasis: Nail pitting, well-demarcated pink plaques with silvery scales on extensor surfaces, Auspitz sign.
3. Signs of systemic lupus erythematosus (SLE): Discoid and/or malar rash, oral ulcers, serositis, photosensitivity, neurologic symptoms (seizures, lupus cerebritis).
4. AP X-ray: Anteroposterior view.
5. ds-DNA: Double-stranded DNA antibody I.
6. DMARDs: Disease-modifying antirheumatic drugs.
7. Sacroiliac (SI) joint abnormalities: SI joint fusion, vertebral fusion ("bamboo spine"), erosions, sclerosis, joint width changes.
Chronic Inflammatory Polyarticular Joint Pain
Presence of pain, redness, warmth, swelling for >6 months
Age >16
Age <16
Juvenile Idiopathic Arthritis
NSAIDs or steroids
Symmetric
RF, anti-CCP, ANA[1]
+ANA, –RF, –anti-CCP
Signs of SLE[3]
See Rheumatologic Serologies, pp. 298–299
ds-DNA[5] and/or anti-Smith antibodies, UA for proteinuria
SLE Arthritis
NSAIDs, prednisone
+RF, +anti-CCP, –ANA
Rheumatoid Arthritis
DMARDs (methotrexate)[6]
Asymmetric
Signs of psoriasis[2]
Presence of inflammatory bowel disease
IBD-Associated Arthritis
NSAIDs; treat underlying IBD
Back pain predominant
HLA-B27, AP pelvic X-ray[4]
+HLA-B27, sacroiliac joint abnormalities[7]
Ankylosing Spondylitis
Exercise (postural training, stretching, ROM exercises, PT); NSAIDs
Psoriatic Arthritis
NSAIDs
A
Distal interphalangeal joint
Proximal interphalangeal joint
Metacarpophalangeal joint
Hamate
Capitate
Triquetrum
Pisiform
Lunate
Ulna styloid process
Ulna
Distal phalanx
Middle phalanx
Phalanges
Proximal phalanx
Metacarpals
Trapezoid
Trapezium
Scaphoid
Carpals
Radial styloid process
Radius
B
DIP: OA, psoriatic or reactive arthritis
PIP: OA, SLE, RA, psoriatic arthritis
MCP: RA, pseudogout, hemochromatosis
Wrist: RA, pseudogout, gonococcal arthritis
1st CMC: OA

Ulnar deviation of MCP joints in rheumatoid arthritis.
Figure 8.2.2

Classic "bamboo" appearance of the spine in ankylosing spondylitis resulting from fusion of the vertebral bodies and posterior elements.
Figure 8.2.3

Sites of hand or wrist involvement and their potential disease associations.
Figure 8.2.1

FIGURE 8.2

8-2 Chronic Inflammatory Polyarticular Joint Pain

RHEUMATOID ARTHRITIS (RA)

A 39-year-old F with PMH of tobacco use disorder presents with 2 months of fatigue and bilateral hand and wrist pain that is worse in the morning. Her **exam** reveals a low-grade fever, swelling and tenderness of the PIP and MCP joints, ulnar deviation of the fingers and boutonniere deformities, and multiple arm nodules. **Labs** show elevated ESR and CRP and are positive for RF and anti-ACPA antibody. Synovial fluid is inflammatory. On **imaging**, her hand X-ray shows joint space narrowing, periarticular osteopenia, and marginal erosions.

Management:

1. Disease-modifying antirheumatic drugs (DMARDs) (eg, methotrexate, hydroxychloroquine, sulfasalazine).
2. NSAIDs, glucocorticoids. TNF-α inhibitors (eg, infliximab, etanercept) for active inflammation.
3. Analgesics.
4. Surgery in severe cases that do not respond to medical therapy.

Complications:

- Systemic symptoms: Fever, malaise, weight loss.
- Hand deformities (eg, swan neck, boutonniere), nodules.
- Compressive neuropathies (eg, carpal tunnel syndrome).
- Atlantoaxial joint instability → cervical myelopathy.
- Extra-articular manifestations: Uveitis, pericarditis, interstitial lung disease, exudative pleural effusions, amyloidosis.

HYF: Predominantly affects the PIP, MCP, and wrist joints. Associated with HLA-DR4 and smoking. Can present with extra-articular manifestations such as 1) Felty syndrome (splenomegaly, neutropenia, increased risk of bacterial infections) due to autoantibodies against neutrophil components and G-CSF, and 2) Caplan's syndrome (pulmonary fibrosis, pneumoconiosis). Associated with Sjögren's disease. RA is the most common cause of AA amyloidosis in the United States. Treatment with TNF-α inhibitors can cause guttate psoriasis. A potentially devastating complication is atlantoaxial subluxation causing cord compression: The initial symptom is usually cervical pain followed by progressive weakness and UMN signs; urgent MRI of the cervical spine will show separation of C1–C2, for which neurosurgery will need to perform a cervical fixation.

ANKYLOSING SPONDYLITIS

A 24-year-old M presents with 4 months of low back pain that is worse in the morning and relieved with exercise. The **exam** shows limited forward spine flexion and tenderness over the bilateral sacroiliac (SI) joints. **Labs** show ↑ ESR and CRP. He is HLA-B27+. On **imaging**, hip X-rays show sacroiliitis and fused SI joints. His spine X-ray shows squaring of the vertebral bodies.

Management:

1. Exercise, physical therapy.
2. NSAIDs.
3. Anti-TNF-α agent (eg, adalimumab) or IL-17 inhibitor.

Complications:

- Restrictive lung disease due to ↓ chest wall expansion.
- Spinal cord injury (eg, cauda equina).
- Osteoporosis (mediated by TNF-α and IL-6).
- Enthesitis, dactylitis.
- Extra-articular manifestations: Pulmonary fibrosis, amyloidosis, uveitis, aortitis with aortic regurgitation.

HYF: Most commonly in men age <40. Associated with inflammatory bowel disease (IBD), psoriasis, uveitis, and positive HLA-B27. Can present as pain at tendon insertion sites. The classic spine X-ray finding is "bamboo spine" due to formation of syndesmophytes.

JUVENILE IDIOPATHIC ARTHRITIS

An 11-year-old F presents with 2 months of fatigue and joint pain that is worse in the morning. On **exam**, she has swollen and tender knee; pink, macrash; and fever. **Labs** show ↑ ESR, positive ANA, and negative RF.

Management:

1. NSAIDs or corticosteroids.
2. Methotrexate.
3. IL-1 or IL-6 inhibitors (anakinra, tocilizumab).
4. Refractory disease: DMARDs.

Complications:

- Macrophage activation syndrome.
- Uveitis leading to blindness.
- Joint damage, growth issues.
- Pericarditis.

HYF: Present for >6 weeks in patients aged <16 years. There are many subtypes, including:

- Pauciarticular: Asymmetric + <4 joints. ↑ risk of iridocyclitis.
- Polyarticular: Symmetric with >5 joints. Less risk of iridocyclitis.
- Systemic (ie, Still disease): Daily, spiking fevers and maculopapular, salmon-colored rash, ± hepatosplenomegaly.

PSORIATIC ARTHRITIS

A 63-year-old F with PMH of psoriasis and chronic back pain presents with joint pain and stiffness in the hands, which is worse in the morning. The **exam** shows swelling of DIP joints in her left hand, several sausage-shaped fingers, nail pitting, and silvery plaques on her skin. **Labs** are negative for any serologies. On **imaging**, her hand X-ray shows a "pencil-in-cup" deformity of the DIP joints.

Management:

1. Psoriasis management (see Dermatology, p. 309).
2. Mild: NSAIDs.
3. Moderate to severe: DMARDs (eg, methotrexate), anti-TNF-α agents (eg, infliximab, etanercept).
4. Lifestyle modifications: Weight loss, exercise, PT/OT.

Complications:

- Arthritis mutilans (ie, joint deformities), enthesopathy.
- Cardiovascular disease, aortic aneurysms.
- Uveitis.

HYF: Associated with HLA-B27. It is a seronegative spondyloarthropathy; patients must have negative RF to be diagnosed. There is often DIP involvement, asymmetric oligoarticular or symmetric polyarticular involvement, spondyloarthritis (eg, sacroiliitis), enthesitis, nail pitting, dactylitis ("sausage digit"), ocular inflammation, and pitting edema. Arthritis can precede psoriatic skin lesions.

8-3 Rheumatologic Serologies

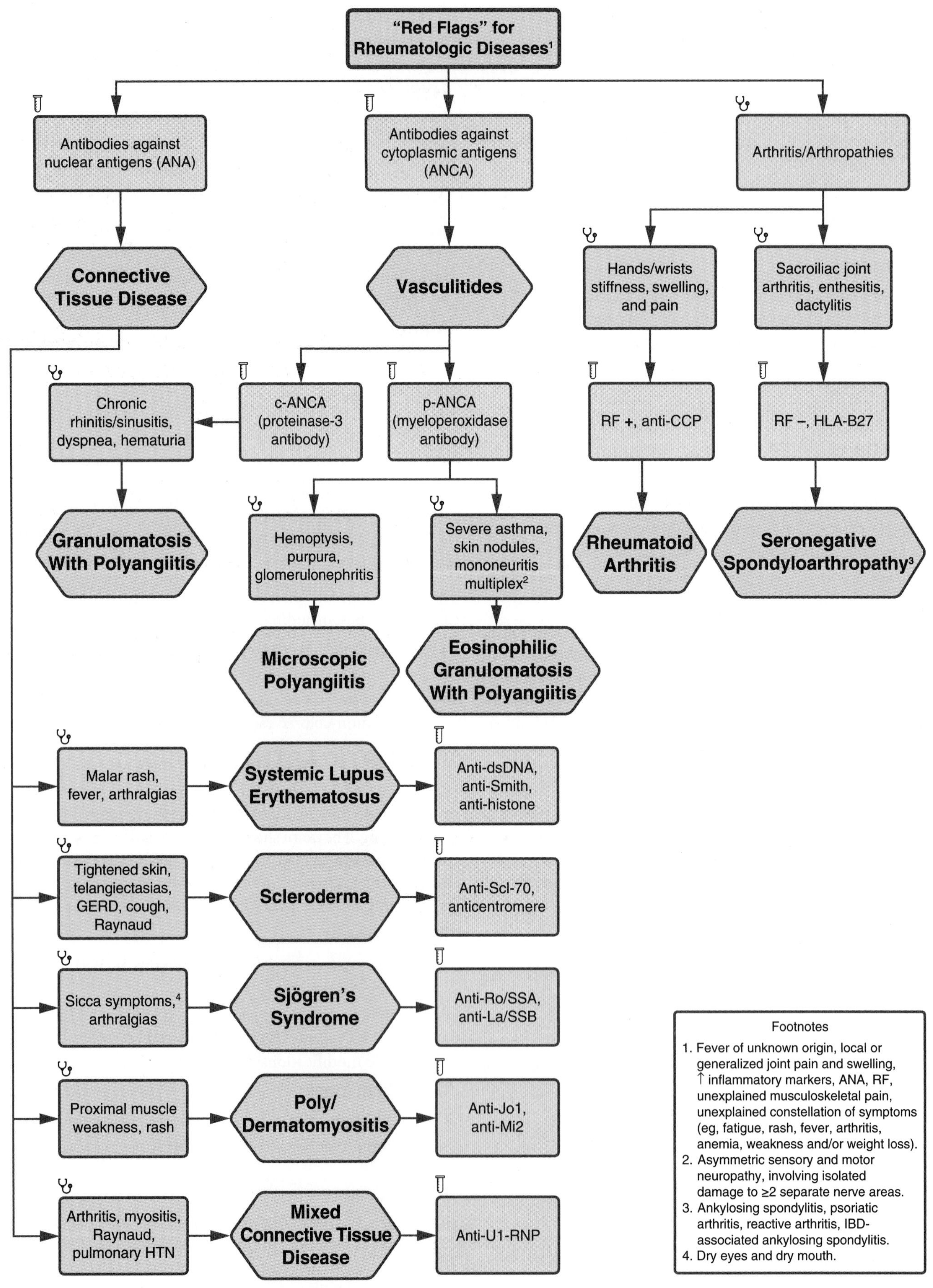
"Red Flags" for Rheumatologic Diseases[1]
Antibodies against nuclear antigens (ANA)
Antibodies against cytoplasmic antigens (ANCA)
Arthritis/Arthropathies
Connective Tissue Disease
Vasculitides
Hands/wrists stiffness, swelling, and pain
Sacroiliac joint arthritis, enthesitis, dactylitis
Chronic rhinitis/sinusitis, dyspnea, hematuria
c-ANCA (proteinase-3 antibody)
p-ANCA (myeloperoxidase antibody)
RF +, anti-CCP
RF –, HLA-B27
Granulomatosis With Polyangiitis
Hemoptysis, purpura, glomerulonephritis
Severe asthma, skin nodules, mononeuritis multiplex[2]
Rheumatoid Arthritis
Seronegative Spondyloarthropathy[3]
Microscopic Polyangiitis
Eosinophilic Granulomatosis With Polyangiitis
Malar rash, fever, arthralgias
Systemic Lupus Erythematosus
Anti-dsDNA, anti-Smith, anti-histone
Tightened skin, telangiectasias, GERD, cough, Raynaud
Scleroderma
Anti-Scl-70, anticentromere
Sicca symptoms,[4] arthralgias
Sjögren's Syndrome
Anti-Ro/SSA, anti-La/SSB
Proximal muscle weakness, rash
Poly/ Dermatomyositis
Anti-Jo1, anti-Mi2
Arthritis, myositis, Raynaud, pulmonary HTN
Mixed Connective Tissue Disease
Anti-U1-RNP

Footnotes

1. Fever of unknown origin, local or generalized joint pain and swelling, ↑ inflammatory markers, ANA, RF, unexplained musculoskeletal pain, unexplained constellation of symptoms (eg, fatigue, rash, fever, arthritis, anemia, weakness and/or weight loss).
2. Asymmetric sensory and motor neuropathy, involving isolated damage to ≥2 separate nerve areas.
3. Ankylosing spondylitis, psoriatic arthritis, reactive arthritis, IBD-associated ankylosing spondylitis.
4. Dry eyes and dry mouth.

FIGURE 8.3

8-3 Rheumatologic Serologies

Rheumatologic Diagnosis	Labs
Systemic Lupus Erythematosus (SLE)	• ANA: Best initial test for SLE, high sensitivity, low specificity. Can be positive in other autoimmune diseases. • Anti-dsDNA: Positive in 70% of patients with SLE, high specificity. Deposited in glomeruli in lupus nephritis → indicates renal disease. Can correlate with disease activity. • Anti-Smith: High specificity, low sensitivity. • Low complements: C3, C4 • Anti-histone: Present in drug-induced SLE.
Scleroderma	• Anti-Scl-70 (anti-topoisomerase antibody I): Present in 30–70% of patients with scleroderma (diffuse). • Anticentromere antibody: CREST syndrome.
Sjögren's Syndrome	• Anti-Ro/SSA: Neonatal heart block. • Anti-La/SSB: Neonatal heart block. Can be positive in SLE.
Polymyositis/Dermatomyositis	• Anti-Jo1: Present in 20–30% of patients. Can be positive in antisynthetase syndrome. • Anti-Mi2: Present in 10–30% of patients, most commonly dermatomyositis. • Anti-SRP.
Polymyalgia Rheumatica	• ESR, CRP
Mixed Connective Tissue Disease	• Anti-U1 RNP: Can also be positive in SLE.
Microscopic Polyangiitis	• p-ANCA: 70% of patients are ANCA positive, most of them p-ANCA.
Granulomatosis with Polyangiitis	• 90% of patients are c-ANCA positive.
Eosinophilic Granulomatosis with Polyangiitis	• p-ANCA or c-ANCA.
Rheumatoid Arthritis	• ANA: Positive in <50% patients. • Anti-ACPA are specific (formally anti-CCP). • RF is sensitive. RF is an IgM antibody that targets the Fc portion of IgG. RF positive patients are more likely to develop extra-articular manifestations. Not correlated with disease activity. • 20% of patients are seronegative. • Often positive HLA-DR4.
Seronegative Spondyloarthropathies	• RF negative, ANA negative. • Often positive HLA-B27.
Goodpasture Syndrome	• Anti-GBM antibody.
Autoimmune Hepatitis	• Anti-smooth muscle.
Primary Biliary Cirrhosis	• Anti-mitochondrial.
Lambert-Eaton Myasthenic Syndrome (LEMS)	• Antibodies to presynaptic calcium channel.
Myasthenia gravis	• Antibodies to postsynaptic ACh receptor.

*c-ANCA is also known as PR3-ANCA. p-ANCA is also known as MPO-ANCA.

8-4 Petechiae

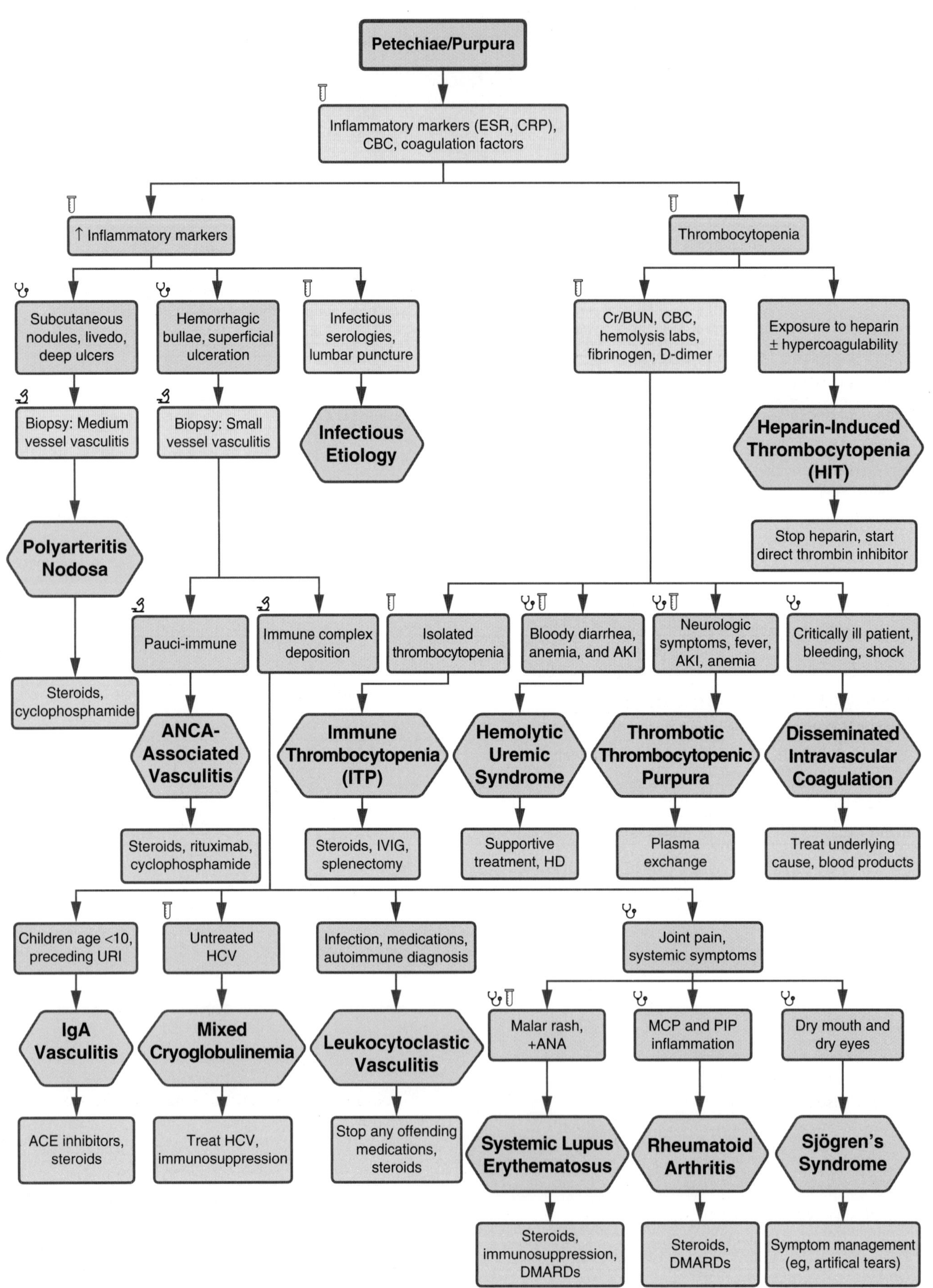

Petechiae/Purpura
Inflammatory markers (ESR, CRP), CBC, coagulation factors
↑ Inflammatory markers
Thrombocytopenia
Subcutaneous nodules, livedo, deep ulcers
Hemorrhagic bullae, superficial ulceration
Infectious serologies, lumbar puncture
Cr/BUN, CBC, hemolysis labs, fibrinogen, D-dimer
Exposure to heparin ± hypercoagulability
Biopsy: Medium vessel vasculitis
Biopsy: Small vessel vasculitis
Infectious Etiology
Heparin-Induced Thrombocytopenia (HIT)
Stop heparin, start direct thrombin inhibitor
Polyarteritis Nodosa
Steroids, cyclophosphamide
Pauci-immune
Immune complex deposition
Isolated thrombocytopenia
Bloody diarrhea, anemia, and AKI
Neurologic symptoms, fever, AKI, anemia
Critically ill patient, bleeding, shock
ANCA-Associated Vasculitis
Immune Thrombocytopenia (ITP)
Hemolytic Uremic Syndrome
Thrombotic Thrombocytopenic Purpura
Disseminated Intravascular Coagulation
Steroids, rituximab, cyclophosphamide
Steroids, IVIG, splenectomy
Supportive treatment, HD
Plasma exchange
Treat underlying cause, blood products
Children age <10, preceding URI
Untreated HCV
Infection, medications, autoimmune diagnosis
Joint pain, systemic symptoms
IgA Vasculitis
Mixed Cryoglobulinemia
Leukocytoclastic Vasculitis
Malar rash, +ANA
MCP and PIP inflammation
Dry mouth and dry eyes
ACE inhibitors, steroids
Treat HCV, immunosuppression
Stop any offending medications, steroids
Systemic Lupus Erythematosus
Rheumatoid Arthritis
Sjögren's Syndrome
Steroids, immunosuppression, DMARDs
Steroids, DMARDs
Symptom management (eg, artifical tears)

FIGURE 8.4

8-4 Petechiae

POLYARTERITIS NODOSA (PAN)

A 65-year-old M with PMH of HBV and cirrhosis presents with fever, arthralgias, palpable purpura, orchitis, asymmetric neuropathy, and abdominal pain. **Imaging** shows renal arterial aneurysms and renal infarcts.

Management:

1. Corticosteroids +/– cyclophosphamide.

Complications:

- Rupture of renal arterial aneurysms, coronary artery disease.
- Polyneuropathy, stroke, mesenteric arteritis.

HYF: "**PAN** s**P**ares **P**ulm" (lungs). Systemic necrotizing vasculitis of medium-sized vessels. Associated with HBV (most common) and HCV, hairy cell leukemia. Patients are usually middle-aged males and often present with skin lesions and GI bleeding. ANCA –.

IMMUNE THROMBOCYTOPENIC PURPURA (ITP)

A 28-year-old F at 28 weeks' gestation presents with easy bruising and petechiae. **Labs** show a platelet count of 25,000.

Management:

1. Platelets >30,000 and no bleeding: Observation.
2. Platelets <30,000 or significant bleeding: Corticosteroids or IVIG.
3. Refractory: Rituximab, thrombopoietin receptor agonist, splenectomy.
4. Platelet transfusion only in life-threatening bleed.

Complications:

- In pregnant patients, fetus may have thrombocytopenia.
- Intracranial hemorrhage, GI bleed.

HYF: Due to IgG antibodies against platelets. Increased megakaryocytes in bone marrow are commonly seen. Patients are often asymptomatic or may have minor mucocutaneous bleeding, easy bruising, hematuria, or melena. There is usually no splenomegaly. Associated with SLE, HIV, HCV, and hematologic malignancies. May be acute (children after viral illness) or chronic (adults age 20–40). Diagnosis of exclusion.

THROMBOTIC THROMBOCYTOPENIC PURPURA (TTP)

A 33-year-old F with PMH of SLE presents with fever, jaundice, and petechiae. She has a seizure in the ER. **Labs** show an ↑ Cr consistent with an AKI, as well as anemia, ↑ LDH, and ↓ haptoglobin consistent with hemolysis.

Management:

1. Urgent plasma exchange ± corticosteroids.

Complications:

- Stroke, seizures, paresis, coma.
- Hemorrhagic colitis, bowel necrosis.
- Hypertension, chronic kidney disease.

HYF: Deficiency of the vWF-cleaving enzyme (ADAMTS-13) results in abnormally large vWF multimers that aggregate platelets and create platelet microthrombi, which block small blood vessels and cause end-organ damage. Classic pentad: Anemia, neurologic changes, impaired renal function, and fever (suspect if ≥3 out of 5). Associated with SLE, malignancy, pregnancy, HIV.

DISSEMINATED INTRAVASCULAR COAGULATION

A 29-year-old F is hospitalized with a new diagnosis of acute promyelocytic leukemia and is now developing **exam** findings of ecchymosis and purpura. Blood is oozing from gingivae and intravenous lines.

Management:

1. Treat underlying cause. Supportive care.
2. FFP, cryoprecipitate, pRBC, and/or platelet transfusion as indicated.

Complications:

- Widespread thrombosis, ischemia, necrosis.
- Microangiopathic hemolytic anemia. Life-threatening bleeding.
- Acute kidney failure, ARDS, shock.

HYF: An abnormal systemic activation of clotting cascade leads to bleeding and paradoxical thrombosis. Causes: Obstetric complications (amniotic emboli, abruptio placentae, preeclampsia, retained fetal products), infection/sepsis (usually Gram-negative pathogens), acute pancreatitis, autoimmune diseases, malignancy (prostate, pancreas, lung, stomach), trauma, critical illness, snakebites, and burns. Labs can show thrombocytopenia, ↓ fibrinogen and clotting factors, ↑ PT/PTT and D-dimer, and schistocytes.

MICROSCOPIC POLYANGIITIS

A 34-year-old M presents with palpable purpura and skin ulcers, hemoptysis, and hematuria. Kidney biopsy is consistent with rapidly progressive glomerulonephritis, with immunofluorescence (IF) revealing a pauci-immune pattern. **Labs** show the following serologies: MPO-ANCA+/pANCA+.

Management:

1. Corticosteroids and cyclophosphamide.

Complications: Renal failure.

HYF: Necrotizing vasculitis of small vessels. No granulomas. Nasopharynx usually not affected (no sinusitis or rhinitis).

GRANULOMATOSIS WITH POLYANGIITIS

A 60-year-old M with PMH of HTN presents with hemoptysis, fever, diffuse arthralgias, weight loss, dyspnea, and bloody nasal discharge. **Labs** show ↑ ESR and CRP, Cr 4.2, and PR3-ANCA+/cANCA+. On **imaging**, CXR shows pulmonary nodules.

(Continued)

8-4 Petechiae

Management:

1. Corticosteroids + methotrexate, cyclophosphamide, or rituximab.

Complications:

- Rapidly progressive glomerulonephritis.
- Recurrent otitis media, perforation of nasal septum, gingival hyperplasia.
- Pulmonary (fibrosis, hypertension, hemorrhage) and cardiac complications.

HYF: Small- to medium-sized vessel necrotizing vasculitis with granuloma formation. Affects upper (nasopharynx) and lower respiratory tracts (lungs), as well as kidneys. Positive PR3–ANCA/cANCA in 90% of patients.

EOSINOPHILIC GRANULOMATOSIS WITH POLYANGIITIS

A 38-year-old M with PMH of severe asthma presents with tender subcutaneous nodules, numbness and weakness of the right upper extremity, and sinusitis. **Labs** show ↑ eosinophils and MPO-ANCA+/pANCA+.

Management:

1. Corticosteroids + cyclophosphamide or azathioprine.

Complications:

- Necrotizing glomerulonephritis.
- Eosinophilic infiltration of organs.
- Coronary arteritis, myocarditis, alveolar hemorrhage.

HYF: Small- and medium-sized vessel necrotizing vasculitis. Patients may present with peripheral neuropathy (mononeuritis multiplex), peripheral eosinophilia, adult-onset severe asthma, allergic rhinitis, nasal polyps (typically no epistaxis), and GI and skin involvement.

IgA VASCULITIS (HENOCH-SCHONLEIN PURPURA)

A 6-year-old boy presents with colicky abdominal pain, lower extremity rash up to his buttocks, ankle and knee pain, and hematuria. He had an upper respiratory infection (URI) 2 weeks ago. No thrombocytopenia on **labs**.

Management:

1. Supportive care. Expect spontaneous resolution within 4 weeks.
2. Glucocorticoids if persistent renal disease.

Complications: Intussusception or renal disease (rare).

HYF: IgA immune complex deposition in small vessels and triad of palpable purpura, arthralgias, and abdominal pain. Most common childhood vasculitis. Look for a preceding URI, especially group A *Streptococcus*. Clinical diagnosis.

MIXED CRYOGLOBULINEMIA (CRYOGLOBULINEMIC VASCULITIS)

A 48-year-old M with PMH of untreated HCV presents with fatigue, weight loss, purpuric rash, and arthritis. **Labs** show proteinuria, hematuria, and low serum complement levels.

Management:

1. HCV treatment.
2. Corticosteroids and rituximab if severe.
3. Plasmapheresis if refractory to the above steps.

Complications: Renal failure, cardiovascular disease.

HYF: Temperature-dependent deposition of immunoglobulins in blood vessels. Frequently RF+. Associated with HCV. Patients may present with skin lesions, acrocyanosis, polyneuropathy, and glomerulonephritis.

CUTANEOUS SMALL CELL VASCULITIS (HYPERSENSITIVITY)

A 44-year-old F with PMH of SLE and cellulitis on cephalexin, presents with **exam** findings of lower-extremity palpable purpura, vesicles, and skin nodules.

Management:

1. Investigation of underlying cause. Consider skin biopsy.
2. Corticosteroids, (topical vs. oral).

Complications: Visceral involvement (GI, kidneys).

HYF: Due to immune-complex deposition as a result of hypersensitivity reaction to drugs (eg, penicillin, sulfa), infections, malignancy, or autoimmune disease. 50% of cases are idiopathic. Skin is predominantly affected.

8-4 Petechiae

HEMOLYTIC UREMIC SYNDROME (HUS)

A 5-year-old M presents with jaundice, abdominal pain, and petechiae. **Labs** show thrombocytopenia, anemia, and severe acute kidney injury. The mother reports he had bloody diarrhea 1 week ago.

Management:

1. Supportive care. Hemodialysis if needed.

Complications:

- Hypertension, chronic kidney disease.
- Seizures, stroke, coma.

HYF: Most commonly seen in children and caused by *E. coli* O157:H7 (EHEC) due to *Shiga*-like toxin, *S. pneumoniae* or *Shigella* spp. infection. Triad of thrombocytopenia, non-immune microangiopathic hemolytic anemia, and acute kidney failure. No fever or neurologic symptoms. Use of antimotility agents or antibiotics in EHEC diarrhea are risk factors.

Heparin-Induced Thrombocytopenia (HIT): See pp. 106–107.

Systemic Lupus Erythematosus: See p. 328.

Rheumatoid Arthritis: See pp. 296–298.

Sjögren's Syndrome: See pp. 298, 304.

8-5 Additional Rheumologic Diagnoses

SYSTEMIC LUPUS ERYTHEMATOSUS

A 23-year-old F presents with several months of fatigue, bilateral pain, and swelling in her wrists and knees. **Exam** is notable for a fever (38°C) and reveals an erythematous rash on her face, oral ulcers, and enlarged, mildly tender joints. **Labs** show ↑ ESR and creatinine; ↓ C3 and C4 with pancytopenia; and a (+) ANA and the presence of anti-double-stranded DNA (anti-dsDNA) antibodies. Urinalysis is positive for +2 protein.

Management:

1. Non-pharmacologic management: Sunscreen, immunizations, smoking cessation.
2. Long-term: Hydroxychloroquine or chloroquine ± prednisone.
3. Antimalarials.
4. DMARDs.
5. For arthralgias: NSAIDs.
6. Flare: Prednisolone or hydroxychloroquine.
7. Lupus nephritis/cerebritis: Cyclophosphamide.

Complications:

- Renal disease.
- Infections.
- Libman-Sacks endocarditis.
- Fetal heart block in pregnancy.
- Antiphospholipid antibody syndrome.

HYF: Renal disease, cardiovascular disease, and infections are the most common causes of death. Anti-Smith antibodies are specific and indicate poor prognosis. Anti-dsDNA antibodies are also specific and often seen in patients with lupus nephritis. If UA shows signs of proteinuria/hematuria, a kidney biopsy is indicated prior to treatment. Anti-histone antibodies are seen in drug-induced lupus and are associated with medications like hydralazine, procainamide, isoniazid, and TNF-α inhibitors; stop the offending medication.

SJÖGREN'S SYNDROME

A 45-year-old F presents with several months of a gritty sensation in both eyes and feeling like her mouth is dry. **Exam** shows dry mucous membranes, bilateral enlargement of the parotid glands, and multiple dental caries with halitosis. **Labs** show ↑ ESR, (+) ANA, and the presence of anti-Ro and anti-La antibodies.

Management:

1. Artificial tears for dry eyes.
2. Increased oral hygiene.
3. Saliva stimulants: Pilocarpine or cevimeline.

Complications:

- Dental caries.
- Increased risk for non-Hodgkin B-cell lymphoma.
- Fetal heart block in pregnancy.

HYF: In patients with a (–) ANA or low antibody titers, you can consider a minor salivary gland biopsy, which should show a periductal lymphoid infiltrate of the exocrine glands. Associated with HLA-DR5. ~50% of patients with Sjögren also have extraglandular symptoms (eg, polyarthritis, purpura, vasculitis), which can be treated with steroids or hydroxychloroquine.

SCLERODERMA/CREST

A 33-year-old F with PMH of severe GERD refractory to PPIs presents with months of fatigue and stiffening of her joints. She also endorses pain and discoloration of her hands when cold and shortness of breath with exertion. On **exam**, she has SpO_2 93% on room air, end-inspiratory crackles, digital ulcerations, and puffiness of the hands and face.

Management: Treatment is usually dictated by organ system involvement and disease severity.

1. Skin: Methotrexate, mycophenolate.
2. Kidney: ACE inhibitors (captopril), dialysis.
3. Lung: Mycophenolate, cyclophosphamide, azathioprine.
4. GI: PPIs, metoclopramide.
5. Raynaud: Keeping warm, CCBs (nifedipine).
6. Musculoskeletal: NSAIDs, hydroxychloroquine, methotrexate.

Complications:

- Lung: Interstitial lung disease, fibrosis, pulmonary hypertension.
- Kidney: Hypertension, renal crisis, renal failure.
- Heart: Fibrosis, pericarditis, pericardial effusion.

HYF: Associated with anti-topoisomerase (anti-Scl-70), anti-centromere, and anti-RNA polymerase III antibodies. Systemic sclerosis can be either diffuse or limited (CREST syndrome). Diffuse scleroderma has widespread skin involvement, early visceral involvement, and association with the anti-Scl-70 antibody. CREST syndrome is associated with the anti-centromere antibody. **CREST** syndrome (**C**alcinosis cutis/anti-**C**entromere, **R**aynaud, **E**sophageal dysmotliity, **S**clerodactyly, **T**elangiectasia) is associated with anti-centromere antibody.

TAKAYASU ARTERITIS

A 23-year-old F presents with several months of pain and numbness in both arms. She works at a grocery store and notices the symptoms worsen when she stocks books on high shelves. She also notes joint stiffness and night sweats. **Exam** shows weak bilateral upper extremity pulses and a bruit in the base of the neck. Blood pressure in her right arm is 145/92 and 100/50 in her left. **Labs** show ↑ ESR.

Management:

1. Prednisone ± methotrexate.
2. Surgical revascularization.
3. Aortic valvular surgery.

Complications:

- Hypertension.
- Heart failure, heart attack.
- Stroke, TIA.
- Aortic aneurysm.

8-5 Additional Rheumologic Diagnoses

BEHÇET'S SYNDROME

A 50-year-old M presents with painful mouth ulcers, genital lesions, and blurry vision. Exam shows multiple ulcers of the oral mucosa and around his penis and redness of the eyes. When poked with a needle, a red papule forms. Labs are within normal limits.

Management: Treatment is usually dictated by organ system involvement and disease severity.

1. Ocular: Steroids ± azathioprine.
2. Mucocutaneous: Triamcinolone cream, colchicine.
3. Musculoskeletal: Steroids, NSAIDs.
4. Vascular: Steroids.
5. Neurologic: Azathioprine.
6. GI: Steroids ± azathioprine.

Complications:

- Blindness.
- Thrombus.
- Arterial aneurysm and rupture.
- Pregnancy loss.

HYF: Behçet's syndrome can also present with erythema nodosum. A pathergy test as described in the vignette above (presence of exaggerated skin ulceration after minor trauma) can help in diagnosis.

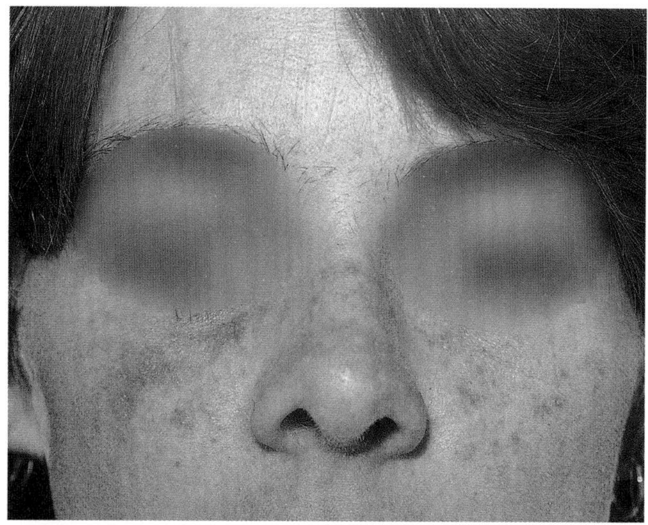

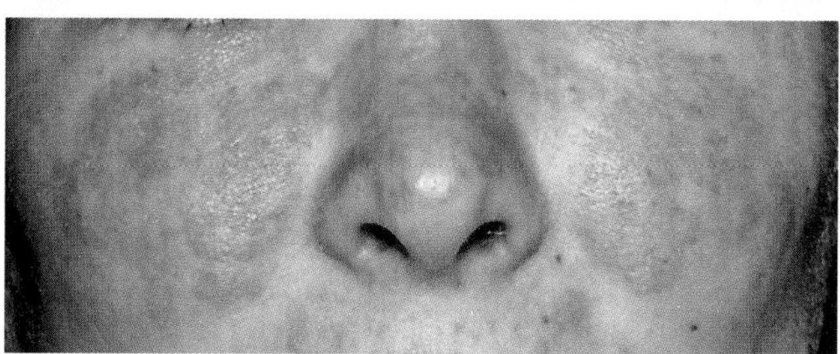

Malar rash of acute lupus erythematosus.

COMPLEX REGIONAL PAIN SYNDROME

A 33-year-old M presents with severe, constant, burning pain in his right arm 1 month after previously spraining his wrist. Previously his sprain had been healing well. Exam shows an erythematous, edematous, and warm arm with no hair. While examining his arm, the patient experiences severe pain with light touch. His left arm shows no abnormalities. On imaging, X-ray of the arm shows patchy demineralization.

Management:

1. Physical and occupational therapy.
2. NSAIDs.
3. Gabapentin, TCAs.

Complications:

- Impaired cognitive executive function.
- Dystonia.
- Muscle atrophy.

HYF: Complex regional pain syndrome is also called reflex sympathetic dystrophy. It usually presents 4–6 weeks after trauma or surgery. The associated pain is neuropathic and follows a non-dermatomal pattern. It is worse with light tough (allodynia) or movement. Bone scintigraphy can show increased uptake.

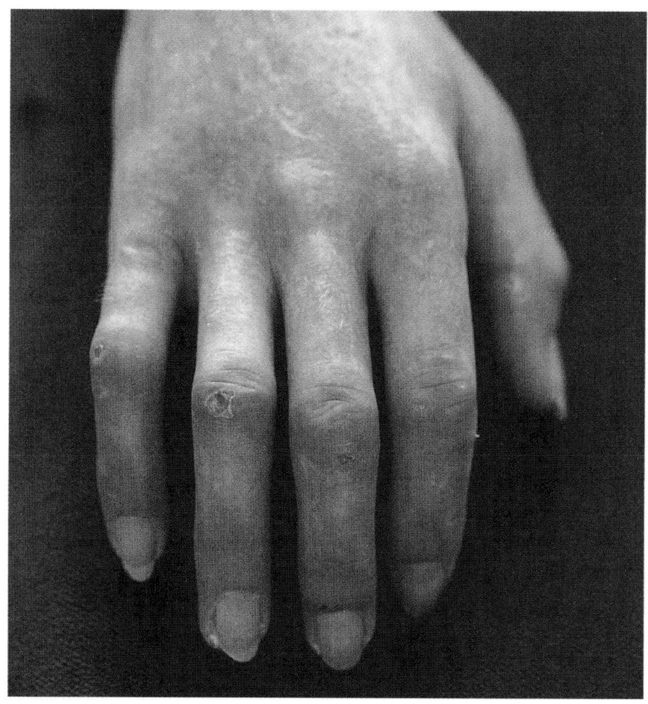

Sclerodactyly in systemic sclerosis.

8-6 Progressive Generalized Weakness

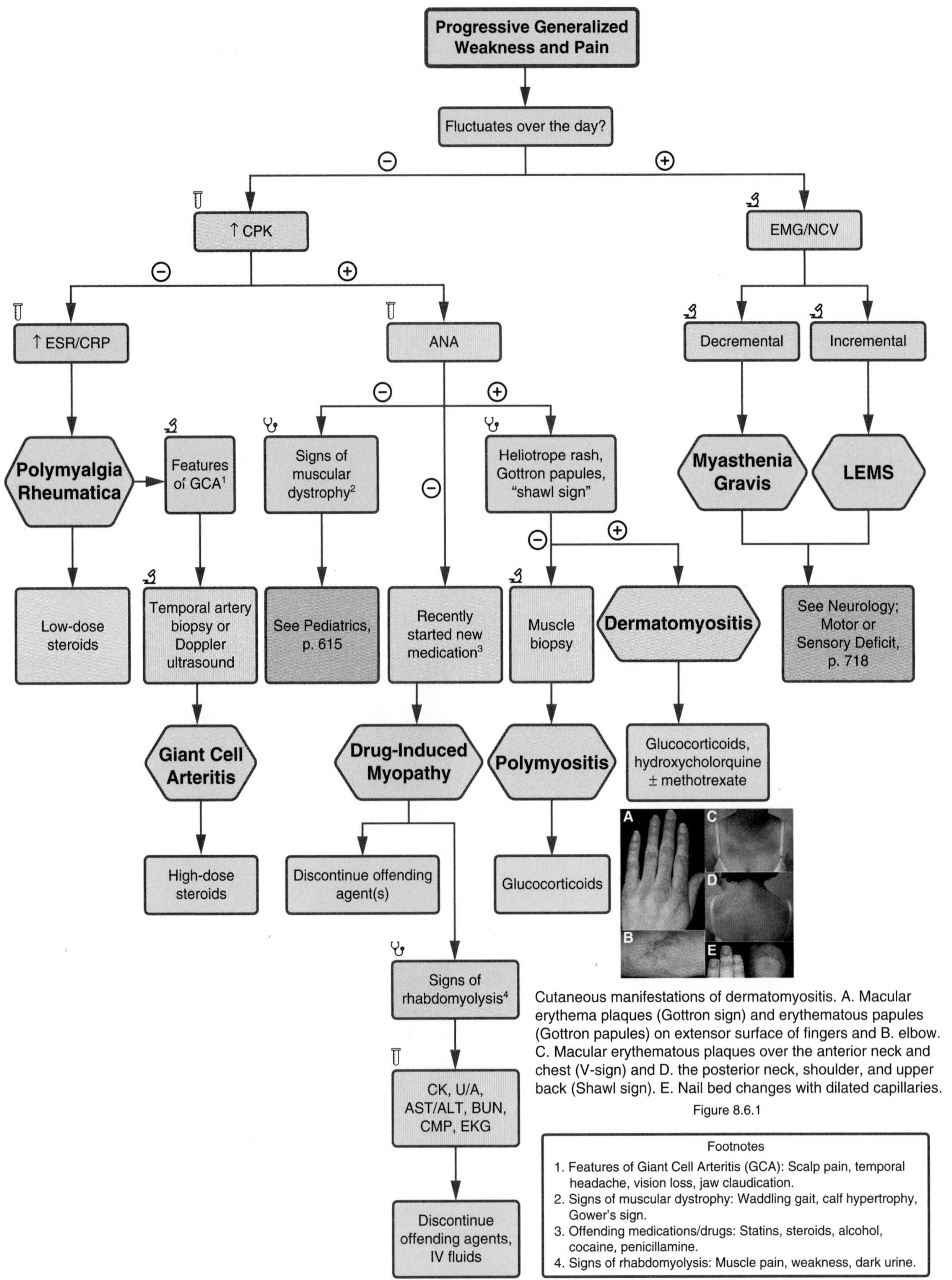

Progressive Generalized Weakness and Pain
Fluctuates over the day?
⊖
⊕
↑ CPK
EMG/NCV
⊖
⊕
↑ ESR/CRP
ANA
Decremental
Incremental
⊖
⊕
Polymyalgia Rheumatica
Features of GCA[1]
Signs of muscular dystrophy[2]
⊖
Heliotrope rash, Gottron papules, "shawl sign"
Myasthenia Gravis
LEMS
⊖
⊕
Low-dose steroids
Temporal artery biopsy or Doppler ultrasound
See Pediatrics, p. 615
Recently started new medication[3]
Muscle biopsy
Dermatomyositis
See Neurology; Motor or Sensory Deficit, p. 718
Giant Cell Arteritis
Drug-Induced Myopathy
Polymyositis
Glucocorticoids, hydroxycholorquine ± methotrexate
A
B
C
D
E
High-dose steroids
Discontinue offending agent(s)
Glucocorticoids
Signs of rhabdomyolysis[4]
CK, U/A, AST/ALT, BUN, CMP, EKG
Discontinue offending agents, IV fluids

Cutaneous manifestations of dermatomyositis. A. Macular erythema plaques (Gottron sign) and erythematous papules (Gottron papules) on extensor surface of fingers and B. elbow. C. Macular erythematous plaques over the anterior neck and chest (V-sign) and D. the posterior neck, shoulder, and upper back (Shawl sign). E. Nail bed changes with dilated capillaries.

Figure 8.6.1

Footnotes

1. Features of Giant Cell Arteritis (GCA): Scalp pain, temporal headache, vision loss, jaw claudication.
2. Signs of muscular dystrophy: Waddling gait, calf hypertrophy, Gower's sign.
3. Offending medications/drugs: Statins, steroids, alcohol, cocaine, penicillamine.
4. Signs of rhabdomyolysis: Muscle pain, weakness, dark urine.

FIGURE 8.6

8-6 Progressive Generalized Weakness

POLYMYALGIA RHEUMATICA (PMR)

A 72-year-old F presents with bilateral pain and stiffness in her shoulders, hips, and neck, which are worse in the morning. The **exam** shows low-grade fever, ↓ ROM in shoulders and hips, diffuse tenderness in her shoulders, and 5/5 strength throughout. **Labs** show ↑ ESR and CRP.

Management:

1. Low-dose corticosteroids for an extended course (eg, 24 months). Taper if improvement is seen.
2. If corticosteroids are not working or contraindicated: Methotrexate.

Complications:

- Blindness caused by giant cell arteritis (GCA).
- Complications from long-term steroids.
- Aortic aneurysm.

HYF: PMR resolves quickly with low-dose steroids. Usually seen at age >50. Associated with GCA, which can present with jaw claudication, headache, and visual disturbance. If GCA is suspected, perform an urgent temporal artery biopsy and give high-dose corticosteroids prior to receiving biopsy results. PMR and GCA are both associated with HLA-DR4.

DRUG-INDUCED MYOPATHY

A 57-year-old M with PMH of T2DM, HTN, and recently diagnosed HLD presents with crampy bilateral thigh and calf pain. He recently started atovastatin. The **exam** shows low-grade fever, as well as bilateral proximal muscle weakness and tenderness. **Labs** show ↑ CK.

Management:

1. Cessation or dose reduction of the offending agent.
2. If due to statin: Switch to pravastatin or fluvastatin, which are less associated with statin-associated myopathy.

Complications:

- Rhabdomyolysis with acute renal failure.

HYF: Most commonly associated drugs are statins, glucocorticoids, alcohol, and cocaine. Symptoms usually occur weeks to months after drug initiation. With glucocorticoid-induced myopathy, patients can present with painless proximal muscle weakness and normal ESR/CRP.

POLYMYOSITIS

A 49-year-old F presents with several months of unintentional weight loss, increased weakness, trouble combing hair, and dyspnea. **Exam** shows proximal muscle weakness but normal ROM, strength, and reflexes. **Labs** show ↑ ESR, CK, aldolase, and LDH. Muscle biopsy shows an endomysial cellular infiltrate and patchy necrosis.

Management:

1. Systemic glucocorticoids (eg, prednisone).
2. ±Glucocorticoid-sparing agents (methotrexate, azathioprine, mycophenolate mofetil).
3. Age-appropriate cancer screenings.

Complications:

- Same as dermatomyositis.

HYF: Resembles dermatomyositis but without skin manifestations.

DERMATOMYOSITIS

A 63-year-old F presents with several months of generalized muscle weakness. She has difficulty climbing stairs or combing her hair. **Exam** shows an erythematous rash on her face (periorbital, nasolabial folds), upper chest and shoulders, papules over the bony areas of her hands, elbows, and knees, "dirty"-appearing marks on her fingertips, as well as symmetric proximal muscle weakness. **Labs** show ↑ ESR, CK, LDH, and aldolase, as well as presence of anti-Jo-1, anti-SRP, and anti-Mi-2 antibodies. Muscle biopsy shows an endomysial cellular infiltrate and patchy necrosis.

Management:

1. Systemic glucocorticoids (eg, prednisone).
2. ± Glucocorticoid-sparing agents (eg, methotrexate, azathioprine, mycophenolate mofetil).
3. Dermatologic manifestations: Topical corticosteroids and/or calcineurin inhibitors, hydroxychloroquine ± methotrexate, avoidance of the sun, antipruritic agents.
4. Age-appropriate cancer screenings.

Complications:

- Dyspnea (interstitial lung disease).
- Dysphagia (esophageal dysmotility, pharyngeal dysfunction).
- Myocarditis, AV block.
- Increased risk of occult malignancy.

HYF: Due to autoantibodies associated with poly- and dermatomyositis: anti-Jo-1, anti-SRP, and anti-Mi-2. Dermatomyositis classically presents with a heliotrope rash, malar rash, shawl rash, Gottron papules, and "mechanic's hands." It can be a paraneoplastic manifestation of multiple malignancies (especially breast, lung, ovaries, colon, non-Hodgkin lymphoma).

MYASTHENIA GRAVIS

A 33-year-old F presents with intermittent episodes of blurry vision, difficulty swallowing, and fatigue in the evenings. **Exam** shows bilateral mild ptosis, diplopia, normal DTRs, and initially normal strength that diminishes with repetition. **Labs** are positive for anti-AChR antibody. On **imaging**, CT chest shows a thymoma.

Management:

1. Acetylcholinesterase inhibitors (eg, pyridostigmine).
2. Persistent symptoms: Corticosteroids (eg, prednisone) and immunosuppressants (eg, cyclosporine, azathioprine)
3. Evaluation for underlying thymoma: Thymectomy if found on CT can be curative.
4. Myasthenic crisis: Respiratory support (ie, intubation), plasmapheresis or IVIG, corticosteroids.

(Continued)

8-6 Progressive Generalized Weakness

Complications:

- Myasthenic crises can be precipitated by illness, pregnancy, surgery, drugs (eg, aminoglycosides, penicillamine, β-blockers, procainamide, fluoroquinolones, magnesium) leading to respiratory failure and/or aspiration.

HYF: Due to postsynaptic ACh receptor autoantibodies from the thymus, leading to worsening weakness with repetitive use. If labs are negative for acetycholine receptor antibodies but clinical suspicion is high, check for muscle-specific tyrosine kinase (MuSK) antibodies. EMG studies can also be helpful in establishing the diagnosis.

LAMBERT-EATON MYASTHENIC SYNDROME (LEMS)

A 67-year-old M with an extensive smoking history presents with unintentional weight loss, dry mouth, and several weeks of progressive weakness in his limbs. The **exam** shows orthostatic hypotension, bilateral proximal weakness, and diminished DTRs. His strength improves with repeated testing. On **imaging**, CXR shows a left lung mass.

Management:

1. Evaluation for underlying malignancy; treat if present (most commonly small-cell lung cancer).
2. Mild weakness: Aminopyridines (eg, 3,4-diaminopyridine, amifampridine) or low-dose guanidine ± pyridostigmine.
3. Moderate/severe weakness: IVIG, immunosuppressive agents (eg, steroids, azathioprine).

Complications: Respiratory failure in later stages of disease.

HYF: LEMS is a paraneoplastic syndrome due to autoantibodies against the presynaptic calcium channels in the NMJ, which ↓ Ach release due to ↓ presynaptic vesicle fusion. Antibodies against voltage-gated calcium channels may also be present. Obtain imaging (eg, CT) to evaluate for occult malignancy. Weakness improves with repetitive muscle use (Lambert sign).

Fibromyalgia: See pp. 294-295.
Giant Cell Arteritis: See pp. 306, 615, 750, 767, 769.
Muscular Dystrophies: See pp. 615-616.

9
Internal Medicine: Dermatology

9-1 Hyperpigmented Macules

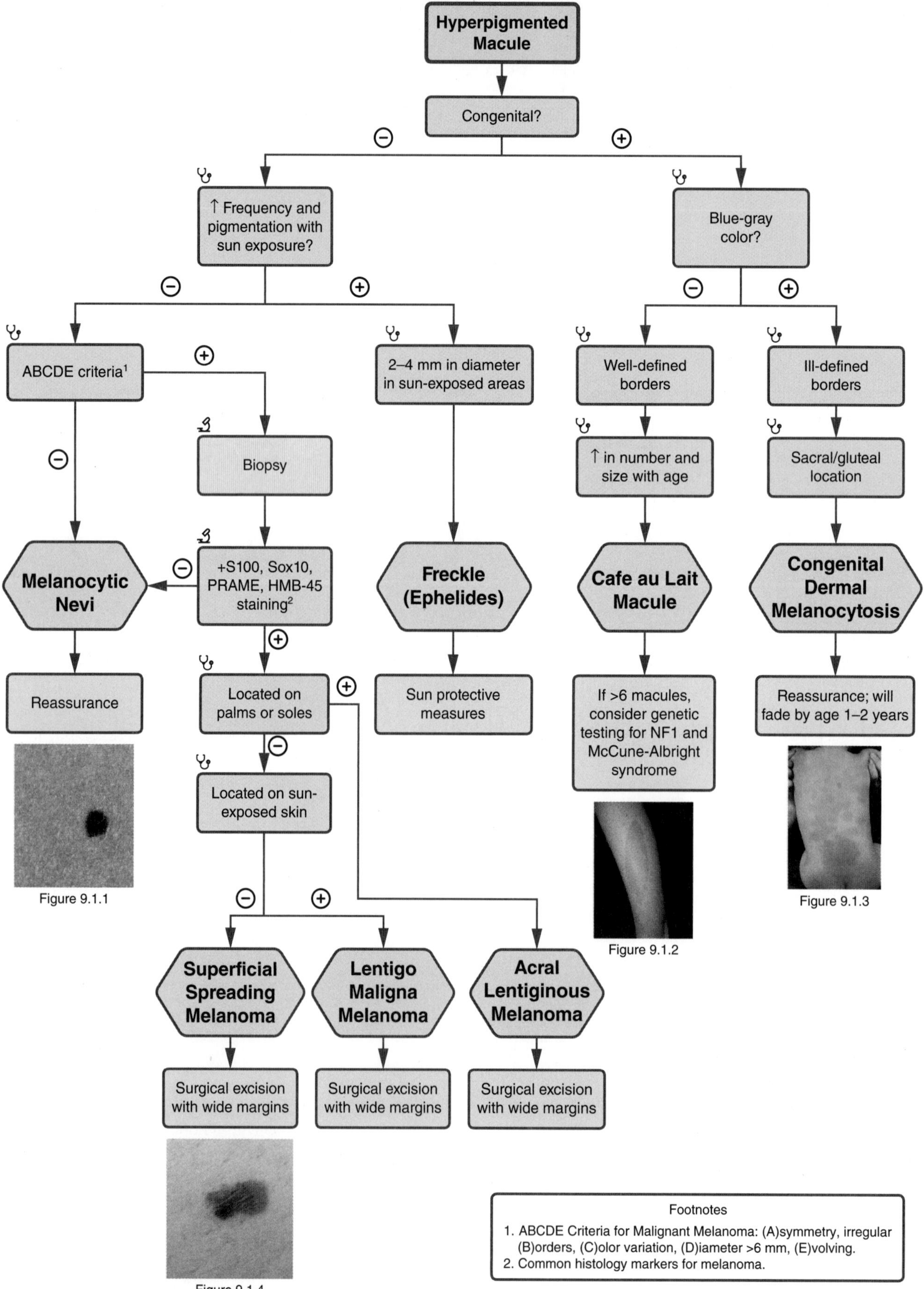
Hyperpigmented Macule
Congenital?
↑ Frequency and pigmentation with sun exposure?
Blue-gray color?
ABCDE criteria[1]
2–4 mm in diameter in sun-exposed areas
Well-defined borders
Ill-defined borders
Biopsy
↑ in number and size with age
Sacral/gluteal location
Melanocytic Nevi
+S100, Sox10, PRAME, HMB-45 staining[2]
Freckle (Ephelides)
Cafe au Lait Macule
Congenital Dermal Melanocytosis
Reassurance
Located on palms or soles
Sun protective measures
If >6 macules, consider genetic testing for NF1 and McCune-Albright syndrome
Reassurance; will fade by age 1–2 years
Located on sun-exposed skin
Figure 9.1.1
Figure 9.1.2
Figure 9.1.3
Superficial Spreading Melanoma
Lentigo Maligna Melanoma
Acral Lentiginous Melanoma
Surgical excision with wide margins
Surgical excision with wide margins
Surgical excision with wide margins
Figure 9.1.4
Footnotes
1. ABCDE Criteria for Malignant Melanoma: (A)symmetry, irregular (B)orders, (C)olor variation, (D)iameter >6 mm, (E)volving.
2. Common histology markers for melanoma.

FIGURE 9.1

9-1 Hyperpigmented Macules

MELANOCYTIC NEVI

A 45-year-old Caucasian M who works as a farmer presents with a 6-month history of a 3-mm, non-itching, and non-painful hyperpigmented macule on his back. On exam, the macule has well-defined borders, a smooth flat surface, and is uniformly dark brown in color.

Management:

1. Observation, sun protection.
2. If multiple acquired nevi, periodic total-body skin exams.

Complications: Associated with increased melanoma risk.

HYF: Melanocytic nevi lack ABCDE criteria for malignant melanoma. More common in patients with light skin tones and history of significant sun exposure.

FRECKLE (EPHELIDES)

A 7-year-old girl presents for a well-child visit in August and is noted to have macules on the face and dorsal hands. On exam, macules are hyperpigmented, 2–4 mm, and confluent in some areas.

Management:

1. Encourage sun protective measures.
2. For cosmetic purposes: laser/phototherapy.

Complications: None.

HYF: Benign. Most common in patients with lighter skin tones. Develop in sun-exposed areas, increase in number and pigmentation with sun exposure.

CAFÉ AU LAIT MACULE

A 10-year-old boy with PMH of optic pathway gliomas and ADHD presents with 8 hyperpigmented macules found on his trunk and extremities that have been increasing in number and size throughout childhood. Labs: Genetic testing is positive for *NF1* mutation.

Management:

1. If >6 lesions, genetic testing for neurofibromatosis type 1 (*NF1* gene) and McCune-Albright syndrome (*GNAS* gene).
2. Laser/phototherapy for cosmetic purposes.

Complications:

- *NF1*-related sequelae: Lisch nodules in the iris, optic gliomas, cutaneous neurofibromas, hypertension, and cognitive deficits/learning disabilities.
- McCune-Albright syndrome: Precocious puberty, fibrous dysplasia of bone.

HYF: Café au lait macules in McCune-Albright syndrome are unilateral with irregular borders ("coast of Maine"). In *NF1*, they have well-defined borders and are found bilaterally.

CONGENITAL DERMAL MELANOCYTOSIS

A 2-day-old Asian-American newborn presents with macule in the sacral-gluteal region. On exam, the macule has ill-defined borders and appears blue-gray in color.

Management:

1. Reassurance; these typically will fade by age 1–2 years.

Complications: None.

HYF: Caused by the delayed disappearance of dermal melanocytes. Most commonly found in Asian and Black newborns in the sacral-gluteal region.

SUPERFICIAL SPREADING MELANOMA

A 35-year-old F presents with new, rapidly growing macule on her left calf. On exam, the macule is 1 cm in diameter with irregular borders and color variegation. Biopsy is obtained. Immunohistochemistry is (+)S100, Sox10, HMB-45 staining.

Management:

1. Full-thickness excisional biopsy and staging.
2. Monitor with skin exam every 3–6 months for the first 2 years, biannually for 3 years, then annually thereafter.
3. If depth is >0.8–1.0 mm, consider sentinel lymph node biopsy.

Complications:

- Recurrence.
- Metastasis.

HYF: **ABCDEs of melanoma:** Asymmetry, irregular Borders, multi-Color, Diameter >6 mm, Evolving.

LENTIGO MALIGNA (LM) MELANOMA

A 70-year-old Caucasian F with a history of frequent tanning in her 20–30s presents with a macule on her right cheek. The lesion has been present for many years but began to enlarge over the past few months. On exam, the macule is 6 cm in diameter; multicolored with brown, red, and black hues; raised in some areas; and has poorly defined borders. On labs/imaging, histology shows neoplastic melanocytes along the dermoepidermal junction and epidermal atrophy consistent with solar elastosis.

Management:

1. Biopsy to confirm diagnosis.
2. Excision with 5–10 mm margins. If >1.0 cm, consider 1–2 cm margins and sentinel lymph node biopsy.
3. Total-body skin exam every 3–6 months for the first 2 years, biannually for 3 years, then annually thereafter.

(*Continued*)

9-1 Hyperpigmented Macules

Complications:

- Recurrence.
- Regional and distant metastasis.

HYF: LM melanoma has a predilection for sun-exposed sites like the head and neck in older patients.

ACRAL LENTIGINOUS MELANOMA

A 60-year-old Asian M presents with an ulcerating and non-healing lesion on the sole of his foot. The lesion is an irregularly shaped, unevenly pigmented, dark brown-black macule that bleeds.

Management:

1. Full-thickness excisional biopsy for diagnosis.
2. Surgical excision. Consider sentinel lymph node biopsy.
3. Skin exam every 3–6 months for the first 2 years, biannually for 3 years, then annually thereafter.

Complications:

- Recurrence.
- Regional and distant metastasis.

HYF: Acral lentiginous melanoma most commonly occurs on the palms, soles, or nail beds in Asian and Black populations.

9-2 Hypopigmented Lesions

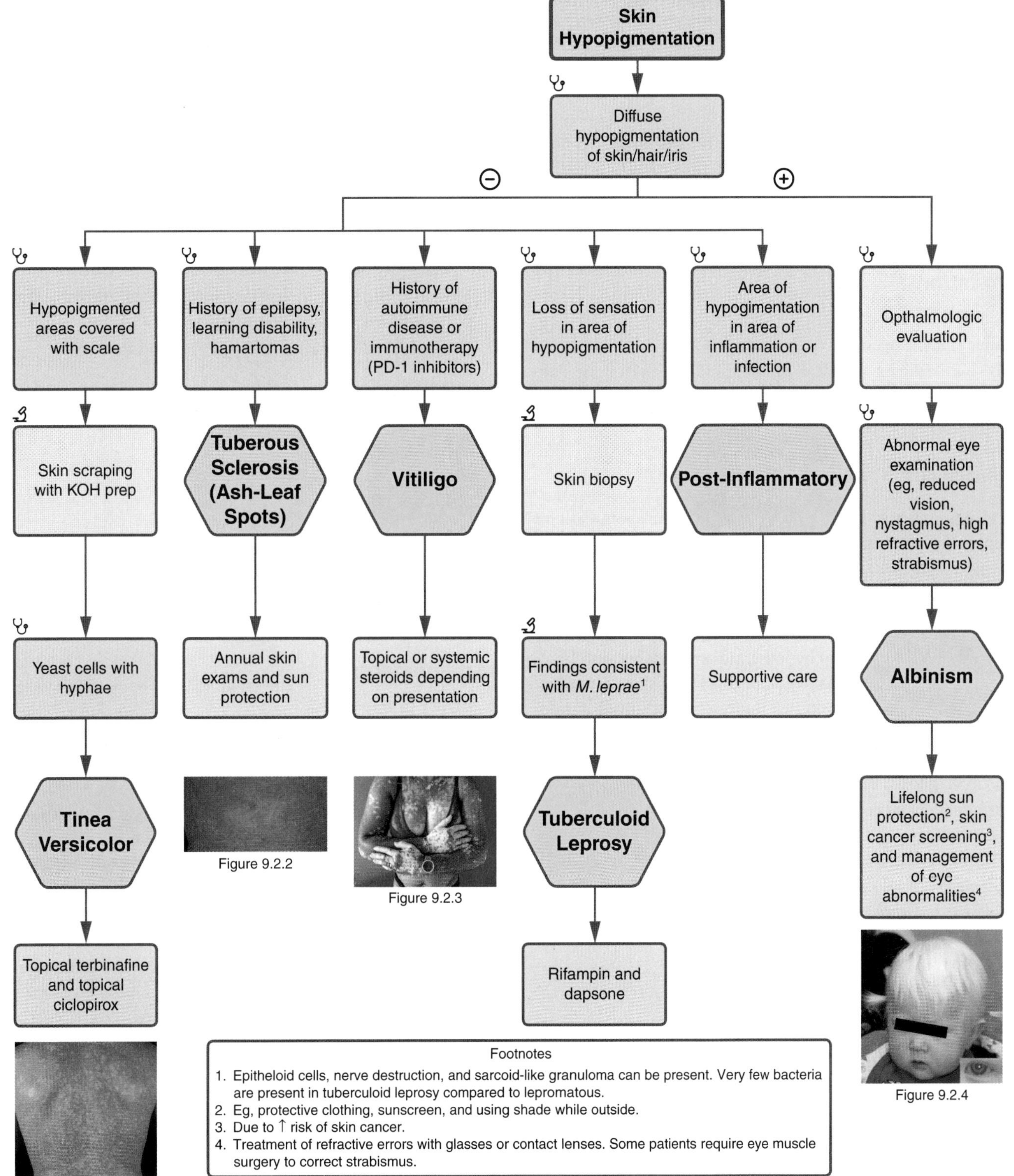

Skin Hypopigmentation
Diffuse hypopigmentation of skin/hair/iris
Hypopigmented areas covered with scale
History of epilepsy, learning disability, hamartomas
History of autoimmune disease or immunotherapy (PD-1 inhibitors)
Loss of sensation in area of hypopigmentation
Area of hypogimentation in area of inflammation or infection
Opthalmologic evaluation
Skin scraping with KOH prep
Tuberous Sclerosis (Ash-Leaf Spots)
Vitiligo
Skin biopsy
Post-Inflammatory
Abnormal eye examination (eg, reduced vision, nystagmus, high refractive errors, strabismus)
Yeast cells with hyphae
Annual skin exams and sun protection
Topical or systemic steroids depending on presentation
Findings consistent with M. leprae1
Supportive care
Albinism
Tinea Versicolor
Tuberculoid Leprosy
Lifelong sun protection2, skin cancer screening3, and management of eye abnormalities4
Topical terbinafine and topical ciclopirox
Rifampin and dapsone

Figure 9.2.1

Figure 9.2.2

Figure 9.2.3

Figure 9.2.4

Footnotes

1. Epitheloid cells, nerve destruction, and sarcoid-like granuloma can be present. Very few bacteria are present in tuberculoid leprosy compared to lepromatous.
2. Eg, protective clothing, sunscreen, and using shade while outside.
3. Due to ↑ risk of skin cancer.
4. Treatment of refractive errors with glasses or contact lenses. Some patients require eye muscle surgery to correct strabismus.

FIGURE 9.2

9-2 Hypopigmented Lesions

TUBEROUS SCLEROSIS (TS)

A 7-year-old boy with PMH of epilepsy, learning disability, and brain hamartomas presents with a hypopigmented macule. **Exam** shows a hypopigmented macule that accentuates with Wood's lamp, as well as angiofibromas in the malar distribution and patches of thickened skin.

Management:

1. Annual skin examinations.
2. Sun protection.

Complications:

- Susceptible to sunburn.
- Cardiac rhabdomyoma.
- Brain hamartomas (cortical glioneuronal hamartomas, subependymal nodules).
- Angiomyolipoma (eg, renal).
- Seizures.
- Intellectual disability.

HYF: Hypopigmented lesions are known as ash-leaf spots. Patients also commonly have angiofibromas and shagreen patches. TS is an AD disease due to mutation of the *TSC1* or *TSC2* gene.

VITILIGO

A 25-year-old F with PMH of hypothyroidism presents with lightening of her skin over the past few months. **Exam** shows symmetrical patches of depigmentation that fluoresce with Wood's lamp.

Management:

1. Clinical diagnosis. Biopsy may help if presentation is unusual.
2. Treatment depends on surface involvement and if disease is stable or active.
   a. Active: systemic steroids and phototherapy.
   b. Stable
      - Localized: topical steroids or calcineurin inhibitors. Consider Ruxolitinib.
      - Disseminated: phototherapy.

Complications:

- More prone to sunburn and skin cancer.
- Social stigmatization and mental stress.

HYF: Associated with autoimmune thyroiditis. T-cell–mediated destruction of melanocytes.

POST-INFLAMMATORY

A 6-month-old male infant with recent diaper dermatitis presents with pelvic hypopigmentation. **Exam** shows a patch of hypopigmentation that matches the shape and distribution of his previous inflammatory lesion.

Management:

1. Treat underlying cause of hypopigmentation and stimulation of melanogenesis.

Complications: Permanent depigmentation or hypopigmentation.

HYF: Clinical diagnosis. Typically resolves spontaneously over weeks to months.

TINEA VERSICOLOR

A 23-year-old M lifeguard presents with lightening of skin. **Exam** shows macules of depigmentation covered with fine scales on the torso. **Labs** show hyphae and yeast cells on KOH preparation.

Management:

1. Topical antifungals, topical selenium sulfide, and topical zinc pyrithione are first-line therapies.
2. Oral azole antifungals if refractory to topicals.

Complications: Hypopigmentation and hyperpigmentation can persist for months.

HYF: Caused by *Malassezia* species.

TUBERCULOID LEPROSY

A 60-year-old F who recently immigrated from India presents with skin concerns. **Exam** shows diffuse hypopigmented plaques with decreased sensation. **Labs** show *M. leprae* from full-thickness skin biopsy culture.

Management:

1. Biopsy of skin lesion.
2. If histology is not convincing, PCR.
3. Treat with dapsone and rifampicin for 12 months.

Complications: Peripheral neuropathy.

HYF: Skin biopsies may demonstrate acid-fast bacilli with granulomatous infiltration (epithelioid and Langhans giant cells).

ALBINISM

A 2-year-old boy presents for a well-child visit and is found to have hypopigmentation of the skin, hair, and iris. Ophthalmologic **exam** shows photophobia and reduced visual acuity.

Management:

1. Photoprotection and skin cancer surveillance.
2. Management of eye abnormalities.

Complications:

- Increased risk for skin cancer.
- Vision abnormalities.

HYF: Albinism with recurrent pyogenic infections is concerning for Chediak-Higashi syndrome.

9-3 Papular Skin Lesions

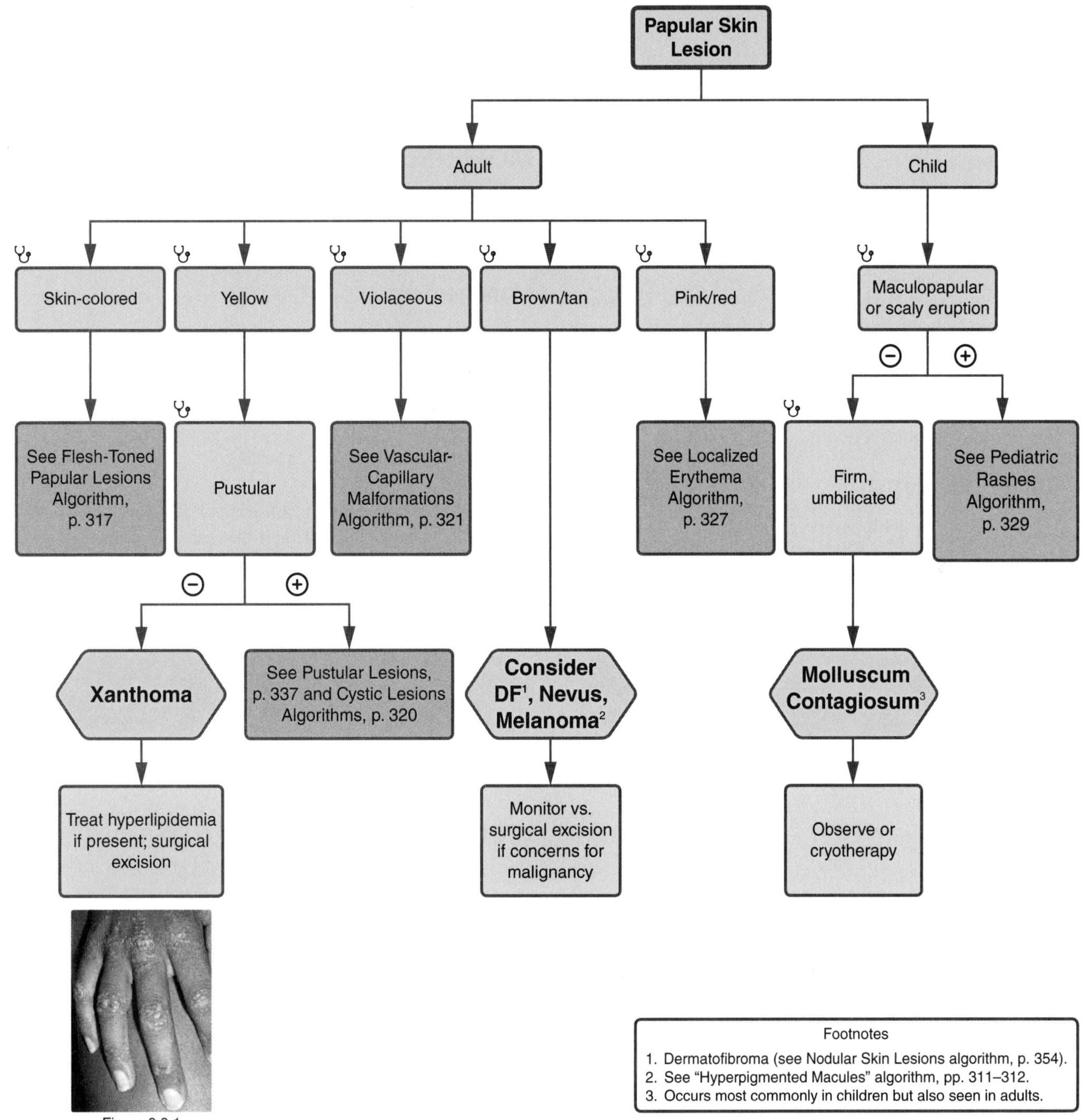
Papular Skin Lesion
Adult
Child
Skin-colored
Yellow
Violaceous
Brown/tan
Pink/red
Maculopapular or scaly eruption
See Flesh-Toned Papular Lesions Algorithm, p. 317
Pustular
See Vascular-Capillary Malformations Algorithm, p. 321
See Localized Erythema Algorithm, p. 327
Firm, umbilicated
See Pediatric Rashes Algorithm, p. 329
Xanthoma
See Pustular Lesions, p. 337 and Cystic Lesions Algorithms, p. 320
Consider DF[1], Nevus, Melanoma[2]
Molluscum Contagiosum[3]
Treat hyperlipidemia if present; surgical excision
Monitor vs. surgical excision if concerns for malignancy
Observe or cryotherapy
Figure 9.3.1
Footnotes
1. Dermatofibroma (see Nodular Skin Lesions algorithm, p. 354).
2. See "Hyperpigmented Macules" algorithm, pp. 311–312.
3. Occurs most commonly in children but also seen in adults.

FIGURE 9.3

9-3 Papular Skin Lesions

XANTHOMAS

A 44-year-old M with PMH of HLD presents with exam findings of yellowish plaques and papules on his eyelids.

Management:

1. Treat HLD if present.
2. Surgical excision of lesions if wanted.

HYF: Often but not always associated with HLD. Multiple clinical variants exist:

- **Eruptive:** Acute onset, red-yellow papules arising in crops. Koebnerization may be present (appearance of xanthomas at sites of trauma).
- **Xanthelasma:** Planar xanthomas often found near eyelids.
- **Tendinous:** Firm, mobile lesions that form over tendons/ligaments (usually Achilles tendon).

MELANOCYTIC NEVI

A 15-year-old M presents with several moles. On exam, they are all brown/black, 3–5.5 mm in size, and have sharply demarcated borders.

Management:

1. Longitudinal observation.
2. Use of sun protection.

Complications: Progression to melanoma.

HYF: Watch out for atypical melanocytic nevi. See Hyperpigmented Macules algorithm for further details, p. 310.

MOLLUSCUM CONTAGIOSUM

An 8-year-old boy presents with a pruritic rash on his neck and trunk. On exam, he has skin tone, firm, waxy, umbilicated, dome-shaped papules 2–5 mm in diameter.

Management:

1. Usually optional as lesions usually resolve spontaneously in 12 months, though some persist for years.
2. If treatment is preferred, can use curettage, cryotherapy, or topical agents (cantharidin, podophyllotoxin).

Complications: Risk of scarring.

HYF: Most often seen in children or in immunocompromised patients. Consider HIV testing if the rash is diffuse, widespread, or severe (ie, lesion >10 mm).

Neurofibroma: See Flesh-Toned Papular Lesions, p. 318.

9-4 Flesh-Toned Papular Lesions

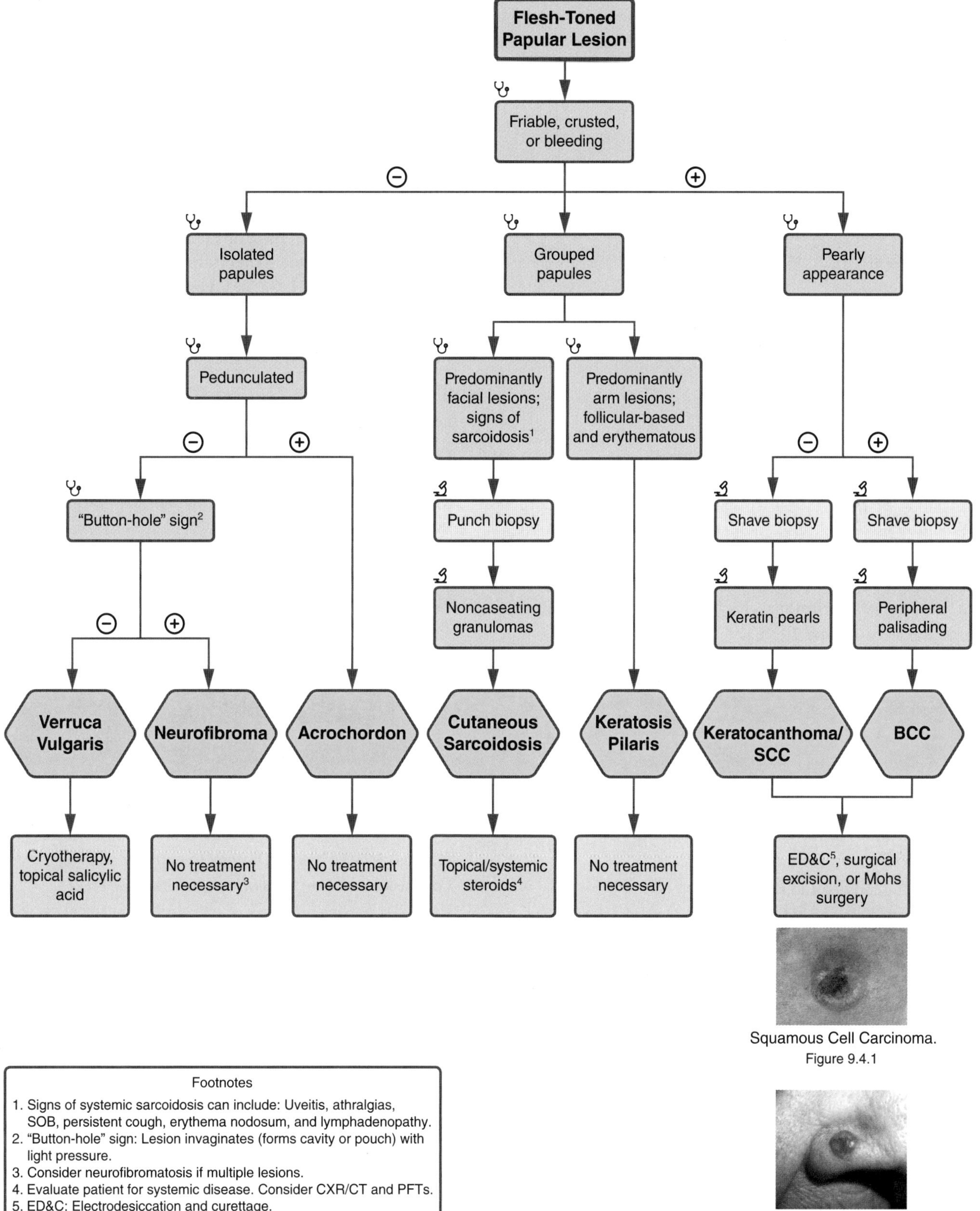

Flesh-Toned Papular Lesion
Friable, crusted, or bleeding
⊖
⊕
Isolated papules
Grouped papules
Pearly appearance
Pedunculated
Predominantly facial lesions; signs of sarcoidosis[1]
Predominantly arm lesions; follicular-based and erythematous
⊖
⊕
"Button-hole" sign[2]
Punch biopsy
Noncaseating granulomas
⊖
⊕
Shave biopsy
Keratin pearls
Shave biopsy
Peripheral palisading
⊖
⊕
Verruca Vulgaris
Neurofibroma
Acrochordon
Cutaneous Sarcoidosis
Keratosis Pilaris
Keratocanthoma/ SCC
BCC
Cryotherapy, topical salicylic acid
No treatment necessary[3]
No treatment necessary
Topical/systemic steroids[4]
No treatment necessary
ED&C[5], surgical excision, or Mohs surgery

Squamous Cell Carcinoma.
Figure 9.4.1

Basal Cell Carcinoma.
Figure 9.4.2

Footnotes

1. Signs of systemic sarcoidosis can include: Uveitis, athralgias, SOB, persistent cough, erythema nodosum, and lymphadenopathy.
2. "Button-hole" sign: Lesion invaginates (forms cavity or pouch) with light pressure.
3. Consider neurofibromatosis if multiple lesions.
4. Evaluate patient for systemic disease. Consider CXR/CT and PFTs.
5. ED&C: Electrodesiccation and curettage.

FIGURE 9.4

9-4 Flesh-Toned Papular Lesions

VERRUCA VULGARIS (WARTS)

A 10-year-old M presents with new skin-colored lesions on his fingers. On exam, there are five 3–4 mm papules that are rough to touch. There is no itching or tenderness.

Management:

1. Topical salicylic acid/imiquimod or cryotherapy.
2. Refractory: topical immunotherapy.

HYF: Most commonly on hands, feet, and elbows. Caused by HPV. Many can regress spontaneously, especially in children.

NEUROFIBROMA

A 25-year-old M presents with 5-mm skin-colored lesion on the left forearm. No other symptoms. On exam, the lesion invaginates on palpation.

Management:

1. No treatment necessary. Can be surgically resected if symptomatic or for cosmetic reasons.

HYF: 90% of lesions are solitary, but assess for autosomal dominant systemic causes:

- **Neurofibromatosis type 1 (NF1)**: Can presents with 6+ café au lait spots, freckling (axillary/inguinal), Lisch nodules, 2+ neurofibromas.
- **Neurofibromatosis type 2 (NF2)**: Often presents with hearing loss, vertigo due to bilateral acoustic neuromas, and possibly neurofibromas, meningiomas, gliomas, or seizures.

ACROCHORDON (SKIN TAG)

A 60-year-old F with PMH of DM2 presents with a small cutaneous growth on her neck. Exam shows a 2-mm, pedunculated, and skin-colored lesion.

Management:

1. Removal using forceps and scissors.
2. Cryosurgery utilizing liquid nitrogen or electrodessication.

HYF: Usually occurs in high-friction areas: neck, axilla, and inframammary regions. Can bleed if caught on/rub against items. Perianal skin tags can be seen in patients with Crohn's disease.

KERATOSIS PILARIS

A 24-year-old M presents with rough, bumpy skin on the bilateral extensor areas of her proximal arms. Exam shows diffuse follicular papules and erythema.

Management:

1. No treatment necessary.

HYF: Lactic acid, salicylic acid, or topical urea can help.

SQUAMOUS CELL CARCINOMA (SCC)

A 68-year-old F with PMH of kidney transplant presents with a pruritic, slow-growing lesion on the scalp. On exam, the lesion is erythematous, scaly, and crusting.

Management:

1. Skin biopsy and histopathology to confirm diagnosis and stage.
2. Low-risk lesions on trunk or extremities: electrodessication and curettage (ED&C).
3. High-risk lesions on trunk or extremities: surgical excision with 4–6 mm margins ± chemotherapy or radiation.
4. Lesion on face, hands, feet or groin: Mohs micrographic surgery.

Complications: Metastases in 2% of patients, higher risk in immunocompromised/transplant patients.

HYF: Second most common type of skin cancer with 2–5% chance of metastasizing. Risk factors: UV light, smoking, immunosuppression, HPV, actinic keratosis, scarring, arsenic exposure.

- **Cutaneous SCC in situ (Bowen disease):** Erythematous, scaly, well-demarcated plaque/patch in sun-exposed areas. Grows slowly over years and can ulcerate.
- **Keratoacanthoma:** A rapidly growing dome-shaped lesion with a keratotic core that spontaneously regresses.
- **Marjolin ulcer:** A quickly growing nodule with excessive granulation tissue that forms at sites of chronic wounds or scars (burn scars most common).

BASAL CELL CARCINOMA (BCC)

A 62-year-old M gardener with PMH of 2 severe childhood sunburns presents with exam findings of a pink, pearly lesion with central ulceration on his cheek.

Management: Depends on size, depth, histology, and location.

1. Skin biopsy and histopathology to confirm and stage.
2. Low-risk lesions on trunk or extremities: ED&C.
3. High-risk lesions on trunk or extremities: Surgical excision with 4–5 mm margins.
4. Lesion on face, hands, feet or groin: Mohs micrographic surgery.

HYF: Most common skin malignancy. Slow-growing lesions with little to no metastatic potential, rolled borders, and/or peripheral telangiectasias. Risk factors: UV light exposure, prior radiation.

Molluscum Contagiosum: See Papular Skin Lesions, p. 316.

9-5 Cystic Skin Lesions

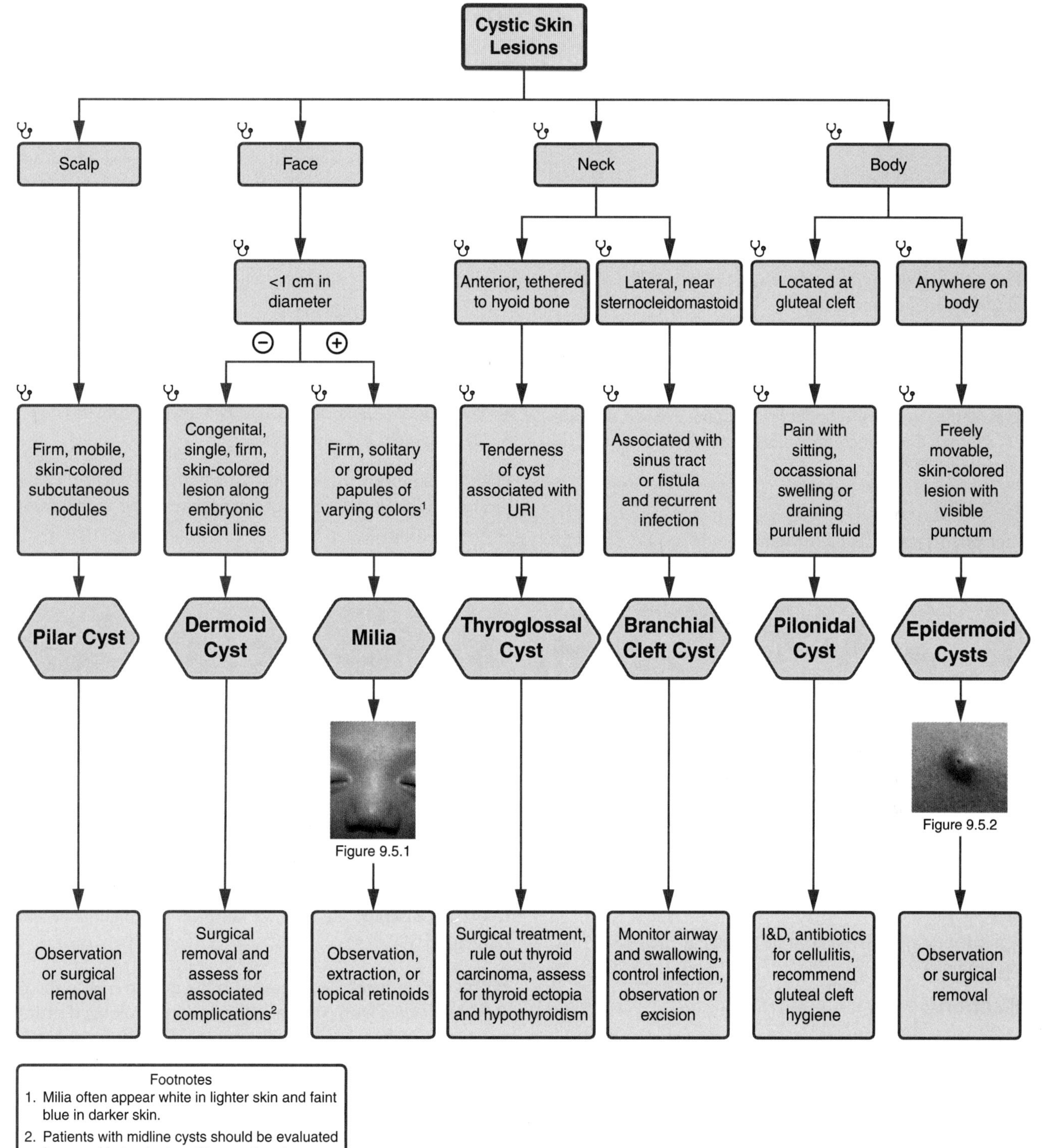
Cystic Skin Lesions
Scalp
Face
Neck
Body
<1 cm in diameter
Anterior, tethered to hyoid bone
Lateral, near sternocleidomastoid
Located at gluteal cleft
Anywhere on body
Firm, mobile, skin-colored subcutaneous nodules
Congenital, single, firm, skin-colored lesion along embryonic fusion lines
Firm, solitary or grouped papules of varying colors[1]
Tenderness of cyst associated with URI
Associated with sinus tract or fistula and recurrent infection
Pain with sitting, occassional swelling or draining purulent fluid
Freely movable, skin-colored lesion with visible punctum
Pilar Cyst
Dermoid Cyst
Milia
Thyroglossal Cyst
Branchial Cleft Cyst
Pilonidal Cyst
Epidermoid Cysts
Figure 9.5.1
Figure 9.5.2
Observation or surgical removal
Surgical removal and assess for associated complications[2]
Observation, extraction, or topical retinoids
Surgical treatment, rule out thyroid carcinoma, assess for thyroid ectopia and hypothyroidism
Monitor airway and swallowing, control infection, observation or excision
I&D, antibiotics for cellulitis, recommend gluteal cleft hygiene
Observation or surgical removal
Footnotes
1. Milia often appear white in lighter skin and faint blue in darker skin.
2. Patients with midline cysts should be evaluated for neural heterotopias with neuroimaging.

FIGURE 9.5

9-5 Cystic Skin Lesions

PILAR CYST

A 55-year-old M presents with a skin-colored nodule on his scalp. The patient is unsure when he first noticed the bump but guesses it has been present for 5 years. On exam, the nodule is firm but mobile and smooth. No punctum is present.

Management:

1. Observation or surgical removal.

Complications: None.

HYF: Firm, slow-growing cysts derived from hair follicles. They are classically located on the scalp.

DERMOID CYST

A 2-year-old F presents for an annual checkup and is found to have a 3-cm cyst on the lateral aspect of her right upper eyelid. On exam, the cyst is rubbery and noncompressible. Parents confirm that the lesion was present at birth.

Management:

1. Monitor vs. surgical excision. Imaging should be performed for surgical planning.

Complications:

- Dermal sinus tracts may cause cutaneous infections or meningitis.
- Cyst may adhere to periosteum and erode skull.

HYF: Congenital lesions are distributed along embryonic fusion lines and can be associated with several complications, particularly if midline.

MILIA

A 34-year-old F presents with grouped small, white papules on her face. On exam, the papules are firm and non-compressible.

Management:

1. None needed. May self-resolve or be treated by incision or topical retinoids.

Complications: None.

HYF: Small, keratin cysts that arise from pilosebaceous units. They classically present as firm, white papules. Observed in all ages and common in newborns.

THYROGLOSSAL CYST

A 15-year-old M presents with tender mass on his neck. Patient recently recovered from URI. Physical exam reveals a midline mass of the anterior neck just below the hyoid bone. The mass moves up when the patient swallows.

Management:

1. CT scan to confirm diagnosis.
2. Surgical treatment. Histopathological examination to rule out thyroid carcinoma.

Complications: Rarely hypothyroidism secondary to thyroid ectopia.

HYF: Most common type of congenital neck mass. Remnant of thyroglossal tract; classically presents as a midline mass closely associated with the hyoid bone.

BRANCHIAL CLEFT CYST

A 17-year-old M presents with a lump on his neck. Physical exam reveals a cyst anterior to his sternocleidomastoid muscle on the lateral aspect of the neck.

Management:

1. Assess for infection before treating mass.
2. Observation or excision.

Complications:

- Recurrent infections can complicate surgical removal.
- Pharyngeal edema, airway and swallowing problems.
- Development of fistula to skin.

HYF: Arise from the 1st and 2nd branchial arches. Classically located on the lateral aspect of the neck, anterior to the sternocleidomastoid muscle.

PILONIDAL CYST

A 21-year-old M truck driver presents with a painful lesion on his gluteal cleft. The lesion becomes swollen during long drives, and he occasionally notices fluid seeping out of the wound. Physical exam reveals an erythematous nodule with surrounding edema and erythema.

Management:

1. Prompt incision and drainage. Wound care.
2. Antibiotics for cellulitis.
3. Encourage patient to practice regular gluteal cleft shaving and perineal hygiene.

Complications: Recurrence. Surgical treatment is necessary if refractory.

HYF: Due to mechanical forces on the skin overlying the gluteal cleft. Associated with occupations requiring prolonged sitting.

EPIDERMOID CYST

A 61-year-old M presents with a skin-colored nodule with a central punctum on his chest. On exam, the nodule is freely movable and does not produce pain with palpation.

Management:

1. Okay to monitor stable/uninfected cyst. Removal per patient request when not inflamed.

Complications:

- Inflamed/ruptured cysts.
- Infection requiring incision and drainage.
- Recurrence.

HYF: Cysts can occur anywhere on body. Classically present as skin-colored dermal nodules with central punctum.

9-6 Vascular Malformations

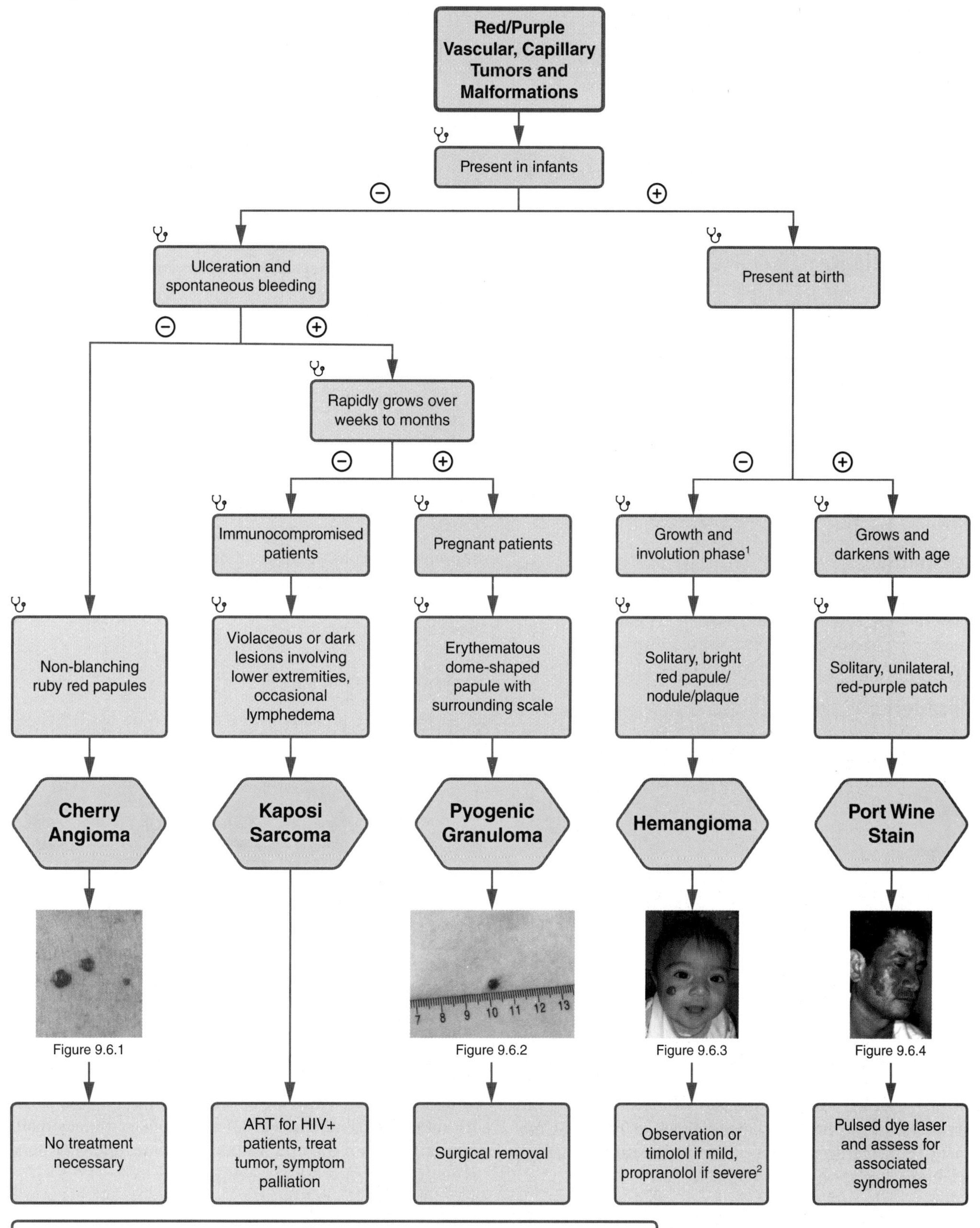
Red/Purple Vascular, Capillary Tumors and Malformations
Present in infants
Ulceration and spontaneous bleeding
Present at birth
Rapidly grows over weeks to months
Immunocompromised patients
Pregnant patients
Growth and involution phase[1]
Grows and darkens with age
Non-blanching ruby red papules
Violaceous or dark lesions involving lower extremities, occasional lymphedema
Erythematous dome-shaped papule with surrounding scale
Solitary, bright red papule/nodule/plaque
Solitary, unilateral, red-purple patch
Cherry Angioma
Kaposi Sarcoma
Pyogenic Granuloma
Hemangioma
Port Wine Stain
Figure 9.6.1
Figure 9.6.2
Figure 9.6.3
Figure 9.6.4
No treatment necessary
ART for HIV+ patients, treat tumor, symptom palliation
Surgical removal
Observation or timolol if mild, propranolol if severe[2]
Pulsed dye laser and assess for associated syndromes

Footnotes

1. During the proliferation phase, hemangiomas rapidly grow into dark red nodules over the first year. After proliferation, hemangiomas plateau and involute. During the involution phase, hemangiomas flatten, decrease in size, and become paler in color over a variable number of years.
2. Treatment options should consider size, morphology, location, and potential for scarring/complications. Severe hemangiomas are large, cause ulcerations, or are located in high-risk areas (eg, eye, airway).

FIGURE 9.6

9-6 Vascular Malformations

CHERRY ANGIOMA

A 62-year-old M presents with multiple ruby red papules on his chest. The patient denies pain or bleeding unless they get caught in clothing.

Management:

1. Advise that new lesions will likely arise, and there is no way to prevent recurrence.
2. Removal for cosmetic reasons via electrocautery or laser.

Complications: None.

HYF: Benign capillary proliferations common in middle-aged and older adults.

KAPOSI SARCOMA (KS)

A 45-year-old M with PMH of HIV not managed with ART presents with nodules on the back, left lower leg, and foot that have grown rapidly for the last month. On exam, the lesions are violaceous to brown patches, plaques, and nodules. Lower extremity edema is also noted.

Management:

1. Biopsy, PCR for HHV-8, and staging.
2. Initiate ART and consider intralesional vs. systemic chemotherapy, excision or cryotherapy of lesions, and radiation.

Complications: Visceral involvement in advanced stages of KS.

HYF: Vascular tumor that develops from infection with HHV-8. Immunosuppressed populations are at higher risk.

PYOGENIC GRANULOMA

A 22-year-old pregnant F presents with a papule on her chest for 2 months, which bleeds profusely when bumped. Exam demonstrates an erythematous, pedunculated papule that is ulcerated.

Management:

1. Surgical removal and histopathologic confirmation to exclude malignancies.

Complications: Risk of recurrence.

HYF: Benign vascular tumor of the skin or mucous membranes often associated with pregnancy, medications, or trauma. Commonly on gingiva of pregnant women. Surgical treatment is usually required due to ulcerations and profuse bleeding.

INFANTILE HEMANGIOMA

A 1-month-old F infant presents with a bright red periocular plaque. Parents state that they first noticed the lesion about 1 week after birth and were told that it is benign. They are seeking medical advice as the lesion has been growing quickly since it was first identified.

Management:

1. Patient has a high-risk hemangioma due to periocular location. Initiate propranolol if there are no contraindications. Monitor patient for 1–3 hours after administration of first dose of propranolol.
2. Follow up at 1- to 3-month intervals to assess progress.

Complications:

- High-risk infantile hemangiomas have risk of scarring or disfigurement.
- Functional impairments if located in airway or periocular areas.
- Rarely associated with symptomatic visceral hemangiomas if solitary (<5). Consider liver ultrasound if 5+ hemangiomas.

HYF: Benign tumors of vascular endothelium, marked by growth and involution phase. Observation and administering timolol are reasonable management methods for uncomplicated, localized hemangioma. Propranolol is first-line treatment for high-risk hemangiomas (large, ulcerated, high-risk sites).

PORT WINE STAIN

A 13-year-old F presents with a red patch on her left cheek. Her family confirms that the lesion has been present since birth, but it has grown, darkened, and thickened with age. The patient denies pain with palpation. On exam, there is a pink/red, blanching patch.

Management:

1. Treat with pulsed dye laser.

Complications:

- Will become thicker, darker, and nodular if untreated.
- Associated with certain abnormalities (eg, glaucoma) or malformation syndromes.

HYF: Congenital vascular malformations. These lesions grow proportionally with child's growth and, unlike infantile hemangiomas, do not have an involution phase. Associated with Sturge-Weber syndrome (SWS), which is characterized by a port wine stain in the trigeminal distribution (V1/V2) and capillary-venous malformations in the brain and eyes leading to seizures and glaucoma; SWS is due to a mutation in the *GNAQ* gene.

9-7 Erythroderma

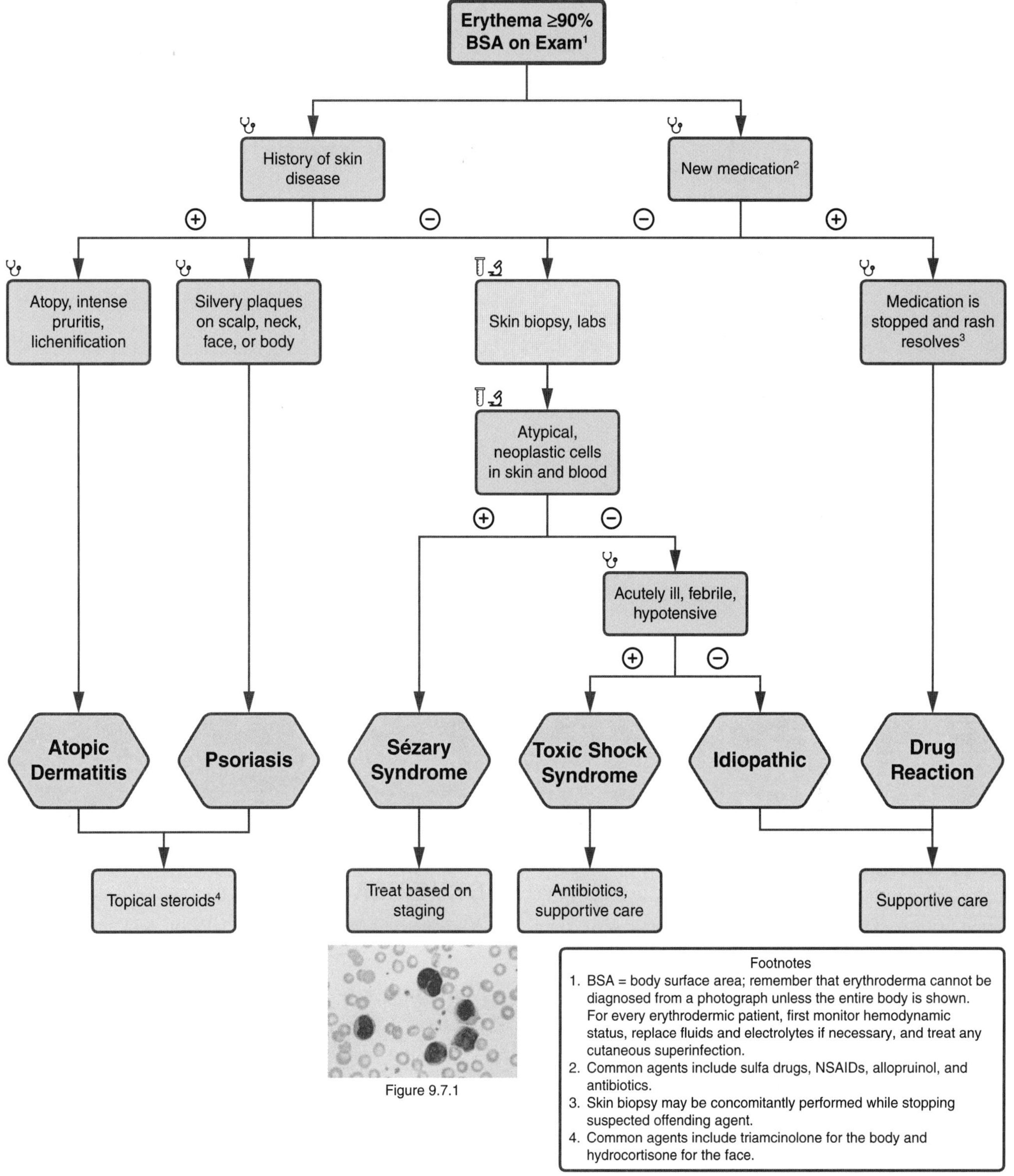
Erythema ≥90% BSA on Exam[1]
History of skin disease
New medication[2]
Atopy, intense pruritis, lichenification
Silvery plaques on scalp, neck, face, or body
Skin biopsy, labs
Medication is stopped and rash resolves[3]
Atypical, neoplastic cells in skin and blood
Acutely ill, febrile, hypotensive
Atopic Dermatitis
Psoriasis
Sézary Syndrome
Toxic Shock Syndrome
Idiopathic
Drug Reaction
Topical steroids[4]
Treat based on staging
Antibiotics, supportive care
Supportive care

Figure 9.7.1

Footnotes

1. BSA = body surface area; remember that erythroderma cannot be diagnosed from a photograph unless the entire body is shown. For every erythrodermic patient, first monitor hemodynamic status, replace fluids and electrolytes if necessary, and treat any cutaneous superinfection.
2. Common agents include sulfa drugs, NSAIDs, allopruinol, and antibiotics.
3. Skin biopsy may be concomitantly performed while stopping suspected offending agent.
4. Common agents include triamcinolone for the body and hydrocortisone for the face.

FIGURE 9.7

9-7 Erythroderma

ATOPIC DERMATITIS

A 32-year-old M with PMH of allergies and asthma presents with a pruritic rash. **Exam** shows diffuse erythema and lichenified patches. **Labs** show increased serum IgE and eosinophilia.

Management:

1. Topical steroids and antihistamines. Consider steroid wet wraps.
2. Systemic non-biologics, including methotrexate or cyclosporine.
3. Dupilumab and JAK inhibitors.

Complications: No specific complications.

HYF: Avoidance of irritants and frequent emollient use are mainstays in preventing flares. Use caution with PO steroids, as they cause rebound flares.

PSORIASIS

A 55-year-old F with PMH of previously well-controlled plaque psoriasis on methotrexate and topical steroids presents with diffuse rash after stopping all medications weeks ago. **Exam** shows diffuse erythema and nail pitting with oil spots.

Management:

1. Topical steroids, calcipotriene, retinoid.
2. Systemic non-biologics, including methotrexate or cyclosporine.
3. Biologics.

Complications: Increased risk of cardiac and cerebrovascular diseases.

HYF: Psoriasis is the #1 cause of erythroderma in otherwise healthy patients, usually due to abrupt medication discontinuation.

SÉZARY SYNDROME

A 72-year-old F with PMH of DM2 presents with widespread erythema and pruritus. On **exam**, she is erythrodermic with lymphadenopathy. **Labs** show atypical neoplastic T cells in the skin and blood.

Management:

1. Stratification by stage to determine treatment.

Complications: Increased risk of secondary malignancies.

HYF: Compared to mycosis fungoides (which is indolent), Sézary syndrome is more aggressive and can be fatal. Five-year survival rate is around 50%.

STAPHYLOCOCCAL TOXIC SHOCK SYNDROME

A 24-year-old F with no PMH presents with sudden onset of fever and hypotension, vomiting, and diarrhea. **Exam** shows diffuse maculopapular rash involving the palms and soles and altered mental status. **Labs** show elevated Cr, thrombocytopenia, and elevated LFTs.

Management:

1. Treatment of shock.
2. Removal of any foreign body.
3. Antibiotics (eg, clindamycin + vancomycin).

Complications: Palmoplantar desquamation 1–3 weeks after symptom onset.

HYF: Certain strains of *S. aureus* produce an exotoxin (toxic shock syndrome toxin-1), which acts as a superantigen, binding to TCR and causing nonspecific activation of T cells. Associated with tampon use, nasal packing, surgical wound infection.

IDIOPATHIC

An 87-year-old M with PMH of HTN and CAD presents with a 4-year history of a scaly red rash covering >80% BSA. **Exam** shows lymphadenopathy.

Management:

1. Supportive skin care, topical steroids, and antihistamines.

Complications: No specific complications.

HYF: Etiology may become apparent over time, so patients require close monitoring.

DRUG REACTION

A 45-year-old M with PMH of HIV on ART presents with rash. **Exam** shows erythroderma with lymphadenopathy.

Management:

1. Withdrawal of any suspected offending agent.
2. Supportive care, topical or PO steroids, and antihistamines.

Complications: No specific complications.

HYF: Most common in HIV patients. Classic offending agents are ART, antiepileptics, allopurinol, and sulfa drugs.

*For every erythrodermic patient, first monitor hemodynamic status, replace fluids and electrolytes if necessary, and treat any cutaneous superinfection.

9-8 Generalized Erythema

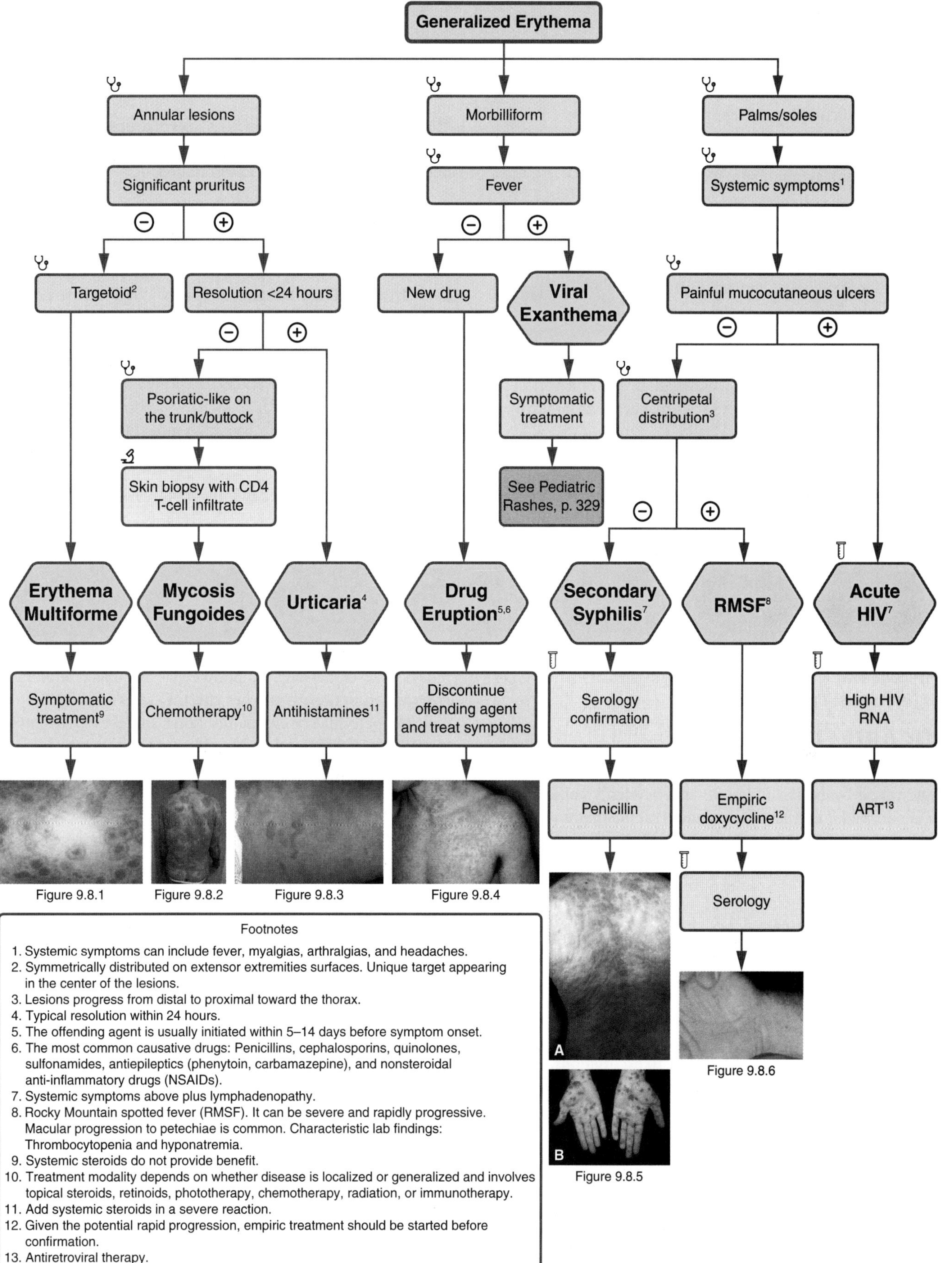

Generalized Erythema
Annular lesions
Significant pruritus
Targetoid[2]
Resolution <24 hours
Psoriatic-like on the trunk/buttock
Skin biopsy with CD4 T-cell infiltrate
Morbilliform
Fever
New drug
Viral Exanthema
Symptomatic treatment
See Pediatric Rashes, p. 329
Palms/soles
Systemic symptoms[1]
Painful mucocutaneous ulcers
Centripetal distribution[3]
Erythema Multiforme
Mycosis Fungoides
Urticaria[4]
Drug Eruption[5,6]
Secondary Syphilis[7]
RMSF[8]
Acute HIV[7]
Symptomatic treatment[9]
Chemotherapy[10]
Antihistamines[11]
Discontinue offending agent and treat symptoms
Serology confirmation
High HIV RNA
Penicillin
Empiric doxycycline[12]
ART[13]
Serology
A
B

Figure 9.8.1 Figure 9.8.2 Figure 9.8.3 Figure 9.8.4 Figure 9.8.5 Figure 9.8.6

Footnotes

1. Systemic symptoms can include fever, myalgias, arthralgias, and headaches.
2. Symmetrically distributed on extensor extremities surfaces. Unique target appearing in the center of the lesions.
3. Lesions progress from distal to proximal toward the thorax.
4. Typical resolution within 24 hours.
5. The offending agent is usually initiated within 5–14 days before symptom onset.
6. The most common causative drugs: Penicillins, cephalosporins, quinolones, sulfonamides, antiepileptics (phenytoin, carbamazepine), and nonsteroidal anti-inflammatory drugs (NSAIDs).
7. Systemic symptoms above plus lymphadenopathy.
8. Rocky Mountain spotted fever (RMSF). It can be severe and rapidly progressive. Macular progression to petechiae is common. Characteristic lab findings: Thrombocytopenia and hyponatremia.
9. Systemic steroids do not provide benefit.
10. Treatment modality depends on whether disease is localized or generalized and involves topical steroids, retinoids, phototherapy, chemotherapy, radiation, or immunotherapy.
11. Add systemic steroids in a severe reaction.
12. Given the potential rapid progression, empiric treatment should be started before confirmation.
13. Antiretroviral therapy.

FIGURE 9.8

9-8 Generalized Erythema

ERYTHEMA MULTIFORME

A 33-year-old M with recent URI symptoms presents with a new skin lesion on both arms and legs. Exam shows well-demarcated targetoid lesions with some small blisters on the dorsum of his hands without mucosal involvement. Nikolsky negative.

Management:

1. Reassurance and symptomatic treatment.

Complications: None, usually self-limited.

HYF: Targetoid lesions are usually on extensor surfaces. Presence of blisters is common. Systemic symptoms and mucosal involvement are red flags for SJS/TEN. Often precipitated by HSV infection.

MYCOSIS FUNGOIDES (CUTANEOUS T-CELL LYMPHOMA)

A 76-year-old M presents with 2 years of severely pruritic back lesions. Exam shows 3 erythematous scaly plaques, with largest 6 cm.

Management:

1. Skin biopsy with immunophenotyping.
2. Treatment depends on the degree of invasion (cutaneous vs. systemic disease; ranges from local treatment with phototherapy/radiation to systemic chemotherapy/immunotherapy to stem cell transplant).

Complications: Progression to systemic disease (Sézary syndrome).

HYF: This is a cutaneous mature CD4+ T-cell lymphoma. Lesions are psoriatic-like, typically on the back and buttocks and in elderly patients. Skin biopsy shows epidermal aggregates of mature CD4+ T cells (ie, Pautrier microabscesses).

URTICARIA

A 34-year-old F presents with 2 episodes over the past 3 days of multiple raised oval pruritic lesions that suddenly come and go. Exam is notable for erythematous plaques on the thighs with signs of linear superficial scratches. She asks for medication to help with the intense itchiness during the episodes. She denies fever or chills.

Management:

1. Avoid triggers when identifiable.
2. Antihistamines.
3. Omalizumab or oral steroids if severe or refractory.

Complications:

- Anaphylaxis.
- Secondary skin bacterial infection due to excoriations.

HYF: Intense pruritis associated with rapid (usually <24-hour) resolution. Topical steroids are ineffective.

DRUG ERUPTION

A 43-year-old F with a recently treated cellulitis presents with diffuse rash. She denies fever, myalgias, or arthralgias. Exam shows a diffuse, symmetric maculopapular rash without mucosal involvement.

Management:

1. Review recent (5–14 days) medication exposure.
2. Discontinue offending agent.
3. Antihistamines if pruritus is present. Can consider topical and/or oral steroids if severe.

Complications: Severe cases involve systemic manifestations and can lead to DRESS, SJS, and TEN.

HYF: Usually occurs within 5–14 days of drug exposure. Drug eruptions are unlikely within 2 days of exposure. Typically self-limited once the offending agent is discontinued.

SECONDARY SYPHILIS

A 28-year-old M presents with 2 days of low-grade fever, lymphadenopathy, and rash after returning from a camping trip. On exam, he has bilateral axillary lymphadenopathy and a diffuse non-pruritic and painless maculopapular rash on all extremities.

Management:

1. Specific treponemal tests (eg, Treponemal IgG), reflex to non-treponemal test (RPR).
2. Benzathine penicillin 2.4 million units IM (single dose).

Complications:

- Progression to tertiary syphilis if untreated.
- Chronic granulomas.

HYF: Characterized by mild systemic symptoms associated with lymphadenopathy. Rash is non-pruritic and involves palms/soles.

ROCKY MOUNTAIN SPOTTED FEVER

A 31-year-old F who recently hiked in Massachusetts presents with 3 days of fever, headache, and myalgias associated with a progressive rash from the arms to her chest. Exam shows diffuse macular rash and petechiae on her palms, arms, and chest. Labs reveal normal WBC, 70,000 platelets, Na 128, and mild transaminitis.

Management:

1. Empiric doxycycline.
2. Rickettsia serology.

Complications: Severe vasculitis with intravascular hemolysis and shock.

HYF: Severe tick bite disease caused by *Rickettsia rickettsii.* Rash typically progresses centripetally. Associated with thrombocytopenia and hyponatremia.

ACUTE HIV INFECTION

A 26-year-old M with PMH of syphilis presents with 2 days of fever and diffuse rash. Exam shows a painful posterior oropharyngeal ulcer, diffuse maculopapular rash involving his palms, and lymphadenopathy. Initial labs are unremarkable.

Management:

1. HIV screening Abs, followed by RNA levels if positive.
2. ART.

Complications: Progression to AIDS if left untreated.

HYF: Acute HIV typically presents with mononucleosis-like symptoms and is differentiated from mononucleosis and secondary syphilis by the presence of painful mucocutaneous ulcers.

9-9 Localized Erythema

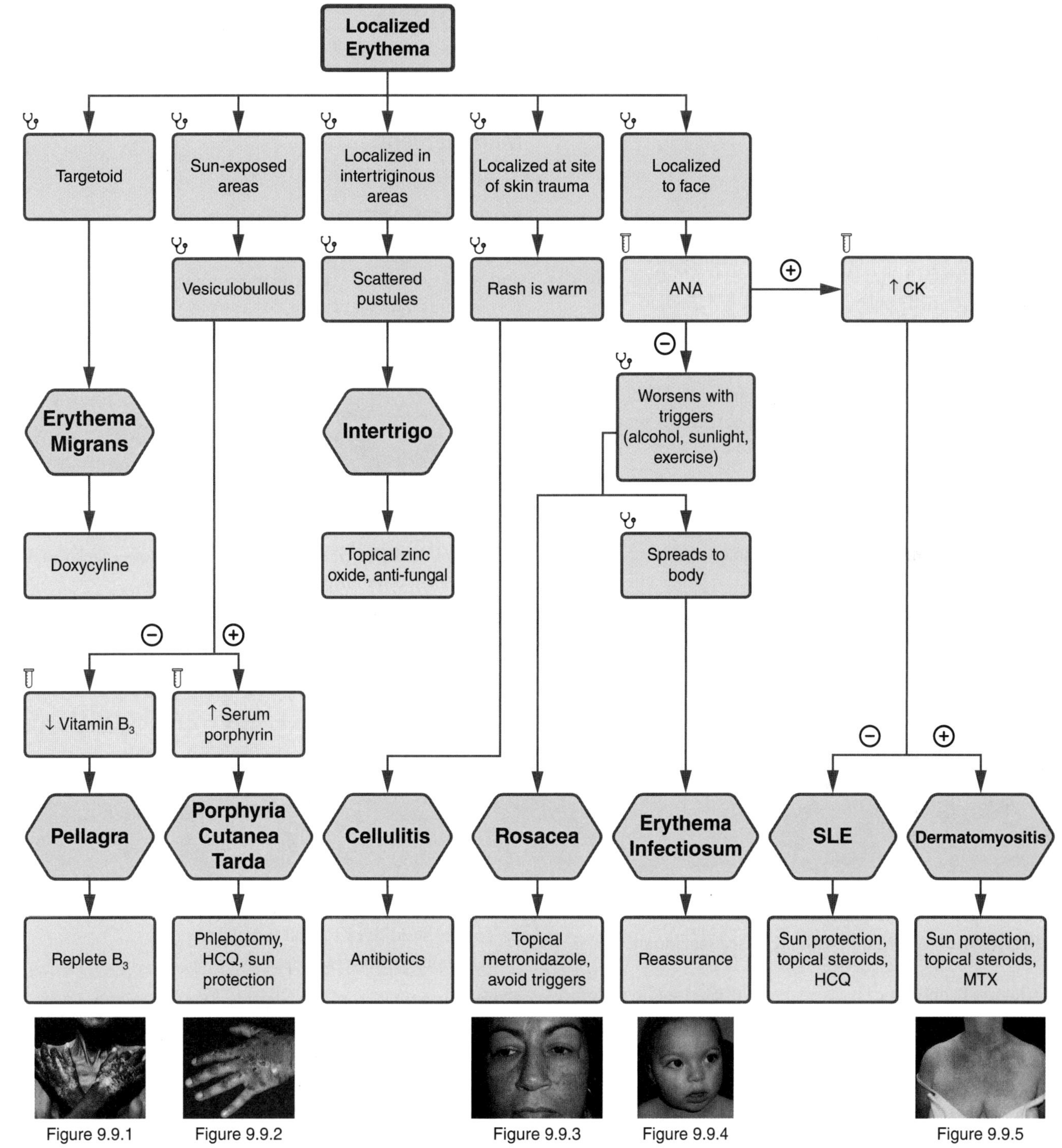

Localized Erythema
Targetoid
Sun-exposed areas
Localized in intertriginous areas
Localized at site of skin trauma
Localized to face
Vesiculobullous
Scattered pustules
Rash is warm
ANA
↑ CK
Worsens with triggers (alcohol, sunlight, exercise)
Erythema Migrans
Intertrigo
Doxycyline
Topical zinc oxide, anti-fungal
Spreads to body
↓ Vitamin B_3
↑ Serum porphyrin
Pellagra
Porphyria Cutanea Tarda
Cellulitis
Rosacea
Erythema Infectiosum
SLE
Dermatomyositis
Replete B_3
Phlebotomy, HCQ, sun protection
Antibiotics
Topical metronidazole, avoid triggers
Reassurance
Sun protection, topical steroids, HCQ
Sun protection, topical steroids, MTX
Figure 9.9.1
Figure 9.9.2
Figure 9.9.3
Figure 9.9.4
Figure 9.9.5

FIGURE 9.9

9-9 Localized Erythema

ERYTHEMA MIGRANS

A 25-year-old M in Vermont presents with 1 week of fatigue, myalgia, and rash on his lower leg. On exam, there is a single erythematous circular plaque with central clearing.

Management:

1. Oral doxycycline.

Complications: Disseminated Lyme disease.

HYF: Symptoms of disseminated Lyme disease can include heart block, arthropathy, Bell's palsy, and multiple EM lesions.

CANDIDA/INTERTRIGO

A 40-year-old F with PMH of obesity presents with painful rashes underneath her breasts and pannus. On exam, there are tender erythematous patches with scattered pustules in these areas.

Management:

1. Keep area clean and dry.
2. Topical zinc oxide and topical ketoconazole.

Complications: Recurrence is common.

HYF: Can be caused by irritant/contact dermatitis, bacteria, or yeast. Satellite pustules are characteristic of *Candida*.

PELLAGRA

A 45-year-old M with PMH of gastric bypass 8 months ago presents with diarrhea, confusion, and rash on his chest. On exam, there is a large hyperpigmented erythematous plaque on his upper chest.

Management:

1. Sun protection and vitamin B_3 repletion.

Complications: Associated with increased melanoma risk.

HYF: Vitamin B_3 deficiency is associated with carcinoid syndrome, alcohol use disorder, and malabsorption.

PORPHYRIA CUTANEA TARDA (PCT)

A 50-year-old M with PMH of untreated hepatitis C presents with a new rash on both hands. On exam, the dorsum of bilateral hands have multiple erythematous bulla. **Labs** show elevated serum porphyrins.

Management:

1. Phlebotomy and/or hydroxychloroquine.
2. Decrease risk factors (alcohol use, liver dz, sun protection).

Complications: Increased risk of developing hepatocellular carcinoma.

HYF: PCT is caused by a deficiency in uroporphyrinogen decarboxylase (UROD), an enzyme in heme synthesis, which causes accumulation of photosensitizing porphyrins in skin.

CELLULITIS

A 10-year-old M with PMH of atopic dermatitis presents with 3 days of fever and new rash on his right leg. On exam, there is an edematous and erythematous plaque that is warm to the touch.

Management:

1. Antibiotics.

Complications: Development of abscess or sepsis.

HYF: Most common organisms are beta-hemolytic *Streptococcus* and MSSA. Suspect MRSA if the patient has systemic symptoms (fever, chills, tachycardia) or abscess/pus formation.

ROSACEA

A 25-year-old F presents with 3 months of erythematous rash on the nose and bilateral cheeks that worsens with cold weather and exercise.

Management:

1. Avoidance of triggers, sun protection.
2. Topical therapies (metronidazole gel, dapsone, azelaic acid) mostly effective for papulopustular rosacea.
3. Can consider laser for erythrotelangectatic (ET) rosacea.

HYF: Common triggers include extreme temperatures, alcohol, exercise, and sunlight.

SYSTEMIC LUPUS ERYTHEMATOSUS (SLE)

A 20-year-old F presents with a month of fatigue, joint pain, and facial rash. On exam, the rash spares the nasolabial folds and telangiectasis are noted. **Labs** show (+)ANA, (+)anti-dsDNA, and (+) anti-Smith.

Management:

1. Encourage sun protective measures.
2. Topical steroids or topical tacrolimus.
3. Systemic hydroxychloroquine.

Complications: Renal, neurologic, and hematologic involvement.

HYF: For suspected SLE, initial workup includes CBC, BMP, UA, and ANA with reflex ENA serology.

DERMATOMYOSITIS

A 40-year-old F presents with proximal muscle weakness and new rash on her face and trunk. On exam, she has violaceous erythema on her eyelids and a confluent erythematous plaque covering her neck and upper chest. **Labs** show ↑ CK, ESR, (+)ANA, and (+)anti-RNP.

Management:

1. Sun protection.
2. Topical steroids and tacrolimus.
3. Systemic hydroxychloroquine or methotrexate.

Complications: Can be associated with underlying malignancy.

HYF: All patients should undergo workup to rule out malignancy.

9-10 Pediatric Rashes

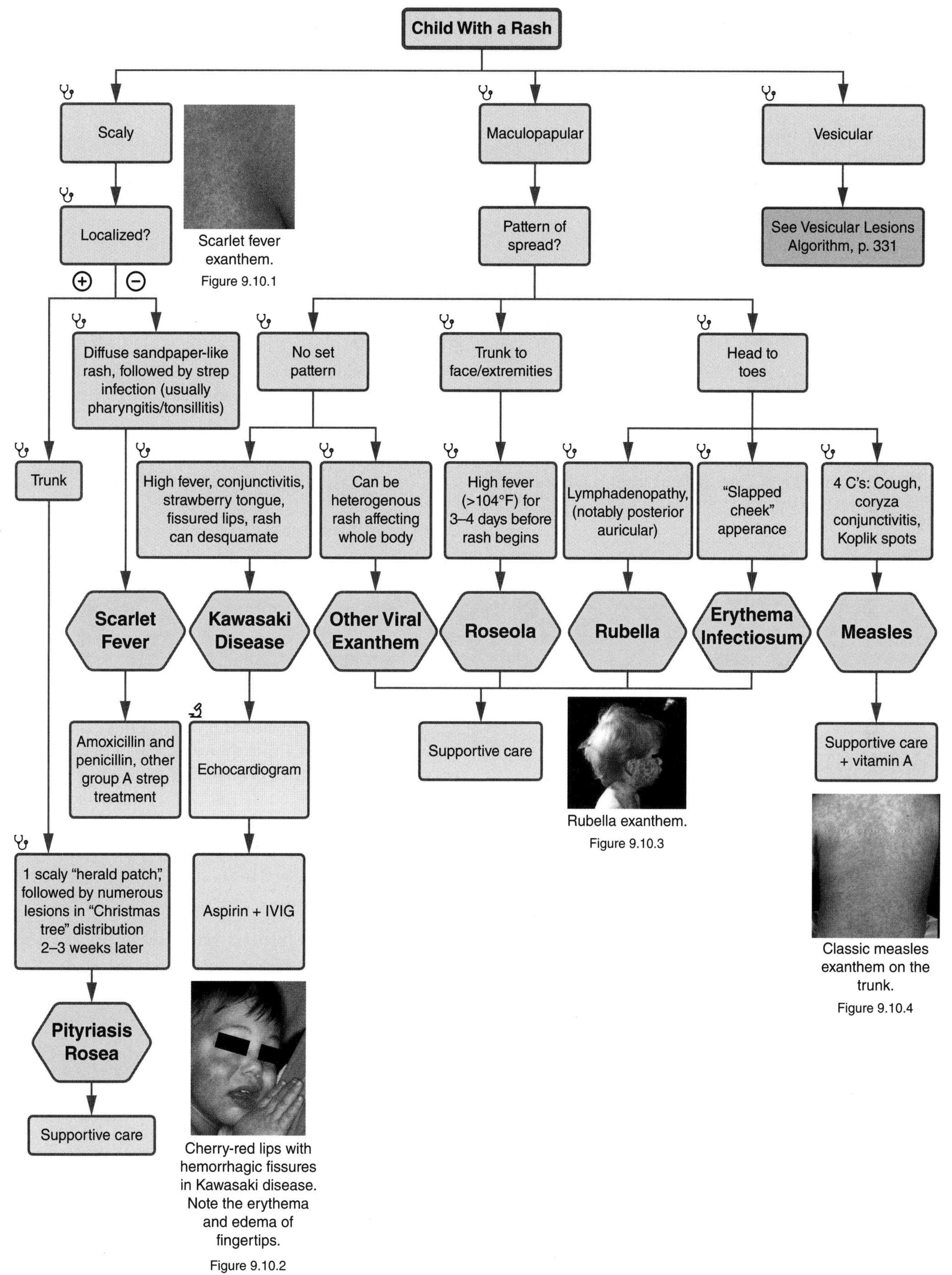
Child With a Rash
Scaly
Localized?
+
−
Trunk
1 scaly "herald patch", followed by numerous lesions in "Christmas tree" distribution 2–3 weeks later
Pityriasis Rosea
Supportive care
Diffuse sandpaper-like rash, followed by strep infection (usually pharyngitis/tonsillitis)
Scarlet Fever
Amoxicillin and penicillin, other group A strep treatment
Maculopapular
Pattern of spread?
No set pattern
High fever, conjunctivitis, strawberry tongue, fissured lips, rash can desquamate
Kawasaki Disease
Echocardiogram
Aspirin + IVIG
Can be heterogenous rash affecting whole body
Other Viral Exanthem
Trunk to face/extremities
High fever (>104°F) for 3–4 days before rash begins
Roseola
Head to toes
Lymphadenopathy, (notably posterior auricular)
Rubella
"Slapped cheek" apperance
Erythema Infectiosum
4 C's: Cough, coryza conjunctivitis, Koplik spots
Measles
Supportive care
Supportive care + vitamin A
Vesicular
See Vesicular Lesions Algorithm, p. 331

Scarlet fever exanthem.
Figure 9.10.1

Cherry-red lips with hemorrhagic fissures in Kawasaki disease. Note the erythema and edema of fingertips.
Figure 9.10.2

Rubella exanthem.
Figure 9.10.3

Classic measles exanthem on the trunk.
Figure 9.10.4

FIGURE 9.10

9-10 Pediatric Rashes

SCARLET FEVER

A 5-year-old fully vaccinated M presents with sore throat and diffuse rash. Exam is significant for sandpaper-like rash on the trunk, purulent tonsillar exudate, "strawberry tongue," and anterior cervical lymphadenopathy.

Management:

1. ASO titers/rapid strep test.
2. Treat group A strep (amoxicillin).

Complications: Rheumatic fever.

HYF: Do not delay treatment while awaiting laboratory confirmation. Less commonly precipitated by group A *Streptococcus* skin or other non-pharyngeal infection.

KAWASAKI DISEASE

A 3-year-old fully vaccinated M presents with 5 days of fever and malaise. No sick contacts. On exam, he has bilateral non-purulent conjunctivitis, tongue erythema, fissured lips, an erythematous rash on the abdomen and groin, and swelling in his hands and feet.

Management:

1. High-dose ASA and IVIG.

Complications: Coronary artery aneurysms → must obtain echocardiogram at time of diagnosis, at 2 weeks, and at 6–8 weeks.

HYF: Clinical diagnosis. Medium-vessel vasculitis. This is the rare case where you can give aspirin to a child; otherwise, it is contraindicated due to risk for Reye syndrome. Must have cardiology referral due to coronary artery aneurysm risk.

VIRAL EXANTHEM

An 11-year-old fully vaccinated F presents with general malaise and sore throat for several days. On exam, she is afebrile and has mild tonsillar erythema and a diffuse maculopapular rash on the trunk. She does not have lymphadenopathy.

Management:

1. Symptomatic treatment.

Complications: Virus-specific.

HYF: Rash can have a range of appearances: maculopapular, reticulated, vesicular, and purpuric.

ROSEOLA

A 5-year-old fully vaccinated M presents with high-grade fever for 3 days and a recent rash for the last few hours. Exam is significant for maculopapular rash on the trunk; he is afebrile at this time.

Management:

1. Symptomatic treatment.

Complications: Febrile seizures due to high fever.

HYF: Rash usually occurs AFTER the fever breaks. Caused by HHV-6/HHV-7.

RUBELLA

A 3-year-old unvaccinated M presents with a rash on his entire body. It spread from his head to his toes over the last 2 days. On exam, he has a maculopapular rash affecting the entire body and notable postauricular lymphadenopathy.

Management:

1. Symptomatic treatment.

Complications: Arthritis.

HYF: Similar to measles, but less ill-presenting. Postauricular lymphadenopathy is a defining clue. Prevention is vaccination.

MEASLES

A 5-year-old unvaccinated F presents with 3 days of fever, cough, maculopapular rash over the entire body, and conjunctivitis.

Management:

1. Supportive care.
2. Vitamin A supplementation.

Complications: Subacute sclerosing panencephalitis (rare).

HYF: Caused by paramyxovirus and causes the "4 C's": Cough, Coryza, Conjunctivitis, Koplik spots. Treatment with vitamin A decreases mortality. Prevention is vaccination.

ERYTHEMA INFECTIOSUM (FIFTH DISEASE)

A 3-year-old fully vaccinated M presents with a rash on his entire body for several days. Exam shows a diffuse maculopapular rash with prominent erythema of the cheeks.

Management:

1. Symptomatic treatment.

Complications:

- Arthropathy.
- Aplastic crisis in patients with sickle cell or hereditary spherocytosis.

HYF: "Slapped-cheek appearance." Caused by parvovirus B19.

PITYRIASIS ROSEA

An 11-year-old fully vaccinated M presents with a rash on his back for the last few weeks. Exam is significant for numerous erythematous scaly patches on the back.

Management:

1. Symptomatic treatment, resolves in 6–8 weeks.

Complications: None.

HYF: Presents as 1 "herald patch," then develops numerous similar lesions a few weeks later in a "Christmas tree" distribution on the back. Hypothesized reaction to HHV-7.

9-11 Vesicular Lesions

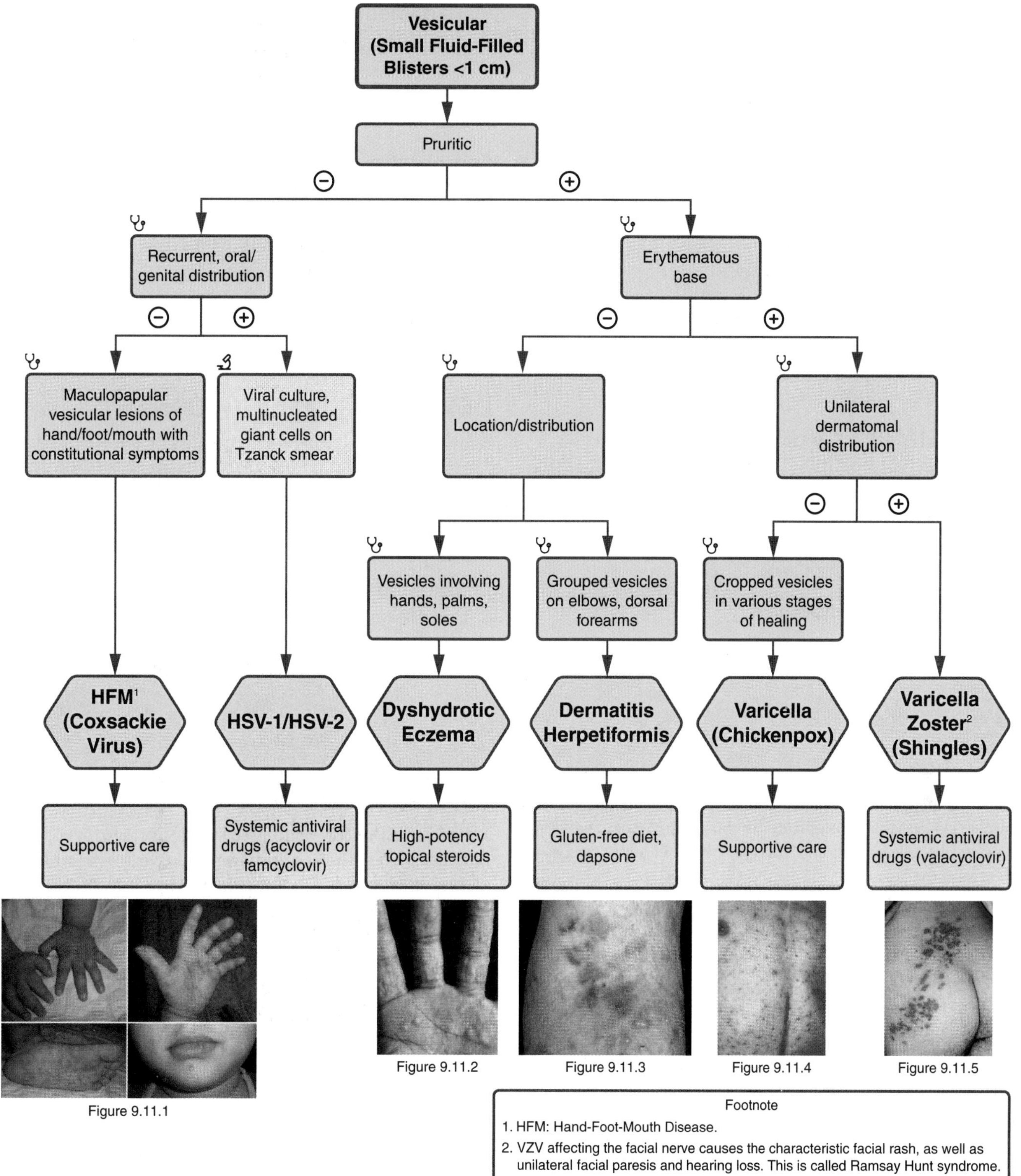
Vesicular
(Small Fluid-Filled Blisters <1 cm)
Pruritic
Recurrent, oral/ genital distribution
Erythematous base
Maculopapular vesicular lesions of hand/foot/mouth with constitutional symptoms
Viral culture, multinucleated giant cells on Tzanck smear
Location/distribution
Unilateral dermatomal distribution
Vesicles involving hands, palms, soles
Grouped vesicles on elbows, dorsal forearms
Cropped vesicles in various stages of healing
HFM[1] (Coxsackie Virus)
HSV-1/HSV-2
Dyshydrotic Eczema
Dermatitis Herpetiformis
Varicella (Chickenpox)
Varicella Zoster[2] (Shingles)
Supportive care
Systemic antiviral drugs (acyclovir or famcyclovir)
High-potency topical steroids
Gluten-free diet, dapsone
Supportive care
Systemic antiviral drugs (valacyclovir)

Figure 9.11.1

Figure 9.11.2

Figure 9.11.3

Figure 9.11.4

Figure 9.11.5

Footnote

1. HFM: Hand-Foot-Mouth Disease.
2. VZV affecting the facial nerve causes the characteristic facial rash, as well as unilateral facial paresis and hearing loss. This is called Ramsay Hunt syndrome.

FIGURE 9.11

9-11 Vesicular Lesions

HAND-FOOT-MOUTH DISEASE

A 4-year-old presents with refusal to take PO, increased fussiness, and mild fever. Exam shows maculopapular and vesicular lesions with a surrounding ring of erythema located on the buccal mucosa, palms, and soles.

Management:

1. Supportive care.
2. IV fluids if severe dehydration.

Complications: Highly contagious.

HYF: This is a clinical diagnosis. Children should be excluded from daycare/childcare settings until open blisters have crusted and symptomatic improvement is observed. Hand hygiene is key.

HERPES SIMPLEX VIRUS (HSV)

A 21-year-old F with recent unprotected sexual intercourse presents with dysuria, mild fever, and tender groin lymphadenopathy. Genital exam shows several grouped vesicles on an erythematous base involving the vulva. **Labs:** UA shows sterile pyuria. Viral culture and PCR testing for HSV DNA are positive.

Management:

1. Oral antiviral therapy (valacyclovir, acyclovir). Treatment should be initiated in the first 24 hours if possible.
2. Consider suppressive therapy for severe or frequent recurrences.

Complications:

- Vertical transmission in pregnancy from mother to fetus.
- Rarely, extragenital complications can occur, such as HSV encephalitis (see below) and HSV retinitis (slit lamp: dendritic lesions on the cornea).
- Acute urinary retention.
- Associated with Bell's palsy (HSV-1).
- Eczema herpeticum (superimposed HSV-1 on eczema).

HYF: Diagnosis is clinical, but Tzanck smear (multinucleated giant cells) and viral PCR are available. HSV-1 typically causes oral lesions; HSV-2 typically causes genital lesions. HSV encephalitis presents with acute-onset neurologic symptoms (eg, seizures, ataxia, behavioral changes such as hypersexuality), temporal lobe abnormalities on brain MRI, and CSF with +RBCs and otherwise viral pattern; treat with IV acyclovir immediately after obtaining CSF.

DYSHIDROTIC ECZEMA

A 22-year-old F with PMH of seasonal allergies presents with recurrent episodes of intensely itchy vesicles on the fingers and palms. Exam shows pruritic vesicles on the lateral aspects of both hands along with some fissuring. She describes symptom recurrence, typically in warmer weather.

Management:

1. First-line: Emollients, high-potency topical steroids (clobetasol, betamethasone), phototherapy. Topical calcineurin inhibitors if above are ineffective.
2. Systemic corticosteroids in severe cases.

Complications:

- Desquamation, chronic dermatitis, secondary infection.
- Persistent symptoms beyond 4 weeks after appropriate treatment warrant testing for fungal infections with KOH prep and/or skin biopsy to confirm diagnosis.

HYF: Also known as pompholyx or acute palmoplantar eczema. This is a clinical diagnosis; biopsy is usually not needed. Both hands and feet can be involved.

DERMATITIS HERPETIFORMIS

A 29-year-old F with PMH of celiac disease presents with pruritic papules and vesicles on her elbows. Exam shows heavily excoriated, grouped papulovesicles on both elbows as well as her back and knees.

Management:

1. Gluten-free diet.
2. Oral dapsone.

Complications: Resumption of gluten diet can lead to recurrence of symptoms.

HYF: Dermal manifestation of celiac disease mediated by subepidermal anti-transglutaminase IgA autoantibodies.

VZV (CHICKENPOX)

A 7-year-old presents with fever, sore throat, loss of appetite, and itchy rash. Exam shows pruritic, red macular lesions with pustular and crusted vesicles, all in different stages of healing.

Management:

1. Typically self-limited. Those at high risk of developing complications can be treated with acyclovir.
2. Prophylactic vaccination is recommended.

Complications:

- Skin and soft tissue infections.
- Less commonly encephalitis.
- Shingles in the future.

HYF: Post-exposure prophylaxis is recommended for immunocompromised patients, pregnant women, and newborns using VZV immune globulin within 10 days of exposure. Immunocompetent adults should receive varicella vaccine within 5 days of exposure.

VZV (SHINGLES/HERPES ZOSTER)

A 67-year-old F with PMH of childhood chickenpox presents with intense pain and blistering on her right flank. Exam shows grouped vesicles on the erythematous base in a unilateral dermatomal distribution.

9-11 Vesicular Lesions

Management:

1. Treatment depends on duration of presenting symptoms. Antiviral therapy (acyclovir, valacylovir, famcyclovir) can be initiated within 72 hours of clinical symptoms.
2. Pain management: NSAIDs, analgesics in the acute phase.

Complications:

- Disseminated herpes zoster in immunocompromised patients.
- Post-herpetic neuralgia.

HYF: Caused by reactivation of VZV in a dorsal root ganglion. Neuritic symptoms (eg, allodynia) can precede onset of rash. Post-herpetic neuralgia (ie, persistent pain >4 months after rash resolution) can be treated with anticonvulsants, TCAs, or gabapentin. Prevent shingles with vaccination in at-risk populations (eg, the elderly). Ramsay Hunt syndrome (ie, herpes zoster oticus) is marked by a triad: ear pain, facial paralysis, and rash over the external auditory canal (EAC). It is caused by reactivation of latent VZV in the geniculate ganglion, leading to CN VII involvement (facial paralysis), a rash in the EAC, and CN VIII involvement (auditory and vestibular disturbances).

9-12 Bullous Lesions

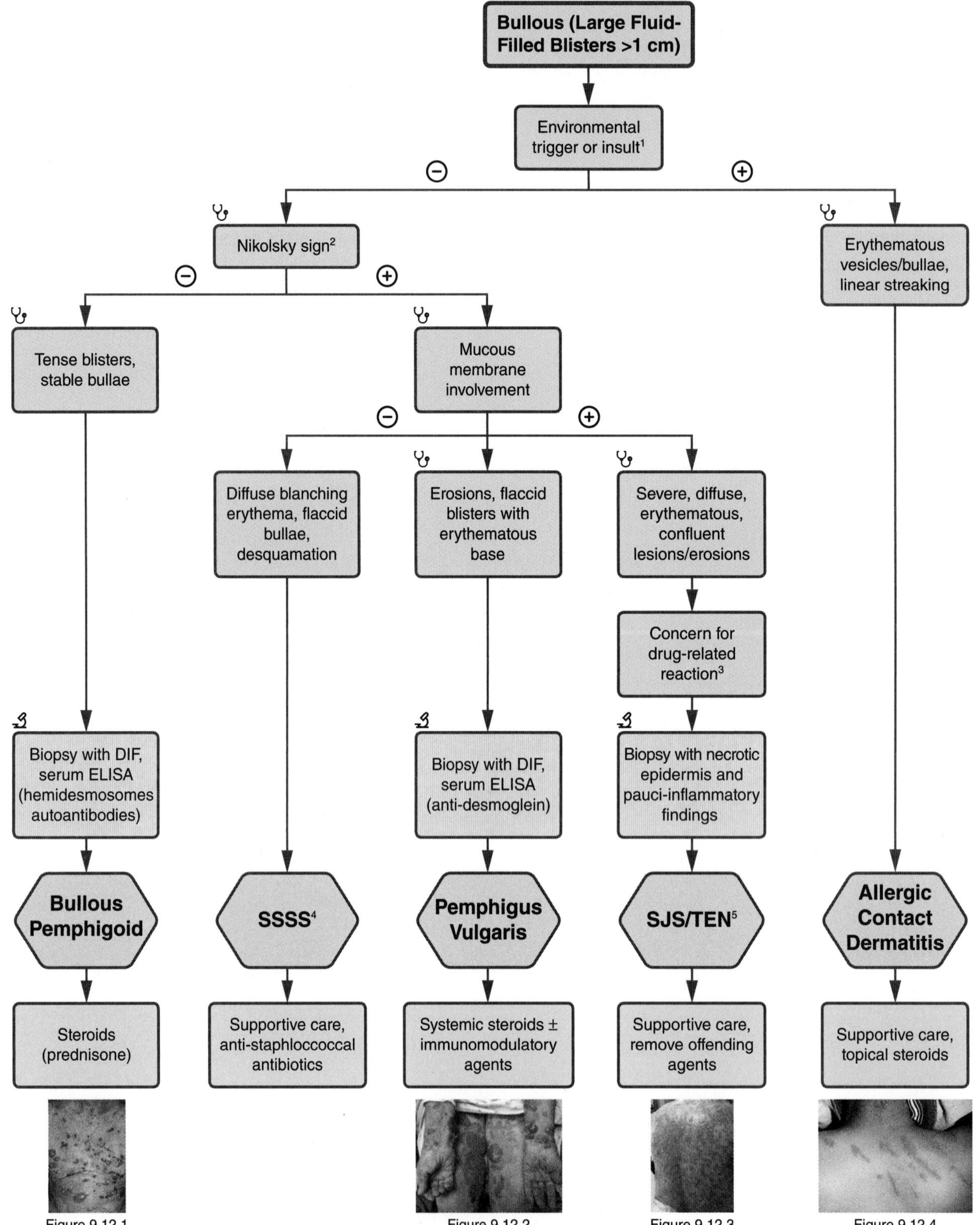
Bullous (Large Fluid-Filled Blisters >1 cm)
Environmental trigger or insult[1]
⊖
⊕
Nikolsky sign[2]
Erythematous vesicles/bullae, linear streaking
⊖
⊕
Tense blisters, stable bullae
Mucous membrane involvement
⊖
⊕
Diffuse blanching erythema, flaccid bullae, desquamation
Erosions, flaccid blisters with erythematous base
Severe, diffuse, erythematous, confluent lesions/erosions
Concern for drug-related reaction[3]
Biopsy with DIF, serum ELISA (hemidesmosomes autoantibodies)
Biopsy with DIF, serum ELISA (anti-desmoglein)
Biopsy with necrotic epidermis and pauci-inflammatory findings
Bullous Pemphigoid
SSSS[4]
Pemphigus Vulgaris
SJS/TEN[5]
Allergic Contact Dermatitis
Steroids (prednisone)
Supportive care, anti-staphloccoccal antibiotics
Systemic steroids ± immunomodulatory agents
Supportive care, remove offending agents
Supportive care, topical steroids
Figure 9.12.1
Figure 9.12.2
Figure 9.12.3
Figure 9.12.4

Footnotes

1. Exposure to an environmental trigger such as an allergenic plant (eg, toxicodendron radicans).
2. Positive Nikolsky sign: Skin blistering with gentle applied traction/pressure.
3. Common offending drugs include sulfonamide antibiotics, antiepileptics (phenytoin, carbamazepine, lamotrigene), NSAIDS, allopurinol, and cephalosporins.
4. SSSS: Staphylococcal scalded skin syndrome.
5. SJS/TEN: Stevens-Johnson syndrome/toxic epidermal necrolysis.

FIGURE 9.12

9-12 Bullous Lesions

BULLOUS PEMPHIGOID

A 75-year-old M with PMH of Parkinson's disease presents with multiple blisters involving the trunk that are acutely painful. Preceding the blister formation, the patient described associated pruritus. Exam shows multiple confluent tense bullae on an erythematous base and (–) Nikolsky sign.

Management:

1. High-potency topical steroids (clobetasol).
2. Oral steroids (prednisone).
3. Tetracyclines + niacinamide for long-term mild-moderate disease, immunosuppressants (eg, mycophenolate) for more severe disease.

Complications: Refractory disease and risk of relapse.

HYF: Mediated by autoantibodies against hemidesmosome proteins in the epidermal basement membrane (hemidesmosomes are down "bullow"). The course is typically milder compared to pemphigus vulgaris. Mucosal involvement is uncommon. Skin biopsy shows subepidermal cleavage; IF shows IgG deposits in a linear pattern at the basement membrane. Most commonly affects patients age >60.

STAPHYLOCOCCAL SCALDED SKIN SYNDROME (SSSS)

A 6-month-old M with no PMH presents with fever, reduced PO intake, and irritability in the setting of a diffuse rash. On exam, there is diffuse blanchable erythema with flaccid bullae, thick crusted lesions surrounding the mouth and eyes, and (+) Nikolsky sign.

Management:

1. Hospital admission for IV fluids and IV antistaphylococcal antibiotics (oxacillin, nafcillin).
2. Test for MRSA and broaden antibiotics if indicated.

Complications:

- Systemic infection/sepsis.
- Hypovolemia, dehydration, and electrolyte disturbances.
- Pneumonia.

HYF: Diagnosis is clinical. Usually presents with superficial flaccid bullae, followed by extensive skin exfoliation due to exfoliative toxins produced by some strains of *S. aureus*. Primary site of infection may be difficult to discern (perform full-body skin exam). Most common in infants and rare after age 5. Can also occur in the elderly and patients with reduced renal function. Bullous impetigo is a localized form of SSSS.

PEMPHIGUS VULGARIS

A 45-year-old F with PMH of SLE presents with multiple erosive lesions on her back and several blisters involving the oral mucosa that are acutely painful. Exam shows flaccid bullae and ulcers on the back and several mucosal blisters that bleed easily with (+) Nikolsky sign. These symptoms were noted after the patient started captopril.

Management:

1. High-dose steroids and/or immunomodulatory therapy (azathioprine, mycophenolate mofetil, IVIG, rituximab).

Complications:

- Skin/soft tissue infection, sepsis.

HYF: Mediated by autoantibodies targeting desmogleins 1 and 3. Common medication triggers include ACEis, penicillamine, phenobarbital, and penicillin. Exam shows (+) Nikolsky sign, flaccid bullae, and ulcers with mucosal involvement. Skin biopsy would show intraepidermal cleavage, acantholysis, and "tombstone" cells along the basal layer. IF shows IgG and C3 deposits in a net-like pattern. Most commonly affects patients aged 40–60.

STEVENS-JOHNSON SYNDROME / TOXIC EPIDERMAL NECROLYSIS

A 65-year-old M with PMH of seizure disorder (on carbamazepine) presents with diffuse erythematous rash with sloughing of skin. On exam, there are confluent hemorrhagic bullae with severe mucosal erosions and (+)Nikolsky sign. On labs, skin biopsy shows degeneration of the basal layer of the epidermis.

Management:

1. Discontinue offending agents. Common precipitating drugs: sulfonamides, penicillin, phenytoin, carbamazepine, quinolones, cephalosporins, steroids, NSAIDs.
2. Correct electrolyte disturbances, IV fluids.

Complications:

- Superimposed infections (bacteremia, septic shock).
- Pneumonia.

HYF: SJS involves <10% BSA; TEN involves >30% BSA.

ALLERGIC CONTACT DERMATITIS (POISON IVY)

A 40-year-old F gardener with no PMH presents with 1 day of intense itchiness on her arm. Exam shows a linear streak of erythematous papules and associated bulla on the right lateral forearm.

Management:

1. Supportive measures: removal of affected clothing and calamine lotion.
2. For limited mild disease, topical corticosteroids.
3. For severe disease, systemic glucocorticoids.

Complications: Skin/soft tissue infection.

9-13 Pustular Lesions

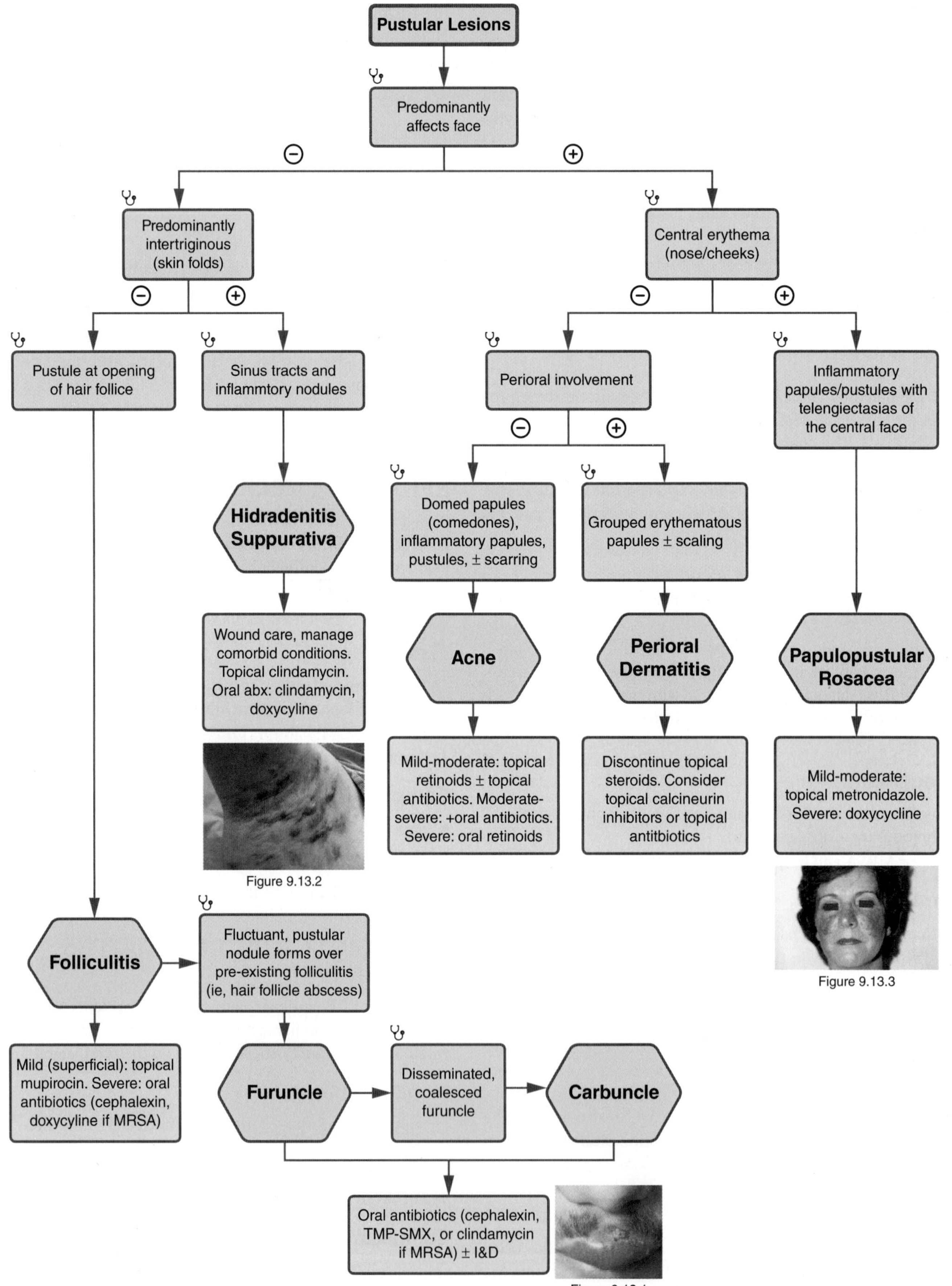
Pustular Lesions
Predominantly affects face
Predominantly intertriginous (skin folds)
Central erythema (nose/cheeks)
Pustule at opening of hair follice
Sinus tracts and inflammtory nodules
Perioral involvement
Inflammatory papules/pustules with telengiectasias of the central face
Hidradenitis Suppurativa
Domed papules (comedones), inflammatory papules, pustules, ± scarring
Grouped erythematous papules ± scaling
Wound care, manage comorbid conditions. Topical clindamycin. Oral abx: clindamycin, doxycyline
Acne
Perioral Dermatitis
Papulopustular Rosacea
Mild-moderate: topical retinoids ± topical antibiotics. Moderate-severe: +oral antibiotics. Severe: oral retinoids
Discontinue topical steroids. Consider topical calcineurin inhibitors or topical antitbiotics
Mild-moderate: topical metronidazole. Severe: doxycycline
Figure 9.13.2
Figure 9.13.3
Folliculitis
Fluctuant, pustular nodule forms over pre-existing folliculitis (ie, hair follicle abscess)
Mild (superficial): topical mupirocin. Severe: oral antibiotics (cephalexin, doxycyline if MRSA)
Furuncle
Disseminated, coalesced furuncle
Carbuncle
Oral antibiotics (cephalexin, TMP-SMX, or clindamycin if MRSA) ± I&D
Figure 9.13.1

FIGURE 9.13

9-13 Pustular Lesions

HIDRADENITIS SUPPURATIVA

A 46-year-old F with PMH of T2DM and tobacco use disorder presents with a recurring irritating skin rash underneath her left axilla. Exam shows intertriginous papules/pustules with sinus tracts and scarring in the left axilla.

Management:

1. Supportive wound care.
2. Smoking cessation and weight loss.
3. Topical clindamycin, oral doxycycline.
4. Combined clindamycin and rifampin can be used as initial treatment for more severe disease.
5. Intralesional corticosteroid injections.
6. For severe and refractory cases, consider TNF-α inhibitors (infliximab, adalimumab).

Complications: Skin contractures, strictures, lymphedema. Sinus tract and fistula formation. Superimposed infection.

HYF: HS is characterized by recurrent, painful nodules in the intertriginous areas (eg, axilla, groin, perineum).

ACNE

A 16-year-old M with no significant PMH presents with red pimples over his face and upper back. Exam shows inflammatory papules and pustules over the face and upper back with underlying closed comedones.

Management: Depending on severity:

1. Mild-moderate: Topical retinoids or benzoyl peroxide, ± topical antibiotics (clindamycin, erythromycin).
2. Moderate-severe: In addition to above, oral antibiotics (doxycycline or minocycline).
3. Severe: Oral retinoids (isotretinoin).

Complications: Acne can lead to psychological comorbidity. Individuals treated chronically with doxycycline for acne may be at higher risk of developing bacterial folliculitis. Acne fulminans may be provoked with use of isotretinoin.

HYF: Monitor LFTs and lipids in patients on isotretinoin. Isotretinoin is teratogenic; obtain pregnancy tests for female patients and counsel on 2 forms of contraception.

PERIORAL DERMATITIS

A 45-year-old F with recent use of topical triamcinolone presents with a red rash around her lips associated with an occasional burning sensation. Exam shows perioral, grouped erythematous papules with mild scaling and sparing of a small region around the vermilion border of the lips.

Management:

1. Cessation of all topical corticosteroids and other irritants (skin care products, cosmetics) to the affected areas.
2. Topical calcineurin inhibitors (tacrolimus) or topical antibiotics (erythromycin) can be considered.
3. Oral antibiotics (tetracyclines such as doxycycline or minocycline) can be considered in more severe cases.

Complications: Symptoms may persist for months to years.

HYF: This condition can improve spontaneously with cessation of topical corticosteroids and other irritants.

ROSACEA

A 55-year-old F with PMH of T2DM presents with chronic red rash over her cheeks exacerbated by alcohol and spicy foods. Exam shows central facial erythema with associated telangiectasias.

Management: Depending on subtype:

1. Papulopustular: topical metronidazole, azelaic acid, or ivermectin is 1st-line. Consider oral doxycycline for 2nd-line therapy.
2. Erythematotelangiectatic: Laser or pulsed light therapy.
3. Phymatous: oral isotretinoin, laser therapy.
4. Ocular: Ocular lubricants, topical or systemic antibiotics (eg, metronidazole).

HYF: There are multiple subtypes: Erythematotelangiectatic (this patient), papulopustular (papules and pustules on central face), phymatous (irregular skin thickening), and ocular (conjunctival hyperemia, eyelid telangiectasias, corneal ulcers, keratitis, blepharitis; requires referral to ophthalmology).

FOLLICULITIS

A 26-year-old M presents with an itchy tender red lesion over his neck. The lesion is a tiny inflamed erythematous pustule at the opening of a hair follicle.

Management: Depends on severity, as below.

1. For mild disease, topical antibiotics such as mupirocin.
2. For more severe disease, PO antibiotics (eg, cephalexin, dicloxacillin, or clindamycin if MRSA is suspected).

Complications:

- Furuncle/carbuncle/skin abscess, sepsis.

HYF: Folliculitis barbae is a bacterial folliculitis typically caused by *Staphylococcus aureus* affecting regions of the face/neck/beard.

FURUNCLE/CARBUNCLE

A 26-year-old M presents with a tender circular nodule at the nape of his neck. Exam shows a well-circumscribed, indurated, pustular nodule over the posterior neck that is inflamed and erythematous.

Management:

1. Anti-staphylococcal antibiotics (eg, cephalexin or dicloxacillin for MSSA, TMP/SMX or clindamycin for MRSA).
2. Consider I&D for drainable abscesses.

Complications: Persistent symptoms can lead to systemic symptoms, including bacteremia/sepsis.

HYF: Furuncle = deeper infection of a hair follicle often with associated abscess. Carbuncle = larger inflammatory plaque with pustules from coalescing of several inflamed follicles. Usually due to *S. aureus*.

9-14 Lichenified Plaque Lesions

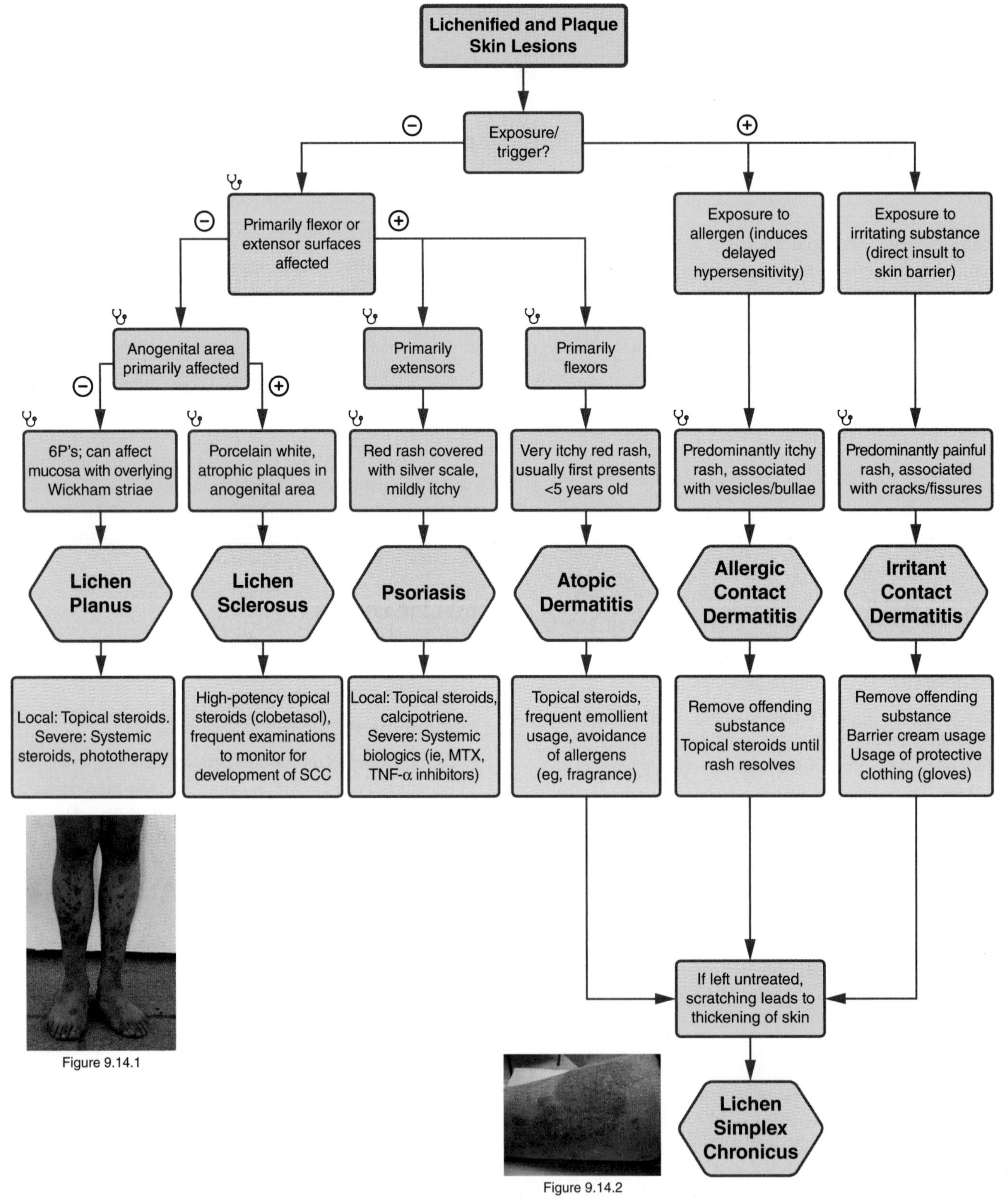

Lichenified and Plaque Skin Lesions
Exposure/ trigger?
⊖
⊕
Primarily flexor or extensor surfaces affected
Exposure to allergen (induces delayed hypersensitivity)
Exposure to irritating substance (direct insult to skin barrier)
Anogenital area primarily affected
Primarily extensors
Primarily flexors
6P's; can affect mucosa with overlying Wickham striae
Porcelain white, atrophic plaques in anogenital area
Red rash covered with silver scale, mildly itchy
Very itchy red rash, usually first presents <5 years old
Predominantly itchy rash, associated with vesicles/bullae
Predominantly painful rash, associated with cracks/fissures
Lichen Planus
Lichen Sclerosus
Psoriasis
Atopic Dermatitis
Allergic Contact Dermatitis
Irritant Contact Dermatitis
Local: Topical steroids. Severe: Systemic steroids, phototherapy
High-potency topical steroids (clobetasol), frequent examinations to monitor for development of SCC
Local: Topical steroids, calcipotriene. Severe: Systemic biologics (ie, MTX, TNF-α inhibitors)
Topical steroids, frequent emollient usage, avoidance of allergens (eg, fragrance)
Remove offending substance Topical steroids until rash resolves
Remove offending substance Barrier cream usage Usage of protective clothing (gloves)
If left untreated, scratching leads to thickening of skin
Lichen Simplex Chronicus

Figure 9.14.1

Figure 9.14.2

FIGURE 9.14

9-14 Lichenified Plaque Lesions

LICHEN PLANUS

A 45-year-old F presents with itchy spots on her leg. On exam, she has flat purple papules on her right shin.

Management:

1. Ask about medication history and history of HCV.
2. Start topical steroids.
3. If refractory, treat with systemic steroids or phototherapy.

Complications: None

HYF: 6 P's – purple, planar, polygonal, pruritic, papules, and plaques. Wickham striae (lacy white lines) may be present on the lesions. Most classically affects flexural sites (eg, wrists) but can affect any part of the body, including mucosa and nails. Associated with numerous medications and HCV.

LICHEN SCLEROSUS

A 65-year-old F presents with a groin rash. On exam, she has atrophied, shiny white plaques on her labia minora and perineum and mild obliteration of her clitoris.

Management:

1. Empiric trial of topical clobetasol.
2. Yearly gynecology examination to rule out malignancy.

Complications: Development of vulvar SCC.

HYF: LS has biomodal distribution (pre-pubertal and post-menopausal). More commonly in groin ("figure 8 pattern"), less commonly affects men and extra-genital sites. Typically does not affect mucosa. Monitor for vulvar SCC.

PSORIASIS

A 27-year-old M with PMH of tobacco use disorder presents with rash. On exam, he has erythematous plaques with overlying silver scale on the elbows, knees, and lower back and pitting of the fingernails.

Management:

1. Topical steroids.
2. Counsel on smoking cessation and weight loss.
3. If resistant to topicals, consider MTX, apremilast, UV light, or biologics (TNF-α inhibitors, IL-12/17/23 blockers).

Complications:

- Psoriatic arthritis – need to be on DMARD.
- Higher risk of cardiovascular disease.

HYF: Bimodal distribution (develops in 20s or 50s). Associated with smoking and obesity.

ATOPIC DERMATITIS

A 4-year-old M with PMH of seasonal allergy and asthma presents with itchy rash. Exam shows erythematous patches on the antecubital/popliteal fossa, with notable excoriations.

Management:

1. Empiric trial of topical steroids (max 2 weeks at a time to prevent atrophy, striae, and dyspigmentation).
2. Frequent emollient usage.
3. Start sensitive skin regimen (unscented detergent, no dryer sheets, unscented soaps, etc.).
4. If treatment resistant, consider bleach baths, occluding steroid with plastic wrap, and dupilimab.

Complications: Secondary infection (*S. aureus*, molluscum, HSV).

HYF: Flexural distribution. Patients may have the atopic triad (allergies, atopic dermatitis, asthma).

CONTACT DERMATITIS

A 25-year-old M who works in construction presents with a painful rash on his hands. Exam shows erythematous rash on his palmar hands with associated fissuring.

Management:

1. Avoid triggers.
2. Frequent barrier cream usage.
3. Barrier clothing (eg, gloves).
4. Topical steroids if there is an allergic component.

Complications: Psychosocial distress.

HYF: Irritant contact dermatitis is more painful than itchy. Allergic contact dermatitis is more itchy than painful and can have vesicles/bullae.

LICHEN SIMPLEX CHRONICUS

An 8-year-old F with PMH of atopic dermatitis presents with an itchy rash untreated for years. Exam shows thickened erythematous plaques with numerous surrounding excoriations, notably on the antecubital fossa and lower legs.

Management:

1. Treat underlying disease.
2. Break itch-and-scratch cycle.

Complications: Residual pigment changes even after treatment that may last months to years.

HYF: LSC is usually secondary to another disease. It results from chronic itching and scratching → thickening of the skin in the area.

9-15 Scaling and Crusted Lesions

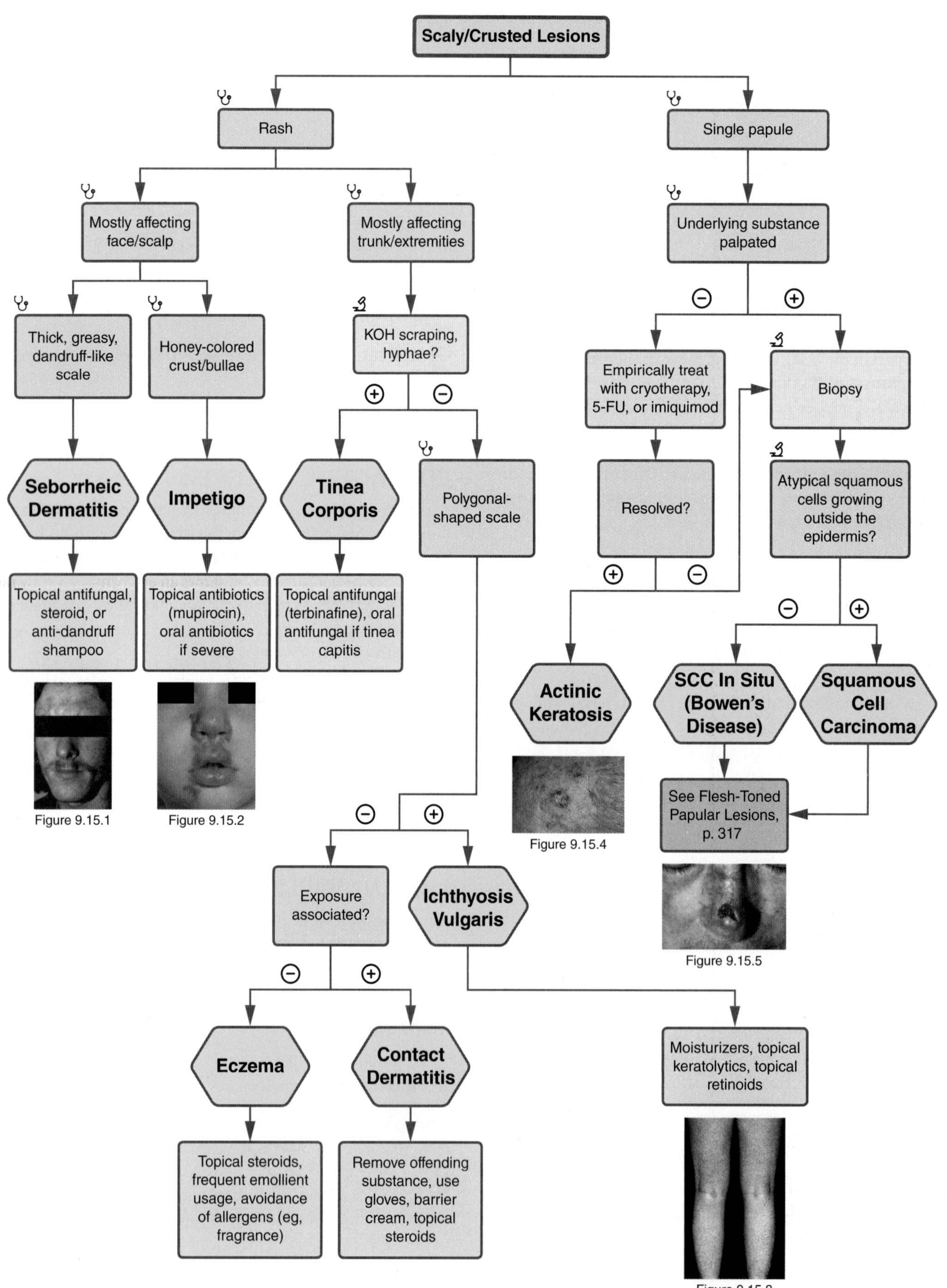
Scaly/Crusted Lesions
Rash
Single papule
Mostly affecting face/scalp
Mostly affecting trunk/extremities
Underlying substance palpated
Thick, greasy, dandruff-like scale
Honey-colored crust/bullae
KOH scraping, hyphae?
Empirically treat with cryotherapy, 5-FU, or imiquimod
Biopsy
Seborrheic Dermatitis
Impetigo
Tinea Corporis
Polygonal-shaped scale
Resolved?
Atypical squamous cells growing outside the epidermis?
Topical antifungal, steroid, or anti-dandruff shampoo
Topical antibiotics (mupirocin), oral antibiotics if severe
Topical antifungal (terbinafine), oral antifungal if tinea capitis
Actinic Keratosis
SCC In Situ (Bowen's Disease)
Squamous Cell Carcinoma
See Flesh-Toned Papular Lesions, p. 317
Exposure associated?
Ichthyosis Vulgaris
Eczema
Contact Dermatitis
Moisturizers, topical keratolytics, topical retinoids
Topical steroids, frequent emollient usage, avoidance of allergens (eg, fragrance)
Remove offending substance, use gloves, barrier cream, topical steroids
Figure 9.15.1
Figure 9.15.2
Figure 9.15.3
Figure 9.15.4
Figure 9.15.5

FIGURE 9.15

9-15 Scaling and Crusted Lesions

SEBORRHEIC DERMATITIS

A 27-year-old M with PMH of HIV/AIDS presents with a scaly rash on his face and scalp. Exam shows erythematous patches with overlying greasy scale on the scalp, eyebrows, and nasolabial folds.

Management:

1. OTC anti-dandruff shampoos (eg, selenium sulfide, zinc pyrithione), topical antifungals, or topical steroids.

Complications: Secondary bacterial or fungal infections.

HYF: Severe disease more common in HIV/AIDS and neurologic disease (eg, Parkinson's disease). Associated with *Malassezia* species, vitamin B_2 and B_6 deficiency. Can be seen in "seborrheic distribution" of scalp, central face, behind ears, and chest. In infants, can present as a cradle cap or diaper rash.

IMPETIGO

A 3-year-old previously healthy M presents with a painful rash on his face. A child at day care had a similar rash on her arms. On exam, he has erythematous patches with overlying honey-colored crust and a few bullae surrounding his lips.

Management:

1. For limited disease, topical antibiotics (mupirocin).
2. For more disseminated disease, oral anti-staphylococcal antibiotics (eg, cephalexin, dicloxacillin, clindamycin).

Complications: Systemic infection, scarlet fever, post-streptococcal glomerulonephritis.

HYF: Non-bullous impetigo = group A strep or *S. aureus*; painful, non-pruritic pustules and honey-crusted lesions. Bullous impetigo = *S. aureus* typically; enlarging flaccid bullae; can progress to staphylococcal scalded skin syndrome.

TINEA CORPORIS/PEDIS

A 15-year-old M with no PMH presents with itchy, scaly rash on his feet. He notes others on his wrestling team have had similar rashes. Exam shows erythematous scaly plaque between the toes and on the soles of both feet.

Management:

1. KOH scraping, evaluate under microscope for hyphae.
2. If positive, treat with topical antifungal (eg, allylamine agents: terbinafine; azoles: miconazole).

Complications: Cellulitis if left untreated.

HYF: Tinea is caused by dermatophytes, most commonly *Trichophyton rubrum*. Can affect the body (tinea corporis), feet (tinea pedis), scalp (tinea capitis), and groin (tinea cruris). Mild/early TP often follows an interdigital pattern (ie, between toes), but in more chronic cases, it extends to the soles and sides of the feet ("moccasin pattern"). Tinea capitis needs to be treated with an oral antifungal agent. Poorly controlled diabetes is a major risk factor.

ACTINIC KERATOSIS

A 65-year-old M with history of numerous sunburns presents with scaly spots on his forehead. Exam shows numerous erythematous, scaly papules along the hairline.

Management:

1. Cryosurgery (liquid nitrogen), topical 5-FU or imiquimod, phototherapy, dermabrasion.

Complications: 0.5% risk of developing into squamous cell carcinoma per lesion per year.

HYF: Clinical diagnosis. If lesion recurs despite being treated, biopsy is required, as it may be squamous cell carcinoma.

ICHTHYOSIS VULGARIS

A 15-year-old M with PMH of atopic dermatitis presents with a rash on his arms and legs. His father had a similar rash growing up, which improved as he got older. Exam shows an erythematous scaly rash on arms, legs, and abdomen; the scale has a polygonal appearance.

Management:

1. Frequent emollient usage, keratolytics (ammonium lactate/urea cream), topical retinoids.

Complications: Skin infections.

HYF: Inherited in AD fashion due to loss-of-function mutations in the filaggrin (*FLG*) gene. Patients commonly have a history of atopic dermatitis. Presents in childhood, improves with age, and then worsens again in old age. "Ikhthýs" is Greek for fish (scales).

NUMMULAR ECZEMA

A 65-year-old F with no PMH presents with an itchy rash on her lower left leg. Exam shows a nummular erythematous scaly plaque on the dorsal right shin with surrounding excoriations.

Management:

1. Trial of topical steroids (eg, betamethasone), regular emollient usage, and sensitive skin care routine.

Complications: Bacterial or viral (HSV) superinfection.

HYF: Eczema is a reaction pattern, rather than a specific diagnosis. Types of eczema include atopic dermatitis (children), asteatotic dermatitis (as in this patient), and dyshidrotic dermatitis. If lesions are resistant to topical steroids, consider other diagnoses.

9-16 Ulcerous Lesions

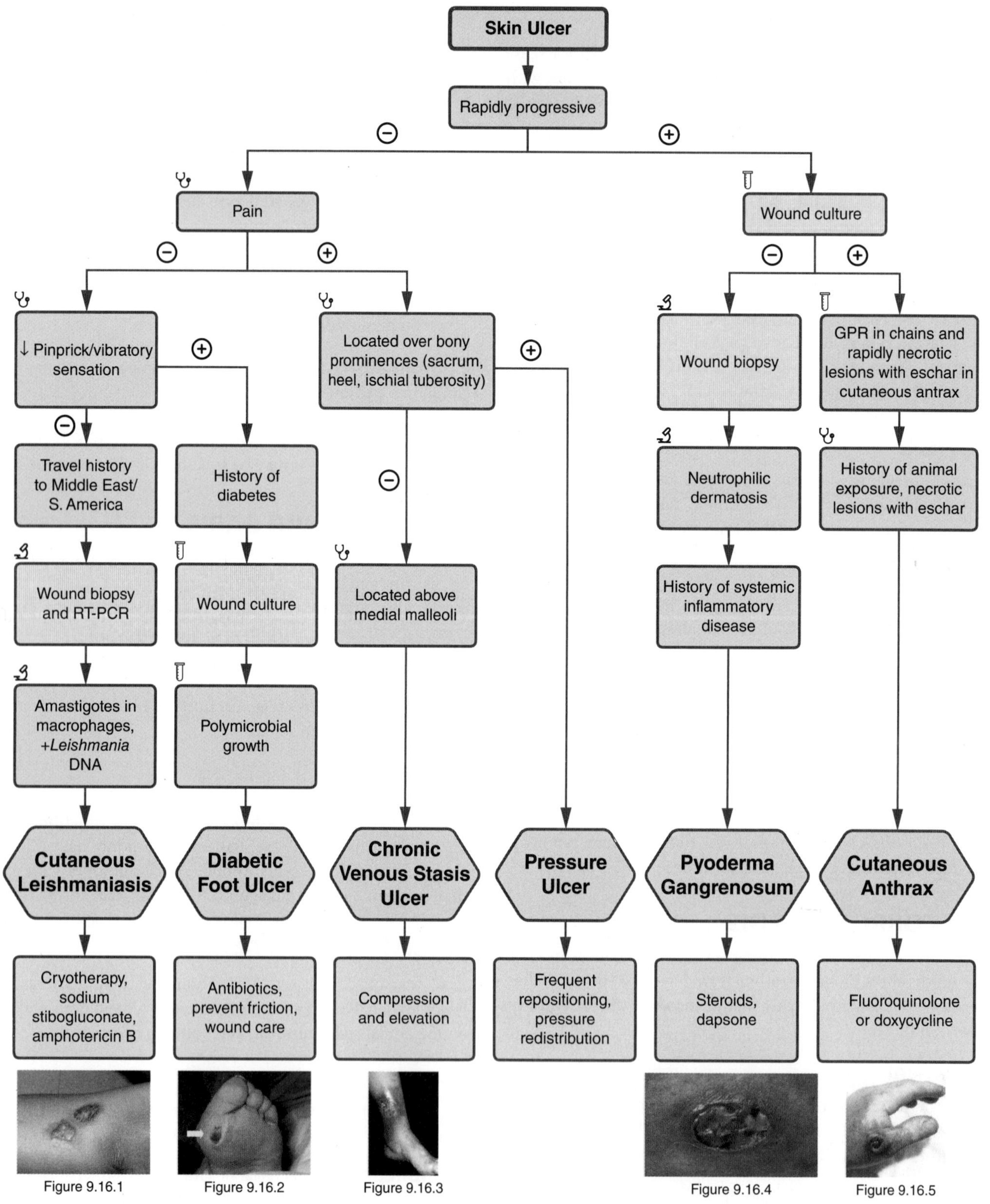

Skin Ulcer
Rapidly progressive
⊖
⊕
Pain
⊖
⊕
↓ Pinprick/vibratory sensation
⊕
⊖
Travel history to Middle East/ S. America
Wound biopsy and RT-PCR
Amastigotes in macrophages, +*Leishmania* DNA
Cutaneous Leishmaniasis
Cryotherapy, sodium stibogluconate, amphotericin B
History of diabetes
Wound culture
Polymicrobial growth
Diabetic Foot Ulcer
Antibiotics, prevent friction, wound care
Located over bony prominences (sacrum, heel, ischial tuberosity)
⊕
⊖
Located above medial malleoli
Chronic Venous Stasis Ulcer
Compression and elevation
Pressure Ulcer
Frequent repositioning, pressure redistribution
Wound culture
⊖
⊕
Wound biopsy
Neutrophilic dermatosis
History of systemic inflammatory disease
Pyoderma Gangrenosum
Steroids, dapsone
GPR in chains and rapidly necrotic lesions with eschar in cutaneous antrax
History of animal exposure, necrotic lesions with eschar
Cutaneous Anthrax
Fluoroquinolone or doxycycline
Figure 9.16.1
Figure 9.16.2
Figure 9.16.3
Figure 9.16.4
Figure 9.16.5

FIGURE 9.16

9-16 Ulcerous Lesions

CUTANEOUS LEISHMANIASIS

A 21-year-old F who returned from a trip in Brazil 4 weeks ago presents with an ulcer on her right forearm. On **exam**, the ulcer is painless and surrounded by 3 satellite papules. **Labs/imaging:** Biopsy of the ulcer border with Giemsa stain shows amastigotes within macrophages, and RT-PCR confirms the presence of *Leishmania* DNA.

Management:

1. Local cryotherapy.
2. Sodium stibogluconate or amphotericin B.

Complications:

- Secondary bacterial infection.
- Mucosal involvement.
- Disseminated infection.

HYF: Sand flies are the vectors for CL. Endemic areas include Afghanistan, Algeria, Brazil, and Colombia.

DIABETIC/NEUROPATHIC FOOT ULCER

A 70-year-old M with PMH of poorly controlled T2DM presents with a several week history of an ulcer on his right foot. On **exam**, there is an ulcer under the metatarsal head of the big toe and decreased sensation to vibration, pain, and temperature. **Labs:** Wound culture is (+) GPCs, GNRs, and anaerobes.

Management:

1. Prevent pressure, friction, trauma.
2. Wound care and debridement.
3. Antimicrobial therapy based on cultures and sensitivities.

Complications:

- Osteomyelitis requiring amputation.
- Recurrent cellulitis.

HYF: High-risk diabetic/neuropathic foot ulcers (>2 cm, present for >1 week, systemic symptoms) almost always have polymicrobial infections that can extend to the bone and cause osteomyelitis. Antibiotic coverage should include GPCs with MRSA, GNRs with *Pseudomonas*, and anaerobic coverage (ie, vancomycin + cefepime).

CHRONIC VENOUS STASIS ULCER

A 65-year-old M with PMH of obesity and lower extremity DVT presents with chronic bilateral ulcers above the medial malleolus. On **exam**, he has 2+ pitting edema in the bilateral lower extremities, varicose veins, and brownish discoloration of the skin surrounding the ulcers. On **imaging**, venous duplex ultrasound confirms venous hypertension and reflux.

Management:

1. Compression stockings or boots and elevation.
2. Wound care.

Complications: Cellulitis, osteomyelitis, sepsis.

HYF: Typically bilateral and symmetric, unlike cellulitis.

PRESSURE ULCER

An 80-year-old M with PMH of metastatic prostate cancer to spine presents with a progressive ulcer on his sacrum. On **exam**, there is a painful ulcer showing full-thickness skin loss with visible subcutaneous fat in the sacral area. **Labs** shows low pre-albumin and albumin levels.

Management:

1. Pressure redistribution.
2. Wound care and debridement.
3. Nutritional support.

Complications:

- Secondary bacterial infection and osteomyelitis.
- Formation of sinus tracts connecting to bowel/bladder.
- Squamous cell carcinoma.

HYF: Immobility and malnutrition are 2 major risk factors for developing pressure ulcers. Key prevention measures include frequent repositioning, continuous rotation, and nutritional support to promote wound healing.

PYODERMA GANGRENOSUM

A 45-year-old F with PMH of Crohn's disease and rheumatoid arthritis presents with a new ulcer on the right leg. On **exam**, the ulcer has a purulent base with an irregular gunmetal gray border. On **labs**, biopsy of the ulcer margin shows a neutrophilic infiltrate, and tissue cultures are negative for bacteria and fungi.

Management:

1. Local or systemic steroids.
2. Dapsone.
3. Immunomodulatory/biologic therapy (eg, TNF-α inhibitor).

Complications:

- Infection.
- Cushing's disease secondary to steroid treatment.
- Infusion reactions, increased infection risk, heart failure secondary to anti-TNFa therapy.

HYF: Associated with pathergy, systemic inflammatory disorders, hematologic malignancy.

CUTANEOUS ANTHRAX (NO SYSTEMIC INVOLVEMENT)

A 40-year-old M with exposure to sheep hides presents with a rapidly progressive ulcer on hand. On **exam**, the ulcer is painless, black, and necrotic and is surrounded by edema. On **labs**, wound culture grows GPRs in chains.

Management:

1. Fluoroquinolones or doxycycline or clindamycin.

Complications:

- Pulmonary anthrax.
- GI anthrax.
- Meningitis.

HYF: Caused by *Bacillus anthracis* spore entry into subcutaenous tissues. Exposure risks include working with infected animals and animal products.

9-17 Nodular Skin Lesions

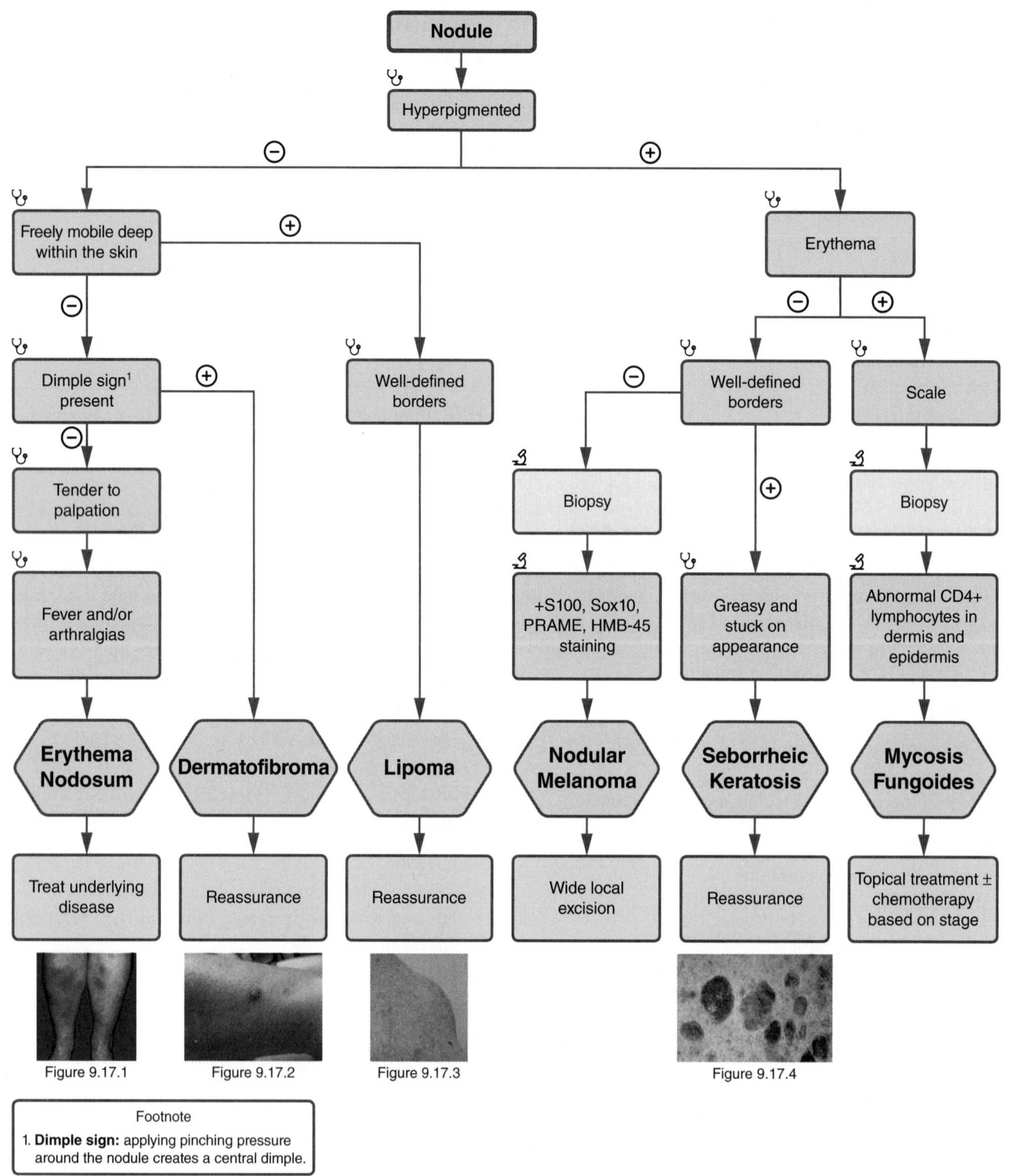
Nodule
Hyperpigmented
Freely mobile deep within the skin
Erythema
Dimple sign[1] present
Well-defined borders
Well-defined borders
Scale
Tender to palpation
Biopsy
Biopsy
Fever and/or arthralgias
+S100, Sox10, PRAME, HMB-45 staining
Greasy and stuck on appearance
Abnormal CD4+ lymphocytes in dermis and epidermis
Erythema Nodosum
Dermatofibroma
Lipoma
Nodular Melanoma
Seborrheic Keratosis
Mycosis Fungoides
Treat underlying disease
Reassurance
Reassurance
Wide local excision
Reassurance
Topical treatment ± chemotherapy based on stage
Figure 9.17.1
Figure 9.17.2
Figure 9.17.3
Figure 9.17.4
Footnote
1. Dimple sign: applying pinching pressure around the nodule creates a central dimple.

FIGURE 9.17

9-17 Nodular Skin Lesions

ERYTHEMA NODOSUM

A 20-year-old F with a recent history of self-resolving pharyngitis presents with a 4-day history of fever and painful nodules on shins. On exam, the nodules have ill-defined borders and are palpable deep in the skin. Labs show (+) anti-streptolysin O titer.

Management:

1. Evaluate for and treat the underlying disease.
2. NSAIDs for symptomatic treatment.
3. Glucocorticoids for pain refractory to NSAIDs.

Complications: None. Self-limiting, resolves in 3–6 weeks.

HYF: Often associated with underlying disease, including streptococcal infection, sarcoidosis, IBD, tuberculosis, fungal infections, and lymphoma.

DERMATOFIBROMA

A 30-year-old F presents with a nodule on her posterior calf. On exam, there is a 4-mm uniformly brown hyperpigmented nodule. Pinching the nodule causes dimpling in the center of the lesion.

Management:

1. Reassurance: benign lesion.

Complications: None.

HYF: A positive "dimple sign" (central dimpling when pinching the lesion) is characteristic and would be rare in any other skin lesion. Often arises in sites of trauma.

LIPOMA

A 65-year-old F presents with a chronic nodule on her trunk. On exam, the nodule is skin-colored with no overlying changes, soft and mobile with distinct borders, and palpable deep in the skin.

Management:

1. Reassurance: benign lesion.
2. Consider biopsy if lesion grows in size.

Complications: None.

HYF: Due to its location in subcutaneous fat, a lipoma will be freely movable and most easily felt with deep palpation of the skin.

NODULAR MELANOMA

A 50-year-old M presents with a rapidly growing nodule on his upper back. On exam, the nodule is discrete and brown, blue, and black in color. On labs, biopsy shows dermal invasion of cells staining positive for S100, HMB45, and Sox10.

Management:

1. Full-thickness biopsy and staging.
2. For melanomas >1 mm in depth and clinically negative LN, sentinel lymph node mapping and biopsy are warranted to assess for metastatic disease.
3. Monitor with biannual skin exams.

Complications:

- Recurrence.
- Metastasis.

HYF: Nodular melanomas skip the radial growth phase within the epidermis and immediately enter the vertical growth phase and invade into the dermis.

SEBORRHEIC KERATOSIS

A 65-year-old M presents with 2 new stable nodules on his back that have been present for several months. On exam, they are hyperpigmented, appearing greasy and "stuck on" the skin.

Management:

1. Reassurance: benign lesions.
2. Cryotherapy for cosmetic removal.

Complications: Lesions can become irritated/inflamed with friction and excoriation.

HYF: Rapid increase in frequency and size of seborrheic keratoses and pruritus is characteristic of Leser-Trelat sign, which is a paraneoplastic syndrome found in adenocarcinomas.

MYCOSIS FUNGOIDES

A 65-year-old M presents with a new nodule that has developed in the area of a pruritic and scaly plaque. On exam, the nodule is ulcerated and surrounded by several asymmetrical erythematous plaques. On labs, biopsy shows atypical lymphocytes within the epidermis and dermis with cerebriform nuclei.

Management:

1. Biopsy of ≥ 2 sites and staging.
2. CBC with differential and flow cytometry to assess for presence of atypical CD4+ in blood (Sézary syndrome).
3. If systemic symptoms are present, assess possible metastasis with full-body CT with contrast.
4. Topical treatment (steroids, phototherapy) for skin disease or chemotherapy + topicals for systemic disease.

Complications: Metastasis.

HYF: Mycosis fungoides is a cutaneous CD4+ T-cell lymphoma that initially presents in the skin. Abnormal T cells first proliferate in the dermis and invade into the epidermis over time, which manifests as a patch or plaque that becomes elevated and nodular over time.

9-18 Skin Necrosis

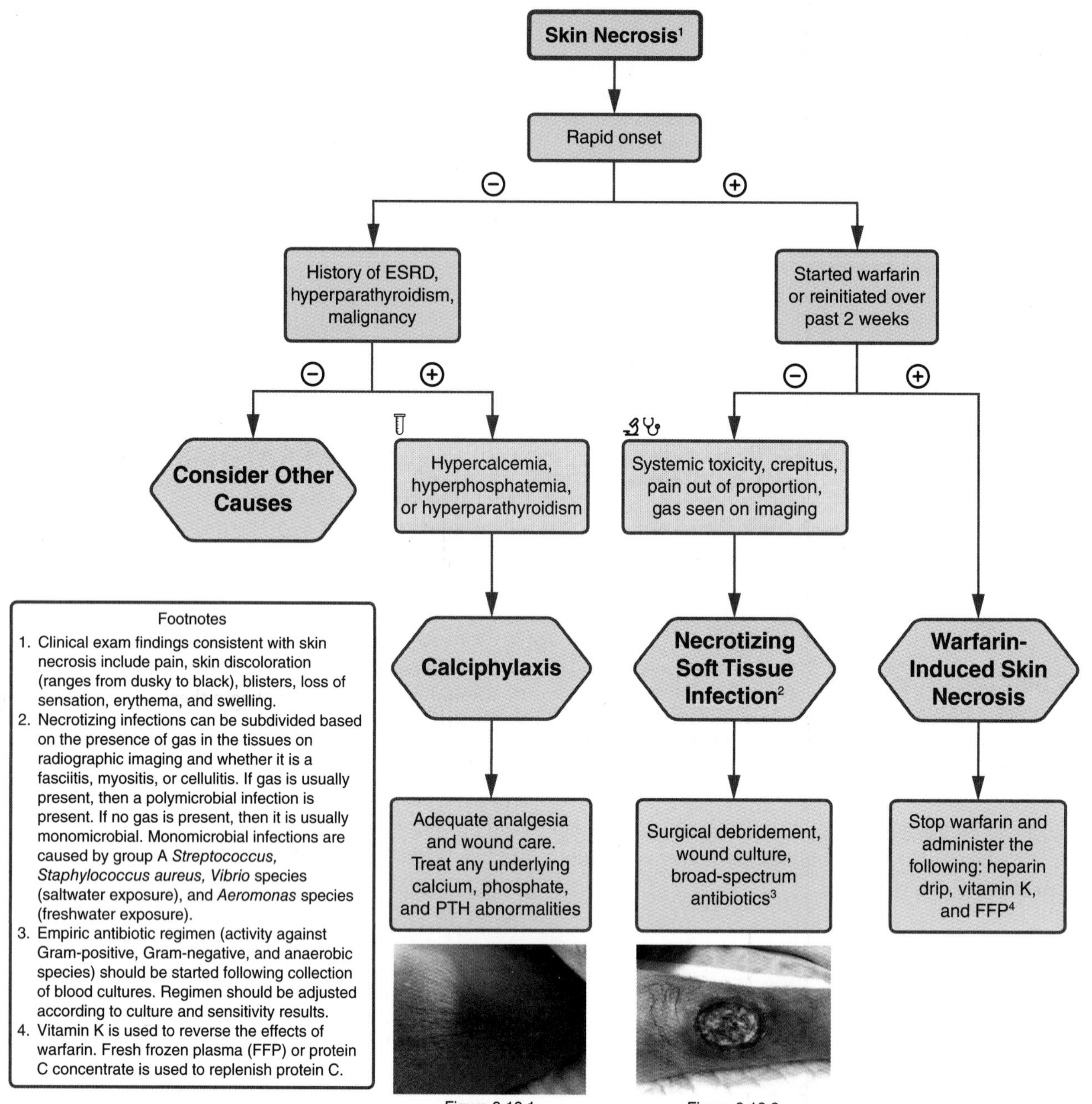

Skin Necrosis[1]
Rapid onset
⊖
⊕
History of ESRD, hyperparathyroidism, malignancy
Started warfarin or reinitiated over past 2 weeks
⊖
⊕
⊖
⊕
Consider Other Causes
Hypercalcemia, hyperphosphatemia, or hyperparathyroidism
Systemic toxicity, crepitus, pain out of proportion, gas seen on imaging
Calciphylaxis
Necrotizing Soft Tissue Infection[2]
Warfarin-Induced Skin Necrosis
Adequate analgesia and wound care. Treat any underlying calcium, phosphate, and PTH abnormalities
Surgical debridement, wound culture, broad-spectrum antibiotics[3]
Stop warfarin and administer the following: heparin drip, vitamin K, and FFP[4]

Footnotes

1. Clinical exam findings consistent with skin necrosis include pain, skin discoloration (ranges from dusky to black), blisters, loss of sensation, erythema, and swelling.
2. Necrotizing infections can be subdivided based on the presence of gas in the tissues on radiographic imaging and whether it is a fasciitis, myositis, or cellulitis. If gas is usually present, then a polymicrobial infection is present. If no gas is present, then it is usually monomicrobial. Monomicrobial infections are caused by group A *Streptococcus, Staphylococcus aureus, Vibrio* species (saltwater exposure), and *Aeromonas* species (freshwater exposure).
3. Empiric antibiotic regimen (activity against Gram-positive, Gram-negative, and anaerobic species) should be started following collection of blood cultures. Regimen should be adjusted according to culture and sensitivity results.
4. Vitamin K is used to reverse the effects of warfarin. Fresh frozen plasma (FFP) or protein C concentrate is used to replenish protein C.

Figure 9.18.1

Figure 9.18.2

FIGURE 9.18

9-18 Skin Necrosis

CALCIPHYLAXIS (CALCIFIC UREMIC ARTERIOLOPATHY)

A 59-year-old M with PMH of DM2 and ESRD on dialysis presents with 4 months of pain and discoloration on his abdomen. **Exam** shows a tender black eschar on the abdomen, painful subcutaneous nodules on his right thigh and left calf, and intact peripheral pulses. **Labs** show normocalcemia, hyperphosphatemia, and high PTH.

Management:

1. Pain management and wound care.
2. Treatment of infected wounds if applicable.
3. Treatment of calcium, phosphorus, and parathyroid hormone abnormalities.
4. Trial of sodium thiosulfate.

Complications:

- Infection.
- High mortality (approximately 50% survival at 1 year).

HYF: Calciphylaxis is usually a clinical diagnosis in patients with ESRD; if unsure, biopsy the lesion. Due to arteriolar calcification and soft tissue calcium deposition → tissue ischemia and necrosis most commonly in high-adiposity tissue. Normal serum calcium levels do not rule out calciphylaxis, as tissue calcium can be much higher. Risk factors: ESRD on dialysis, history of renal transplant, hyperparathyroidism, oral anticoagulants (eg, warfarin), obesity, diabetes, hypercalcemia, hyperphosphatemia.

NECROTIZING SOFT TISSUE INFECTION

A 65-year-old M presents with progressively worsening pain in his LLE that began earlier in the day. On **exam**, he is hypotensive and febrile, and there is erythematous swelling in his left lower extremity with severe pain to palpation and crepitus. **Labs** show leukocytosis. On **imaging**, CT of his leg demonstrates subcutaneous gas collection and fat stranding.

Management:

1. Obtain blood cultures and begin broad-spectrum antibiotics. Volume expansion with IV fluids.
2. Urgent surgical exploration/debridement is the gold standard for diagnosis and treatment. Obtain specimen for Gram stain/culture.

Complications:

- Loss of limb.
- Shock.
- Death.

HYF: If a necrotizing soft tissue infection involves the perineum, it is also known as Fournier gangrene.

WARFARIN-INDUCED SKIN NECROSIS

A 50-year-old M diagnosed with DVT and started on warfarin 3 days ago presents with painful skin lesions. **Exam** shows large, painful, red plaque on the buttocks. **Labs** show decreased protein C and S activity on functional assay.

Management:

1. Immediately discontinue warfarin.
2. Administer vitamin K and begin therapeutic heparin drip.
3. Administer protein C concentrate (eg, FFP).
4. Debridement of necrotic tissue and possible skin grafting.

Complications:

- Infection.
- Uncontrolled pain.

HYF: This is a clinical diagnosis. Skin necrosis is usually seen in the first 2–5 days after warfarin initiation due to decreased protein C compared to clotting factors. Individuals with protein C or S deficiency are especially susceptible. A heparin bridge is necessary for individuals started on warfarin.

9-19 Genital Lesions

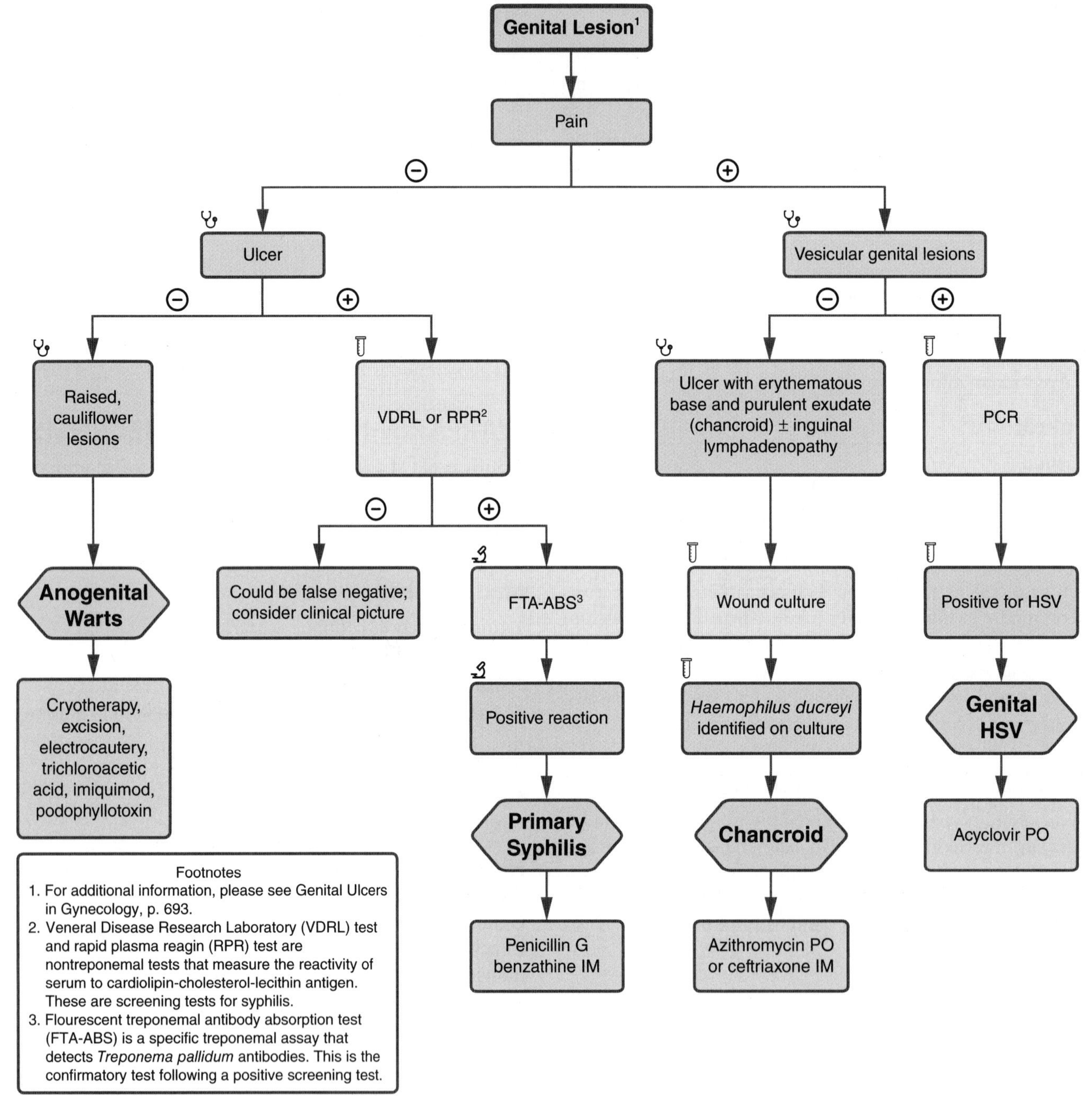
Genital Lesion[1]
Pain
⊖
⊕
Ulcer
Vesicular genital lesions
⊖
⊕
⊖
⊕
Raised, cauliflower lesions
VDRL or RPR[2]
Ulcer with erythematous base and purulent exudate (chancroid) ± inguinal lymphadenopathy
PCR
⊖
⊕
Anogenital Warts
Could be false negative; consider clinical picture
FTA-ABS[3]
Wound culture
Positive for HSV
Cryotherapy, excision, electrocautery, trichloroacetic acid, imiquimod, podophyllotoxin
Positive reaction
Haemophilus ducreyi identified on culture
Genital HSV
Primary Syphilis
Chancroid
Acyclovir PO
Penicillin G benzathine IM
Azithromycin PO or ceftriaxone IM

Footnotes

1. For additional information, please see Genital Ulcers in Gynecology, p. 693.
2. Veneral Disease Research Laboratory (VDRL) test and rapid plasma reagin (RPR) test are nontreponemal tests that measure the reactivity of serum to cardiolipin-cholesterol-lecithin antigen. These are screening tests for syphilis.
3. Flourescent treponemal antibody absorption test (FTA-ABS) is a specific treponemal assay that detects *Treponema pallidum* antibodies. This is the confirmatory test following a positive screening test.

FIGURE 9.19

9-19 Genital Lesions

ANOGENITAL WARTS

A 27-year-old M with PMH of HIV presents with anal pruritis. **Exam** shows multiple non-tender irregular anal papules. On **labs**, biopsy shows koilocytosis and is negative for malignancy.

Management:

1. Clinical diagnosis. Biopsy if uncertain or atypical features (bleeding, ulceration).
2. 1st-line therapies include cryotherapy, electrocautery, excision, trichloroacetic acid, imiquimod, and podophyllotoxin. Treatment depends on the number and size of warts in addition to patient preference.
3. Review need for testing for other sexually transmitted infections and concomitant internal involvement (eg, Pap smear).

Complications: Anogenital intraepithelial neoplasms, coinfection with high-risk HPV genotypes.

HYF: HPV genotypes 16 and 18 cause ~70% of all cervical cancers and ~90% of anal cancers. Genotypes 6 and 11 cause ~90% of anogenital warts. Three different vaccines are available for prevention of HPV.

PRIMARY SYPHILIS

A 22-year-old M with no PMH presents with a non-painful penile lesion. **Exam** shows an indurated, non-painful penile ulcer with non-painful inguinal lymphadenopathy. **Labs** show positive VDRL and RPR.

Management:

1. Nontreponemal test (VDRL, RPR) or dark-field microscopy of the lesion. If positive, confirm with treponemal test (FTA-ABS).
2. Treat with penicillin G benzathine. Doxycycline is used if allergic to penicillin.

Complications:

- If untreated, can lead to secondary and tertiary syphilis, leading to cardiac and neurologic complications.
- Treatment can lead to Jarisch-Herxheimer reaction.

HYF: Caused by *Treponema pallidum*. Lesion is called a chancre and is non-painful. Tertiary syphilis can cause tabes dorsalis, gummas, Argyll Robertson pupil, and aortitis. VDRL/RPR can falsely be negative in the first 2–4 weeks due to seroconversion. False-positive tests can occur in patients with SLE.

CHANCROID

A 25-year-old M presents with a painful penile lesions for the past 3 days. **Exam** shows 2 non-indurated, painful penile lesions and painful, fluctuant inguinal lymphadenopathy. **Labs** show culture positive for *Haemophilus ducreyi*.

Management:

1. Confirm diagnosis with culture or probable diagnosis if an individual has 1 or more painful genital ulcers, regional lymphadenopathy, and no evidence of *T. pallidum* or HSV.
2. Treat with azithromycin or ceftriaxone. If contraindications to other regimens, treat with ciprofloxacin.
3. Drain any buboes with needle aspiration.

Complications:

- Large abscess and fistula formation.
- Bacterial superinfection.
- Enhanced HIV transmission.

HYF: *H. ducreyi* causes chancroid, whereas primary syphilis causes a chancre. Chancroid is painful (think "ducreyi" = "you will cry"), whereas chancre is non-painful.

GENITAL HSV

A 35-year-old F presents with malaise, fever, painful genital ulcers, and dysuria for 2 days. **Exam** shows grouped vulvar vesicles with surrounding erythema and tender inguinal lymphadenopathy. **Labs** show viral culture positive for HSV-2.

Management:

1. If clinical suspicion for genital HSV, confirm with laboratory testing. Options include viral culture (low sensitivity), PCR (more sensitive than culture), and Tzanck smear (low sensitivity and specificity).
2. After confirming diagnosis, start antiviral therapy (eg, acyclovir, famciclovir, or valacyclovir).
3. For recurrent infections, consider episodic or chronic suppressive therapy.

Complications:

- Aseptic meningitis.
- Urinary bladder retention secondary to sacral radiculitis.
- Recurrent infection.
- Transmission to sexual partners and infant during delivery.

HYF: Genital lesions can be caused by HSV-1 and -2.

9-20 Scalp Pathologies

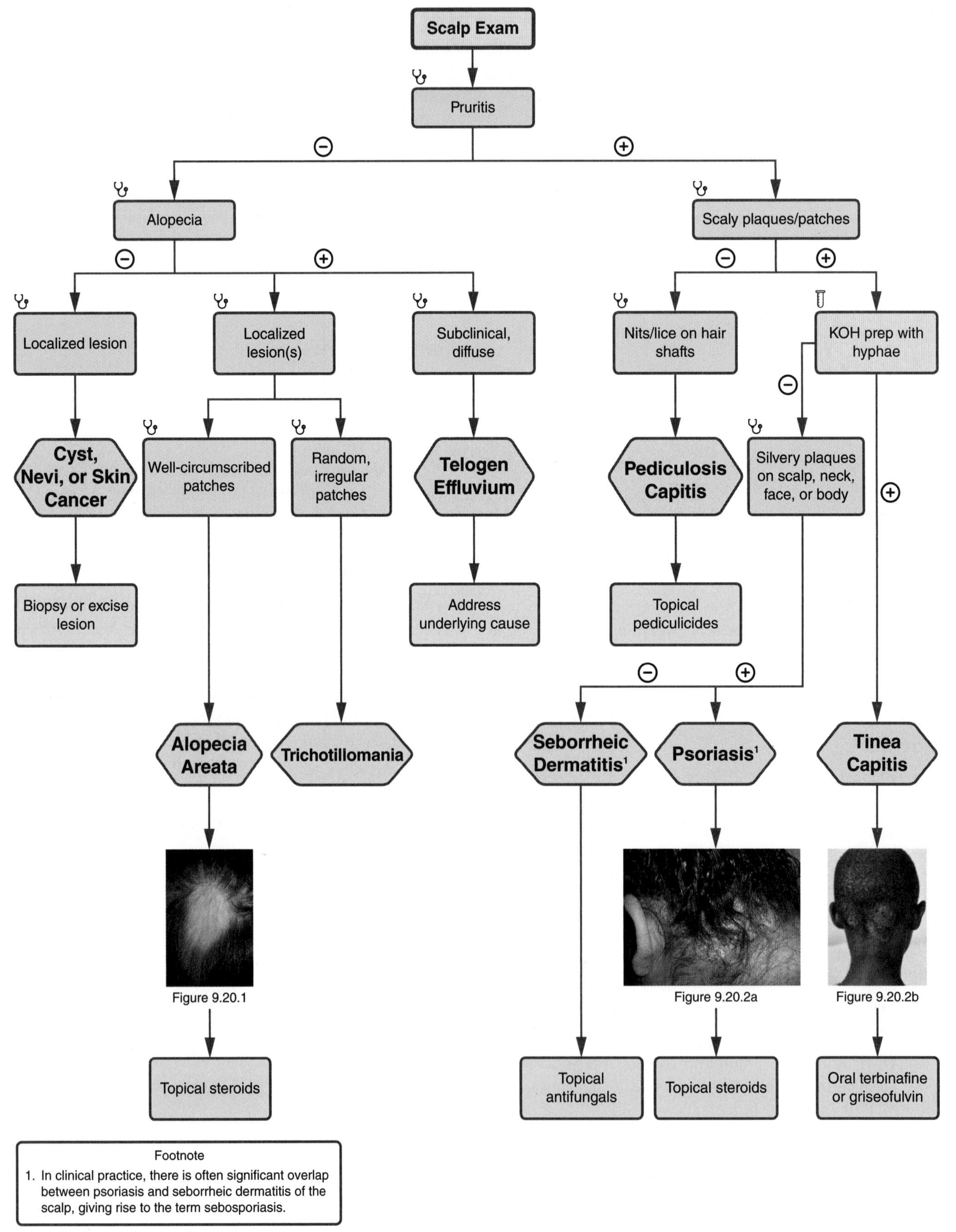

Scalp Exam
Pruritis
⊖
⊕
Alopecia
Scaly plaques/patches
⊖
⊕
⊖
⊕
Localized lesion
Localized lesion(s)
Subclinical, diffuse
Nits/lice on hair shafts
KOH prep with hyphae
⊖
Cyst, Nevi, or Skin Cancer
Well-circumscribed patches
Random, irregular patches
Telogen Effluvium
Pediculosis Capitis
Silvery plaques on scalp, neck, face, or body
⊕
Biopsy or excise lesion
Address underlying cause
Topical pediculicides
⊖
⊕
Alopecia Areata
Trichotillomania
Seborrheic Dermatitis[1]
Psoriasis[1]
Tinea Capitis
Figure 9.20.1
Figure 9.20.2a
Figure 9.20.2b
Topical steroids
Topical antifungals
Topical steroids
Oral terbinafine or griseofulvin

Footnote

1. In clinical practice, there is often significant overlap between psoriasis and seborrheic dermatitis of the scalp, giving rise to the term sebospoiasis.

FIGURE 9.20

9-20 Scalp Pathologies

CYST, NEVI, OR SKIN CANCER

A 79-year-old M presents with a bleeding, scaly lesion on the scalp. Exam shows diffuse alopecia with scaly red plaques and a pink, pearly papule on the vertex of the scalp.

Management:

1. Shave biopsy.
2. Mohs surgery.

HYF: For papules or nodules on the scalp, consider pilar cysts, benign nevi, or skin cancer.

TELOGEN EFFLUVIUM

A 35-year-old F who is 3 months postpartum presents with hair loss. Exam shows no obvious alopecia or inflammation of scalp.

Management:

1. Treat underlying cause.
2. Reassurance.

HYF: A positive hair pull test can aid in the diagnosis.

PEDICULOSIS CAPITIS (HEAD LICE)

A 7-year-old F presents with itchy scalp. Exam shows multiple nits firmly attached to hair shafts and numerous excoriations.

Management:

1. Topical pediculicides like permethrin, malathion, or ivermectin.
2. Wet combing.

HYF: Caused by head louse, *Pediculus humanus*. Can cause conjunctivitis from eyelash infestation, secondary bacterial infection at site of excoriations, and psychosocial distress.

ALOPECIA AREATA

A 34-year-old F with PMH of hypothyroidism presents with hair loss. Exam shows multiple small patches of hair loss on the scalp.

Management:

1. Topical or intralesional steroids.

HYF: Alopecia areata can be associated with other autoimmune diseases, including thyroid disease and vitiligo. Patients may also have nail pitting.

TRICHOTILLOMANIA

A 12-year-old F with PMH of anxiety and depression presents with hair loss. On exam, she has large, irregular patches on the scalp.

Management:

1. Behavior modification therapy.
2. SSRIs.

HYF: Associated with OCD and obsessive-compulsive personality disorder. Ingestion of hair can cause a trichobezoar.

SEBORRHEIC DERMATITIS

A 41-year-old M with PMH of eczema and rheumatoid arthritis presents with dandruff. Exam shows pink-yellow patches with a greasy scalp on his scalp, eyebrows, and nasolabial folds.

Management:

1. Topical ketoconazole.
2. Topical ciclopirox, corticosteroids, or selenium sulfide.

HYF: See Scaling and Crusted Lesions, p. 341.

PSORIASIS

A 52-year-old M with PMH of HTN and CAD presents with concerns of a rash and dandruff. Exam shows erythematous plaques with overlying scale on his elbows, knees, and scalp.

Management:

1. Topical steroids, topical vitamin D analogs, tazarotene.
2. Various non-biologics like methotrexate and phototherapy.
3. Biologics.

HYF: Associated with increased risk of cardiovascular disease and metabolic syndrome. Psoriatic arthritis affects up to 35% of psoriasis patients.

TINEA CAPITIS

A 10-year-old M with PMH of asthma presents with severe dandruff and itchy scalp. Exam shows a scaly patch on the scalp with associated hair loss and cervical adenopathy.

Management:

1. Oral antifungals: griseofulvin, terbinafine.

HYF: Kerion is a severe form that presents with a tender, crusted, boggy plaque on the scalp. There is a high risk of tinea capitis (97% in Black children) if a patient presents with a scalp patch and postauricular lymphadenopathy. Permanent hair loss can result if there is a severe, prolonged course.

9-21 Oral Lesions

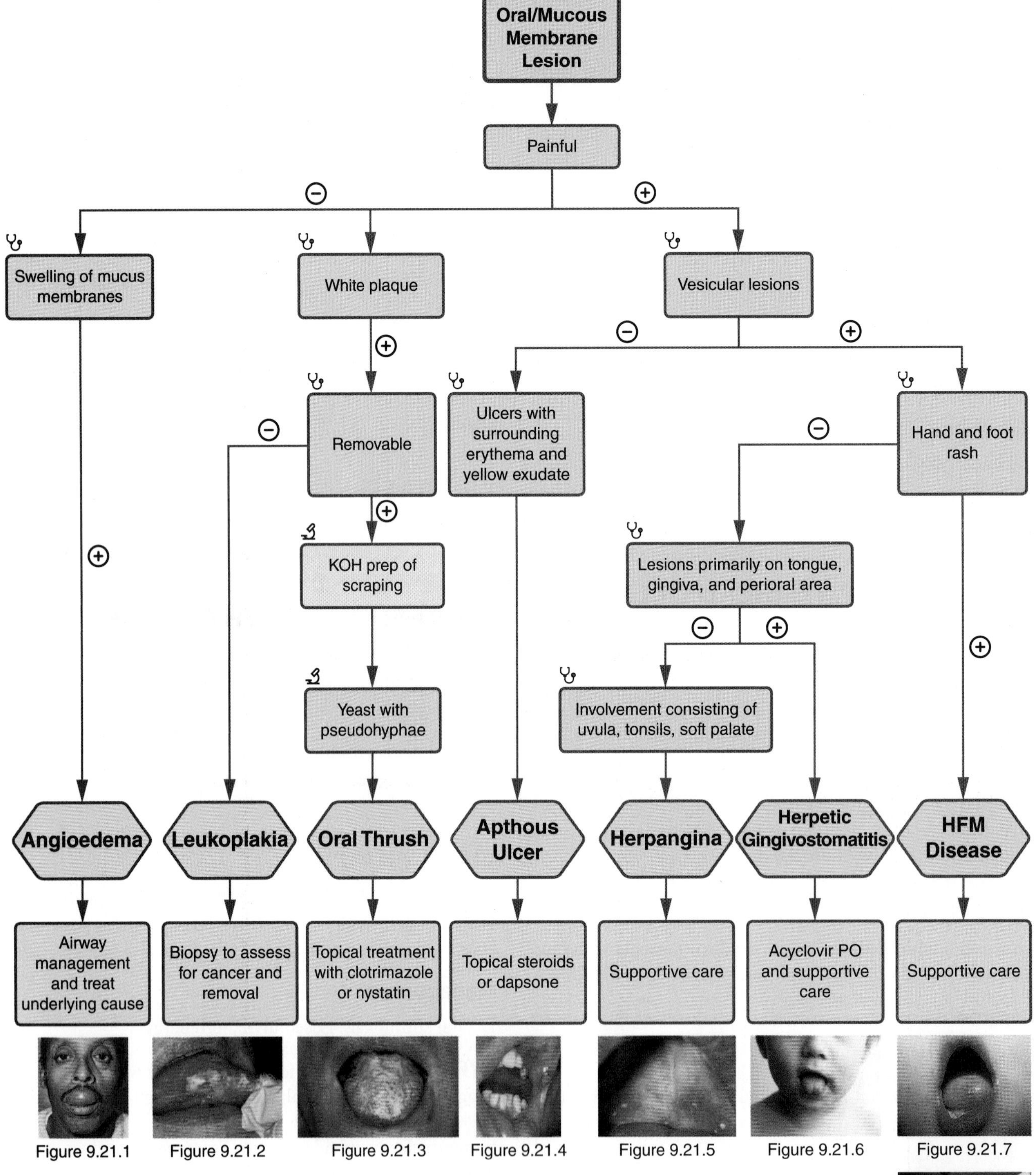
Oral/Mucous Membrane Lesion
Painful
Swelling of mucus membranes
White plaque
Vesicular lesions
Removable
Ulcers with surrounding erythema and yellow exudate
Hand and foot rash
KOH prep of scraping
Lesions primarily on tongue, gingiva, and perioral area
Yeast with pseudohyphae
Involvement consisting of uvula, tonsils, soft palate
Angioedema
Leukoplakia
Oral Thrush
Apthous Ulcer
Herpangina
Herpetic Gingivostomatitis
HFM Disease
Airway management and treat underlying cause
Biopsy to assess for cancer and removal
Topical treatment with clotrimazole or nystatin
Topical steroids or dapsone
Supportive care
Acyclovir PO and supportive care
Supportive care
Figure 9.21.1
Figure 9.21.2
Figure 9.21.3
Figure 9.21.4
Figure 9.21.5
Figure 9.21.6
Figure 9.21.7
Figure 9.21.8

FIGURE 9.21

9-21 Oral Lesions

ANGIOEDEMA

A 50-year-old F who recently started an ACEi presents with tongue swelling. On exam, significant tongue swelling is present with no signs of urticaria.

Management:

1. Airway management.
2. Further management is dictated by underlying etiology:
   a. Discontinue offending agent (eg, ACEi).
   b. Epinephrine if allergic reaction.
   c. Treat with C1 inhibitor concentrate if hereditary angioedema.

Complications: Can be life-threatening due to airway obstruction.

HYF: Can be hereditary, allergic, acquired, or idiopathic. A hereditary cause is deficiency of C1 esterase inhibitor.

LEUKOPLAKIA

A 65-year-old M with PMH of tobacco use disorder presents with a white oral lesion. Exam shows a lingual non-tender white plaque that cannot be wiped off.

Management:

1. Definitive diagnosis requires a biopsy to assess for underlying malignancy.
2. Treatment goal is to prevent/decrease risk of oral cancer. Options include surgical excision, laser ablation, and medical therapies.
3. Lifetime monitoring.

Complications: Progression to cancer.

HYF: Erythroplakia is like leukoplakia, but it is erythematous and more likely to have underlying dysplasia or carcinoma. Recurrence or progression to malignancy is common despite treatment.

ORAL THRUSH

A 55-year-old F with PMH of breast cancer on chemotherapy presents with painful oral white lesions and odynophagia. On exam, the white lesions are scraped off with a tongue depressor. Labs show KOH preparation with pseudohyphae and budding yeast.

Management:

1. If the patient does not have risk factors for oral thrush, discuss HIV testing.
2. Use topical treatments (eg, clotrimazole, nystatin) for mild disease. Treat patients with severe disease and concomitant esophageal candidiasis with fluconazole.

Complications: Dissemination of infection (eg, bloodstream, esophagus).

HYF: Associated with immunocompromised patients and patients treated with antibiotics or inhaled corticosteroids.

APHTHOUS ULCERS

A 45-year-old F presents with 2 days of a painful oral lesion. She has had similar prior episodes. On exam, there is a tender 3-mm round ulcer with surrounding erythema and central yellow exudate.

Management:

1. Supportive care: oral hygiene, avoidance of exacerbating factors, pain control.
2. Topical corticosteroids can assist with healing.

Complications: Secondary infection.

HYF: Aphthous ulcers with urogenital and cutaneous lesions are seen in Behçet's syndrome.

HERPANGINA

A 3-year-old M presents with fever, anorexia, and sore throat. On exam, papulovesicular lesions are present on the uvula and tonsils.

Management:

1. Supportive care.

Complications:

- Inadequate PO intake.
- Rhombencephalitis, acute flaccid paralysis, and aseptic meningitis.

HYF: Caused by coxsackievirus and enterovirus.

HAND-FOOT-MOUTH DISEASE

A 4-year-old F presents with with throat pain and a rash on the feet and hands. On exam, there are multiple superficial tongue ulcers and a maculopapular rash on the hands and feet.

Management:

1. Supportive care: hydration, symptom control.

Complications:

- Decreased PO intake.
- Rhombencephalitis, acute flaccid paralysis, aseptic meningitis.
- Myocarditis.

HYF: Caused by the coxsackievirus and enterovirus.

PRIMARY HERPETIC GINGIVOSTOMATITIS

A 3-year-old F presents with fever, anorexia, and oral and perioral lesions. On exam, there are gingival ulcerative lesions and perioral vesicular lesions. Labs are positive for HSV-1 on PCR.

Management:

1. Oral acyclovir if within 96 hours of onset.
2. Supportive care: Hydration, pain control, and barrier cream on lip lesions.

Complications:

- Dehydration.
- Secondary bacterial infection.
- Dissemination of HSV (herpetic whitlow, HSV esophagitis, HSV encephalitis).

HYF: Typically caused by HSV-1.

9-22 Pruritis

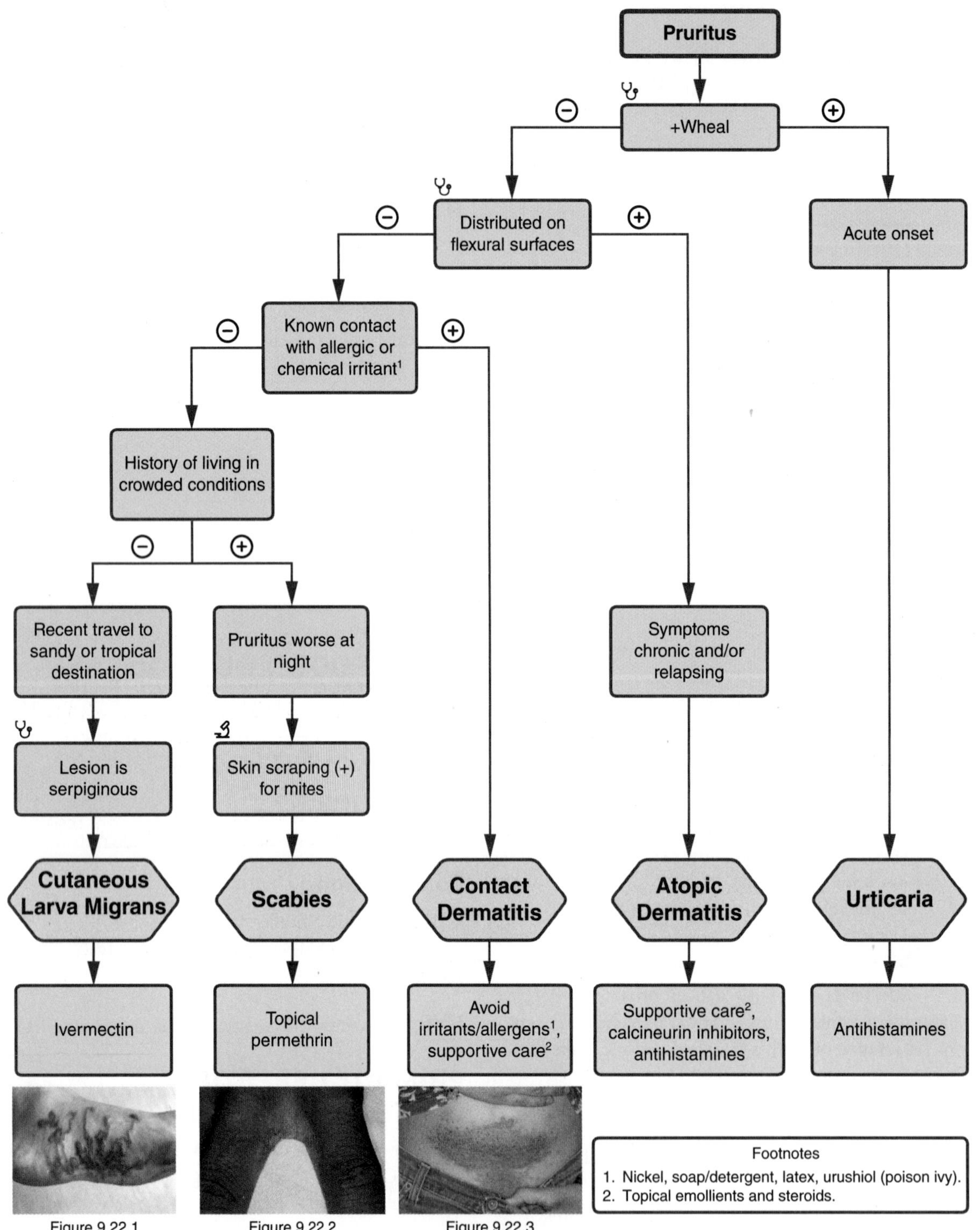
Pruritus
+Wheal
Distributed on flexural surfaces
Acute onset
Known contact with allergic or chemical irritant[1]
History of living in crowded conditions
Recent travel to sandy or tropical destination
Pruritus worse at night
Symptoms chronic and/or relapsing
Lesion is serpiginous
Skin scraping (+) for mites
Cutaneous Larva Migrans
Scabies
Contact Dermatitis
Atopic Dermatitis
Urticaria
Ivermectin
Topical permethrin
Avoid irritants/allergens[1], supportive care[2]
Supportive care[2], calcineurin inhibitors, antihistamines
Antihistamines

Figure 9.22.1

Figure 9.22.2

Figure 9.22.3

Footnotes

1. Nickel, soap/detergent, latex, urushiol (poison ivy).
2. Topical emollients and steroids.

FIGURE 9.22

9-22 Pruritis

CUTANEOUS LARVA MIGRANS

A 30-year-old M with recent travel to the Caribbean presents with new-onset pruritus on his right foot. On exam, there is an elevated and serpiginous red track with excoriation on his right foot. Labs show eosinophilia.

Management:

1. Ivermectin or albendazole.
2. Antihistamines for pruritus management.

Complications: Hematogenous dissemination to the lungs.

HYF: Most commonly caused by hookworm *Ancylostoma*, which are typically found on sandy beaches.

SCABIES

A 25-year-old M who recently enlisted in the military complains of new-onset itching of hands and wrists. On exam, his wrists and interdigital spaces have multiple erythematous papules with excoriations and several 5-mm red linear marks. Labs/Imaging: Dermoscopy of a linear mark shows a dark triangular shape. CBC shows eosinophilia.

Management:

1. Skin scraping of the site to confirm presence of scabies mites, eggs, and feces.
2. Topical permethrin and oral ivermectin are 1st-line agents.

Complications:

- Secondary infections (staph/strep).
- If immunocompromised, can develop crusted scabies, which is characterized by rapid spread and thick, crusted plaques with fissuring.

HYF: Pruritus is caused by a delayed hypersensitivity reaction to mite antigens. Typical locations include finger webs, wrists, axillary folds, male genitalia, and periareolar skin (in females). The head is spared. Symptoms are worse at night. Risk factors include living in crowded conditions (eg, military barracks, nursing homes).

CONTACT DERMATITIS (ALLERGIC VS. IRRITANT)

A 30-year-old F who works as a hairstylist presents with bilateral hand pruritus associated with burning pain that began 2 weeks ago. On exam, both hands are erythematous with oozing vesicles. The erythema is sharply demarcated at her wrists.

Management:

1. Avoid irritants and/or allergens.
2. Emollients and moisturizer to repair skin barrier.
3. Topical corticosteroids to control inflammation.

Complications: Should self-resolve after removal of the irritants.

HYF: Irritant contact dermatitis (ICD) is a non-immunological reaction, whereas allergic contact dermatitis (ACD) is caused by a delayed hypersensitivity reaction. ACD can be diagnosed through positive allergy patch testing.

ATOPIC DERMATITIS (AD)

A 5-year-old F with asthma presents with itching on her elbows and knees that has been worsening over several months. On exam, the antecubital and popliteal fossa are covered with erythematous and lichenified plaques that appear weepy. Labs showed an elevated serum IgE level.

Management:

1. Eliminate exacerbating factors (heat, exposures).
2. Maintain skin barrier with emollients and moisturizers.
3. Topical corticosteroids or calcineurin inhibitors, oral antihistamines for controlling pruritis.
4. For refractory disease, consider biologics like dupilumab (anti-IL-4/IL-13) or upadactinib (JAKi).

Complications:

- Secondary infection (bacterial, viral, and/or fungal).
- Associated with asthma and allergic rhinitis.

HYF: Must meet the following criteria: Pruritus, typical morphology and location, and chronic or relapsing history. Acute flares are characterized by erythematous papules and vesicles that are weeping. Chronic disease will show lichenification and dry skin. In infants, AD presents on extensor surfaces and the face. In children and teens, AD is distributed in flexural locations and the neck.

URTICARIA

A 35-year-old F recently treated for pneumonia with antibiotics presents with a new itchy rash on her trunk. On exam, there are circular and raised erythematous weals with central pallor diffusely distributed over the trunk.

Management:

1. Address exacerbating factors (allergens, environment, infection).
2. Antihistamines for pruritus.
3. If symptoms persist, consider systemic glucocorticoids or omalizumab.

Complications: Typically self-limited and resolving.

HYF: Causes of urticaria are numerous and include allergic reactions, arthropod bites, environmental and physical factors, infection, serum sickness, blood transfusion reactions, and cholinergic urticaria (following exercise, excitement, or hot showers). Drugs (eg, opioids) also cause urticaria through direct mast cell activation. Allergic drug reactions are common with beta-lactam antibiotics and NSAIDs. Urticaria of pregnancy can occur, possibly due to allergic sensitization to endogenous hormones. Systemic disorders can also have urticaria on initial presentation, including autoimmune disease, malignancy, uremia, and polycythemia vera.

9-23 Nail Pathologies

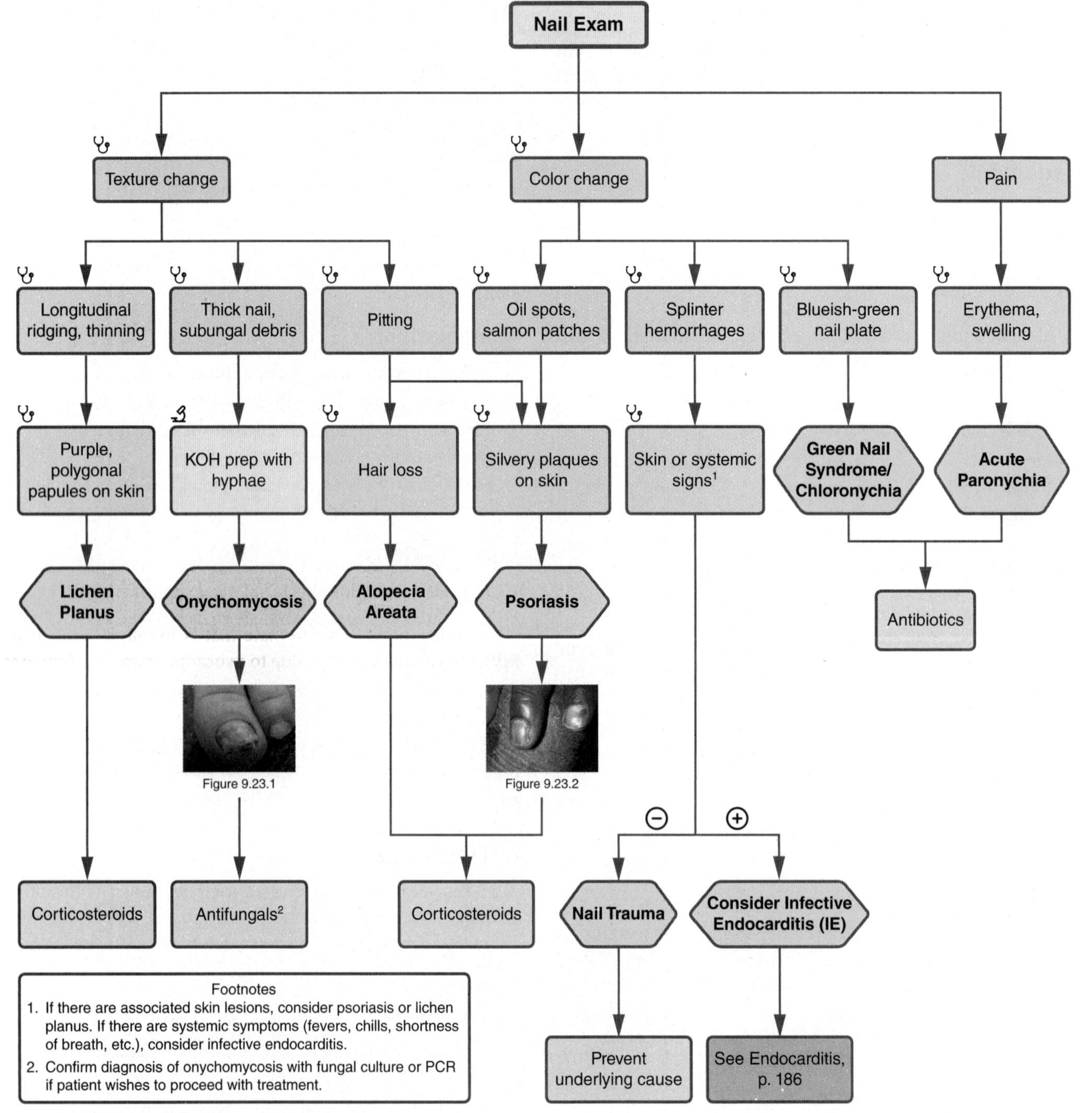

Nail Exam
Texture change
Color change
Pain
Longitudinal ridging, thinning
Thick nail, subungal debris
Pitting
Oil spots, salmon patches
Splinter hemorrhages
Blueish-green nail plate
Erythema, swelling
Purple, polygonal papules on skin
KOH prep with hyphae
Hair loss
Silvery plaques on skin
Skin or systemic signs¹
Green Nail Syndrome/ Chloronychia
Acute Paronychia
Lichen Planus
Onychomycosis
Alopecia Areata
Psoriasis
Antibiotics
Figure 9.23.1
Figure 9.23.2
Corticosteroids
Antifungals²
Corticosteroids
Nail Trauma
Consider Infective Endocarditis (IE)
Prevent underlying cause
See Endocarditis, p. 186

Footnotes

1. If there are associated skin lesions, consider psoriasis or lichen planus. If there are systemic symptoms (fevers, chills, shortness of breath, etc.), consider infective endocarditis.
2. Confirm diagnosis of onychomycosis with fungal culture or PCR if patient wishes to proceed with treatment.

FIGURE 9.23

9-23 Nail Pathologies

LICHEN PLANUS

A 32-year-old M with no PMH presents with rash and cracked nails. Exam shows purple polygonal papules on his wrist and longitudinal ridging and fissuring of all fingernails.

Management:

1. Systemic or intralesional corticosteroids.

Complications:

- Nail loss.
- Psychosocial distress.

HYF: Most patients have oral lesions. Look for Wickham striae.

ONYCHOMYCOSIS

A 69-year-old M with PMH of DM2 presents with thick, deformed toenails on exam.

Management:

1. Oral terbinafine.
2. Topical azole or ciclopirox.

Complications:

- Thick, deformed nails can be difficult to trim and cause pain with ambulation.
- High rate of recurrence, especially with topical treatment.

HYF: There are many causes of nail dystrophy, so always confirm fungal infection with KOH, culture, or PAS stain prior to treatment.

ALOPECIA AREATA

A 14-year-old M presents with hair loss. Exam shows round patches of non-scarring hair loss on his scalp and small, regularly distributed superficial pits along most nail plates.

Management:

1. Observation. Usually self-resolves.
2. If chronic or severe disease, consider topical or intralesional corticosteroids.

Complications: Additional nail pathologies like onychorrhexis (fissuring of nail plate), onycholysis (separate of distal nail plate from bed), and onychomadesis (separate of proximal plate from bed) are possible and often indicate more severe disease.

HYF: Screen patients for thyroid disease, given association with other autoimmune conditions.

PSORIASIS

A 49-year-old F with PMH of HTN and psoriasis presents with nail changes. On exam, she has superficial pitting, onycholysis, and salmon-colored patches on half her fingernails.

Management:

1. Topical corticosteroid or vitamin D analogs.
2. Biologics if severe/refractory.

Complications:

- Psychosocial distress.
- Strong association between psoriatic arthritis and nail psoriasis.

HYF: See Erythroderma, p. 324; Lichenified Plaque Lesions, p. 339; and Scalp Pathologies, p. 351.

GREEN NAIL SYNDROME

A 22-year-old M who works as a dish cleaner presents with concerns for discolored nails. Exam shows greenish discoloration of the right thumbnail and onycholysis of numerous other nails.

Management:

1. Antibiotics.
2. Antiseptic soaks.
3. Avoid excessive water exposure.

Complications: Recurrence.

HYF: Infection of the nail plate that is usually restricted to 1-2 nails. Green appearance is due to pyocanin from *Pseudomonas.*

ACUTE PARONYCHIA

A 39-year-old F with PMH of anxiety and depression presents with a painful, swollen left index finger. On exam, she has erythema and edema around the nail fold.

Management:

1. Antibiotics.
2. Antiseptic soaks.

Complications: Rarely, infection spreads to nail bed or bone and requires I&D.

HYF: Usually caused by trauma leading to *S. aureus* or *Streptococcus pyogenes* infection.

NAIL TRAUMA

An 8-year-old F who bites her nails presents with discolored nails. Exam shows multiple thin, black longitudinal streaks on most nails.

Management:

1. Avoid trauma to nails.

Complications: Increased risk of bacterial or fungal nail infections.

HYF: Splinter hemorrhages are most often due to trauma but can also be a sign of other skin diseases (psoriasis, lichen planus) or systemic diseases (infective endocarditis, chronic renal failure).

10
Surgery: Trauma

10-1 Trauma ABCs

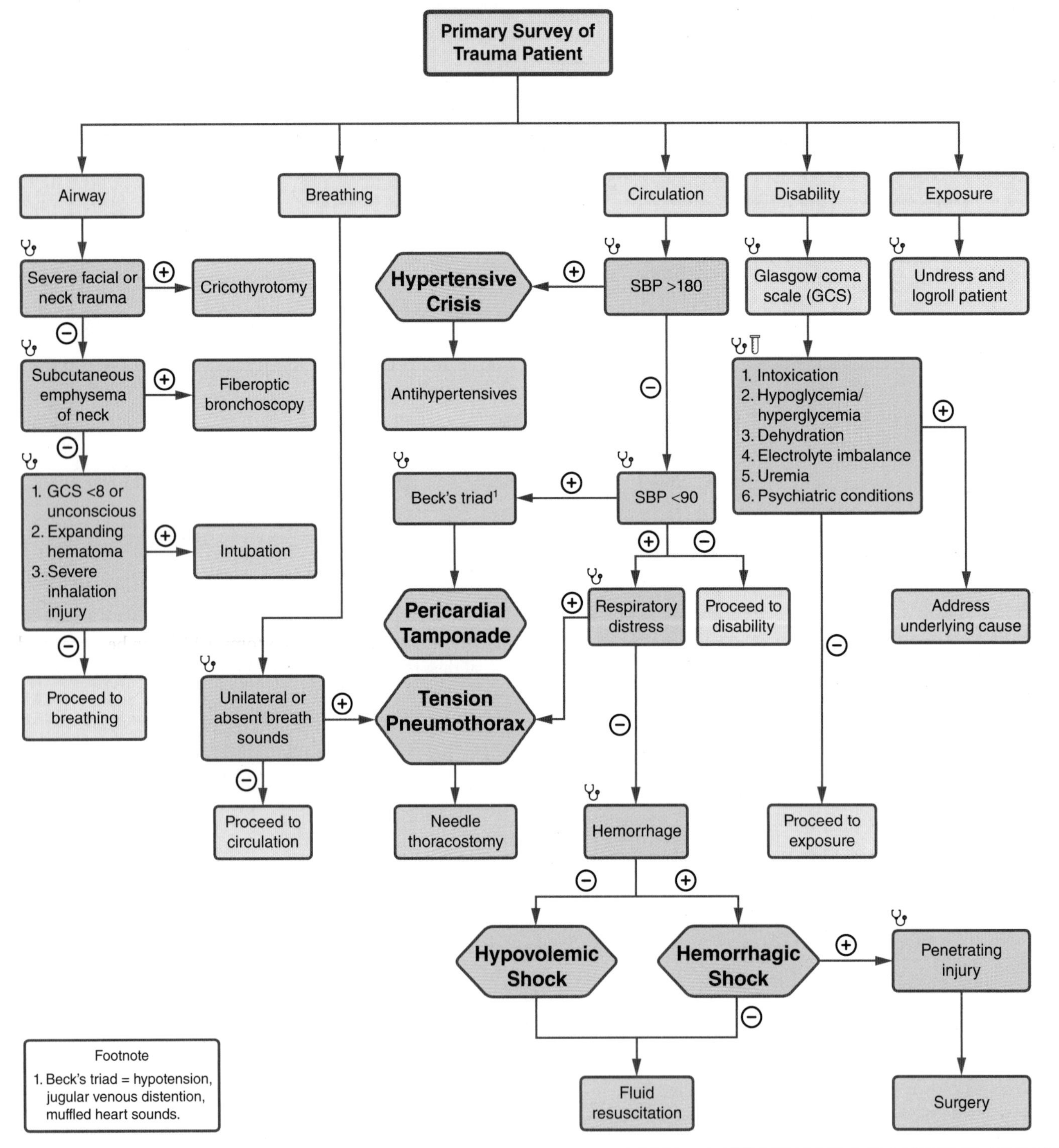
Primary Survey of Trauma Patient
Airway
Breathing
Circulation
Disability
Exposure
Severe facial or neck trauma
Cricothyrotomy
Subcutaneous emphysema of neck
Fiberoptic bronchoscopy
1. GCS <8 or unconscious
2. Expanding hematoma
3. Severe inhalation injury
Intubation
Proceed to breathing
Hypertensive Crisis
Antihypertensives
SBP >180
SBP <90
Beck's triad[1]
Pericardial Tamponade
Respiratory distress
Proceed to disability
Unilateral or absent breath sounds
Tension Pneumothorax
Proceed to circulation
Needle thoracostomy
Hemorrhage
Hypovolemic Shock
Hemorrhagic Shock
Fluid resuscitation
Penetrating injury
Surgery
Glasgow coma scale (GCS)
1. Intoxication
2. Hypoglycemia/ hyperglycemia
3. Dehydration
4. Electrolyte imbalance
5. Uremia
6. Psychiatric conditions
Proceed to exposure
Undress and logroll patient
Address underlying cause
Footnote
1. Beck's triad = hypotension, jugular venous distention, muffled heart sounds.

FIGURE 10.1

10-1 Trauma ABCs

HYPERTENSIVE CRISIS

A 55-year-old M with PMH of HTN and medication non-adherence is brought to the ED by ambulance after he developed a headache, blurry vision, and confusion. On **exam**, his vital signs are notable for BP 230/110 and HR 55. The patient is oriented to self only and endorses blurry vision. **Labs/Imaging:** EKG, CXR, D-dimer, and troponin are normal. Fundoscopy shows bilateral papilledema. CT head shows no acute hemorrhage or infarct.

Management:

1. Admit to ICU.
2. IV antihypertensives.
   a. β-blockers: Esmolol, labetalol.
   b. Nitrates: Nitroprusside, nitroglycerin.
   c. Calcium channel blockers: Clevidipine, nicardipine.
   d. Dopamine-1 agonist: Fenoldopam.
   e. Other: Hydralazine, phentolamine, enalaprilat.
3. Serial examinations.
4. Transition to PO antihypertensives when BP is within goal range. For most hypertensive emergencies, mean arterial pressure should be reduced gradually by approximately 10–20% in the first hour and by a further 5–15% over the next 23 hours.

Complications:

- Stroke.
- Acute coronary syndrome.
- Flash pulmonary edema.
- Retinopathy.
- Acute renal failure.

HYF: Can be caused by primary hypertension (as in this case), or pre-existing disease such as pheochromocytoma (must give irreversible α-antagonists such as phenoxybenzamine before β-blockers to avoid hypertensive crisis), hyperthyroidism, thyrotoxicosis, preeclampsia, or adverse drug event (eg, eating tyramine-rich foods while taking an MAO inhibitor).

CARDIAC TAMPONADE

A 22-year-old M previously healthy football player presents with sudden-onset chest pain and dyspnea after being tackled in the chest. He endorses worsening dyspnea when lying flat. On **exam**, he has BP 80/55, distant heart sounds, elevated JVP, pulsus paradoxus, and narrow pulse pressure. On **imaging**, CXR shows multiple broken ribs and a large cardiac silhouette with a "water bottle" appearance. EKG shows sinus tachycardia, low-amplitude QRS complexes, and electrical alternans. TTE confirms the diagnosis, revealing a large hypoechoic pericardial fluid collection, decreased ventricular compliance, and decreased ejection fraction.

Management:

1. Aggressive volume expansion with IV fluids.
2. If stable, urgent pericardiocentesis ("pericardiotomy"). If unstable (as in this case), emergent pericardial window.
3. Fluid studies to determine etiology (eg, cultures).
4. If recurrent case, consider pericardial window.

Complications:

- Hypotension.
- Shock.
- Death.
- Iatrogenic injury during pericardiocentesis (eg, pneumothorax, thoracic vasculature).

HYF: Classically presents with Beck's triad: Hypotension, distant heart sounds, and JVD. Pulsus paradoxus (exaggerated decrease in systolic BP with inspiration) and EKG with electrical alternans are also strongly suggestive of the diagnosis. Associated with pericarditis, malignancy, autoimmune disease (eg, SLE), and trauma (eg, stab wounds medial to left nipple).

TENSION PNEUMOTHORAX

A 19-year-old F presents to ED after being stabbed in the chest with a knife. She appears anxious and short of breath. On **exam**, BP 78/55, HR 120, RR 22, SpO_2 85% on room air. She has elevated JVP, distant breath sounds, and hyperresonance to percussion on the right lung. She has a visible stab wound between the 7th and 8th ribs on the right midclavicular line. On **imaging**, CXR shows a right-sided pneumothorax and laterally displaced mediastinal contents toward the left.

Management:

1. Immediate needle thoracostomy, which can be performed at the 5th intercostal space in midaxillary line or in the midclavicular line through the 2nd intercostal space. Of note, needle decompression should be performed before CXR if tension pneumothorax is suspected.
2. Chest tube placement after the pneumothorax has been decompressed.

Complications:

- Obstructive shock.
- Death.
- Fistula
- Damage to nerves and lymphatics (secondary to primary injury, needle thoracostomy, or chest tube).

HYF: Due to creation of a "one-way valve" in which air enters the pleural space during inspiration (negative pressure) and cannot leave the pleural space during expiration (positive pressure that closes the "valve"). Tension pneumothorax can be due to open pneumothorax, which should be treated with an occlusive dressing closed on 3 sides. If high suspicion for tension pneumothorax, treatment should be initiated immediately and not delayed for CXR.

HYPOVOLEMIC SHOCK

A 33-year-old F with no significant PMH is brought by her friend after being found in a confused state at her house. She returned from Mexico last week and has had several days of intractable vomiting, diarrhea, and decreased PO intake. On **exam**, BP 82/55, HR 120, RR 12, SpO_2 98% on room air. She has dry mucous membranes, delayed capillary refill, and skin tenting, and is experiencing ongoing watery diarrhea. **Labs** are consistent with a pre-renal AKI.

(Continued)

10-1 Trauma ABCs

Management:

1. Manage airway, breathing, circulation.
2. IV fluid resuscitation.
3. Labs to assess perfusion (lactate, creatinine, AST/ALT, troponin).
4. Treat underlying disease process (eg, profuse diarrhea).

Complications: End-organ damage (AKI, ACS, stroke, shock liver).

HYF: Initial management should focus on airway, breathing, and circulation. Assess end-organ perfusion with appropriate labs. It is important to identify and treat the underlying cause, as there are many different etiologies for hypovolemic shock (eg, dehydration from decreased PO intake or diarrhea, hemorrhage, burn injury).

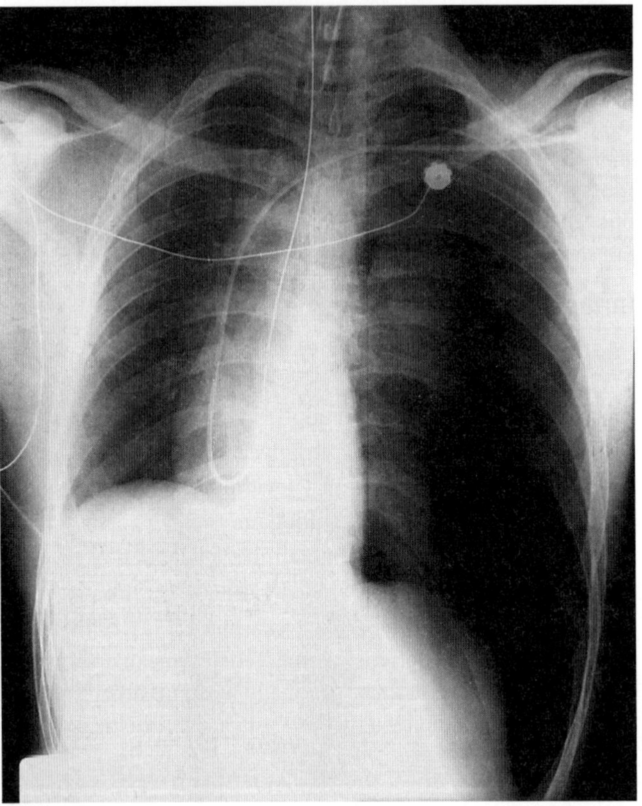

Tension pneumothorax.

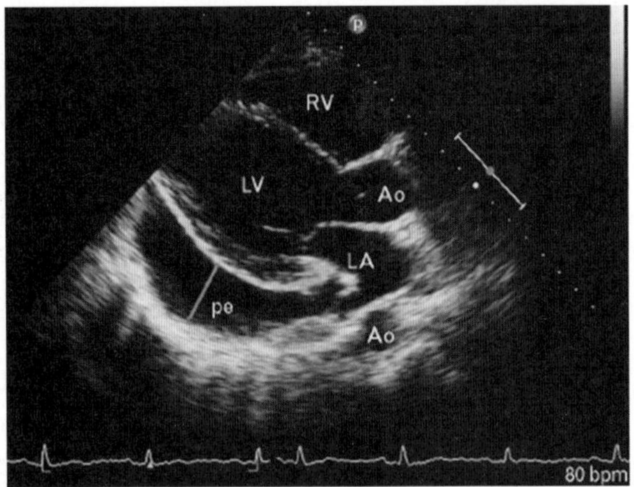
RV
LV
Ao
LA
pe
Ao
80 bpm

Large pericardial effusion.

HEMORRHAGIC SHOCK

A 44-year-old M with no significant PMH presents with a gunshot wound to the abdomen. On exam, BP is 65/45, HR 125, RR 22, SpO_2 95% on room air. He is stuporous, diaphoretic, and pale. He has a bullet wound above the umbilicus that is bleeding actively.

Management:

1. Emergent exploratory laparotomy.
2. Blood transfusion with type O (do not wait to order type and crossmatch as this is an emergency).
3. IV fluid resuscitation via 2 large-bore IVs.

Complications:

- End-organ failure.
- Death.

HYF: Immediate goals of care include identifying and stopping the source of bleeding and replenishing intravascular fluid with blood products. Do not give pressors to patients in hemorrhagic shock, because this can cause systemic vasoconstriction that exacerbates end-organ damage. Hemorrhagic shock is a type of hypovolemic shock.

10-2 Head Trauma

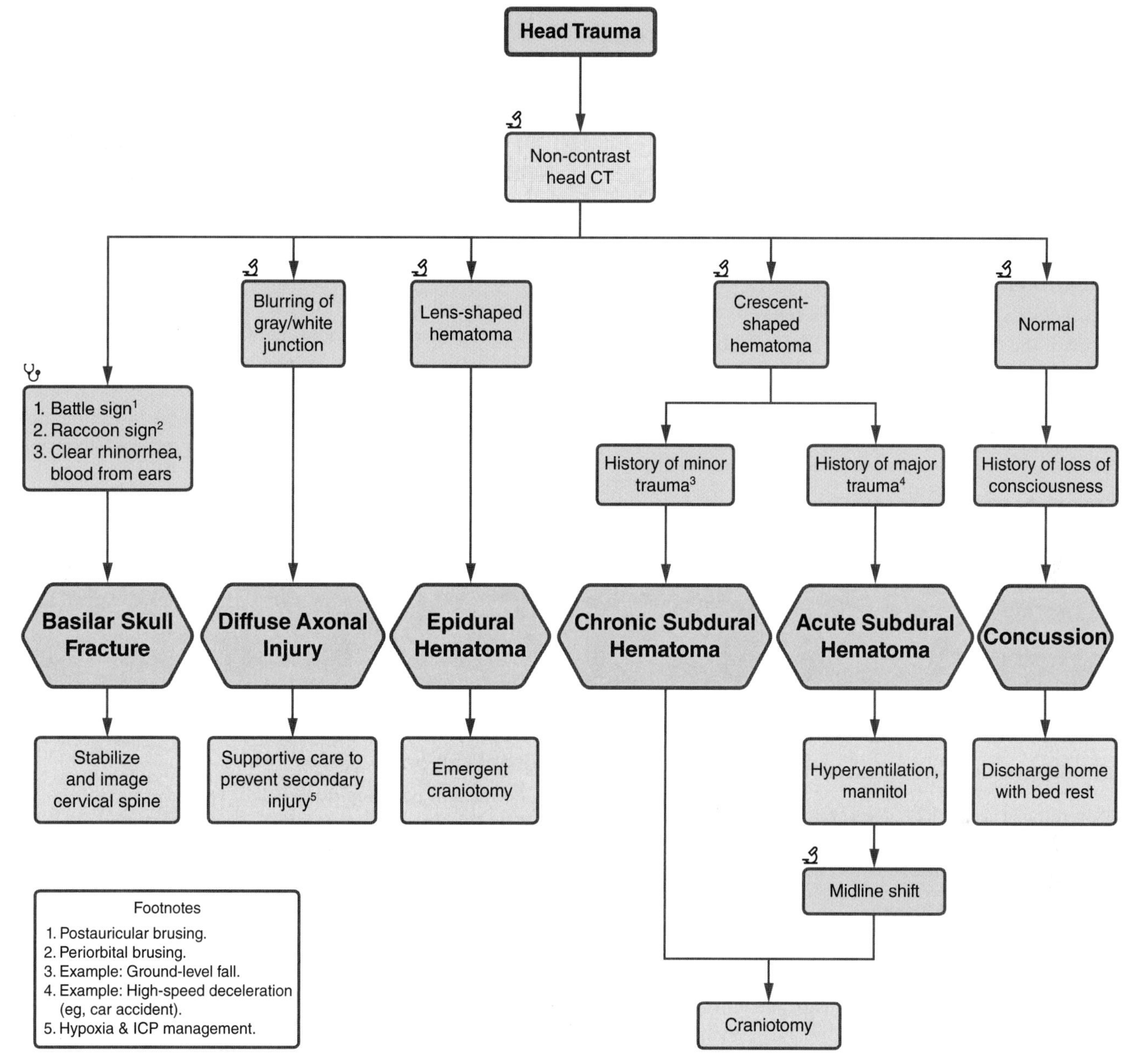
Head Trauma
Non-contrast head CT
1. Battle sign1
2. Raccoon sign2
3. Clear rhinorrhea, blood from ears
Blurring of gray/white junction
Lens-shaped hematoma
Crescent-shaped hematoma
Normal
History of minor trauma3
History of major trauma4
History of loss of consciousness
Basilar Skull Fracture
Diffuse Axonal Injury
Epidural Hematoma
Chronic Subdural Hematoma
Acute Subdural Hematoma
Concussion
Stabilize and image cervical spine
Supportive care to prevent secondary injury5
Emergent craniotomy
Hyperventilation, mannitol
Discharge home with bed rest
Midline shift
Craniotomy
Footnotes
1. Postauricular brusing.
2. Periorbital brusing.
3. Example: Ground-level fall.
4. Example: High-speed deceleration (eg, car accident).
5. Hypoxia & ICP management.

FIGURE 10.2

10-2 Head Trauma

BASILAR SKULL FRACTURE

A 25-year-old M presents with head trauma after a high-speed, high-impact injury (eg, car accident). On **exam**, he has periorbital hematomas ("raccoon eyes") and mastoid or postauricular ecchymosis (Battle sign), as well as CSF rhinorrhea.

Management:

1. Stat head CT without contrast, CT c-spine.
2. Close inpatient monitoring. Expectant management.

Complications:

- Associated with severe traumatic brain injury.
- Anosmia if the cribriform plain is fractured and compromises the olfactory nerve.

HYF: Do NOT perform nasotracheal intubation or nasogastric tube placement. Associated with risk of cribriform plate disruption, which can lead to inadvertent intracranial passage of the tube.

DIFFUSE AXONAL INJURY

A 35-year-old M presents with unresponsiveness after a high-speed car accident. On **exam**, he is comatose. On **imaging**, stat head CT without contrast shows numerous minute punctate hemorrhages with blurring of the gray-white interface.

Management:

1. Craniotomy can reduce cerebral edema. Brain MRI is more sensitive than head CT for diagnosis. CT scan can be normal.

Complications: Persistent vegetative state.

HYF: Severe, rapid acceleration/deceleration causes shearing of axons at the microscopic level. Patient loses consciousness instantaneously. Most significant cause of morbidity in traumatic brain injury.

EPIDURAL HEMATOMA

A 25-year-old M who was struck in the head presents with a brief loss of consciousness followed by lucid interval and now has impaired consciousness, headache, nausea, and emesis. On **imaging**, stat head CT without contrast shows a lens-shaped, biconvex hematoma that does not cross suture lines.

Management:

1. Emergent craniotomy.

Complications:

- Expanding hematoma can lead to uncal herniation (ipsilateral pupil dilation due to CN III palsy, ipsilateral hemiparesis due to contralateral crus cerebri compression).

HYF:

- Refer to Neurology, p. 734.
- Classically occurs after traumatic injury to the sphenoid bone and/or fracture in the pterion region → laceration of the middle meningeal artery.
- Known as the "talk and die syndrome" (patients have a loss of consciousness followed by a lucid interval). A commonly presented scenario is a young boy hit in the head with a baseball bat who is walking and talking and then deteriorates.

CHRONIC SUBDURAL HEMATOMA

An elderly or alcoholic patient with PMH of recurrent falls presents with weeks of progressive altered mental status, personality change, headache, or cognitive or motor deficits. On **imaging**, stat head CT shows crescent-shaped hypodensity crossing suture lines.

Management: Similar to acute subdural hematoma.

Complications: Similar to acute subdural hematoma.

HYF:

- Similar to acute subdural hematoma.
- Commonly presents in the elderly and alcoholics due to increased cerebral atrophy and fall risk.
- Subdural hematomas commonly rebleed, leading to radiographic findings consistent with hemorrhages of varying age.
- In elderly patients, subdural bleeding is the "great imitator" due to its variable and subtle presentation (eg, gait abnormalities, seizures, somnolence, memory loss).

ACUTE SUBDURAL HEMATOMA

A 45-year-old M with PMH of head trauma 1–2 days ago presents with altered mental status, headache, nausea, and vomiting. On **imaging**, stat head CT shows a crescent-shaped hyperdensity.

Management:

1. Craniotomy for symptomatic or large bleeds.
2. Small, asymptomatic hematomas may regress spontaneously and are thus managed conservatively.

Complications:

- Permanent neurological deficits
- Large hematomas can cause transtentorial herniation with decreased consciousness and pupillary abnormalities.

HYF:

- Refer to Neurology, p. 734.
- Results from sheared bridging veins.
- Do NOT perform an LP in patients with subdural hematoma due to increased risk of herniation.

CONCUSSION

A 22-year-old athlete with PMH of recent head trauma presents with difficulty concentrating, disorientation, and mood disturbance. On **imaging**, head CT without contrast shows no structural abnormalities.

Management:

1. Rest for >24 hours.
2. Remove temporarily from sports. Gradual return to normal activity if symptoms do not worsen.
3. Symptoms usually resolve in weeks to months.

Complications:

- Premature return to sports increases risk of more concussions and long-term sequelae (eg, chronic traumatic encephalopathy).
- Patients with mild TBI are at increased risk of developing epilepsy.

HYF: Head imaging is only required for those who are considered high-risk (eg, focal neurologic deficits, signs of skull fracture, amnesia >30 minutes prior to injury). In the absence of risk factors, no imaging is required.

10-3 Shock

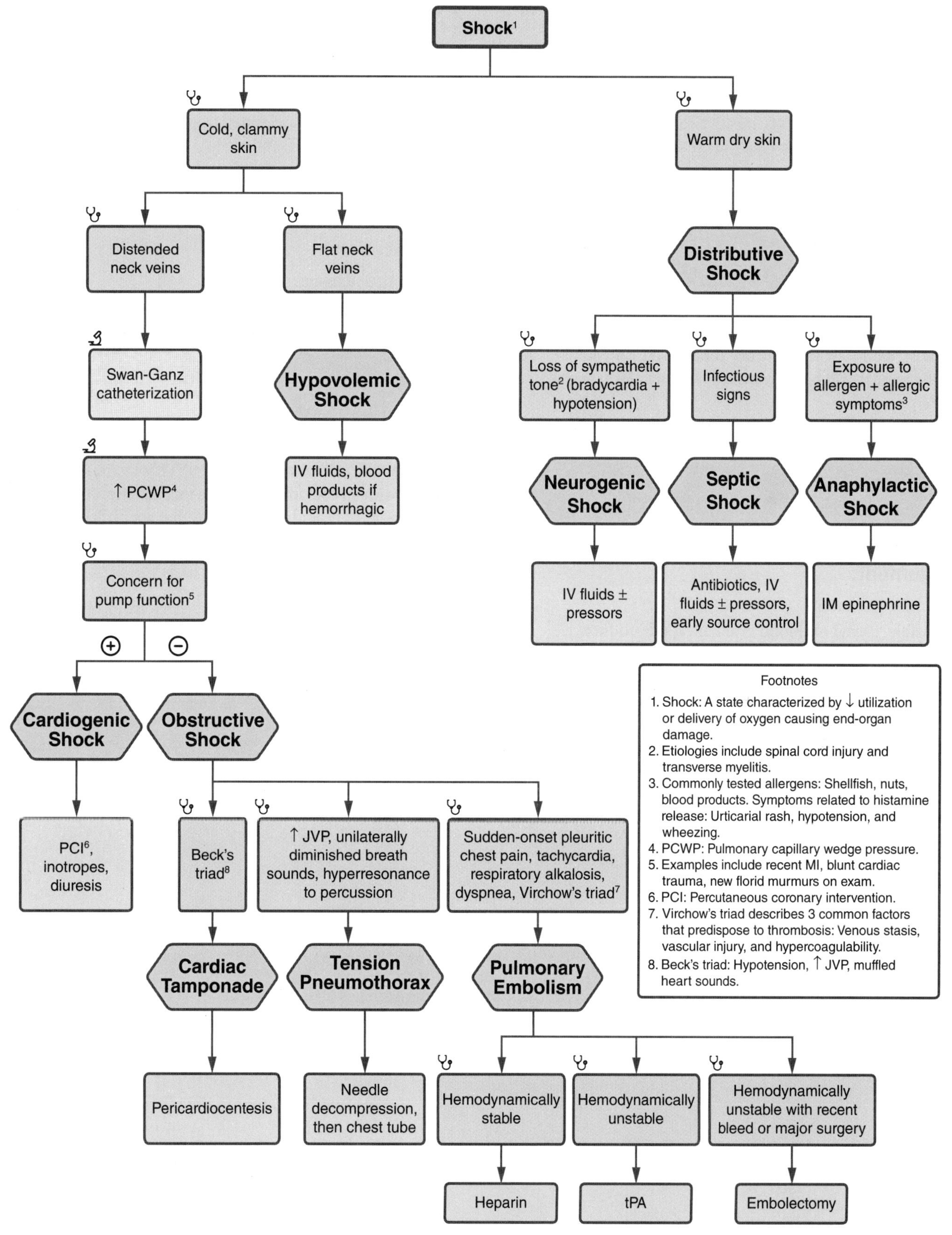
Shock[1]
Cold, clammy skin
Warm dry skin
Distended neck veins
Flat neck veins
Distributive Shock
Swan-Ganz catheterization
Hypovolemic Shock
Loss of sympathetic tone[2] (bradycardia + hypotension)
Infectious signs
Exposure to allergen + allergic symptoms[3]
↑ PCWP[4]
IV fluids, blood products if hemorrhagic
Neurogenic Shock
Septic Shock
Anaphylactic Shock
Concern for pump function[5]
IV fluids ± pressors
Antibiotics, IV fluids ± pressors, early source control
IM epinephrine
⊕
⊖
Cardiogenic Shock
Obstructive Shock
PCI[6], inotropes, diuresis
Beck's triad[8]
↑ JVP, unilaterally diminished breath sounds, hyperresonance to percussion
Sudden-onset pleuritic chest pain, tachycardia, respiratory alkalosis, dyspnea, Virchow's triad[7]
Cardiac Tamponade
Tension Pneumothorax
Pulmonary Embolism
Pericardiocentesis
Needle decompression, then chest tube
Hemodynamically stable
Hemodynamically unstable
Hemodynamically unstable with recent bleed or major surgery
Heparin
tPA
Embolectomy

Footnotes

1. Shock: A state characterized by ↓ utilization or delivery of oxygen causing end-organ damage.
2. Etiologies include spinal cord injury and transverse myelitis.
3. Commonly tested allergens: Shellfish, nuts, blood products. Symptoms related to histamine release: Urticarial rash, hypotension, and wheezing.
4. PCWP: Pulmonary capillary wedge pressure.
5. Examples include recent MI, blunt cardiac trauma, new florid murmurs on exam.
6. PCI: Percutaneous coronary intervention.
7. Virchow's triad describes 3 common factors that predispose to thrombosis: Venous stasis, vascular injury, and hypercoagulability.
8. Beck's triad: Hypotension, ↑ JVP, muffled heart sounds.

FIGURE10.3

10-3 Shock

DISTRIBUTIVE SHOCK

A 56-year-old F with PMH of breast cancer s/p chemotherapy with port placement presents with T 39°C and BP 78/55. On exam, she has warm and dry skin. **Labs** show a WBC 22, Cr 1.7, and BUN 35. Preliminary blood cultures are positive for Gram-positive cocci in clusters. Since admission, she has only made 50 mL of urine.

Management:

1. Aggressive IV fluid resuscitation.
2. Treat underlying etiology (eg, sepsis).
3. If the above fails, use vasopressors.

Complications: End-organ damage (eg, AKI with oliguria).

HYF: Distributive or vasodilatory shock is the only kind of shock where the patient will have vasodilation, which leads to warm and dry skin.

HYPOVOLEMIC SHOCK

A previously healthy 25-year-old M presents with a gunshot wound to the thigh. On exam, BP is 70/45, HR 135. There is a profusely bleeding wound on his right lower extremity.

Management:

1. IV fluid resuscitation.
2. If possible, use whole blood or other blood products.
3. Hemorrhage control (direct pressure, surgical intervention).

Complications: End-organ damage.

HYF: 1:1:1 ratio of whole blood and platelets to packed RBCs to fresh frozen plasma is preferred because 1) resuscitation with crystalloid fluids is associated with hypercoagulable state due to dilution of clotting factors, 2) hypothermia can occur because room temperature liquids are cooler than body temperature, and 3) crystalloid solutions can cause non-anion gap metabolic acidosis.

CARDIOGENIC SHOCK

A 65-year-old M with PMH of T2DM, HLD, and a 40-pack-year smoking history presents with chest pain radiating up to the chin and down the left arm. On exam, he is diaphoretic, and skin is cold and clammy. **Labs** show elevated troponin. EKG shows ST-segment elevation in leads II, III, and aVF.

Management:

1. PCI or CABG depending on cardiac vessels involved.

Complications:

- End-organ damage.
- Classic complications of MI (eg, free wall rupture, pericarditis).

HYF: Three-vessel or left main coronary artery disease needs CABG. Inferior infarcts should not get nitrates, as they are preload-dependent. For more information, see cardiology, pp. 15–17.

OBSTRUCTIVE SHOCK

A 40-year-old M with PMH of NSTEMI s/p PCI 5 days ago presents with an episode of syncope this morning. On exam, he has hypotension, JVD, and heart sounds that are difficult to auscultate. EKG shows low-voltage QRS complexes and electrical alternans.

Management:

1. Remove obstruction (in this case, pericardiocentesis).

Complications: End-organ damage.

HYF: Specifically for cardiac tamponade, look for Beck's triad (JVD, hypotension, distant heart sounds), equalization of diastolic pressures across all 4 heart chambers, and electrical alternans on EKG.

10-4 Chest Trauma

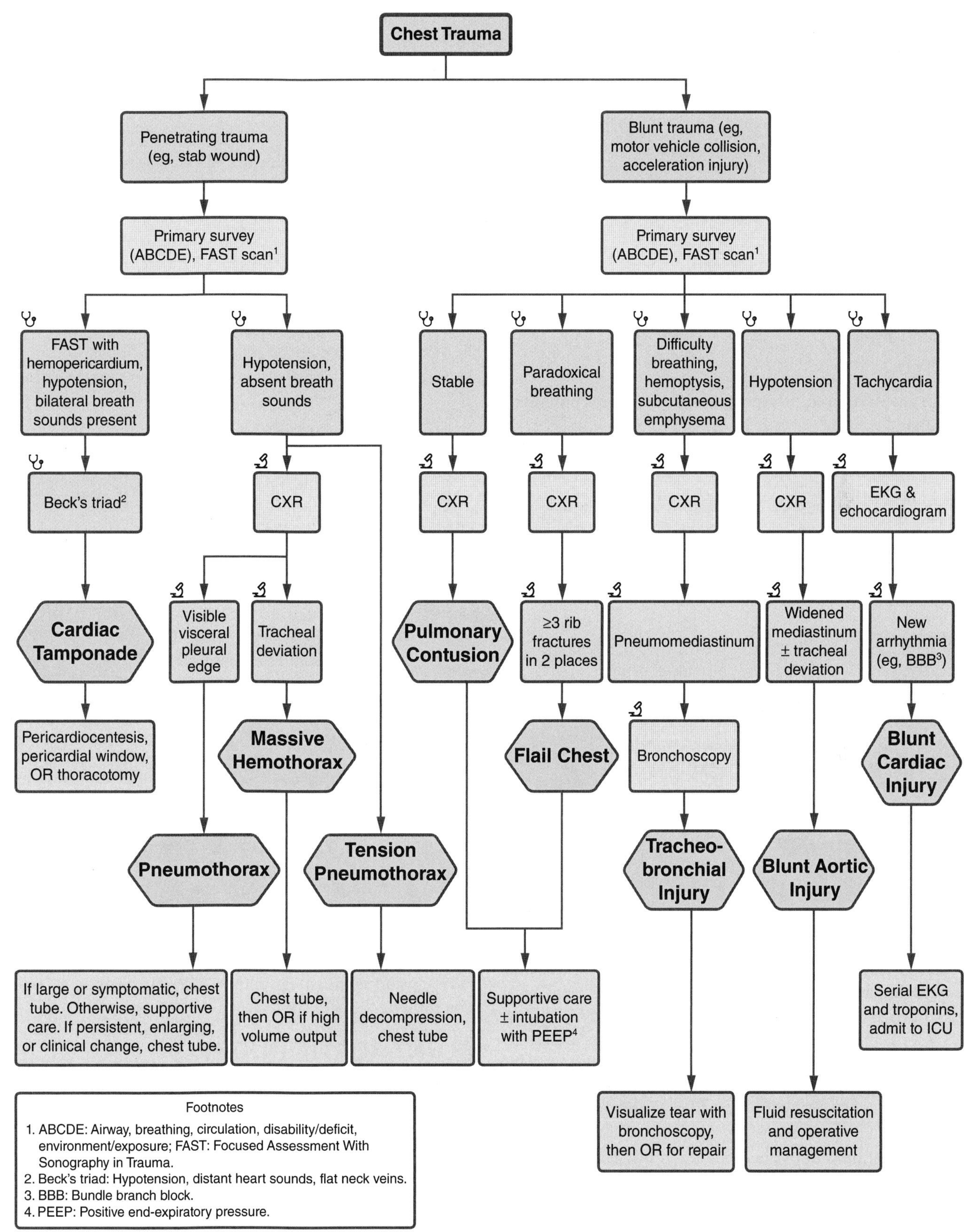

Chest Trauma
Penetrating trauma (eg, stab wound)
Blunt trauma (eg, motor vehicle collision, acceleration injury)
Primary survey (ABCDE), FAST scan[1]
Primary survey (ABCDE), FAST scan[1]
FAST with hemopericardium, hypotension, bilateral breath sounds present
Hypotension, absent breath sounds
Stable
Paradoxical breathing
Difficulty breathing, hemoptysis, subcutaneous emphysema
Hypotension
Tachycardia
Beck's triad[2]
CXR
CXR
CXR
CXR
CXR
EKG & echocardiogram
Cardiac Tamponade
Visible visceral pleural edge
Tracheal deviation
Pulmonary Contusion
≥3 rib fractures in 2 places
Pneumomediastinum
Widened mediastinum ± tracheal deviation
New arrhythmia (eg, BBB[3])
Pericardiocentesis, pericardial window, OR thoracotomy
Massive Hemothorax
Flail Chest
Bronchoscopy
Blunt Cardiac Injury
Pneumothorax
Tension Pneumothorax
Tracheo-bronchial Injury
Blunt Aortic Injury
If large or symptomatic, chest tube. Otherwise, supportive care. If persistent, enlarging, or clinical change, chest tube.
Chest tube, then OR if high volume output
Needle decompression, chest tube
Supportive care ± intubation with PEEP[4]
Serial EKG and troponins, admit to ICU
Visualize tear with bronchoscopy, then OR for repair
Fluid resuscitation and operative management
Footnotes
1. ABCDE: Airway, breathing, circulation, disability/deficit, environment/exposure; FAST: Focused Assessment With Sonography in Trauma.
2. Beck's triad: Hypotension, distant heart sounds, flat neck veins.
3. BBB: Bundle branch block.
4. PEEP: Positive end-expiratory pressure.

FIGURE 10.4

10-4 Chest Trauma

PULMONARY CONTUSION

A 42-year-old M presents to the ED after a motor vehicle collision in which he was a restrained passenger. On **exam**, he was initially stable but has since developed respiratory distress, worsened by fluid resuscitation. On **imaging**, chest X-ray shows patchy alveolar infiltrate over the right lung.

Management:

1. Supportive care with oxygen and pain control.
2. Intubation as needed for respiratory failure.

Complications:

- ARDS.
- Respiratory failure.
- Pneumonia.

HYF: Can have a delayed presentation with symptoms progressing over time.

PNEUMOTHORAX

A 45-year-old M presents to the ED with a stab wound to his right lateral chest. On **exam**, he is tachycardic and tachypneic, with decreased breath sounds and hyperresonance to percussion on the right side. On **imaging**, a FAST exam is negative for hemopericardium, and a chest X-ray shows increased lucency on the right.

Management:

1. Supportive care with oxygen and close monitoring.
2. Thoracostomy chest tube.
3. Serial chest X-rays to monitor progression.

Complications:

- Pneumonia.
- Tension pneumothorax if open wound or tracheobronchial injury.

HYF: These can be spontaneous or secondary to trauma.

MASSIVE HEMOTHORAX

A 30-year-old M presents to the ED with multiple stab wounds to his anterior chest. On **exam**, he is tachycardic, tachypneic, and hypotensive despite fluid resuscitation, with flat neck veins and dullness to percussion on the left side. On **imaging**, a FAST exam is negative for hemopericardium, and chest X-ray shows increased opacity on the right, blunting of the costophrenic angle, and left tracheal deviation.

Management:

1. Initial stabilization with oxygen and fluid resuscitation.
2. Drainage via large-bore thoracostomy.
3. Emergency thoracotomy if continued drainage or hemodynamic instability.

Complications:

- Hemorrhagic shock and death.
- Pneumothorax.
- Infection.

HYF: Chest trauma leads to bleeding in the pleural cavity, which prevents normal lung expansion and leads to acute systemic blood loss. Associated with rib fractures, pericardial tamponade, pulmonary contusion, tracheobronchial injury, and/or aortic injury.

FLAIL CHEST

A 33-year-old M present to the ED with worsening shortness of breath after a motor vehicle accident where he was ejected from the vehicle. On **exam**, he is tachypneic, tachycardic, and hypotensive, with right-sided chest expansion on expiration. On **imaging**, chest X-ray shows multiple fractures in 3 adjacent ribs on the right side.

Management:

1. Supportive care with oxygen and close monitoring.
2. Aggressive pain control; consider regional block.
3. Surgical rib fracture fixation if patient is in respiratory failure.

Complications:

- Pneumothorax from fractured rib.
- Respiratory failure.
- Pneumonia.

HYF: Defined as 3 adjacent ribs with ≥2 fractures per rib.

TRACHEOBRONCHIAL INJURY

A 68-year-old M presents to the ED after a motor vehicle accident where he was an unrestrained driver. He was initially diagnosed with a pneumothorax and a chest tube was placed, which has had a persistent air leak. On **imaging**, follow-up chest X-ray shows persistent pneumothorax and pneumomediastinum.

Management:

1. Secure the airway, if possible, with fiberoptic bronchoscopic intubation.
2. Surgical repair.

Complications:

- Death.
- Pneumothorax.
- Pneumonia.

HYF: Securing the airway in these cases can be difficult, as intubation must be distal to the tear.

BLUNT AORTIC INJURY

A 26-year-old F presents to the ED after a fall from a height >10 feet. On **exam**, she is hypotensive and tachycardic. On **imaging**, chest X-ray shows a widened mediastinum.

Management:

1. Aggressive blood pressure control.
2. Surgical repair.

Complications:

- Hemorrhagic shock and death.

HYF: Depending on severity of injury or tear, many die at the scene.

10-4 Chest Trauma

BLUNT CARDIAC INJURY

A 62-year-old M presents to the ED after a motor vehicle accident in which he was a restrained passenger. On **exam**, he is tachycardic and hypotensive, with significant bruising over his left chest. On **imaging**, a FAST exam is negative for hemopericardium, a transthoracic echocardiogram shows LV dysfunction, and EKG shows a new bundle branch block.

Management:

1. Supportive care with fluid resuscitation.
2. Antiarrhymics.

Complications:

- Life-threatening arrhythmias.
- Embolic events.

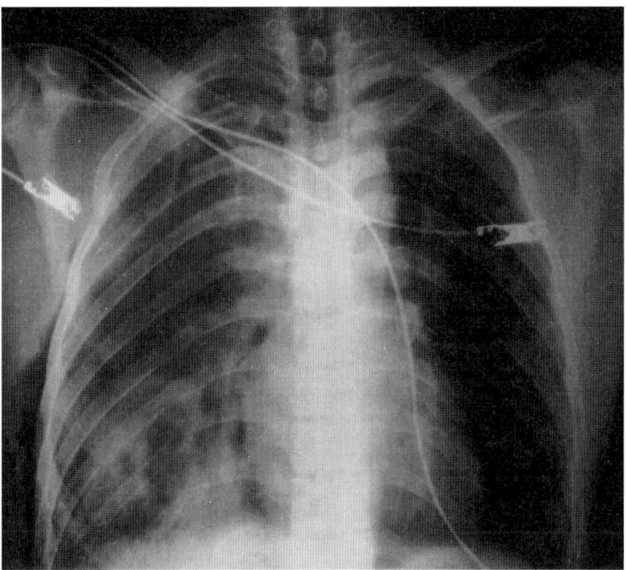

Pulmonary contusion.

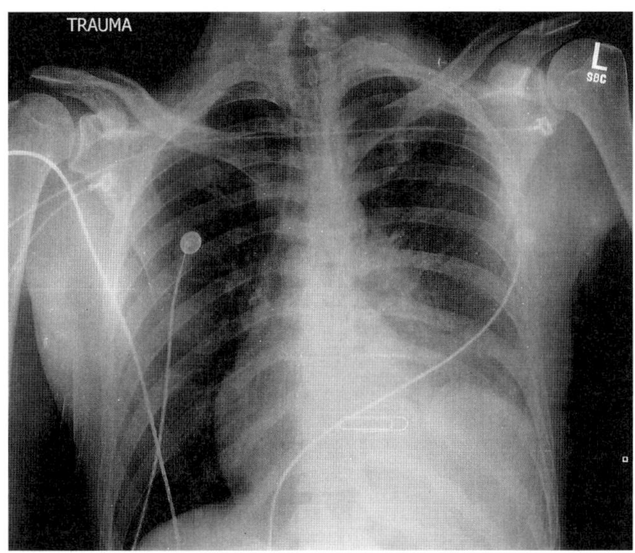
TRAUMA
L

Hemothorax.

HYF: Bundle branch block is a commonly seen arrhythmia in this clinical scenario.

Cardiac Tamponade: See p. 39.

Tension Pneumothorax: See p. 561.

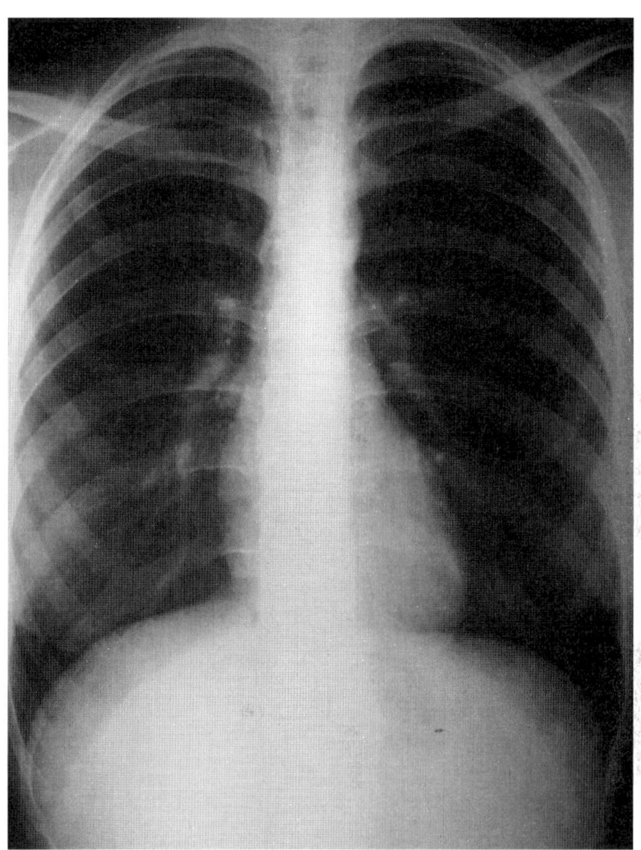

Pneumothorax.

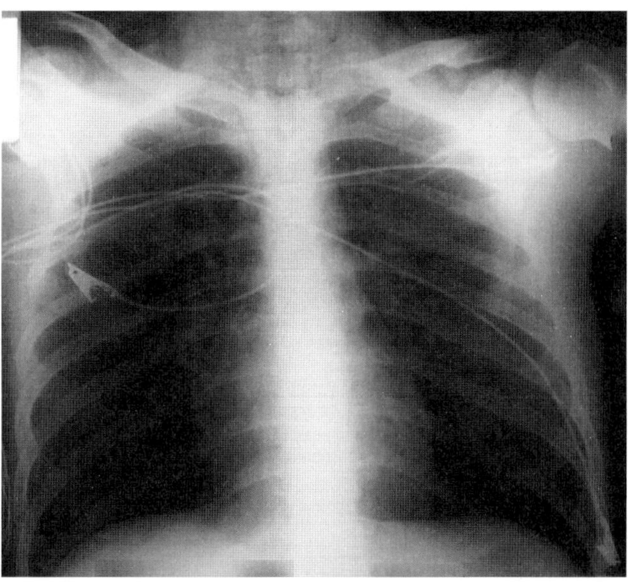

Pneumomediastinum.

10-5 Abdominal Trauma

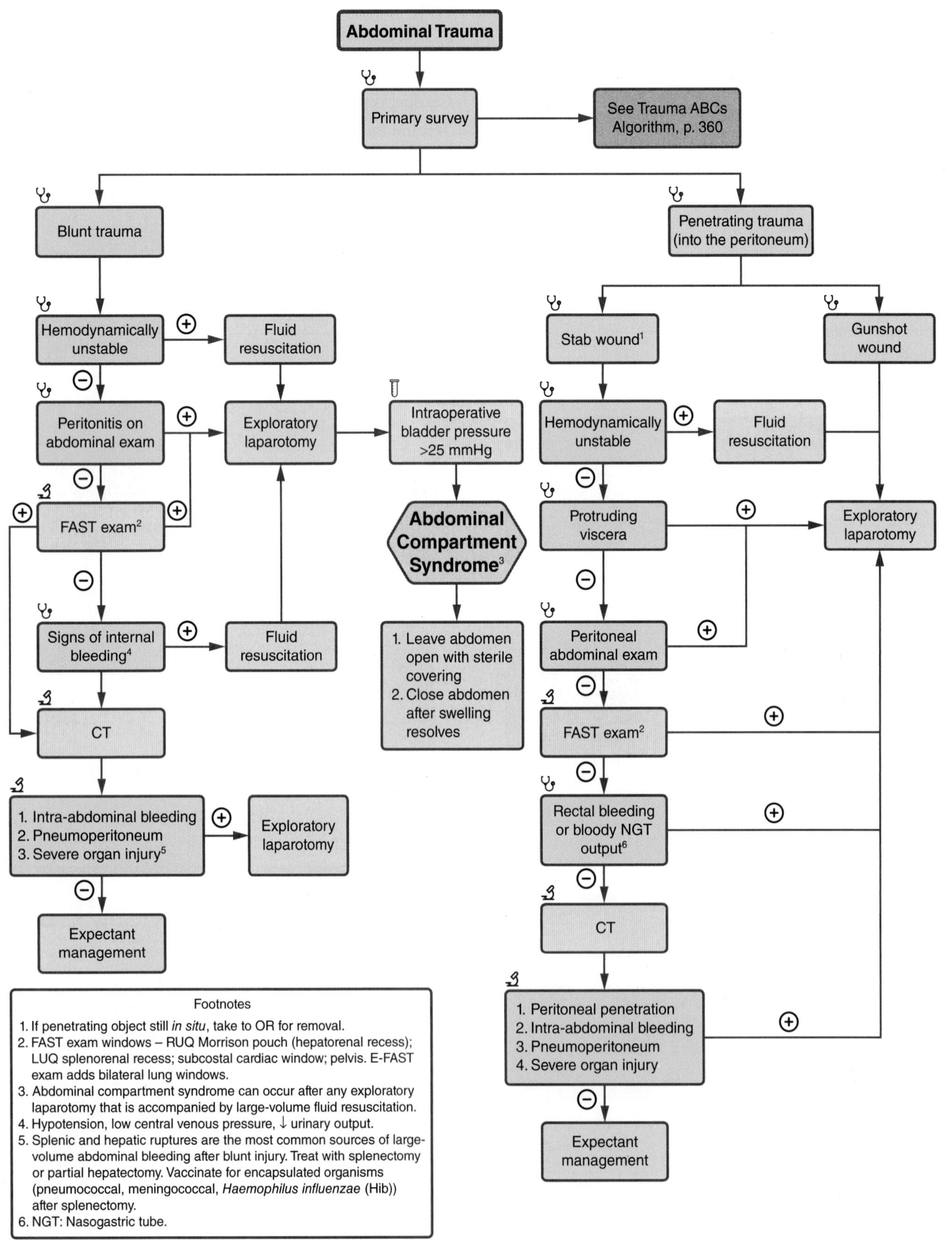
Abdominal Trauma
Primary survey
See Trauma ABCs Algorithm, p. 360
Blunt trauma
Penetrating trauma (into the peritoneum)
Hemodynamically unstable
Fluid resuscitation
Peritonitis on abdominal exam
Exploratory laparotomy
Intraoperative bladder pressure >25 mmHg
Abdominal Compartment Syndrome[3]
FAST exam[2]
Signs of internal bleeding[4]
Fluid resuscitation
CT
1. Intra-abdominal bleeding
2. Pneumoperitoneum
3. Severe organ injury[5]
Exploratory laparotomy
Expectant management
1. Leave abdomen open with sterile covering
2. Close abdomen after swelling resolves
Stab wound[1]
Gunshot wound
Hemodynamically unstable
Fluid resuscitation
Protruding viscera
Exploratory laparotomy
Peritoneal abdominal exam
FAST exam[2]
Rectal bleeding or bloody NGT output[6]
CT
1. Peritoneal penetration
2. Intra-abdominal bleeding
3. Pneumoperitoneum
4. Severe organ injury
Expectant management

Footnotes

1. If penetrating object still *in situ*, take to OR for removal.
2. FAST exam windows – RUQ Morrison pouch (hepatorenal recess); LUQ splenorenal recess; subcostal cardiac window; pelvis. E-FAST exam adds bilateral lung windows.
3. Abdominal compartment syndrome can occur after any exploratory laparotomy that is accompanied by large-volume fluid resuscitation.
4. Hypotension, low central venous pressure, ↓ urinary output.
5. Splenic and hepatic ruptures are the most common sources of large-volume abdominal bleeding after blunt injury. Treat with splenectomy or partial hepatectomy. Vaccinate for encapsulated organisms (pneumococcal, meningococcal, *Haemophilus influenzae* (Hib)) after splenectomy.
6. NGT: Nasogastric tube.

FIGURE 10.5

10-6 Pelvic Injury

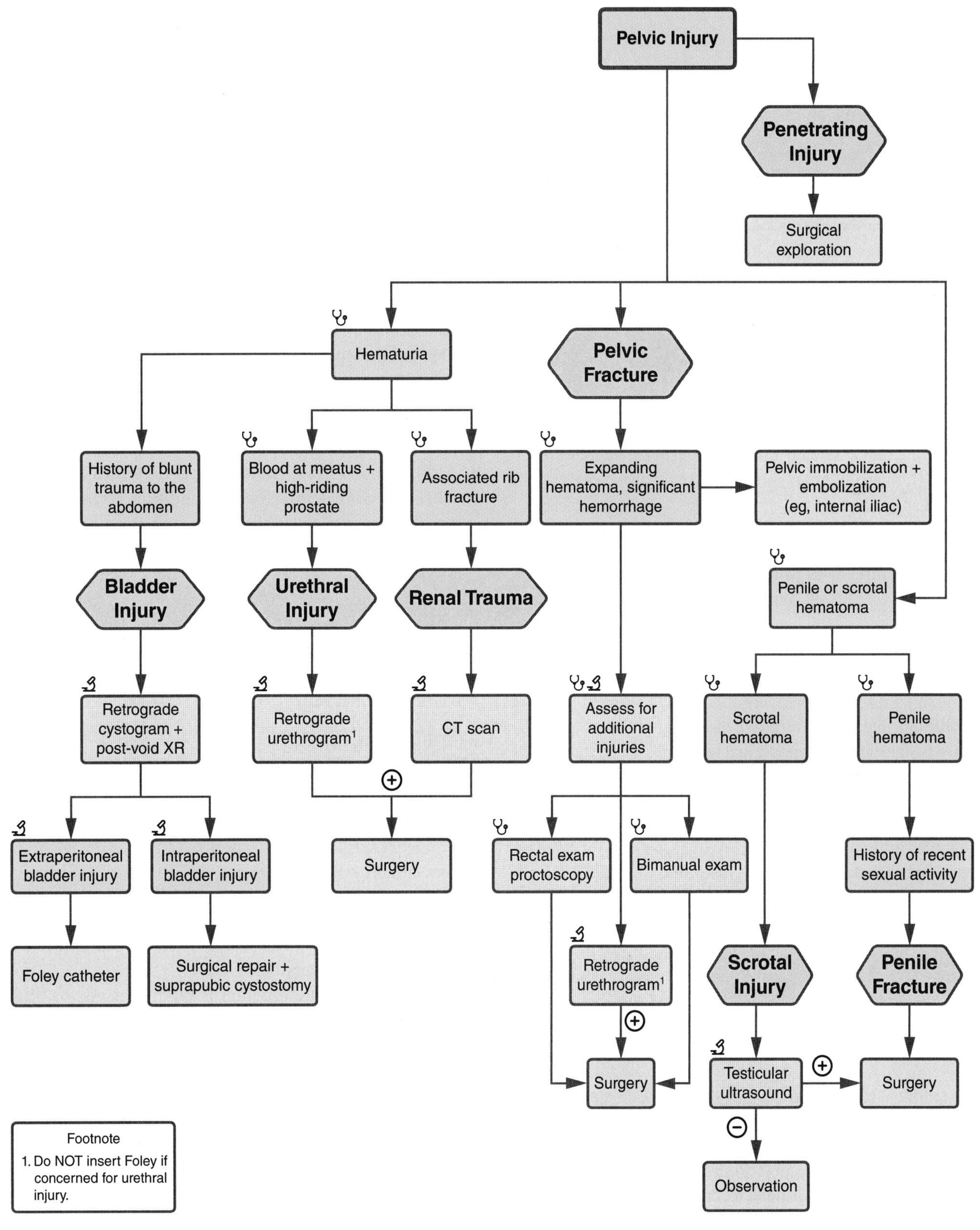
Pelvic Injury
Penetrating Injury
Surgical exploration
Hematuria
Pelvic Fracture
History of blunt trauma to the abdomen
Blood at meatus + high-riding prostate
Associated rib fracture
Expanding hematoma, significant hemorrhage
Pelvic immobilization + embolization (eg, internal iliac)
Bladder Injury
Urethral Injury
Renal Trauma
Penile or scrotal hematoma
Retrograde cystogram + post-void XR
Retrograde urethrogram[1]
CT scan
Assess for additional injuries
Scrotal hematoma
Penile hematoma
Extraperitoneal bladder injury
Intraperitoneal bladder injury
Surgery
Rectal exam proctoscopy
Bimanual exam
History of recent sexual activity
Foley catheter
Surgical repair + suprapubic cystostomy
Retrograde urethrogram[1]
Scrotal Injury
Penile Fracture
Surgery
Testicular ultrasound
Surgery
Observation
Footnote
1. Do NOT insert Foley if concerned for urethral injury.

FIGURE 10.6

10-6 Pelvic Injury

PELVIC FRACTURE

A 62-year-old M presents after falling off the roof. On **exam**, his right leg appears shorter than his left and his pelvis is unstable. **Labs** are significant for Hgb 9.6. On **imaging**, pelvic X-ray demonstrates open-book pelvic fracture.

Management:

1. Non-expanding pelvic hematoma and hemodynamically stable: Monitor. No intervention necessary if not expanding.
2. Significant hemorrhage: Pelvic immobilization with binder followed by vascular embolization.

Complications:

- Rectal injury: Assess with rectal exam and proctoscopy.
- Vaginal injury: Assess with bimanual exam.
- Bladder and urethral injuries.
- Erectile dysfunction.
- Hypovolemic shock: Usually due to tearing of the venous plexus (presacral, lumbar) but may rarely involve the iliac vessels.
- Fat embolism.
- Injury to the femoral nerve.

HYF: Pelvic fractures tend to occur in multiples instead of single fractures. A significant number of patients require blood transfusion.

BLADDER INJURY

A 32-year-old F presents with severe abdominal pain after a motor vehicle collision where the steering wheel impacted her lower abdomen. **Exam** is significant for abdominal tenderness and guarding in all 4 quadrants.

Management:

1. Retrograde cystogram with post-void X-ray to assess for extra vs. intraperitoneal bladder injury. Extraperitoneal [ie, FAST (-)] for intraperitoneal free fluid: Place Foley catheter. Intraperitoneal [ie, FAST (+)]: Surgical repair protected with suprapubic cystostomy.

Complications:

- Urinary ascites, chemical peritonitis.
- Infection, abscess.

HYF:

- Extraperitoneal bladder injury: Due to injury of the neck, anterior wall, or anterolateral bladder wall. Urine extravasation → localized pain in the suprapubic region.
- Intraperitoneal bladder injury: Rupture of the bladder dome (superior, lateral walls). Urine extravasation → peritonitis and referred shoulder pain (Kehr sign). Labs can show increased BUN and creatinine from peritoneal reabsorption of urine.

URETHRAL INJURY

A 50-year-old M presents after a car accident and is found to have a pelvic fracture. On **exam**, he is hypotensive, tachycardic, and complaining of considerable pelvic pain. He has blood at the penile meatus, distended bladder, hematuria, and a high-riding prostate.

Management:

1. Retrograde urethrogram.
2. Suprapubic catheterization to decompress the bladder.
3. Urethrography or urethroscopy.
4. Anterior urethral injuries require urgent surgical repair. Posterior urethral injuries are treated with suprapubic catheterization for temporary urinary diversion, followed by delayed surgical repair.

Complications:

- Do NOT insert Foley catheter if urethral injury is suspected, as it can convert a partial urethral tear into a complete urethral laceration or cause infection of periurethral hematoma.
- Delayed presentation of anterior urethral injury can be complicated by sepsis due to urine extravasation into the scrotum, perineum, and/or abdominal wall.

HYF:

- Most common in men due to longer urethral length.
- Abrupt upward shifting of the bladder and prostate can lead to urethral tearing, especially at the bulbomembranous junction (transition point between anterior and posterior urethra).

RENAL TRAUMA

A 25-year-old F presents after a motorcycle accident with significant separation from the bike. On **exam**, she has severe tenderness to palpation over bilateral flanks and flank ecchymosis. On **imaging**, CXR reveals lower rib fractures. Urine dipstick is significant for blood.

Management:

1. CT abdomen/pelvis with contrast.
2. Most blunt renal injuries can be managed non-operatively. If there is severe renal injury and/or ongoing bleeding, go to emergent surgical repair and/or selective renal angiography and embolization.

Complications:

- Severe renal injury can cause retroperitoneal bleeding and hemodynamic instability.
- Retrograde cystourethrogram is used to assess for bladder or urethral injuries.
- AV fistula development → congestive heart failure.
- Renal artery stenosis → renovascular hypertension.

SCROTAL INJURY

A teenage M presents after falling off his bike and landing straddled on the bike's frame. He complains of severe pelvic pain. **Exam** shows an expanding scrotal hematoma.

Management:

1. Testicular US.
2. Surgery only if testicle is ruptured.

Complications:

- Testicular necrosis if ruptured and not surgically repaired.
- Anterior urethral injury.

10-6 Pelvic Injury

HYF: Patients may present with impressive swelling, but only testicular rupture warrants surgical intervention

PENILE FRACTURE

A 27-year-old M presents with severe penile pain after an "accident" during sexual intercourse. He describes a snapping sound during intercourse, followed by sudden-onset penile pain. **Exam** shows a large hematoma on his penile shaft but a normal-appearing glans.

Management:

1. If high clinical suspicion for concomitant urethral injury (eg, blood at the meatus, dysuria, urinary retention), obtain an emergent retrograde urethrogram prior to Foley catheter insertion.
2. Focal penile soft tissue injury without skin loss or injury to the tunica albuginea of the corporal bodies can generally be managed non-operatively. Otherwise, emergent surgical repair.

Complications:

- Anterior urethral injury.
- If not surgically repaired, painful erections or erectile dysfunction can result due to AV shunt development.

HYF: The corpora cavernosa or tunica albuginea is the structure damaged.

10-7 Neck Trauma

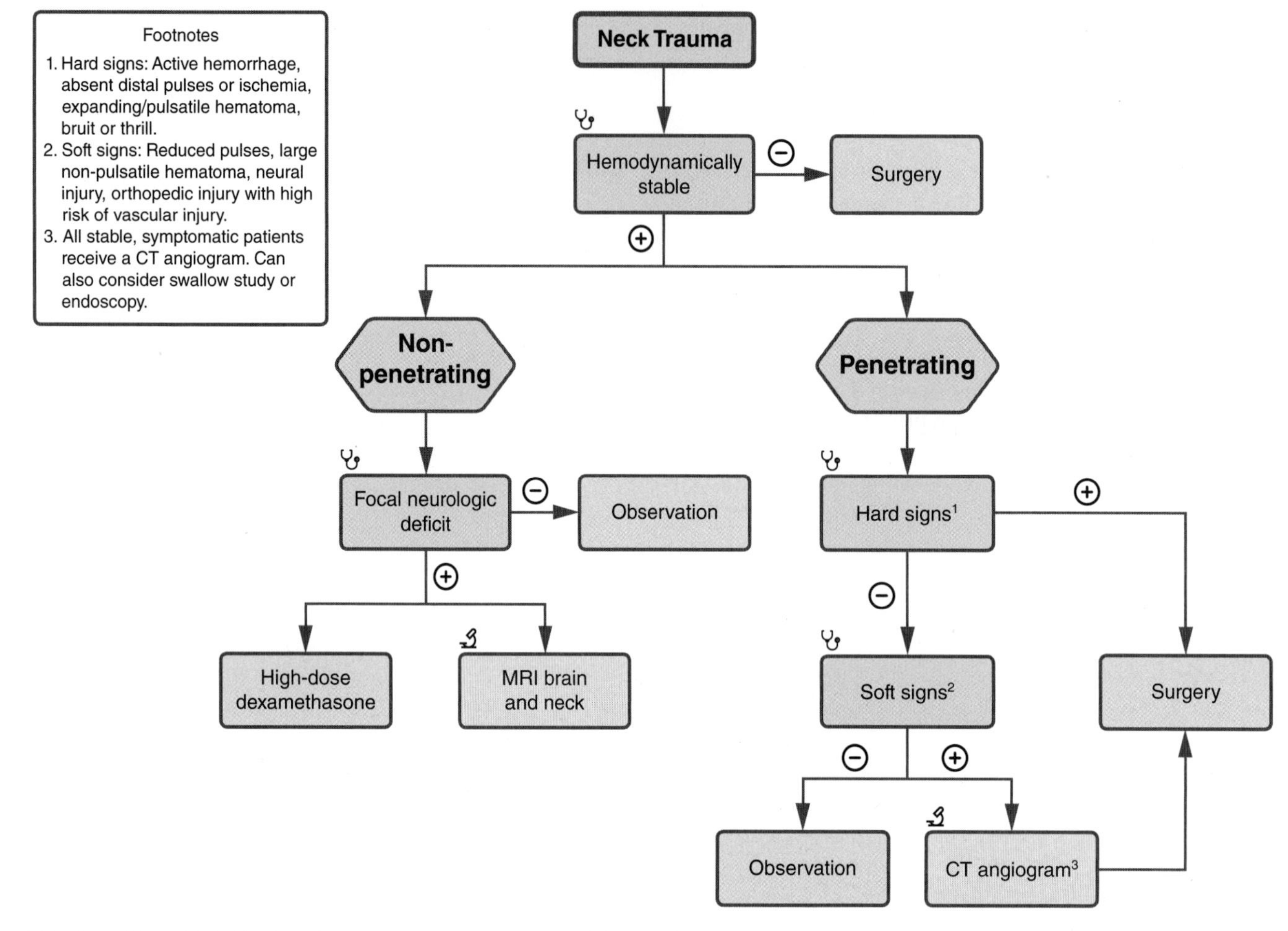
Footnotes
1. Hard signs: Active hemorrhage, absent distal pulses or ischemia, expanding/pulsatile hematoma, bruit or thrill.
2. Soft signs: Reduced pulses, large non-pulsatile hematoma, neural injury, orthopedic injury with high risk of vascular injury.
3. All stable, symptomatic patients receive a CT angiogram. Can also consider swallow study or endoscopy.
Neck Trauma
Hemodynamically stable
Surgery
Non-penetrating
Penetrating
Focal neurologic deficit
Observation
Hard signs1
High-dose dexamethasone
MRI brain and neck
Soft signs2
Surgery
Observation
CT angiogram3

FIGURE 10.7

10-7 Neck Trauma

NON-PENETRATING NECK TRAUMA

A patient presents with severe blunt neck trauma after a car accident.

Management:

1. Manage ABCs.
2. Stat CT cervical spine.
3. High-dose dexamethasone.
4. MRI brain to assess for stroke and/or MRI neck to assess for spinal cord injury.

Complications:

- Permanent neurologic deficits.
- Blunt injury to the carotid artery or vertebral artery (eg, from overstretching the vessel, direct trauma, or cervical spine fracture) can easily be missed and lead to neurologic deficits not explained by head CT. CTA neck can rule out injury.

HYF: Neurologic deficits that develop after blunt spinal cord injuries are usually due to cord edema; therefore, they are managed with high-dose steroids rather than surgery.

PENETRATING NECK TRAUMA

A patient presents with a stab or gunshot wound to the neck.

Management:

1. Manage ABCs.
2. If injury does not violate the platysma, conservative management.
3. If injury violates the platysma:
   a. If hemodynamically unstable or has presence of hard signs (gurgling, stridor, apnea, expanding hematoma, arterial bleeding, stroke, shock, or frank mediastinitis), then surgical exploration.
   b. If hard signs are absent and soft signs (dysphonia, crepitus, stable hematoma, blood oozing, or dysphagia) are present, a CTA is indicated. Positive CTA findings go to surgery; negative CTAs are managed with observation.
4. Depending on sequelae of neck trauma (eg, mediastinitis, dysphonia), other radiologic studies include cervical X-ray, CT cervical spine, carotid Doppler US, EGD, esophagram, CTA, or bronchoscopy may be indicated.
5. Prophylactic antibiotics may be indicated due to increased risk of contamination by oropharyngeal flora (anaerobic coverage).

Complications:

- Airway compromise.
- Neurologic deficits.

HYF: Patients can initially present without obvious airway compromise due to the thick fascial layers of the neck, which limit outward displacement of tissue. Internal compressible structures can become affected without external signs of hematoma, leading to rapid clinical decompensation.

10-8 Extremity Trauma

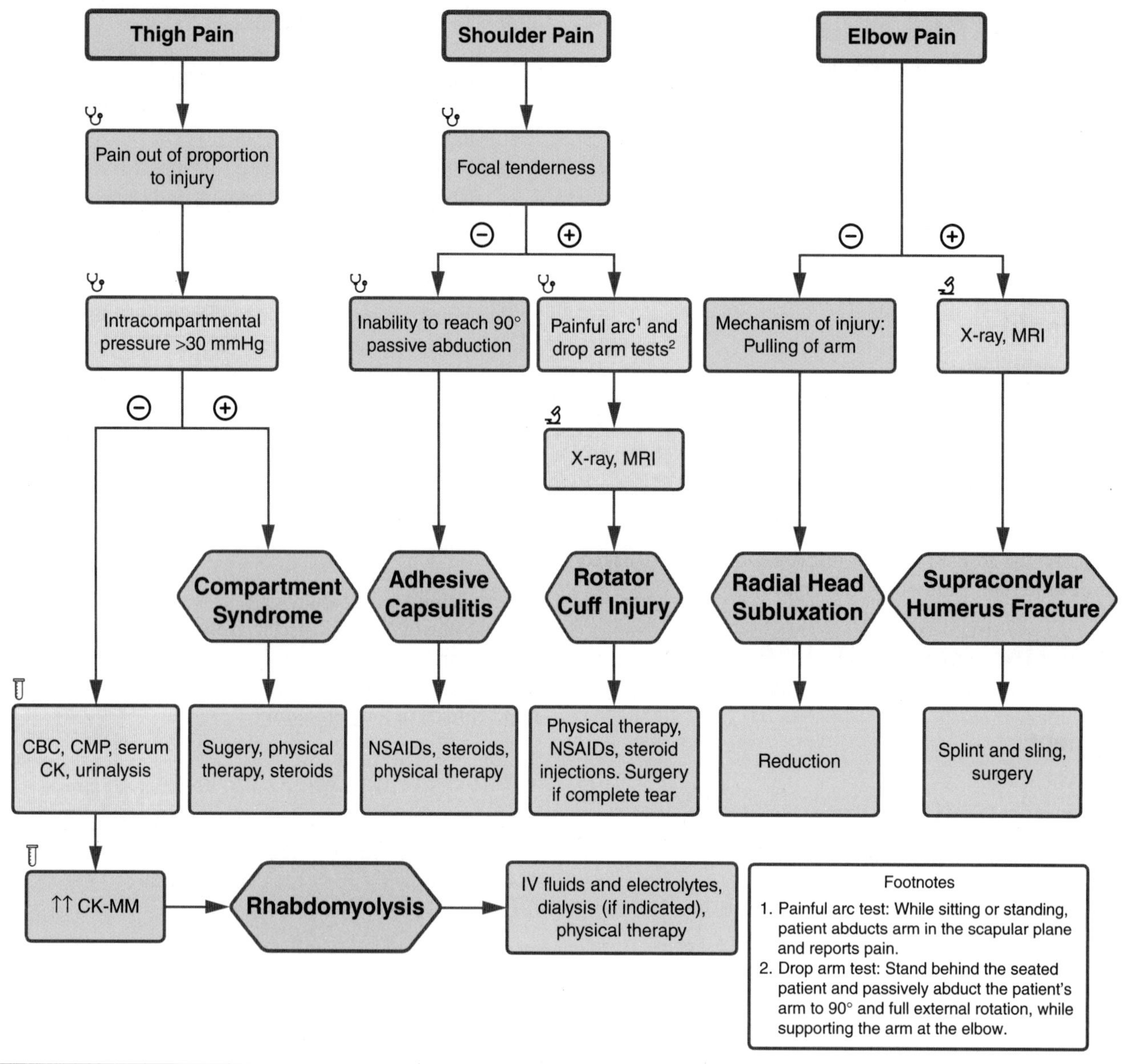
Thigh Pain
Pain out of proportion to injury
Intracompartmental pressure >30 mmHg
⊖
⊕
Compartment Syndrome
CBC, CMP, serum CK, urinalysis
Sugery, physical therapy, steroids
↑↑ CK-MM
Rhabdomyolysis
IV fluids and electrolytes, dialysis (if indicated), physical therapy
Shoulder Pain
Focal tenderness
⊖
⊕
Inability to reach 90° passive abduction
Painful arc[1] and drop arm tests[2]
X-ray, MRI
Adhesive Capsulitis
Rotator Cuff Injury
NSAIDs, steroids, physical therapy
Physical therapy, NSAIDs, steroid injections. Surgery if complete tear
Elbow Pain
⊖
⊕
Mechanism of injury: Pulling of arm
X-ray, MRI
Radial Head Subluxation
Supracondylar Humerus Fracture
Reduction
Splint and sling, surgery
Footnotes
1. Painful arc test: While sitting or standing, patient abducts arm in the scapular plane and reports pain.
2. Drop arm test: Stand behind the seated patient and passively abduct the patient's arm to 90° and full external rotation, while supporting the arm at the elbow.

FIGURE 10.8

10-8 Extremity Trauma

COMPARTMENT SYNDROME

A 27-year-old M presents with severe thigh pain after being in a car crash 7 hours prior with no apparent injuries. On exam, the pain is localized to the anterior compartment. Muscles are firm and swollen on palpation. He endorses significant pain that is out of proportion to exam. Intra-compartmental pressure is >30 mmHg.

Management:

1. Place limb at level of the heart without elevation.
2. Analgesics and supplementary oxygen.
3. Emergent fasciotomy.

Complications:

- Volkmann contracture.
- Acute kidney injury.

HYF: Most common cause is a tibial fracture. While compartment syndrome can occur in the thigh, it is more commonly seen in the calves, requiring 4 compartment fasciotomies.

ADHESIVE CAPSULITIS

A 43-year-old F presents with prolonged unilateral shoulder stiffness. She has mild pain with movement. On exam, she has decreased active and passive range of motion. She is unable to reach 90° with passive abduction.

Management:

1. NSAIDs.
2. Physical therapy.
3. Oral corticosteroids or injections.

Complications: Persistent pain and stiffness.

HYF: Associated with diabetes mellitus, thyroid disease, trauma, scleroderma, and Dupuytren's disease.

ROTATOR CUFF INJURY

A 59-year-old M presents with complaints of shoulder pain at rest and with overhead motions. On exam, there is focal tenderness over the right anterolateral shoulder. Painful arc and drop arm tests are positive. On imaging, MRI shows partial supraspinatus tear.

Management:

1. If partial tear, supportive care: Rest, NSAIDs, physical therapy, glucocorticoid injections.
2. If complete tear, surgery.

Complications:

- Recurrence.
- Acromioclavicular (AC) joint pain.
- Axillary/suprascapular nerve injury.
- Impingement syndrome.

HYF: The supraspinatus muscle is most commonly injured.

RADIAL HEAD SUBLUXATION

A 4-year-old M presents with elbow pain. Mother reports she forcefully pulled him onto the curb to avoid getting hit by an oncoming car. On exam, pain and tenderness are localized to the lateral aspect of the elbow.

Management:

1. Reduction.

Complications: Recurrence.

HYF: Uncommon in children ≥5 years of age. Point tenderness over the distal posterior humerus can be a sign of an associated fracture requiring further evaluation.

SUPRACONDYLAR HUMERUS FRACTURE

A 6-year-old F presents with elbow pain. Mother reports she fell on her outstretched arm while jumping off the kitchen counter. On exam, she is unable to move her elbow due to pain. Significant swelling of the elbow is noted. On imaging, X-ray shows a supracondylar humerus fracture.

Management:

1. Cast immobilization.
2. If significantly displaced, closed reduction with cutaneous pinning.

Complications:

- Malunion.
- Neurovascular injury (brachial artery, median nerve, radial nerve).
- Brachial artery entrapment.
- Compartment syndrome.
- Volkmann contracture of the wrist and fingers.

HYF: Risk of injury to the brachial artery and median nerve. Volkmann contracture of the wrist and fingers is caused by compartment syndrome from injury to the brachial artery → ischemia and muscle fibrosis.

RHABDOMYOLYSIS

A 21-year-old M presents with severe thigh pain. He reports drunkenly spending the night asleep on the floor. On exam, he endorses muscle tenderness. Labs show elevated serum creatine kinase-MM. Urinalysis is positive for blood but no RBCs.

Management:

1. IV fluids and electrolyte management (titrate resuscitation to a goal of UOP >1 mL/kg/hr).
2. Dialysis if severe renal failure.
3. Physical therapy.

Complications:

- Acute kidney injury.
- Cardiac arrest from hyperkalemia.

HYF: Classic triad: Myalgia, weakness, and pigmenturia. Myalgia, pigmenturia, and myoglobinuria are absent in up to 50% of patients. When myalgia is present, it is usually severe. Urine dipstick will be positive for large amounts of "blood" (because dipstick cannot distinguish myoglobin from hemoglobin), but UA microscopy will show lack of RBCs.

See Upper Extremity Injuries table for complete list of diagnoses, pp. 458, 474–475.

10-9 Burns

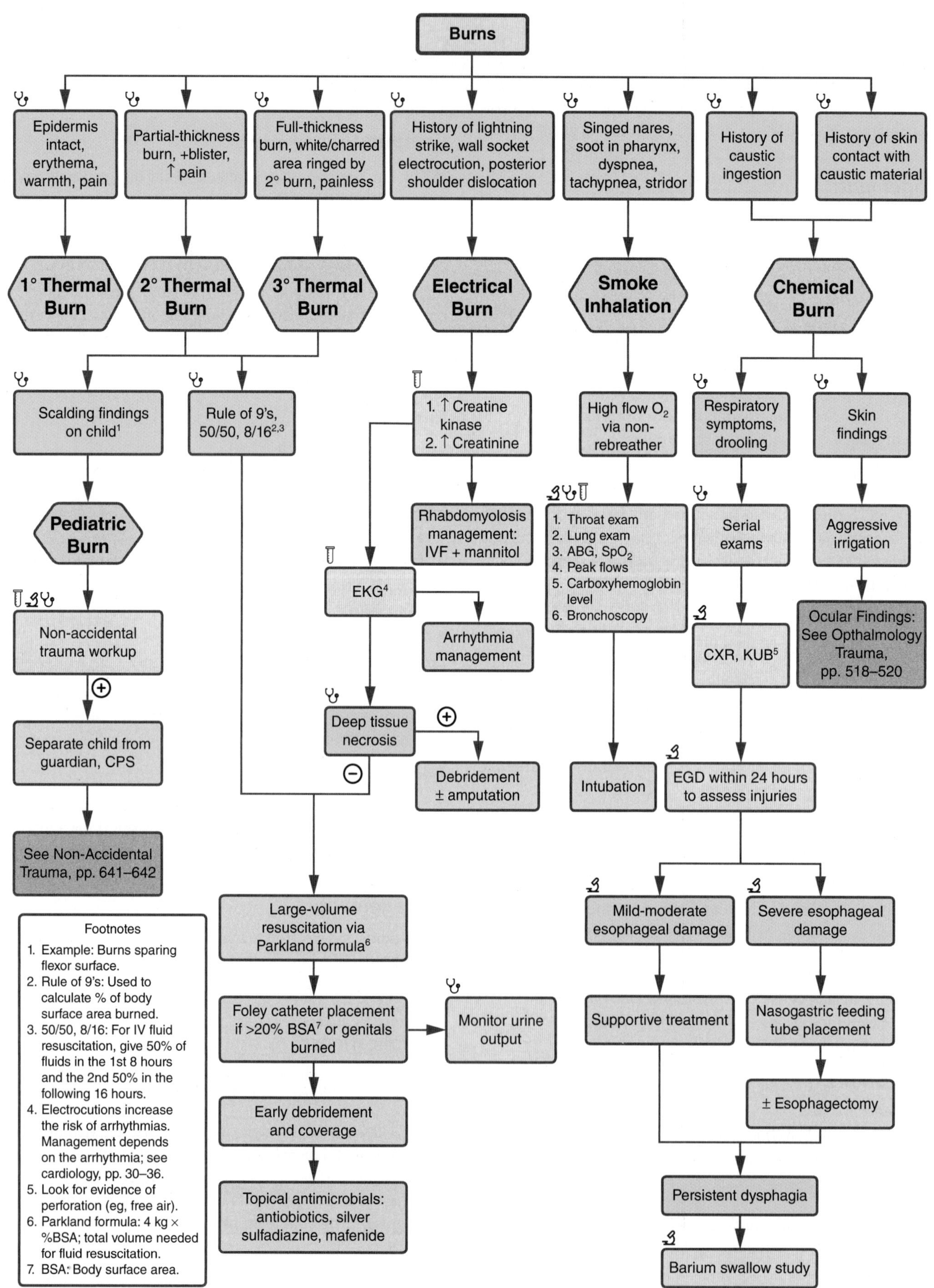
Burns
Epidermis intact, erythema, warmth, pain
Partial-thickness burn, +blister, ↑ pain
Full-thickness burn, white/charred area ringed by 2° burn, painless
History of lightning strike, wall socket electrocution, posterior shoulder dislocation
Singed nares, soot in pharynx, dyspnea, tachypnea, stridor
History of caustic ingestion
History of skin contact with caustic material
1° Thermal Burn
2° Thermal Burn
3° Thermal Burn
Electrical Burn
Smoke Inhalation
Chemical Burn
Scalding findings on child[1]
Rule of 9's, 50/50, 8/16[2,3]
1. ↑ Creatine kinase
2. ↑ Creatinine
High flow O_2 via non-rebreather
Respiratory symptoms, drooling
Skin findings
Pediatric Burn
Rhabdomyolosis management: IVF + mannitol
1. Throat exam
2. Lung exam
3. ABG, SpO_2
4. Peak flows
5. Carboxyhemoglobin level
6. Bronchoscopy
Serial exams
Aggressive irrigation
EKG[4]
Non-accidental trauma workup
Arrhythmia management
CXR, KUB[5]
Ocular Findings: See Opthalmology Trauma, pp. 518–520
+
Separate child from guardian, CPS
Deep tissue necrosis
+
−
Debridement ± amputation
Intubation
EGD within 24 hours to assess injuries
See Non-Accidental Trauma, pp. 641–642
Large-volume resuscitation via Parkland formula[6]
Mild-moderate esophageal damage
Severe esophageal damage
Foley catheter placement if >20% BSA[7] or genitals burned
Monitor urine output
Supportive treatment
Nasogastric feeding tube placement
Early debridement and coverage
± Esophagectomy
Topical antimicrobials: antiobiotics, silver sulfadiazine, mafenide
Persistent dysphagia
Barium swallow study
Footnotes
1. Example: Burns sparing flexor surface.
2. Rule of 9's: Used to calculate % of body surface area burned.
3. 50/50, 8/16: For IV fluid resuscitation, give 50% of fluids in the 1st 8 hours and the 2nd 50% in the following 16 hours.
4. Electrocutions increase the risk of arrhythmias. Management depends on the arrhythmia; see cardiology, pp. 30–36.
5. Look for evidence of perforation (eg, free air).
6. Parkland formula: 4 kg × %BSA; total volume needed for fluid resuscitation.
7. BSA: Body surface area.

FIGURE 10.9

10-9 Burns

CHEMICAL BURN

A 6-year-old M presents with his father after complaining of severe abdominal pain and pain with swallowing. His father found all the bottles pulled out from under the kitchen sink. On exam, he is drooling and has significant voice hoarseness. EGD shows significant inflammation in his esophagus.

Management:

1. Manage ABCs.
2. Serial CXR and KUB to look for perforation.
3. If suspected perforation, obtain upper GI X-ray with water-soluble contrast.
4. Once perforation is ruled out, obtain EGD within 24 hours to assess severity of injury.
   a. No or mild esophageal injury: Supportive care.
   b. Significant injury: Place nasogastric feeding tube for tube feeds under endoscopy, refer for possible esophagectomy.
5. For significant injury or persistent dysphagia, perform barium swallow in 2–3 weeks to assess for strictures.

Complications:

- Ulcers, esophageal or gastric perforation (mediastinitis, peritonitis), pyloric stenosis, esophageal strictures, upper airway compromise, esophageal squamous cell carcinoma.

HYF:

- Alkaline ingestions (eg, lye) cause liquefactive necrosis and are worse than acidic ingestions (eg, battery acid) that cause coagulative necrosis.
- Do NOT try to neutralize ingestions (eg, vinegar); buffer reactions generate heat and further damage.
- Do NOT induce vomiting (eg, nasogastric lavage, activated charcoal, water, ipecac, milk).

THERMAL AND SMOKE INHALATION INJURY

A 34-year-old F presents to the ED after being in a house fire. On exam, she has normal breath sounds bilaterally, denies dyspnea, and has a small amount of black dust on her nares. After an initial exam, the patient is left to rest. When her nurse returns, the patient is markedly dyspneic. Bronchoscopy shows mucosal erythema and blistering.

Management:

1. All burn patients must be treated initially with high-flow oxygen via a non-rebreather mask.
2. Oropharyngeal and lung exam. If singed nares are present or soot is detected in the larynx, proceed to intubation, as impending edema may comprise the airway.
3. Obtain ABG, SpO_2, and peak flows. Monitor the level of carboxyhemoglobin in the blood; elevated levels can be treated with 100% FiO_2.
4. Bronchoscopy is the gold standard for diagnosis.

Complications:

- Laryngeal edema caused by the chemical injury from smoke inhalation leading to airway obstruction.
- Carbon monoxide, cyanide, or arsenic poisoning.
- Tracheobronchitis and pneumonitis from direct toxic injury.

HYF: 100% oxygen both displaces carbon monoxide from hemoglobin and shortens its half-life.

ELECTRICAL BURN

A 32-year-old M presents after being struck by lightning. On exam, he has a branching pattern of erythema on his right thigh and severe left shoulder pain with obvious deformity. On labs, urinalysis shows high levels of blood but no RBCs.

Management:

1. For deep tissue necrosis, debridement and possible amputation.
2. Assess for arrhythmias with EKG.
3. IV fluids to address myoglobinuria-induced nephropathy.

Complications:

- Early: Rhabdomyolysis, muscle necrosis, cardiac arrhythmias, posterior shoulder dislocation.
- Late: Demyelination syndromes and cataracts.

HYF:

- The 2 most common causes of posterior shoulder dislocation are seizure and electrocution.
- High voltage heats bone and causes significant soft tissue necrosis that can be delayed in presentation.
- Electrocution can cause a characteristic skin finding known as "ferning" caused by leaky capillaries.

THERMAL BURN

A firefighter presents to the ED after being trapped in a house fire. Exam shows hypotension, tachycardia, right hemithorax, significant pain, and erythema over her right leg and left arm, with scattered black eschars.

Management:

1. Manage ABCs.
2. IV fluids (lactated Ringer's): Rule of 9's, 50/50, 8/16. Use body diagram to calculate % body surface area burned. Use the Parkland formula (4 kg × %BSA) to calculate the volume of lactated Ringer's to administer in the first 24 hours. Give 50% of the total fluid requirement in the first 8 hours and the remaining 50% in the following 16 hours. Afterwards, titrate IV fluids to maintain adequate urine output.
3. In patients who have genital burns or burns >20% total BSA, place Foley catheter to monitor fluid resuscitation and urine output. Delay in Foley placement can lead to urethral edema that obstructs catheterization.

(Continued)

10-9 Burns

4. Copious irrigation and debridement of affected areas.
   Apply topical antimicrobial agents and non-stick dressings.
   Prophylaxis with silver sulfadiazine, mafenide (penetrates eschar), or antibiotics.

Complications:

- Major cause of mortality is hypovolemic shock, followed by septic shock due to wound infection or pneumonia.
- Wound infection: Immediately after a severe burn, the most common cause of wound infection is Gram-positive skin flora (*Staphylococcus aureus*). After >5 days, most infections are due to Gram-negative organisms (*Pseudomonas aeruginosa*) and fungi (*Candida*). Earliest sign of wound infection is a change in wound appearance (partial-thickness burn progressing to full thickness) or loss of viable skin graft. Diagnose with quantitative wound culture (>10^5 bacteria/g of tissue) and biopsy for histopathology to determine tissue invasion depth. Treat with broad-spectrum antibiotics.
- Hypermetabolic response in the 1st week (hyperglycemia, muscle wasting, hyperthermia, increased energy expenditure, nutritional deficiencies). Supplement with a high-calorie, high-nitrogen diet.
- Circumferential, full-thickness (3rd-degree) burns can cause compartment syndrome if on limb and respiratory compromise if on chest. Treat with escharotomy or fasciotomy at bedside.
- Marjolin ulcer: Squamous cell carcinoma arising from burn; has increased risk of metastases.

HYF:

- Scalding burns with sharp lines of demarcation and uniform depth and sparing flexor surfaces on children raise concern for child abuse.
- Large-volume resuscitation is only considered in second- and third-degree burns.
- Do NOT put ice on wounds, which can cause frostbite and hypothermia.
- Lactated Ringer's is preferred for fluid resuscitation for burns. Normal saline is associated with hyperchloremic metabolic acidosis and hypercoagulability.

10-10 Bites and Stings

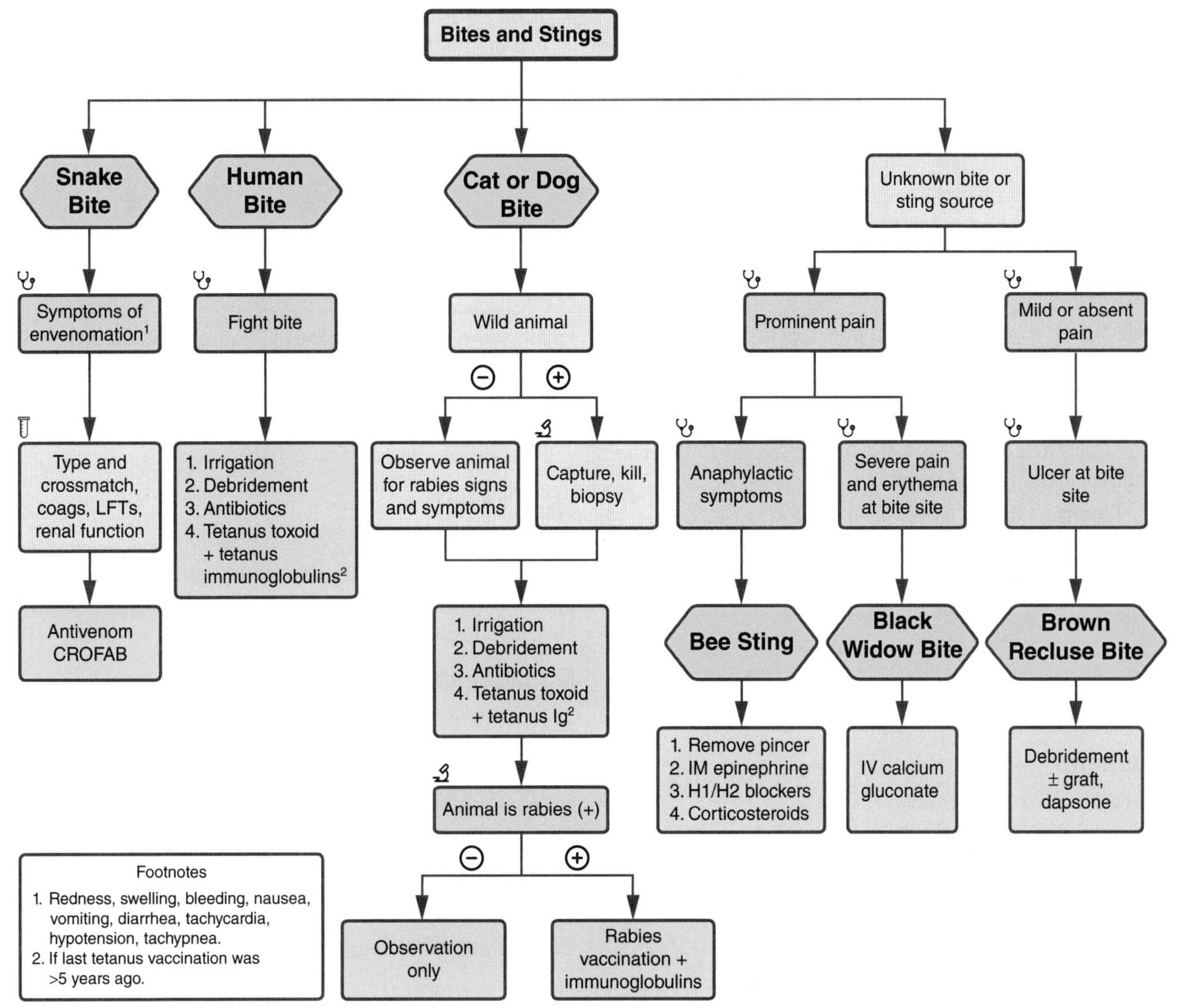
Bites and Stings
Snake Bite
Human Bite
Cat or Dog Bite
Unknown bite or sting source
Symptoms of envenomation[1]
Fight bite
Wild animal
Prominent pain
Mild or absent pain
Type and crossmatch, coags, LFTs, renal function
1. Irrigation
2. Debridement
3. Antibiotics
4. Tetanus toxoid + tetanus immunoglobulins[2]
Observe animal for rabies signs and symptoms
Capture, kill, biopsy
Anaphylactic symptoms
Severe pain and erythema at bite site
Ulcer at bite site
Antivenom CROFAB
1. Irrigation
2. Debridement
3. Antibiotics
4. Tetanus toxoid + tetanus Ig[2]
Bee Sting
Black Widow Bite
Brown Recluse Bite
1. Remove pincer
2. IM epinephrine
3. H1/H2 blockers
4. Corticosteroids
IV calcium gluconate
Debridement ± graft, dapsone
Animal is rabies (+)
Observation only
Rabies vaccination + immunoglobulins
Footnotes
1. Redness, swelling, bleeding, nausea, vomiting, diarrhea, tachycardia, hypotension, tachypnea.
2. If last tetanus vaccination was >5 years ago.

FIGURE 10.10

10-10 Bites and Stings

SNAKE BITE

A 25-year-old F presents with 2 puncture marks on her left calf ringed with marked erythema and edema after hiking in North Carolina. She complains of significant pain and thinks she may have seen a striped red and yellow animal slither through the grass.

Management:

1. Crotalid (rattlesnake) bites: CROFAB.
2. Unspecified snake: Antivenin.
3. Debridement of any nonviable tissue.

Complications: Compartment syndrome. Need for fasciotomy is rare.

HYF:

- Coral snakes: **"Red on yellow, kill a fellow."** Their venom contains a neurotoxin that can be fatal.
- Do NOT apply ice or tourniquet to bitten limb.

HUMAN BITE

A 25-year-old M presents with hand pain. On exam, he has marked erythema, tenderness, and swelling surrounding a 2-cm laceration over his 3rd and 4th MCP joints of his right hand. He declines to say how he hurt his hand and seems uncomfortable answering further questions.

Management:

1. Extensive irrigation and debridement.
2. Send for blood AND wound cultures.
3. Empiric antibiotics (amoxicillin/clavulanate).
4. Surgical debridement if necessary. Leave wounds open to heal by secondary intention unless they are on the face.
5. Tetanus shot, if not up-to-date.

Complications: Infection. After I&D, leave the wound open for drainage.

HYF:

- Most common presentation of a human bite is a "fight bite" over the 3rd, 4th, or 5th MCP joints.
- Most common organisms: *Streptococcus, S. aureus, Eikenella corrodens, H. influenzae*, and β-lactamase–producing anaerobes.

CAT OR DOG BITE

A 25-year-old M presents with a large laceration on his right arm after suffering a dog or cat bite. He complains of significant pain but is otherwise stable.

Management:

1. Irrigation, debridement, prophylactic antibiotics.
2. If the last tetanus vaccine >5 years ago, tetanus toxoid + tetanus immunoglobulin.
3. If the animal is rabies (+), give rabies vaccination and immunoglobulin. If the animal is wild and cannot be caught, mandatory prophylaxis. If the animal is available for observation and asymptomatic, observe it for 10 days or test it to determine need for post-exposure prophylaxis.
4. Avoid wound closure. Leave wounds open to heal by secondary intention unless they are on the face.

Complications:

- Tenosynovitis from deep bites (more common with cats).
- Bites to the face risk infection near the brain.
- Rabies from dog bites.
- Rapid-onset cellulitis (within 1–2 days) and necrotizing fasciitis due to *Pasteurella multocida*.

HYF:

- Most common bug: *P. multocida* → give prophylactic amoxicillin/clavulanate.
- Cat bites can transmit *Bartonella henselae* (cat-scratch disease), causing a papular skin lesion at the site of injury and ipsilateral subacute-chronic cervical lymphadenopathy.

BEE STING

A 25-year-old M presents with wheezing and an expanding rash over his abdomen. His friend says they were at a picnic when the patient complained of a pinching bite and collapsed shortly after. On exam, his BP is 90/60 and HR 110.

Management:

1. If no allergic reaction, simply remove pincer.
2. If mild allergic reaction (ie, local reaction): Supportive care (eg, antihistamines, steroids).
3. If concern for anaphylaxis:
   a. IM epinephrine 1:1000, H1/H2 blockers, corticosteroids.
   b. IV fluids.
   c. Airway support.

Complications: Anaphylaxis, vasomotor shock.

HYF: Anaphylaxis is a type I hypersensitivity reaction (First and Fast).

SPIDER BITE

A 25-year-old F presents with a small ulcer on her left hand that is moderately painful. She was bitten by a spider while cleaning her attic yesterday.

Management:

1. If brown recluse: Avoid debridement until lesion is stable and well-demarcated, then go for I&D. Grafting as needed, dapsone.
2. If black widow: IV calcium gluconate and muscle relaxants.

Complications:

- Brown recluse spider bite: Deep ulcer with erythematous halo and necrotic center that progresses to eschar. Bite can cause significant delayed necrosis → amputation.
- Black widow spider bite: Local and systemic symptoms including muscle pain, abdominal rigidity, nausea, vomiting.

HYF:

- Brown recluse spiders are common in the southern US. Black widow spiders have a characteristic red hourglass on the thorax.

10-11 Toxicology

CYANIDE POISONING

A 30-year-old M with no PMH presents with a headache, confusion, nausea, and vomiting after escaping from a factory fire. On **exam**, he is hypoxic and tachycardic with bright red mucous membranes. His hypoxia does not respond to supplemental oxygen. **Labs** are consistent with an elevated anion gap metabolic acidosis.

Management:

1. Assess and secure airway, breathing, and circulation.
2. Hydroxycobalamin and sodium thiosulfate.
3. Sodium nitrate.

Complications:

- Acute: Dependent on route of exposure. Commonly CNS and cardiovascular symptoms.
- Chronic: Severe poisoning is linked to parkinsonism and ataxia.

HYF: Contrary to CO poisoning, cyanide poisoning does not respond to supplemental oxygen. The pathognomonic "cherry red" skin is only found in a minority of patients.

CARBON MONOXIDE POISONING

A 42-year-old F with PMH of alcohol use disorder is found unconscious in her mobile home next to a running kerosene heater. She complains of a headache, dizziness, and confusion. On **exam**, she has flushed skin and normal pulse oximetry. **Labs** show elevated carboxyhemoglobin levels.

Management:

1. Assess and secure airway, breathing, and circulation.
2. 100% inhaled oxygen.
3. Hyperbaric oxygen (for severe poisoning).

Complications

- Acute: Pulmonary edema, ventricular arrhythmias, myocardial ischemia, and seizures.
- Chronic: Severe poisoning is linked to long-term neuropsychiatric sequelae (eg, memory impairments, depression, parkinsonism).

HYF: Carbon monoxide (CO) binds with higher affinity to hemoglobin than oxygen and shifts the oxy-hemoglobin dissociation curve to the left. This prevents hemoglobin from releasing oxygen as readily to the tissues.

TOXIC ALCOHOL INGESTION (METHANOL, ETHYLENE GLYCOL)

Methanol: A 22-year-old M presents with blurry vision, headache, and sedation after drinking moonshine he bought from a stranger. On **exam**, he has Kussmaul respirations (deep rapid breathing) and decreased visual acuity bilaterally. **Labs** show elevated anion gap metabolic acidosis and negative urine toxicology.

Ethylene glycol: A 22-year-old M presents with seizures, photophobia, ataxia, and altered mental status after drinking antifreeze on a dare. On **exam**, he is tachypneic with Kussmaul respirations, not oriented to place, and has bilateral flank pain. **Labs** show elevated anion gap metabolic acidosis, hypocalcemia, and hematuria with calcium oxalate crystals on urinalysis.

Management:

1. Assess and secure airway, breathing, and circulation.
2. IV fomepizole (or IV ethanol) to inhibit alcohol dehydrogenase (ADH).
3. IV sodium bicarbonate to maintain pH >7.3.
4. Hemodialysis for severe cases or refractory to ADH inhibitors.

Complications:

- Methanol: Blindness.
- Ethylene glycol: Multi-organ failure from widespread calcium oxalate deposition. Most commonly renal failure and CNS toxicity.

HYF: Toxic alcohol ingestion causes toxicity via the production of metabolic by-products such as formic acid (from methanol ingestion) and oxalic acid (from ethylene glycol ingestion). Treatment aims to stop production of these by-products by inhibiting ADH.

ORGANOPHOSPHATE POISONING

A 45-year-old M farm worker presents with dyspnea, nausea, and vomiting after spilling and unintendedly inhaling an opened container of pesticides. On **exam**, he is diaphoretic, with excess lacrimation and sialorrhea. An audible wheeze can be heard with each breath. Eye exam is notable for miosis and decreased visual acuity. **Labs** and **imaging** are non-revealing.

Management:

1. Assess and secure airway, breathing, and circulation.
2. IV atropine and pralidoxime.
3. Benzodiazepines for concomitant seizures.
4. Decontamination for topical exposure.

Complications:

- Acute: Arrhythmias, myocardial ischemia, respiratory failure.
- Chronic: Neuropathy, paresthesias, parkinsonism.

HYF: Organophosphate poisoning results from the inhibition (often irreversible) of the enzyme acetylcholinesterase, which leads to an acute cholinergic excess. The major clinical features are related to cholinergic overactivation and can be remembered by the mnemonic **DUMBELS:** **D**efecation, **U**rination, **M**iosis, **B**ronchospasm, **E**mesis, **L**acrimation, **S**alivation. The nicotinic signs include muscle fasciculations, weakness, and paralysis. Atropine competes with acetylcholine at the muscarinic receptor, while pralidoxime reactivates the acetylcholinesterase enzyme.

(Continued)

10-11 Toxicology

Specific Toxic Syndromes and Poisonings

Toxic Agent	Antidote
Acetaminophen	PO activated charcoal if early presentation; *N*-Acetylcysteine
Anticholinergics (eg, atropine; mushrooms and plants including *Amanita muscaria* and *A. pontherina,* nightshade)	Physostigmine
Anticholinesterases (eg, organophosphates, sarin nerve gas)	Atropine, pralidoxime (reactivates acetylcholinesterase)
Benzodiazepines	Flumazenil (rarely used because it can induce seizures in certain high-risk patients for which benzodiazepines will not be effective)
β-blockers	Glucagon
Calcium channel blockers (eg, nifedipine, diltiazem, verapamil)	Calcium, glucagon
Carbon monoxide	Oxygen
Cardiac glycosides (eg, digoxin, foxglove)	Digoxin-specific Fab antibodies
Cesium, thallium (radioactive incident)	Prussian blue
Copper	Penicillamine
Cyanide	Sodium nitrite, sodium thiosulfate; hydroxocobalamin
Heavy metals (eg, lead, mercury, iron) and arsenic	Specific chelating agents: -Arsenic: Succimer, dimercaprol, penicillamine -Gold: Succimer, dimercaprol, penicillamine -Lead: EDTA, succimer, dimercaprol, penicillamine -Mercury: Succimer, dimercaprol
Heparin	Protamine sulfate, argatroban
Iron	Deferoxamine
Isoniazid	Pyridoxine (vitamin B6)
Methanol, ethylene glycol (antifreeze)	Fomepizole, ethanol
Methemoglobin inducers (eg, dapsone, local anesthetics, primaquine-type antimalarials, sulfonamides)	High-dose oxygen; IV methylene blue
Opioids	Naloxone
Salicylate	IV hydration and supplemental glucose; urine alkalization; sodium bicarbonate to correct acidemia; hemodialysis
Serotonin syndrome	Benzodiazepines for agitation or signs of stimulation; cyproheptadine (serotonin receptor antagonist) for severe cases
Sulfonylurea oral hypoglycemic drugs	Glucose, octreotide
Tricyclic antidepressants (eg, amitriptyline, doxepin, imipramine)	Hypertonic sodium bicarbonate (or hypertonic saline) for ventricular tachyarrhythmias associated with QRS prolongation.
tPA, streptokinase	Aminocaproic acid
Warfarin	FFP (immediate); Vitamin K (long-term)

10-12 Major Drug Reactions

Major Drug Side Effects by Organ System

Organ System	Drug	Side Effects
Cardiovascular	ACEIs	Cough, hyperkalemia, angioedema, rash, proteinuria, teratogenicity (renal agenesis)
	Acetazolamide	Hyperammonemia, metabolic acidosis, paresthesias
	Amiodarone	Pulmonary fibrosis, thyroid disease, hepatotoxicity (elevated LFTs), blue-gray skin discoloration, corneal deposits, bradycardia, AV block, QTc prolongation, peripheral neuropathy
	β-blockers	Asthma exacerbation, CHF, hypoglycemia, bradycardia, AV block, impotence, fatigue, depression
	Calcium channel blockers	Dihydropyridines (eg, nifedipine, amlodipine): Peripheral edema, worsening bradyarrhythmias Non-dihydropyridines (eg, verapamil, diltiazem): Constipation, ↓ cardiac output
	Clonidine	CNS depression, respiratory depression, severe rebound headache and hypertension
	Digoxin	Yellow-green visual changes, GI upset, arrhythmias (eg, SVT, junctional tachycardia)
	Furosemide	Ototoxicity, hypokalemia, gout, interstitial nephritis
	Hydrochlorothiazide	Hyponatremia, hypokalemia, hyperglycemia, hypercalcemia, hyperuricemia
	HMG-CoA reductase inhibitors (statins)	Myopathy (check CPK and LFTs)
	Hydralazine	Drug-induced lupus, tachycardia
	Methyldopa	Coombs ⊕ hemolytic anemia, drug-induced lupus
	Niacin	Cutaneous flushing
	Nitroglycerin	Hypotension, headache, tolerance
	Nitroprusside	Hypotension, cyanide toxicity
	Procainamide	Drug-induced lupus, QTc prolongation
	Quinidine	Cinchonism, QTc prolongation, arrhythmias (eg, torsades de pointes), thrombocytopenia
	Salicylates (aspirin)	Aspirin (high doses): Tinnitus, fever, nephrotoxicity, hyperventilation with respiratory alkalosis (early) and metabolic acidosis (late), dyspepsia, gastric ulcers, Reye syndrome in children
	Spironolactone	Hyperkalemia, gynecomastia
Gastroenterology	Bile acid sequestrants (eg, cholestyramine, colestipol, colesevelam)	GI upset, malabsorption of drugs and vitamins (esp. fat-soluble vitamins)
	Fibrates (eg, fenofibrate, gemfibrozil)	Myopathy, elevated LFTs, cholesterol gallstones
	Metoclopramide	Extrapyramidal syndrome, GI upset, hyperprolactinemia
	Proton pump inhibitors (eg, omeprazole)	Decreased Vitamin B_{12} levels (chronic), osteoporosis, acute interstitial nephritis
	5-HT3 antagonists (eg, ondansetron, granisetron)	QTc prolongation, elevated LFTs, GI upset, headaches, risk of serotonin syndrome
Hematology-Oncology	Anastrozole	Osteoporosis, bone fractures
	Bleomycin	Pulmonary fibrosis, myelosuppression
	Busulfan	Pulmonary fibrosis, myelosuppression
	Carboplatin, cisplatin	Nephrotoxicity, ototoxicity (acoustic nerve damage)
	Cyclophosphamide	Myelosuppression, myelodysplasia, hemorrhagic cystitis (prophylaxis with mesna), bladder carcinoma, GI upset, pulmonary fibrosis, hypogammaglobulinemia, opportunistic infections
	Doxorubicin	Cardiomyopathy, reddish urine discoloration
	Flutamide	GI upset, gynecomastia

(Continued)

10-12 Major Drug Reactions

Major Drug Side Effects by Organ System (Continued)

Organ System	Drug	Side Effects
Hematology-Oncology (cont.)	Tamoxifen	Increased risk of endometrial carcinoma (partial estrogen agonist), increased bone density, growth plate fusion
	Vinblastine	Peripheral neuropathy, neurotoxicity, severe myelosuppression
	Vincristine	Peripheral neuropathy, hair loss, paralytic ileus
Endocrinology	Corticosteroids	Cushingoid features, diabetes, hypertension, osteoporosis, myopathy, avascular necrosis of bone, cataracts, glaucoma, opportunistic infections, psychosis, pancreatitis
	Meglitinides (eg, repaglinide)	Hypoglycemia
	Metformin	GI upset, lactic acidosis (esp. in patients with renal insufficiency)
	Propylthiouracil	Pruritic rash, agranulocytosis, aplastic anemia, ANCA-associated vasculitis
	Sulfonylureas (eg, glipizide, glyburide)	Hypoglycemia, disulfiram effects, renal failure
	Thioglitazones (eg, pioglitazone, troglitazone, rosiglitazone)	Heart failure, hepatotoxicity, weight gain
Infectious diseases	Acyclovir	Crystalline nephropathy → acute renal failure
	Amantadine	Ataxia, livedo reticularis
	Aminoglycosides (eg, amikacin, gentamicin)	Nephrotoxicity (esp. when administered with other nephrotoxic agents such as vancomycin, NSAIDs, and cyclosporine), ototoxicity (esp. when administered with diuretics), neuromuscular blockade, teratogenicity
	Amphotericin	Febrile infusion reaction; renal tubular injury (accompanied by severe potassium and magnesium wasting, nephrogenic diabetes insipidus, and metabolic acidosis); potential cardiotoxicity leading to life-threatening arrhythmias; cytopenias
	Atovaquone	GI upset, rash
	Azoles (eg, fluconazole)	QTc prolongation, hepatotoxicity, extensive drug-drug interactions due to inhibition of cytochrome P450 system
	Cephalosporins	Hemolytic anemia. Cefepime is associated with neurotoxicity in elderly patients with renal insufficiency
	Carbapenems (eg, imipenem, meropenem)	Seizures, GI upset, CNS toxicity
	Chloramphenicol	Grey baby syndrome, aplastic anemia
	Dapsone	Methemoglobinemia, agranulocytosis, hemolytic anemia in G6PD deficiency
	Daptomycin	GI upset; rhabdomyolysis and creatine kinase elevations (obtain baseline CK level prior to initiation and then serial monitoring thereafter for duration of antibiotic therapy)
	Ethambutol	Optic neuropathy
	Fluoroquinolones (eg, ciprofloxacin, levofloxacin)	Tendinopathy (esp. Achilles tendon rupture in adults), QTc prolongation, rash, cartilage damage in children
	INH	Peripheral neuropathy (prevent with pyridoxine/vitamin B6), hepatotoxicity, anion gap metabolic acidosis, drug-induced lupus, seizures with toxic dose, hemolysis in G6PD deficiency, inhibition of cytochrome P450 enzymes
	Macrolides (eg, azithromycin)	QTc prolongation (obtain baseline EKG before administration), GI upset, hepatitis, cholestatic jaundice, pancreatitis
	Metronidazole	Disulfiram-like reaction, metallic taste, vestibular dysfunction
	Monobactams (eg, aztreonam)	GI upset
	Nitrofurantoin	Pulmonary fibrosis, hemolytic anemia in G6PD deficiency

(Continued)

10-12 Major Drug Reactions

Major Drug Side Effects by Organ System (Continued)

Organ System	Drug	Side Effects
Infectious diseases (cont.)	Lincosamides (eg, clindamycin)	Diarrhea (esp. *Clostridium difficile* colitis); rash
	Linezolid	GI upset, cytopenias, peripheral neuropathy, serotonin syndrome (esp. in patients taking SSRIs)
	Penicillins/β-lactams	Allergic and hypersensitivity reactions (eg, fever, rash, anaphylaxis), acute interstitial nephritis, hemolytic anemia
	Pentamidine	Nephrotoxicity, neutropenia, arrhythmias, pancreatitis, hepatotoxicity
	Primaquine	Methemoglobinemia, hemolytic anemia in G6PD deficiency
	Pyrazinamide	Hepatotoxicity, hyperuricemia
	Rifampin	Red-orange body secretions (benign), induction of cytochrome P450 enzymes
	Sulfonamides (eg, trimethoprim-sulfamethoxazole)	Hyperkalemia, cytopenias, megaloblastic anemia, hemolytic anemia in G6PD deficiency, rash (SJS/TEN)
	Tetracyclines (eg, doxycycline)	Teeth discoloration, photosensitivity, GI upset, Fanconi syndrome, pill esophagitis
	Trimethoprim	Megaloblastic anemia, neutropenia, hyperkalemia, elevated LFTs
	Vancomycin	Nephrotoxicity (esp. when used with other nephrotoxic agents such as piperacillin-tazobactam), infusion-related flushing ("red man syndrome", caused by histamine release and not a true allergy), ototoxicity, DRESS syndrome
	Zidovudine	Severe megaloblastic anemia, thrombocytopenia
Rheumatology	Azathioprine	GI upset, myelosuppression, hepatotoxicity, hypersensitivity, opportunistic infections
	Cyclosporine	Nephrotoxicity, neurotoxicity, opportunistic infection, gum hyperplasia
	Hydroxychloroquine	GI distress, retinopathy (requires routine ophthalmologic exam for long-term use), hemolysis in G6PD deficiency
	Methotrexate	Myelosuppression, megaloblastic anemia, GI upset, hepatotoxicity (leading to cirrhosis), mucositis/stomatitis, pneumonitis, pulmonary fibrosis
	Mycophenolate mofetil	Myelosuppression, GI upset, opportunistic infections
	Rituximab	Infusion reactions, HBV reactivation, progressive multifocal leuko-encephalopathy, mucocutaneous reactions, hypogammaglobulinemia, neutropenia, opportunistic infections
	Sulfasalazine	Acute megaloblastic anemia, SJS/TEN
Neurology	Carbamazepine	Agranulocytosis, aplastic anemia, rash (SJS/TEN), hepatotoxicity, autoinduction of the cytochrome P450 system
	Phenytoin	Horizontal nystagmus, cerebellar ataxia, diplopia, gingival hyperplasia, rash (SJS/TEN), folic acid deficiency, hirsutism, arrhythmia (in toxic doses), teratogenicity (limb and cardiac anomalies)
	Valproic acid	Teratogenicity (neural tube defects), tremor, weight gain, hepatotoxicity
Psychiatry	Antihistamines (eg, diphenhydramine)	Anticholinergic side effects (eye and oropharyngeal dryness, mydriasis, constipation, urinary retention) and antihistaminic side effects (drowsiness, confusion)
	1st-generation antipsychotics	Low potency (eg, chlorpromazine, thioridazine): Extrapyramidal syndrome, anticholinergic side effects, NMS, hyperprolactinemia, corneal (chlorpromazine) and retinal (thioridazine) deposits, gray-metallic skin and jaundice (chlorpromazine) High potency (eg, haloperidol, fluphenazine): Extrapyramidal syndrome, anticholinergic side effects, NMS, hyperprolactinemia, QTc prolongation
	2nd-generation antipsychotics (eg, clozapine, olanzapine, risperidone, quetiapine, aripiprazole, lurasidone)	Agranulocytosis (clozapine), metabolic syndrome (weight gain, diabetes, hyperlipidemia), extrapyramidal syndrome, anticholinergic side effects, QTc prolongation, hyperlipidemia (olanzapine), hyperprolactinemia (risperidone), cataracts (quetiapine)
	Barbiturates (eg, phenobarbital, thiopental)	Respiratory depression, induction of cytochrome P450 enzymes

(*Continued*)

10-12 Major Drug Reactions

Major Drug Side Effects by Organ System (Continued)

Organ System	Drug	Side Effects
Psychiatry (cont.)	Benzodiazepines (eg, diazepam, lorazepam)	Sedation, dependence, tolerance, respiratory depression
	Bupropion	Lowers seizure threshold, headache, tachycardia, NO sexual dysfunction (unlike many other psychiatric medications)
	Lithium	Nephrogenic diabetes insipidus, hypothyroidism, seizures, tremor, ataxia, teratogenicity (Ebstein anomaly)
	MAOIs (eg, Isocarboxazid, phenelzine, tranylcypromine)	Hypertensive crisis with tyramine consumption (eg, wine and cheese), serotonin syndrome (if taken with TCAs, SNRIs, SSRIs)
	SNRIs (eg, venlafaxine, duloxetine)	↑ BP and stimulant effects (most common), sedation (less common), GI upset
	SSRIs (eg, escitalopram fluoxetine, sertraline)	GI upset, sexual dysfunction, serotonin syndrome (if taken with MAOIs, TCAs, SNRIs), SIADH
	TCAs (eg, amitryptyline, imipramine)	Anticholinergic effects, coma, seizures, cardiotoxicity (QTc prolongation, arrhythmias)
	Traza**done**	Priapism ("Traza**BONE**")
Anesthesiology	Halothane	Hepatotoxicity, malignant hyperthermia
	Ketamine	Hallucinations, nystagmus, disorientation, laryngospasm
	Lidocaine	Seizures, cardiotoxicity (heart block, bradycardia)
	Propofol	Hypotension
	Rocuronium	Tachycardia, respiratory depression
	Succinylcholine	Malignant hyperthermia, hyperkalemia
Urology	Prazosin	Hypotension, priapism
	Sildenafil	Hypotension (esp. in combination with nitrates), ischemic optic neuropathy
Toxicology	Isopropyl alcohol	Altered mental status, coma, diabetic ketoacidosis ("fruity breath")
	Ethylene glycol	Altered mental status, hallucinations, seizures, calcium oxalate deposition in the kidneys, hypocalcemia (leading to tetany), sweet smelling breath
	Methanol	GI upset, CNS depression, optic neuropathy, anion-gap metabolic acidosis

10-12 Major Drug Reactions

Common Drug Interactions and Reactions

Interaction/Reaction	Drugs
Cytochrome P450 inducers (↓ warfarin efficacy)	Antimicrobials: Rifampin, griseofulvin Anti-epileptics: Carbamazepine, barbiturates, phenytoin Miscellaneous: Sulfonylureas, OCPs, St. John's wort, ginseng, green vegetables, alcohol (chronic)
Cytochrome P450 inhibitors (↑ warfarin efficacy)	Antimicrobials: INH, macrolides except azithromycin (erythromycin), metronidazole, ketoconazole, fluconazole, chloramphenicol Cardiac: Amiodarone, quinidine Miscellaneous: Valproic acid, SSRIs (eg, duloxetine), sulfonamides, thyroid hormone, omeprazole, cimetidine, acetaminophen, NSAIDs, cranberry juice, grapefruit juice, Vitamin E, *Ginkgo biloba,* alcohol (acute)
Cytochrome P450 substrates	Cardiac: β-blockers, calcium channel blockers, warfarin, quinidine Anti-epileptics: Phenytoin, carbamazepine, barbiturates, benzodiazepines Miscellaneous: Amide anesthetics (eg, lidocaine, bupivacaine, ropivacaine), statins, theophylline, OCPs, corticosteroids, TCAs
Competition for albumin-binding sites	Warfarin, phenytoin, salicylates (aspirin), sulphonamides
Dilated cardiomyopathy	**D**oxorubicin, **D**aunorubicin, Trastuzumab
Torsades de pointes	Class IA antiarrhythmics (procainamide, disopyramide, quinidine), Class III antiarrhythmics (amiodarone, sotalol), lithium, chloroquine, azithromycin, clarithromycin, antipsychotics (haloperidol, thioridazine, ziprasidone)
Increased risk of digoxin toxicity	Amiodarone, calcium channel blockers, quinidine
Pulmonary fibrosis	Amiodarone, hydralazine, tocainide, bleomycin, busulfan, methotrexate, cyclophosphamide
Hepatic necrosis	Halothane, valproic acid, carbon tetrachloride, acetaminophen toxicity, *Amanita phalloides*
Hepatitis	INH, phenytoin, methyldopa
Interstitial nephritis	NSAIDs, acetaminophen, furosemide, allopurinol
Hemorrhagic cystitis	Cyclophosphamide, ifosfamide (prevent with mesna)
Megaloblastic anemia	Phenytoin, methotrexate, sulfonamides, cytosine arabinoside, 6-mercaptopurine
Aplastic anemia	NSAIDs, carbamazepine, phenytoin, chloramphenicol, propylthiouracil, methimazole, benzene
Hemolysis in G6PD deficiency	INH, aspirin, nitrofurantoin, dapsone, sulfonamides, primaquine, chloroquine, pyrimethamine, methylene blue
Agranulocytosis	Clozapine, carbamazepine, cephalosporins, dapsone, colchicine, propylthiouracil, methimazole
Stevens-Johnson syndrome	Lamotrigine, ethosuximide, carbamazepine, phenytoin, phenobarbital, sulfonamides, penicillins, fluoroquinolones, furosemide, allopurinol
Photosensitivity	Amiodarone, sulfonamides, tetracyclines, fluoroquinolones
Gingival hyperplasia	Phenytoin, lamotrigine, valproic acid, tacrolimus, topiramate, phenobarbitone, primidone, nifedipine
Hypothyroidism	Amiodarone, lithium
Gynecomastia	Spironolactone, kétoconazole, cimetidine, clomiphene, busulfan, vincristine, estrogens, finasteride
Gout	Furosemide, thiazides, levodopa
Osteoporosis	Corticosteroids, proton pump inhibitors, lithium
Drug-induced lupus	Hydralazine, procainamide, INH, phenytoin, carbamazepine
Disulfiram-like reaction	Metronidazole, sulfonylurea
Ototoxicity	Aminoglycosides (neomycin), loop diuretics (furosemide, bumetanide, ethacrynate), cisplatin

10-13 Spinal Cord Trauma

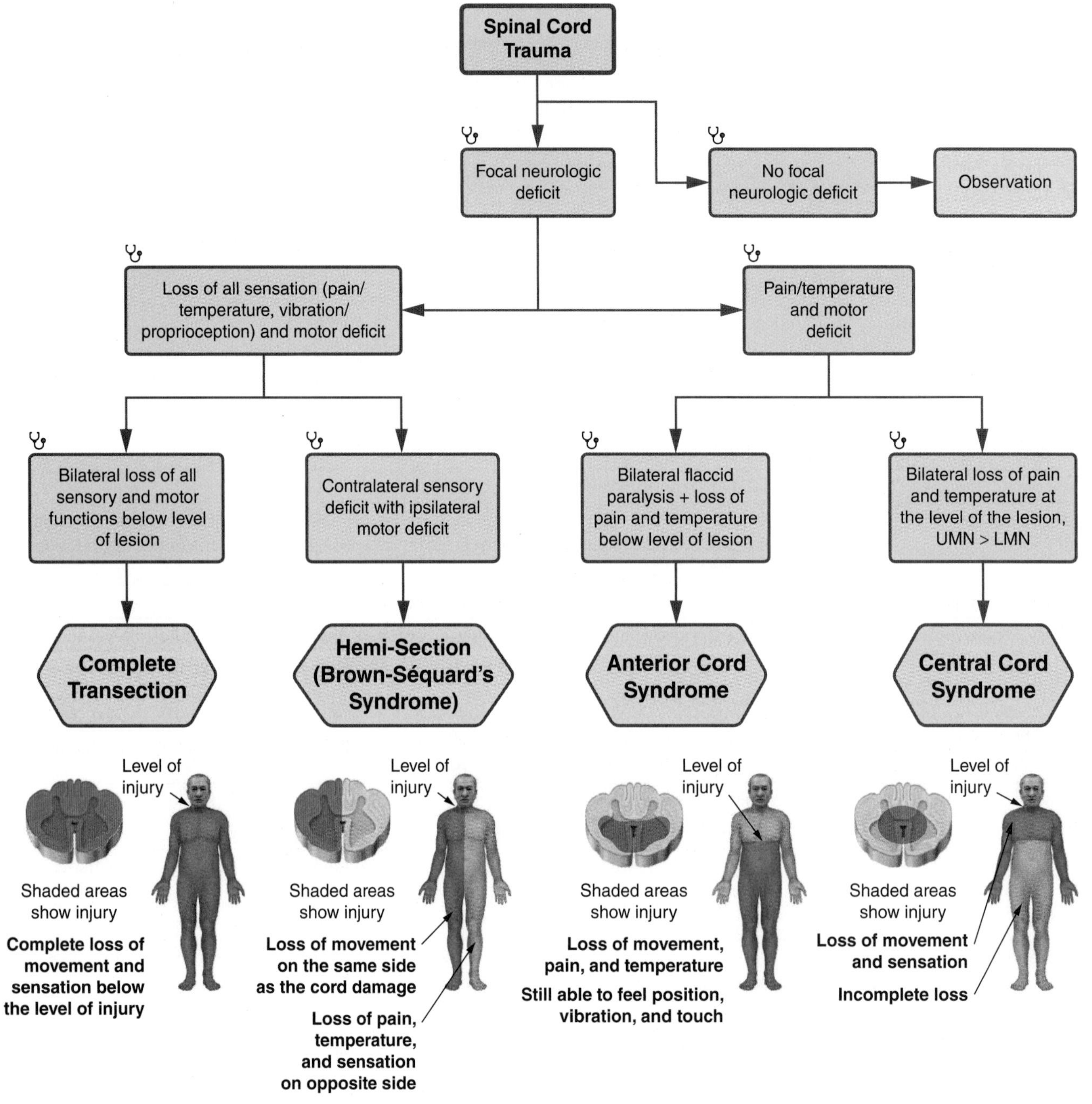
Spinal Cord Trauma
Focal neurologic deficit
No focal neurologic deficit
Observation
Loss of all sensation (pain/temperature, vibration/proprioception) and motor deficit
Pain/temperature and motor deficit
Bilateral loss of all sensory and motor functions below level of lesion
Contralateral sensory deficit with ipsilateral motor deficit
Bilateral flaccid paralysis + loss of pain and temperature below level of lesion
Bilateral loss of pain and temperature at the level of the lesion, UMN > LMN
Complete Transection
Hemi-Section (Brown-Séquard's Syndrome)
Anterior Cord Syndrome
Central Cord Syndrome
Level of injury
Shaded areas show injury
Complete loss of movement and sensation below the level of injury
Level of injury
Shaded areas show injury
Loss of movement on the same side as the cord damage
Loss of pain, temperature, and sensation on opposite side
Level of injury
Shaded areas show injury
Loss of movement, pain, and temperature
Still able to feel position, vibration, and touch
Level of injury
Shaded areas show injury
Loss of movement and sensation
Incomplete loss

Figure 10.13.1

FIGURE 10.13

10-13 Spinal Cord Trauma

COMPLETE SPINAL CORD TRANSECTION

A patient after a motor vehicle collision presents with complete loss of all sensation and movement below a certain spinal cord level.

Management:

1. Irreversible, but give IV steroids to reduce complications.

Complications: Permanent focal deficits.

HYF: At the level of the lesion, there will be bilateral LMN signs. Below the level of the lesion, there will be bilateral UMN signs.

HEMI-SECTION OF SPINAL CORD (BROWN-SÉQUARD'S SYNDROME)

A patient presents with stab wound to the back. On exam, he has hemipsilateral hemiparesis; ipsilateral diminished proprioception, vibration, and light touch; and contralateral diminished pain and temperature sensation.

Management:

1. Irreversible, but give IV steroids to reduce complications.

Complications: Permanent focal deficits.

HYF:

- At the level of the lesion, there is ipsilateral loss of all sensation and LMN signs (eg, flaccid paresis). Below the level of the lesion, there are ispilateral UMN signs (corticospinal tract) and ipsilateral loss of proprioception, vibration, and light 2-point touch (dorsal column). Two levels below the lesion, there is contralateral loss of pain, temperature, and crude non-discriminative touch (lateral spinothalamic tract).
- If lesion occurs above T1, patient may present with ipsilateral Horner's syndrome (ptosis, miosis, anhidrosis) due to damage of the oculosympathetic pathway.

ANTERIOR CORD SYNDROME

A patient presents after a motor vehicle collision with weakness and sensory deficits. On exam, he has complete paralysis and diminished bilateral pain and temperature sensation below a certain spinal cord level. He has intact bilateral proprioception, vibration, and light touch.

Management:

1. Stat spine MRI to assess the extent of neurological damage.
2. Decompressive surgery to regain neurological function but likely irreversible.

Complications:

- Permanent focal deficits.
- Bowel/bladder dysfunction (eg, urinary retention).

HYF:

- Usually due to injury of anterior spinal artery (classically the artery of Adamkiewicz) due to aortic surgery, descending aortic dissection, or vertebral burst fracture, which infarcts the anterior 2/3rds of the spinal cord. Proprioception and vibratory sense are preserved as they are on the posterior 1/3 of the spinal cord.
- Risk of anterior spinal cord ischemia is greatest at T10–T12 levels, where blood flow is lowest.
- At the level of the lesion, there is bilateral hemiparesis. Below the level of the lesion, there are bilateral hemiparesis and diminished bilateral pain and temperature sensation (lateral spinothalamic tract).
- Bilateral proprioception, vibration, and light touch (dorsal column) remain intact because they receive blood flow from the posterior spinal arteries arising from the vertebral artery PICA.
- Patients initially present with flaccid paresis due to spinal shock. UMN signs such as spastic paresis and hyperreflexia subsequently develop over days to weeks.

POSTERIOR/DORSAL CORD SYNDROME

A patient presents after direct fall on the neck with weakness and sensory deficits. On exam, he has loss of proprioception and vibration sensation, ataxic gait, positive Romberg sign, hypotonia, and abolition of deep tendon reflexes.

Management:

1. Irreversible, but give IV steroids to reduce complications.

Complications: Permanent focal deficits.

HYF: Classically associated with trauma (neck hyperflexion), vitamin B_{12} deficiency, or syphilis. Can also be caused by occlusion of spinal arteries, tumors, disc compression, or multiple sclerosis.

SPINAL CORD COMPRESSION (CERVICAL SPONDYLOTIC MYELOPATHY)

A patient presents with a focal neurologic deficit and is found to have a tumor compressing on the spinal cord on **imaging**.

Management:

1. Relieve compressing mass if possible.
2. IV steroids to reduce long-term complications.

Complications: Permanent focal deficits.

HYF: Classically associated with a mass compressing the spinal cord. Can also be caused by trauma applying pressure to the spinal cord. Because any mass or traumatic pressure can cause spinal cord compression, it can present with a diverse array of focal neurologic deficits.

(Continued)

10-13 Spinal Cord Trauma

CENTRAL CORD SYNDROME

An elderly patient with PMH of cervical spondylotic myelopathy presents after he hyperextended his neck during a rear-end motor vehicle collision. On exam, he has bilateral weakness and loss of pain and temperature sensation predominantly in the arms compared to his legs.

Management:

1. Irreversible, but give IV steroids to reduce complications.

Complications:

- Permanent focal deficits.
- Associated with bladder dysfunction.

HYF: Classically associated with a syrinx (cystic cavity expanding with the central canal) or trauma (hyperextension of neck in an elderly patient with pre-existing cervical spine disease, usually due to rear-end collision or fall).

11
Surgery: Pre- & Post-Op Care

11-1 Post-Op Abdominal Distention

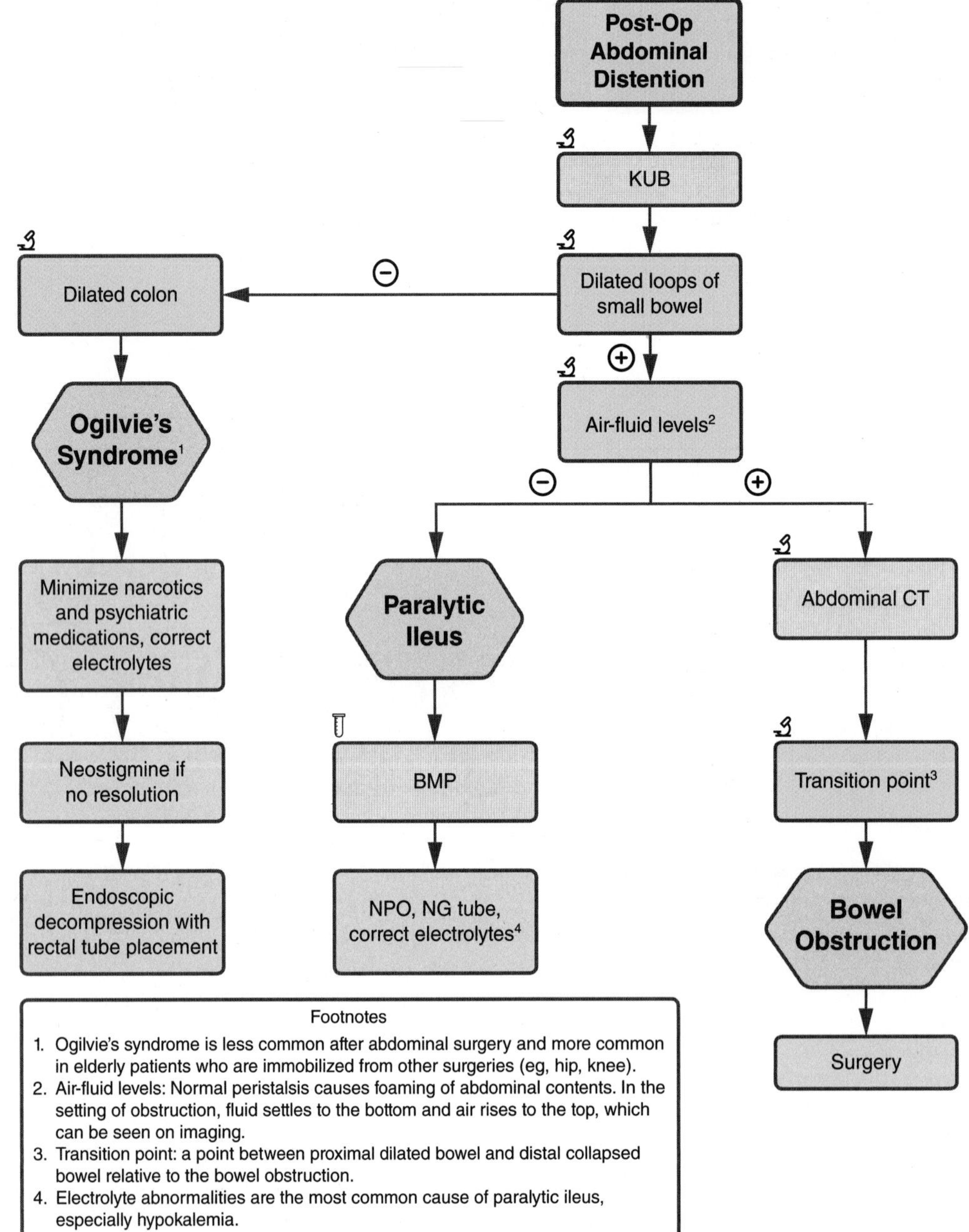
Post-Op Abdominal Distention
KUB
Dilated loops of small bowel
Dilated colon
Ogilvie's Syndrome[1]
Minimize narcotics and psychiatric medications, correct electrolytes
Neostigmine if no resolution
Endoscopic decompression with rectal tube placement
Air-fluid levels[2]
Paralytic Ileus
BMP
NPO, NG tube, correct electrolytes[4]
Abdominal CT
Transition point[3]
Bowel Obstruction
Surgery

Footnotes

1. Ogilvie's syndrome is less common after abdominal surgery and more common in elderly patients who are immobilized from other surgeries (eg, hip, knee).
2. Air-fluid levels: Normal peristalsis causes foaming of abdominal contents. In the setting of obstruction, fluid settles to the bottom and air rises to the top, which can be seen on imaging.
3. Transition point: a point between proximal dilated bowel and distal collapsed bowel relative to the bowel obstruction.
4. Electrolyte abnormalities are the most common cause of paralytic ileus, especially hypokalemia.

FIGURE 11.1

11-1 Post-Op Abdominal Distention

OGILVIE'S SYNDROME (COLONIC PSEUDO-OBSTRUCTION)

An 82-year-old M with PMH of diabetes, chronic kidney disease, atherosclerosis, coronary artery disease, and arthritis of the right hip is 2 days post-op from a right hip replacement. Today, he is complaining of progressive abdominal pain for the last 12 hours. He denies nausea, vomiting, flatus, fevers, chills, and radiation of the pain to the back. On **labs**, his CMP is significant for hypokalemia, hypomagnesemia, and hypocalcemia. On **imaging**, abdominal XR shows distention of the entire colon with small bowel decompression.

Management:

1. Abdominal X-ray: Screening test and used for serial monitoring. In this clinical situation, it can show massive colonic dilation with greatest diameter in the cecum.
2. Discontinue medications that inhibit bowel function (eg, narcotics, anticholinergic medications).
3. 1st line: Order a basic metabolic panel to assess electrolytes and treat with IV fluids, electrolyte repletion, and nasogastric tube for decompression.
4. 2nd line: Neostigmine if no resolution with 48 hours of conservative care.
5. 3rd line: Colonic decompression via rectal tube.

Complications: Risk of intestinal perforation with prolonged dilation.

HYF: Ogilvie's syndrome involves acute dilation of the large intestine (most commonly the cecum and right colon) without an associated mechanical obstruction, possibly due to autonomic nervous system dysfunction. Most often occurs in the elderly with the following risk factors: Narcotics or anticholinergic medications, recent surgery, infection, or malignancy.

PARALYTIC ILEUS

A 56-year-old F with PMH of perforated diverticulitis is now 2 days post-op. She initially was doing well but now complains of generalized abdominal pain and nausea. She denies fevers, chills, flatulence, and emesis. On **exam**, her abdomen is diffusely tender and tympanic. On **labs**, her electrolytes are within normal limits except for hypomagnesemia. On **imaging**, abdominal XR shows dilated loops of small bowel throughout without air-fluid levels.

Management:

1. Abdominal XR is the best initial test and will show dilated loops of small bowel throughout.
2. Correct electrolyte derangements.
3. Consider parenteral nutrition if patient is expected to be NPO for a prolonged period of time.

Complications: Patients with ileus are at risk of aspiration due to backup of gastrointestinal fluid. If the patient is getting increasingly nauseated and distended, treat with a nasogastric tube (NGT).

HYF: Return of bowel function is promoted by activity; thus patient ambulation should be encouraged.

BOWEL OBSTRUCTION

A 77-year-old M with PMH of diabetes, colon cancer, and multiple exploratory laparotomies presents with progressive abdominal pain, nausea, and vomiting over the past 48 hours. On **exam**, he is diffusely tender without rebound or guarding. His **labs** are notable for hypochloremia. On **imaging**, KUB shows air-fluid levels with a transition point in the colon.

Management:

1. Abdominal XR is the best initial screening test and will reveal air-fluid levels +/– dilated loops of bowel with a transition point.
2. Abdominal CT with contrast is the best test to characterize a bowel obstruction.
3. Small bowel obstructions can be managed conservatively at first with oral Gastrografin and serial abdominal XRs to track the contrast through the small bowel to the colon. If the contrast reaches the colon in the first 24 hours, the obstruction is likely to resolve on its own.
4. Small bowel obstructions that do not resolve with conservative management and large bowel obstructions are managed surgically.
5. Early post-operative small bowel obstruction is typically managed non-operatively for longer than a small bowel obstruction unrelated to recent surgery.
6. Patients who present with peritonitis or concerning labs or vital signs should undergo urgent surgical exploration.

Complications: Bowel necrosis. Bowel perforation. Peritonitis.

HYF: Adhesions are the most common cause of bowel obstruction. A history of prior abdominal surgeries is suggestive of this etiology.

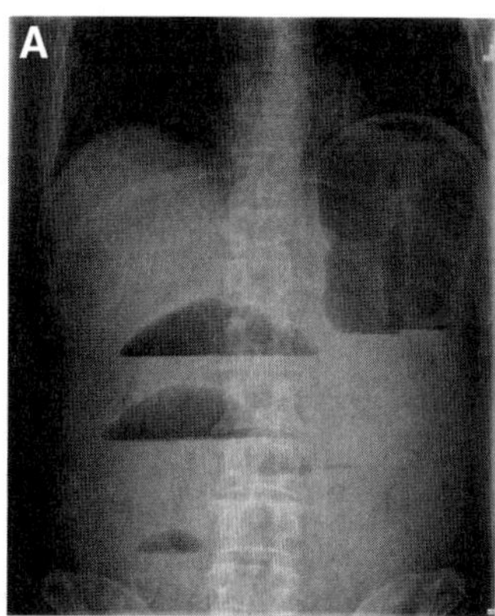
A

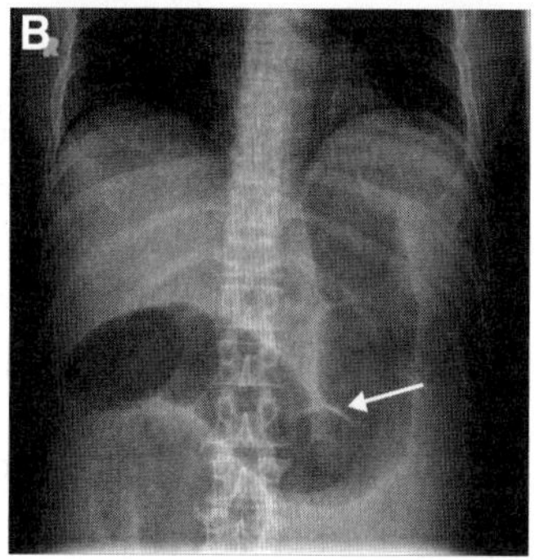
B

Bowel obstruction with air-fluid levels and a dilated portion of colon with transition point to decompressed bowel.

11-2 Peri-Op Chest Pain

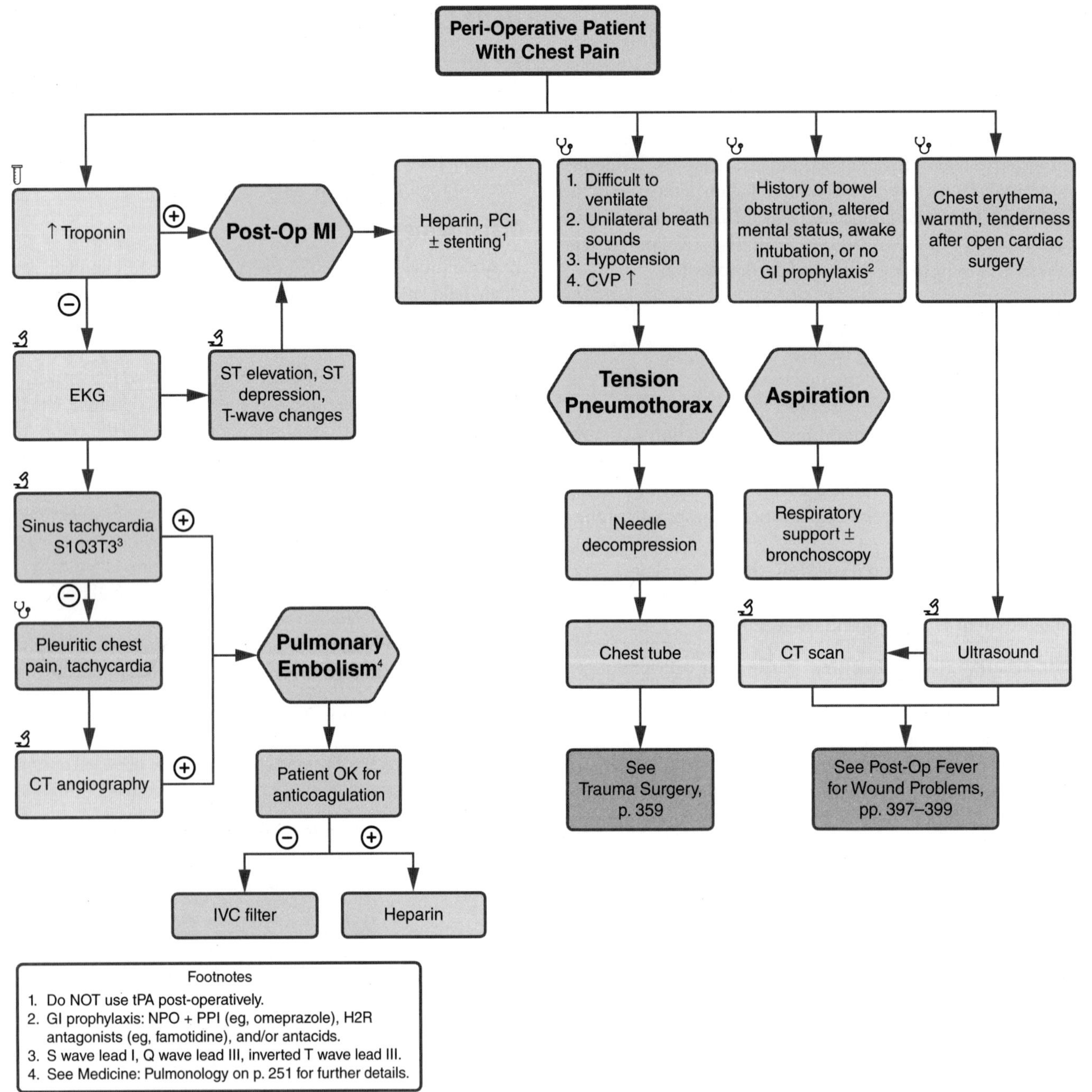
Peri-Operative Patient With Chest Pain
↑ Troponin
Post-Op MI
Heparin, PCI ± stenting[1]
1. Difficult to ventilate
2. Unilateral breath sounds
3. Hypotension
4. CVP ↑
History of bowel obstruction, altered mental status, awake intubation, or no GI prophylaxis[2]
Chest erythema, warmth, tenderness after open cardiac surgery
EKG
ST elevation, ST depression, T-wave changes
Tension Pneumothorax
Aspiration
Sinus tachycardia S1Q3T3[3]
Needle decompression
Respiratory support ± bronchoscopy
Pleuritic chest pain, tachycardia
Pulmonary Embolism[4]
Chest tube
CT scan
Ultrasound
CT angiography
Patient OK for anticoagulation
See Trauma Surgery, p. 359
See Post-Op Fever for Wound Problems, pp. 397–399
IVC filter
Heparin

Footnotes

1. Do NOT use tPA post-operatively.
2. GI prophylaxis: NPO + PPI (eg, omeprazole), H2R antagonists (eg, famotidine), and/or antacids.
3. S wave lead I, Q wave lead III, inverted T wave lead III.
4. See Medicine: Pulmonology on p. 251 for further details.

FIGURE 11.2

11-3 Post-Op Fever

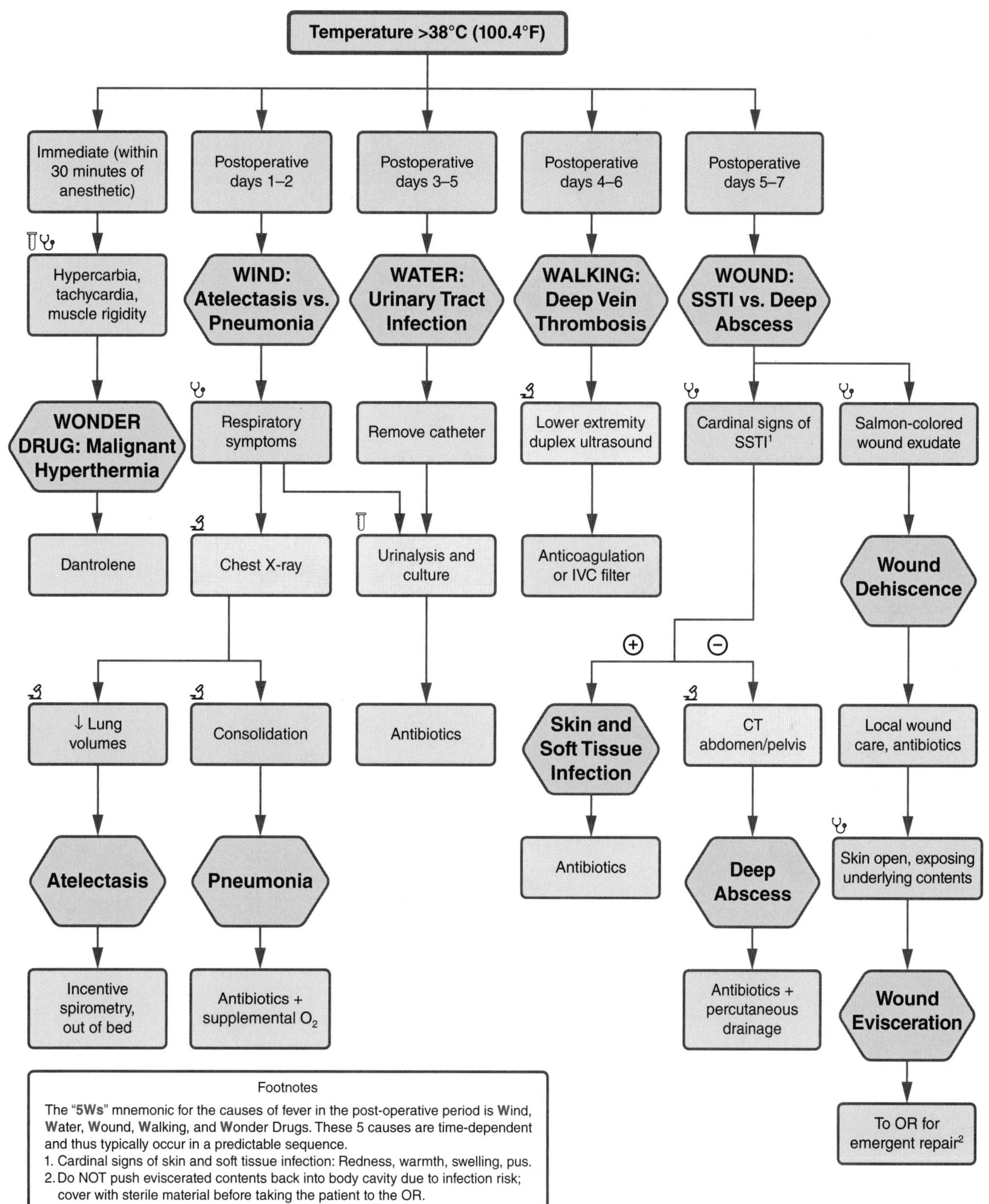
Temperature >38°C (100.4°F)
Immediate (within 30 minutes of anesthetic)
Postoperative days 1–2
Postoperative days 3–5
Postoperative days 4–6
Postoperative days 5–7
Hypercarbia, tachycardia, muscle rigidity
WIND: Atelectasis vs. Pneumonia
WATER: Urinary Tract Infection
WALKING: Deep Vein Thrombosis
WOUND: SSTI vs. Deep Abscess
WONDER DRUG: Malignant Hyperthermia
Respiratory symptoms
Remove catheter
Lower extremity duplex ultrasound
Cardinal signs of SSTI[1]
Salmon-colored wound exudate
Dantrolene
Chest X-ray
Urinalysis and culture
Anticoagulation or IVC filter
Wound Dehiscence
⊕
⊖
↓ Lung volumes
Consolidation
Antibiotics
Skin and Soft Tissue Infection
CT abdomen/pelvis
Local wound care, antibiotics
Atelectasis
Pneumonia
Antibiotics
Deep Abscess
Skin open, exposing underlying contents
Incentive spirometry, out of bed
Antibiotics + supplemental O_2
Antibiotics + percutaneous drainage
Wound Evisceration
To OR for emergent repair[2]

Footnotes

The "**5Ws**" mnemonic for the causes of fever in the post-operative period is **W**ind, **W**ater, **W**ound, **W**alking, and **W**onder Drugs. These 5 causes are time-dependent and thus typically occur in a predictable sequence.

1. Cardinal signs of skin and soft tissue infection: Redness, warmth, swelling, pus.
2. Do NOT push eviscerated contents back into body cavity due to infection risk; cover with sterile material before taking the patient to the OR.

FIGURE 11.3

11-3 Post-Op Fever

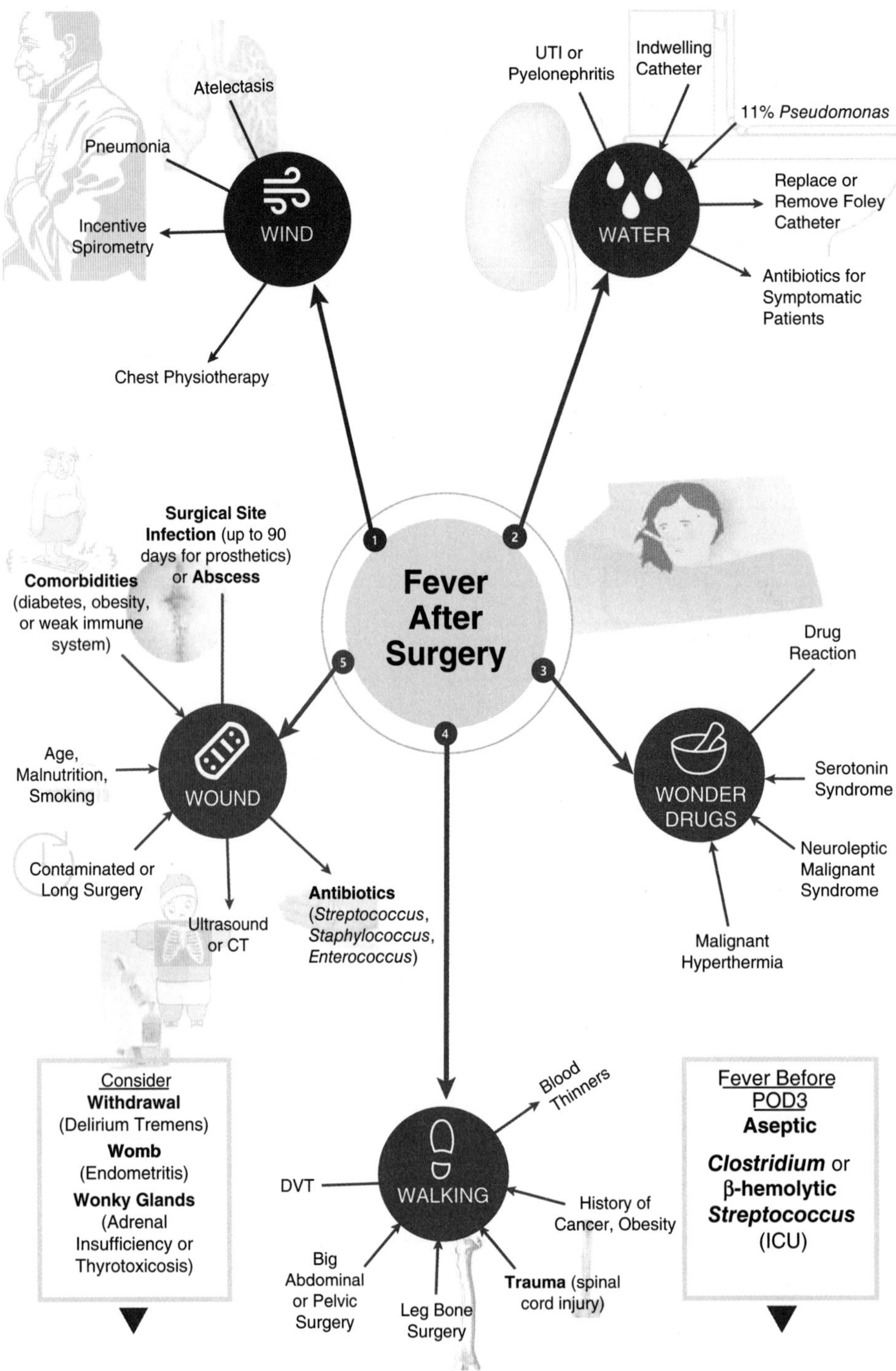
Fever After Surgery
WIND
Atelectasis
Pneumonia
Incentive Spirometry
Chest Physiotherapy
WATER
UTI or Pyelonephritis
Indwelling Catheter
11% Pseudomonas
Replace or Remove Foley Catheter
Antibiotics for Symptomatic Patients
WONDER DRUGS
Drug Reaction
Serotonin Syndrome
Neuroleptic Malignant Syndrome
Malignant Hyperthermia
WALKING
Blood Thinners
DVT
History of Cancer, Obesity
Big Abdominal or Pelvic Surgery
Leg Bone Surgery
Trauma (spinal cord injury)
WOUND
Surgical Site Infection (up to 90 days for prosthetics) or Abscess
Comorbidities (diabetes, obesity, or weak immune system)
Age, Malnutrition, Smoking
Contaminated or Long Surgery
Ultrasound or CT
Antibiotics (Streptococcus, Staphylococcus, Enterococcus)
Consider
Withdrawal (Delirium Tremens)
Womb (Endometritis)
Wonky Glands (Adrenal Insufficiency or Thyrotoxicosis)
Fever Before POD3
Aseptic
Clostridium or β-hemolytic Streptococcus (ICU)

Infographic: Postoperative fever.

11-3 Post-Op Fever

MALIGNANT HYPERTHERMIA

A 15-year-old M undergoing appendectomy develops increasing temperature, acidosis, and muscle rigidity 20 minutes after administration of succinylcholine.

Management:

1. Pause surgery and discontinue the triggering agent.
2. Administer IV dantrolene.
3. Cool patients with core temperature >39°C.

Complications:

- Rhabdomyolysis.
- Disseminated intravascular coagulation.

HYF: Causes include succinylcholine and volatile anesthetics. Associated with genetic mutations in the ryanodine receptor.

ATELECTASIS

A 45-year-old F with PMH of Crohn's disease on postoperative day 1 from small bowel resection presents with fever of 38.1°C and SpO_2 95%.

Management:

1. Supplemental oxygen to maintain SpO_2 >90%.
2. Incentive spirometry.

Complications: Pneumonia.

HYF: Most mild cases will self-resolve. For further details, see Pulmonology, p. 251.

PNEUMONIA

A 51-year-old M with PMH of recently diagnosed colon cancer on postoperative day 2 from partial colectomy presents with fever of 38.5°C and SpO_2 92%. He is found to have leukocytosis on **labs**. On **imaging**, CXR shows a right middle lobe infiltrate.

Management:

1. Supplemental oxygen.
2. Antibiotics.

Complications:

- Bacteremia and sepsis.
- Respiratory failure.

HYF: Pneumonia can be due to aspiration during intubation or associated with ventilator use if the patient remains intubated.

URINARY TRACT INFECTION

A 62-year-old F with PMH of hepatocellular carcinoma on postoperative day 3 from open hepatectomy presents with fever of 38.5°C. On **labs**, urinalysis performed after removal of her indwelling catheter shows 2+ nitrite and 2+ leukocyte esterase.

Management:

1. Remove catheter if possible.
2. Antibiotics.

Complications:

- Pyelonephritis.
- Acute renal failure.
- Bacteremia and sepsis.

HYF: *E. coli* and *Candida* species are common causes. For further details, see Infectious Diseases, p. 163.

DEEP VEIN THROMBOSIS

A 74-year-old F on postoperative day 5 from ventral hernia repair presents with fever of 38.2°C and right calf tenderness.

Management:

1. Lower extremity duplex ultrasound.
2. Anticoagulation or IVC filter, depending on patient's bleeding risk and comorbidities.

Complications: Pulmonary embolism.

HYF: Virchow's triad: Stasis, endothelial injury, hypercoagulability.

SKIN AND SOFT TISSUE INFECTION

A 67-year-old M on postoperative day 6 from exploratory laparotomy presents with fever of 38.6°C, leukocytosis, and yellow drainage from his surgical incision.

Management:

1. Drain and debride wound.
2. Antibiotics.

Complications:

- Fascial dehiscence.
- Bacteremia and sepsis.

HYF: Common bacterial culprits include *Staphylococcus*, *Streptococcus*, and *Pseudomonas.*

INTRA-ABDOMINAL ABSCESS

A 67-year-old M on postoperative day 6 from exploratory laparotomy presents with fever of 38.6°C. He is found to have leukocytosis on **labs**. On **imaging**, CT abdomen/pelvis reveals a deep intra-abdominal abscess.

Management:

1. Antibiotics.
2. Percutaneous drainage.

Complications: Bacteremia and sepsis.

HYF: *E. coli* is the most common bacterial cause.

11-4 Post-Op Altered Mental Status

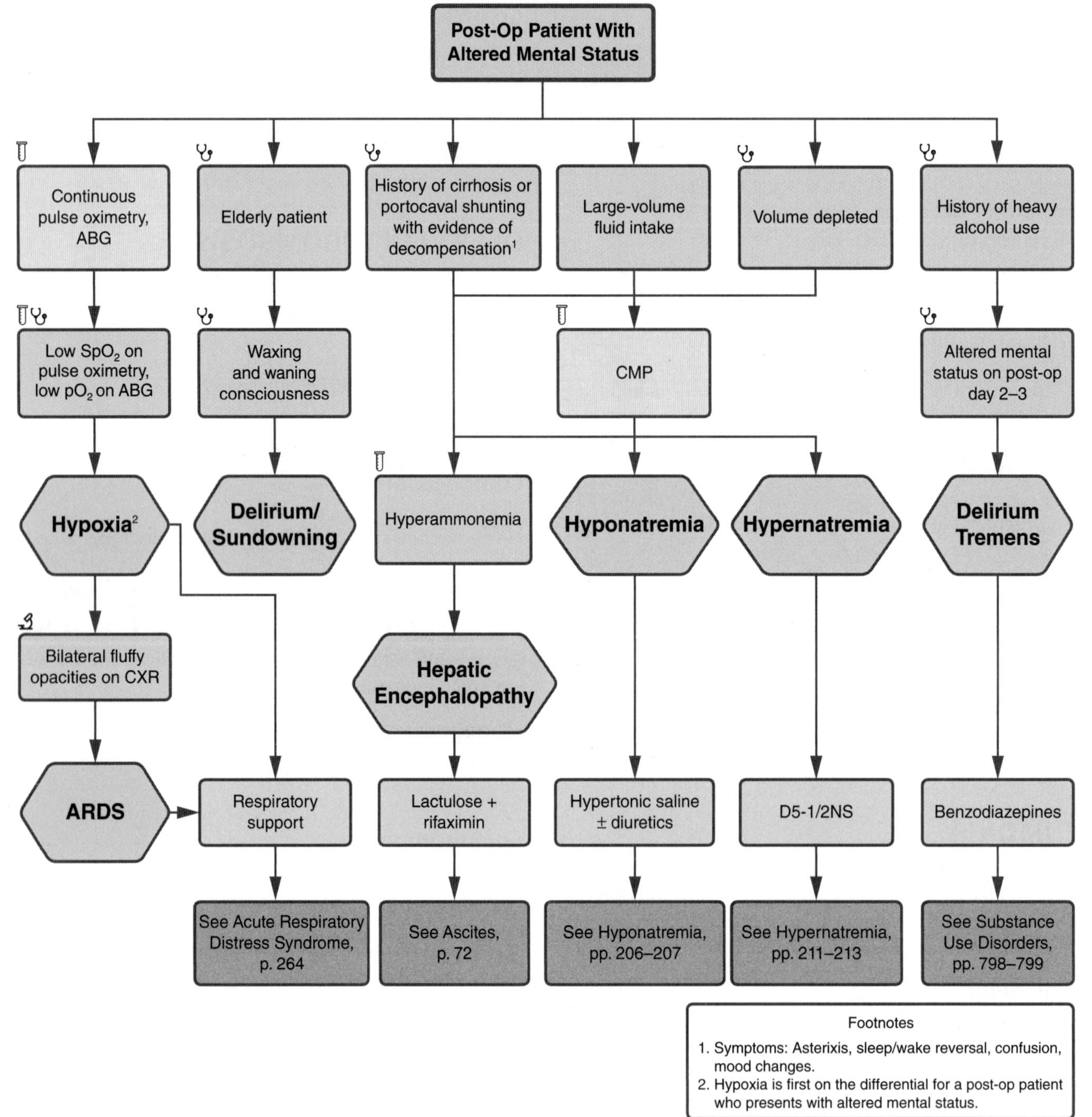

Post-Op Patient With Altered Mental Status
Continuous pulse oximetry, ABG
Elderly patient
History of cirrhosis or portocaval shunting with evidence of decompensation[1]
Large-volume fluid intake
Volume depleted
History of heavy alcohol use
Low SpO_2 on pulse oximetry, low pO_2 on ABG
Waxing and waning consciousness
CMP
Altered mental status on post-op day 2–3
Hypoxia[2]
Delirium/ Sundowning
Hyperammonemia
Hyponatremia
Hypernatremia
Delirium Tremens
Bilateral fluffy opacities on CXR
Hepatic Encephalopathy
ARDS
Respiratory support
Lactulose + rifaximin
Hypertonic saline ± diuretics
D5-1/2NS
Benzodiazepines
See Acute Respiratory Distress Syndrome, p. 264
See Ascites, p. 72
See Hyponatremia, pp. 206–207
See Hypernatremia, pp. 211–213
See Substance Use Disorders, pp. 798–799
Footnotes
1. Symptoms: Asterixis, sleep/wake reversal, confusion, mood changes.
2. Hypoxia is first on the differential for a post-op patient who presents with altered mental status.

FIGURE 11.4

12 Surgery: Gastrointestinal

12-1 Esophagus

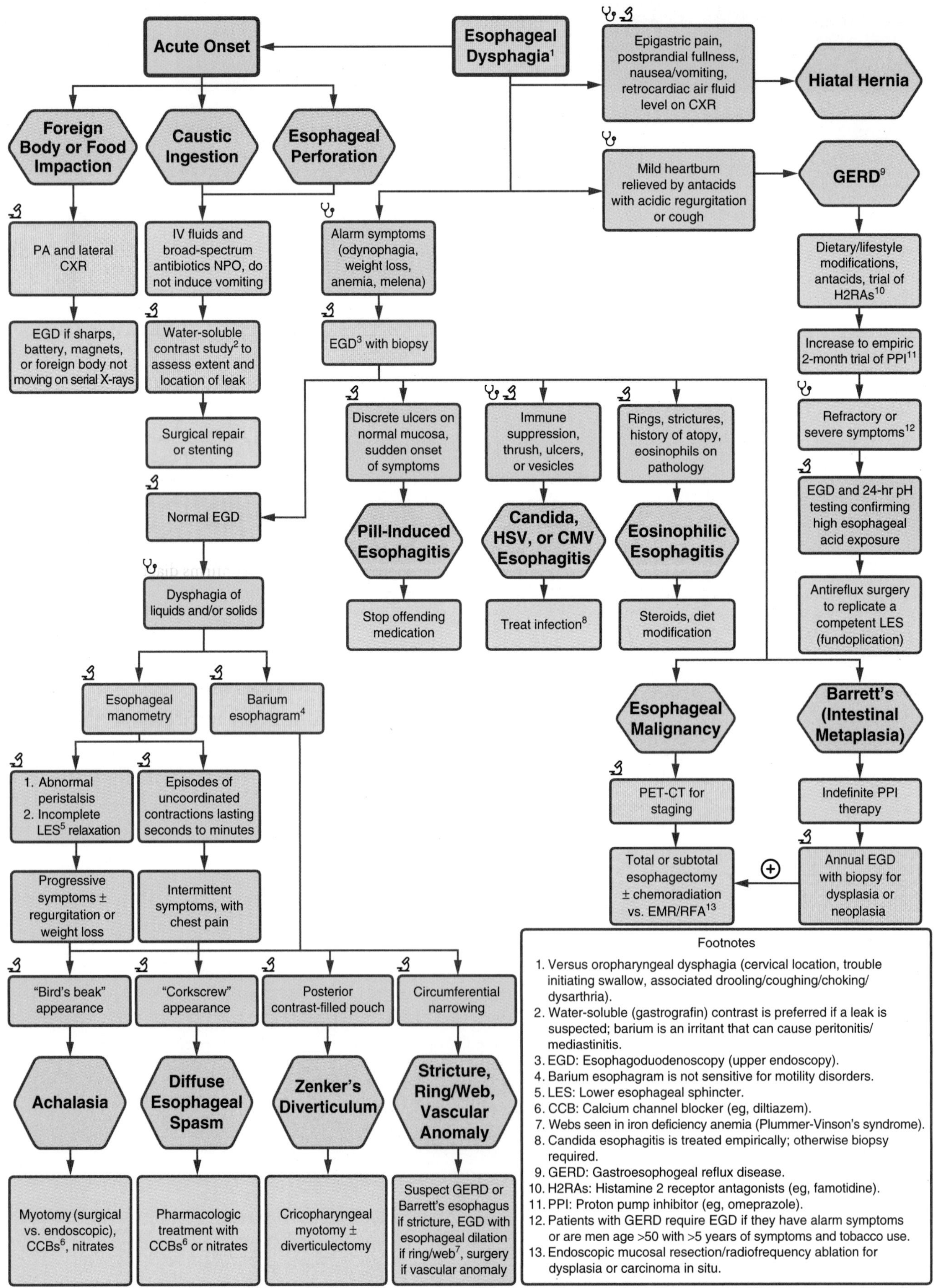

Acute Onset
Esophageal Dysphagia[1]
Epigastric pain, postprandial fullness, nausea/vomiting, retrocardiac air fluid level on CXR
Hiatal Hernia
Mild heartburn relieved by antacids with acidic regurgitation or cough
GERD[9]
Foreign Body or Food Impaction
Caustic Ingestion
Esophageal Perforation
PA and lateral CXR
IV fluids and broad-spectrum antibiotics NPO, do not induce vomiting
Alarm symptoms (odynophagia, weight loss, anemia, melena)
Dietary/lifestyle modifications, antacids, trial of H2RAs[10]
EGD if sharps, battery, magnets, or foreign body not moving on serial X-rays
Water-soluble contrast study[2] to assess extent and location of leak
EGD[3] with biopsy
Increase to empiric 2-month trial of PPI[11]
Surgical repair or stenting
Discrete ulcers on normal mucosa, sudden onset of symptoms
Immune suppression, thrush, ulcers, or vesicles
Rings, strictures, history of atopy, eosinophils on pathology
Refractory or severe symptoms[12]
EGD and 24-hr pH testing confirming high esophageal acid exposure
Normal EGD
Pill-Induced Esophagitis
Candida, HSV, or CMV Esophagitis
Eosinophilic Esophagitis
Dysphagia of liquids and/or solids
Stop offending medication
Treat infection[8]
Steroids, diet modification
Antireflux surgery to replicate a competent LES (fundoplication)
Esophageal manometry
Barium esophagram[4]
Esophageal Malignancy
Barrett's (Intestinal Metaplasia)
1. Abnormal peristalsis
2. Incomplete LES[5] relaxation
Episodes of uncoordinated contractions lasting seconds to minutes
PET-CT for staging
Indefinite PPI therapy
Progressive symptoms ± regurgitation or weight loss
Intermittent symptoms, with chest pain
Total or subtotal esophagectomy ± chemoradiation vs. EMR/RFA[13]
+
Annual EGD with biopsy for dysplasia or neoplasia
"Bird's beak" appearance
"Corkscrew" appearance
Posterior contrast-filled pouch
Circumferential narrowing
Achalasia
Diffuse Esophageal Spasm
Zenker's Diverticulum
Stricture, Ring/Web, Vascular Anomaly
Myotomy (surgical vs. endoscopic), CCBs[6], nitrates
Pharmacologic treatment with CCBs[6] or nitrates
Cricopharyngeal myotomy ± diverticulectomy
Suspect GERD or Barrett's esophagus if stricture, EGD with esophageal dilation if ring/web[7], surgery if vascular anomaly
Footnotes
1. Versus oropharyngeal dysphagia (cervical location, trouble initiating swallow, associated drooling/coughing/choking/dysarthria).
2. Water-soluble (gastrografin) contrast is preferred if a leak is suspected; barium is an irritant that can cause peritonitis/mediastinitis.
3. EGD: Esophagoduodenoscopy (upper endoscopy).
4. Barium esophagram is not sensitive for motility disorders.
5. LES: Lower esophageal sphincter.
6. CCB: Calcium channel blocker (eg, diltiazem).
7. Webs seen in iron deficiency anemia (Plummer-Vinson's syndrome).
8. Candida esophagitis is treated empirically; otherwise biopsy required.
9. GERD: Gastroesophogeal reflux disease.
10. H2RAs: Histamine 2 receptor antagonists (eg, famotidine).
11. PPI: Proton pump inhibitor (eg, omeprazole).
12. Patients with GERD require EGD if they have alarm symptoms or are men age >50 with >5 years of symptoms and tobacco use.
13. Endoscopic mucosal resection/radiofrequency ablation for dysplasia or carcinoma in situ.

FIGURE 12.1

12-1 Esophagus

ESOPHAGEAL PERFORATION

A 37-year-old F presents 1 day after an EGD with odynophagia, fevers, and chills. On **exam**, chest palpation reveals crepitus. **Labs** show leukocytosis. On **imaging**, CXR shows pneumomediastinum.

Management:

1. Water-soluble contrast (Gastrografin) esophagography to confirm diagnosis.
2. NPO, IV fluids, broad-spectrum antibiotics (with antifungal coverage).
3. Surgical repair or esophagectomy.

Complications:

- If intra-abdominal perforation, peritonitis/acute abdomen.
- If intrathoracic perforation, mediastinitis, empyema, pericardial tamponade.
- Sepsis and death (overall mortality rate of 20%).

HYF: Most esophageal perforations are iatrogenic (instrumentation). Other etiologies are spontaneous rupture (eg, Boerhaave syndrome from excessive vomiting/coughing), penetrating trauma, caustic ingestion (especially if alkaline such as drain cleaners or lye), and malignancy. If esophageal perforation is suspected, never induce vomiting even if something was ingested. Contrast this with a Mallory-Weiss tear, which is associated with hematemesis and characterized by a mucosal tear rather than a transmural rupture.

GASTROESOPHAGEAL REFLUX DISEASE (GERD)

A 58-year-old M with PMH of tobacco use presents with 6 years of postprandial epigastric pain with occasional acidic regurgitation that is worse at night. The symptoms improve with antacids.

Management:

1. In males age >50 with >5 years of symptoms and a smoking history, EGD with biopsy must be performed to rule out Barrett's esophagus or adenocarcinoma.
2. Lifestyle changes (eg, weight loss, avoid eating at bedtime, avoid acidic foods), H2RAs.
3. PPI (eg, omeprazole) for severe symptoms, erosive esophagitis on EGD, or laryngeal involvement (eg, cough).

Complications:

- Erosive esophagitis → fibrotic healing → peptic stricture.
- Barrett's esophagus (salmon-colored mucosa on EGD) → adenocarcinoma.

HYF: Patients can present with GERD s/p surgical treatment of achalasia (myotomy disrupts lower esophageal sphincter). A complication of chronic GERD is Barrett's esophagus, which is associated with an increased risk of esophageal adenocarcinoma.

ESOPHAGEAL MALIGNANCY

A 67-year-old M with PMH of Barrett's esophagus and obesity presents with 2 months of dysphagia, chest pain, and weight loss. **Labs** show anemia. On **imaging**, barium swallow shows asymmetric esophageal narrowing. On EGD, the endoscope is difficult to advance past the narrowing into the stomach.

Management:

1. EGD with biopsy (fine-needle aspiration) for diagnosis.
2. PET-CT for staging.
3. Total vs. subtotal esophagectomy with neoadjuvant or adjuvant chemotherapy ± radiation.

HYF: Esophageal adenocarcinoma commonly arises from Barrett's esophagus (columnar metaplasia of the distal esophagus 2/2 chronic GERD), so patients with known Barrett's dysplasia require frequent endoscopic surveillance and chronic PPI therapy. High-grade Barrett's dysplasia requires resection. Esophageal squamous cell carcinoma (associated with smoking, alcohol use, and nitrite-containing foods) is far less common and occurs more proximally in the esophagus.

ACHALASIA

A 41-year-old F presents with progressive dysphagia of solids and liquids, occasionally with regurgitation of undigested food. On **imaging**, EGD is normal, but barium swallow shows a dilated esophagus with "bird's beak" narrowing at the distal end.

Management:

1. Esophageal manometry confirms diagnosis and further characterizes the motility disorder.
2. Calcium channel blockers or nitrites to relax lower esophageal sphincter.
3. Repeated endoscopic balloon dilations.
4. Surgical vs. endoscopic myotomy with fundoplication to recreate lower esophageal sphincter and prevent GERD.

Complications:

- Unintentional weight loss.
- Severe esophageal dilation or tortuosity requiring esophagectomy.
- Increased risk of esophageal squamous cell carcinoma.

HYF: Achalasia is caused by degeneration of myenteric plexus ganglion cells. EGD is not sensitive for motility disorders but is performed to rule out malignancy in a patient with dysphagia.

ZENKER'S DIVERTICULUM

An 83-year-old M with PMH of recurrent pneumonia presents with halitosis and dysphagia with gurgling and regurgitation of undigested food. On **exam**, he has a fluctuant neck mass. On **imaging**, barium swallow shows contrast pooling in a posterior esophageal pouch.

Management:

1. Cricopharyngeal myotomy ± diverticulectomy (transcervical open vs. endoscopic).

Complications:

- Recurrent aspiration pneumonia.
- Esophageal ulceration.
- Tracheoesophageal fistula.

(Continued)

12-1 Esophagus

HYF: Zenker's diverticula are false diverticula herniating through the proximal esophagus due to cricopharyngeal motor dysfunction and increased pharyngeal pressure.

Caustic Ingestion: See p. 378.

Hiatal Hernia: See p. 406.

Candida, HSV, or CMV Esophagitis: See p. 175.

Eosinophilic Esophagitis: See p. 55.

Diffuse Esophageal Spasm: See p. 56.

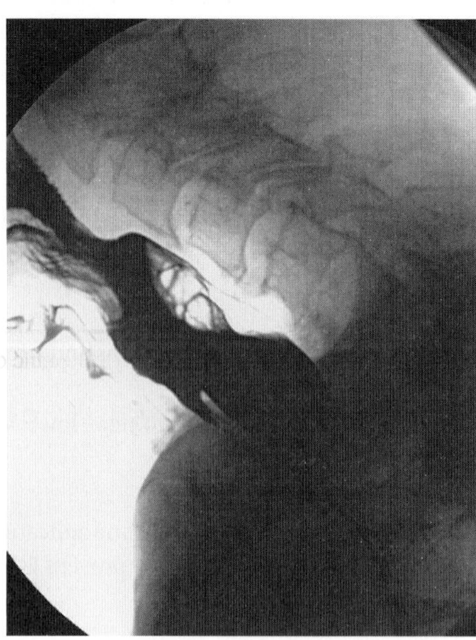

Zenker's diverticula.

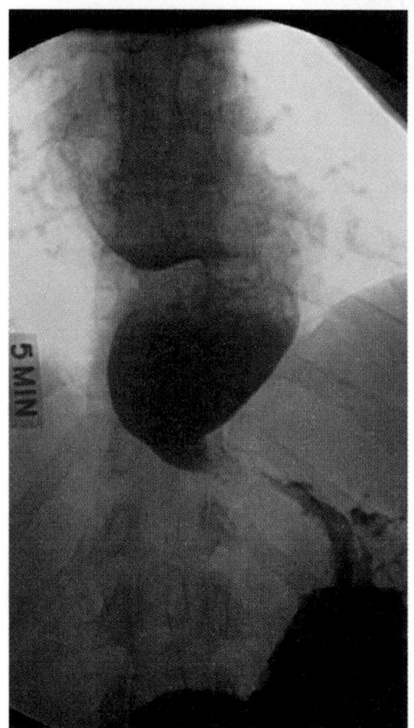
5 MIN

Achalasia.

12-2 Stomach

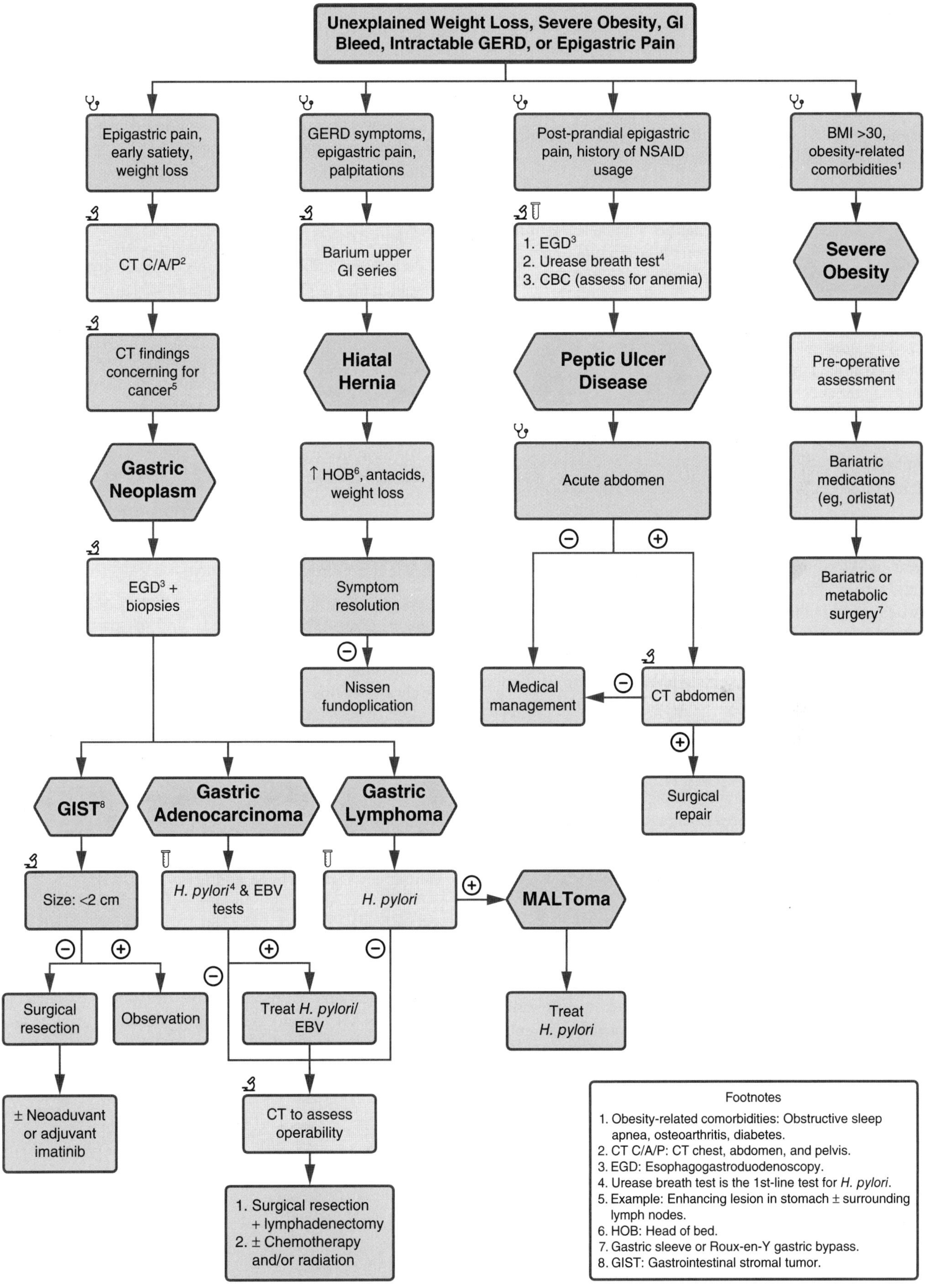
Unexplained Weight Loss, Severe Obesity, GI Bleed, Intractable GERD, or Epigastric Pain
Epigastric pain, early satiety, weight loss
CT C/A/P[2]
CT findings concerning for cancer[5]
Gastric Neoplasm
EGD[3] + biopsies
GIST[8]
Gastric Adenocarcinoma
Gastric Lymphoma
Size: <2 cm
Surgical resection
Observation
± Neoaduvant or adjuvant imatinib
H. pylori[4] & EBV tests
Treat H. pylori/ EBV
CT to assess operability
1. Surgical resection + lymphadenectomy
2. ± Chemotherapy and/or radiation
H. pylori
MALToma
Treat H. pylori
GERD symptoms, epigastric pain, palpitations
Barium upper GI series
Hiatal Hernia
↑ HOB[6], antacids, weight loss
Symptom resolution
Nissen fundoplication
Post-prandial epigastric pain, history of NSAID usage
1. EGD[3]
2. Urease breath test[4]
3. CBC (assess for anemia)
Peptic Ulcer Disease
Acute abdomen
Medical management
CT abdomen
Surgical repair
BMI >30, obesity-related comorbidities[1]
Severe Obesity
Pre-operative assessment
Bariatric medications (eg, orlistat)
Bariatric or metabolic surgery[7]
Footnotes
1. Obesity-related comorbidities: Obstructive sleep apnea, osteoarthritis, diabetes.
2. CT C/A/P: CT chest, abdomen, and pelvis.
3. EGD: Esophagogastroduodenoscopy.
4. Urease breath test is the 1st-line test for H. pylori.
5. Example: Enhancing lesion in stomach ± surrounding lymph nodes.
6. HOB: Head of bed.
7. Gastric sleeve or Roux-en-Y gastric bypass.
8. GIST: Gastrointestinal stromal tumor.

FIGURE 12.2

12-2 Stomach

HIATAL HERNIA

A 55-year old M with PMH of obesity and GERD presents with multiple episodes of palpitations, epigastric pain, and terrible taste in the back of his throat. He works as a contractor and says his symptoms are worst at the end of his workdays. **Exam** is unremarkable. On **imaging**, upper GI series is significant for pooling of barium in an outpouching just above the diaphragm.

Management:

1. Upper GI series: Look for abnormalities at the distal esophagus that could indicate atypical location of the GE junction.
2. Conservative management: Sleep with head of bed elevated, weight loss, antacids.
3. If symptoms are refractory to conservative management, proceed with Nissen fundoplication, wherein the fundus of the stomach is wrapped around the lower esophageal sphincter to keep the stomach in the abdomen and decrease symptoms of GERD.

Complications:

- Dysphagia.
- Malnutrition.

PEPTIC ULCER DISEASE (PERFORATED)

A 30-year-old M with recent ankle sprain presents with black, tarry stools and severe abdominal pain for the last 2 days. He took some of his wife's antacid pills, which improved the pain for a short time before it returned. His medical history is unremarkable aside from an ankle sprain 2 weeks ago, for which he has been taking ibuprofen up to 6 times per day. Abdominal **exam** reveals rebound tenderness and guarding. On **imaging**, KUB reveals pneumoperitoneum. On **labs**, CBC shows Hgb 10 (baseline 13).

Management:

1. This patient's abdominal exam and imaging are concerning for perforation, which requires emergent surgery. Give broad-spectrum IV antibiotics and IV PPI prior to surgery.
2. If no evidence of perforation, manage medically based on etiology of ulcer and severity of symptoms.
   a. For bleeding ulcers, patients will present with melena and, if severe upper GI bleed, hematochezia. Give IV fluids and/or blood transfusions and IV PPI. Patients will require an esophagogastroduodenoscopy (EGD) with endoscopic therapy (eg, electrocautery, endoclip) to address the bleeding lesion. Bleeding ulcers should also be biopsied to differentiate between benign ulcers and malignancy. Obtain urease breath test (best initial test) to assess for presence of *H. pylori*, and treat with triple or quadruple therapy if positive.
   b. For non-bleeding ulcers, obtain urease breath test (best initial test) to assess for presence of *H. pylori* and treat if positive. For all patients, begin an oral PPI. Stop all NSAIDs. Esophagogastroduodenoscopy (EGD) is the gold standard for diagnosis; if there is no symptom improvement following a few weeks of treatment, obtain EGD with biopsy of any lesions to rule out malignancy.
3. If concerned for recurrent ulcerative disease, consider ordering a gastrin level to assess for gastrinoma.

Complications:

- Perforation and hemorrhage, requiring emergent surgery.
- Malignancy (eg, gastric neoplasm).

HYF:

- *H. pylori* infection is a common cause of peptic ulcer disease. If *H. pylori* (+), treat infection with triple therapy (clarithromycin, amoxicillin, and PPI) or quadruple therapy (clarithromycin, amoxicillin, PPI, and metronidazole).
- The most likely etiology of this patient's ulcer is his high NSAID intake. However, if a patient presents with recurrent gastric or duodenal ulcers that are refractory to treatment, consider a gastrinoma (Zollinger-Ellison syndrome).

SEVERE OBESITY

A 50-year-old F with PMH of severe obesity with BMI 50, type 2 diabetes, obstructive sleep apnea, and osteoarthritis presents to clinic to discuss her weight management options. She has struggled with diets for the past 20 years, and though she often loses weight, she always regains it.

Management:

1. If not an operative candidate, medically manage with malabsorptive drugs such as semaglutide (a GLP-1 receptor agonist) or orlistat (inhibits pancreatic lipase and thus breakdown of fat in the GI tract).
2. If operative candidate, consider sleeve gastrectomy or Roux-en-Y gastric bypass surgery.

Complications:

- Malignancy (breast, endometrial, colon cancer) risk is increased by obesity.
- Complications of malabsorptive drugs and bariatric surgery include GI upset, dumping syndrome, steatorrhea, and fat-soluble vitamin deficiencies.

12-2 Stomach

GI STROMAL TUMOR (GIST)

A 65-year-old M with no significant PMH presents with early satiety, increasing abdominal fullness, and intermittent melena over the past 6 months. On **imaging**, CT A/P reveals a 20-cm mass in the LLQ.

Management:

1. CT scan for localization and assessment of malignant features.
2. EGD with biopsy (FNA) for tissue diagnosis.
3. Surgical resection if >2 cm, adjuvant imatinib (tyrosine kinase inhibitor).

Complications:

- Tumor often grows rapidly in size if not resected.
- Tumors >2 cm are more likely to ulcerate, bleed, and lead to mechanical bowel obstructions.

HYF: Can be caused by previous radiation to the abdomen for other cancers. Associated with *c-kit* mutation. GISTs occur in the stomach (60%), small bowel (35%), and colon/rectum/esophagus/omentum (5%)

GASTRIC ADENOCARCINOMA

A 70-year-old M with a 30-pack-year smoking history and PUD presents with early satiety and a 20-lb weight loss over the past month. He notes that he can still eat his favorite smoked salmon. Abdominal **exam** reveals epigastric tenderness. **Labs** are significant for anemia. On **imaging**, EGD reveals a bleeding mass in the antrum of the stomach. Endoscopic ultrasound (EUS) with biopsy confirms the diagnosis.

Management:

1. Test for *H. pylori* and treat if positive.
2. PET scan.
3. Diagnostic laparoscopy to evaluate for occult peritoneal disease.
4. Upfront surgery with lymphadenectomy vs. neoadjuvant chemotherapy followed by surgery and adjuvant chemotherapy ± radiation.

Complications:

- Local invasion and metastatic spread.
- Perforation and sepsis.
- Krukenberg tumor: Metastatic disease with mucin-laden signet ring cells in the ovaries. The most likely primary tumor is in the stomach.
- Virchow node: Stomach cancer metastasis to left supraclavicular node.
- Sister Mary Joseph nodule: Periumbilical metastasis of stomach cancer.

HYF: Risk factors: Smoking, heavy alcohol use, high salt/nitrate intake, history of *H. pylori* or EBV infection.

GASTRIC LYMPHOMA

An 80-year-old F with PMH of *H. pylori* infection presents with severe abdominal pain. History reveals 3 months of weight loss and abnormal fatigue. **Labs** are significant for anemia. Her daughter notes that she took medication for *H. pylori* 2 years ago but is unsure if she finished the course.

Management:

1. CT scan.
2. Endoscopy and biopsies.
3. Test for *H. pylori* and treat if positive; only proceed to surgery if obstruction, bleeding, or perforation.
4. Chemotherapy and radiation, depending on stage.

Complications:

- Metastatic spread.
- Perforation and sepsis.

HYF: If biopsy reveals the tumor is a MALToma (mucosa-associated lymphoid tissue lymphoma) associated with *H. pylori* infection, definitive treatment is *H. pylori* eradication.

MALToma: See p. 119.

12-3 Small Bowel

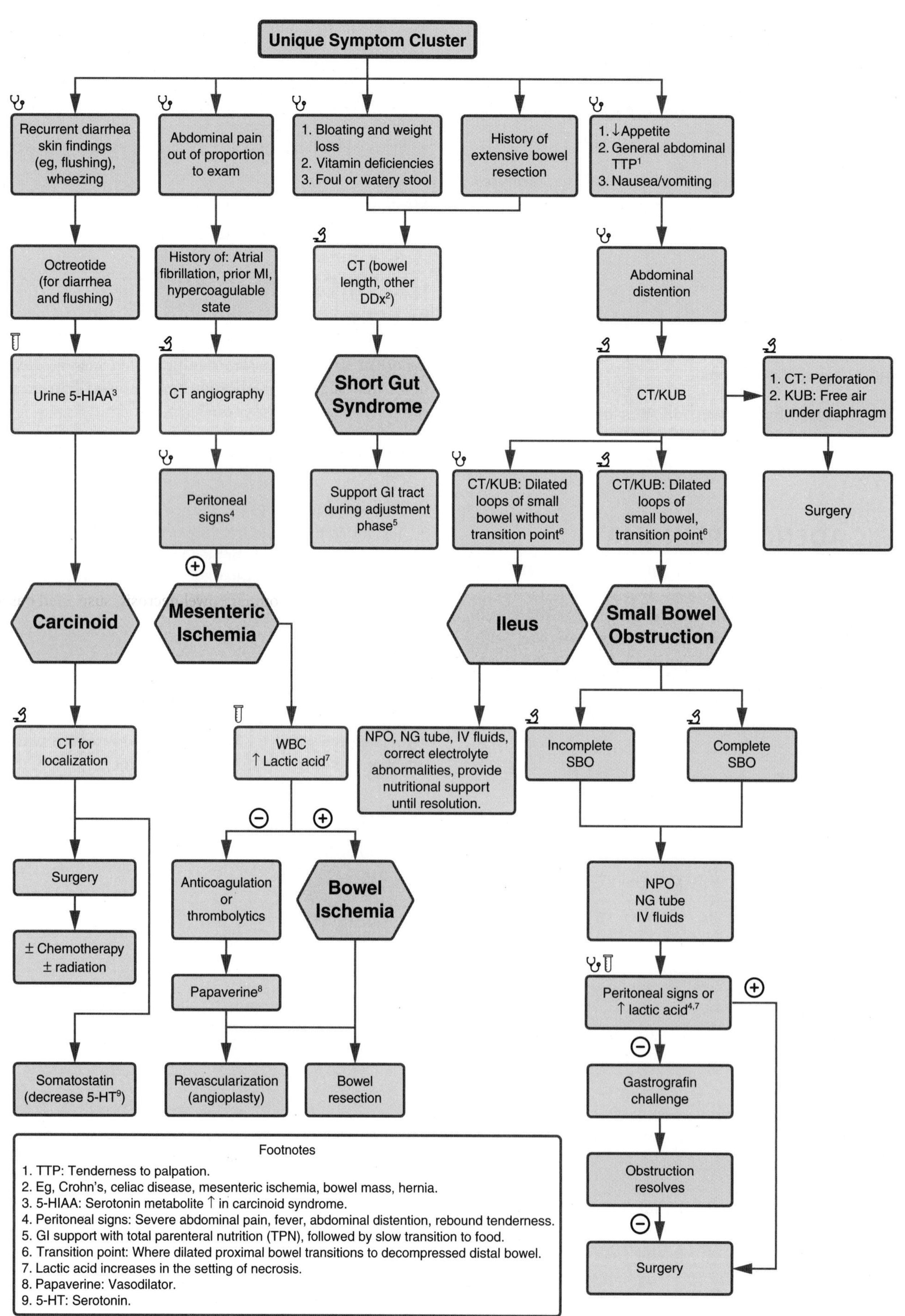

Unique Symptom Cluster
Recurrent diarrhea skin findings (eg, flushing), wheezing
Abdominal pain out of proportion to exam
1. Bloating and weight loss
2. Vitamin deficiencies
3. Foul or watery stool
History of extensive bowel resection
1. ↓Appetite
2. General abdominal TTP[1]
3. Nausea/vomiting
Octreotide (for diarrhea and flushing)
History of: Atrial fibrillation, prior MI, hypercoagulable state
CT (bowel length, other DDx[2])
Abdominal distention
Urine 5-HIAA[3]
CT angiography
Short Gut Syndrome
CT/KUB
1. CT: Perforation
2. KUB: Free air under diaphragm
Peritoneal signs[4]
Support GI tract during adjustment phase[5]
CT/KUB: Dilated loops of small bowel without transition point[6]
CT/KUB: Dilated loops of small bowel, transition point[6]
Surgery
Carcinoid
Mesenteric Ischemia
Ileus
Small Bowel Obstruction
CT for localization
WBC ↑ Lactic acid[7]
NPO, NG tube, IV fluids, correct electrolyte abnormalities, provide nutritional support until resolution.
Incomplete SBO
Complete SBO
Surgery
Anticoagulation or thrombolytics
Bowel Ischemia
NPO NG tube IV fluids
± Chemotherapy ± radiation
Papaverine[8]
Peritoneal signs or ↑ lactic acid[4,7]
Somatostatin (decrease 5-HT[9])
Revascularization (angioplasty)
Bowel resection
Gastrografin challenge
Obstruction resolves
Surgery

Footnotes

1. TTP: Tenderness to palpation.
2. Eg, Crohn's, celiac disease, mesenteric ischemia, bowel mass, hernia.
3. 5-HIAA: Serotonin metabolite ↑ in carcinoid syndrome.
4. Peritoneal signs: Severe abdominal pain, fever, abdominal distention, rebound tenderness.
5. GI support with total parenteral nutrition (TPN), followed by slow transition to food.
6. Transition point: Where dilated proximal bowel transitions to decompressed distal bowel.
7. Lactic acid increases in the setting of necrosis.
8. Papaverine: Vasodilator.
9. 5-HT: Serotonin.

FIGURE 12.3

12-3 Small Bowel

SHORT GUT SYNDROME

A 45-year-old F with PMH of Crohn's disease complicated by multiple strictures requiring bowel resections presents with bloating and watery diarrhea for the past 2 months. Her last bowel resection was 12 weeks ago. Her abdominal exam is benign.

Management:

1. CT scan to rule out other etiologies (eg, active Crohn's flare) and assess remaining bowel length.
2. Support patient's transition back to a normal diet by starting with TPN and weaning as food is added back into the diet.

Complications:

- Mineral (copper, zinc, selenium, iron) and electrolyte deficiencies. Fat-soluble vitamin deficiencies (A, D, E, K). Steatorrhea and diarrhea.

HYF: A similar set of symptoms can be observed in the setting of other malabsorptive pathologies (eg, lactose intolerance, celiac, sprue). This patient's history of multiple bowel resections, however, favors short bowel length over other malabsorptive etiologies for this patient.

CARCINOID SYNDROME (GI TRACT)

A 60-year-old M presents with severe dyspnea and is found on exam to have wheezing bilaterally. He says he has been intermittently unwell for the past 9 months with episodes of severe watery diarrhea and flushing of his face and chest. On **labs**, urine 5-HIAA level is elevated. On **imaging**, CT AP shows a mass in the distal ileum and multiple liver lesions.

Management:

1. Best initial test: Urine 5-HIAA. Serotonin (5-HT) released by the tumor arrives at the liver through portal circulation and is metabolized to 5-HIAA. Elevated levels suggest the presence of a carcinoid tumor.
2. CT and In-111 octreotide scans to localize tumor.
3. First-line treatment: Surgical resection.
4. Chemotherapy and radiation.
5. Octreotide to treat diarrhea and flushing.
6. Somatostatin analogues can treat the elevated serotonin levels to prevent systemic side effects (eg, carcinoid heart disease).

Complications:

- Carcinoid heart disease: Right-sided heart fibrosis without damage to the left heart. Serotonin is metabolized in the lungs, protecting the left heart.
- Pellagra: Resulting from niacin (vitamin B_3) deficiency. All the body's tryptophan is consumed in production of excess 5-HT.

HYF:

- Most common tumor of the small bowel with most found in the terminal ileum or appendix. Serotonin (5-HT) produced by the tumor in the GI tract undergoes first-pass metabolism in the liver. The patient only exhibits symptoms if the tumor has metastasized to the liver, where it releases 5-HT directly into circulation.

MESENTERIC ISCHEMIA

A 72-year-old F with PMH of atrial fibrillation presents with severe, progressive 8/10 generalized abdominal pain. Abdominal exam reveals mild tenderness to palpation in all 4 quadrants and an abdominal bruit. On **imaging**, CT abdomen shows bowel wall edema and air within the bowel wall (*pneumatosis intestinalis*).

Management:

1. Best initial test: CT scan of the abdomen.
2. Gold standard: Mesenteric angiography.
3. CBC and lactate: Leukocytosis and elevated lactate indicate bowel ischemia and possible necrosis.
4. IV fluids, IV antibiotics.
5. Non-occlusive: NG tube, anticoagulation, vasodilator (papaverine).
6. Occlusive: Thrombolytics (tPA) or angioplasty for revascularization.
7. Emergent laparotomy if bowel necrosis, suspected based on clinical exam, WBC, lactate, and vital signs.

Complications:

- Bowel ischemia: Prolonged blood flow obstruction (arterial inflow or venous outflow) will result in bowel ischemia and eventual bowel necrosis. CBC would reveal a leukocytosis; lactate would be elevated.
- Perforation, sepsis, end-organ failure.

HYF: Acute mesenteric ischemia is usually caused by an embolism, while chronic mesenteric ischemia is usually due to atherosclerosis. Most commonly occurs in the proximal SMA.

SMALL BOWEL OBSTRUCTION

A 32-year-old G2P2 woman with PMH of 2 Cesarean section deliveries presents with intermittent, severe abdominal pain for the last 72 hours. She reports constipation for the last week. Abdominal exam reveals generalized tenderness to palpation. On **imaging**, KUB reveals air-fluid levels with dilated loops of small bowel.

Management:

1. CT/KUB: Look for distended loops of small bowel and air-fluid levels on KUB; dilated loops of bowel followed by decompressed bowel on CT; evidence of perforation on CT.
2. Medical management: NPO + NG tube for bowel rest; IV fluids.

(Continued)

12-3 Small Bowel

3. Gastrografin challenge: Patient is given enteric water-soluble contrast and followed with serial KUBs; if the contrast reaches the colon within 24 hours, the obstruction will likely resolve without surgical intervention.
4. If the obstruction resolves, continue medical management.
5. If the obstruction does not resolve, proceed to surgery.
6. If peritonitis or concerning vital signs or labs on initial presentation, proceed immediately to surgery after resuscitation and NG tube placement.

Complications:

- Nausea, vomiting, dehydration.
- Aspiration risk, especially in patients with a history of active alcohol use disorder or elderly patients.
- Intestinal rupture and sepsis.

HYF:

- Adhesions are the most common cause of small bowel obstructions. Hernias are also a common cause of small bowel obstruction. Occasionally small bowel obstruction can be caused by malignancy: Adenocarcinoma, neuroendocrine tumors, lymphoma, metastatic melanoma.

12-4 Colorectal

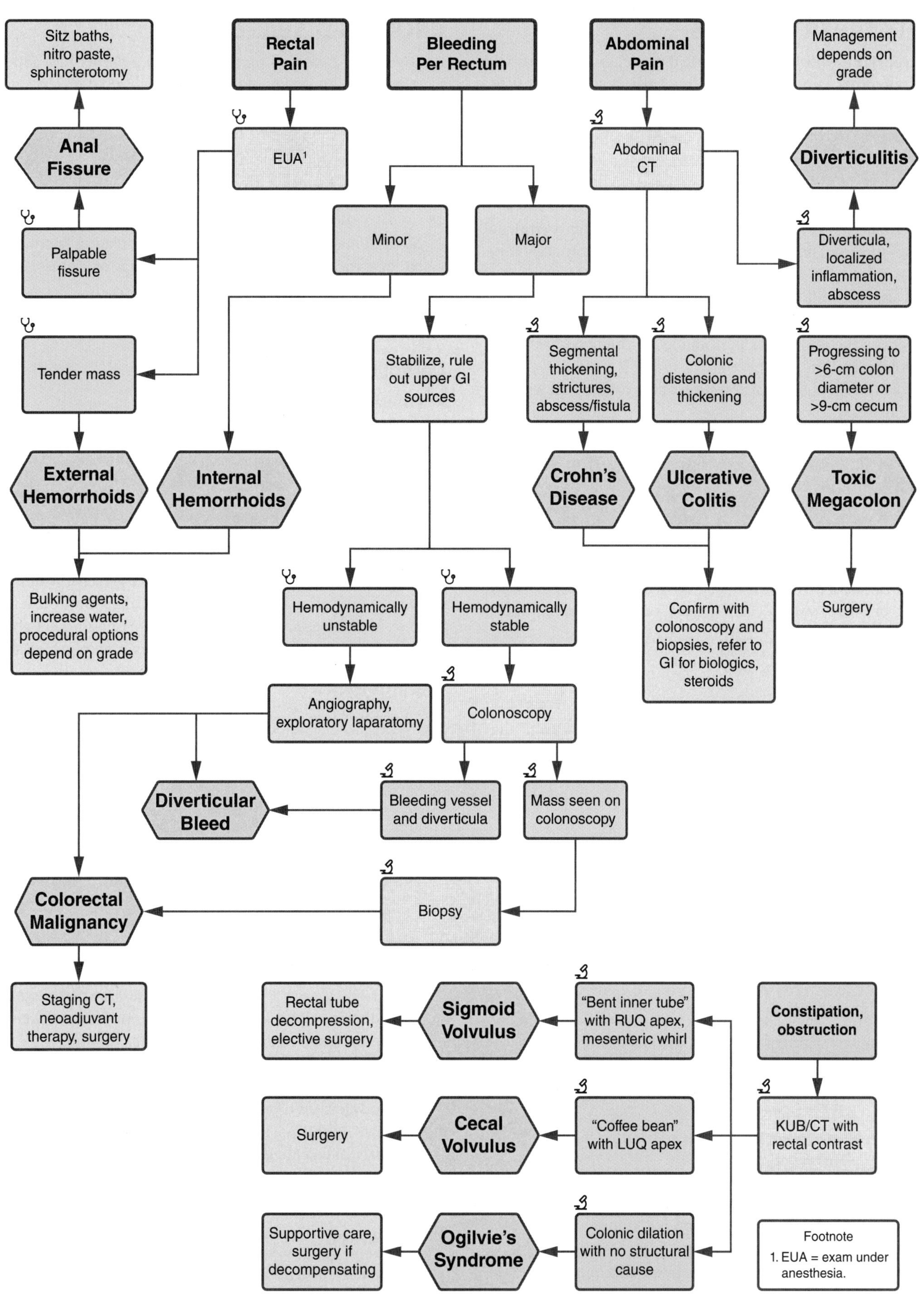

Sitz baths, nitro paste, sphincterotomy
Rectal Pain
Bleeding Per Rectum
Abdominal Pain
Management depends on grade
Anal Fissure
EUA[1]
Abdominal CT
Diverticulitis
Minor
Major
Palpable fissure
Diverticula, localized inflammation, abscess
Tender mass
Stabilize, rule out upper GI sources
Segmental thickening, strictures, abscess/fistula
Colonic distension and thickening
Progressing to >6-cm colon diameter or >9-cm cecum
External Hemorrhoids
Internal Hemorrhoids
Crohn's Disease
Ulcerative Colitis
Toxic Megacolon
Bulking agents, increase water, procedural options depend on grade
Hemodynamically unstable
Hemodynamically stable
Confirm with colonoscopy and biopsies, refer to GI for biologics, steroids
Surgery
Angiography, exploratory laparatomy
Colonoscopy
Diverticular Bleed
Bleeding vessel and diverticula
Mass seen on colonoscopy
Colorectal Malignancy
Biopsy
Staging CT, neoadjuvant therapy, surgery
Rectal tube decompression, elective surgery
Sigmoid Volvulus
"Bent inner tube" with RUQ apex, mesenteric whirl
Constipation, obstruction
Surgery
Cecal Volvulus
"Coffee bean" with LUQ apex
KUB/CT with rectal contrast
Supportive care, surgery if decompensating
Ogilvie's Syndrome
Colonic dilation with no structural cause
Footnote
1. EUA = exam under anesthesia.

FIGURE 12.4

12-4 Colorectal

ACUTE DIVERTICULITIS

A 60-year-old F with PMH of colonic diverticulosis presents with fever, abdominal pain, and constipation. **Labs** show elevated WBC. On **imaging**, CT abdomen shows sigmoid diverticula, mural thickening of the colon, and pericolic fat stranding.

Management:

1. Uncomplicated diverticulitis is managed conservatively with antibiotics, bowel rest (NPO, NG tube placement if severe), and broad-spectrum antibiotics (metronidazole + fluoroquinolone OR a 2nd- or 3rd-generation cephalosporin). Diet advanced as pain and labs improve. Encourage high-fiber diet.
2. If complicated diverticulitis (eg, development of abscess, bowel obstruction, fistula, perforation), address the specific complication:
   a. If perforation, surgical resection of diseased bowel with temporary colostomy.
   b. Percutaneous drainage for localized fluid collections.
   c. If fistulization, surgical resection of fistula.
3. Outpatient colonoscopy after the initial stage.
4. If recurrent, consider resection of diseased bowel.

Complications:

- Fistulization of diverticula to nearby structures (bladder, uterus, small intestine, vagina) can cause fecaluria, pneumaturia, or fecal vaginal discharge.
- Bowel perforation.
- Peritonitis.
- Abscess formation.

HYF: Avoid colonoscopy in the initial stages of diverticulitis due to increased risk of perforation. Right-sided diverticulitis is rare but more common in patients of Asian descent.

HEMORRHOIDS

A 50-year-old M with PMH of constipation presents with pain with defecation, anal pruritus, and blood when wiping after bowel movements.

Management: Depends on type of hemorrhoid (internal or external) and severity of disease (grade). Generally, treatment entails the following:

1. Conservative treatment with fiber and stool softeners.
2. Clinic-based procedures (ligation, banding, ablation) may be indicated for medium-grade disease.
3. Excisional or stapled hemorrhoidectomy reserved for hemorrhoids that are not amenable to banding, high grade, thrombosed, or gangrenous.

Complications: Sepsis may occur if full-thickness rectum is ligated. Postoperative urinary retention is common.

HYF: The 2 types of hemorrhoids are internal hemorrhoids (above the pectinate line, not painful) and external hemorrhoids (below the pectinate line, painful).

CROHN'S DISEASE

A 30-year-old F with no significant PMH presents with abdominal pain, diarrhea, and weight loss. **Labs** reveal iron deficiency anemia, leukocytosis, and elevated CRP. On **imaging**, MRI enterography shows thickened bowel with cobblestoning, as well as an abscess and several pseudodiverticula.

Management:

1. Confirm diagnosis with endoscopy and biopsies.
2. Medical management with immunomodulation (steroids, biologic therapies), percutaneous drainage of abscesses in the setting of flares.
3. Surgery indicated for refractory disease or management of complications.

Complications:

- Fistula.
- Strictures.
- Colon cancer if colonic involvement.

HYF: Most common area of involvement is the ileum.

ULCERATIVE COLITIS

A 30-year-old M with no significant PMH presents with abdominal pain, bloody diarrhea, and tenesmus. **Labs** show iron deficiency anemia, leukocytosis, and elevated CRP. On **imaging**, CT abdomen shows colonic wall thickening with proliferation of perirectal fat.

Management:

1. Confirm diagnosis with endoscopy and biopsies.
2. Medical management with immunomodulation (sulfasalazine, steroids, biologics).
3. Surgery is indicated for refractory disease or management of complications. Unlike Crohn's, surgery can be curative.

Complications:

- Fulminant colitis (toxic megacolon).
- Colon cancer.

COLORECTAL CANCER

A 65-year-old M with PMH of alcohol use disorder presents with abdominal pain, blood in the stool, and unintentional weight loss of 20 lb in the last 3 months. Upon further questioning, he reports decreased stool caliber and needing to strain to have a bowel movement. He has never had a colonoscopy. **Labs** show iron deficiency anemia and elevated CEA. Digital rectal **exam** does not reveal a palpable mass. Stool is positive for occult blood. Diagnostic colonoscopy reveals an ulcerated mass in the sigmoid colon. Biopsy reveals adenocarcinoma. On **imaging**, staging CT reveals metastases in the liver, lungs, and brain.

Management:

1. Depending on staging, tumor resection ± (neo)adjuvant chemotherapy (eg, leucovorin, 5-FU, oxaliplatin, and irinotecan) ± radiation.

12-4 Colorectal

2. If unresectable metastatic disease, palliative chemotherapy ± biologic agent (irinotecan, regorafenib), immunotherapy.

Complications:

- Sequelae of metastases (eg, seizures from brain metastases).
- Iron deficiency anemia.
- GI bleeding.
- Death.

HYF: Iron deficiency anemia in an older adult is an indication for a diagnostic colonoscopy. Similarly, large bowel obstruction in adults is colon cancer unless proven otherwise. Right-sided (ascending) CRC is associated with iron deficiency anemia, occult blood loss, and vague abdominal pain. Left-sided (descending) CRC is associated with obstructive symptoms (eg, "apple core lesion"), change in bowel habits, and hematochezia. Associated with IBD (ulcerative colitis > Crohn's), *Streptococcus bovis* bacteremia, *Clostridium septicum*, acromegaly, and cancer syndromes (below).

Syndromes associated with colorectal cancer	Features
Familial adenomatous polyposis (FAP)	Autosomal dominant mutation in *APC* tumor suppressor gene. Prophylactic total colectomy is recommended due to nearly 100% risk of developing CRC.
Lynch syndrome	Autosomal dominant mutation of DNA mismatch repair (MMR) genes (eg, *MSH2*), leading to microsatellite instability. Associated with colorectal, ovarian, endometrial, and skin cancers.
Gardner syndrome	Germline mutation in the *APC* gene. Supernumerary and impacted teeth, osseous and soft tissue tumors, congenital hypertrophy of retinal pigment epithelium.
Peutz-Jegher syndrome	Autosomal dominant. Patients develop many hamartomas throughout the GI tract and hyperpigmented mouth, lips, hands, genitalia. Associated with GI and breast cancers.
Juvenile polyposis syndrome	Autosomal dominant. Hamartomatous polyps in GI tract in children age <5 years that are initially benign but may become malignant.

SIGMOID VOLVULUS

A 70-year-old F with PMH of dementia presents with nausea, vomiting, abdominal pain, and constipation. On **imaging**, abdominal XR shows the "bent inner tube" sign. CT with contrast enema shows bird's beak deformity.

Management:

1. Endoscopic detorsion (sigmoidoscopy) with rectal tube placement.
2. Elective sigmoid colectomy during the same admission or shortly thereafter.

Complications:

- Perforation.
- Bowel obstruction.
- Bowel necrosis.
- High risk of recurrence if surgical resection is not performed.

HYF: Risk factors: Elderly, redundancy of the sigmoid colon, institutionalized patients with neurologic/psychiatric comorbidities. Surgical resection should be performed soon after endoscopic reduction due to the high risk of recurrence and high mortality rates in patients with recurrent volvulus.

CECAL VOLVULUS

A 30-year-old F presents with nausea, vomiting, abdominal pain, and constipation. On **imaging**, abdominal X-ray shows the "coffee bean" sign.

Management:

1. Surgical reduction: Volvulus detorsion, followed by ileocecal resection or right colectomy OR cecopexy, depending on patient's stability.

Complications:

- Perforation.
- Bowel obstruction.
- Colonic necrosis.

HYF: Unlike sigmoid volvulus, cecal volvulus requires surgical correction as non-operative reduction (eg, barium enema, colonoscopy) is rarely successful and can cause perforation. Caused by a congenital failure of cecal tethering.

Diverticular Bleed: See p. 86.

Ogilvie's Syndrome: See p. 395.

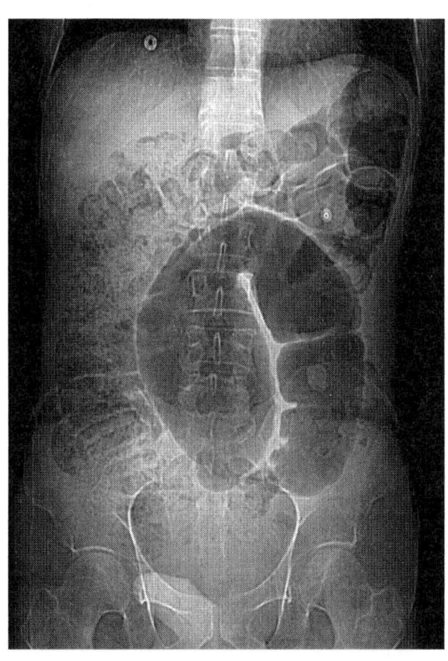

Sigmoid volvulus. Note the characteristic "coffee bean" sign.

12-5 Hepatic Disease

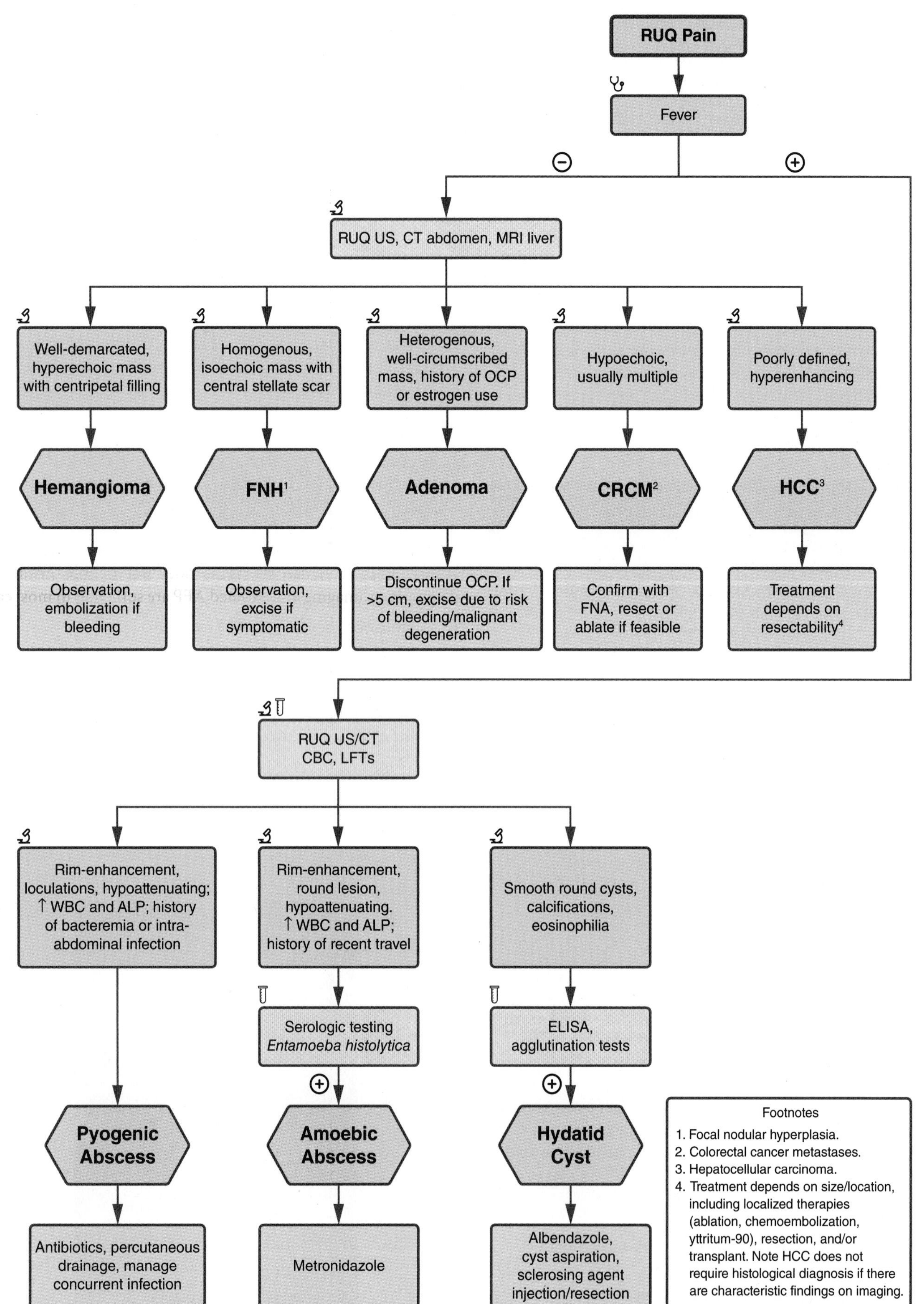
RUQ Pain
Fever
⊖
⊕
RUQ US, CT abdomen, MRI liver
Well-demarcated, hyperechoic mass with centripetal filling
Homogenous, isoechoic mass with central stellate scar
Heterogenous, well-circumscribed mass, history of OCP or estrogen use
Hypoechoic, usually multiple
Poorly defined, hyperenhancing
Hemangioma
FNH[1]
Adenoma
CRCM[2]
HCC[3]
Observation, embolization if bleeding
Observation, excise if symptomatic
Discontinue OCP. If >5 cm, excise due to risk of bleeding/malignant degeneration
Confirm with FNA, resect or ablate if feasible
Treatment depends on resectability[4]
RUQ US/CT CBC, LFTs
Rim-enhancement, loculations, hypoattenuating; ↑ WBC and ALP; history of bacteremia or intra-abdominal infection
Rim-enhancement, round lesion, hypoattenuating. ↑ WBC and ALP; history of recent travel
Smooth round cysts, calcifications, eosinophilia
Serologic testing *Entamoeba histolytica*
ELISA, agglutination tests
⊕
⊕
Pyogenic Abscess
Amoebic Abscess
Hydatid Cyst
Antibiotics, percutaneous drainage, manage concurrent infection
Metronidazole
Albendazole, cyst aspiration, sclerosing agent injection/resection
Footnotes
1. Focal nodular hyperplasia.
2. Colorectal cancer metastases.
3. Hepatocellular carcinoma.
4. Treatment depends on size/location, including localized therapies (ablation, chemoembolization, yttritum-90), resection, and/or transplant. Note HCC does not require histological diagnosis if there are characteristic findings on imaging.

FIGURE 12.5

12-5 Hepatic Disease

HEMANGIOMA

A 28-year-old M bodybuilder with PMH of androgen steroid use presents for follow-up for a liver mass that was incidentally found on imaging. On **imaging**, abdominal US shows a hepatic mass that is hyperechoic with well-demarcated margins and centripetal fill-in. **Labs** are normal.

MANAGEMENT:

1. If asymptomatic, observation.
2. If causing mass effect or pain, consider enucleation vs. resection.
3. If spontaneously bleeding, angioembolization.

Complications: Rupture is exceedingly rare; no potential for malignant degeneration. Risk for CHF in massive hemangiomas or consumptive thrombocytopenia (Kasalbach-Merritt's syndrome).

HYF: Most common benign liver tumor. Associated with high-estrogen states (eg, oral contraceptives) or androgen use. Most are asymptomatic and found incidentally in patients undergoing imaging for other reasons.

FOCAL NODULAR HYPERPLASIA (FNH)

A 25-year-old F with no significant PMH presents for follow-up for a liver mass that was incidentally found on imaging. **Exam** and **labs** are normal. On **imaging**, CT abdomen shows a homogenous mass with a central stellate scar.

Management:

1. If asymptomatic, observation.
2. Consider resection only for attributed symptoms (eg, pain) or for histologic confirmation in the setting of diagnostic uncertainty.

Complications: No malignant potential; rupture is rare.

HYF: Second most common benign liver tumor. Women > men. Consider FNH in a patient without cirrhosis who is found to have a solid liver lesion on imaging.

HEPATIC ADENOMA

A 22-year-old F on OCPs presents for follow-up for a liver mass that was incidentally found on **imaging**. CT abdomen had shown a liver mass with well-demarcated margins. **Labs** and **exam** are normal.

Management:

1. Cessation of hormonal exposure.
2. If <5 cm, surveillance. If >5 cm, symptomatic, or ruptured, excision is the definitive treatment. If a patient is not an operative candidate, can consider transarterial embolization or radiofrequency ablation.

Complications: Risk of malignant transformation to HCC, spontaneous rupture for larger lesions.

HYF: Benign liver tumors that are associated with OCP use. Most are asymptomatic and found incidentally in patients undergoing imaging for other reasons. Biopsies of suspected hepatic adenomas are not routinely performed due to the high risk of bleeding and limited diagnostic benefit. Rupture is more common in men > women.

HEPATOCELLULAR CARCINOMA (HCC)

A 60-year-old M with PMH of alcohol use disorder and cirrhosis presents with unintentional weight loss and vague RUQ pain. **Labs** show elevated LFTs and AFP. On **imaging**, triple-phase CT of the abdomen and pelvis reveals a 5-cm mass in the liver demonstrating arterial phase enhancement and delayed phase washout.

Management: Treatment varies depending on resectability and the patient's baseline liver function:

1. Surgical resection is reserved for patients with good hepatic function and small tumors.
2. Sorafenib is used for advanced disease.
3. Treatment options for patients in between include chemoembolization, ablation, and liver transplant.

HYF: Most common primary hepatic malignancy. Risk factors include all causes of cirrhosis (eg, ETOH, NASH, HBV/HCV). Unlike other malignancies, HCC does not require histological diagnosis, as imaging and elevated AFP are sufficient in most cases.

PYOGENIC ABSCESS

A 50-year-old M with a recent episode of diverticulitis presents with fever and abdominal pain. **Exam** shows tenderness to palpation in the RUQ. **Labs** show elevated WBC and ALP. On **imaging**, CT abdomen shows a rim-enhancing liver lesion.

Management:

1. IV antibiotics + percutaneous drainage.
2. Operative drainage reserved for multiple abscesses or failure of more conversative treatment.

HYF: Arises from hematogenous spread of non-hepatic sources, direct introduction through instrumentation, or biliary-enteric anastomoses. *Esherichia coli* is the most common organism.

AMOEBIC ABSCESS

A 30-year-old M with recent travel to a foreign country presents with fever and RUQ pain. **Labs** show elevated WBC and ALP, as well as positive *E. histolytica* antibodies. On **imaging**, CT abdomen shows a rim-enhancing liver lesion.

Management:

1. Needle aspiration is not routinely necessary but performed if diagnostic uncertainty ("anchovy paste" fluid).
2. Metronidazole × 7–10 days.

Complications: Cyst rupture or erosion into other structures may occur, requiring surgical management.

(Continued)

12-5 Hepatic Disease

HYF: May present with other signs and symptoms of amebiasis such as diarrhea.

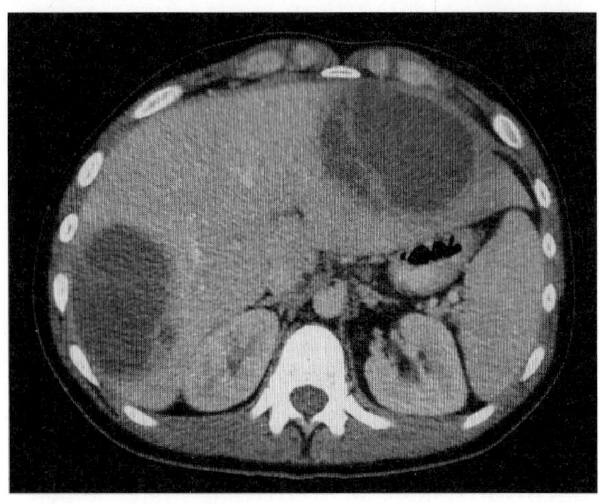

Amoebic abscesses of the liver.

HYDATID CYST

A 40-year-old M sheep farmer presents with fever and RUQ pain. **Labs** show elevated WBC and ALP, eosinophilia, and ELISA positive for *Echinococcus* antibodies.

Management:

1. Albendazole.
2. Percutaneous aspiration + injection of scolicidal agents (alcohol or hypertonic saline).
3. Surgical resection reserved for complicated disease (eg, cyst rupture).

Complications: Avoid diagnostic aspiration, as spillage of cyst contents can cause anaphylaxis.

HYF: Most common hepatic cyst globally.

12-6 Biliary Disease

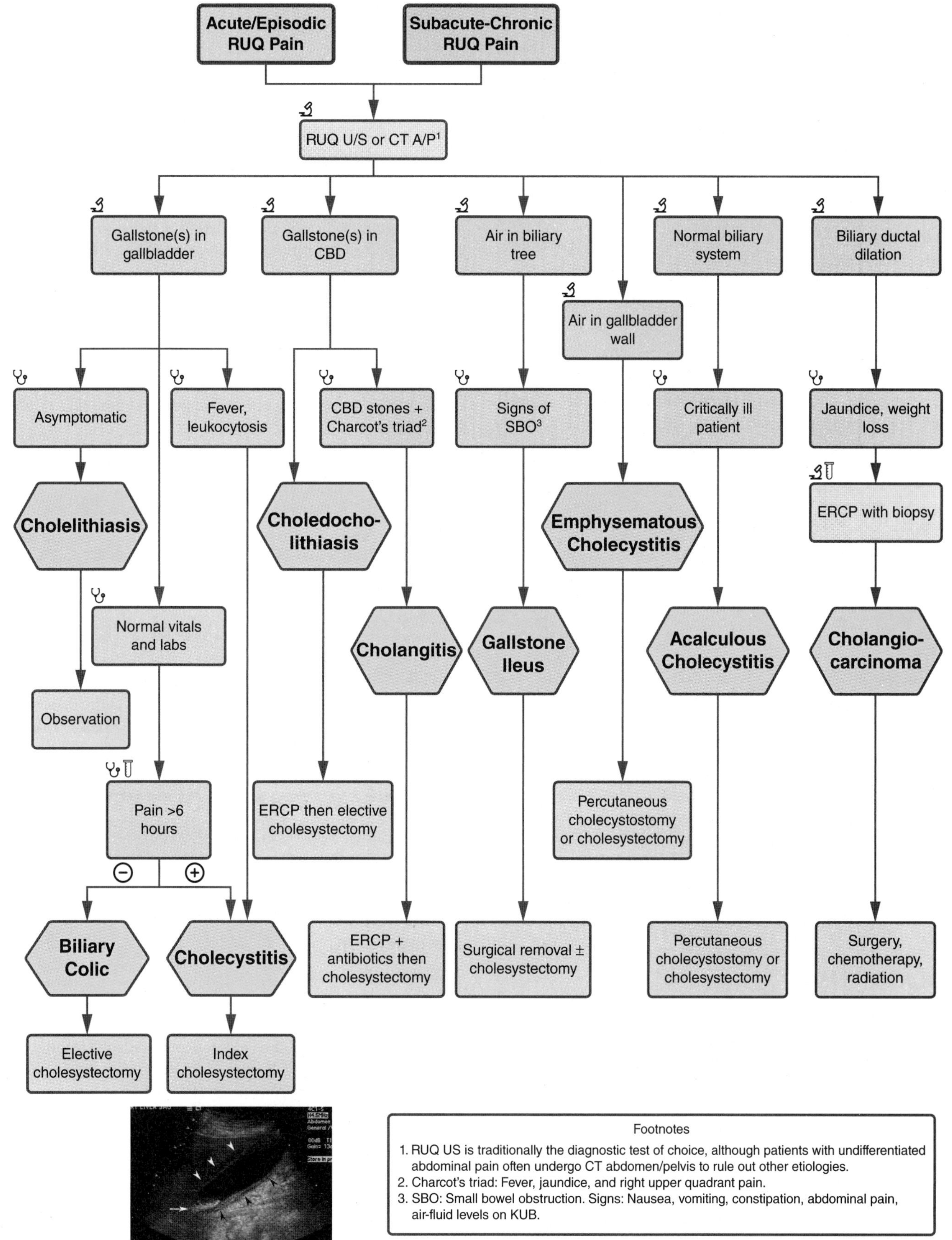
Acute/Episodic RUQ Pain
Subacute-Chronic RUQ Pain
RUQ U/S or CT A/P[1]
Gallstone(s) in gallbladder
Gallstone(s) in CBD
Air in biliary tree
Normal biliary system
Biliary ductal dilation
Air in gallbladder wall
Asymptomatic
Fever, leukocytosis
CBD stones + Charcot's triad[2]
Signs of SBO[3]
Critically ill patient
Jaundice, weight loss
ERCP with biopsy
Cholelithiasis
Choledocho-lithiasis
Emphysematous Cholecystitis
Normal vitals and labs
Cholangitis
Gallstone Ileus
Acalculous Cholecystitis
Cholangio-carcinoma
Observation
Pain >6 hours
ERCP then elective cholesystectomy
Percutaneous cholecystostomy or cholesystectomy
−
+
Biliary Colic
Cholecystitis
ERCP + antibiotics then cholesystectomy
Surgical removal ± cholesystectomy
Percutaneous cholecystostomy or cholesystectomy
Surgery, chemotherapy, radiation
Elective cholesystectomy
Index cholesystectomy

Gallbladder ultrasound in cholecystitis.

Figure 12.6.1

Footnotes

1. RUQ US is traditionally the diagnostic test of choice, although patients with undifferentiated abdominal pain often undergo CT abdomen/pelvis to rule out other etiologies.
2. Charcot's triad: Fever, jaundice, and right upper quadrant pain.
3. SBO: Small bowel obstruction. Signs: Nausea, vomiting, constipation, abdominal pain, air-fluid levels on KUB.

FIGURE 12.6

12-6 Biliary Disease

CHOLELITHIASIS

A 45-year-old F who is healthy at baseline, takes no medications, and undergoes **imaging** CT A/P for unrelated reasons is incidentally found to have gallstones.

Management:

1. Observation.

Complications:

- Biliary colic.
- Acute cholecystitis.
- Choledocholithiasis.
- Cholangitis.
- Gallstone ileus.
- Gallstone pancreatitis.

HYF: 10% of the population has gallstones. Two types of gallstones: Cholesterol stones (obesity, age, IBD) and pigment stones (IBD, chronic hemolysis, alcoholic cirrhosis, biliary infections, total parenteral nutrition).

CHOLEDOCHOLITHIASIS

A 45-year-old F presents with subacute RUQ pain. **Labs** are notable for elevated LFTs, ALP, and GGT. On **imaging**, RUQ US shows a dilated common bile duct and/or a gallstone in the common bile duct.

Management:

1. ERCP.
2. Elective cholecystectomy.

Complications:

- Cholangitis.
- Gallstone pancreatitis.
- Sepsis, multiorgan failure, and death.
- Pyogenic hepatic abscess.

HYF: LFTs are elevated in a cholestatic pattern (ALP, GGT, direct bilirubin). *Chole* = gallbladder; *Docho* = duct; *Lith* = stone.

CHOLANGITIS

A 45-year-old F with known cholelithiasis presents with acute-onset fever, jaundice, and RUQ pain on **exam**. **Labs** are significant for leukocytosis and elevated bilirubin and ALP.

Management:

1. Supportive care (IV fluids, analgesia).
2. Maintain NPO.
3. Blood cultures, followed by empiric antibiotics (gram-negative and anaerobic coverage).
4. Biliary drainage via ERCP.

Complications:

- Bacteremia.
- Pancreatitis (complication of ERCP).
- Pyogenic hepatic abscess.

HYF: LFTs are elevated in a cholestatic pattern. Charcot's triad: Fever, jaundice, RUQ pain. Reynold's pentad: Fever, jaundice, RUQ pain, altered mental status, hypotension. Imaging is not needed if the clinical picture is clear; otherwise, RUQ ultrasound or CT A/P will show common bile duct dilation ± gallstones. Patients with cholangitis can deteriorate quickly; therefore, biliary drainage via ERCP or percutaneous drainage must be done expeditiously.

GALLSTONE ILEUS

An 80-year-old F with PMH of diabetes, HTN, and known cholelithiasis presents with abdominal pain, nausea, vomiting, and obstipation. On **imaging**, CT A/P shows pneumobilia (ie, air in the biliary tree).

Management:

1. Surgical removal of the gallstone (enterolithotomy).
2. Low-risk patients: Cholecystectomy and biliary-enteric fistula closure after enterolithotomy.
3. High-risk patients: Expectant management after enterolithotomy.

Complications: Repeated obstruction.

HYF: Due to fistulization between gallbladder and GI tract; a gallstone stone enters the GI lumen and obstructs at the ileocecal valve (narrowest point). Most common in elderly females with significant comorbidities.

EMPHYSEMATOUS CHOLECYSTITIS

A 60-year-old M with PMH of T2DM presents with severe abdominal pain and fever. **Exam** is notable for positive Murphy's sign. **Labs** show leukocytosis. On **imaging**, CT A/P shows air in the gallbladder wall and lumen.

Management:

1. Blood cultures, followed by empiric antibiotics (gram-negative and anaerobic coverage).
2. Surgical candidate: Cholecystectomy.
3. Non-surgical candidate: Percutaneous cholecystostomy.

Complications:

- Gallbladder perforation.
- Sepsis.

HYF: Commonly isolated organisms include *Clostridium perfringens, Escherichia coli,* and *Bacteroides fragilis.*

12-6 Biliary Disease

ACALCULOUS CHOLECYSTITIS

A 75-year-old M with PMH of T2DM and CAD has been recovering in the ICU after cardiac surgery and now has new abdominal pain and fever. On **exam**, he has a tender, palpable mass in the RUQ. On **imaging**, RUQ US shows gallbladder wall thickening with no evidence of gallstones.

Management:

1. Blood cultures, followed by empiric antibiotics (gram-negative and anaerobic coverage).
2. Surgical candidate: Cholecystectomy.
3. Non-surgical candidate: Percutaneous cholecystostomy.

Complications:

- Gallbladder perforation.
- Gangrenous cholecystitis.
- Sepsis.

HYF: Most common in critically ill patients. Associated with gallbladder stasis, hypoperfusion, and infection (CMV). Lab abnormalities may include leukocytosis and/or elevated LFTs in a cholestatic pattern. Secondary infection with *Escherichia coli, Enterococcus faecalis, Klebsiella, Pseudomonas, Proteus,* and *Bacteroides fragilis* is common.

CHOLANGIOCARCINOMA

A 65-year-old F presents with painless jaundice and unintentional weight loss. **Labs** show direct hyperbilirubinemia and elevated ALP, as well as elevated CA 19–9 and CEA. On **imaging**, RUQ US shows biliary ductal dilation without evidence of gallstones. Cross-sectional MRI demonstrates a malignancy of the intrahepatic bile duct. EUS with tissue biopsy confirms the diagnosis. Staging CT reveals metastases in the liver.

Management: Depends on the staging of disease.

1. Surgical resection ± chemotherapy ± radiation.

Complications: Metastasis (most commonly to the liver), biliary obstruction, pancreatic duct obstruction.

HYF: Cholangiocarcinoma arises from the epithelial cells of the bile ducts, and these cells are grouped based on their site of origin: Intrahepatic, perihilar, or extrahepatic. Klatskin tumors are cholangiocarcinomas that arise from the hilum. Associated with primary sclerosing cholangitis and, in Asia, infection with *Clonorchis sinensis* (liver flukes) transmitted via undercooked fish.

BILIARY COLIC

A 45-year-old F with no significant PMH presents with post-prandial RUQ pain that is intermittent and colicky. She is not currently experiencing abdominal pain. **Exam** and **labs** are normal. On **imaging**, RUQ US shows gallstones.

Management:

1. Limit fatty foods.
2. NSAIDs for pain control.
3. Elective cholecystectomy.

Complications:

- Acute cholecystitis.
- Choledocholithiasis.
- Cholangitis.
- Gallstone ileus.
- Gallstone pancreatitis.

HYF: 1–3% of patients with cholelithiasis will develop biliary colic.

ACUTE CHOLECYSTITIS

A 45-year-old F with PMH of obesity presents with 8 hours of RUQ pain. On **exam**, she has positive Murphy's sign and pain radiating to the right shoulder. Vitals and **labs** are significant for fever and leukocytosis. On **imaging**, RUQ US shows gallbladder wall thickening and a stone in the cystic duct.

Management:

1. Supportive care: IV fluids, analgesia.
2. Maintain NPO.
3. Blood cultures, followed by empiric antibiotics (Gram-negative and anaerobic coverage).
4. Surgical candidate: Perform laparoscopic cholecystectomy as soon as possible.
5. Non-surgical candidate: Perform a drainage procedure such as percutaneous cholecystostomy.
6. Assess for concurrent choledocholithiasis (eg, obtain transaminase and bilirubin levels, diameter of common bile duct on ultrasound).

Complications:

- Gallbladder perforation, biliary fistula, gallstone ileus.
- Choledocolithiasis.
- Gangrenous cholecystitis.
- Pyogenic hepatic abscess.

HYF: 1–3% of patients with biliary colic will develop acute cholecystitis. Risk factors include: Female sex, obesity, history of childbirth, middle-age. Murphy's sign: Pain during inspiration with deep palpation of the gallbladder fossa. Pain may radiate to the right shoulder due to irritation of the phrenic nerve. LFTs are normal in acute cholecystitis that does not involve the common bile duct. Diagnose with abdominal US or cholescintigraphy (HIDA scan); inability to visualize gallbladder on HIDA scan suggests obstruction of the cystic duct. *Chole* = gallbladder; *Itis* = inflammation. Recurrent episodes of acute cholecystitis can lead to chronic cholecystitis and development of porcelain gallbladder; perform prophylactic cholecystectomy for porcelain gallbladder due to increased risk of gallbladder cancer.

12-7 Pancreas

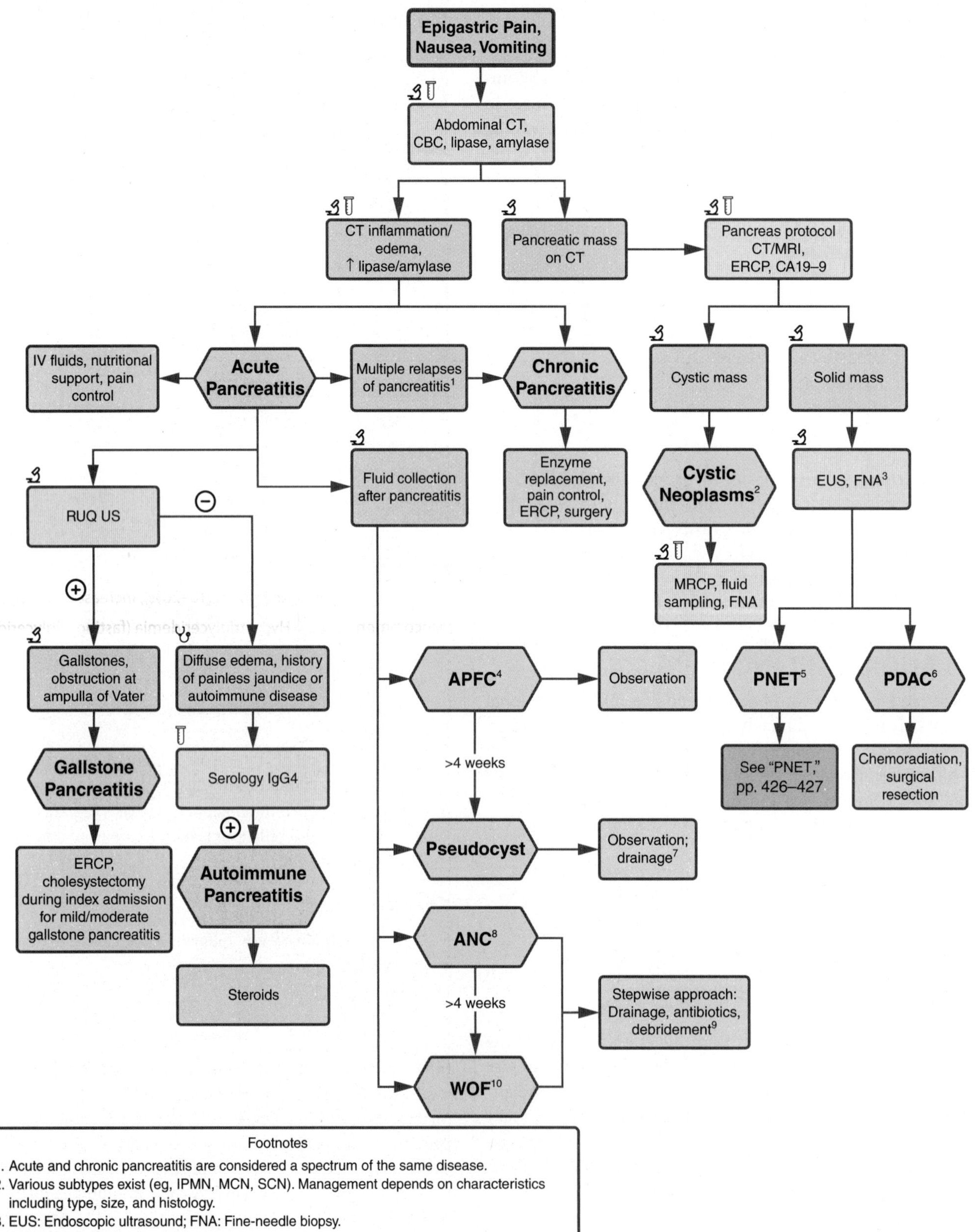

Epigastric Pain, Nausea, Vomiting
Abdominal CT, CBC, lipase, amylase
CT inflammation/ edema, ↑ lipase/amylase
Pancreatic mass on CT
Pancreas protocol CT/MRI, ERCP, CA19–9
IV fluids, nutritional support, pain control
Acute Pancreatitis
Multiple relapses of pancreatitis[1]
Chronic Pancreatitis
Cystic mass
Solid mass
Fluid collection after pancreatitis
Enzyme replacement, pain control, ERCP, surgery
Cystic Neoplasms[2]
EUS, FNA[3]
RUQ US
MRCP, fluid sampling, FNA
Gallstones, obstruction at ampulla of Vater
Diffuse edema, history of painless jaundice or autoimmune disease
APFC[4]
Observation
PNET[5]
PDAC[6]
Gallstone Pancreatitis
Serology IgG4
>4 weeks
See "PNET," pp. 426–427
Chemoradiation, surgical resection
ERCP, cholesystectomy during index admission for mild/moderate gallstone pancreatitis
Autoimmune Pancreatitis
Pseudocyst
Observation; drainage[7]
ANC[8]
Steroids
>4 weeks
Stepwise approach: Drainage, antibiotics, debridement[9]
WOF[10]

Footnotes

1. Acute and chronic pancreatitis are considered a spectrum of the same disease.
2. Various subtypes exist (eg, IPMN, MCN, SCN). Management depends on characteristics including type, size, and histology.
3. EUS: Endoscopic ultrasound; FNA: Fine-needle biopsy.
4. APFC: Acute peripancreatic fluid collection.
5. PNET: Pancreatic neuroendocrine tumors.
6. PDAC: Pancreatic ductal adenocarcinoma.
7. May resolve spontaneously; only intervene if large or symptomatic >4 weeks.
8. ANC: Acute necrotic collection.
9. Stepwise approach begins with drainage, then only add antibiotics if there is evidence of infection (eg, positive cultures). If there is no improvement, then opt for surgical debridement.
10. WOF: Walled-off necrosis.

FIGURE 12.7

12-7 Pancreas

ACUTE PANCREATITIS

A 40-year-old M with PMH of alcohol use disorder presents with epigastric pain. On **exam**, he has periumbilical (Cullen's sign) and flank ecchymoses (Grey-Turner sign). **Labs** show elevated amylase and lipase. On **imaging**, CT A/P shows pancreatic inflammation and peripancreatic fluid.

Management:

1. IV fluids, pain control.
2. Early enteral feeding. If not tolerating oral intake, consider nasoenteric feeding.

Complications:

- Chronic pancreatitis.
- APFC → pseudocyst.
- ANC → WOF.
- Pseudoaneurysm.

HYF: Variety of etiologies—gallstone pancreatitis (most common), alcohol, hypertriglyceridemia, post-ERCP, hereditary (PRSS1, SPINK1), autoimmune.

CHRONIC PANCREATITIS

A 50-year-old M with PMH of multiple previous episodes of pancreatitis presents with epigastric pain and steatorrhea. **Labs** show pancreatic insufficiency. On **imaging**, CT A/P shows pancreatic calcifications and fibrosis, as well as a pancreatic duct stricture.

Management:

1. Pain control.
2. Enzyme replacement, fat-soluble vitamin supplementation.
3. Surgery may be an option for pain control and/or pancreatic duct obstructions.

Complications:

- Pancreatic cancer.
- Metabolic sequelae of pancreatic insufficiency: Diabetes mellitus, metabolic bone disease (osteoporosis).
- Chronic abdominal pain.
- Biliary stricture ± biliary cirrhosis, pancreatic duct stricture, pseudocyst.
- Splanchic venous thrombosis.

PANCREATIC DUCT ADENOCARCINOMA

A 65-year-old M with 40-pack-year smoking history presents with epigastric pain, jaundice, and weight loss. On **exam**, he has mild TTP in the epigastrium. **Labs** show an elevated CA19-9. On **imaging**, CT A/P shows a mass in the head of the pancreas.

Management:

1. Cancer staging with CT/MRI, ERCP/EUS with biopsy.
2. Biliary drainage if obstructed.
3. Chemotherapy, surgery if resectable.

HYF: New-onset diabetes and migratory thrombophlebitis (Trousseau's syndrome) should raise concern for pancreatic cancer. Courvoisier's sign is an enlarged gallbladder secondary to pancreatic malignancy.

Pancreatic Neuroendocrine Tumors: See pp. 426–427.

Causes of Acute Pancreatitis

Common	Gallstones (35–75%) Alcohol (25–35%) Idiopathic (10–20%); increases with age
Uncommon	Hypertriglyceridemia (fasting triglycerides >1000 mg/dL) (1–4%) Endoscopic retrograde cholangiopancreatography Drugs (1.4–2%); usually mild disease
More uncommon (total <8% of cases)	Abdominal trauma Postoperative complications, especially post-cardiopulmonary bypass Hyperparathyroidism Infection (bacterial, viral, or parasitic) Autoimmune disease Tumor (pancreatic, ampullary) Hypercalcemia Cystic fibrosis
Rare	Ischemia Posterior penetrating ulcer Toxin exposure
Unknown	Congenital abnormalities

12-8 Hernia

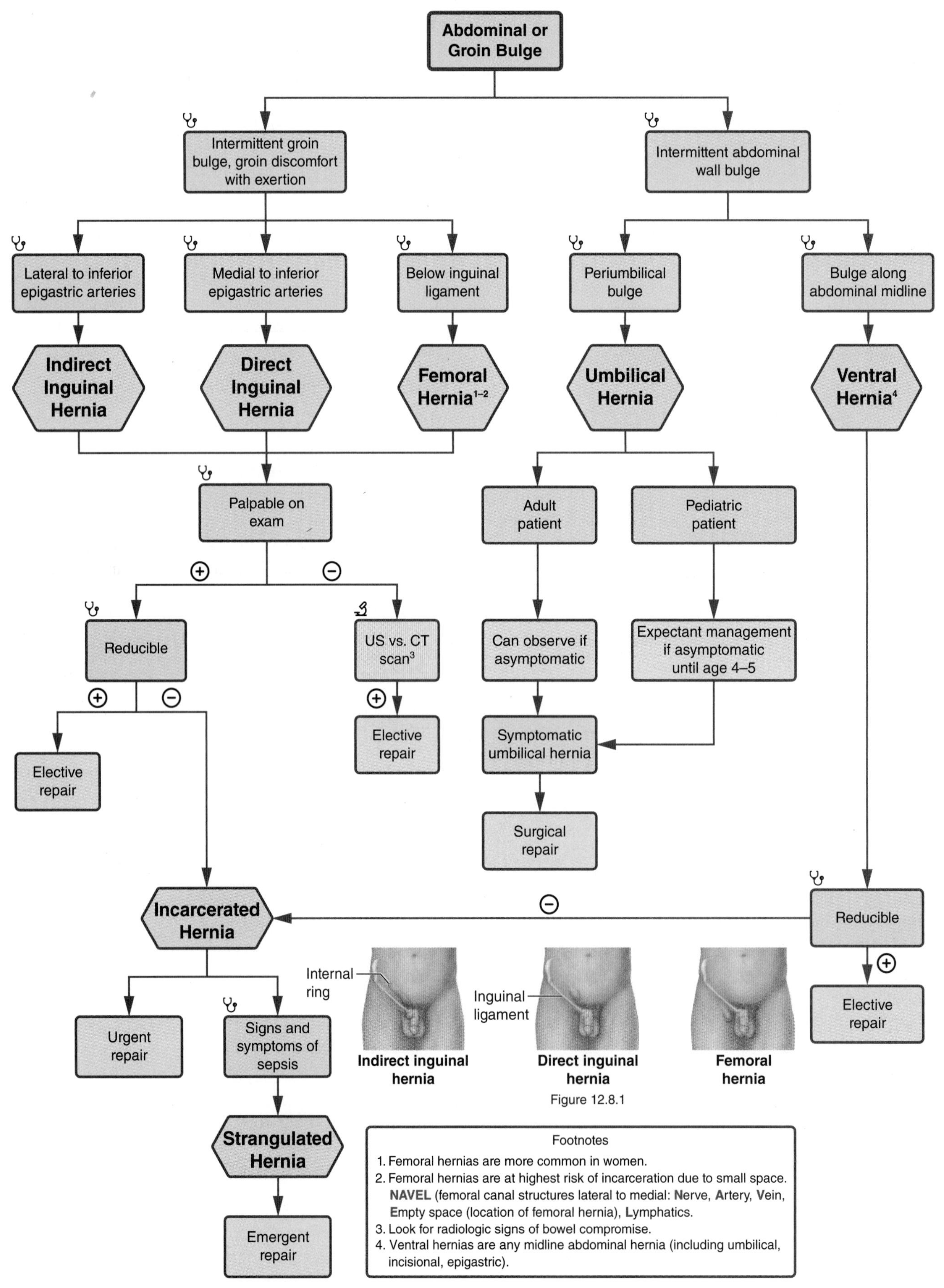
Abdominal or Groin Bulge
Intermittent groin bulge, groin discomfort with exertion
Intermittent abdominal wall bulge
Lateral to inferior epigastric arteries
Medial to inferior epigastric arteries
Below inguinal ligament
Periumbilical bulge
Bulge along abdominal midline
Indirect Inguinal Hernia
Direct Inguinal Hernia
Femoral Hernia[1–2]
Umbilical Hernia
Ventral Hernia[4]
Palpable on exam
Adult patient
Pediatric patient
+
−
Reducible
US vs. CT scan[3]
Can observe if asymptomatic
Expectant management if asymptomatic until age 4–5
+
−
+
Elective repair
Elective repair
Symptomatic umbilical hernia
Surgical repair
Incarcerated Hernia
−
Reducible
+
Elective repair
Urgent repair
Signs and symptoms of sepsis
Strangulated Hernia
Emergent repair
Internal ring
Inguinal ligament
Indirect inguinal hernia
Direct inguinal hernia
Femoral hernia

Figure 12.8.1

Footnotes

1. Femoral hernias are more common in women.
2. Femoral hernias are at highest risk of incarceration due to small space. **NAVEL** (femoral canal structures lateral to medial: **N**erve, **A**rtery, **V**ein, **E**mpty space (location of femoral hernia), **L**ymphatics.
3. Look for radiologic signs of bowel compromise.
4. Ventral hernias are any midline abdominal hernia (including umbilical, incisional, epigastric).

FIGURE 12.8

12-8 Hernia

INGUINAL HERNIA

A 65-year-old M presents with a 4-month history of intermittent left-sided groin pain and bulging. He states these symptoms only bother him while playing tennis and lifting weights. On exam, a non-erythematous bulge can be felt along the left inguinal ligament when the patient is asked to Valsalva. The bulge spontaneously reduces.

Management:

1. Elective surgical repair: Open vs. laparoscopic.
2. Asymptomatic/minimally symptomatic inguinal hernia: Patients may opt for watchful waiting with low associated risk of future complications.

Complications:

- Incarceration: Abdominal contents become trapped within the hernia sac; subsequent bowel obstruction is possible.
- Strangulation: Blood supply to an incarcerated hernia becomes compromised, leading to subsequent ischemia, necrosis, perforation.
- Post-operative complications include hernia recurrence and chronic pain.

HYF:

- Indirect inguinal hernia: Herniation occurs through external and internal rings lateral to the inferior epigastric vessels; due to congenital patent processus vaginalis; most common hernia.
- Direct inguinal hernia: Herniation occurs through the floor of Hesselbach triangle medial to epigastric vessels; due to degeneration of transversalis fascia with age.
- ~10% of patients experience chronic pain following inguinal hernia repair; more common in open repairs.
- Laparoscopic approach is preferred for bilateral hernias to allow for repair of both sides through the same incisions.
- Although inguinal hernias are far more common in males, they also occur in females; there is less likely to be a visible bulge in females, and US or other imaging may be needed for diagnosis.

FEMORAL HERNIA

A 66-year-old F presents with an asymptomatic bulge in her groin that she first noticed 2 weeks ago. On exam, a non-erythematous protrusion can be palpated just below the right inguinal ligament.

Management:

1. Elective surgical repair.
   a. Watchful waiting, while permissible with inguinal hernias, is not recommended with femoral hernias due to the higher risk of complications associated with this hernia type.

Complications: Incarceration, strangulation.

HYF: Herniation occurs below the inguinal ligament through the femoral canal. Risk factors: Weak pelvic floor, increased intra-abdominal pressure. Femoral hernias are more common in females than males, unlike other groin hernias. Femoral hernias have the highest risk for incarceration.

INCISIONAL HERNIA

A 35-year-old M with PMH of exploratory laparotomy for a gunshot wound 3 years ago presents with a protrusion along his surgical scar that appears when he coughs.

Management:

1. Elective surgical repair.
   a. For complex hernias >10 cm in width, preoperative CT imaging is recommended. Complex repair with myofascial flaps and mesh may be required for large defects.

Complications: Incarceration, strangulation, bowel obstruction.

STRANGULATED HERNIA (OF ANY TYPE)

A 46-year-old M presents with 1 day of right-sided groin pain that began suddenly while at a weightlifting tournament. He also complains of nausea. On exam, an erythematous protrusion can be seen along the right inguinal ligament. Localized tenderness is present on palpation, and the bulge is non-reducible. Labs show leukocytosis and elevated lactate. CT imaging confirms the diagnosis.

Management:

1. Urgent surgical hernia repair ± bowel resection of ischemic bowel.
   a. If bowel perforation occurs as a result of strangulation or bowel resection is needed due to necrosis, a non-mesh repair is required due to high risk of mesh infection.
2. NG tube placement if bowel obstruction is suspected.
3. Broad-spectrum antibiotics if there is concern for bowel necrosis/perforation.

Complications: Bowel obstruction, necrosis, and/or perforation.

HYF: Instead of groin pain, patients can present with acute abdomen and an irreducible bulge in the abdominal wall, depending on the type of hernia. Erythema of the skin overlying the hernia raises suspicion for bowel ischemia/necrosis.

13
Surgery: Endocrine

13-1 Pancreatic Neuroendocrine Tumors

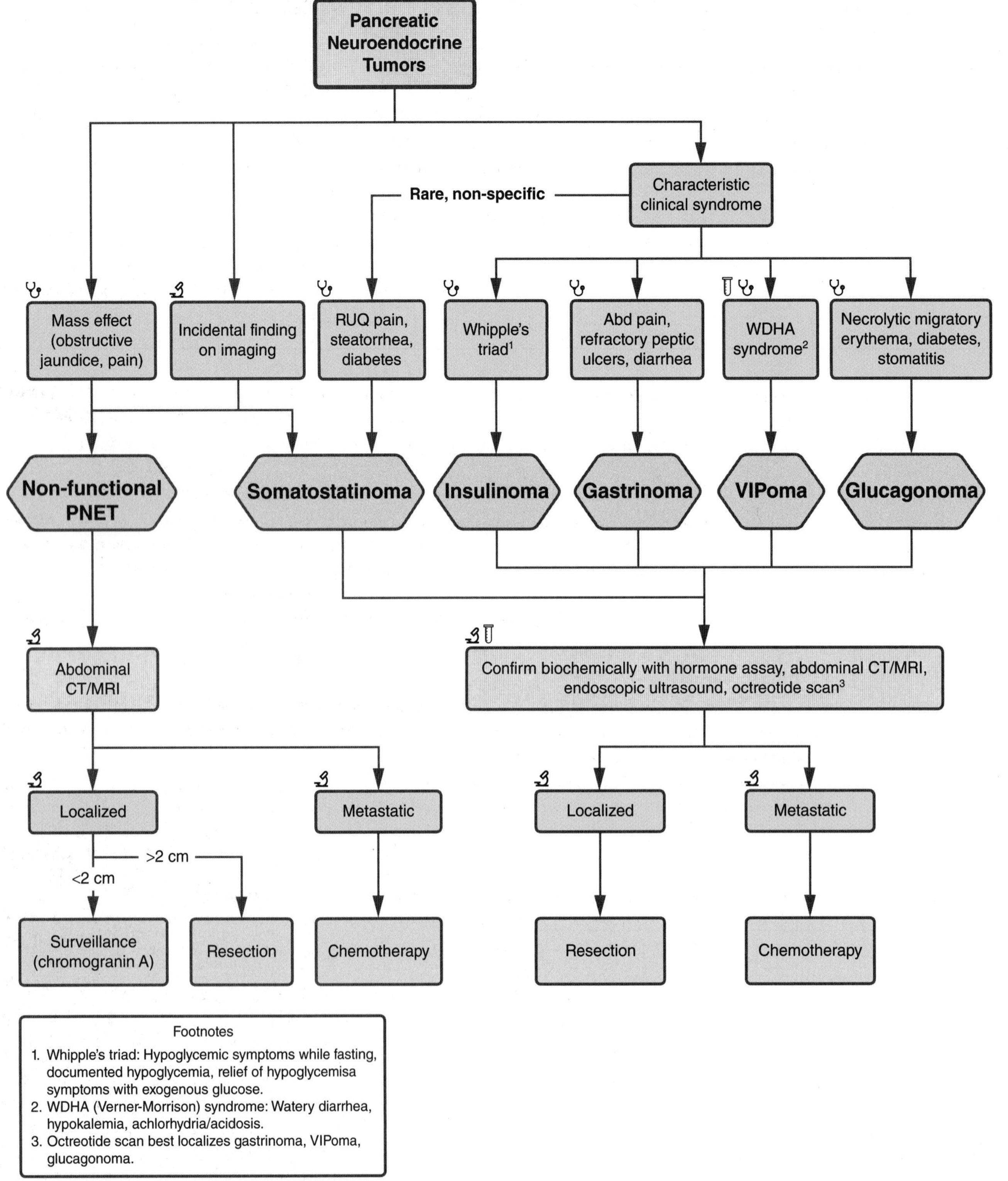
Pancreatic Neuroendocrine Tumors
Rare, non-specific
Characteristic clinical syndrome
Mass effect (obstructive jaundice, pain)
Incidental finding on imaging
RUQ pain, steatorrhea, diabetes
Whipple's triad[1]
Abd pain, refractory peptic ulcers, diarrhea
WDHA syndrome[2]
Necrolytic migratory erythema, diabetes, stomatitis
Non-functional PNET
Somatostatinoma
Insulinoma
Gastrinoma
VIPoma
Glucagonoma
Abdominal CT/MRI
Confirm biochemically with hormone assay, abdominal CT/MRI, endoscopic ultrasound, octreotide scan[3]
Localized
Metastatic
>2 cm
<2 cm
Surveillance (chromogranin A)
Resection
Chemotherapy
Localized
Metastatic
Resection
Chemotherapy
Footnotes
1. Whipple's triad: Hypoglycemic symptoms while fasting, documented hypoglycemia, relief of hypoglycemisa symptoms with exogenous glucose.
2. WDHA (Verner-Morrison) syndrome: Watery diarrhea, hypokalemia, achlorhydria/acidosis.
3. Octreotide scan best localizes gastrinoma, VIPoma, glucagonoma.

FIGURE 13.1

13-1 Pancreatic Neuroendocrine Tumors

NON-FUNCTIONAL PNET

A 45-year-old M with a history of smoking and/or chronic pancreatitis PMH presents with abdominal pain, obstructive jaundice, or weight loss (or may present for incidental finding on imaging). **Labs** and **exam** are normal. EUS with biopsy confirms the diagnosis. Staging CT does not reveal any metastases.

Management:

1. Localization/staging with CT, EUS, DOTA-TATE PET, octreotide scan.
2. Chromogranin A levels.
3. Surveillance vs. surgery vs. chemotherapy.

HYF: Evaluate patient for MEN 1, as most patients with MEN 1 develop PNETs.

SOMATOSTATINOMA

A 50-year-old F presents with new-onset diabetes, steatorrhea, abdominal pain, and weight loss. **Imaging** shows cholelithiasis.

Management:

1. Elevated serum somatostatin levels for confirmation.
2. Localization/staging with CT, EUS, DOTA-TATE PET.
3. Surgery vs. chemotherapy.

HYF: Evaluate patient for NF1. Classic triad of somatostatinoma: Diabetes, steatorrhea, and cholelithiasis.

INSULINOMA

A 45-year-old F presents with recurrent episodes of blurry vision, palpitations, and diaphoresis. She has another episode while in the office. **Labs** show serum plasma glucose of 45. Her symptoms resolve after drinking some juice. A week later, other **labs** come back showing a high insulin level and high C-peptide. Sulfonylurea and meglitinide levels are negative.

Management:

1. Elevated fasting serum insulin and C-peptide.
2. Confirmatory test: 72-hour fasting with symptomatic hypoglycemia with elevated serum insulin level.
3. Localization/staging with CT, EUS, DOTA-TATE PET.
4. Rule out self-administration of exogenous insulin or hypoglycemic agents (eg, serum labs for sulfonylurea, meglitinide).
5. Surgery vs. chemotherapy.

HYF: Evaluate patient for MEN 1. Most cases are benign adenomas.

GASTRINOMA (ZOLLINGER-ELLISON SYNDROME)

A 40-year-old M presents with abdominal pain, GERD, diarrhea, and peptic ulcer disease unresponsive to medical therapy, with multiple or refractory gastric ulcers or ulcers distal to duodenum. **Labs** show elevated gastrin levels.

Management:

1. Fasting serum gastrin concentration and gastric pH level; secretin stimulation test if initial tests negative but high clinical suspicion.
2. Localization/staging with CT, EUS, DOTA-TATE PET.
3. Surgery vs. chemotherapy.

HYF: Evaluate patient for MEN 1 (most common PNET in MEN 1). Most occur in the gastrinoma triangle: Confluence of the cystic and CBD, junction of 2nd and 3rd portions of the duodenum, and junction of head and neck of the pancreas.

VIPOMA (VERNER-MORRISON SYNDROME)

A 50-year-old F presents with persistent high-volume watery diarrhea, flushing episodes, weight loss, lethargy, and nausea. **Labs** show hypokalemia, achlorhydria, and acidosis.

Management:

1. Correction of electrolyte abnormalities.
2. Stool sample: Low stool osmotic gap.
3. Elevated serum VIP level for confirmation.
4. Localization/staging with CT, EUS, DOTA-TATE PET, octreotide scan.
5. Surgery vs. chemotherapy.

HYF: Most are malignant. Octreotide can be used to treat diarrhea by inhibiting VIP secretion. VIP inhibits gastrin secretion, so patients will have achlorhydria on labs.

GLUCAGONOMA

A 45-year-old F presents with pruritic and painful rash, diabetes, depression, chronic diarrhea, stomatitis, and/or weight loss. **Labs** show hyperglycemia. On **imaging**, venous Doppler shows a DVT in one of her legs.

Management:

1. Elevated serum glucagon levels for confirmation.
2. Localization/staging with CT, EUS, DOTA-TATE PET.
3. Surgery vs. chemotherapy.

HYF: High suspicion in older patient losing weight with new-onset diabetes and dermatological complaints. Pathognomonic rash is necrolytic migratory erythema.

13-2 Adrenals

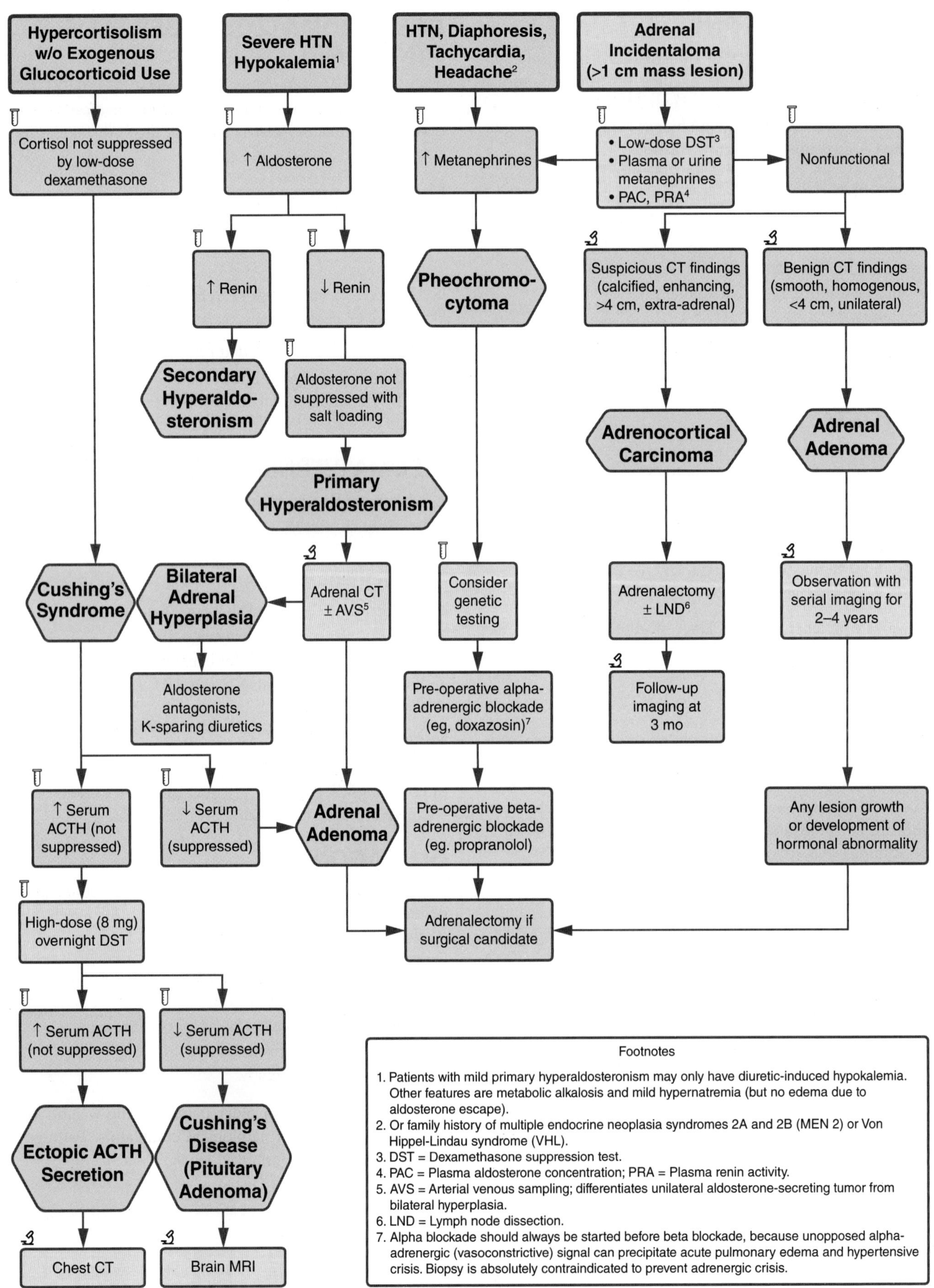
Hypercortisolism w/o Exogenous Glucocorticoid Use
Cortisol not suppressed by low-dose dexamethasone
Severe HTN Hypokalemia[1]
↑ Aldosterone
↑ Renin
↓ Renin
Secondary Hyperaldosteronism
Aldosterone not suppressed with salt loading
Primary Hyperaldosteronism
HTN, Diaphoresis, Tachycardia, Headache[2]
↑ Metanephrines
Pheochromocytoma
Adrenal Incidentaloma (>1 cm mass lesion)
• Low-dose DST[3]
• Plasma or urine metanephrines
• PAC, PRA[4]
Nonfunctional
Suspicious CT findings (calcified, enhancing, >4 cm, extra-adrenal)
Benign CT findings (smooth, homogenous, <4 cm, unilateral)
Adrenocortical Carcinoma
Adrenal Adenoma
Cushing's Syndrome
Bilateral Adrenal Hyperplasia
Adrenal CT ± AVS[5]
Consider genetic testing
Adrenalectomy ± LND[6]
Observation with serial imaging for 2–4 years
Aldosterone antagonists, K-sparing diuretics
Pre-operative alpha-adrenergic blockade (eg, doxazosin)[7]
Follow-up imaging at 3 mo
↑ Serum ACTH (not suppressed)
↓ Serum ACTH (suppressed)
Adrenal Adenoma
Pre-operative beta-adrenergic blockade (eg. propranolol)
Any lesion growth or development of hormonal abnormality
High-dose (8 mg) overnight DST
Adrenalectomy if surgical candidate
↑ Serum ACTH (not suppressed)
↓ Serum ACTH (suppressed)
Ectopic ACTH Secretion
Cushing's Disease (Pituitary Adenoma)
Chest CT
Brain MRI

Footnotes

1. Patients with mild primary hyperaldosteronism may only have diuretic-induced hypokalemia. Other features are metabolic alkalosis and mild hypernatremia (but no edema due to aldosterone escape).
2. Or family history of multiple endocrine neoplasia syndromes 2A and 2B (MEN 2) or Von Hippel-Lindau syndrome (VHL).
3. DST = Dexamethasone suppression test.
4. PAC = Plasma aldosterone concentration; PRA = Plasma renin activity.
5. AVS = Arterial venous sampling; differentiates unilateral aldosterone-secreting tumor from bilateral hyperplasia.
6. LND = Lymph node dissection.
7. Alpha blockade should always be started before beta blockade, because unopposed alpha-adrenergic (vasoconstrictive) signal can precipitate acute pulmonary edema and hypertensive crisis. Biopsy is absolutely contraindicated to prevent adrenergic crisis.

FIGURE 13.2

13-2 Adrenals

PHEOCHROMOCYTOMA

A 56-year-old M with HTN and family history of thyroid cancer presents with **exam** findings of pallor and tachycardia after induction of anesthesia for elective surgery. BP is 242/139.

Management:

1. Urine or plasma fractionated metanephrines are highly sensitive markers of catecholamine overproduction, but abdominal imaging is needed to confirm tumor location.
2. Pre-operative alpha-adrenergic antagonists prior to beta-blockers (do not give unopposed beta-blockers to avoid hypertensive emergency).
3. Laparoscopic or open adrenalectomy.

Complications:

- Severe hypertensive episodes precipitated by tumor palpation, surgical manipulation, or anesthesia.
- Cardiomyopathy from catecholamine excess.
- Malignant potential with risk of metastasis.

HYF: Medullary thyroid carcinoma should raise suspicion for MEN 2 syndromes; affected patients should get *RET* mutation testing and hormonal screening for pheochromocytoma.

10% Rule: 10% of pheochromocytomas are malignant, 10% are bilateral, 10% are extra-adrenal, 10% are familial (MEN 2/VHL).

BENIGN ADRENAL ADENOMA

A 51-year-old F who is otherwise healthy presents for further evaluation of a 3-cm adrenal mass identified incidentally on CT A/P. She is asymptomatic. **Exam** and **labs** are normal.

Management:

1. Consider biopsy or excision if there are malignant features on CT (eg, high density, irregular, heterogenous, poor contrast washout).
2. Exclude subclinical hormonal hyperfunction.
3. Re-image in 1 year if imaging appearance is benign.

Complications:

- Mass effect of a benign lesion.
- Development of hormonal hyperfunctionality.
- Interval growth of previously undetected malignant lesion.

HYF: Pheochromocytoma must be excluded before needle biopsy or surgical excision.

CUSHING'S SYNDROME DUE TO ADRENAL ADENOMA

A 37-year-old F with PMH of osteoporosis and HTN presents with weight gain. On **exam**, she has facial plethora. **Labs** show hyperglycemia. 24-hour urine free cortisol is elevated. Serum ACTH is low.

Management:

1. Low-dose dexamethasone test to confirm diagnosis of Cushing's Syndrome (AM cortisol is not suppressed).
2. Adrenal CT to rule out cortisol-producing carcinoma.
3. Unilateral adrenalectomy (curative surgery).

Complications:

- Mortality from cardiovascular, thromboembolic, and infectious complications in untreated Cushing's Syndrome.
- Post-op adrenal insufficiency from prolonged HPA axis suppression (may require long-term steroid replacement).

HYF: Do not forget exogenous glucocorticoid use as a cause of Cushing's syndrome.

ADRENAL ALDOSTERONOMA

A 29-year-old M with no PMH presents with muscle cramps. BP is 157/95. **Labs** show potassium of 2.8.

Management:

1. Elevated plasma aldosterone/renin ratio (>20) confirms primary hyperaldosteronism.
2. Adrenal CT to characterize lesion; arterial venous sampling distinguishes adenoma from bilateral adrenal hyperplasia if imaging is equivocal.
3. Adrenalectomy for unilateral aldosteronoma.
4. Mineralocorticoid receptor antagonists (K-sparing diuretics, eg, spironolactone) for bilateral hyperplasia.

Complications:

- Cardiovascular morbidity from untreated hypertension.
- Muscle cramps/weakness from severe hypokalemia.

HYF: If renin is also elevated, consider secondary hyperaldosteronism. Etiologies are either hypertensive (renovascular HTN, renin-secreting tumors) or normotensive (excessive vomiting/diuretics, Bartter/Gitelman's syndromes).

13-3 Parathyroids

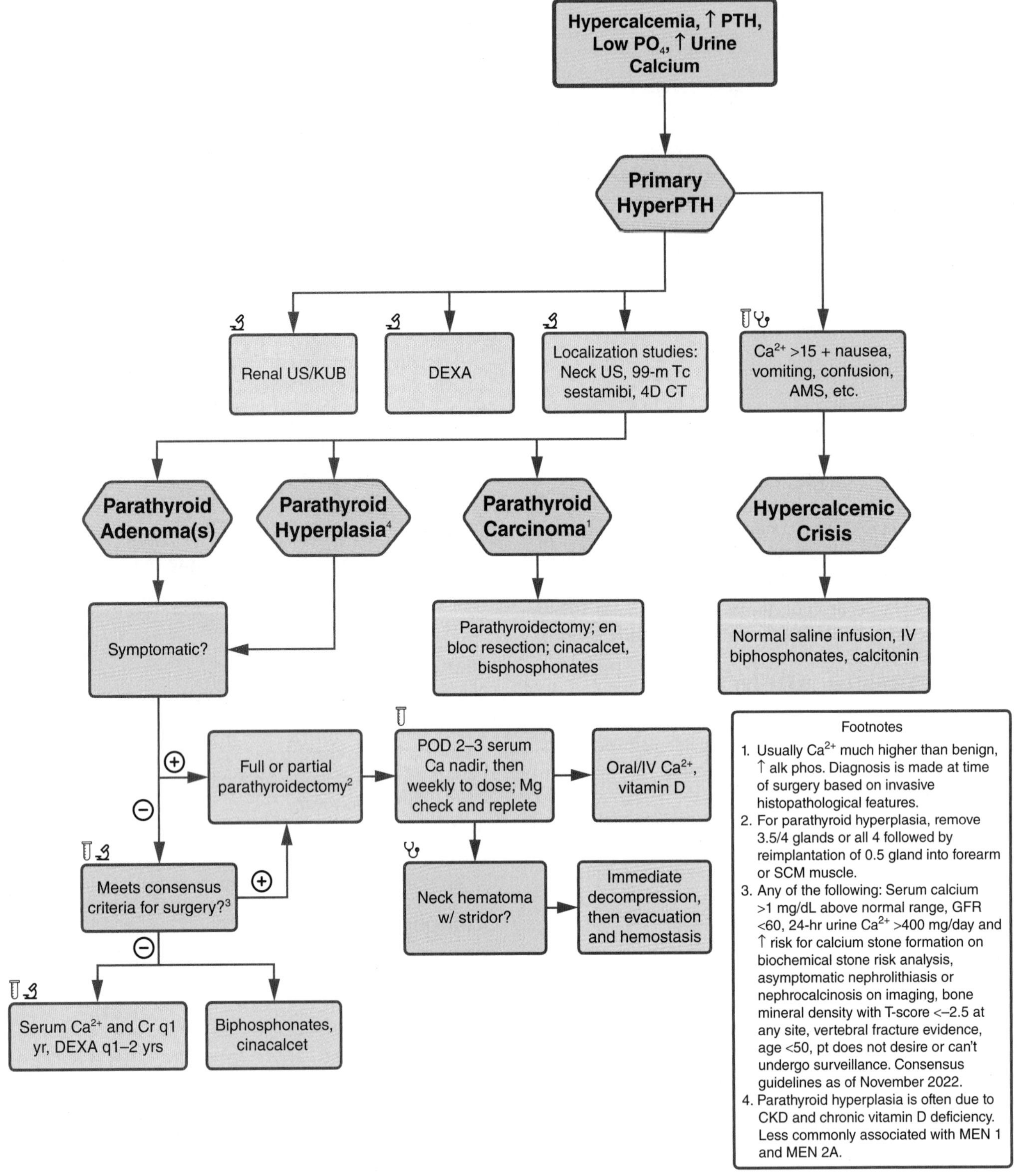
Hypercalcemia, ↑ PTH, Low PO4, ↑ Urine Calcium
Primary HyperPTH
Renal US/KUB
DEXA
Localization studies: Neck US, 99-m Tc sestamibi, 4D CT
Ca2+ >15 + nausea, vomiting, confusion, AMS, etc.
Parathyroid Adenoma(s)
Parathyroid Hyperplasia4
Parathyroid Carcinoma1
Hypercalcemic Crisis
Symptomatic?
Parathyroidectomy; en bloc resection; cinacalcet, bisphosphonates
Normal saline infusion, IV biphosphonates, calcitonin
+
−
Full or partial parathyroidectomy2
POD 2–3 serum Ca nadir, then weekly to dose; Mg check and replete
Oral/IV Ca2+, vitamin D
Meets consensus criteria for surgery?3
+
Neck hematoma w/ stridor?
Immediate decompression, then evacuation and hemostasis
−
Serum Ca2+ and Cr q1 yr, DEXA q1–2 yrs
Biphosphonates, cinacalcet
Footnotes
1. Usually Ca2+ much higher than benign, ↑ alk phos. Diagnosis is made at time of surgery based on invasive histopathological features.
2. For parathyroid hyperplasia, remove 3.5/4 glands or all 4 followed by reimplantation of 0.5 gland into forearm or SCM muscle.
3. Any of the following: Serum calcium >1 mg/dL above normal range, GFR <60, 24-hr urine Ca2+ >400 mg/day and ↑ risk for calcium stone formation on biochemical stone risk analysis, asymptomatic nephrolithiasis or nephrocalcinosis on imaging, bone mineral density with T-score <–2.5 at any site, vertebral fracture evidence, age <50, pt does not desire or can't undergo surveillance. Consensus guidelines as of November 2022.
4. Parathyroid hyperplasia is often due to CKD and chronic vitamin D deficiency. Less commonly associated with MEN 1 and MEN 2A.

FIGURE 13.3

14
Surgery: Urology

14-1 Lower Urinary Tract Symptoms

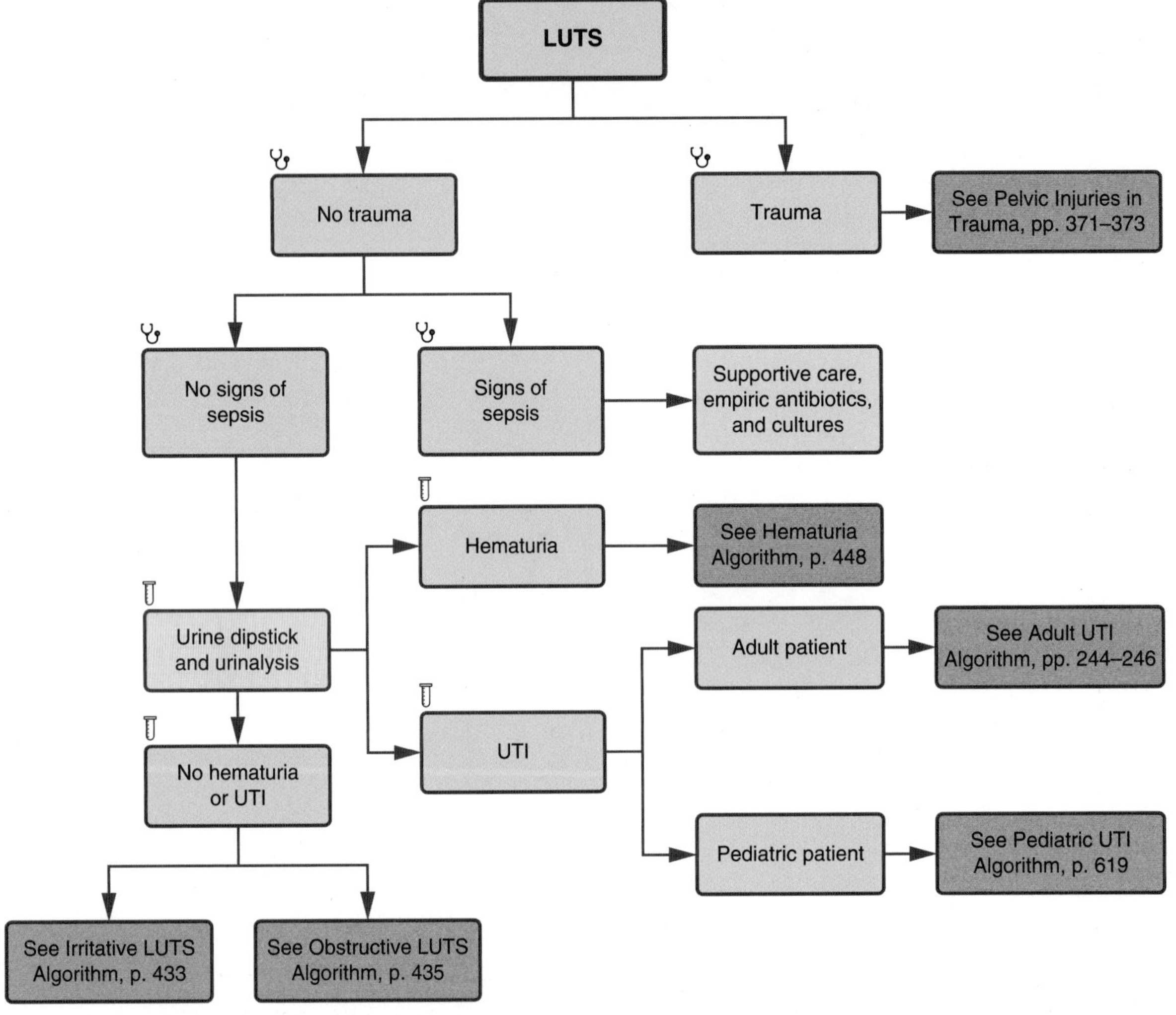
LUTS
No trauma
Trauma
See Pelvic Injuries in Trauma, pp. 371–373
No signs of sepsis
Signs of sepsis
Supportive care, empiric antibiotics, and cultures
Hematuria
See Hematuria Algorithm, p. 448
Urine dipstick and urinalysis
Adult patient
See Adult UTI Algorithm, pp. 244–246
UTI
No hematuria or UTI
Pediatric patient
See Pediatric UTI Algorithm, p. 619
See Irritative LUTS Algorithm, p. 433
See Obstructive LUTS Algorithm, p. 435

Lower urinary tract symptoms (LUTS) is a term reserved for nonspecific symptoms that often coincide with, and should raise suspicion for, pathology affecting the lower urinary tract. There are 2 main types of LUTS: Irritative and obstructive. Irritative LUTS include urinary frequency, small voids, dysuria, urgency with or without urge incontinence, nocturia, enuresis, and hematuria. Obstructive LUTS include straining or hesitating to initiate a urinary stream, weak stream, incomplete bladder emptying, urinary intermittency, and overflow incontinence. There are many etiologies for LUTS; some originate from the lower urinary tract (eg, cystitis, urethritis, urethral stricture, BPH), and some originate from the upper urinary tract (eg, nephrolithiasis, ureterolithiasis, upper tract malignancy). Importantly, a single etiology can cause both irritative and obstructive LUTS in a patient simultaneously; for example, BPH can cause urinary retention that leads to nocturia with frequent, small voids.

FIGURE 14.1

14-2 Lower Urinary Tract Symptoms (Irritative)

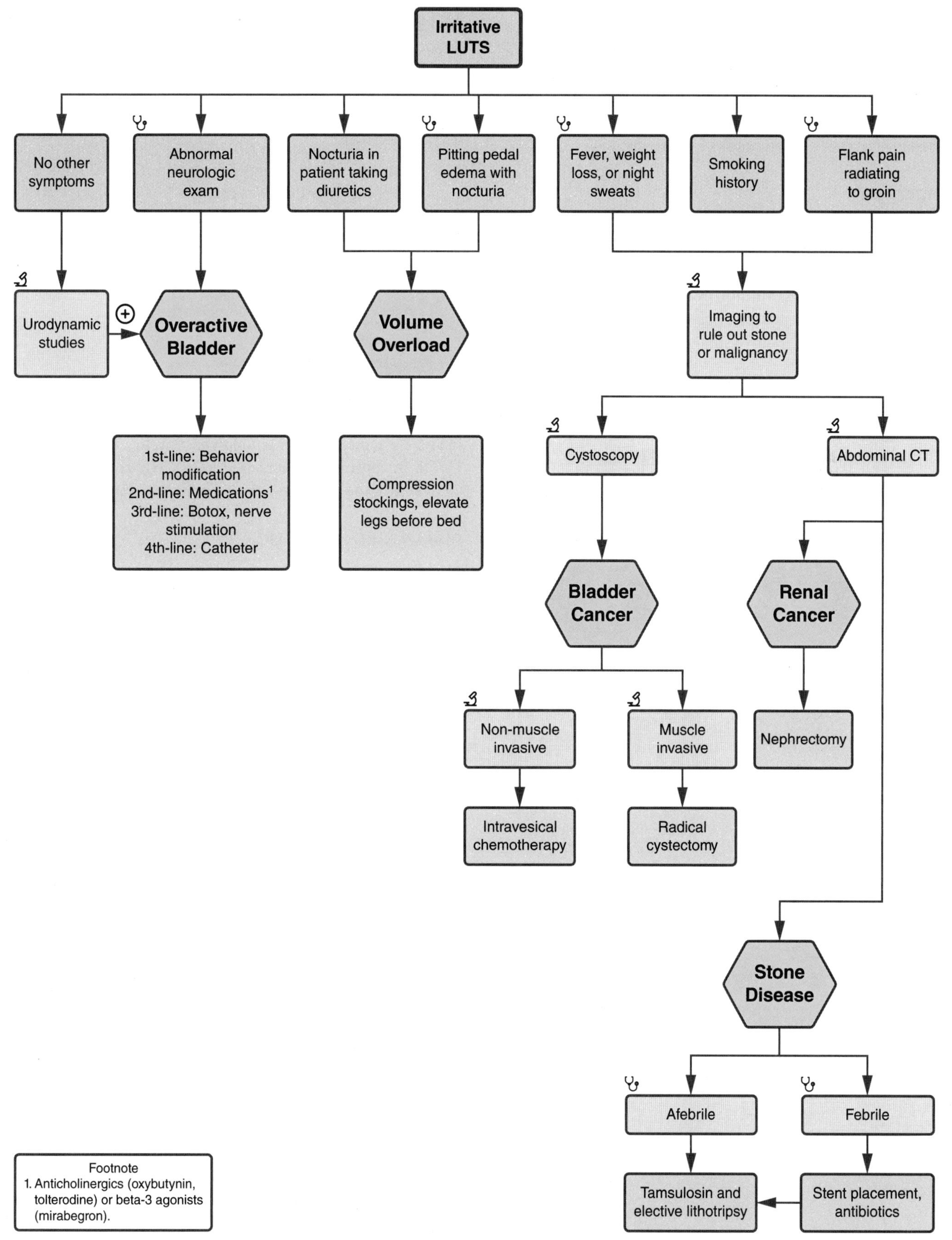
Irritative LUTS
No other symptoms
Abnormal neurologic exam
Nocturia in patient taking diuretics
Pitting pedal edema with nocturia
Fever, weight loss, or night sweats
Smoking history
Flank pain radiating to groin
Urodynamic studies
+
Overactive Bladder
Volume Overload
Imaging to rule out stone or malignancy
1st-line: Behavior modification
2nd-line: Medications[1]
3rd-line: Botox, nerve stimulation
4th-line: Catheter
Compression stockings, elevate legs before bed
Cystoscopy
Abdominal CT
Bladder Cancer
Renal Cancer
Non-muscle invasive
Muscle invasive
Nephrectomy
Intravesical chemotherapy
Radical cystectomy
Stone Disease
Afebrile
Febrile
Tamsulosin and elective lithotripsy
Stent placement, antibiotics
Footnote
1. Anticholinergics (oxybutynin, tolterodine) or beta-3 agonists (mirabegron).

FIGURE 14.2

14-2 Lower Urinary Tract Symptoms (Irritative)

OVERACTIVE BLADDER

A 36-year-old F with PMH of T2DM and multiple sclerosis presents with urinary frequency, urge incontinence, and nocturia. Her GU **exam** is normal, but neurologic exam shows hyperreflexia. **Labs** show Hgb A1c of 8.2. On **imaging**, MRI head/neck shows white matter changes consistent with multiple sclerosis.

Management:

1. Behavioral interventions: Pelvic floor exercises, avoidance of bladder irritants (coffee, red wine, tomato juice), and bladder retraining with a voiding diary.
2. Anticholinergics (eg, oxybutinin) or beta-3 agonists (eg, mirabegron).
3. Intravesical Botox, tibial nerve stimulation, or sacral neuromodulation.
4. 4th-line is indwelling catheter +/− surgical bladder augmentation.

Complications: Patients taking anticholinergics (eg, tolterodine, oxybutinin) may experience anticholinergic toxicity such as urinary retention, constipation, and altered mental status.

HYF: Choose mirabegron over oxybutinin if a patient has contraindications to anticholinergics (eg, elderly patient with dementia, history of acute angle closure glaucoma).

VOLUME OVERLOAD

A 59-year-old F with PMH of HFrEF on furosemide presents with nocturia ×8–10 episodes per night. On **exam**, she has JVD and pitting pedal edema. On **labs**, UA is normal.

Management:

1. Continue HFrEF drug regimen—nocturia won't kill the patient but stopping their diuretics might!
2. Behavior change: Fluid restriction >2 hours before bed; wear compression stockings and elevate legs 1–2 hours before bed (nocturia is caused by redistribution of pedal edema to dependent areas while lying flat during sleep).

Complications:

- Poor sleep quality.
- CHF exacerbation in patients who try to discontinue their furosemide.

HYF: By increasing urine volume, diuretics are associated with LUTS. In those with nocturia due to CHF, continue treating the CHF even if the diuretics are causing worsening LUTS.

Bladder Cancer: See p. 436.

Renal Cancer: See p. 449.

Stone Disease: See pp. 441–442.

14-3 Lower Urinary Tract Symptoms (Obstructive)

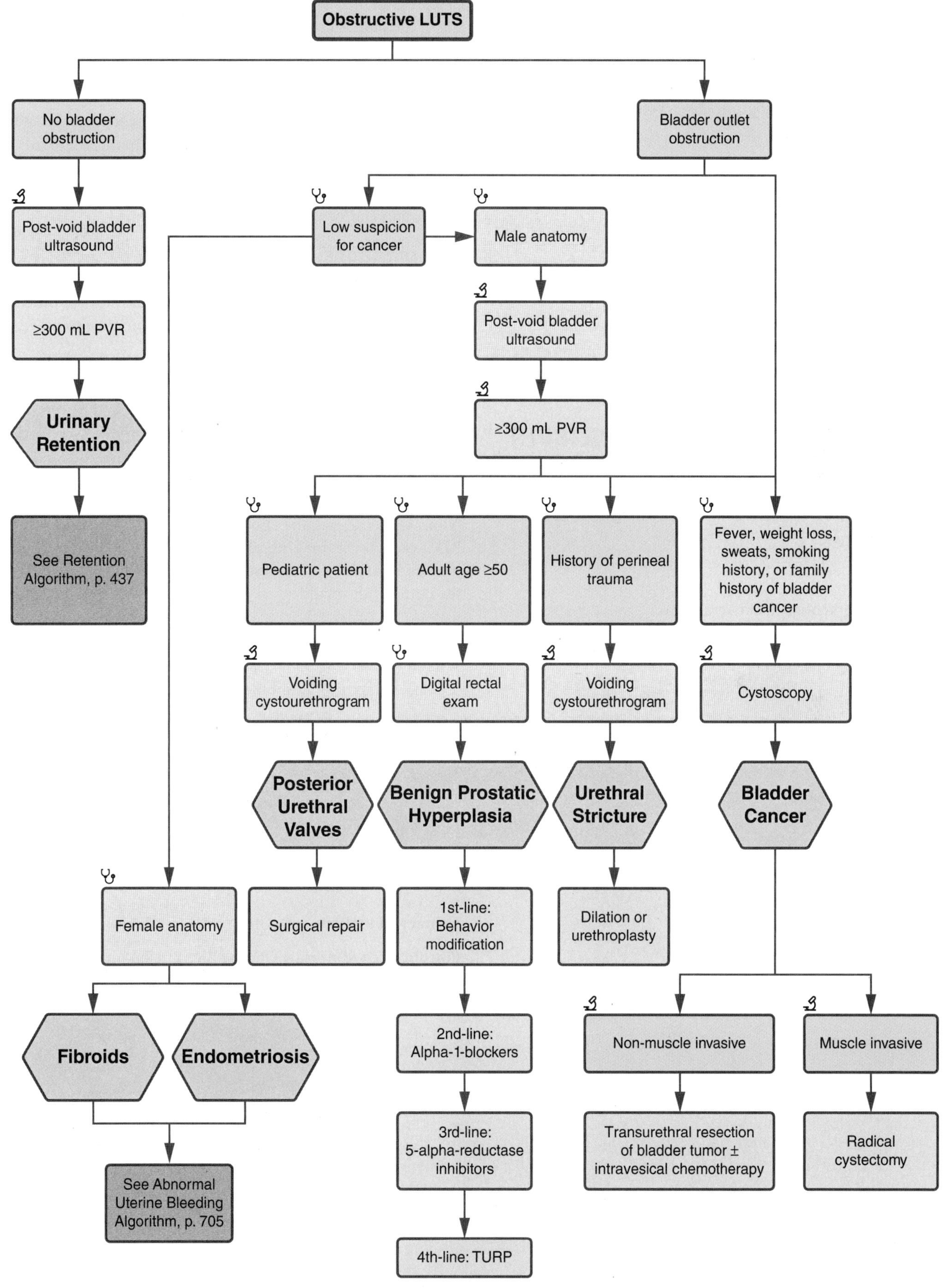
Obstructive LUTS
No bladder obstruction
Bladder outlet obstruction
Post-void bladder ultrasound
≥300 mL PVR
Urinary Retention
See Retention Algorithm, p. 437
Low suspicion for cancer
Male anatomy
Post-void bladder ultrasound
≥300 mL PVR
Pediatric patient
Adult age ≥50
History of perineal trauma
Fever, weight loss, sweats, smoking history, or family history of bladder cancer
Voiding cystourethrogram
Digital rectal exam
Voiding cystourethrogram
Cystoscopy
Posterior Urethral Valves
Benign Prostatic Hyperplasia
Urethral Stricture
Bladder Cancer
Female anatomy
Surgical repair
1st-line: Behavior modification
Dilation or urethroplasty
Fibroids
Endometriosis
2nd-line: Alpha-1-blockers
Non-muscle invasive
Muscle invasive
See Abnormal Uterine Bleeding Algorithm, p. 705
3rd-line: 5-alpha-reductase inhibitors
Transurethral resection of bladder tumor ± intravesical chemotherapy
Radical cystectomy
4th-line: TURP

FIGURE 14.3

14-3 Lower Urinary Tract Symptoms (Obstructive)

POSTERIOR URETHRAL VALVES

A newborn male with Potter sequence and ARDS is found to have abdominal distension on **exam**. On **imaging**, prenatal ultrasound had shown bilateral hydroureteronephrosis and oligohydramnios. Postnatal voiding cystourethrogram shows vesicoureteral reflux.

Management:

1. As temporizing measure, place a catheter to prevent postrenal AKI.
2. Definitive treatment: Surgical ablation of the pathologic valve.

Complications:

- Prenatal: Oligohydramnios with Potter sequence.
- Postnatal: Chronic renal failure.

HYF: Posterior urethral valves are the most common cause of postrenal obstruction and chronic renal failure in newborn males.

BENIGN PROSTATIC HYPERPLASIA (BPH)

A 62-year-old M with no significant PMH presents with nocturia ×7 episodes per night, straining to urinate, and weak stream. On digital rectal **exam**, he appears comfortable and has a uniformly enlarged, soft prostate.

Management:

1. Alpha-1-blockers (tamsulosin, terazosin).
2. 5-Alpha-reductase inhibitors (finasteride).
3. Surgical intervention (eg, TURP).

Complications: Urinary retention → UTI → urosepsis.

HYF: BPH can be associated with mildly elevated PSA. Not a risk factor for prostate cancer. Hyperplasia occurs at the transition zone of the prostate, which surrounds the urethra and causes obstructive LUTS (unlike prostate cancer, which occurs in the peripheral zone and does not typically cause urinary symptoms). Alpha-1-blockers are a common cause of orthostatic hypotension in elderly males with BPH.

URETHRAL STRICTURE

A 22-year-old M gymnast presents with 2-month history of weak stream and straining to void after falling with split legs on the balance beam. **Exam** is unremarkable. On **imaging**, retrograde urethrogram and voiding cystourethrogram demonstrate narrowing of the bulbar urethra.

Management:

1. Perform retrograde urethrogram to confirm diagnosis and characterize the location and length of the urethral stricture.
2. If there is urinary retention, place a suprapubic tube (to prevent postrenal AKI) and schedule an elective surgical repair.
3. Definitive treatment is elective repair with either urethral dilation and/or urethroplasty.

Complications: Urinary retention → urosepsis.

HYF: Urethral dilation and urethroplasty are elective procedures; as a temporizing measure, place a suprapubic tube to prevent urinary retention.

BLADDER CANCER

A 60-year-old M with a 30-pack-year smoking history who works with aniline dyes (eg, textile industry) and/or pesticides presents with subacute painless hematuria, suprapubic pain, and straining while urinating. Physical **exam** demonstrates mild suprapubic tenderness. **Labs** show elevated creatinine and numerous RBCs on UA. On **imaging**, abdominal US shows bilateral hydronephrosis. Cystoscopy shows several friable, pedunculated masses on the dome of the bladder.

Management:

1. Non-muscle-invasive: TURBT +/– intravesical chemotherapy.
2. Muscle-invasive: Radical cystectomy.

Complications:

- Urosepsis.
- Bilateral postrenal AKI.

HYF: If the tumor is muscle-invasive, perform a radical cystectomy. Otherwise, can do TURBT +/– intravesical chemotherapy with active surveillance (schedule repeated cystoscopies).

Urinary Retention: See p. 438.

Fibroids: See Abnormal Uterine Bleeding on pp. 705–707.

Endometriosis: See Abnormal Uterine Bleeding on pp. 705–707.

14-4 Retention

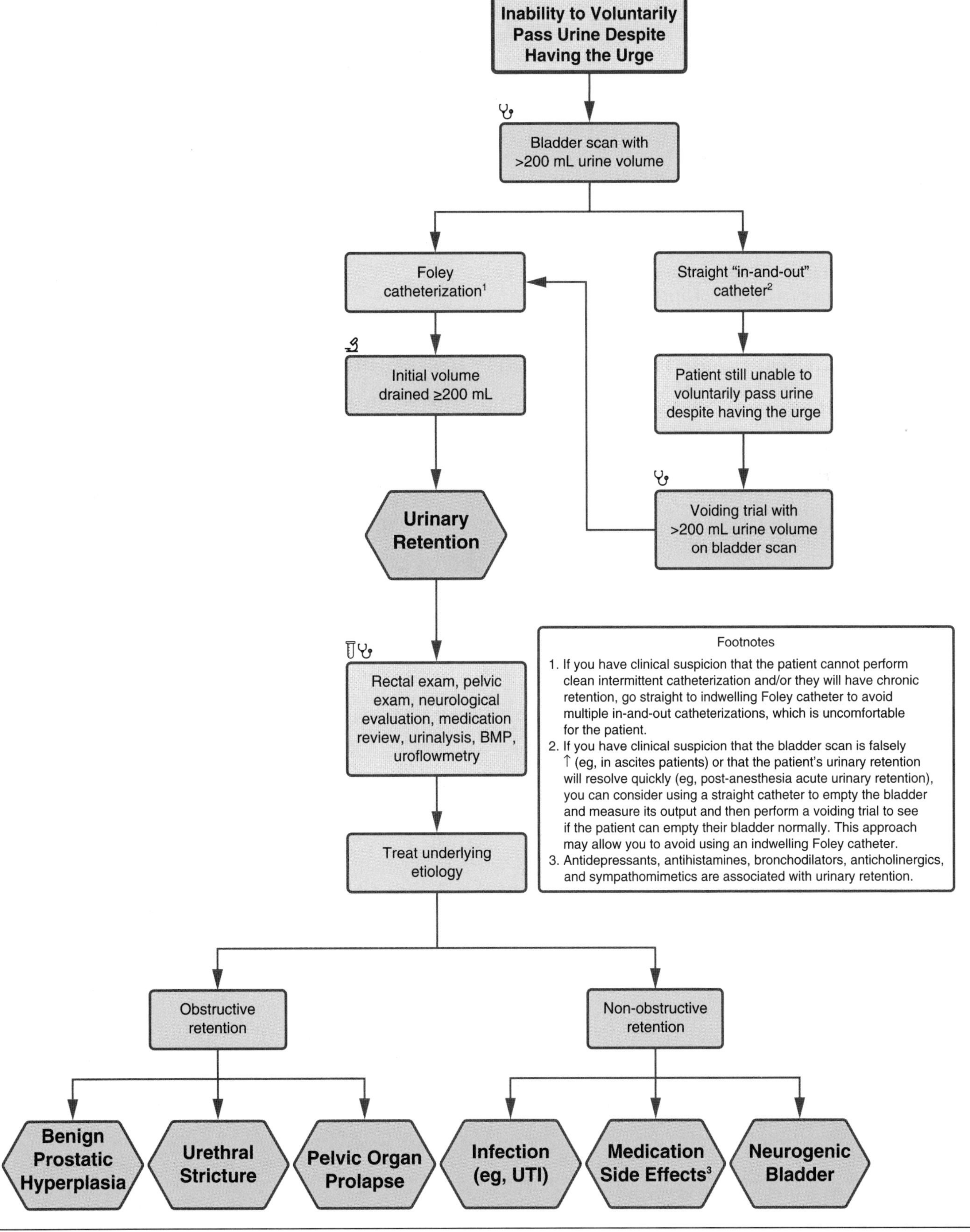
Inability to Voluntarily Pass Urine Despite Having the Urge
Bladder scan with >200 mL urine volume
Foley catheterization[1]
Straight "in-and-out" catheter[2]
Initial volume drained ≥200 mL
Patient still unable to voluntarily pass urine despite having the urge
Voiding trial with >200 mL urine volume on bladder scan
Urinary Retention
Rectal exam, pelvic exam, neurological evaluation, medication review, urinalysis, BMP, uroflowmetry
Treat underlying etiology
Obstructive retention
Non-obstructive retention
Benign Prostatic Hyperplasia
Urethral Stricture
Pelvic Organ Prolapse
Infection (eg, UTI)
Medication Side Effects[3]
Neurogenic Bladder
Footnotes
1. If you have clinical suspicion that the patient cannot perform clean intermittent catheterization and/or they will have chronic retention, go straight to indwelling Foley catheter to avoid multiple in-and-out catheterizations, which is uncomfortable for the patient.
2. If you have clinical suspicion that the bladder scan is falsely ↑ (eg, in ascites patients) or that the patient's urinary retention will resolve quickly (eg, post-anesthesia acute urinary retention), you can consider using a straight catheter to empty the bladder and measure its output and then perform a voiding trial to see if the patient can empty their bladder normally. This approach may allow you to avoid using an indwelling Foley catheter.
3. Antidepressants, antihistamines, bronchodilators, anticholinergics, and sympathomimetics are associated with urinary retention.

FIGURE 14.4

14-4 Retention

URINARY RETENTION

A 74-year-old M with PMH of BPH presents with inability to pass urine and abdominal discomfort. On **exam**, he has a palpable suprapubic mass. On **imaging**, bladder US shows a volume of 450 mL.

Management:

1. Ultrasound is the preferred initial test followed by catheterization, but if the patient is in severe distress, then catheterization can be done immediately. Catheterization is both therapeutic and diagnostic when the initial volume drained is >200 mL.
2. Next steps are to treat the urinary retention and underlying etiology. Options for management of urinary retention are clean intermittent or straight catheterization. Underlying etiology such as BPH in males or pelvic organ prolapse in females is common (digital rectal exam and pelvic examination are key).
3. Management of BPH is complex, but for increased likelihood of passing void trial, alpha-1 antagonists (tamsulosin, terazosin, doxazosin) are typically given. In addition, 5-alpha-reductase inhibitors (finasteride) may be added. If medication fails, consider referral to a specialist for surgical intervention.

Complications:

- Urinary retention and stasis predispose to infection. Obtain a urinalysis to assess for UTI.
- Increased pressure from the bladder can predispose to kidney damage and hydronephrosis. Obtain a BMP to assess for renal function.
- Retention can also be a complication of surgery. For these patients, a post-void residual should be obtained for diagnosis.

HYF: Urinary retention is characterized by the inability to pass urine and can present acutely (usually in men) or chronically (usually in women). For bladder volume showing >300 mL, treat with either Foley catheterization or clean intermittent catheterization. Identify and treat the underlying cause.

Benign Prostatic Hyperplasia: See p. 436.

Obstruction: See pp. 435–436.

Urethral Stricture: See p. 436.

14-5 Incontinence

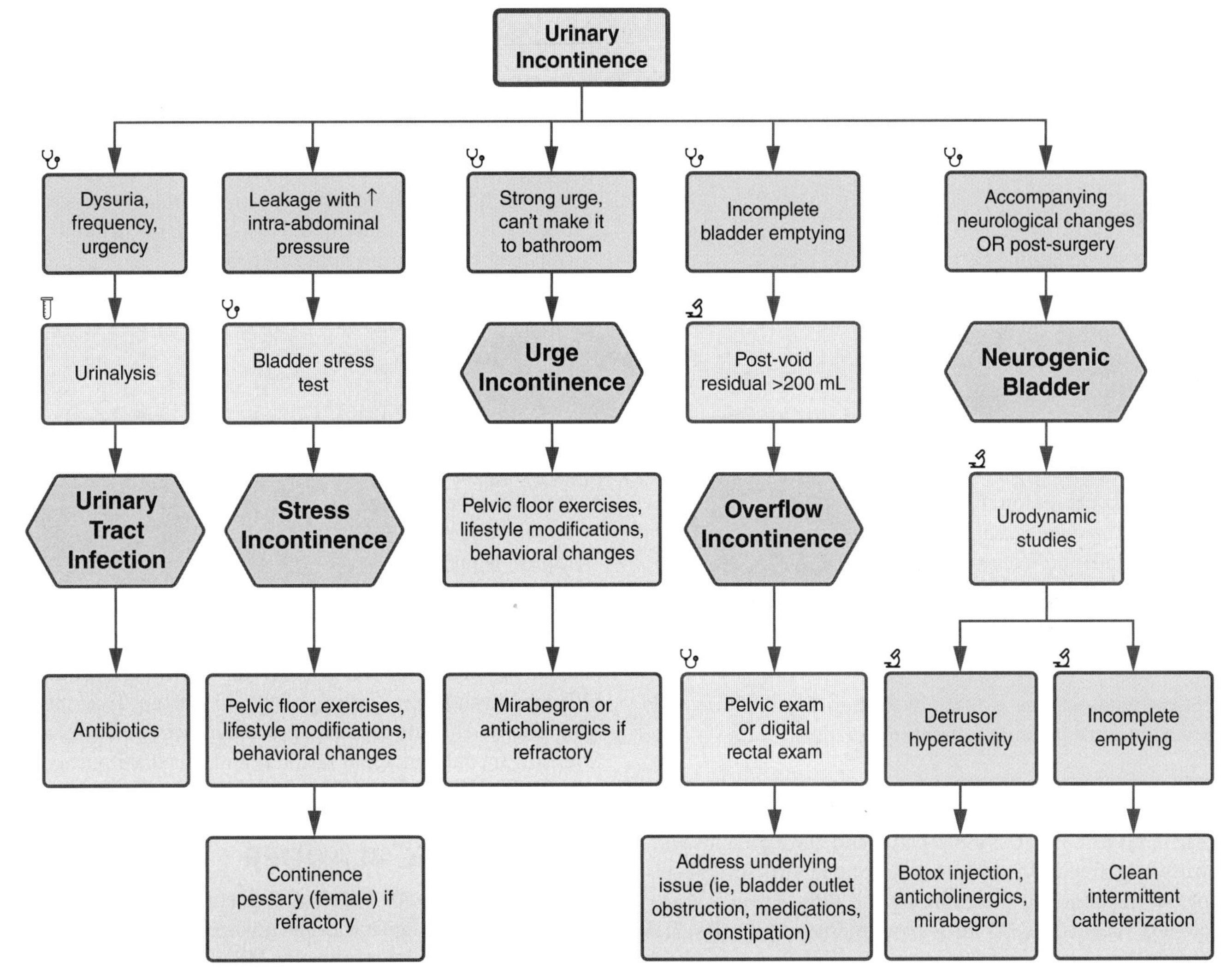
Urinary Incontinence
Dysuria, frequency, urgency
Leakage with ↑ intra-abdominal pressure
Strong urge, can't make it to bathroom
Incomplete bladder emptying
Accompanying neurological changes OR post-surgery
Urinalysis
Bladder stress test
Urge Incontinence
Post-void residual >200 mL
Neurogenic Bladder
Urinary Tract Infection
Stress Incontinence
Pelvic floor exercises, lifestyle modifications, behavioral changes
Overflow Incontinence
Urodynamic studies
Antibiotics
Pelvic floor exercises, lifestyle modifications, behavioral changes
Mirabegron or anticholinergics if refractory
Pelvic exam or digital rectal exam
Detrusor hyperactivity
Incomplete emptying
Continence pessary (female) if refractory
Address underlying issue (ie, bladder outlet obstruction, medications, constipation)
Botox injection, anticholinergics, mirabegron
Clean intermittent catheterization

FIGURE 14.5

14-5 Incontinence

STRESS INCONTINENCE

A 68-year-old F with PMH of obesity and multi-parity presents with urine leakage. On **exam**, with patient upright, Valsalva maneuver elicits urine leakage from the urethra. On **labs**, UA is (–) for leukocyte esterase, nitrites, and blood.

Management:

1. Pelvic floor strengthening exercises (Kegels), lifestyle modifications (drink less coffee and alcohol, lose weight).
2. If above fails, consider placement of a continence pessary to strengthen pelvic floor muscles.
3. If above fails, consider surgical intervention with a mid-urethral sling.

Complications:

- This is the most common type of incontinence. Chronic incontinence can potentially cause perineal infections from moisture retention or falls and fractures.
- Pelvic organ prolapse can be a potential cause of stress incontinence. Surgical management (eg, anterior vaginal wall repair) can be offered.

HYF: Stress incontinence is more likely to occur in those with increased abdominal pressure (obesity, pregnancy).

URGE INCONTINENCE

A 69-year-old F with PMH of multi-parity and DM2 presents with urinary urgency, frequency, and nocturia. She reports several episodes of not making it to the bathroom on time. **Exam** is unremarkable. On **labs**, UA is (–) for leukocyte esterase, nitrites, and blood.

Management:

1. Pelvic floor strengthening exercises (Kegels), lifestyle modifications (drink less coffee and alcohol, weight loss).
2. Behavioral changes with bladder training.
3. If above measures fail, consider bladder relaxants: Anticholinergics (oxybutynin, tolterodine) or beta-3 agonists (mirabegron).

Complications: Like stress incontinence, this can cause perineal infections and falls/fractures.

HYF: Urge incontinence is increased urgency and frequency with patients commonly complaining of being unable to make it to the bathroom on time. Be sure to obtain a UA to distinguish it from UTI and implement behavioral changes such as voiding diaries. Etiology of urgency incontinence can be multifactorial; be sure to also evaluate for neurologic disorders such as spinal cord injury.

OVERFLOW INCONTINENCE

A 70-year-old M with PMH of BPH presents with weak urinary stream, sensation of incomplete bladder emptying, and continuous urine leakage. On digital rectal **examination**, he has a symmetrically, mildly enlarged prostate and palpable suprapubic mass. On **labs**, UA is (–) for leukocyte esterase, nitrites, and blood.

Management:

1. Assess for urinary retention via bladder scan (≥200 mL) or straight catheterization yielding ≥200 mL urine output.
2. Identify underlying etiology. For men, this is commonly due to benign prostatic hypertrophy or, rarely, urethral strictures. For women, it is usually due to pelvic organ prolapse or detrusor underactivity. In children (and less commonly in adults), constipation can result in incontinence.
3. Treat underlying etiology (see other topics and especially "Urinary Retention" on p. 437), and perform clean intermittent catheterization.

Complications:

- Urinary stasis seen in overflow incontinence can predispose to UTIs, hydronephrosis, or pyelonephritis.
- Straight catheterization can be performed, but long-term catheter use can predispose to infection. Clean intermittent catheterization is preferred, but patient education and compliance are required. Suprapubic catheterization is another option if urethral access is difficult.

HYF: The most common etiology for overflow incontinence is BPH in men and pelvic organ prolapse in women. Treat the underlying issue and be sure to drain the bladder to prevent urinary stasis. Overflow incontinence can result as an immediate post-operative complication, which is usually self-limiting.

NEUROGENIC BLADDER

A 24-year-old M with PMH of a recent motor vehicle accident presents with involuntary urine leakage. On **exam**, he has wet undergarments. On **imaging**, spine MRI shows T8–T10 spinal cord injury.

Management:

1. Identify underlying etiology. Neurogenic bladder is always a secondary complication. Common causes: Spinal cord damage from trauma or spinal stenosis (look for patient with lower back pain and bladder changes), normal pressure hydrocephalus and stroke (which alter micturition centers in the brain), diabetes (damages the peripheral nerves connecting to the bladder, interfering with sensation and motor function), and post-operative complication.
2. Presentation of neurogenic bladder varies and can commonly involve both urinary retention and urgency.
3. Thorough neurologic evaluation is necessary.

Complications: Treatment typically involves both clean intermittent catheterization and detrusor relaxants for hyperactivity. Complications from usage of both of these treatments can be seen.

HYF: Neurogenic bladder can be seen as a complication of other central nervous system pathologies or diabetes. Treatment involves addressing both hyperactivity and underactivity of the detrusor.

Urinary Tract Infection: See pp. 247, 439, 683.

14-6 Kidney Stone Types

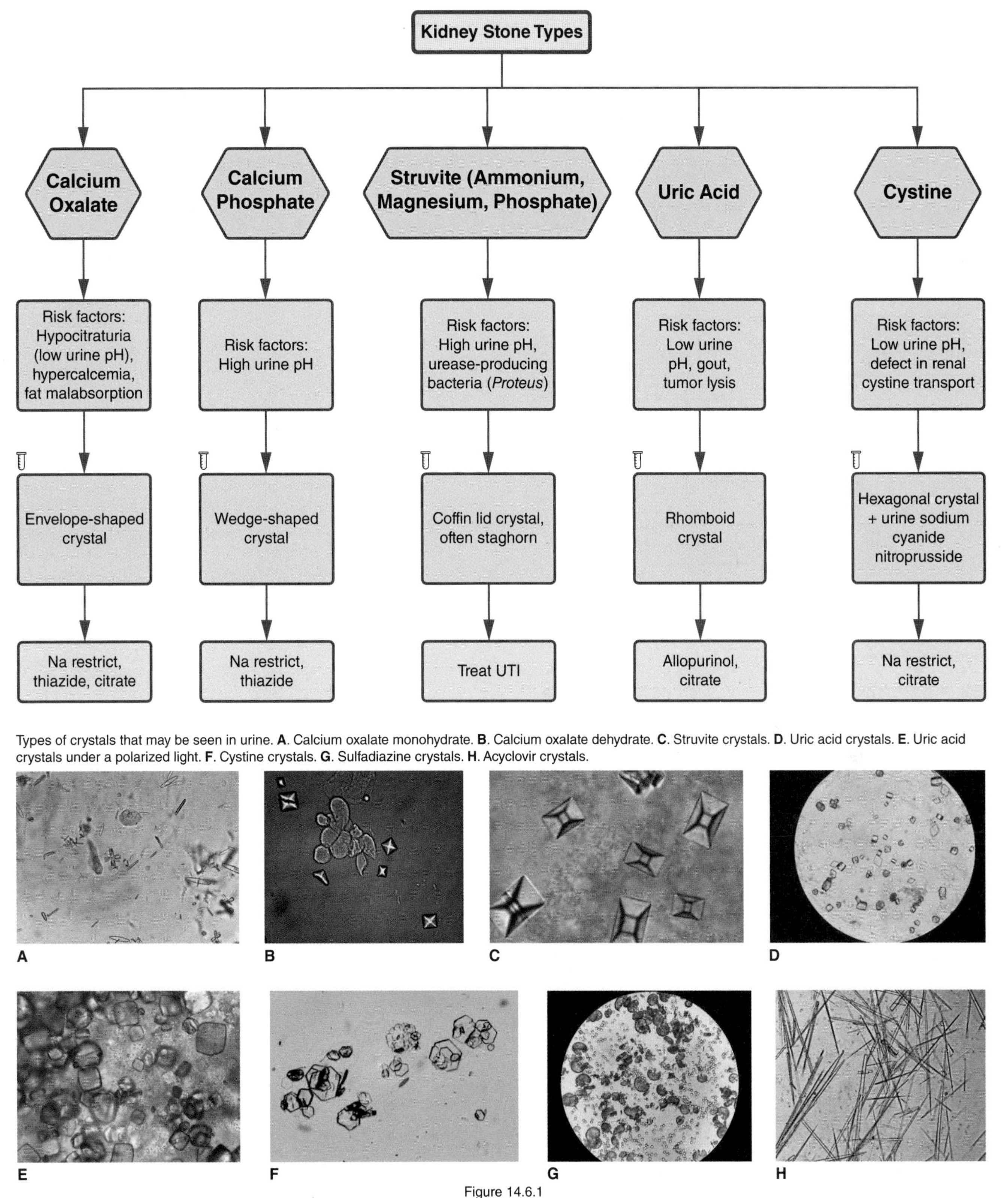
Kidney Stone Types
Calcium Oxalate
Calcium Phosphate
Struvite (Ammonium, Magnesium, Phosphate)
Uric Acid
Cystine
Risk factors: Hypocitraturia (low urine pH), hypercalcemia, fat malabsorption
Risk factors: High urine pH
Risk factors: High urine pH, urease-producing bacteria (Proteus)
Risk factors: Low urine pH, gout, tumor lysis
Risk factors: Low urine pH, defect in renal cystine transport
Envelope-shaped crystal
Wedge-shaped crystal
Coffin lid crystal, often staghorn
Rhomboid crystal
Hexagonal crystal + urine sodium cyanide nitroprusside
Na restrict, thiazide, citrate
Na restrict, thiazide
Treat UTI
Allopurinol, citrate
Na restrict, citrate
A
B
C
D
E
F
G
H

Types of crystals that may be seen in urine. **A**. Calcium oxalate monohydrate. **B**. Calcium oxalate dehydrate. **C**. Struvite crystals. **D**. Uric acid crystals. **E**. Uric acid crystals under a polarized light. **F**. Cystine crystals. **G**. Sulfadiazine crystals. **H**. Acyclovir crystals.

Figure 14.6.1

FIGURE 14.6

14-7 Kidney Stone Management

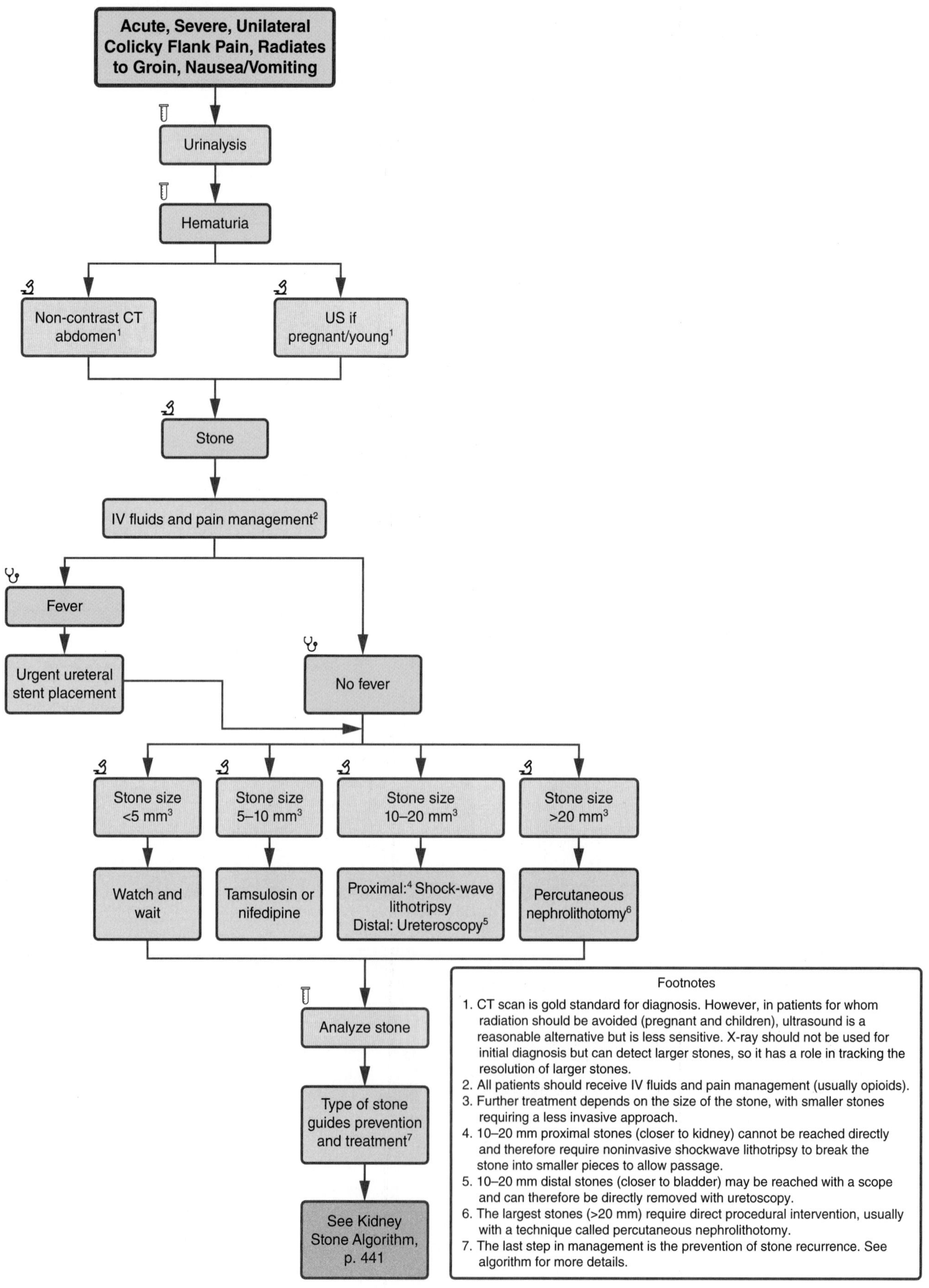
Acute, Severe, Unilateral Colicky Flank Pain, Radiates to Groin, Nausea/Vomiting
Urinalysis
Hematuria
Non-contrast CT abdomen[1]
US if pregnant/young[1]
Stone
IV fluids and pain management[2]
Fever
Urgent ureteral stent placement
No fever
Stone size <5 mm[3]
Stone size 5–10 mm[3]
Stone size 10–20 mm[3]
Stone size >20 mm[3]
Watch and wait
Tamsulosin or nifedipine
Proximal:[4] Shock-wave lithotripsy
Distal: Ureteroscopy[5]
Percutaneous nephrolithotomy[6]
Analyze stone
Type of stone guides prevention and treatment[7]
See Kidney Stone Algorithm, p. 441
Footnotes
1. CT scan is gold standard for diagnosis. However, in patients for whom radiation should be avoided (pregnant and children), ultrasound is a reasonable alternative but is less sensitive. X-ray should not be used for initial diagnosis but can detect larger stones, so it has a role in tracking the resolution of larger stones.
2. All patients should receive IV fluids and pain management (usually opioids).
3. Further treatment depends on the size of the stone, with smaller stones requiring a less invasive approach.
4. 10–20 mm proximal stones (closer to kidney) cannot be reached directly and therefore require noninvasive shockwave lithotripsy to break the stone into smaller pieces to allow passage.
5. 10–20 mm distal stones (closer to bladder) may be reached with a scope and can therefore be directly removed with uretoscopy.
6. The largest stones (>20 mm) require direct procedural intervention, usually with a technique called percutaneous nephrolithotomy.
7. The last step in management is the prevention of stone recurrence. See algorithm for more details.

FIGURE 14.7

14-8 Urologic Emergencies

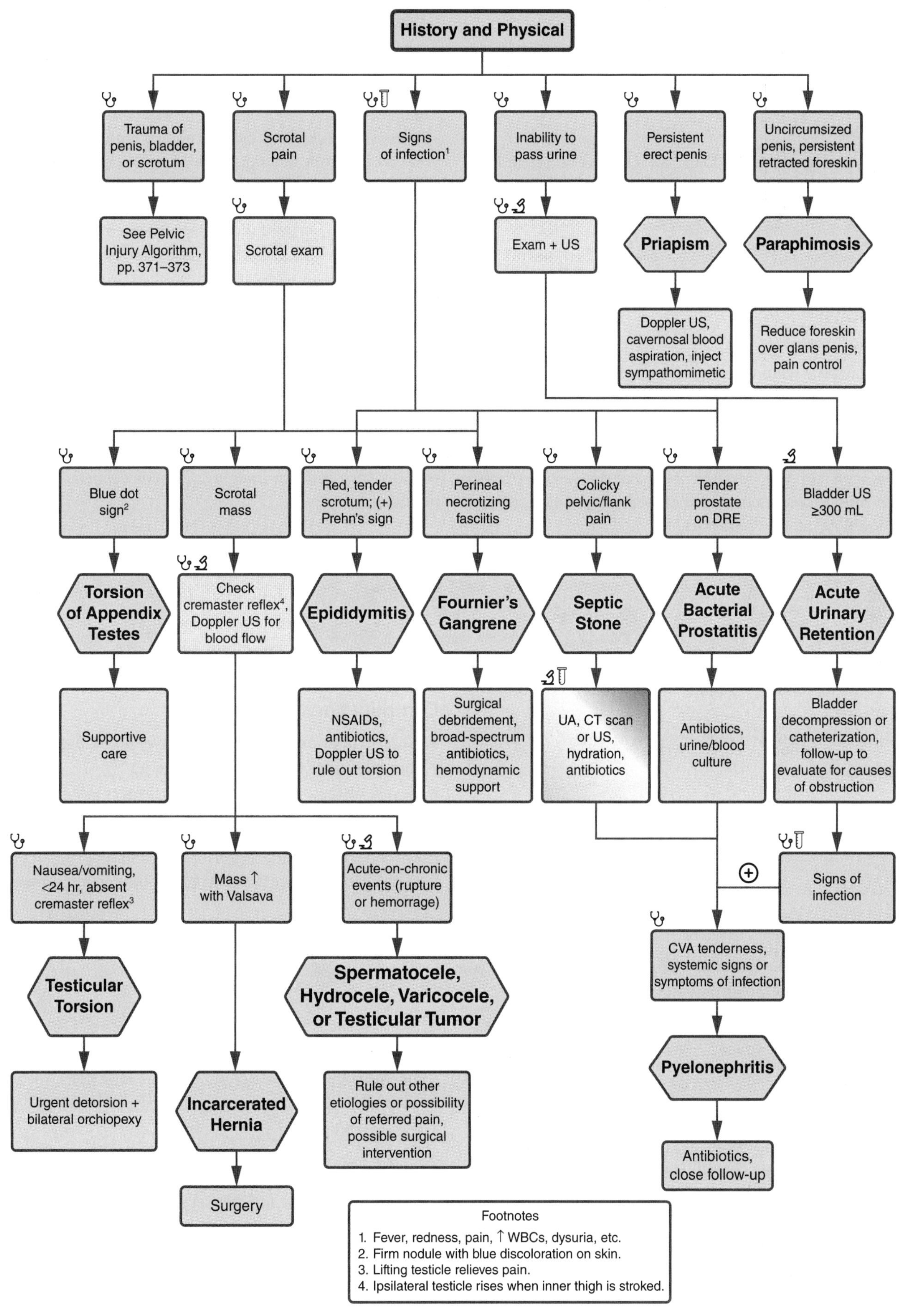
History and Physical
Trauma of penis, bladder, or scrotum
See Pelvic Injury Algorithm, pp. 371–373
Scrotal pain
Scrotal exam
Signs of infection[1]
Inability to pass urine
Exam + US
Persistent erect penis
Priapism
Doppler US, cavernosal blood aspiration, inject sympathomimetic
Uncircumsized penis, persistent retracted foreskin
Paraphimosis
Reduce foreskin over glans penis, pain control
Blue dot sign[2]
Torsion of Appendix Testes
Supportive care
Scrotal mass
Check cremaster reflex[4], Doppler US for blood flow
Red, tender scrotum; (+) Prehn's sign
Epididymitis
NSAIDs, antibiotics, Doppler US to rule out torsion
Perineal necrotizing fasciitis
Fournier's Gangrene
Surgical debridement, broad-spectrum antibiotics, hemodynamic support
Colicky pelvic/flank pain
Septic Stone
UA, CT scan or US, hydration, antibiotics
Tender prostate on DRE
Acute Bacterial Prostatitis
Antibiotics, urine/blood culture
Bladder US ≥300 mL
Acute Urinary Retention
Bladder decompression or catheterization, follow-up to evaluate for causes of obstruction
Nausea/vomiting, <24 hr, absent cremaster reflex[3]
Testicular Torsion
Urgent detorsion + bilateral orchiopexy
Mass ↑ with Valsava
Incarcerated Hernia
Surgery
Acute-on-chronic events (rupture or hemorrage)
Spermatocele, Hydrocele, Varicocele, or Testicular Tumor
Rule out other etiologies or possibility of referred pain, possible surgical intervention
Signs of infection
+
CVA tenderness, systemic signs or symptoms of infection
Pyelonephritis
Antibiotics, close follow-up
Footnotes
1. Fever, redness, pain, ↑ WBCs, dysuria, etc.
2. Firm nodule with blue discoloration on skin.
3. Lifting testicle relieves pain.
4. Ipsilateral testicle rises when inner thigh is stroked.

FIGURE 14.8

14-8 Urologic Emergencies

PRIAPISM

A 15-year-old M with PMH of sickle cell disease presents with erected penis for over 4 hours. **Imaging** shows minimal blood flow on Doppler ultrasonography.

Management:

1. Nonischemic priapism due to high flow: Observe and treat with arteriography/embolization or ligation if needed.
2. Ischemic priapism: More common. Treat with cavernosal aspiration +/− saline irrigation +/− injection of sympathomimetic (eg, phenylephrine). If no improvement, perform a cavernosal shunt.

Complications:

- Necrosis due to ischemia.
- Recurrent priapism (common for SCD or hematologic disorders).

HYF: Most common cause of ischemic priapism in adults is sildenafil toxicity. In children, sickle cell is the most common cause. Ischemic priapism is more common than non-ischemic priapism. Treatment with intracorporal phenylephrine helps by causing smooth muscle constriction in the penile vasculature, which reduces blood flow into the cavernosa.

PARAPHIMOSIS

A 10-year-old M presents with severe penile pain. On **exam**, he has a swollen glans penis with retracted foreskin.

Management:

1. Reduce foreskin: Manual reduction or dorsal slit procedure.
2. Pain control.
3. Counseling on hygiene and preventing recurrence.

Complications:

- Ischemia of glans penis causing necrosis.
- Urinary obstruction.
- Recurrent paraphimosis.

HYF: Can only occur in uncircumcised males.

EPIDIDYMITIS

A 25-year-old M with no significant PMH presents with unilateral testicular pain, dysuria, and urinary frequency. He has multiple sexual partners and inconsistently uses barrier protection. On **exam**, he has a temperature of 38.3°C, as well as a swollen, tender, and erythematous left testicle with moderate induration. Cremasteric reflex is intact. Prehn's sign is positive. **Labs/imaging**: UA reveals positive leukocyte esterase and numerous WBCs. Urethral swab is obtained and shows WBCs on Gram stain. PCR testing for chlamydia is positive. Testicular US with Doppler shows an enlarged, thick epididymis with increased blood flow; testicular torsion is ruled out.

Management:

1. If concern for sexually transmitted etiology, treat with ceftriaxone and doxycycline. Otherwise, treat as a complicated UTI with fluoroquinolones for coverage of enteric pathogens.
2. For symptom management, NSAIDs and scrotal support.

Complications: Urosepsis, testicular atrophy.

HYF: Inflammation of the epididymis due to retrograde ascent of pathogen from an STI or UTI. Most common pathogens are *Chlamydia trachomatis* and *Neisseria gonorrhoeae* in men age <35 years and *Esherichia coli* and enteric pathogens in men age >35 years. Risk factors: Bladder outlet obstruction (BPH, urethral stricture), high-risk sexual activity. Distinguish from testicular torsion (a urologic emergency), which also presents with unilateral testicular pain: Cremasteric reflex is present in epididymitis but absent in testicular torsion, Prehn's sign (decrease in pain with scrotal elevation) is positive with epididymitis and negative with testicular torsion, and testicular US would show increased blood flow with epididymitis compared to absent blood flow with testicular torsion.

FOURNIER'S GANGRENE

A 42-year-old M with PMH of poorly controlled diabetes and HTN presents with severe genital pain. On **exam**, he has fever, chills, discoloration of the perineum with crepitus, and swelling. **Labs** show leukocytosis. On **imaging**, CT shows subcutaneous air in the perineum.

Management:

1. Emergent surgical debridement.
2. Broad-spectrum antibiotics + cultures.
3. IV fluids + electrolyte corrections.
4. Possible diverting colostomy and/or Foley catheter during healing.

Complications:

- Sepsis, multi-organ failure, thromboembolic events.
- Complications from multiple surgeries.
- Severe disease, fecal incontinence, urinary retention.
- Psychological complications.

HYF: Fournier's gangrene is rapid and life-threatening. Risk factors: Diabetes, hypertension, and immunocompromised status.

SEPTIC STONE

A 66-year-old M presents with colicky flank pain. On **exam**, he has fevers and flank pain. On **imaging**, CT shows a stone in the left ureter.

Management:

1. Emergent decompression with ureteral stent or percutaneous nephrostomy tube (to prevent post-renal AKI).
2. IV antibiotics + urine culture.
3. Elective lithotripsy.

Complications:

- Pyelonephritis, bacteremia/sepsis.
- Renal failure.

HYF: Risks for stones include male gender, high-protein diet, dehydration, diabetes, gout, recurrent UTI, hypercalcemia, Lesch-Nyhan's syndrome, and certain medications. Obtain US instead of CT if patient is a pregnant woman or child.

14-8 Urologic Emergencies

ACUTE BACTERIAL PROSTATITIS

A 75-year-old M with PMH of BPH presents with dysuria, fever, and perineal pain. Digital rectal **exam** reveals a firm, edematous, and tender prostate. **Labs** show leukocytosis. UA reveals pyuria.

Management:

1. Obtain urine culture. Also obtain imaging if abscess is suspected and blood culture if sepsis is suspected.
2. Antibiotics with fluoroquinolones (eg, ciprofloxacin) or TMP-SMX. Tailor to culture results and local sensitivity data.

Complications:

- Bacteremia, metastatic infection.
- Acute urinary retention, prostatic abscess.

HYF: Most common cause is chlamydia or gonorrhea in young men (age <35) and *E. coli* in older men (age >35). Avoid vigorous prostate massage, which can cause bacteremia. Prostatitis can occur with cystitis, urethritis, or other urogenital infections. Also consider prostate infections in patients with recent urogenital or colorectal instrumentation or recent procedures.

TESTICULAR TORSION

A 14-year-old M presents with acute testicular pain. On **exam**, he has warm erythematous scrotum, high-riding testis, and negative cremaster reflex. **Imaging** shows diminished blood flow to the testes on Doppler US.

Management:

1. Scrotal exploration (consider manual detorsion in select cases).
2. Surgical detorsion; if testical can be salvaged ("turns pink after detorsing"), perform bilateral orchiopexy. If testicle is grossly necrotic, perform ipsilateral orchiectomy with contralateral orchipexy.
3. UA should be ordered to rule out UTI or orchitis.

Complications: Extended ischemia may require orchiectomy.

HYF: Ideally, the testicle should be detorsed within 6 hours of symptom onset. Most common in neonates and adolescents undergoing puberty. Must perform orchiopexy on the unaffected testis, since torsion in the contralateral testis is common. Congenital bell clapper deformity increases risk.

VARICOCELE

A 30-year-old M with PMH of infertility presents with left-sided scrotal pain and distension for the past 6 months. He describes the pain as a dull ache that worsens with prolonged standing or exercise and improves when lying down. He and his wife have been struggling with infertility. A prior semen analysis showed low sperm concentrations with decreased sperm motility and abnormal morphology. On **exam**, his scrotum appears distended, and the spermatic cord veins are noted to feel like a "bag of worms" on Valsalva. Transillumination test is negative. **Labs** are normal. On **imaging**, scrotal US with Doppler shows dilatation of vessels of the pampiniform plexus and retrograde scrotal vein flow with Valsalva.

Management:

1. If asymptomatic, conservative management: Scrotal support, NSAIDs, and annual exams.
2. If symptomatic (eg, pain, infertility), consider surgical ligation or embolization.

Complications: Testicular atrophy, infertility.

HYF: Most common cause of scrotal enlargement in adults. Due to increased venous pressure causing dilation of veins in the pampiniform plexus and venous reflux. Most are left-sided due to increased resistance from the left gonadal vein draining into the left renal vein. On the right, the gonadal vein drains directly into the IVC; thus, right-sided varicoceles are uncommon and should be evaluated for retroperitoneal neoplasm causing obstruction. In patients with varicoceles, send for semen analysis to assess for infertility.

HYDROCELE

A 30-year-old M with no significant PMH presents with left-sided scrotal swelling. The scrotal swelling began several months ago and has progressively worsened. On **exam**, he has a tense, non-tender mass in the scrotum. Transillumination test is positive. On **imaging**, scrotal US shows a simple fluid collection along the spermatic cord and does not reveal any testicular neoplasm or other acute inflammatory scrotal conditions.

Management:

1. If asymptomatic, no need for follow-up. If symptomatic, consider surgical excision of the hydrocele sac.

Complications: Pyocele, scrotal pain, chronic irritation leading to scrotal skin compromise.

HYF: In adults, most hydroceles are idiopathic and accumulate over a long period of time. Sometimes, inflammatory conditions (epididymitis, testicular torsion, trauma) and testicular neoplasms can cause an acute reactive hydrocele. Consider a scrotal US if the diagnosis is unclear to rule out more serious conditions such as malignancy. Distinguish hydroceles from varicoceles with the transillumination test; hydroceles transilluminate, whereas varicoceles do not.

Acute Urinary Retention: See p. 438.

Incarcerated Hernia: See p. 423.

Pyelonephritis: See pp. 245, 443, 620.

14-9 Male GU Cancers

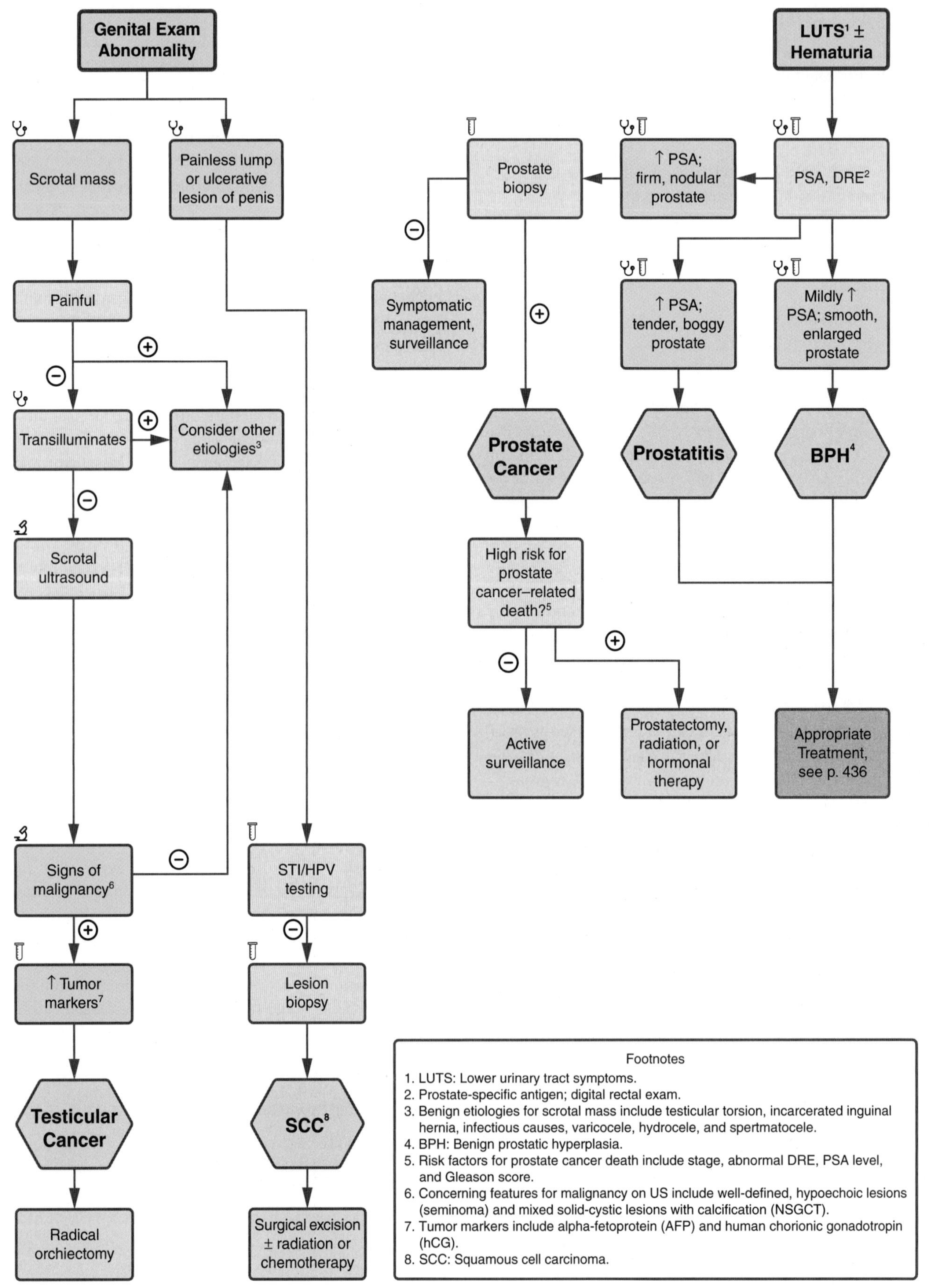

Genital Exam Abnormality
Scrotal mass
Painless lump or ulcerative lesion of penis
Painful
Transilluminates
Consider other etiologies[3]
Scrotal ultrasound
Signs of malignancy[6]
↑ Tumor markers[7]
Testicular Cancer
Radical orchiectomy
STI/HPV testing
Lesion biopsy
SCC[8]
Surgical excision ± radiation or chemotherapy
LUTS[1] ± Hematuria
PSA, DRE[2]
↑ PSA; firm, nodular prostate
Prostate biopsy
Symptomatic management, surveillance
Prostate Cancer
High risk for prostate cancer–related death?[5]
Active surveillance
Prostatectomy, radiation, or hormonal therapy
↑ PSA; tender, boggy prostate
Prostatitis
Mildly ↑ PSA; smooth, enlarged prostate
BPH[4]
Appropriate Treatment, see p. 436
Footnotes
1. LUTS: Lower urinary tract symptoms.
2. Prostate-specific antigen; digital rectal exam.
3. Benign etiologies for scrotal mass include testicular torsion, incarcerated inguinal hernia, infectious causes, varicocele, hydrocele, and spertmatocele.
4. BPH: Benign prostatic hyperplasia.
5. Risk factors for prostate cancer death include stage, abnormal DRE, PSA level, and Gleason score.
6. Concerning features for malignancy on US include well-defined, hypoechoic lesions (seminoma) and mixed solid-cystic lesions with calcification (NSGCT).
7. Tumor markers include alpha-fetoprotein (AFP) and human chorionic gonadotropin (hCG).
8. SCC: Squamous cell carcinoma.

FIGURE 14.9

14-9 Male GU Cancers

PROSTATE CANCER

A 60-year-old M with no PMH presents with elevated PSA on asymptomatic primary care screening. On digital rectal exam (DRE), he has a firm prostate with a discrete left-sided nodule.

Management:

1. Prostate biopsy.
2. If positive, consider active surveillance, prostatectomy, radiation, or androgen deprivation therapy.
3. If negative, continue PSA screening.

Complications:

- LUTS.
- Hematuria.
- Metastatic spread.
- Surgical treatment (eg, prostatectomy) can cause sexual and reproductive dysfunction (eg, erectile, ejaculatory).

HYF: Most prostate cancers occur in the peripheral zone of the prostate, which is why they may be palpable on DRE and do not cause obstructive symptoms (unlike BPH, which occurs in the transition zone and causes obstructive LUTS). However, even patients with advanced prostate cancer may have normal DRE. Prostatitis, BPH, and other prostate conditions may lead to a false elevation in PSA. Prostate cancer metastases commonly occur in the skeleton and are predominately osteoblastic.

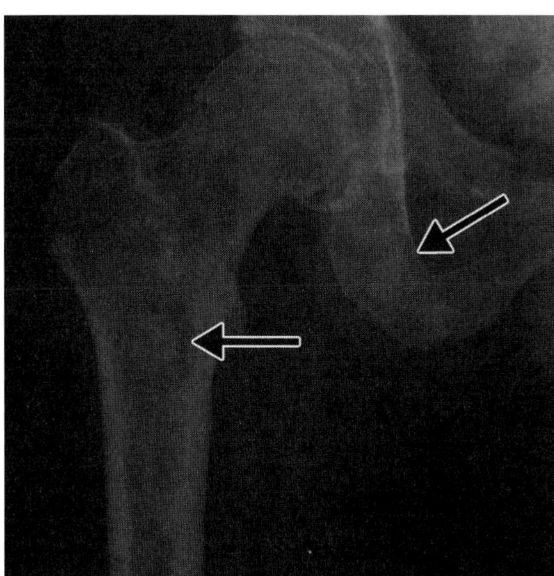

Osteoblastic lesions in metastatic prostate cancer

TESTICULAR CANCER

A 26-year-old M with no PMH presents with a testicular mass found while showering. On exam, he has a firm nodule in the left testicle that does not transilluminate. On imaging, scrotal US shows a solid, hypoechoic lesion.

Management:

1. Assess serum tumor markers.
2. Discuss sperm cryopreservation.
3. Radical inguinal orchiectomy.
4. Consider adjuvant radiation or chemotherapy.

Complications:

- Metastatic spread.
- Impaired fertility (both from cancer and orchiectomy).

HYF: Testicular cancer incidence peaks from ages 15–35, usually presenting with a painless mass. If testicular cancer is suspected, biopsy should NEVER be done due to risk of tumor seeding. 95% of testicular cancers are germ cell tumors, of which most are seminomas. Sertoli and Leydig cell tumors represent ~5%. Tumor markers are often elevated in non-seminoma germ cell tumors (embryonal carcinoma, yolk sac tumor, choriocarcinoma, mixed).

Tumor Markers in Testicular Cancer

Classification	Type	Primary Tumor Marker
Germ Cell Tumors	Seminoma	Usually none. ↑ β-hCG in some cases.
	Choriocarcinoma	↑↑ β-hCG
	Yolk Sac	↑↑ AFP
	Embryonal	↑ AFP, β-hCG
	Teratoma	Usually none. ↑ AFP and/or ↑β-hCG in some cases, depending on what components are present.
Non-Germ Cell Tumors	Sertoli Cell	Usually none. ↑ estrogen in some cases.
	Leydig Cell	↑↑ Testosterone ↑ Estrogen, progesterone, corticosteroids.
Secondary Testicular Tumors	Lymphoma (most commonly diffuse large B-cell lymphoma)	None.

SQUAMOUS CELL CARCINOMA (SCC)

A 64-year-old M with PMH of HIV and a 40-pack-year smoking history presents with a painless ulcerated lesion on the glans of the penis. On exam, he has inguinal lymphadenopathy. On labs, HPV PCR is positive for HPV-16.

Management:

1. Excisional biopsy.
2. Resection of remaining disease.
3. Adjuvant chemotherapy/radiation if indicated.

Complications:

- Infection.
- Metastatic spread.
- Radiation → Peyronie's disease.

HYF: HIV and HPV infection are 2 important risk factors for squamous cell carcinoma of the penis, along with tobacco use. Bowen's disease and erythroplasia of Queyrat are 2 precancerous lesions that may progress to SCC.

Prostatitis: See pp. 245, 445.

Benign Prostatic Hyperplasia (BPH): See p. 436.

14-10 Hematuria

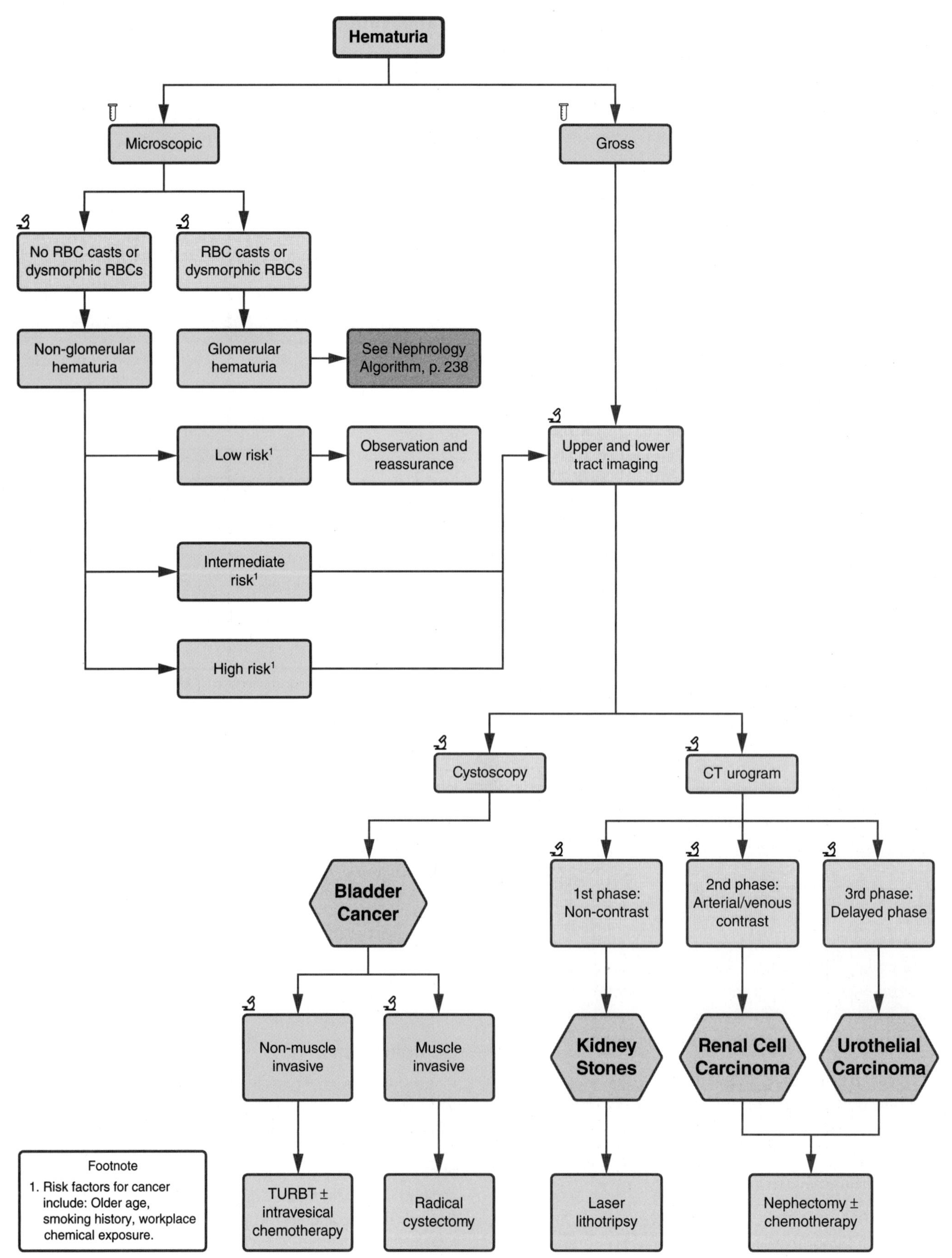
Hematuria
Microscopic
Gross
No RBC casts or dysmorphic RBCs
RBC casts or dysmorphic RBCs
Non-glomerular hematuria
Glomerular hematuria
See Nephrology Algorithm, p. 238
Low risk[1]
Observation and reassurance
Upper and lower tract imaging
Intermediate risk[1]
High risk[1]
Cystoscopy
CT urogram
Bladder Cancer
1st phase: Non-contrast
2nd phase: Arterial/venous contrast
3rd phase: Delayed phase
Non-muscle invasive
Muscle invasive
Kidney Stones
Renal Cell Carcinoma
Urothelial Carcinoma
Footnote
1. Risk factors for cancer include: Older age, smoking history, workplace chemical exposure.
TURBT ± intravesical chemotherapy
Radical cystectomy
Laser lithotripsy
Nephectomy ± chemotherapy

FIGURE 14.10

14-10 Hematuria

BLADDER CANCER (UROTHELIAL CARCINOMA)

A 56-year-old M with a 40-pack-year smoking history who works in a textile factory with aniline dyes and/or pesticides presents with painless hematuria and urinary hesitancy. On **labs**, UA shows numerous RBCs. On **imaging**, cystoscopy shows several friable, pedunculated masses on the dome of the bladder.

Management:

1. Non-muscle-invasive: TURBT, biopsy, and intravesical chemotherapy.
2. Muscle-invasive: Radical cystectomy.
3. Follow-up surveillance cystoscopy.

Complications:

- Metastatic spread.
- Bladder irritation with TURBT.
- UTI from instrumentation.
- Postrenal AKI if the tumor obstructs the ureter or bladder outlet.

HYF: Smoking is the single most important risk factor for urothelial carcinoma, which is by far the most common bladder cancer. Bladder cancer usually presents with hematuria throughout urination. Other risk factors include pesticides, working in a textile factory, and aniline dye exposure.

RENAL CELL CARCINOMA

A 67-year-old F with a 35-pack-year smoking history presents with 15-lb weight loss and hematuria. On **exam**, she has a left flank mass. On **imaging**, CT shows an irregular, enhancing mass in the left kidney.

Management:

1. Workup for metastatic spread.
2. Surgical resection of tumor.

Complications:

- Metastatic spread.
- Impaired renal function.
- Secondary hypercortisolism (ectopic ACTH production).
- Secondary polycythemia (ectopic EPO production).
- Hypertension (excessive renin production).
- Hypercalcemia (PTHrP production).

HYF: Classic triad is hematuria, flank pain, and palpable mass, but this is only present in 10–15% of patients. RCCs can be a part of hereditary cancer syndromes (eg, Von Hippel-Lindau's syndrome, tuberous sclerosis). Chemotherapy is NOT used to treat RCC, as it is highly resistant. It is the most common type of renal malignancy; localized disease has excellent prognosis after nephrectomy (>90% survival). More common in men. Tobacco and obesity are risk factors.

UPPER TRACT UROTHELIAL CARCINOMA

A 73-year-old M with 45-pack-year smoking history presents with right flank pain and hematuria. **Exam** does not show any palpable mass. On **imaging**, CT urogram shows a filling defect in the right renal pelvis.

Management:

1. Staging.
2. Radical nephroureterectomy.
3. Surveillance cystoscopy and cytology.

Complications:

- Metastatic spread.
- Impaired renal function/hydronephrosis.
- UTI.

HYF: Less invasive treatments may be indicated for those with impaired renal function or solitary kidney. Associated with Lynch's syndrome.

NEPHROLITHIASIS (KIDNEY STONES)

A 60-year-old M from Texas with CHF on furosemide presents with severe colicky right flank pain radiating to the groin associated with nausea, vomiting, and hematuria. On **exam**, he is writhing in pain. **Labs/imaging**: UA shows numerous RBCs. Non-contrast CTAP shows a hyperdense mass in the right ureter with right-sided hydronephrosis.

Management:

1. Analgesia.
2. If patient is febrile: Stent placement to prevent postrenal AKI, IV antibiotics.
3. If patient is afebrile: Tamsulosin, elective lithotripsy.

Complications:

- Postrenal AKI.
- Ascending UTI with pyelonephritis.
- Sepsis.

HYF: CT abdomen/pelvis without contrast is the gold standard for diagnosis. More common in men. Associated with furosemide use due to calcium excretion. Thiazides can prevent stone formation due to resorption of calcium in distal convoluted tubule. Occurs in patients with hypercalcemia (eg, hyperparathyroidism). More common in southern USA due to hot weather and dehydration (the "stone belt" of America).

14-11 Erectile Dysfunction

Erectile dysfunction (ED), or impotence, is inability to attain or main an erection during sexual activity. Etiologies can be endocrinologic, psychological, medication-induced, neurologic, and/or vascular. Risk factors include diabetes, atherosclerosis, hypertension, history of depression or anxiety disorder, medications (β-blockers, SSRIs, TCAs, diuretics), spinal cord injury, chronic prostatitis, or history of surgery or radiation for prostate cancer. Distinguish between psychological and organic ED based on the presence of nocturnal or early-morning erections. If the patient reports ongoing nocturnal or early-morning erections, the endocrinologic and neurologic pathways for penile tumescence remain intact, and the ED is non-organic. In cases of non-organic ED, consider situation dependence (ie, occurring with one partner) and other psychogenic causes of ED (mood disorders, performance anxiety). If nocturnal tumescence is absent, the ED is classified as organic. Evaluate for neurologic dysfunction (eg, loss of lower extremity sensation) and hypogonadism (eg, small testes, loss of secondary sexual characteristics). For patients who report loss of libido, depression, or loss of secondary sexual characteristics, initial labs include TSH, morning testosterone, estradiol, LH, prolactin, hemoglobin A1c, lipid panel, and basic metabolic panel. Treatment depends on the etiology.

ERECTILE DYSFUNCTION

A 65-year-old M man with PMH of T2DM, HTN, HLD, and BPH s/p transurethral resection of the prostate (TURP) presents with erectile dysfunction. He has been having difficulty attaining and maintaining an erection for the past 6 months. He does not have any nocturnal or early-morning erections and states that he is still sexually attracted to his partner. His blood pressure is well-controlled with carvedilol. **Exam** is normal. On **labs**, TSH, morning testosterone, estradiol, LH, prolactin, hemoglobin A1c, lipid panel, and basic metabolic panel are normal.

Management:

1. Trial oral phosphodiesterase type 5 (PDE-5) inhibitors (sildenafil, vardenafil, tadalafil).
2. If ongoing symptoms, consider intracavernosal prostaglandin injections, vacuum pumps, and surgical implantation of penile prostheses.

Complications: Anxiety, depression.

HYFs: PDEs inactivate cGMP, resulting in smooth muscle contraction; PDE-5 inhibitors mediate smooth muscle relaxation and thus increase blood flow in the corpora cavernosa. Of note, use of PDE-5 inhibitors with nitrates (eg, for angina) is contraindicated due to risk of profound hypotension. Testosterone is *only* indicated for treatment of ED in the setting of hypogonadism; it is not recommended for patients with normal testosterone levels. Common medications associated with ED: β-blockers, SSRIs, and TCAs. If patients on these medications present with ED, consider transitioning to alternative medications if possible.

***Peyronie's disease** is characterized by erections with penile angulation due to acquired fibrosis of the tunica albuginea that surrounds the corpora cavernosa. Associated with connective tissue disorders. Patients can have penile pain with erections and/or difficulty attaining erections. Penile ultrasound would reveal scar tissue in the tunica albuginea. Treatment is limited pharmacologically; surgical treatment via the Nesbit operation is difficult and used only in extreme cases.

15 Surgery: Otolaryngology–Head and Neck

15-1 ENT: Neck Masses – Lymphadenopathy

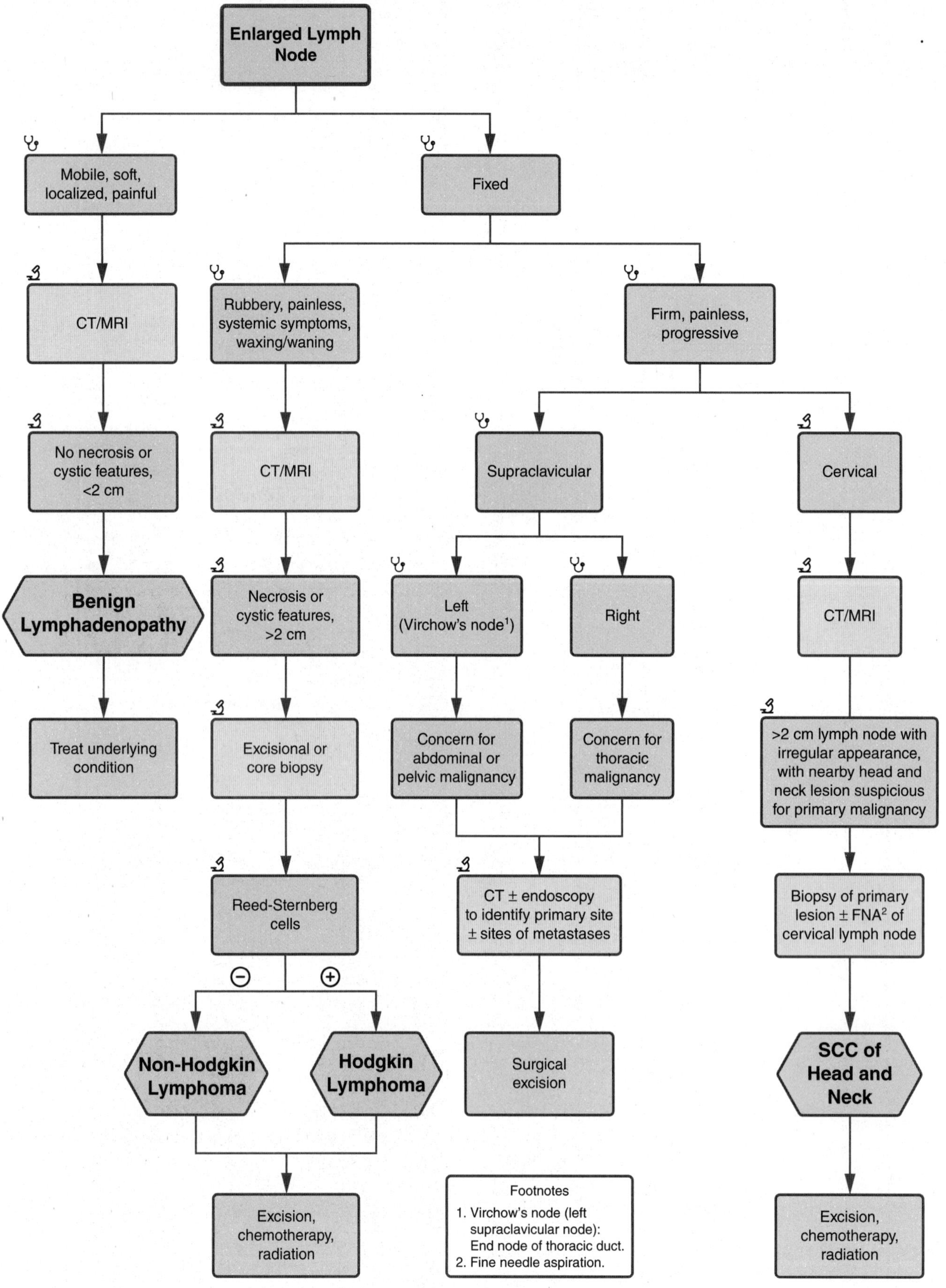
Enlarged Lymph Node
Mobile, soft, localized, painful
Fixed
CT/MRI
Rubbery, painless, systemic symptoms, waxing/waning
Firm, painless, progressive
No necrosis or cystic features, <2 cm
CT/MRI
Supraclavicular
Cervical
Benign Lymphadenopathy
Necrosis or cystic features, >2 cm
Left (Virchow's node[1])
Right
CT/MRI
Treat underlying condition
Excisional or core biopsy
Concern for abdominal or pelvic malignancy
Concern for thoracic malignancy
>2 cm lymph node with irregular appearance, with nearby head and neck lesion suspicious for primary malignancy
Reed-Sternberg cells
CT ± endoscopy to identify primary site ± sites of metastases
Biopsy of primary lesion ± FNA[2] of cervical lymph node
⊖
⊕
Non-Hodgkin Lymphoma
Hodgkin Lymphoma
Surgical excision
SCC of Head and Neck
Excision, chemotherapy, radiation
Footnotes
1. Virchow's node (left supraclavicular node): End node of thoracic duct.
2. Fine needle aspiration.
Excision, chemotherapy, radiation

FIGURE 15.1

15-1 ENT: Neck Masses – Lymphadenopathy

LYMPHOMA

An 18-year-old M with PMH of HIV on antiretroviral therapy presents with night sweats, fatigue, and weight loss. On **exam**, he has multiple rubbery, enlarged cervical lymph nodes. **Labs** show elevated LDH and anemia.

Management:

1. Excisional lymph node biopsy with flow cytometric immunophenotyping.
2. Treatment is category-specific and can range from active surveillance to a combination of chemotherapy, radiation, biologic therapy, and/or immunotherapy.

Complications:

- Pancytopenia (lymphomas can present with ↑ or ↓ WBCs).
- Hepatosplenomegaly.
- Tumor lysis syndrome.

HYF: See Hematology/Oncology Lymphoma algorithm on page 121.

BENIGN (REACTIVE) LYMPHADENOPATHY

A 52-year-old F with PMH of DM2 presents with 1 week of sore throat and conjunctivitis. **Exam** reveals a tender, mobile cervical lymph node. On **imaging**, US shows it is 0.5 cm in diameter, homogenous, and hypoechoic.

Management:

1. Observation. Follow-up in 3–4 weeks.
2. Symptom relief ± antiviral therapy as indicated.

Complications: Typically self-limiting.

HYF: Painful lymphadenopathy (LAD) is generally caused by lymphadenitis, which is a benign proliferation of immune cell clusters in response to an inflammatory process such as a bacterial or viral infection (eg, mycobacterial cervical lymphadenitis). Of note, EBV infection can cause a reactive LAD that mimics malignant lymphoma on histological evaluation.

MYCOBACTERIAL CERVICAL LYMPHADENITIS

A 36-year-old M with PMH of HIV/AIDS presents with 1 week of fever and a painful nodule in the right lateral neck. **Exam** shows a tender, warm area of unilateral cervical lymphadenopathy with overlying violaceous skin discoloration. **Labs** show leukocytosis. FNA is performed but inconclusive. Excisional lymph node biopsy reveals the presence of caseating granulomas, and acid-fast bacilli are revealed on smear and culture. Interferon-Gamma Release Assay (IGRA) is positive. On **imaging**, CXR shows apical fibrosis and pleural thickening.

Management:

1. Use nucleic acid amplification testing (NAAT) if lymph node biopsy and cultures are inconclusive.
2. Antimicrobial treatment based on culture speciation, antimicrobial sensitivities, and HIV status (eg, rifampicin, isoniazid, ethambutol, and pyrazinamide for immunocompetent adults with drug-susceptible *M. tuberculosis* lymphadenitis). Consider lymph node excision.

Complications: Ulceration, fistula, or abscess formation. Patients may have concomitant systemic findings related to the mycobacterial infection, including fever, sweats, weight loss, and pulmonary symptoms.

HYF: Most commonly seen in children and immunocompromised patients. Most tuberculous lymphadenitis is caused by *M. tuberculosis* and atypical mycobacteria, especially *M. scrofulosum* and *M. avium* complex (MAC). Antimicrobial therapy may cause a paradoxical reaction with an increase in lymph node size and/or involvement of additional lymph nodes during or after treatment; these reactions typically do not indicate treatment failure. Skin overlying the lymph node has a characteristic violaceous discoloration and may be indurated.

HEAD AND NECK SQUAMOUS CELL CARCINOMA

A 58-year-old M with PMH of GERD, tobacco use disorder, alcohol use disorder, and dental caries presents with mouth pain and dysphagia. **Exam** shows an ulcerative oral lesion and painless, hard cervical lymph nodes. On **imaging**, MRI head and neck shows hyperintensity and uneven peripheral enhancement.

Management:

1. Biopsy of primary site ± FNA of pathologically enlarged cervical lymph node.
2. CT to assess for distant metastases.
3. Single-modality treatment with surgery, radiation, or immuno-/chemotherapy vs. multimodal treatment.

Complications:

- Fistula formation,
- Airway compromise.
- Radiation therapy → tissue fibrosis, xerostomia, dysgeusia, dysphagia, or osteoradionecrosis.
- Salivary gland damage from radiation → dental comorbidities.

HYF: Cervical lymph node FNA may reveal carcinoma of unknown primary, which would require CT ± endoscopy to identify the primary site. Associated with HPV (especially types 16, 18, 31). Due to differing disease course, oropharyngeal cancers are staged and treated differently if they are HPV positive or negative.

METASTATIC SPREAD TO SUPRACLAVICULAR NODES

A 65-year-old M with PMH of obesity presents with postprandial epigastric pain refractory to PPI treatment. **Exam** shows a fixed, hard, painless lymph node in the left supraclavicular region. FNA is performed; mucinous cells are seen on histological evaluation concerning for malignancy.

Management:

1. CT for diagnosis and staging. Endoscopy (laryngoscopy, esophagoscopy, and/or bronchoscopy) ± biopsy.
2. Treatment is site- and category-specific, but usually treatment options include combinations of surgery, radiation, and chemotherapy.

Complications: Virchow's node enlargement can cause thoracic outlet syndrome via mass effect.

HYF: Virchow's node is a left supraclavicular lymph node that is a common site for metastases of abdominal (eg, gastric) and pelvic cancers.

15-2 ENT: Other Masses

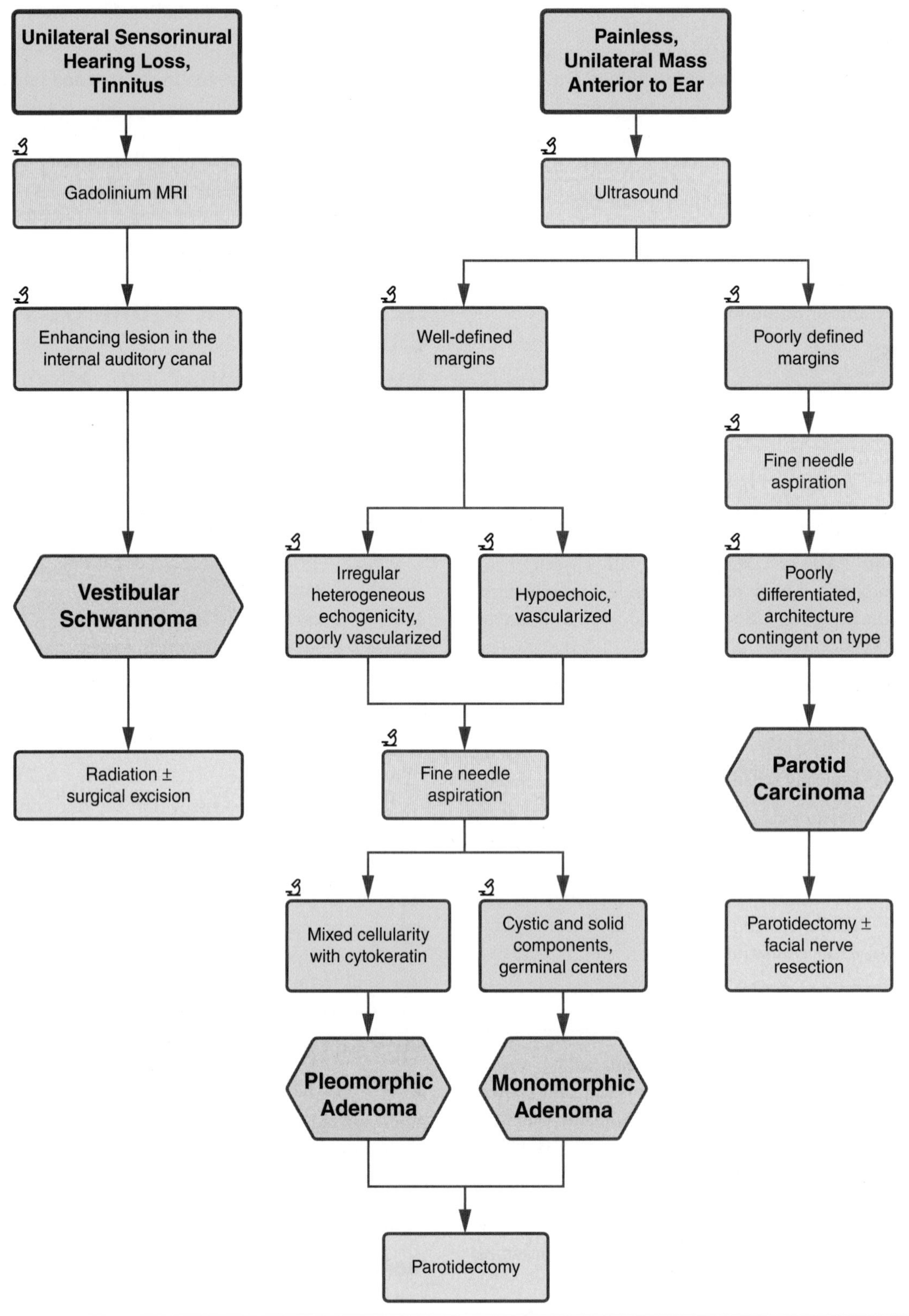
Unilateral Sensorinural Hearing Loss, Tinnitus
Gadolinium MRI
Enhancing lesion in the internal auditory canal
Vestibular Schwannoma
Radiation ± surgical excision
Painless, Unilateral Mass Anterior to Ear
Ultrasound
Well-defined margins
Poorly defined margins
Fine needle aspiration
Irregular heterogeneous echogenicity, poorly vascularized
Hypoechoic, vascularized
Poorly differentiated, architecture contingent on type
Fine needle aspiration
Parotid Carcinoma
Mixed cellularity with cytokeratin
Cystic and solid components, germinal centers
Parotidectomy ± facial nerve resection
Pleomorphic Adenoma
Monomorphic Adenoma
Parotidectomy

FIGURE 15.2

15-2 ENT: Other Masses

VESTIBULAR SCHWANNOMA/ ACOUSTIC NEUROMA

A 65-year-old M with PMH of DM2 and HTN presents with progressive unilateral hearing loss, tinnitus, and loss of balance. Exam shows unilateral sensorineural hearing loss. On **imaging**, MRI brain with contrast shows an enhancing lesion in the internal auditory canal.

Management:

1. Surgical excision of tumor or radiation.

Complications:

- Hearing loss, facial weakness, vestibular disturbances.
- Cerebrospinal fluid (CSF) leak.

HYF: Bilateral vestibular schwannomas are a classic feature of neurofibromatosis type 2 (autosomal dominant mutation in tumor suppressor gene *NF2*; Merlin [schwannomin] protein).

PAROTID TUMOR

A 65-year-old M with PMH of tobacco use disorder presents with painless preauricular swelling. Exam shows a unilateral, mobile mass. On **imaging**, US shows a parotid mass with well-defined borders.

Management:

1. US of parotid gland with fine needle aspiration.
2. If malignant, obtain further imaging (CT, MRI) prior to excision to determine oncologic staging and extent of metastasis.
3. If growth involves the facial nerve, may require facial nerve resection ± facial nerve repair intraoperatively.

Complications:

- Facial nerve involvement/resection → facial nerve palsy.
- Benign parotid adenomas can undergo malignant transformation or can recur if not fully resected during parotidectomy.

HYF: Parotid monomorphic adenomas can be bilateral. After diagnosis is made, the contralateral side must be imaged. The most common benign parotid tumors are pleomorphic adenomas and papillary cystadenodenoma lymphomatosum (Warthin tumor—associated with smoking). The most common malignancies are mucoepidermoid carcinoma and adenoid cystic carcinoma.

15-3 ENT: Emergencies

LUDWIG'S ANGINA

A 35-year-old M with PMH of DM2, poor dentition, and recent dental surgery presents with fever, malaise, mouth pain, and macroglossia. On **exam**, he has tender, symmetric, "woody" induration in the submandibular area, and he cannot close his mouth. On **labs**, he has leukocytosis. Blood cultures are drawn and pending. On **imaging**, CT neck with contrast shows soft tissue thickening, loss of fat in the submandibular plane, and gas bubbles.

Management:

1. Airway management: If concern for airway compromise, fiberoptic intubation via the nasal route. If emergent clinical scenario and intubation is not possible, perform tracheostomy first, followed by intubation once able.
2. IV antibiotics (ampicillin-sulbactam or ceftriaxone).
3. If minimal response to IV antibiotics, repeat CT neck to assess for a fluid collection. If there is a fluid collection, needle aspiration or I&D under general anesthesia. If a decayed tooth is the source of infection, perform tooth extraction for source control.

Complications:

- Airway compromise leading to death.
- Aspiration pneumonia.
- Mediastinitis.

HYF: Emergent and rapidly spreading polymicrobial infection. Immediate IV antibiotics that have broad-spectrum activity against oral flora aerobes and anaerobes are necessary. The most common organisms are viridans streptococci (eg, *Streptococcus anginosus*) and oral anaerobes. Gram-negative aerobes and *Staphylococcus aureus*, including methicillin-resistant *S. aureus* (MRSA), have also been implicated in immunocompromised patients and in pediatric patients.

BELL'S PALSY

A previously healthy 35-year-old F presents with sudden-onset unilateral facial paralysis. On **exam**, she has the inability to close 1 eye with associated ipsilateral eyebrow sagging, disappearance of nasolabial fold, and mouth drooping. This is a clinical diagnosis; **labs** are not necessary at the initial visit.

Management:

1. Glucocorticoids (prednisone 60–80 mg/day).
2. Oral valacyclovir or acyclovir if severe.
3. Artificial tears if affected eye does not fully close.

Complications:

- Synkenisis.
- Facial contracture.
- Recurrent Bell's palsy.

HYF: Most common cause of peripheral facial nerve palsy. Differentiate from stroke because stroke spares the forehead, whereas Bell's palsy affects the entire half of the face. Associated with HSV.

EPISTAXIS

A 65-year-old F with PMH of atrial fibrillation on apixaban presents with persistent nosebleed. After application of a vasoconstrictive nose spray and compression, bleeding continues.

Management:

1. If pediatric, phenylephrine spray and compression until bleeding stops.
   a. If bleeding continues, visualize posterior canal to evaluate for mass.
   b. If there is a mass, resection.
2. If adult, nasal packing and bacitracin.
   a. If bleeding continues, use balloon catheter to stop posterior bleed.

Complications:

- Synechiae.
- Aspiration.
- Hypovolemia if blood loss is severe (rare).

HYF: With the exception of a juvenile nasopharyngeal angiofibroma, bleeding should stop with compression as long as there is no coagulation disorder.

16
Surgery: Orthopedic

16-1 Adult Fractures

Upper Extremity

Injury Type	Characteristics	Treatment
Scaphoid fracture 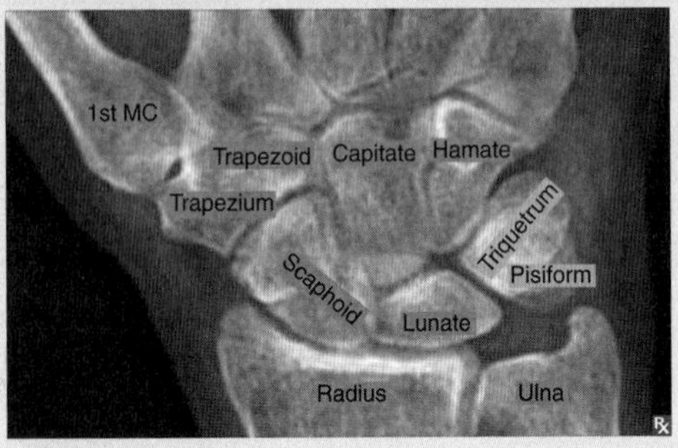 1st MC, Trapezoid, Capitate, Hamate, Trapezium, Triquetrum, Pisiform, Scaphoid, Lunate, Radius, Ulna	Common fracture from fall onto an outstretched hand (FOOSH). Initial radiographs can be negative; repeat in 2-3 weeks if high suspicion. Presents with tenderness at anatomic snuffbox and pain with resisted pronation.	Spica thumb cast immobilization for stable non-displaced fractures. Operative repair otherwise. Risk of non-union and avascular necrosis involving the proximal pole.
Boxer's fracture	Fracture of the neck of the 5th metacarpal. Often from trauma to a closed fist (ie, punching a blunt object).	Immobilization versus operative treatment depending on fracture characteristics.
Lunate dislocation	From direct trauma to an extended and ulnar deviated wrist. Can cause median nerve symptoms due to lunate dislocating into the carpal tunnel.	Urgent closed reduction versus ORIF. Can perform proximal row carpectomy if median nerve compression.
Colles fracture	Distal radius fracture leading to wrist swelling and deformity. Often from fall on an outstretched hand in female patients with osteoporosis.	Closed reduction and immobilization, followed by possible operative management depending on fracture characteristics. DEXA is often indicated given association with osteoporosis.
Galleazi fracture	Radial shaft fracture and associated dislocation of the distal radioulnar joint (DRUJ). From fall on an outstretched hand or high velocity trauma.	Open reduction and internal fixation (ORIF) of the radius in adults and stabilization of the DRUJ. In children, closed reduction can be considered.
Monteggia fracture	Fracture of the proximal ulna with dislocation of the radial head. From fall on an outstretched hand with a pronated forearm.	Adult patients often require ORIF of the ulnar shaft with reduction of the radial head.
Nightstick fracture	Isolated fracture of the ulnar shaft. Often from trauma from a blunt object (ie, nightstick) while in a defensive position.	Degree of displacement determines treatment. ORIF if displacement is significant.
Supracondylar (humerus) fracture	Frequently in young patients with direct trauma. Can present with radial nerve injury.	Non-operative (more common): Coaptation splint followed by functional brace. Operative: ORIF.
Rotator cuff tear 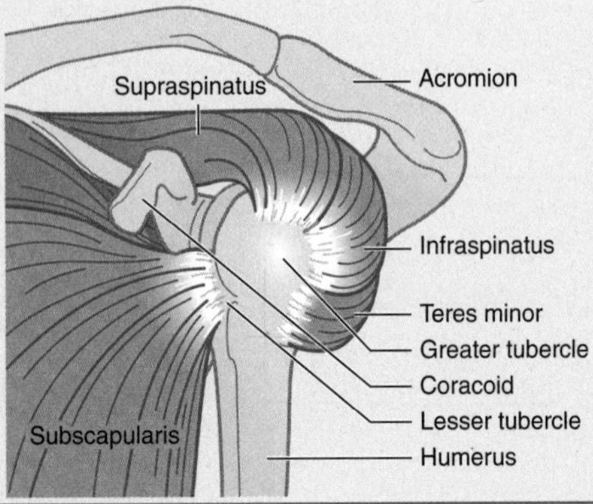 Supraspinatus, Acromion, Infraspinatus, Teres minor, Greater tubercle, Coracoid, Lesser tubercle, Subscapularis, Humerus	Traumatic injury in younger patients. Can be chronic degeneration in older patients. Deltoid pain and weakness with abduction and external rotation.	Ranges from rest, physical therapy, and NSAIDs to surgical repair versus shoulder replacement, depending on tear classification and patient factors.
Clavicular fracture	Most commonly fractures of the middle 3rd of the clavicle from a fall onto the lateral shoulder. Can be associated with pneumothorax, hemothorax or neurovascular injury.	Consists of either sling vs. surgery depending on fracture displacement and shortening, as well as patient factors. Assess for neurovascular compromise given risk of brachial plexus, subclavian or axillary vessel injury.

16-1 Adult Fractures

Lower Extremity Injuries

Injury Type	Characteristics	Treatment
Hip dislocation	Posterior dislocation (90%): Occurs due to force that is directed posteriorly towards an adducted, internally rotated, and flexed hip ("dashboard injury"). On exam, the leg is shortened, flexed, adducted, and internally rotated. Risk of sciatic nerve and femoral artery injury. Anterior dislocation (10%): Occurs due to direct blow on the posterior hip and/or abducted hip. On exam, the leg is lengthened, flexed, abducted, and externally rotated. Risk of femoral nerve and femoral artery injury. Complications: If combined with femoral head fracture, there is increased risk of avascular necrosis of the femoral head. Associated with post-traumatic osteoarthritis.	Closed reduction (as long as there is no associated femoral neck fracture), followed by abduction pillow/bracing. Evaluate with CT after reduction. If closed reduction fails or there are incarcerated intra-articular fragments, open reduction.
Hip fracture	Involves the acetabulum and/or the proximal intracapsular femur. Classified based on anatomical location as intracapsular (fractures involving the femoral head and neck) or extracapsular (intertrochanteric, trochanteric, and subtrochanteric fractures). Associated with osteoporosis. Patients often report groin pain, and the leg is shortened and externally rotated on exam. On imaging, hip x-rays can be negative; obtain CT or MRI if an occult fracture is suspected based on clinical signs. Complications: Associated with DVTs. Displaced femoral neck fractures are associated with sciatic nerve injury and increased risk of avascular necrosis of the femoral head.	ORIF. Femoral neck fractures in older adults may require total hip replacement or hemiarthroplasty. Anticoagulation to prevent DVT.
Femoral Neck Fracture	Due to direct trauma. Associated with osteoporosis. Complications: Avascular necrosis of the femoral head. Fat emboli can present with fever, dyspnea, hypoxia, altered mental status, petechiae, anemia, and thrombocytopenia.	ORIF. Open fractures are considered an orthopedic emergency and require irrigation and debridement. If bilateral and comminuted, severe internal blood loss can lead to hemorrhagic shock; consider external fixation while the patient is being stabilized.
Tibial and/or fibular fractures	May occur proximally (tibial plateau fracture), at the shaft, or distally and can involve solely the tibia, fibula, or both. Usually due to direct trauma. Complications: -Neurovascular injury: Peroneal nerve injury (foot drop). Tibial plateau fractures are associated with popliteal artery injury. -DVTs. -Fat embolism. -Compartment syndrome: The lower leg is at high risk for compartment syndrome; if there is pain under the cast, remove the cast to examine the site.	Casting vs. intramedullary nailing vs. ORIF.
Achilles tendon rupture	Presents with a sudden snap or "pop", followed immediately by a sharp pain in the back of the ankle. Usually caused by sudden dorsiflexion of a plantarflexed foot. Risk factors: physical deconditioning, oral fluoroquinolones, and local glucocorticoid injections. On exam, there is loss of plantar flexion and a ⊕ Thompson test (squeezing the gastrocnemius leads to absent foot plantar flexion). On palpation of the tendon, there is a gap. Obtain MRI for definitive diagnosis. Complications: Re-rupture. Contractures can lead to permanent decreased range of motion. Sural nerve injury if percutaneous tendon repair.	Treatment can be non-operative with brace/cast in resting equinus position (20° of plantar flexion) vs. operative with open end-to-end or percutaneous tendon repair.
Popliteal (Baker's) cyst rupture	Can present with posterior knee pain and/or decreased knee flexion, or may be discovered incidentally on imaging or physical exam. Large or ruptured cysts can cause calf pain and swelling and mimic the signs and symptoms of DVT (pseudothrombophlebitis syndrome). Risk factors: osteoarthritis, other underlying conditions (eg, meniscal tear). Usually a clinical diagnosis, but US is often obtained to exclude DVT. Complications: Neurovascular compression (eg, DVT due to venous compression, tibial nerve injury). Cyst infection.	Conservative measures (eg, NSAIDs, cyst drainage, intra-articular steroid injection). Consider surgical resection if the cyst is persistent and symptomatic or complications (eg, neurovascular compression) develop.
Ankle fracture	Caused by fall onto an everted or inverted foot leading to an isolated, bi- or tri-malleolar fracture. X-ray is the study of choice. Complications: Neurovascular injury (peroneal nerve, saphenous nerve).	Can be managed operatively or nonoperatively, depending on fracture and patient characteristics.

16-2 Knee Injuries

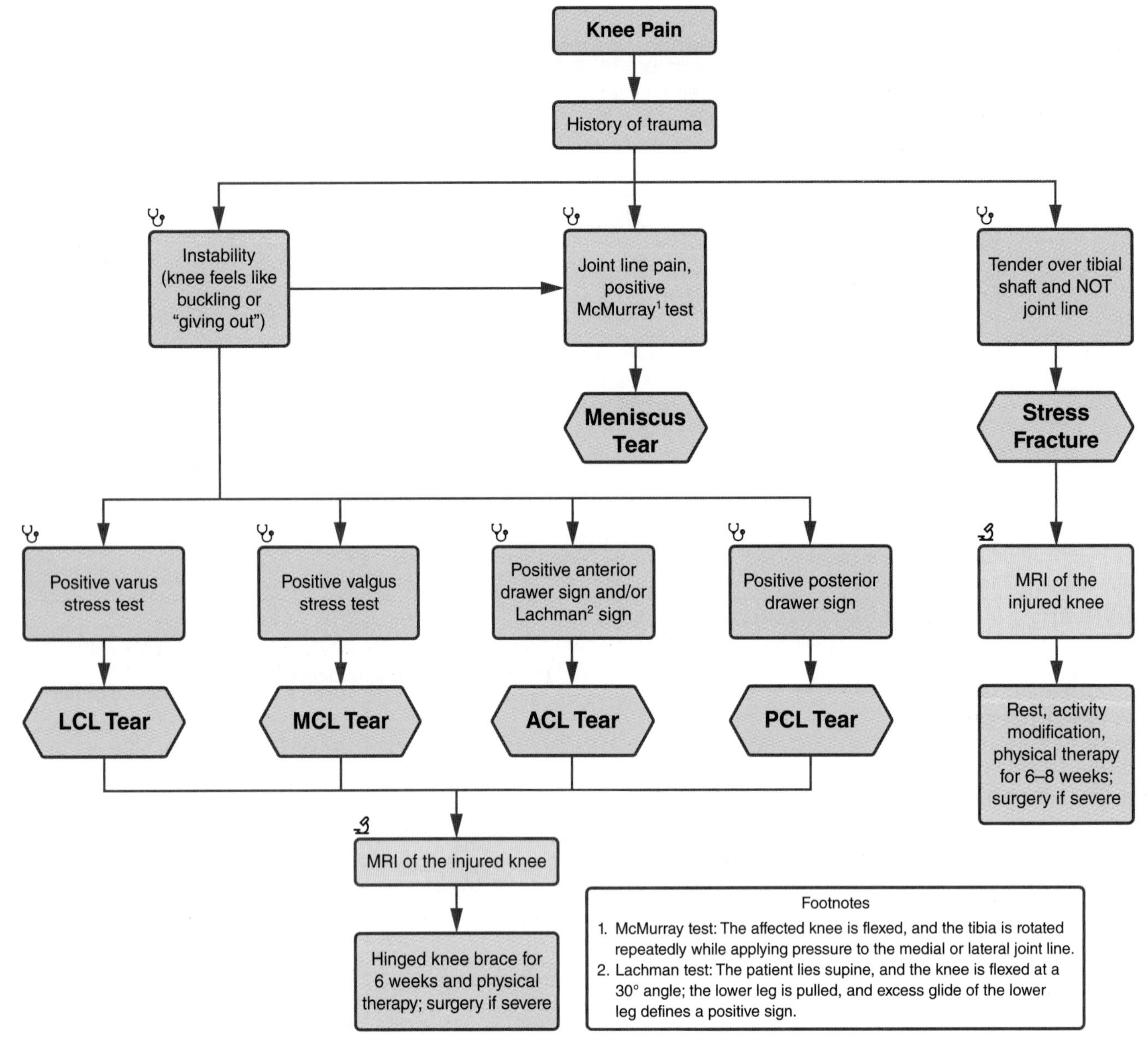
Knee Pain
History of trauma
Instability (knee feels like buckling or "giving out")
Joint line pain, positive McMurray[1] test
Tender over tibial shaft and NOT joint line
Meniscus Tear
Stress Fracture
Positive varus stress test
Positive valgus stress test
Positive anterior drawer sign and/or Lachman[2] sign
Positive posterior drawer sign
MRI of the injured knee
LCL Tear
MCL Tear
ACL Tear
PCL Tear
Rest, activity modification, physical therapy for 6–8 weeks; surgery if severe
MRI of the injured knee
Hinged knee brace for 6 weeks and physical therapy; surgery if severe
Footnotes
1. McMurray test: The affected knee is flexed, and the tibia is rotated repeatedly while applying pressure to the medial or lateral joint line.
2. Lachman test: The patient lies supine, and the knee is flexed at a 30° angle; the lower leg is pulled, and excess glide of the lower leg defines a positive sign.

FIGURE 16.2

16-2 Knee Injuries

MENISCUS TEAR

A 46-year-old F presents with left knee pain, swelling, catching, and locking that began 1 month ago after she twisted her knee while running. On **exam**, she has tenderness to palpation over the medial joint line and is unable to extend her knee fully; McMurray sign is positive. On **imaging**, MRI confirms the diagnosis of a medial meniscus tear.

Management:

1. Conservative management: physical therapy, cortisone injections.
2. Partial meniscectomy or meniscus repair is recommended in younger patients with reparable tears, as well as for injury that is severe (eg, bucket handle) and/or does not respond to conservative treatment.

Complications: Chronic knee pain, tear enlargement, early osteoarthritis.

HYF: Results from a twisting injury in young patients or degenerative tear in elderly patients. Medial meniscus tears are more common than lateral tears (which present similarly after a twisting injury but with pain along the lateral joint line). McMurray test: The affected knee is flexed and tibia is rotated repeatedly while applying pressure to the medial or lateral joint line.

TIBIAL STRESS FRACTURE

A 25-year-old F presents with left shin pain for the past week. She just started training for a marathon and ran roughly 50 miles last week. On **exam**, there is focal tenderness to palpation directly over the anterior shin. On **imaging**, X-ray shows a transverse fracture of the tibial shaft.

Management:

1. If the fracture is well-aligned and not extensive, it will likely heal on its own within 2 months with conservative treatment (cast, crutches, minimize weight-bearing activity).
2. Intramedullary nailing vs. ORIF is indicated for displaced fractures or fractures involving the articular surface.

Complications: Chronic pain, compartment syndrome.

HYF: Stress fractures result from excessive, chronic force applied to a bone. Shin splints are a form of a stress fracture called medial tibial stress syndrome. Common in runners.

LATERAL COLLATERAL LIGAMENT TEAR

A 28-year-old M presents with right knee pain. He was practicing grappling in Brazilian jiu-jitsu, and his opponent quickly pressed into his knee medially, resulting in a pop. On **exam**, there is pain along the lateral joint line and instability with walking. Varus (adduction) stress test is (+). MRI knee confirms the diagnosis.

Management:

1. Hinged knee brace for 6 weeks.
2. Physical therapy.
3. Consider surgery for a full tear or if multiple ligaments are injured.

Complications: Chronic knee laxity, early osteoarthritis.

HYF: Least common ligament injury of the knee. Often part of posterolateral corner injury.

MEDIAL COLLATERAL LIGAMENT TEAR

A 16-year-old F presents with right knee pain while walking on the beach with her dog. Her dog ran toward her, colliding into her knee laterally, and she felt a pop. On **exam**, there is profuse swelling throughout the knee, with pain presenting medially along the joint line. Her knee feels unstable with walking. Valgus stress test is (+). MRI knee confirms the diagnosis.

Management:

1. Hinged knee brace for 6 weeks.
2. Physical therapy.
3. Consider surgery for a full tear or if multiple ligaments are injured or refractory to therapy.

Complications: Chronic knee pain and laxity, early osteoarthritis.

HYF: Most commonly injured knee ligament. Part of the "Terrible Triad": ACL, MCL, and meniscus tears.

ANTERIOR CRUCIATE LIGAMENT TEAR

A 21-year-old M presents with left knee pain while playing rugby. He collided with another player while planting his left foot into the ground and he pivoted his left knee, resulting in a pop. He was unable to continue playing. On **exam**, there is profuse swelling and pain throughout the knee, and the knee buckles with ambulation. Anterior drawer sign, as well as Lachman test, are (+). Left knee MRI confirms the diagnosis.

Management:

1. Immobilization and PT to regain range of motion.
2. In active patients, surgery with graft from the patellar or hamstring tendons is usually recommended. Younger patients = autograft; older patients = allograft.
3. In sedentary patients, immobilization and rehabilitation can be an alternative to surgical repair.

Complications: Chronic knee laxity, early osteoarthritis, tearing of the ipsilateral meniscus.

HYF: For the anterior drawer test, the patient lies with feet on table, hips flexed, and knee bent at 90 degrees; the examiner pulls the tibia forward with both hands, and there is abnormal laxity. For the Lachman test (more sensitive), the patient lies with the knee bent 30°; the examiner places a hand on the thigh and pulls the tibia forward with the other hand. Part of the "Terrible Triad": ACL, MCL, and meniscus tears (lateral more common in acute injuries).

(Continued)

16-2 Knee Injuries

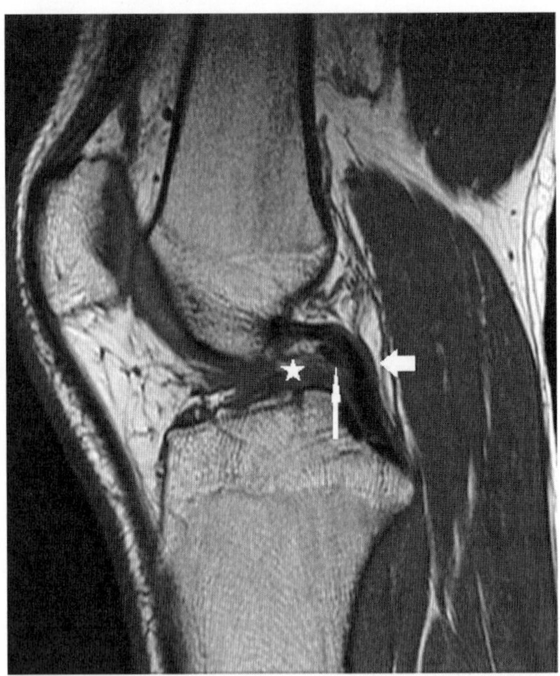

MRI knee demonstrates absence of the anterior cruciate ligament, indicating a chronic complete ACL tear with resorption (star). The posterior cruciate ligament (wide arrow) is intact but buckled, which is an associated imaging finding of an ACL tear. Immediately anterior to the PCL is a normal variant meniscofemoral ligament of Humphrey (thin arrow).

POSTERIOR CRUCIATE LIGAMENT TEAR

A 32-year-old M presents with right knee pain and instability following a car accident 3 weeks ago. He was riding as a passenger in the front seat and his knee collided with the dashboard, causing a loud pop. He has noted difficulty walking, as well as knee swelling. Exam reveals a (+) posterior drawer sign. MRI knee confirms the diagnosis.

Management:

1. Hinged knee brace with a PCL bolster for 6 weeks.
2. Surgical PCL reconstruction is usually only recommended for competitive athletes with severe injury and/or multiple torn ligaments.
3. Physical therapy.

Complications: Chronic knee laxity, early osteoarthritis, associated with popliteal tendon injury (during posterolateral corner knee injuries).

HYF: Known as a "dashboard injury"; typically results from either colliding the knee into a dashboard while in a flexed position or falling directly onto the knee in a flexed position. The majority of isolated PCL injuries can be treated non-operatively.

16-3 Ankle Injuries

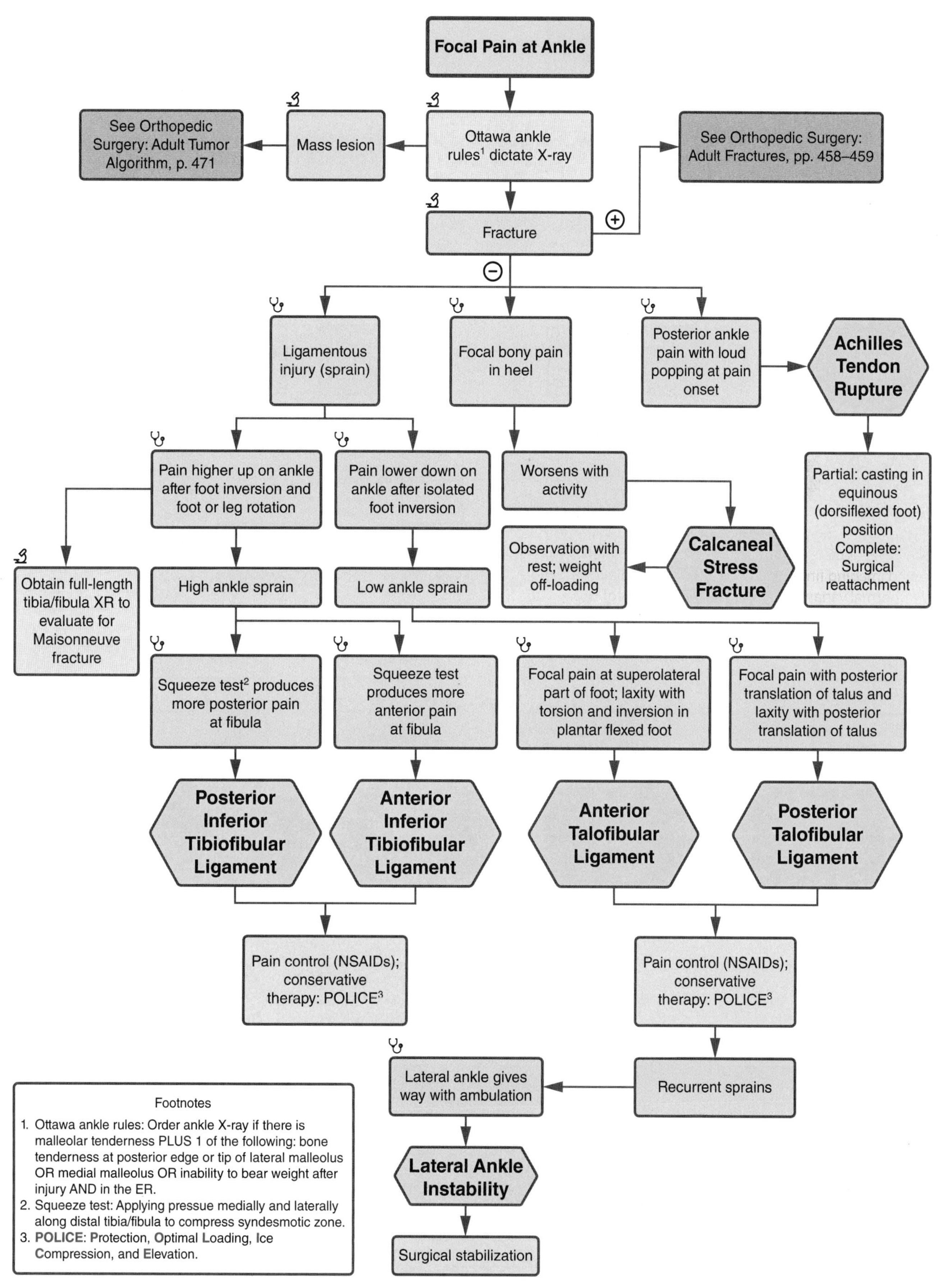
Focal Pain at Ankle
Ottawa ankle rules[1] dictate X-ray
Mass lesion
See Orthopedic Surgery: Adult Tumor Algorithm, p. 471
Fracture
See Orthopedic Surgery: Adult Fractures, pp. 458–459
Ligamentous injury (sprain)
Focal bony pain in heel
Posterior ankle pain with loud popping at pain onset
Achilles Tendon Rupture
Partial: casting in equinous (dorsiflexed foot) position
Complete: Surgical reattachment
Pain higher up on ankle after foot inversion and foot or leg rotation
Pain lower down on ankle after isolated foot inversion
Worsens with activity
Calcaneal Stress Fracture
Observation with rest; weight off-loading
Obtain full-length tibia/fibula XR to evaluate for Maisonneuve fracture
High ankle sprain
Low ankle sprain
Squeeze test[2] produces more posterior pain at fibula
Squeeze test produces more anterior pain at fibula
Focal pain at superolateral part of foot; laxity with torsion and inversion in plantar flexed foot
Focal pain with posterior translation of talus and laxity with posterior translation of talus
Posterior Inferior Tibiofibular Ligament
Anterior Inferior Tibiofibular Ligament
Anterior Talofibular Ligament
Posterior Talofibular Ligament
Pain control (NSAIDs); conservative therapy: POLICE[3]
Pain control (NSAIDs); conservative therapy: POLICE[3]
Recurrent sprains
Lateral ankle gives way with ambulation
Lateral Ankle Instability
Surgical stabilization
Footnotes
1. Ottawa ankle rules: Order ankle X-ray if there is malleolar tenderness PLUS 1 of the following: bone tenderness at posterior edge or tip of lateral malleolus OR medial malleolus OR inability to bear weight after injury AND in the ER.
2. Squeeze test: Applying pressue medially and laterally along distal tibia/fibula to compress syndesmotic zone.
3. POLICE: Protection, Optimal Loading, Ice Compression, and Elevation.

FIGURE 16.3

16-4 Hand Injuries

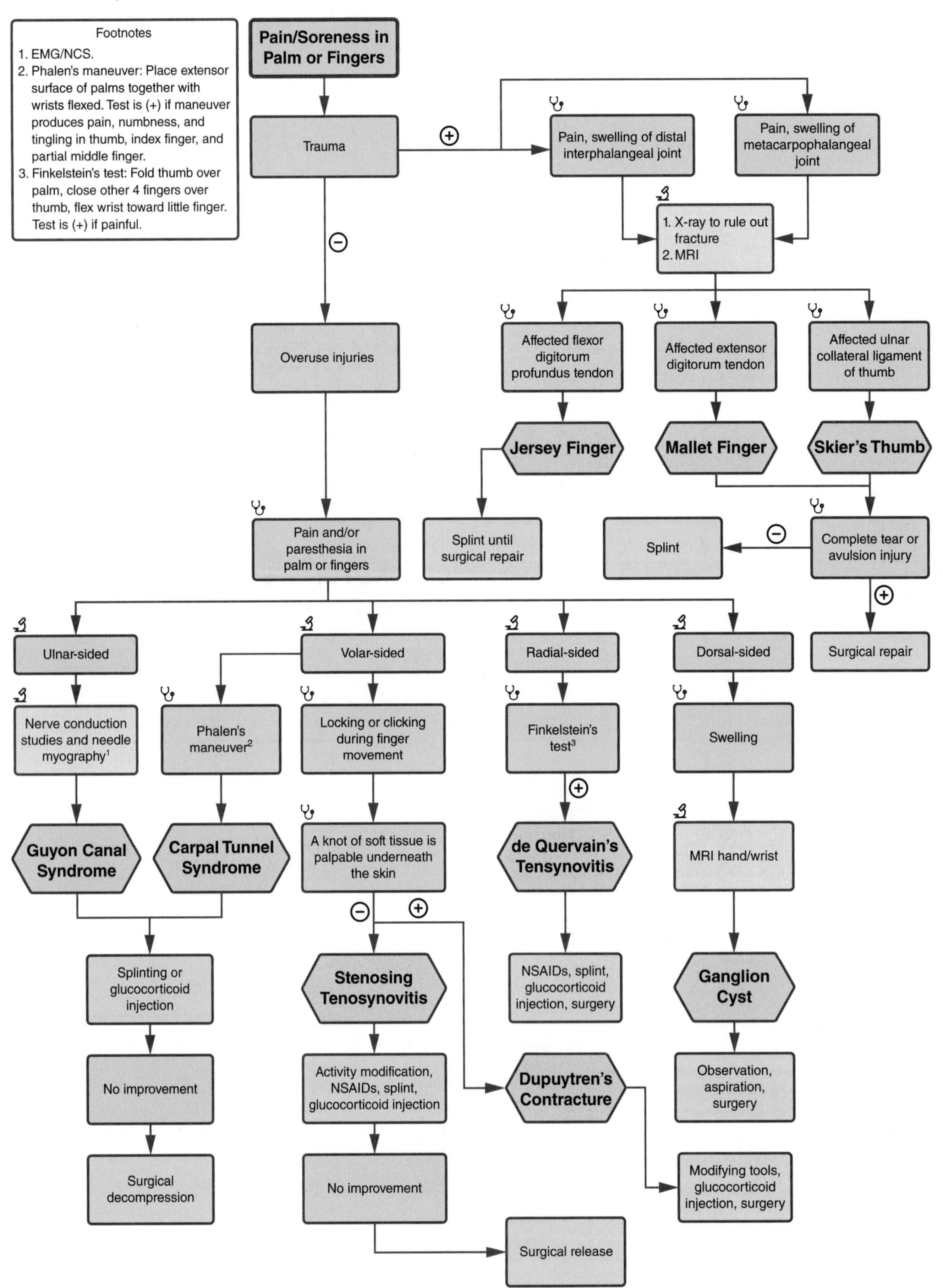
Footnotes
1. EMG/NCS.
2. Phalen's maneuver: Place extensor surface of palms together with wrists flexed. Test is (+) if maneuver produces pain, numbness, and tingling in thumb, index finger, and partial middle finger.
3. Finkelstein's test: Fold thumb over palm, close other 4 fingers over thumb, flex wrist toward little finger. Test is (+) if painful.
Pain/Soreness in Palm or Fingers
Trauma
+
Pain, swelling of distal interphalangeal joint
Pain, swelling of metacarpophalangeal joint
1. X-ray to rule out fracture
2. MRI
Affected flexor digitorum profundus tendon
Affected extensor digitorum tendon
Affected ulnar collateral ligament of thumb
Jersey Finger
Mallet Finger
Skier's Thumb
Splint until surgical repair
Splint
Complete tear or avulsion injury
Surgical repair
−
Overuse injuries
Pain and/or paresthesia in palm or fingers
Ulnar-sided
Volar-sided
Radial-sided
Dorsal-sided
Nerve conduction studies and needle myography[1]
Phalen's maneuver[2]
Locking or clicking during finger movement
Finkelstein's test[3]
Swelling
Guyon Canal Syndrome
Carpal Tunnel Syndrome
A knot of soft tissue is palpable underneath the skin
de Quervain's Tensynovitis
MRI hand/wrist
Splinting or glucocorticoid injection
Stenosing Tenosynovitis
NSAIDs, splint, glucocorticoid injection, surgery
Ganglion Cyst
No improvement
Activity modification, NSAIDs, splint, glucocorticoid injection
Dupuytren's Contracture
Observation, aspiration, surgery
Surgical decompression
No improvement
Modifying tools, glucocorticoid injection, surgery
Surgical release

FIGURE 16.4

16-4 Hand Injuries

GANGLION CYST

A 52-year-old F presents with complaints of left wrist pain. On **exam**, there is swelling on the dorsal side of the wrist, which is firm, smooth, rounded, rubbery, and tender. On **imaging**, MRI shows a cyst.

Management:

1. Observation.
2. Needle aspiration rarely indicated.
3. Surgical excision if refractory and symptomatic.

Complications:

- Infection.
- Guyon canal syndrome.

HYF: Benign tumors found in adults, usually on the dorsum of the wrist.

DE QUERVAIN'S TENOSYNOVITIS

A 46-year-old M golfer presents with complaints of left wrist pain. Patient reports pain when gripping objects. On **exam**, there is pain on the radial side of the wrist, which is more notable with thumb and wrist movement. Finkelstein's test is positive. On **imaging**, X-ray is unremarkable.

Management:

1. NSAIDs and thumb spica splint.
2. Glucocorticoid injection.
3. de Quervain's tendon release surgery if refractory to conservative management.

Complications: High recurrence rate.

HYF: Stenosing tenosynovial inflammation of the 1st dorsal compartment. Not considered an inflammatory condition. Most common among women between ages 30 and 50 in the dominant wrist.

DUPUYTREN'S CONTRACTURE

A 59-year-old M presents with complaints of loss of extension in the 4th finger. On **exam**, there is skin puckering of dermal tissue over the flexor tendon just proximal to the flexor crease of finger. There is a presence of a palpable cord running longitudinally, which puckers the skin.

Management:

1. Activity modification, steroid injection, injection of *Clostridium histolyticum* collagenase, needle aponeurotomy.
2. If refractory to non-operative management, consider Dupuytren's contracture surgery (fasciectomy).

Complications: Recurrence after treatment.

HYF: Autosomal dominant with variable penetrance. Mostly affects those of northern European ancestry. Men > women. Ring > small > middle > index fingers affected. Associated with alcohol use, HIV, diabetes, anti-epileptic medications.

STENOSING TENOSYNOVITIS (TRIGGER FINGER)

A 63-year-old F presents with complaints of finger locking and pain. She reports difficulty extending the affected digit. On **exam**, there is pain over the volar aspect of the MCP joint that radiates into the palm. Flexion and extension of the digit reproduce symptoms.

Management:

1. Activity modification, NSAIDs, splinting.
2. Glucocorticoid injection.
3. Surgical release of A1 pulley.

Complications: None.

HYF: Trigger finger is most common among women in the 5th or 6th decade of life. Associated with carpal tunnel syndrome, diabetes, rheumatoid arthritis, hypothyroidism, and gout.

CARPAL TUNNEL SYNDROME

A 30-year-old F with PMH of type 1 diabetes presents with complaints of numbness and tingling in her first 3 digits and the radial half of the 4th digit. She is a computer programmer who spends hours every day typing. She reports that her symptoms worsen at night and awaken her from sleep. On **exam**, she has numbness in the distribution of median nerve, the thenar eminence is atrophic, and wrist flexion is weak. Phalen's maneuver and Tinel's sign are positive. **Labs** are normal. Nerve conduction studies and electromyography (EMG) confirm the diagnosis.

Management:

1. Activity modification, NSAIDs, splinting.
2. Glucocorticoid injection.
3. Median nerve decompression surgery.

Complications: Permanent loss of hand strength and sensation, decreased fine motor skills.

HYF: Most common entrapment neuropathy in the upper extremity. Due to entrapment of the median nerve in the carpal tunnel between the transverse carpal ligament and carpal bones; sensation is spared because the palmar cutaneous branch enters the hand external to the carpal tunnel. Dislocation of lunate may cause acute carpal tunnel syndrome. Associated with pregnancy, diabetes, rheumatoid arthritis, hypothyroidism, acromegaly, dialysis-related amyloidosis, and repetitive use.

(*Continued*)

16-4 Hand Injuries

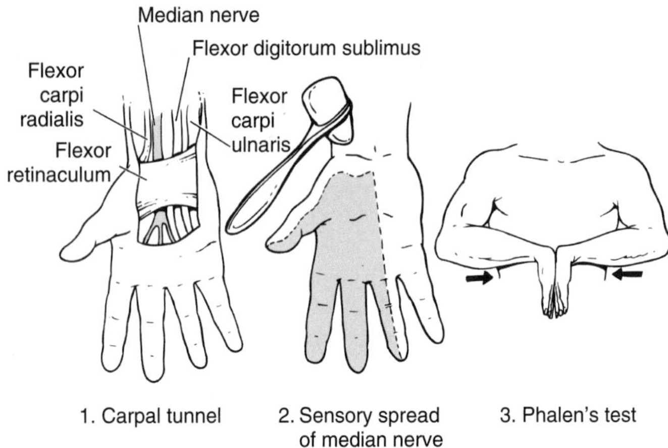
Median nerve
Flexor digitorum sublimus
Flexor carpi radialis
Flexor carpi ulnaris
Flexor retinaculum
1. Carpal tunnel
2. Sensory spread of median nerve
3. Phalen's test

GUYON CANAL SYNDROME

A 52-year-old M cyclist presents with complaints of paresthesias over the little finger and ulnar half of the 4th finger and ulnar dorsum of the hand, as well as hand weakness. He reports that the symptoms worsen at night and awaken him from sleep. On **exam**, he has decreased sensation in ulnar 1-1/2 digits, weak grasp and pincer strength, and a claw-hand deformity. Tinel's sign is positive over the Guyon canal. **Labs** are normal. On **imaging**, nerve conduction studies and EMG confirm the diagnosis.

Management:

1. Activity modification, NSAIDs, splinting.
2. Glucocorticoid injection.
3. Ulnar nerve decompression surgery.

Complications: Permanent loss of hand strength and sensation, decreased fine motor skills.

HYF: Most commonly due to ganglion cyst. Distinguish GCS from cubital tunnel syndrome (ulnar nerve compression at the elbow), which presents with the same ulnar distribution of hand paresthesias and weakness but, in addition, presents with sensory deficit to the dorsum of the hand, weakness of ulnar-innervated extrinsic muscles, positive elbow flexion test, and Tinel's sign at the elbow.

SKIER'S THUMB

A 16-year-old M presents with thumb pain after falling while skiing. On **exam**, there is pain and swelling along the ulnar aspect of the thumb MCP joint. On **imaging**, X-ray shows a condylar fracture. MRI shows an ulnar collateral ligament (UCL) tear.

Management:

1. Immobilization (thumb spica splinting) for 4–6 weeks.
2. If varus/valgus, surgical ligament repair.

Complications: Persistent joint instability, MCP and IP stiffness, superficial radial neuropraxia.

HYF: Skiing accidents in which the thumb strikes a fixed ski pole and other athletic injuries involving thumb abduction are the most common cause. The UCL is most commonly affected in this injury, but the radial collateral ligament (RCL) can also be torn; management is similar.

MALLET FINGER

A 32-year-old M presents after jamming his finger while trying to grab the basketball during a game. On **exam**, there is pain and swelling over the dorsum of the DIP joint of his index finger. Patient is unable to actively extend his DIP joint. On **imaging**, XR reveals a bony avulsion of distal phalanx.

Management:

1. Extension splinting of DIP joint for 6–8 weeks
2. If volar subluxation of the distal phalanx, significant arthritis, or chronic injury, consider surgical repair (closed reduction percutaneous pinning vs. open reduction internal fixation).

Complications:

- Chronic stiffness of DIP joint.
- Extensor lag.
- Swan neck deformity.

HYF: Most common closed tendon injury of the finger, usually work or sports-related, due to injury of the terminal extensor tendon distal to DIP joint.

JERSEY FINGER

An 18-year-old M presents after hyperextending his finger while trying to tackle another player during football. On **exam**, there is pain and swelling over the volar aspect of the DIP joint of his ring finger, which lies in slight extension at the DIP relative to other fingers. He is unable to flex his DIP joint. On **imaging**, XR shows an avulsion fragment. MRI shows flexor digitorum profundus tendon rupture.

Management:

1. Tendon repair or open reduction and internal fixation based on size and presence of bony avulsion.

Complications:

- Development of DIP flexion contracture.
- Instability of DIP joint.

HYF: Traumatic flexor tendon injury due to avulsion injury of the FDP from its insertion at the base of the distal phalanx. Occurs in the ring finger in the majority of cases.

16-5 Foot Pain

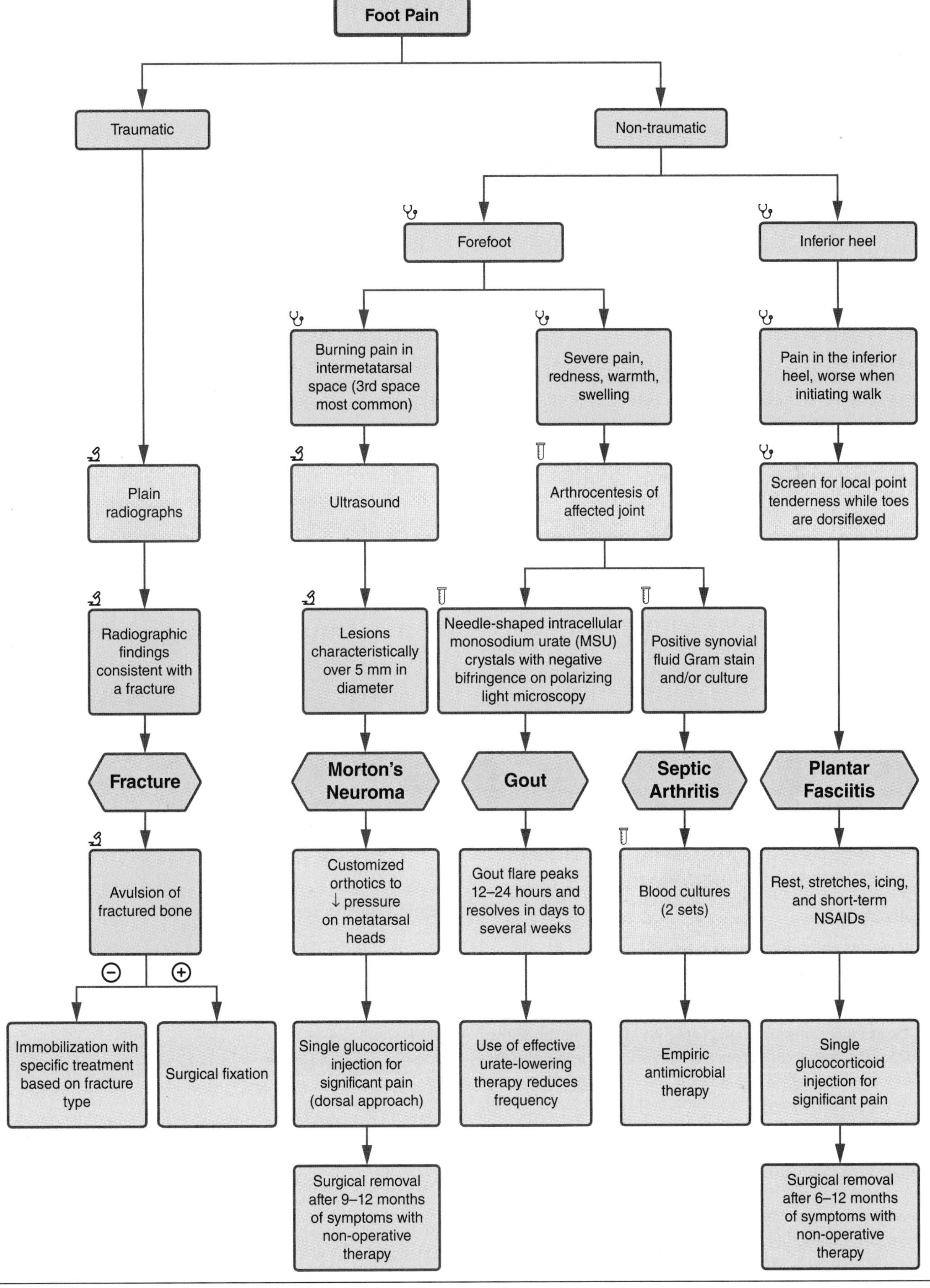
Foot Pain
Traumatic
Non-traumatic
Forefoot
Inferior heel
Burning pain in intermetatarsal space (3rd space most common)
Severe pain, redness, warmth, swelling
Pain in the inferior heel, worse when initiating walk
Plain radiographs
Ultrasound
Arthrocentesis of affected joint
Screen for local point tenderness while toes are dorsiflexed
Radiographic findings consistent with a fracture
Lesions characteristically over 5 mm in diameter
Needle-shaped intracellular monosodium urate (MSU) crystals with negative bifringence on polarizing light microscopy
Positive synovial fluid Gram stain and/or culture
Fracture
Morton's Neuroma
Gout
Septic Arthritis
Plantar Fasciitis
Avulsion of fractured bone
Customized orthotics to ↓ pressure on metatarsal heads
Gout flare peaks 12–24 hours and resolves in days to several weeks
Blood cultures (2 sets)
Rest, stretches, icing, and short-term NSAIDs
⊖
⊕
Immobilization with specific treatment based on fracture type
Surgical fixation
Single glucocorticoid injection for significant pain (dorsal approach)
Use of effective urate-lowering therapy reduces frequency
Empiric antimicrobial therapy
Single glucocorticoid injection for significant pain
Surgical removal after 9–12 months of symptoms with non-operative therapy
Surgical removal after 6–12 months of symptoms with non-operative therapy

FIGURE 16.5

16-5 Foot Pain

MORTON'S NEUROMA

A 55-year-old F runner presents with burning pain in her forefoot. The pain worsens when she wears high-heeled shoes. On **exam**, she has pain in the 3rd intermetatarsal space that radiates toward her toes. Palpating the joint space elicits a clicking sensation. On **imaging**, US reveals a lesion measuring 6.5 mm.

Management:

1. Customized orthotics to decrease pressure on metatarsal heads.
2. Single glucocorticoid injection for significant pain.
3. If symptoms persist despite 9–12 months of non-operative therapy, surgical removal.

Complications: Metatarsal fat pad atrophy after glucocorticoid injection.

HYF: More common in females than males. Due to neuropathic degeneration of nerves, most commonly between the 3rd and 4th toes, leading to pain and paresthesias. Symptoms worsen when metatarsals are squeezed together (eg, wearing tight shoes).

GOUT

A 55-year-old M presents with redness, pain, and swelling of his big toe. He is on a loop diuretic and ACE inhibitor. He says the pain started 2 days ago but has improved. On **imaging**, XR shows a punched-out erosion with a sclerotic rim and overhanging edge ("rat-bite" erosions). Arthrocentesis of the inflamed joint is performed, and intracellular needle-shaped monosodium urate (MSU) crystals with negative birefringence are seen on polarizing light microscopy.

Management:

1. For acute gout flares: NSAIDs, colchicine, or oral glucocorticoids.
2. For maintenance therapy: allopurinol, probenecid.
3. Do not use urate-lower therapy unless there are recurrent gout flares or severe disease (eg, tophi). In patients with recurrent flares, 1st-line treatment is allopurinol.

Complications:

- Joint damage and deformity.
- Colchicine can cause diarrhea and bone marrow suppression (neutropenia).

HYF: Gout most commonly affects the 1st MTP joint (podagra). Thiazides and diuretics can increase serum uric acid levels, increasing risk of developing gout. Commonly tested causes of hyperuricemia: cyclosporine, diabetes insipidus, diet (alcohol, red meats), diuretics, lead poisoning, salicylates, and tumor lysis. In a child with gout and self-harming injuries, consider Lesch-Nyhan syndrome (hypoxanthine-guanine phosphoribosyltransferase [HGPRT] deficiency). In contrast to gout, pseudogout (CPPD) presents with predominant knee and wrist involvement and is associated with hemochromatosis and hyperparathyroidism; its crystals are rhomboid-shaped with positive birefringence on polarizing light microscopy.

PLANTAR FASCIITIS

A 40-year-old M presents with heel pain that is worse when walking after prolonged inactivity (eg, first steps in the morning) and improves gradually with use. He is an active runner. On **exam**, with toes dorsiflexed, he has focal tenderness to palpation at the plantar surface of the heel.

Management:

1. Rest, ice, and NSAIDs for pain relief.
2. Stretching exercises and footwear modification.
3. Glucocorticoid injections of sites of tenderness.
4. If disease is refractory to the above, surgical plantar fascia release.

Complications: Glucocorticoid injections can cause heel pad atrophy.

HYF: Characterized by pain that is worst when initiating walking.

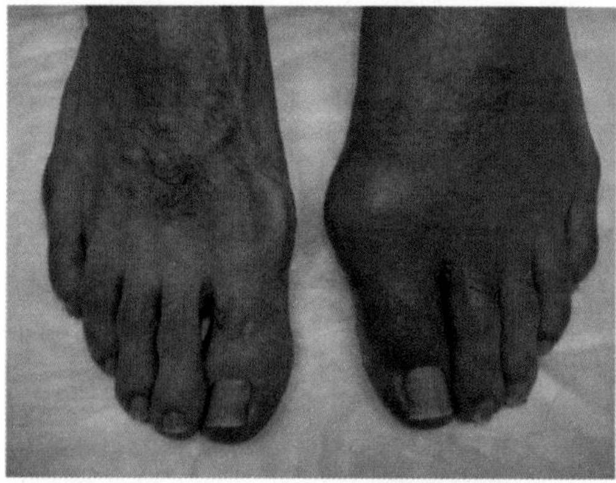

Gout (podagra). The left 1st MTP joint is swollen, erythematous, and tender.

Septic Arthritis: See pp. 295, 632.

16-6 Emergencies

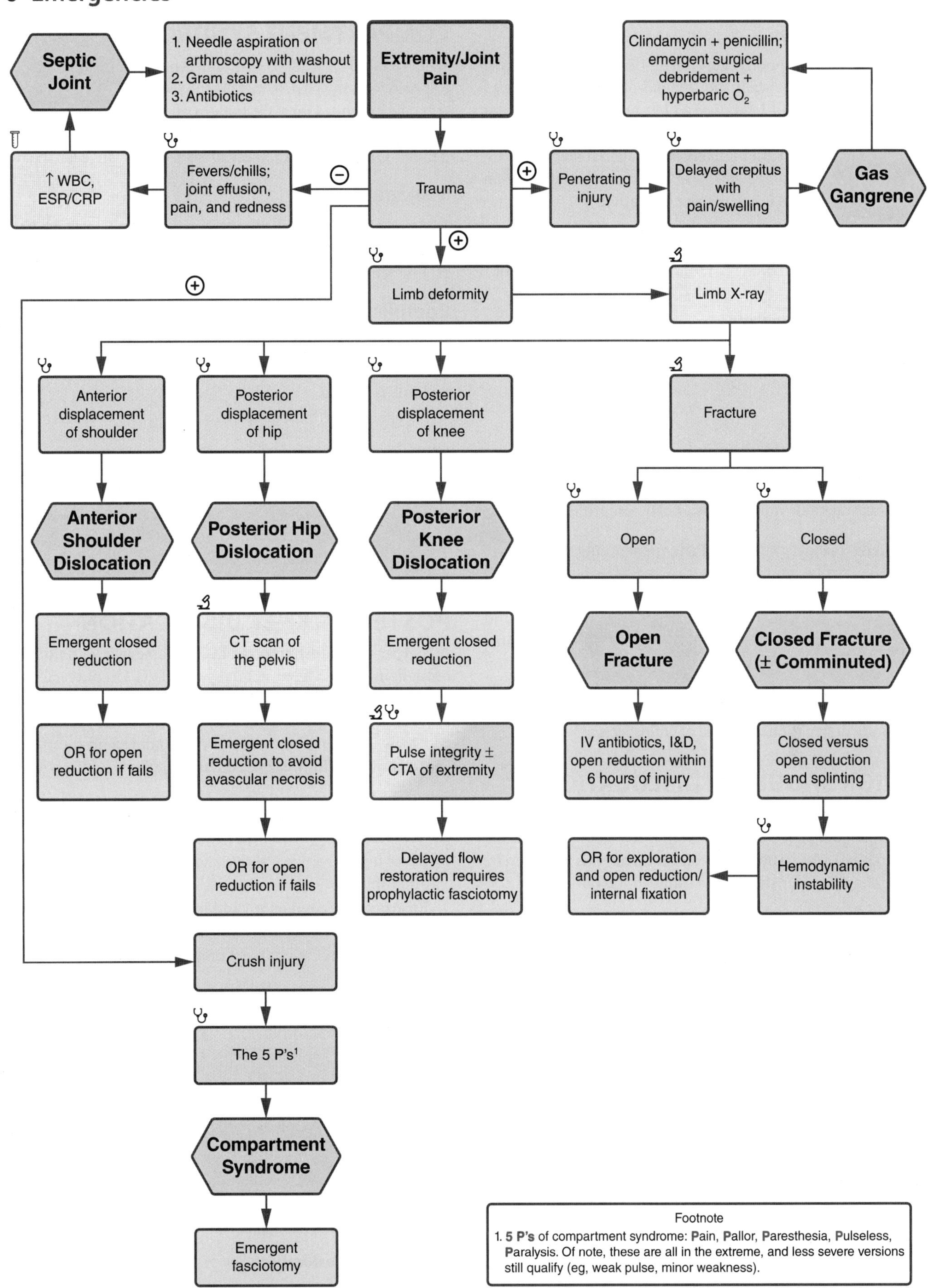
Septic Joint
1. Needle aspiration or arthroscopy with washout
2. Gram stain and culture
3. Antibiotics
Extremity/Joint Pain
Clindamycin + penicillin; emergent surgical debridement + hyperbaric O_2
↑ WBC, ESR/CRP
Fevers/chills; joint effusion, pain, and redness
Trauma
Penetrating injury
Delayed crepitus with pain/swelling
Gas Gangrene
Limb deformity
Limb X-ray
Anterior displacement of shoulder
Posterior displacement of hip
Posterior displacement of knee
Fracture
Anterior Shoulder Dislocation
Posterior Hip Dislocation
Posterior Knee Dislocation
Open
Closed
Emergent closed reduction
CT scan of the pelvis
Emergent closed reduction
Open Fracture
Closed Fracture (± Comminuted)
OR for open reduction if fails
Emergent closed reduction to avoid avascular necrosis
Pulse integrity ± CTA of extremity
IV antibiotics, I&D, open reduction within 6 hours of injury
Closed versus open reduction and splinting
OR for open reduction if fails
Delayed flow restoration requires prophylactic fasciotomy
OR for exploration and open reduction/ internal fixation
Hemodynamic instability
Crush injury
The 5 P's[1]
Compartment Syndrome
Emergent fasciotomy
Footnote
1. 5 P's of compartment syndrome: Pain, Pallor, Paresthesia, Pulseless, Paralysis. Of note, these are all in the extreme, and less severe versions still qualify (eg, weak pulse, minor weakness).

FIGURE 16.6

16-6 Emergencies

GAS GANGRENE

A 74-year-old F with poorly controlled diabetes was walking around in her basement when she stepped on a broken piece of glass and suffered a small laceration to her heel. The wound was cleaned and bandaged at a local emergency room. She returns with her husband 4 days later with high fevers and altered mental status. Her heel is now painful and swollen. On exam, palpating the skin produces the sensation of crackling rice beneath it.

Management:

1. ± CT of the affected area to see if underlying collection/extent of injury.
2. Broad-spectrum IV antibiotics.
3. Wound and blood cultures.
4. OR for wound debridement.
5. Hyperbaric O_2.

Complications:

- Sepsis, myositis, rhabdomyolysis.
- Limb amputation.
- Numbness/weakness from neurovascular compromise.

HYF: Presents in a delayed fashion after penetrating injury, often in context of a dirty wound, such as a rusty nail or object covered in mud or manure. Patients can present with altered mental status and possible sepsis with hemodynamic instability, fevers, chills, and diaphoresis. Crepitus, or subcutaneous emphysema, is not specific, but helpful in confirming diagnosis. *C. perfringens* is a common pathogen. Antibiotics with surgical debridement are the first line of therapy. Imaging can help guide surgery by visualizing extent of infection/bony destruction/presence of collections.

ANTERIOR SHOULDER DISLOCATION

A 31-year-old F with no PMH presents to urgent care after falling off her bicycle going over a speed hump a few hours earlier. She has no frank weakness or numbness on exam, but this is limited by pain in her shoulder. Her shoulder is slumped forward.

Management:

1. Axillary X-ray to confirm dislocation.
2. Emergent closed reduction.
3. If closed reduction fails, may require open reduction.
4. Sling post-reduction.

Complications: Necrosis of humeral head. Soft tissue injury (rotator cuff, labrum). Fracture (bony Bankart, Hill-Sachs lesion). Neurovascular compromise. Axillary nerve injury.

HYF: This often occurs in the context of trauma but can occur in more benign circumstances, such as spiking a volleyball or serving in tennis. This injury puts the axillary artery and its branches at risk, which in turn provide a tenuous blood supply to the humeral head. Posterior dislocations are less common and present with an internally rotated and adducted arm often in the context of seizures or electrical injury.

COMPARTMENT SYNDROME

A 22-year-old M with no PMH presents with complaints of severe calf pain with any passive movement. He was playing football earlier that day and ended up at the bottom of a pile. On exam, pulse is normal, and his leg is warm and well-perfused. He has no neurologic deficits. On imaging, an X-ray of his leg is negative for fracture.

Management:

1. Serial physical exams: monitor for tense limb, swelling, pain with passive motion, ± measurement of compartment pressure.
2. Emergent fasciotomy.

Complications:

- Numbness/weakness from neurovascular compromise.
- Rhabdomyolysis with associated AKI.
- Limb ischemia.
- Myopathy and muscle necrosis.

HYF: Compartment syndromes can arise from not only trauma and crush injury but any condition that causes prolonged ischemia with subsequent reperfusion, such as a traumatic vessel dissection that recanalized. Be aware of the associated conditions, such as rhabdomyolysis, which comes with its own host of complications including end-organ injury (eg, acute kidney injury).

POSTERIOR KNEE DISLOCATION

A 25-year-old M restrained front seat passenger with no PMH was brought in by EMS from a high-speed MVC. On physical exam, the patient has gross deformity of the RLE with knee hyperextension beyond 30°. Sensation is diminished over the dorsum of the foot and toes, including between the first and second toes. ABI is 0.8 (normal >0.9), with weak pulses on Doppler.

Management:

1. XR of knee to confirm dislocation.
2. XR of hip and ankle ("above and below joint") to assess for other injuries.
3. Emergent knee reduction and immobilization, with admission for at least 24 hours of neurovascular checks.
4. Avoid pressure on popliteal fossa due to risk of further injuring popliteal artery.
5. Vascular consult after reduction ± arterial Doppler US or CT angiography to evaluate for vascular injury.
6. Delayed ligamentous repair.

Complications: Popliteal nerve and artery injury. Compartment syndrome. Limb ischemia requiring amputation.

HYF: Associated with high-energy injuries ("dashboard injury") imposing force on a flexed knee.

Septic Joint: See pp. 295, 632.

Posterior Hip Dislocation: See p. 459.

16-7 Adult Bone Lesions

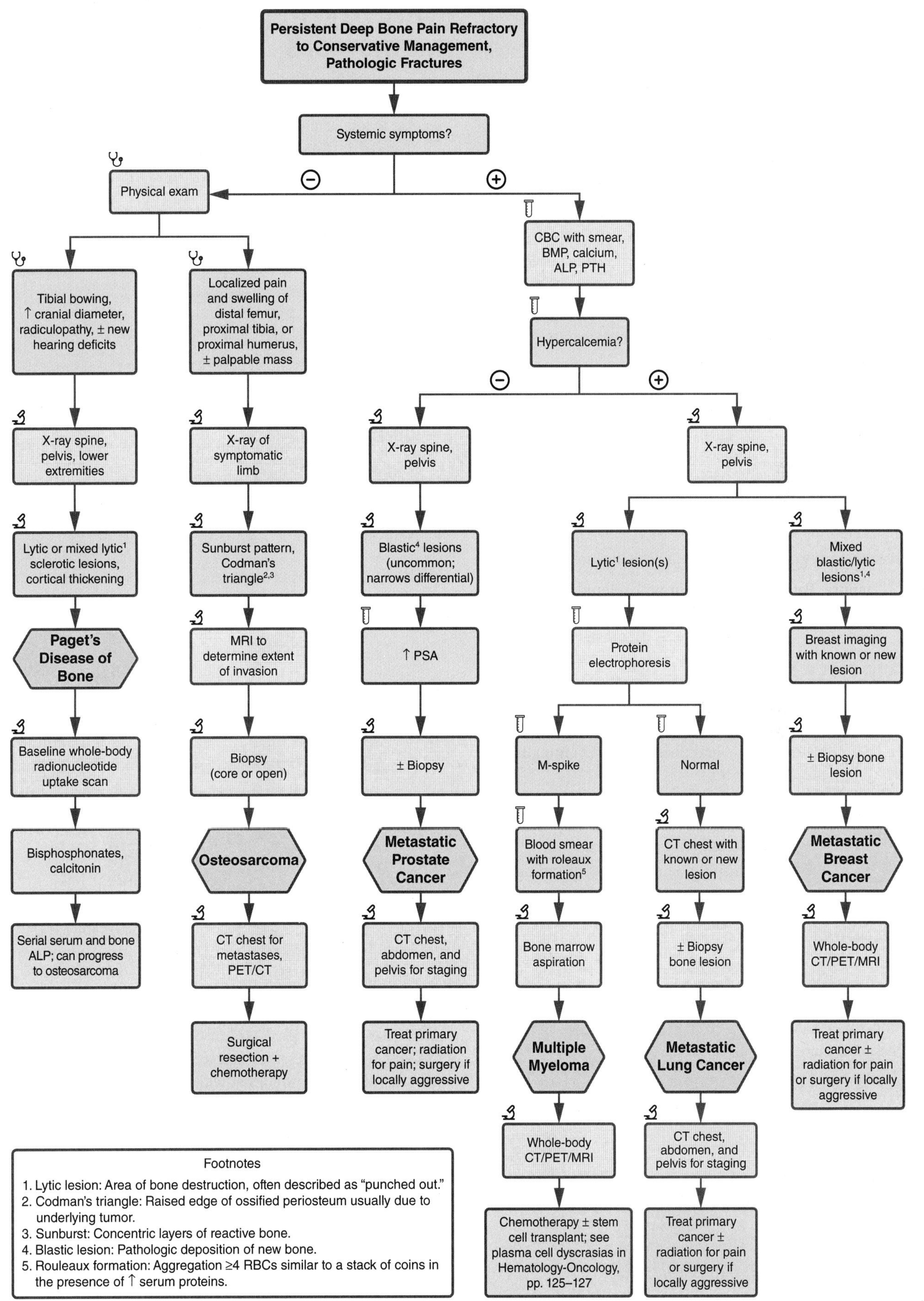
Persistent Deep Bone Pain Refractory to Conservative Management, Pathologic Fractures
Systemic symptoms?
Physical exam
CBC with smear, BMP, calcium, ALP, PTH
Hypercalcemia?
Tibial bowing, ↑ cranial diameter, radiculopathy, ± new hearing deficits
Localized pain and swelling of distal femur, proximal tibia, or proximal humerus, ± palpable mass
X-ray spine, pelvis, lower extremities
X-ray of symptomatic limb
X-ray spine, pelvis
X-ray spine, pelvis
Lytic or mixed lytic[1] sclerotic lesions, cortical thickening
Sunburst pattern, Codman's triangle[2,3]
Blastic[4] lesions (uncommon; narrows differential)
Lytic[1] lesion(s)
Mixed blastic/lytic lesions[1,4]
Paget's Disease of Bone
MRI to determine extent of invasion
↑ PSA
Protein electrophoresis
Breast imaging with known or new lesion
Baseline whole-body radionucleotide uptake scan
Biopsy (core or open)
± Biopsy
M-spike
Normal
± Biopsy bone lesion
Bisphosphonates, calcitonin
Osteosarcoma
Metastatic Prostate Cancer
Blood smear with roleaux formation[5]
CT chest with known or new lesion
Metastatic Breast Cancer
Serial serum and bone ALP; can progress to osteosarcoma
CT chest for metastases, PET/CT
CT chest, abdomen, and pelvis for staging
Bone marrow aspiration
± Biopsy bone lesion
Whole-body CT/PET/MRI
Surgical resection + chemotherapy
Treat primary cancer; radiation for pain; surgery if locally aggressive
Multiple Myeloma
Metastatic Lung Cancer
Treat primary cancer ± radiation for pain or surgery if locally aggressive
Whole-body CT/PET/MRI
CT chest, abdomen, and pelvis for staging
Chemotherapy ± stem cell transplant; see plasma cell dyscrasias in Hematology-Oncology, pp. 125–127
Treat primary cancer ± radiation for pain or surgery if locally aggressive

Footnotes

1. Lytic lesion: Area of bone destruction, often described as "punched out."
2. Codman's triangle: Raised edge of ossified periosteum usually due to underlying tumor.
3. Sunburst: Concentric layers of reactive bone.
4. Blastic lesion: Pathologic deposition of new bone.
5. Rouleaux formation: Aggregation ≥4 RBCs similar to a stack of coins in the presence of ↑ serum proteins.

FIGURE 16.7

16-7 Adult Bone Lesions

MULTIPLE MYELOMA

A 65-year-old African-American M with unremarkable PMH presents with 5 weeks of back pain, fatigue, and weight loss. **Exam** shows diffuse vertebral tenderness. **Labs** show elevated ESR, hypercalcemia, elevated creatinine, and normocytic anemia. Blood smear shows RBCs in rouleaux formation. Protein electrophoresis reveals an M-spike. On **imaging**, spine XR shows lytic lesions.

Management:

1. Bone marrow biopsy confirms; >10% clonal plasma cells.
2. Stage with whole-body CT, PET/CT, or MRI.
3. Chemotherapy ± bisphosphonates.
4. Possible hematopoietic stem cell transplant.
5. Infection prophylaxis (eg, 13-valent pneumococcal vaccine).
6. Long-term maintenance therapy.

Complications:

- Renal insufficiency (nephrotic syndrome ± ATN).
- Vulnerable to encapsulated bacteria (esp. *S. pneumoniae*).
- Priapism.
- Pathologic fractures.
- Spinal cord compression.
- Hypercalcemia resulting in pathologic calcification, depression, and constipation.

HYF: Look for hypercalcemia, lytic lesions, and M-spike.

PAGET'S DISEASE OF BONE

A 65-year-old M with PMH of hearing loss presents for his annual physical. On **exam**, he has frontal bossing. **Labs** show elevated ALP and procollagen with normal calcium and phosphorus. On **imaging**, XR shows mixed lytic and blastic lesions.

Management:

1. Stage with whole-body bone radionucleotide scan.
2. Follow up with plain film imaging of areas of increased uptake.
3. Long-term bisphosphonates if symptomatic.

Complications: Hearing loss. Increased risk of osteosarcoma. Bowing deformities of long bone. Early arthritis. Pathologic fractures, osteoarthritis. Spinal stenosis ± radiculopathy.

HYF: Look for absence of systemic symptoms, frontal bossing, hearing loss, and increase in hat size.

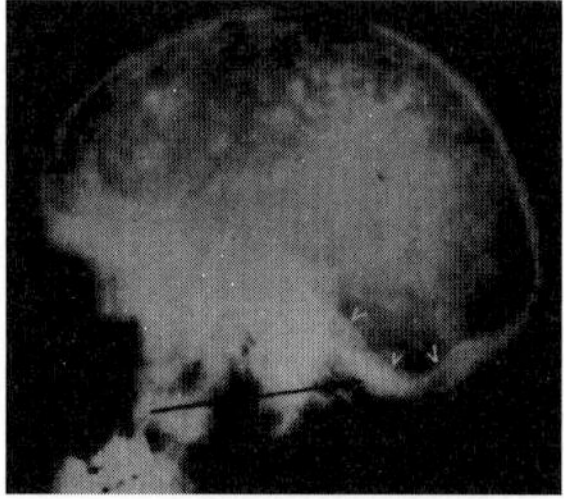

Skull with "cotton wool" areas of fluffy sclerosis and skull base thickening (arrowheads) in a patient with Paget's disease of bone.

NON-SMALL CELL LUNG CANCER METASTASES

A 65-year-old F with PMH of HTN, DM2, and 30-pack-year smoking history presents with progressively worsening back pain for 5 weeks, worse at night and unrelieved with rest. Her **exam** reveals focal vertebral tenderness at T10. **Labs** show hypercalcemia. On **imaging**, spine XR suggests lytic lesions at T9 and T10.

Management:

1. MRI spine (more sensitive than XR).
2. CT chest, abdomen, and pelvis with contrast to assess for primary tumor and metastases.
3. Stage with FDG-PET/CT.
4. Biopsy most accessible lesion.
5. Bisphosphonates for hypercalcemia.
6. Radiation ± surgical resection.

Complications:

- Pathologic fractures.
- Radiculopathy.
- Spinal cord compression.
- Neurologic dysfunction.

HYF: Only lytic lesions are seen with this diagnosis. Patients will usually have hypercalcemia.

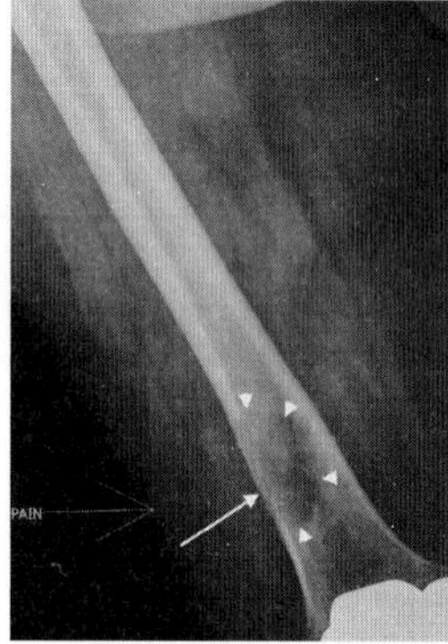

Lucent lytic lesion (arrowheads) in distal femoral diaphysis with adjacent cortical thinning (arrow).

PROSTATE CANCER METASTASES

A 65-year-old M with PMH of prostate cancer s/p prostatectomy presents with progressively worsening "aching" back pain ×8 weeks, worse at night and unrelieved with rest. **Exam** reveals focal vertebral tenderness at T10. **Labs** show elevated ALP. On **imaging**, spine XR suggests blastic lesions at T9 and T10.

Management:

1. MRI spine (more sensitive than XR).
2. Whole-body bone scan for additional mets.
3. Biopsy usually unnecessary if known cancer dx.
4. PSA.
5. Treat primary cancer.
6. Radiation ± surgical resection.

16-7 Adult Bone Lesions

Complications:

- Radiculopathy.
- Spinal cord compression.
- Neurologic dysfunction.

HYF: Present with blastic lesions only. Patients have elevated ALP.

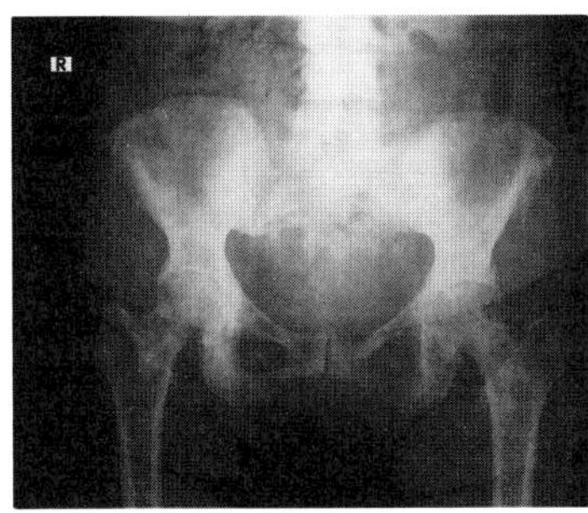

Extensive sclerotic (osteoblastic) metastases in lower lumbar spine, pelvis, and bilateral femurs.

BREAST CANCER METASTASES

A 65-year-old F with PMH of breast cancer s/p lumpectomy and radiation presents with progressively worsening back pain ×5 weeks, worse at night and unrelieved with rest. **Exam** reveals focal vertebral tenderness at T10. **Labs** show hypercalcemia. Spine XR suggests mixed lytic/blastic lesions at T9 and T10.

Management:

1. MRI spine (more sensitive than XR).
2. Whole-body bone scan.
3. Biopsy usually unnecessary if known prior cancer diagnosis.
4. Treat primary cancer.
5. Bisphosphonates.
6. Radiation ± surgical resection.

Complications:

- Pathologic fractures.
- Radiculopathy.
- Spinal cord compression.
- Neurologic dysfunction.

HYF: Mixed lytic/blastic lesions.

OSTEOSARCOMA

A 65-year-old Caucasian M with PMH of Paget's disease presents with 3 months of progressively worsening lower pack and hip pain. On **exam**, there is a large, tender mass in one of his legs. **Labs** show elevated ALP, ESR, and LDH. On **imaging**, pelvic XR shows a sunburst pattern with Codman's triangle.

Management:

1. MRI to evaluate extent of lesion.
2. Biopsy.
3. Stage with CT chest and bone scan vs. PET/CT.
4. Neoadjuvant chemotherapy.
5. Surgical resection.
6. Adjuvant chemotherapy.

Complications: In older adults, osteosarcoma is often "secondary" in the setting of prior causes of bone distortion (eg, Paget's disease), and patients have complications related to the primary process. If secondary, patients have poor prognosis.

HYF: Associated with sunburst periosteal reaction, history of Paget's disease, and radiation exposure.

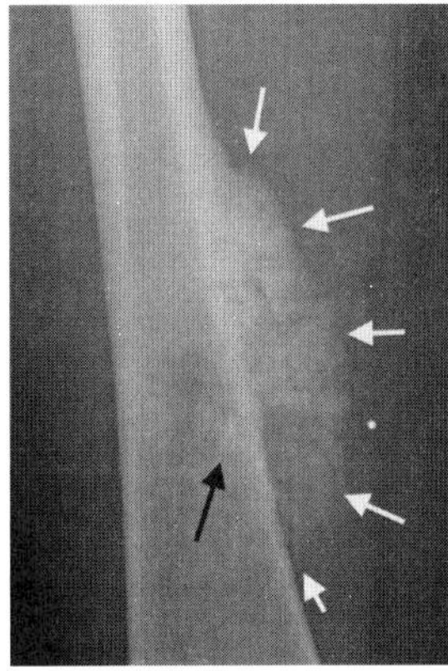

Osteoid matrix (black arrow) and "sunburst" soft tissue ossifications (white arrows).

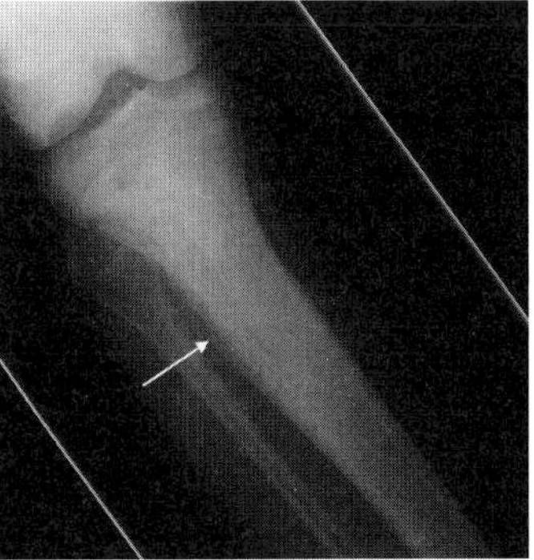

Codman's triangle periosteal reaction seen in various bone lesions, including osteosarcoma (most common) and Ewing's sarcoma.

16-8 Neurovascular Injuries

UPPER EXTREMITY

Brachial Plexus Injuries

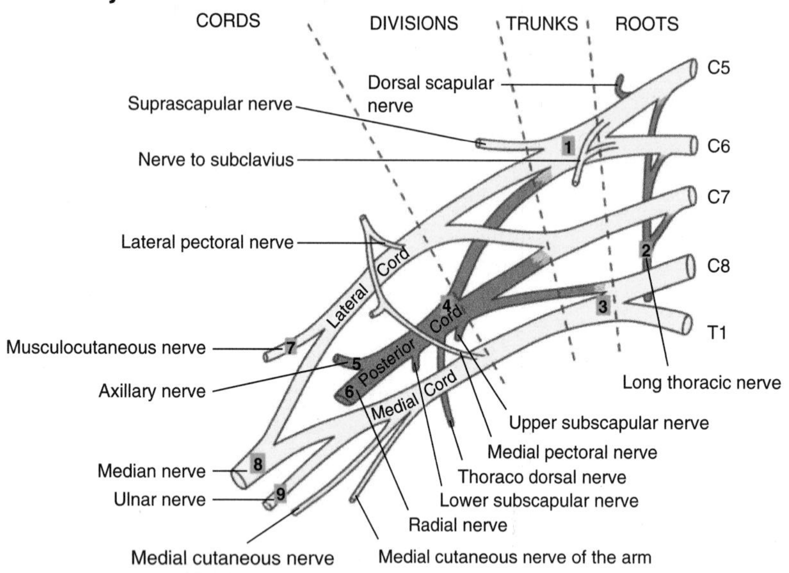
CORDS
DIVISIONS
TRUNKS
ROOTS
C5
C6
C7
C8
T1
Dorsal scapular nerve
Suprascapular nerve
Nerve to subclavius
Lateral pectoral nerve
Lateral Cord
Posterior Cord
Medial Cord
Musculocutaneous nerve
Axillary nerve
Median nerve
Ulnar nerve
Medial cutaneous nerve of the forearm
Medial cutaneous nerve of the arm
Radial nerve
Lower subscapular nerve
Thoraco dorsal nerve
Medial pectoral nerve
Upper subscapular nerve
Long thoracic nerve
1
2
3
4
5
6
7
8
9

1. Erb Palsy.
2. Winged Scapula.
3. Klumpke Palsy.
4. Wrist Drop.
5. Deltoid Paralysis.
6. Wrist Drop.
7. Weakness of elbow flexion, bicep atrophy.
8. Benediction sign, difficulty flexing thumb.
9. Claw hand, decreased grip strength.

Brachial Plexus Injuries

Syndrome	Presentation	Injury	Causes	
Erb Palsy	Arm is adducted, internally rotated and pronated at elbow ("Waiter's tip")	Upper trunk injury C5—Axillary, suprascapular, musculocutaneous C6—Radial	Lateral traction in infants during delivery, or fall onto shoulder in adults	Reproduced with permission from Socolovsky M, Costales JR, et al, Obstetric brachial plexus palsy: reviewing the literature comparing the results of primary versus secondary surgery. Childs Nerv Syst. 32(3): 415-425; 2016, Springer Nature.
Winged Scapula	Elevation and medial protrusion of inferomedial scapula, difficulty abducting arm	Long thoracic nerve injury, C5-C7 causing deficit in serratus anterior	Traction injury or direct nerve damage (radical mastectomy, chest tube placement, blunt trauma)	
Klumpke Palsy	Hyperextended MCP joints, flexed IP joints, weakness of intrinsic hand muscles ("Claw Hand")	Lower trunk injury C8—Ulnar wrist and finger flexors T1—Intrinsic Hand muscles	Traction on an abducted arm (arm presentation in delivery, trauma in adults)	

Upper Extremity Mononeuropathies

Nerve	Nerve Roots	Innervation	Presentation
Suprascapular nerve	C5-C6	Motor: Supraspinatus (upper arm abduction [15–30°]), infraspinatus (upper arm adduction) Sensory: glenohumeral joint, acromioclavicular joint	Dull, posterolateral shoulder pain. Weakness of shoulder abduction and external rotation. Frequently from repeated overhead motion or trauma to the shoulder.
Axillary	C5-C6	Motor: Deltoid (shoulder abduction) Sensory: Lateral shoulder	Commonly presents as weakness on shoulder abduction ± loss of sensation of the lateral shoulder. Seen in glenohumeral joint dislocation, proximal humerus fracture or trauma to deltoid muscle.
Musculocutaneous	C5-T1	Motor: Biceps (elbow flexion, forearm supination) Sensory: Anterolateral forearm	Presents as weakness and atrophy of the bicep, paresthesias or decreased sensation of the anterolateral forearm Rarely seen in isolation. Can be caused by weightlifting, shoulder dislocation or surgery.

16-8 Neurovascular Injuries

Upper Extremity Mononeuropathies (Continued)

Nerve	Nerve Roots	Innervation	Presentation
Radial	C5-T1	Motor: Brachioradialis (elbow flexion of half-pronated forearm), triceps (elbow extension), extensor carpi radialis (wrist extension) Sensory: Lower lateral cutaneous (lateral arm below deltoid), posterior cutaneous arm and forearm, superficial (dorsal surface of lateral 3 ½ fingers and associated dorsum of hand)	Radial neuropathy at the spiral groove ("Saturday night palsy"): Wrist drop with sparing of triceps (elbow extension; loss of finger and thumb extensors; sensory loss in wrist (radial region). Classically precipitated by sleeping on an arm after drinking alcohol.
Posterior interosseous branch of radial nerve	C6-C8	Motor: Supinator (forearm supination), extensor carpi ulnaris (wrist extension), finger extensors Sensory: No cutaneous innervation	Posterior interosseous nerve (PIN) syndrome is a compressive neuropathy. Often presents with insidious onset forearm/wrist pain and weakness on wrist and finger metacarpal extension. More common in manual laborers and with repeated pronation and supination, space occupying lesions, and trauma.
Median	C5-T1	Motor: Pronator teres (forearm pronation), flexor carpi radialis (wrist flexion), finger flexors at the PIP joint, abductor pollicis brevis (thumb abduction), opponens pollicis (thumb to 5th finger), lumbricals 1 and 2 (flexion of index and middle fingers at MCP) Sensory: Palmar cutaneous (lateral palm), palmar digital cutaneous (anterior surface and fingertips of lateral 3 ½ digits)	Carpal tunnel syndrome: Compressive neuropathy at the wrist. Sensory loss in thumb, 2nd, and 3rd fingers; weakness in thenar muscles; positive Tinel sign and Phalen test. Most common neuropathy. Caused by repetitive motion, inflamed synovium, or space occupying lesions. Pronator syndrome: Compressive neuropathy at the elbow. Differentiate from carpal tunnel syndrome by involvement of palmar cutaneous branch and proximal forearm pain.
Ulnar	C5-T1	Motor: Flexor carpi ulnaris (wrist flexion), flexor digitorum profundus 3 and 4 (flexion of 4th and 5th fingers at DIP joint), adductor pollicis (thumb adduction), dorsal interossei (finger abduction), palmar interossei (finger adduction), opponens digiti minimi (5th finger to thumb), lumbricals 3 and 4 (flexion of 4th and 5th fingers at MCP) Sensory: Palmar cutaneous (medial half of palm), dorsal cutaneous (dorsal surface of medial 1 ½ fingers and associated dorsal hand), superficial branch (palmar surface of medial 1 ½ fingers)	Ulnar nerve entrapment (UNE) at cubital fossa (elbow): Sensory loss in the little finger and ulnar half of 4th finger, weakness of the thumb adductor and interossei; claw hand. Frequently due to compression or traction at the elbow. UNE at Guyon's canal (wrist): Similar to UNE at the elbow but sensation is spared in the dorsum of the hand and only select hand muscles are affected. Less common. Seen in cyclists (handlebar palsy), ganglion cysts, and excess traction.

LOWER EXTREMITY

Lower Extremity Mononeuropathies

Nerve	Nerve Roots	Innervation	Presentation
Iliohypogastric	T12-L1	Motor: Lower internal oblique, transversus abdominis. Sensory: Suprapubic region, lateral hip.	Presents after lower abdominal and pelvic surgeries with paresthesias at the incision site and referred pain to the suprapubic and inguinal regions.
Genitofemoral	L1-L2	Motor: Cremaster. Sensory: Labia majora or anterior scrotum, anterior and medial thigh.	↓ cremasteric reflex, sensation in the upper medial/anterior thigh (lateral femoral triangle) after abdominal laparoscopic surgery.
Lateral femoral cutaneous	L2-L3	Motor: None. Sensory: Anterior and lateral thigh.	*Meralgia paresthetica*: Paresthesias on the anterior and lateral thigh due to pelvic surgery or compression at the level of the inguinal ligament (eg, increased intraabdominal pressure in the setting of ascites or obesity, external compression from tight clothes).

(Continued)

16-8 Neurovascular Injuries

LOWER EXTREMITY

Lower Extremity Mononeuropathies (Continued)

Nerve	Nerve Roots	Innervation	Presentation
Femoral	L2-L4	Motor: Iliopsoas, pectineus, rectus femoris, and sartorius (hip flexion); quadriceps (knee extension, patellar reflex). Sensory: Anterior and medial thigh.	↓ leg extension and patellar reflex due to pelvic, abdominal, or spinal surgery; femoral line placement; pelvic fracture; diabetic lumbosacral plexopathy; or aortic or iliac aneurysms. Patients can also present with pain in the inguinal region that relieves with external rotation and flexion of the hip. A lesion of the saphenous nerve (pure sensory branch of the femoral nerve that arises in the femoral triangle and innervates the skin of the medial leg) can cause paresthesias in the medial knee, calf, and foot.
Obturator	L2-L4	Motor: Adductor longus, adductor brevis, gracilis, pectineus, adductor magnus, obturator externus, gracilis, pectineus (thigh adduction). Sensory: Medial thigh.	↓ thigh adduction and medial thigh sensation due to pelvic surgery or pelvic fracture.
Superior gluteal	L4-S1	Motor: Gluteus medius and gluteus minimus (thigh/hip abduction), tensor fascia latae. Sensory: None.	Trendelenburg gait: Lateral pelvic drop because the weight-bearing leg cannot maintain pelvic alignment through hip abduction. The lesion is contralateral to the side that drops. Often due to iatrogenic injury (eg, IM injection to the superomedial gluteal region).
Common peroneal fibular) ("Up and Out")	L4-S2	Superficial peroneal nerve: -Motor: Peroneus longus and brevis (foot eversion). -Sensory: Lateral lower leg, dorsum of the foot and toes except skin between the 1st and 2nd toes. Deep peroneal nerve: -Motor: Tibialis anterior (foot dorsiflexion), extensor hallucis longus and brevis (toe extension), extensor digitorum longus and brevis (toe extension). -Sensory: Skin between the 1st and 2nd toes ("flip flop zone").	Foot drop: loss of dorsiflexion and eversion, steppage gait. Loss of sensation on the dorsum of the foot and toes. Common peroneal nerve injury commonly presents after fibular neck fracture, trauma to the lateral leg, or compression (eg, sitting cross-legged, tight cast). Superficial peroneal nerve injury can present after ankle injury.
Sciatic	L4-S3	Motor: Hamstrings (knee flexion), adductor magnus (hip adduction). Sensory: Lower leg and foot.	Deficits of the common peroneal and tibial nerves. Often presents in the context of posterior hip dislocation, total hip arthroplasty, or herniated disc.
Tibial ("Down and In")	L4-S3	Motor: Gastrocnemius/soleus (foot plantar flexion, ankle reflex), tibialis posterior (foot inversion), flexor digitorum longus and brevis (toe flexion), flexor hallucis longus and brevis (toe flexion) Sensory: Plantar surface of the foot.	Loss of inversion, plantar flexion, ability to stand on or curl toes. Loss of sensation on the sole of the foot. Often occurs in the setting of knee trauma, Baker's cyst (proximal lesion), or tarsal tunnel syndrome (distal lesion due to involvement of the posterior tibial nerve).
Sural	L4-S3	Motor: None. Sensory: Posterior and lateral lower leg, lateral foot, heel.	Sensory nerve that can be injured after Achilles tendon rupture.
Inferior gluteal	L5-S2	Motor: Gluteus maximus (thigh/hip extension). Sensory: None.	Loss of hip extension leading to backward lurching gait ("gluteus maximus lurch"), forward pelvic tilt, and difficulty rising from chairs and climbing stairs. Often due to posterior hip dislocation.
Pudendal	S2-S4	Motor: External urethral sphincter, anal sphincter. Sensory: Perineum.	↓ sensation in the perineum and genitals, which can lead to incontinence. Often due to surgical procedures, childbirth, trauma, or certain repetitive activities (eg, squatting, cycling). During childbirth, a nerve block can be performed using the ischial spine as a landmark for anesthetic injection.

16-8 Neurovascular Injuries

Radiculopathies[a]

Nerve Roots	Reflex	Sensory	Motor	Pain Distribution
C5	Biceps	Lateral deltoid	Rhomboids[b] (elbow extends backward with hand on hip) Infraspinatus[b] (arm rotates externally with elbow flexed at the side) Deltoid[b] (arm raised laterally 30–45° from the side)	Lateral arm, medial scapula
C6	Biceps	Thumb/index finger Dorsal hand/lateral forearm	Biceps[b] (arm flexed at the elbow in supination) Pronator teres (forearm pronated)	Lateral forearm, thumb/index fingers
C7	Triceps	Middle fingers Dorsal forearm	Triceps[b] (forearm extension, flexed at elbow) Wrist/finger extensors[b]	Posterior arm, dorsal forearm, dorsal hand
C8	Finger flexors	Palmar surface of little finger Medial hand and forearm	1st dorsal interosseous (abduction of index finger). Abductor digiti minimi (abduction of little finger)	Fourth and fifth fingers, medial hand and forearm
T1	Finger flexors	Axilla and medial arm	Abductor pollicis brevis (abduction of thumb). 1st dorsal interosseous (abduction of index finger). Abductor digiti minimi (abduction of little finger)	Medial arm, axilla
L2	—	Upper anterior thigh	Psoas (hip flexors)	Anterior thigh
L3	—	Lower anterior thigh and knee	Psoas (hip flexors), Quadriceps (knee extensors)[b] Thigh adductors	Anterior thigh, knee
L4	Quadriceps (knee)	Medial calf	Quadriceps[b] (knee extensors) Thigh adductors	Anterolateral thigh
L5	—	Lateral thigh, lateral calf, dorsum of foot	Peronei[b] (foot evertors), Tibialis anterior (foot dorsiflexors), Gluteus medius (hip abductors). Toe dorsiflexors	Lateral calf, dorsal foot, posterolateral thigh, buttocks
S1	Gastrocnemius/soleus (ankle)	Plantar and lateral aspect of foot, fourth + fifth toes	Gastrocnemius/soleus (foot plantar flexors)[b], Abductor hallucis (toe flexors)[b], Gluteus maximus (hip extensors)	Bottom foot, posterior calf, posterior thigh, buttocks

[a]Disc herniation is a common cause of radiculopathies; the affected nerve is usually *below* the level of herniation (eg, disc herniation at level L3-L4 affects the L4 nerve root).
[b]These muscles receive the majority of innervation from this root.

Nerve and Artery Pairings[a]

Extremity	Location	Nerve	Artery
Upper extremity	Axilla	Long thoracic	Lateral thoracic
	Humerus (surgical neck)	Axillary	Posterior circumflex
	Humerus (midshaft)	Radial	Deep brachial
	Humerus (distal) Cubital fossa	Median	Brachial
Lower extremity	Popliteal fossa	Tibial	Popliteal
	Medial malleolus	Tibial	Posterior tibial

[a]Most nerve and artery pairings have the same name based on anatomical location. Exceptions are noted in this table.

16-8 Neurovascular Injuries

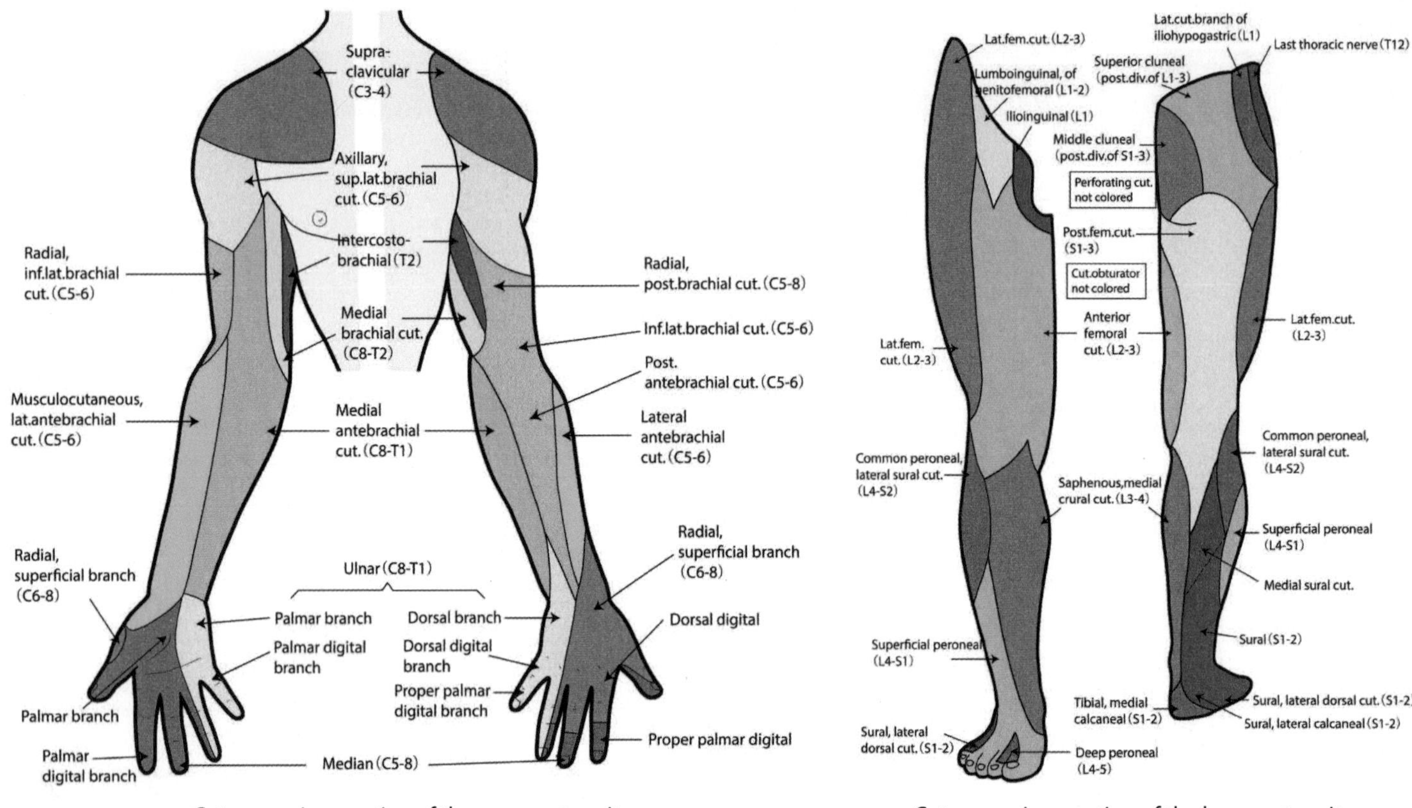
Supra-
clavicular
(C3-4)
Axillary,
sup.lat.brachial
cut. (C5-6)
Intercosto-
brachial (T2)
Radial,
inf.lat.brachial
cut. (C5-6)
Radial,
post.brachial cut. (C5-8)
Medial
brachial cut.
(C8-T2)
Inf.lat.brachial cut. (C5-6)
Post.
antebrachial cut. (C5-6)
Musculocutaneous,
lat.antebrachial
cut. (C5-6)
Medial
antebrachial
cut. (C8-T1)
Lateral
antebrachial
cut. (C5-6)
Radial,
superficial branch
(C6-8)
Ulnar (C8-T1)
Radial,
superficial branch
(C6-8)
Palmar branch
Dorsal branch
Dorsal digital
Palmar digital
branch
Dorsal digital
branch
Proper palmar
digital branch
Palmar branch
Proper palmar digital
Palmar
digital branch
Median (C5-8)
Lat.fem.cut. (L2-3)
Lat.cut.branch of
iliohypogastric (L1)
Last thoracic nerve (T12)
Lumboinguinal, of
genitofemoral (L1-2)
Superior cluneal
(post.div.of L1-3)
Ilioinguinal (L1)
Middle cluneal
(post.div.of S1-3)
Perforating cut.
not colored
Post.fem.cut.
(S1-3)
Cut.obturator
not colored
Anterior
femoral
cut. (L2-3)
Lat.fem.
cut. (L2-3)
Lat.fem.cut.
(L2-3)
Common peroneal,
lateral sural cut.
(L4-S2)
Saphenous,medial
crural cut. (L3-4)
Common peroneal,
lateral sural cut.
(L4-S2)
Superficial peroneal
(L4-S1)
Medial sural cut.
Superficial peroneal
(L4-S1)
Sural (S1-2)
Tibial, medial
calcaneal (S1-2)
Sural, lateral dorsal cut. (S1-2)
Sural, lateral calcaneal (S1-2)
Sural, lateral
dorsal cut. (S1-2)
Deep peroneal
(L4-5)

Cutaneous innervation of the upper extremity.

Cutaneous innervation of the lower extremity.

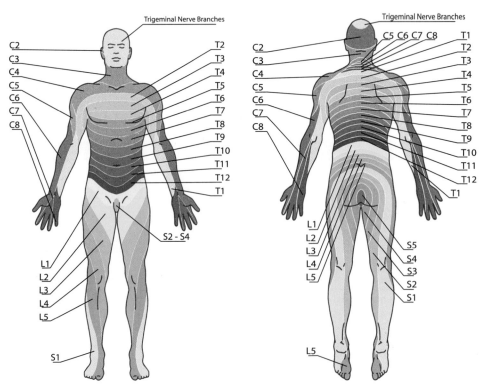

Dermatomes (anterior and posterior views).

17
Surgery: Neurosurgery

17-1 Spinal Disorders

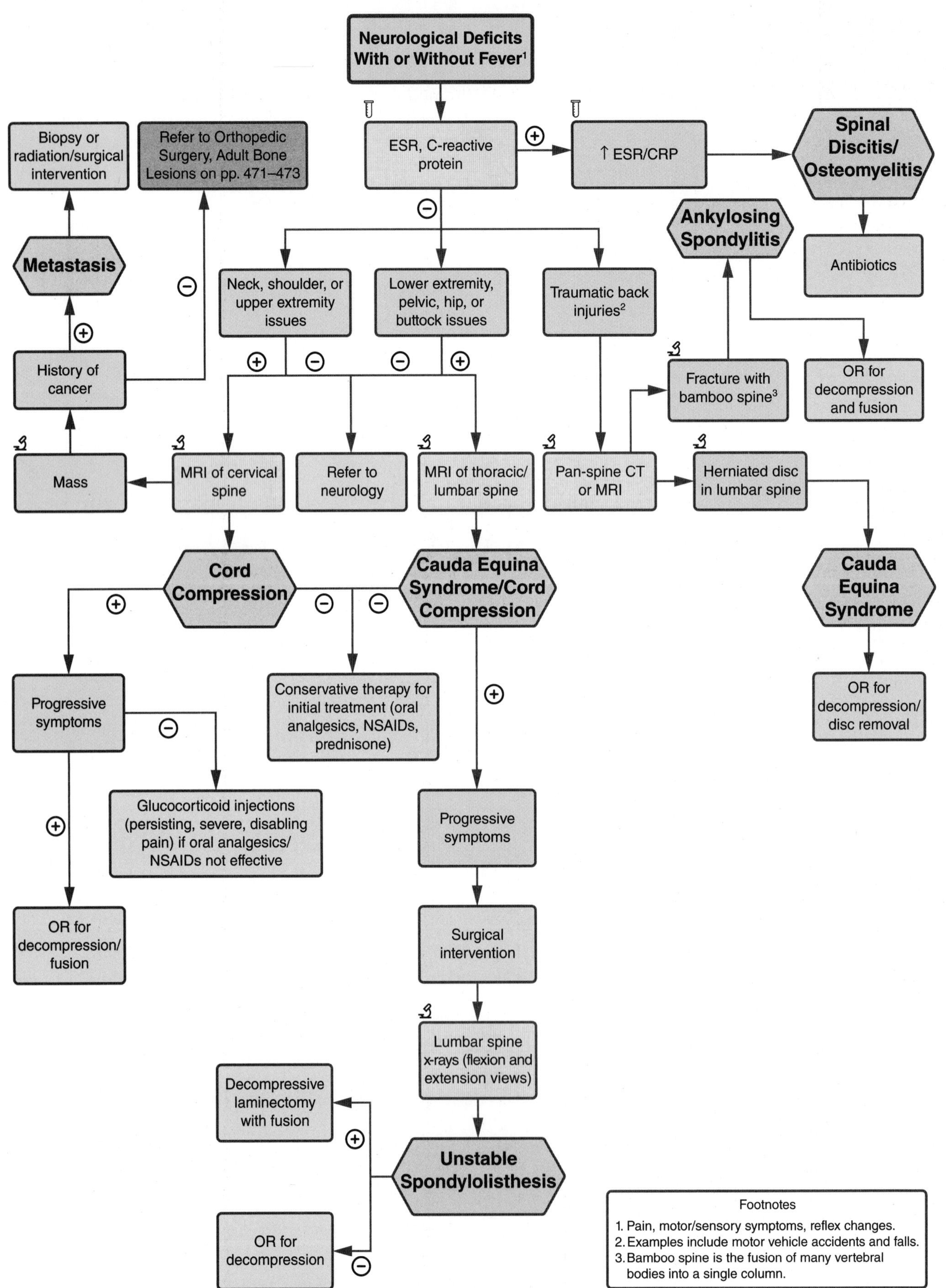
Neurological Deficits With or Without Fever[1]
ESR, C-reactive protein
↑ ESR/CRP
Spinal Discitis/ Osteomyelitis
Antibiotics
Ankylosing Spondylitis
Biopsy or radiation/surgical intervention
Refer to Orthopedic Surgery, Adult Bone Lesions on pp. 471–473
Metastasis
History of cancer
Mass
Neck, shoulder, or upper extremity issues
Lower extremity, pelvic, hip, or buttock issues
Traumatic back injuries[2]
Fracture with bamboo spine[3]
OR for decompression and fusion
MRI of cervical spine
Refer to neurology
MRI of thoracic/ lumbar spine
Pan-spine CT or MRI
Herniated disc in lumbar spine
Cord Compression
Cauda Equina Syndrome/Cord Compression
Cauda Equina Syndrome
Progressive symptoms
Conservative therapy for initial treatment (oral analgesics, NSAIDs, prednisone)
OR for decompression/ disc removal
Glucocorticoid injections (persisting, severe, disabling pain) if oral analgesics/ NSAIDs not effective
Progressive symptoms
OR for decompression/ fusion
Surgical intervention
Lumbar spine x-rays (flexion and extension views)
Decompressive laminectomy with fusion
Unstable Spondylolisthesis
OR for decompression
Footnotes
1. Pain, motor/sensory symptoms, reflex changes.
2. Examples include motor vehicle accidents and falls.
3. Bamboo spine is the fusion of many vertebral bodies into a single column.

FIGURE 17.1

17-1 Spinal Disorders

SPINAL DISCITIS/OSTEOMYELITIS

A 55-year-old M with PMH of poorly controlled DM2 presents with fevers, weakness, and severe back pain. On **exam**, he has decreased reflexes. **Labs** show an increased WBC of 17.

Management:

1. ESR/CRP.
2. MRI spine with and without contrast at affected area; ± CT of that area to assess for endplate erosion.
3. Blood cultures. If negative, may require biopsy with cultures → give appropriate antibiotics based on cultures.
4. Observation.
5. OR for decompression if neurologic deficits from epidural abscess.

Complications:

- Increased systemic infection.
- Sepsis.
- Epidural abscess/phlegmon.
- Weakness/numbness.
- Loss of bowel/bladder function.

HYF: Elevated ESR/CRP with negative imaging with contrast-enhancing disc space is highly suggestive of discitis/osteomyelitis. Clinically, patients have such extreme back pain that movement is limited. Surgery is recommended if epidural abscess is present, regardless of symptoms, in the cervical or thoracic spine. Cultures are needed for diagnosis.

METASTATIC MALIGNANCY

A 60-year-old F with extensive smoking history presents with neck and shoulder pain on the right side with associated weight loss. On **exam**, she has no neurologic deficits but does have dyspnea.

Management:

1. MRI spine with and without contrast in area corresponding to neurologic deficit.
2. CT CAP for metastatic workup.
3. Biopsy of spinal lesion if no other accessible lesion (eg, lung mass).
4. Depending on symptoms and biopsy results, either observe or resect.
5. If resection is too dangerous or not possible, consider radiotherapy.

Complications:

- Progressive and irreversible numbness/weakness.
- Increased bladder/bowel dysfunction.
- Intractable, unremitting back pain.
- Gait dysfunction.
- Compression fractures from loss of vertebral body structure.

HYF: Patients with neurological symptoms, associated significant back pain, and constitutional symptoms should raise suspicion for metastatic spinal disease. Any intervention must be considered in the context of their overall functional status and prognosis. Circumferential decompression with stabilization is the standard of care when there is cord compression or impending cord compression. Isolated vertebral body lesions can be treated with radiotherapy depending on the pathology. Renal cell metastases often require preoperative embolization to prevent massive hemorrhage in surgery.

ANKYLOSING SPONDYLITIS

A 53-year-old F with PMH of lower back pain presents with a fall off a ladder while doing garden work yesterday. On **exam**, she has increasing weakness in her lower extremities and difficulty walking. On **imaging**, CT of the thoracic spine shows fused vertebral bodies without clear fracture.

Management:

1. MRI imaging of target area (eg, thoracic spine).
2. If fracture, stabilize injury with surgical intervention (fusion).
3. If no fracture, bracing is appropriate.
4. Work-up for ankylosing spondylitis with appropriate rheumatologic panel and rheumatology consult.

Complications:

- Increased cord compression.
- Worsening neurological deficits.
- Increased pain.
- Bowel/bladder dysfunction.
- Permanent gait instability.
- Paraplegia.

HYF: When a patient presents without clear fracture, fused vertebral bodies across disc spaces, and progressive neurologic decline, a disc-space fracture in the context of ankylosing spondylitis is the first thought. These are inherently unstable fractures. They require urgent-to-emergent stabilization to prevent further neurologic deterioration. HLA-B27 is the associated genetic abnormality.

CAUDA EQUINA SYNDROME

A 65-year-old M with PMH of underlying spinal stenosis presents with extreme back pain, progressive insidious-onset urinary retention, and weakness. Post-void residual is >300, and he does not have a history of benign prostatic hyperplasia. On **exam**, he is diffusely weak bilaterally from his knees downward with associated numbness. Rectal tone is diminished.

Management:

1. MRI lumbar and thoracic spine without contrast.
2. Surgical intervention emergently if symptom onset is <24 hours and acute; chronic cases can be addressed urgently.

Complications:

- Progressive and irreversible numbness/weakness.
- Increased bladder/bowel dysfunction.
- Intractable, unremitting back pain.
- Gait dysfunction.

(Continued)

17-1 Spinal Disorders

HYF: Trauma is not a prerequisite for this condition. It can occur acutely or chronically. Acute cases often result from a large lumbar disc herniation, whereas chronic cases are often the result of a broad minor-to-moderate disc herniation in the context of spinal stenosis. Back pain is common with symmetric bilateral neurological deficits. Whenever symmetric deficits are identified in the legs, thoracic spine imaging is also required because cord compression from a thoracic disc can also be the cause.

CERVICAL SPINE DISC HERNIATION

A 32-year-old M with no significant PMH presents with progressively worsening pain radiating down his left since a car crash 2 weeks ago. On **exam**, he has weakness in his hand grip and wrist extension. **Imaging** shows a C6 herniated disc.

Management:

1. MRI of cervical spine without contrast, cervical myelogram.
2. Conservative treatment (physical therapy, NSAIDs, observation) if the patient only has radicular pain without motor or sensory deficits.
3. Surgical intervention if evidence of myelopathy (T2 signal in spinal cord, hyperreflexia, difficulty walking) or motor/sensory deficits.

Complications:

- Worsening neurological deficits.
- Worsening pain.
- Progressive spinal cord compression.
- Lhermitte phenomenon: Shock-like paraesthesia with neck flexion, muscular atrophy in hands and neck.

HYF: Neurological symptoms (motor, sensory, reflex changes) with specifically neck, shoulder, and upper extremity issues should clue you into a cervical disc disorder, especially after trauma. If conservative treatments do not work, then surgical options are needed. If an MRI reveals a herniated disc, obtain a CT to look for ossification of the disc. Additionally, look on myelogram for foraminal compression and soft tissue injuries. With imaging, especially cervical XR, get flexion and extension views to see degree of spondylolisthesis.

LUMBAR SPINE DISC HERNIATION

A 65-year-old M with PMH of degenerative disc disease presents with increased weakness in his right leg with a foot drop for the past 3 days. On **exam**, he has weakness with dorsiflexion in his right leg with associated radiating pain down the side of his leg into his medial ankle.

Management:

1. MRI of lumbar spine without contrast.
2. XR lumbar spine with flexion and extension views if spondylolisthesis is present.
3. Conservative treatment if pain is the only symptom: Pain control, steroids, physical therapy.
4. Surgical intervention if the patient has pain and other neurological symptoms (gain instability, increased sensory or motor loss, etc.) or failed conservative management.

Complications:

- Worsening neurological deficits (sensory and motor) to the point of paralysis of specific motor groups.
- Paresthesia that can progress to anesthesia.
- Worsening pain.
- Bowel/bladder dysfunction.
- Gait instability.

HYF: Chronic unilateral symptoms with radicular pain should suggest a lumbar disc herniation in an older patient with underlying degenerative disc disease. There is often accompanying spinal stenosis. In younger patients, this problem often presents acutely with excruciating pain. Pain not responsive to conservative measures, even in the absence of neurologic deficits, can be an indication for surgery. Additionally, it is important to characterize the degree of spondylolisthesis in these patients to see if more involved surgical treatment such as fusion is required.

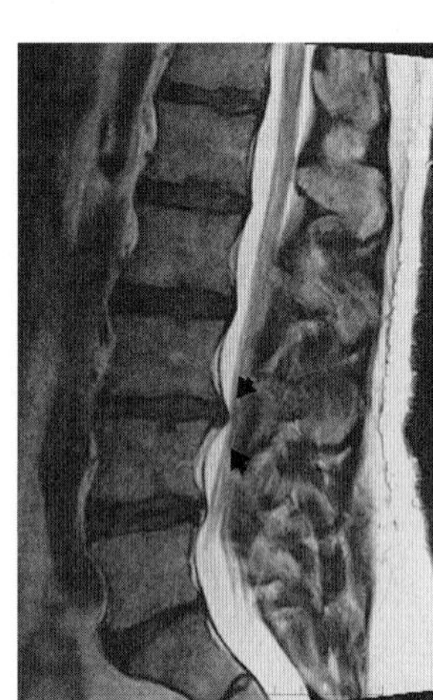

Lumbar disc herniation.

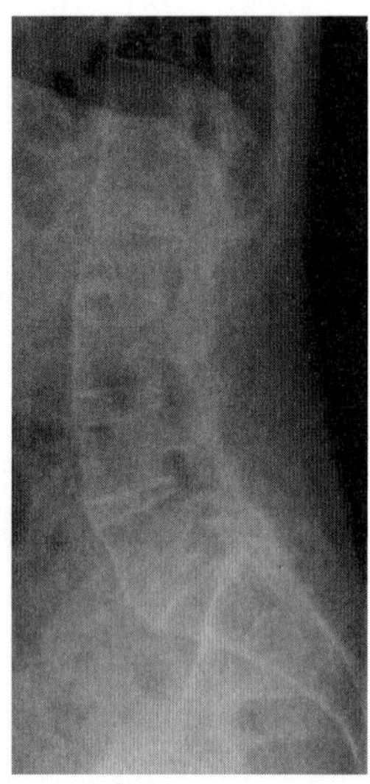

Ankylosing spondylosis.

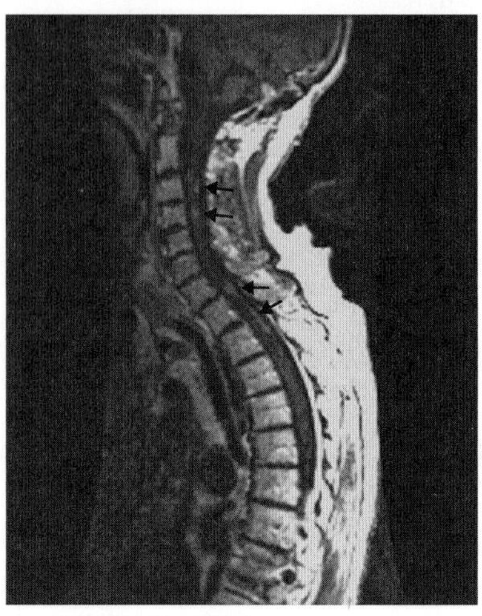

Leptomeningeal metastases.

17-2 Intracranial Hemorrhage

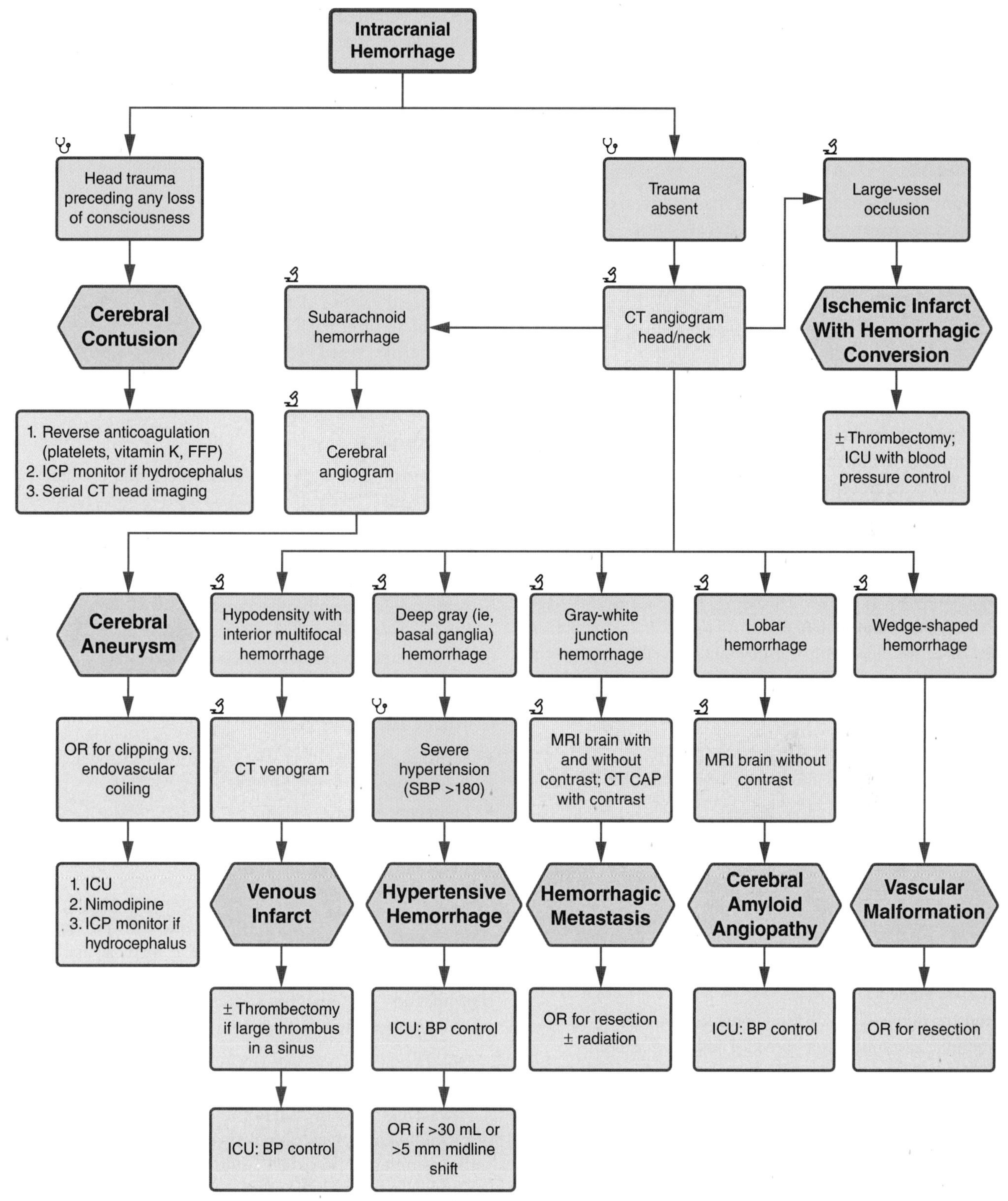
Intracranial Hemorrhage
Head trauma preceding any loss of consciousness
Trauma absent
Large-vessel occlusion
Cerebral Contusion
Subarachnoid hemorrhage
CT angiogram head/neck
Ischemic Infarct With Hemorrhagic Conversion
1. Reverse anticoagulation (platelets, vitamin K, FFP)
2. ICP monitor if hydrocephalus
3. Serial CT head imaging
Cerebral angiogram
± Thrombectomy; ICU with blood pressure control
Cerebral Aneurysm
Hypodensity with interior multifocal hemorrhage
Deep gray (ie, basal ganglia) hemorrhage
Gray-white junction hemorrhage
Lobar hemorrhage
Wedge-shaped hemorrhage
OR for clipping vs. endovascular coiling
CT venogram
Severe hypertension (SBP >180)
MRI brain with and without contrast; CT CAP with contrast
MRI brain without contrast
1. ICU
2. Nimodipine
3. ICP monitor if hydrocephalus
Venous Infarct
Hypertensive Hemorrhage
Hemorrhagic Metastasis
Cerebral Amyloid Angiopathy
Vascular Malformation
± Thrombectomy if large thrombus in a sinus
ICU: BP control
OR for resection ± radiation
ICU: BP control
OR for resection
ICU: BP control
OR if >30 mL or >5 mm midline shift

FIGURE 17.2

17-2 Intracranial Hemorrhage

CEREBRAL CONTUSION

A 54-year-old M with PMH of COPD presents with a bruise on the side of his head after a car accident. He had loss of consciousness in the field. On **exam**, he has a scalp hematoma but no focal neurologic deficits.

Management:

1. Reverse any anticoagulation therapy (vitamin K and plasma infusion, factor replacement, platelet transfusion).
2. Head CT for hemorrhage confirmation.
3. Monitor ICP with mannitol or hypertonic saline (to lower ICP) if GCS ≤8.
4. 24-hour inpatient observation is recommended.

Complications:

- Seizures.
- Mass effect from cerebral edema if a large contusion.
- Intraventricular hemorrhage (IVH).
- Post-traumatic hydrocephalus.

HYF: Occurs after head trauma with or without open lacerations. On imaging, CT angiogram of the head can visualize active bleeding, but this is rare in a contusion. Often, this study is not obtained unless the contusion is rapidly expanding. Reverse any anticoagulation therapy and monitor ICP with mannitol if the patient is obtunded. If active bleed, you will potentially need to evacuate a hematoma via surgery. Look for classic signs of head trauma: Lacerations, vomiting, loss of consciousness, neurological deterioration.

ANEURYSMAL SUBARACHNOID HEMORRHAGE

A 65-year-old M with PMH of tobacco use and HTN presents with sudden-onset headache ("worst headache of his life") with acute loss of consciousness. On **exam**, he has neck pain, neck stiffness, and vomiting.

Management:

1. ICP monitoring with external ventricular drain with Hunt-Hess grade >3.
2. Monitoring in the ICU with blood pressure control.
3. Nimodipine administration to reduce risk of vasospasm.
4. ESR/CRP/WBC with vitals evaluation (in the context of history of IVDU) to rule out mycotic aneurysm.
5. Craniotomy for clipping or endovascular coiling/stenting.

Complications:

- Vasospasm.
- Seizures.
- Post-hemorrhagic hydrocephalus.
- Rebleeding.
- SIADH vs. cerebral salt wasting.
- Neurogenic cardiac abnormalities.

HYF: "Worst headache of the patient's life" or thunderclap, 10/10 headache is a classic clinical presentation. Generally, this is the result of a ruptured saccular or "berry" aneurysm located in the proximal anterior or posterior circulation (like the circle of Willis). A CT angiogram of the head is an initial study required to identify the location of the aneurysm. A diagnostic cerebral angiogram is then often the next step. Depending on the aneurysm morphology, endovascular securing of the aneurysm may be pursued. Otherwise, if unfavorable morphology is encountered, a craniotomy for clipping is recommended. Medical management with antivasospasm agents such as nimodipine is always used.

VENOUS INFARCT

A 65-year-old F with PMH of HTN and visual disturbance presents with focal seizure, papilledema, and loss of consciousness. On **exam**, she has visual field deficits, bitemporal headaches, and hypertension (155/100). **Imaging** shows a hypodense infarct with multifocal hemorrhage.

Management:

1. CT venogram of the head to confirm cerebral venous thrombosis.
2. Consider thrombectomy if there is a large thrombus in a sinus.
3. BP and ICP should be monitored for brain swelling if low GCS.
4. Monitor for seizures.
5. Anticoagulation with subcutaneous low-molecular-weight heparin (LMWH) or heparin drip.
6. Do not surgically resect venous infarction. Decompressive surgery may be required for large infarctions with malignant edema.

Complications:

- Seizures.
- Rebleeding.
- Malignant edema.

HYF: Look out for headaches, papilledema, visual loss, focal/generalized seizures, and loss of consciousness. Main treatments include reversing any underlying causes, controlling symptoms (headaches, seizures), and antithrombotic therapy. Endovascular/surgical intervention may be required if medical management is not sufficient. These thromboses can occur in the context of adjacent infection. Treatment is addressing the underlying infection, NOT anticoagulation.

HYPERTENSIVE HEMORRHAGE

A 75-year-old M with PMH of uncontrolled HTN presents after being found down. On **exam**, BP is 198/110. He is not responsive to verbal commands, flaccid on 1 side to noxious stimulus, and localizes and withdraws on the other.

Management:

1. CT head shows basal ganglia, pontine, thalamic, or cerebellar hemorrhage.
2. BP control in ICU; ICP monitoring if obtunded ± intraventricular hemorrhage.
3. Surgical intervention if significant midline shift.
4. Reverse all anticoagulants and antiplatelet drugs.

17-2 Intracranial Hemorrhage

5. Serial CTs of the head to confirm stability.
6. CT angiogram of the head to identify underlying vascular abnormality.
7. MRI in a delayed fashion to rule out metastasis or primary brain tumor.

Complications:

- Additional bleeding and permanent brain damage.
- Seizures, coma, death.
- Vascular remodeling if left untreated.

HYF: In the absence of trauma, one of the main causes of ICH is severe hypertension. Here, vessel rupture is in the deep gray structures such as the putamen, thalamus, pons, midbrain, and caudate. Medical management involves the reversal of all antiplatelet and anticoagulant medications and BP control.

CEREBRAL AMYLOID ANGIOPATHY

A 65-year-old M with no prior PMH presents with loss of consciousness. On **exam**, he has normal BP. **Imaging** shows multiple lobar/cortical/subcortical hemorrhages.

Management:

1. Admit to ICU for management of BP.
2. Immunosuppressive therapy (methylprednisolone).
3. CT angiogram of the head to rule out vascular cause.
4. MRI for evaluation of underlying causes.
5. Serial CTs of the head for monitoring hemorrhages.
6. Avoid anticoagulants and antiplatelets. Reverse if needed.

Complications:

- Permanent brain damage.
- Malignant edema requiring decompressive surgery.
- Future lobar hemorrhages.
- Seizures.

HYF: Patients are often asymptomatic but have a spontaneous lobar hemorrhage. Generally, patients are age >65. Pathology is used to confirm a diagnosis of cerebral amyloid angiopathy. On MRI, there will be multiple lobar/cortical/subcortical hemorrhages, and, on exam, patients generally do not have hypertension. There is ultimately no good treatment to prevent progression of CAA or hemorrhage risk.

VASCULAR MALFORMATION

A 48-year-old F non-smoker with no prior PMH presents with loss of consciousness. She had a seizure last night. On **exam**, she has normal blood pressure. **Imaging** shows lobar ICH with vascular malformations.

Management:

1. CTA/MRA.
2. All AVMs need to be assessed via the Spetzler-Martin grading scale for medical management vs. surgical intervention.
3. ICP monitoring if accompanying intraventricular hemorrhage and obtundation.
4. Ruptured AVMs should be treated acutely (including those patients with prior ruptured AVMs).
5. Unruptured AVMs may be managed with surgery, endovascular embolization, or radiation therapy depending on the location, size, and venous drainage pattern.
6. Surgical intervention involves surgical excision, embolization, or a combination thereof.

Complications:

- Seizures.
- Rebleeding.
- Permanent brain damage with neurologic impairment.
- Intraventricular hemorrhage (IVH).
- Malignant edema.
- SIADH vs. cerebral salt wasting.

HYF: The patients are generally age <65, female, and non-smokers with no prior history of hypertension who present with lobar ICH. The hemorrhage typically has a "flame" pattern that appears like a wedge traveling to the cortex. Patients will need to be assessed using the Spetzler-Martin grading scale, which uses demographics and clinical and prior medical history data to help determine whether medical vs. surgical management is preferred. Surgical management consists of surgical resection of the AVM, embolization, or radiosurgery. There are 2 big peaks of potential AVM rupture, one in childhood (age <18) and one between the ages of 30 and 50.

Ischemic Infarct: See pp. 492–493, 727–729, 731–732.

17-3 Intracranial Tumors

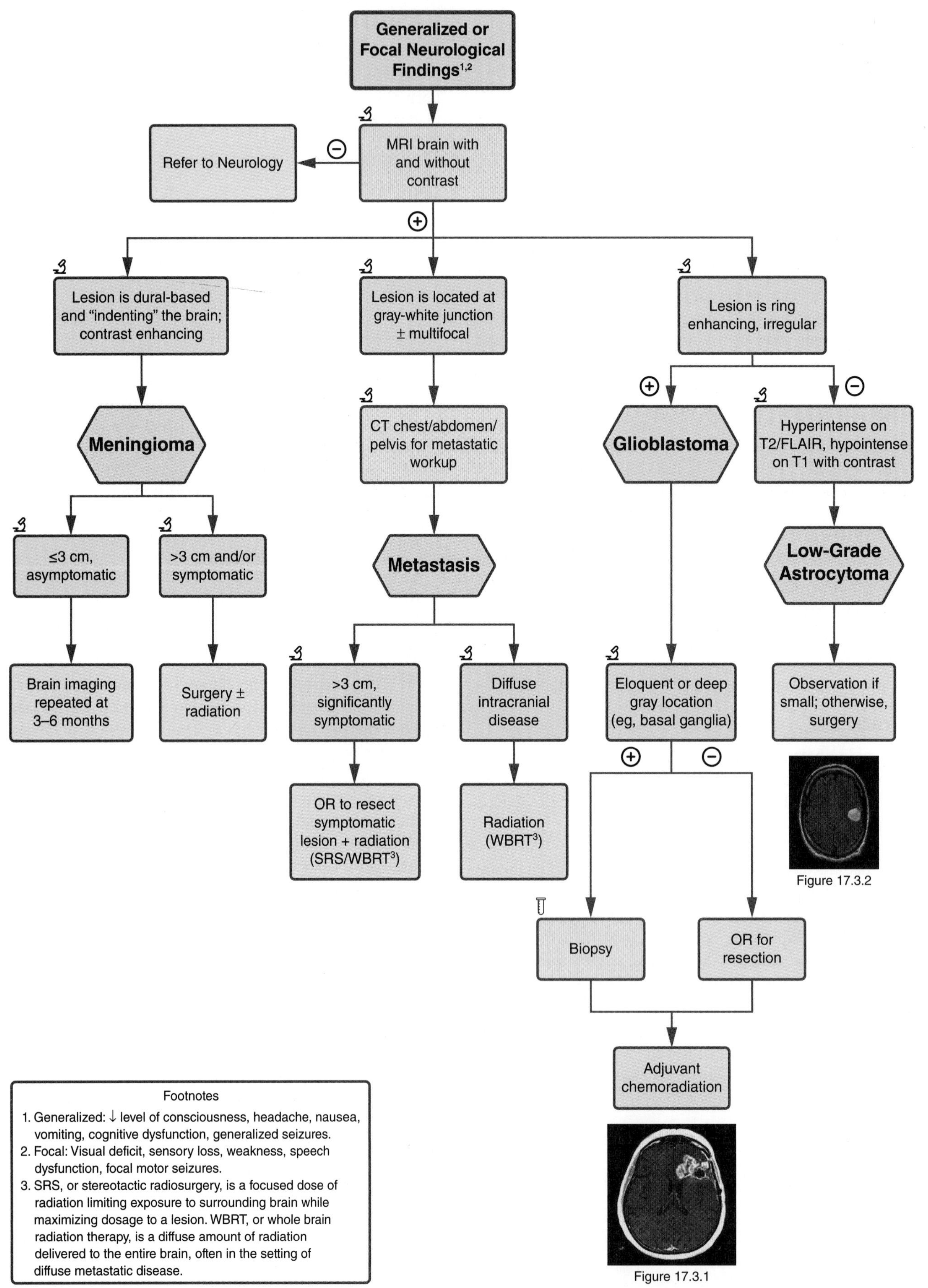

Generalized or Focal Neurological Findings[1,2]
MRI brain with and without contrast
Refer to Neurology
Lesion is dural-based and "indenting" the brain; contrast enhancing
Lesion is located at gray-white junction ± multifocal
Lesion is ring enhancing, irregular
Meningioma
CT chest/abdomen/pelvis for metastatic workup
Glioblastoma
Hyperintense on T2/FLAIR, hypointense on T1 with contrast
≤3 cm, asymptomatic
>3 cm and/or symptomatic
Metastasis
Low-Grade Astrocytoma
Brain imaging repeated at 3–6 months
Surgery ± radiation
>3 cm, significantly symptomatic
Diffuse intracranial disease
Eloquent or deep gray location (eg, basal ganglia)
Observation if small; otherwise, surgery
OR to resect symptomatic lesion + radiation (SRS/WBRT[3])
Radiation (WBRT[3])
Figure 17.3.2
Biopsy
OR for resection
Adjuvant chemoradiation
Figure 17.3.1

Footnotes

1. Generalized: ↓ level of consciousness, headache, nausea, vomiting, cognitive dysfunction, generalized seizures.
2. Focal: Visual deficit, sensory loss, weakness, speech dysfunction, focal motor seizures.
3. SRS, or stereotactic radiosurgery, is a focused dose of radiation limiting exposure to surrounding brain while maximizing dosage to a lesion. WBRT, or whole brain radiation therapy, is a diffuse amount of radiation delivered to the entire brain, often in the setting of diffuse metastatic disease.

FIGURE 17.3

17-3 Intracranial Tumors

MENINGIOMA

A 65-year-old F with PMH of NF2 presents with progressive visual changes and dull headaches upon waking up for the past few months. She denies any recent head trauma; alcohol, tobacco, or drug use; or recent changes in her diet. On **imaging**, head CT shows a well-defined mass that is displacing normal brain tissue. On brain MRI, there is a dural-based contrast-enhancing lesion.

Management:

1. <3 cm and asymptomatic: Observe and repeat imaging every 3–6 months.
2. >3 cm and symptomatic: Surgical resection ± radiation.

Complications:

- Sensory/motor deficits.
- Personality change/memory decline.
- Seizures.
- Cerebral edema, deep vein thrombosis.
- Obstructive hydrocephalus (if in ventricles).

HYF: Head CT usually shows a bright white, extra-axial lesion (hyperdense) indenting the brain itself. Common locations include within the skull, falx cerebri, tentorium cerebelli, and venous sinuses. Calcifications can be seen. The underlying skull can be thick. MRI will show a homogeneously enhancing lesion with the brain deforming around it. Meningiomas may be asymptomatic, so it is important to consider how the patient is doing prior to planning treatments.

METASTASIS

A 58-year-old M with PMH of lung cancer presents with new complaints of headache, memory decline, and a recent seizure. On **imaging** with MRI brain with contrast, there are multiple (8), well-circumscribed lesions with large amounts of vasogenic edema located near the junctions of the gray-white matter.

Management:

1. Biopsy if no previous cancer diagnosis and/or no additional lesion accessible elsewhere in the body.
2. CT of the chest/abdomen/pelvis for workup or repeat staging.
3. If diffuse lesions throughout the brain, consider focal radiation (SRS) vs. general radiation (WBRT).
4. Surgical resection is recommended if there is a solitary lesion >3 cm or if the lesion is symptomatic with significant edema.
5. CNS-penetrating chemotherapy.
6. Steroids for edema.

Complications:

- Cognitive decline.
- Sensory/motor deficits.
- Seizures.
- Cerebral edema.
- Hemorrhage.
- Leptomeningeal disease.
- Imbalance and gait difficulty.
- Hydrocephalus (if periventricular).

HYF: Rounded, well-circumscribed masses that contrast-enhance and are located at the junction of gray-white matter are typical for metastases. In a person with a history of cancer or additional lesions on body imaging, an intracranial metastasis is likely. WBRT has significant neurocognitive sequelae. Patients may have headaches, focal neurological dysfunctions, seizures, or even strokes. It is important to know the diagnosis of the metastasis via a biopsy, plus the number and sizes of all other metastases, prior to making a plan.

HIGH-GRADE GLIOMA (GLIOBLASTOMA)

An 85-year-old M with recent headaches, visual disturbances, and personality changes presents with a seizure. He states that these neurological deficits have been progressive over the past few weeks. He has no cancer history or signs of infection. On **imaging**, MRI shows a diffuse mass in the frontal lobe with severe edema and rim enhancement with central clearing.

Management:

1. Biopsy if in unresectable location (eg, deep gray—ie, basal ganglia).
2. Surgical resection if able.
3. Steroids for edema.
4. ± Anti-epileptic drugs if history of or suspicion for seizure.
5. Adjuvant chemoradiation.
6. If possible, enroll in clinical trials.

Complications:

- Hemorrhage.
- Sensory/motor deficits.
- Speech dysfunction.
- Cognitive decline/memory decline.
- Cerebral edema.
- Seizures.

HYF: Malignant, rapidly progressive tumors. Patients are often older at presentation, as this is the most common primary brain tumor in patients age >65. MRI will show a lesion that enhances heterogeneously after contrast. There is rim enhancement with central necrosis. Treatment should be resection if possible, with follow-up chemoradiation. If not, then biopsy with chemoradiation is the only option. Poor overall prognosis. Patients should be enrolled in clinical trials when possible, with concurrent therapy groups.

17-4 Pituitary Disorders

Pituitary adenomas may be silent (non-secreting) or hormone-producing (secreting). Most adenomas are non-secreting, and they may be clinically silent. Hormone-producing adenomas result from hyperplasia of one type of endocrine cells found in the pituitary gland. Lactotroph adenomas (prolactin, hyperprolactinemia, and infertility) > somatotrophs (growth hormone, acromegaly) > corticotrophs (ACTH, Cushing's disease). Rarely, adenomas present as gonadotrophs (FSH, LH) and thyrotrophs (TSH). Tumors can also present with symptoms of mass effect, including headache, bitemporal hemianopia due to pressure on the optic chiasm, and hypopituitarism. Below, we will cover some presentations of pituitary adenomas; other diagnoses are covered elsewhere in the book.

Summary of Pituitary Hormones

Pituitary Hormone	Cells Responsible for Synthesis	Hypothalamus: Releasing Hormones	Hypothalamus: Inhibiting Factors	Target Gland or Tissue	Function
Adrenocorticotropin hormone (ACTH)	Corticotrophs	Corticotropin-releasing hormone (CRH) Arginine vasopressin (AVP)		Adrenal	Stimulation of corticosteroids and adrenal androgens
Growth hormone (GH)	Somatotrophs	GH-releasing hormone (GHRH)	Somatostatin (somatotropin-release inhibiting hormone, SRIF)	Peripheral tissue, liver	Direct and indirect (insulin-like growth factor 1 [IGF-1]) stimulation of growth, metabolism, homeostasis
Prolactin (PRL)	Lactotrophs	Oxytocin, thyrotropin-releasing hormone (TRH)	Dopamine	Mammary gland	Stimulation of lactation
Thyrotropin or thyroid-stimulating hormone (TSH)	Thyrotrophs	TRH	Somatostatin	Thyroid	Stimulation of thyroid hormone release
Luteinizing hormone (LH)	Gonadotrophs	Gonadotropin-releasing hormone (GnRH)		Ovary, testis	Stimulation of estrogen and testosterone production
Follicle-stimulating hormone (FSH)	Gonadotrophs	GnRH		Ovary, testis	Regulation of theca and Sertoli cell function
Human chorionic gonadotropin (hCG)	Gonadotrophs	GnRH	Unknown	Unknown	Differs from placental and trophoblastic isoforms. The role of pituitary hCG is unknown—it may serve to facilitate some of the LH functions

17-4 Pituitary Disorders

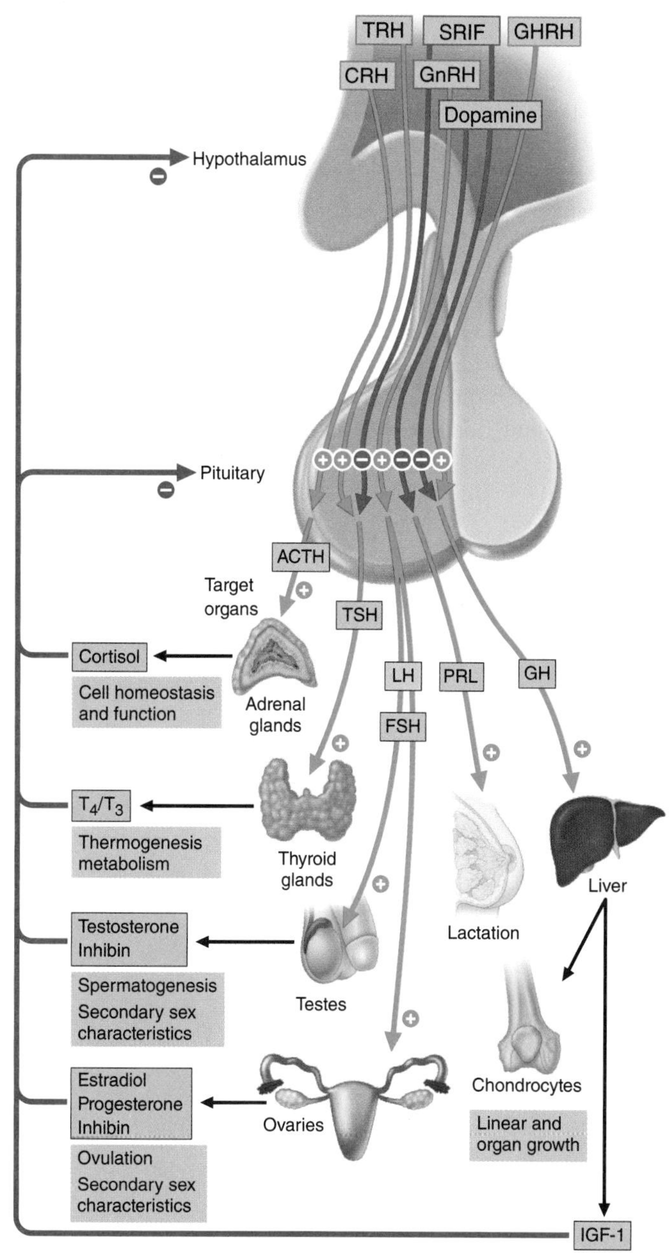
TRH
SRIF
GHRH
CRH
GnRH
Dopamine
Hypothalamus
Pituitary
ACTH
Target organs
TSH
Cortisol
Cell homeostasis and function
Adrenal glands
LH
PRL
GH
FSH
T4/T3
Thermogenesis metabolism
Thyroid glands
Liver
Testosterone Inhibin
Lactation
Spermatogenesis Secondary sex characteristics
Testes
Estradiol Progesterone Inhibin
Chondrocytes
Ovaries
Linear and organ growth
Ovulation Secondary sex characteristics
IGF-1

Diagram of pituitary axes. Hypothalamic hormones regulate anterior pituitary trophic hormones, which in turn regulate target gland secretion in feedback loops.

PROLACTINOMA

A 30-year-old F with PMH of headaches presents with amenorrhea, galactorrhea, and worsening vision for the past 3 months. She is not sexually active. **Exam** shows bilateral milky nipple discharge with no breast masses, as well as visual field deficits consistent with bitemporal hemianopsia. **Labs** are notable for negative beta-hCG, elevated serum prolactin levels >200, low LH and FSH, and normal thyroid function tests. On **imaging**, MRI of the brain reveals a calcified sellar mass.

Management:

1. 1st-line: Dopamine agonist (cabergoline, bromocriptine).
2. If refractory or patient has mass effect (eg, visual deficits), consider tumor resection with transsphenoidal pituitary surgery.

Complications:

- Mass effect.
- Visual deficits (eg, bitemporal hemianopia) due to pressure on optic chiasm.
- Pituitary apoplexy.
- Hyper- or hypopituitarism.
- Increased intracranial pressure from compression of the 3rd ventricle.

HYF: Hyperprolactinemia occurs most commonly in women due to pregnancy to support lactation. Prolactinomas (lactotroph adenomas) are another common cause of hyperprolactinemia and affect women more than men. The larger the tumor, the higher the expected prolactin level; screen patients with large pituitary adenomas for hyperprolactinemia. Elevated prolactin causes amenorrhea, galactorrhea, infertility due to anovulation from low LH and FSH, decreased bone mass in women, and impotence and infertility in men. Associated with multiple endocrine neoplasia (MEN) type 1.

HYPOPITUITARISM

A 55-year-old M with PMH of headaches presents with concerns about erectile dysfunction and low libido. He reports decreased interest in sexual activity, lower energy, constipation, cold intolerance, weight gain particularly in the belly, and vision changes. On **exam**, BP is 95/55, and he has central obesity with numerous violaceous striae, visual field deficits consistent with bitemporal hemianopsia, cold and dry skin, hyporeflexia, and normal genitourinary exam. **Labs** show low testosterone, cortisol, GH, FSH, LH, serum TSH, and free T4; and normal prolactin levels. On **imaging**, MRI brain shows a pituitary mass.

Management:

1. Hormone replacement therapy (eg, testosterone, thyroxine, hydrocortisone).
2. Transsphenoidal pituitary surgery for tumor resection.

Complications:

- Mass effect.
- Visual deficits (eg, bitemporal hemianopia) due to pressure on optic chiasm.
- Pituitary apoplexy.
- Increased intracranial pressure from compression of the 3rd ventricle.

HYF: Hypopituitarism is characterized by insufficient production of several pituitary hormones, leading to secondary hypogonadism, secondary hypothyroidism, secondary hypoadrenalism, growth hormone deficiency, and/or central diabetes insipidus. A common cause is a non-secreting pituitary adenoma (as seen in this patient). Hypopituitarism can also result from traumatic brain injury, Sheehan syndrome (postpartum bleeding leading to infarct of the pituitary gland), empty sella syndrome (gland atrophy or compression, usually idiopathic and seen in women with obesity), pituitary apoplexy (usually due to hemorrhage from fragile blood vessels supplying an existing pituitary adenoma), or craniopharyngioma (usually in children or the elderly).

(Continued)

17-4 Pituitary Disorders

ACROMEGALY

A 39-year-old with PMH of OSA, type 2 diabetes, HTN, and carpal tunnel syndrome presents with arthralgias, enlarging hands and feet, and headache. **Exam** shows coarse facial features with prominent jaw and forehead and bitemporal hemianopsia. **Labs** show elevated IGF-1 levels. Oral glucose tolerance test does not suppress growth hormone levels. On **imaging**, brain MRI shows a pituitary adenoma.

Management:

1. Surgical resection of tumor
2. Medical therapy if not a surgical candidate with somatostatin analogues (eg, octreotide), growth hormone (GH) receptor antagonist (eg, pegvisomant), or dopamine agonist (cabergoline).

Complications:

- Headache, visual field defects, and cranial nerve defects from mass effect of tumor.
- Carpal tunnel syndrome.
- Visceral organ enlargement (eg, tongue, thyroid).
- Concentric myocardial hypertrophy.
- Colorectal polyps and cancer.
- Diabetes mellitus due to effect of growth hormone on insulin receptors.
- Hypertension.
- Hypopituitarism (if pituitary mass grows).

HYF: Caused by excessive GH secretion, usually by a pituitary somatotroph adenoma → increased IGF-1 secretion. Leading cause of death is cardiovascular disease (concentric hypertrophy, heart failure, arrhythmias). If the epiphyses have not yet closed (ie, during childhood), patients present with gigantism rather than acromegaly.

17-5 Vascular Occlusive Diseases

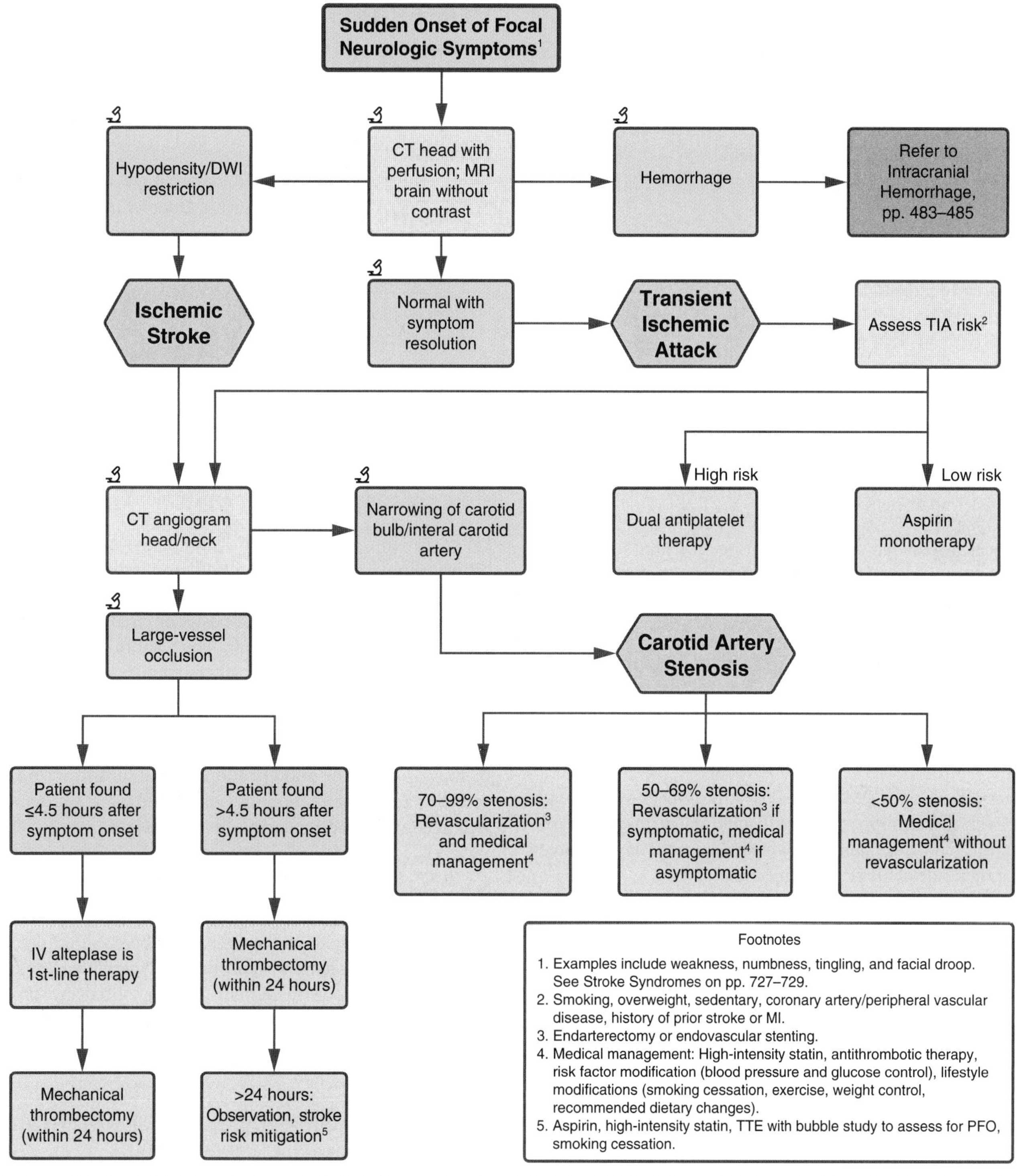
Sudden Onset of Focal Neurologic Symptoms[1]
CT head with perfusion; MRI brain without contrast
Hypodensity/DWI restriction
Hemorrhage
Refer to Intracranial Hemorrhage, pp. 483–485
Normal with symptom resolution
Ischemic Stroke
Transient Ischemic Attack
Assess TIA risk[2]
High risk
Low risk
CT angiogram head/neck
Narrowing of carotid bulb/interal carotid artery
Dual antiplatelet therapy
Aspirin monotherapy
Large-vessel occlusion
Carotid Artery Stenosis
Patient found ≤4.5 hours after symptom onset
Patient found >4.5 hours after symptom onset
70–99% stenosis: Revascularization[3] and medical management[4]
50–69% stenosis: Revascularization[3] if symptomatic, medical management[4] if asymptomatic
<50% stenosis: Medical management[4] without revascularization
IV alteplase is 1st-line therapy
Mechanical thrombectomy (within 24 hours)
Mechanical thrombectomy (within 24 hours)
>24 hours: Observation, stroke risk mitigation[5]
Footnotes
1. Examples include weakness, numbness, tingling, and facial droop. See Stroke Syndromes on pp. 727–729.
2. Smoking, overweight, sedentary, coronary artery/peripheral vascular disease, history of prior stroke or MI.
3. Endarterectomy or endovascular stenting.
4. Medical management: High-intensity statin, antithrombotic therapy, risk factor modification (blood pressure and glucose control), lifestyle modifications (smoking cessation, exercise, weight control, recommended dietary changes).
5. Aspirin, high-intensity statin, TTE with bubble study to assess for PFO, smoking cessation.

FIGURE 17.5

17-5 Vascular Occlusive Diseases

TRANSIENT ISCHEMIC ATTACK (TIA)

A 55-year-old M with PMH of HTN presents with sudden onset of focal neurologic deficits, which his wife says lasted about 12 hours. On **exam**, he has aphasia and transient vision loss. On **imaging**, non-contrast head CT shows a hyperdense infarct. Later, his symptoms self-resolve within 24 hours of onset.

Management:

1. Assess risk for TIA (high vs. low risk).
2. Head imaging (non-contrast CT/brain MRI).
3. High risk = dual antiplatelet therapy; low risk = aspirin monotherapy.
4. Use the ABCDD score to assess high risk; NIHSS score for low risk.

Complications:

- Larger strokes, repeat TIAs.
- Permanent damage to brain regions.
- Cognitive impairment.

HYF: Focal neurologic symptoms lasting <24 hours are classic for a TIA. Assess the risk for stroke and then start dual antiplatelet therapy. CT angiogram of the head will show absent occlusive thrombus but may identify significant atherosclerotic disease or sub-occlusive thrombus, which should raise suspicion for microemboli causing TIA. After a TIA, secondary prevention is key (eg, BP control, statins).

ISCHEMIC STROKE

A 65-year-old M with PMH of HTN and 20-pack-year smoker presents with facial droop, speech difficulty, and right-sided weakness lasting 2 days. On **exam**, he has significant aphasia, inability to move the right side of his face, and memory issues.

Management:

1. Head imaging (non-contrast head CT/brain MRI), cardiac studies for localizing stroke origin.
2. CT angiogram head for identification of thrombus.
3. If found within 4.5 hours, intravenous alteplase. If found within 24 hours, mechanical thrombectomy.
4. Stroke rehabilitation is key for post-stroke care.
5. Secondary prevention with statins and antiplatelet agents.

Complications:

- Larger or repeat strokes.
- Permanent damage to brain regions.
- Hemorrhagic conversion.

HYF: Always assess risk for stroke and get head imaging (non-contrast head CT to rule out hemorrhage), then start on therapy: IV alteplase (within 4.5 hours) or mechanical thrombectomy (within 24 hours). CT perfusion studies can help guide therapy by showing at-risk territories that have not yet fully infarcted. Secondary prevention and post-stroke care (including stroke rehabilitation) are important.

VERTEBRAL/CAROTID ARTERY STENOSIS

A 75-year-old M with PMH of atherosclerosis and HTN presents with dizziness and sensory loss on the right side. On **exam**, he has increased sensory loss as well as weakness on the right side.

Management:

1. Ischemic stroke workup and management, as discussed above.
2. CTA/MRA head/neck or carotid Doppler ultrasound to assess for presence of stenosis and degree of stenosis.
3. 70–99% stenosis: Asymptomatic or symptomatic ≥ revascularization. 50–69% stenosis: Symptomatic ≥ revascularization; asymptomatic ≥ medical management. <50% stenosis = no revascularization, only medical management.

Complications:

- Progressive deficits vs. accruement of deficits.
- Brain stem symptoms such as intermittent or progressive dysphagia, speech difficulty, drooling, vertigo, diplopia, etc.
- Ischemic infarction from hypoperfusion or thrombotic events.

HYF: Patients with high cholesterol, hypertension, and smoking history should raise concern for atherosclerotic disease. This will lead to stenosis, predominantly in the common or internal carotid arteries, but can be seen in the posterior circulation such as vertebral arteries as well. Additionally, you want to get CTA/MRA head and neck or carotid Doppler ultrasound to assess the degree of vessel occlusion. Revascularization, when indicated, can be done endovascularly with stenting or open with endarterectomy. Medical management includes high-intensity statin, antithrombotic therapy, risk factor modification (blood pressure and glucose control), and lifestyle modifications (smoking cessation, exercise, weight control, recommended dietary changes).

CLASSIC TRIGEMINAL NEURALGIA

A 54-year-old F presents to her primary care physician after 2 weeks of intense, shock-like pain in the right side of her face. She describes the episodes as seconds long; however, they are typically back-to-back with as many as 10 episodes in an hour. She has noticed any stimuli (light and hard touch or pressure) to the middle of her face will elicit pain. She reports history of migraines, which are managed by sumatriptan.

Management:

1. For continued pain relief, prescribe oxcarbazepine (300 mg BID) or carbamazepine (100–200 mg BID).
2. If no relief from pharmacological treatment, consider microvascular decompression, partial rhizotomy sparing V1, or gamma-knife radiosurgery (GKS), depending on size and location of lesion.

Complications:

- Tiredness and sleepiness reported from oxcarbazepine and carbamazepine use.
- Risk for infection and stroke or hemorrhage from microvascular decompression and rhizotomy procedures.
- Risk of losing corneal reflex and facial numbness from GKS.

17-5 Vascular Occlusive Diseases

HYF:

- When treating trigeminal neuralgia, 1st-line pharmacological treatment is oxcarbazepine, then carbamazepine. (Put the **OX** before the **CART**.)
- Classic trigeminal neuralgia presents with vascular compression and morphological changes at the root, characterized by electric/shock-like pain.
- Classic trigeminal neuralgia affects women more than men. Previous medical history often includes migraines.

SECONDARY TRIGEMINAL NEURALGIA

A 33-year-old F presents to her neurologist for a routine visit concerning her multiple sclerosis. During the visit, she reports sharp, stabbing pain on the left side of her face. The pain does not last longer than a second or two; however, it has started to increase in frequency over the past 2 weeks.

Management:

1. Given her medical history of multiple sclerosis, her trigeminal neuralgia is likely due to a MS plaque at the CN V entry zone. This is also common in patients with a history of cerebellopontine angle lesions. Oxcarbazepine or carbamazepine is unlikely to provide pain relief.
2. Recommend microvascular decompression, GKS, or percutaneous ganglion lesioning depending on previous medical history.

Complications:

- Risk of stroke, hemorrhage, and infection associated with microvascular decompression and percutaneous ganglion lesioning.
- Risk of hearing loss associated with GKS.

HYF:

- Multiple sclerosis and cerebellopontine lesions are commonly associated with secondary trigeminal neuralgia.
- Oxcarbazepine and carbamazepine are unlikely to provide relief in secondary trigeminal neuralgia.

18
Surgery: Vascular

18-1 Aortic Disease

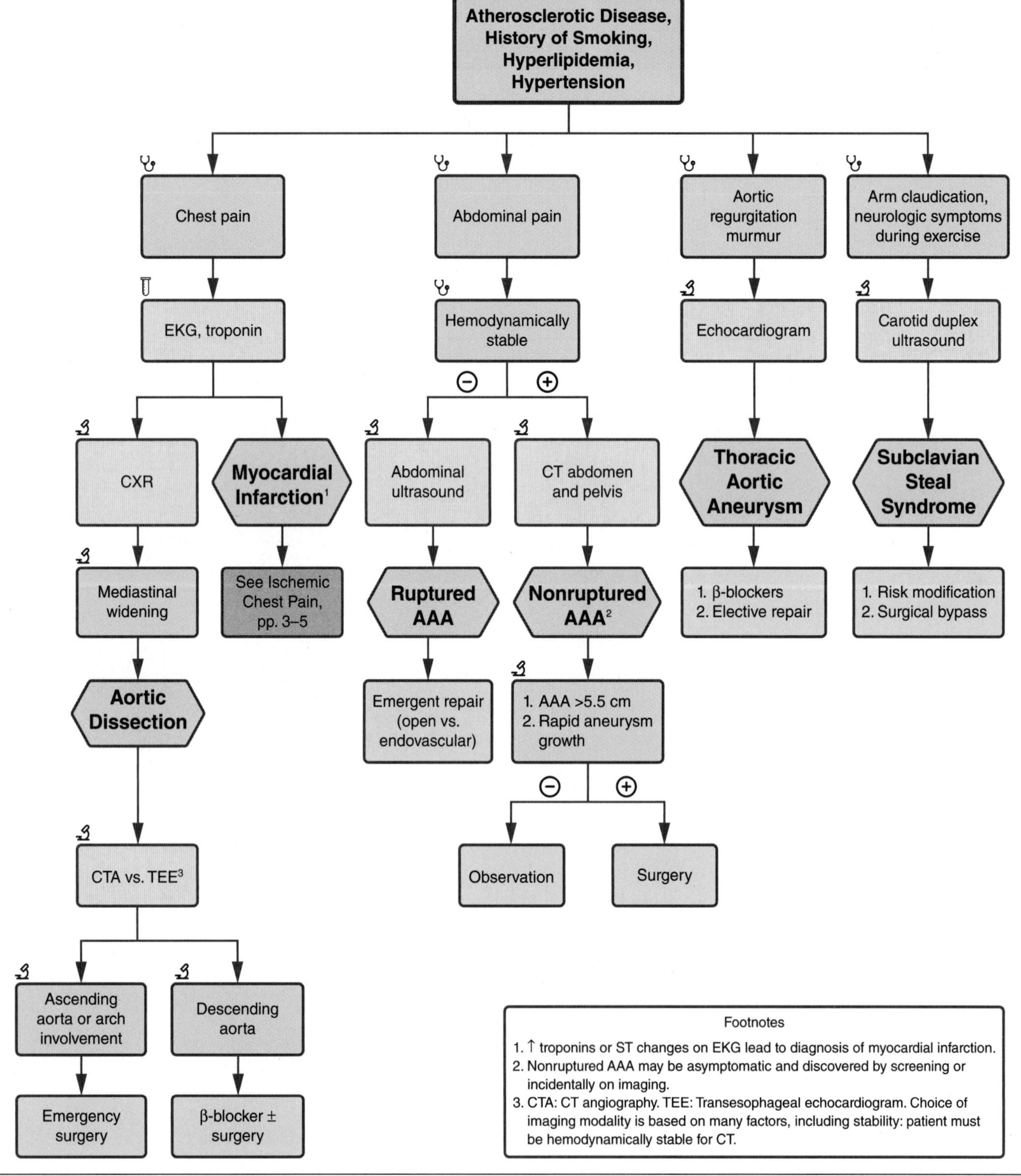
Atherosclerotic Disease, History of Smoking, Hyperlipidemia, Hypertension
Chest pain
EKG, troponin
CXR
Myocardial Infarction[1]
Mediastinal widening
See Ischemic Chest Pain, pp. 3–5
Aortic Dissection
CTA vs. TEE[3]
Ascending aorta or arch involvement
Descending aorta
Emergency surgery
β-blocker ± surgery
Abdominal pain
Hemodynamically stable
⊖
⊕
Abdominal ultrasound
CT abdomen and pelvis
Ruptured AAA
Nonruptured AAA[2]
Emergent repair (open vs. endovascular)
1. AAA >5.5 cm
2. Rapid aneurysm growth
⊖
⊕
Observation
Surgery
Aortic regurgitation murmur
Echocardiogram
Thoracic Aortic Aneurysm
1. β-blockers
2. Elective repair
Arm claudication, neurologic symptoms during exercise
Carotid duplex ultrasound
Subclavian Steal Syndrome
1. Risk modification
2. Surgical bypass
Footnotes
1. ↑ troponins or ST changes on EKG lead to diagnosis of myocardial infarction.
2. Nonruptured AAA may be asymptomatic and discovered by screening or incidentally on imaging.
3. CTA: CT angiography. TEE: Transesophageal echocardiogram. Choice of imaging modality is based on many factors, including stability: patient must be hemodynamically stable for CT.

FIGURE 18.1

18-1 Aortic Disease

AORTIC DISSECTION

A 63-year-old F with PMH of HTN presents with stabbing chest pain that radiates to the back. On exam, her BP is 20 mmHg higher in 1 arm compared to the other, and she has a diastolic decrescendo murmur. On imaging, CXR shows mediastinal widening.

Management:

1. Stanford type A – emergency surgery.
2. Stanford type B (stable) – β-blocker therapy.
3. Stanford type B (unstable) – surgery.

Complications: Dissections involving the ascending aorta can cause aortic regurgitation.

HYF: Tears involving the ascending aorta are Stanford type A; all others are type B. Associated with connective tissue disorders, Turner syndrome, bicuspid aortic valve, and coarctation of the aorta.

ABDOMINAL AORTIC ANEURYSM (AAA)

A 60-year-old M smoker presents with indolent-onset nonspecific back pain. On imaging, abdominal CT shows a 4-cm aortic aneurysm.

Management:

1. If symptomatic or if there is concern for impending rupture, urgent repair (open vs. endovascular) is needed.
2. If asymptomatic, surgery for AAA >5.5 cm or rapidly growing.

Complications: Concern for rupture if aneurysm is large or rapidly growing on repeated scans.

HYF: Most common location is below the renal arteries.

RUPTURED AAA

A 56-year-old M with uncontrolled HTN and 40-pack-year smoking history presents with sudden-onset abdominal pain. Exam reveals hypotension and a pulsatile abdominal mass. Labs show acute anemia.

Management:

1. Emergent endovascular repair if suitable.
2. Emergent open repair otherwise.

Complications: Death if untreated.

HYF: Mortality rate is extremely high.

THORACIC AORTIC ANEURYSM

A 63-year-old F with PMH of aortic regurgitation presents for further cardiac work-up. She is asymptomatic. On imaging, echocardiogram shows an ascending aortic aneurysm.

Management:

1. β-blocker therapy and elective repair if asymptomatic.
2. Surgical repair for symptomatic aneurysms or those risking rupture.
3. Open vs. endovascular surgery assessment based on anatomy.

Complications: Aortic regurgitation.

HYF: Associated with Marfan syndrome, Ehlers-Danlos syndrome, Turner syndrome.

SUBCLAVIAN STEAL SYNDROME

A 65-year-old M with severe atherosclerotic disease and 40-pack-year smoking history presents for his yearly physical. On exam, he is noted to have a lower systolic BP in the left arm than the right by 20 mmHg and a bruit in the neck. He reports intermittent left arm pain during exercise.

Management:

1. Cardiovascular risk modification (eg, lipids, HTN, diabetes).
2. Surgical bypass.
3. Possible endovascular intervention.

Complications: Syncope from vertebrobasilar insufficiency, head injury.

HYF: When symptomatic, upper extremity ischemia most commonly presents before neurologic symptoms.

Myocardial Infarction: See p. 4.

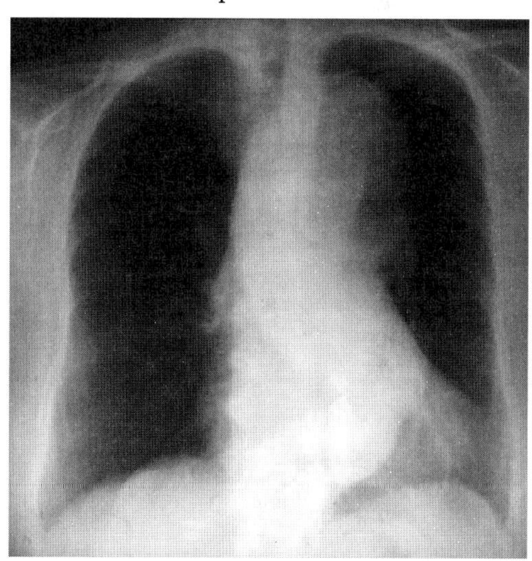

Thoracic aortic aneurysm.

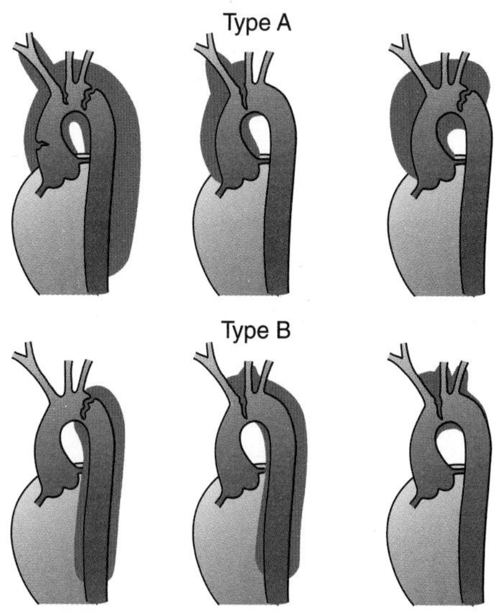
Type A
Type B

Classification of aortic dissections.

18-2 Peripheral Vascular Disease

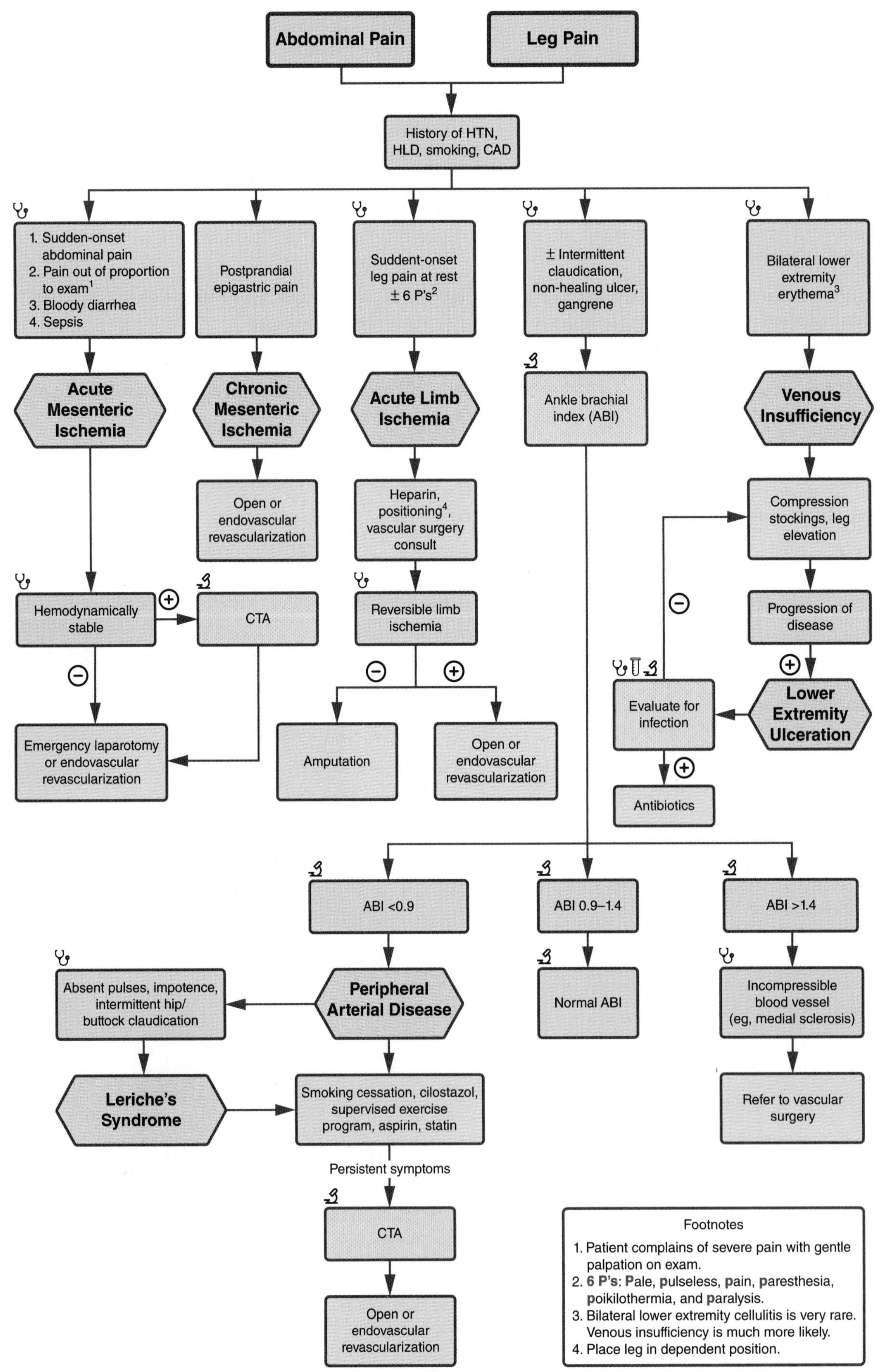

Abdominal Pain
Leg Pain
History of HTN, HLD, smoking, CAD
1. Sudden-onset abdominal pain
2. Pain out of proportion to exam[1]
3. Bloody diarrhea
4. Sepsis
Postprandial epigastric pain
Suddent-onset leg pain at rest ± 6 P's[2]
± Intermittent claudication, non-healing ulcer, gangrene
Bilateral lower extremity erythema[3]
Acute Mesenteric Ischemia
Chronic Mesenteric Ischemia
Acute Limb Ischemia
Ankle brachial index (ABI)
Venous Insufficiency
Open or endovascular revascularization
Heparin, positioning[4], vascular surgery consult
Compression stockings, leg elevation
Hemodynamically stable
CTA
Reversible limb ischemia
Progression of disease
Evaluate for infection
Lower Extremity Ulceration
Emergency laparotomy or endovascular revascularization
Amputation
Open or endovascular revascularization
Antibiotics
ABI <0.9
ABI 0.9–1.4
ABI >1.4
Absent pulses, impotence, intermittent hip/ buttock claudication
Peripheral Arterial Disease
Normal ABI
Incompressible blood vessel (eg, medial sclerosis)
Leriche's Syndrome
Smoking cessation, cilostazol, supervised exercise program, aspirin, statin
Refer to vascular surgery
Persistent symptoms
CTA
Open or endovascular revascularization
Footnotes
1. Patient complains of severe pain with gentle palpation on exam.
2. 6 P's: Pale, pulseless, pain, paresthesia, poikilothermia, and paralysis.
3. Bilateral lower extremity cellulitis is very rare. Venous insufficiency is much more likely.
4. Place leg in dependent position.

FIGURE 18.2

18-2 Peripheral Vascular Disease

ACUTE MESENTERIC ISCHEMIA

A 75-year-old M with PMH of recently diagnosed atrial fibrillation presents with 10/10 LLQ abdominal pain, nausea, and vomiting. On exam, the abdomen is severely tender to palpation throughout without rigidity or rebound.

Management:

1. If there is evidence of perforation or peritonitis, exploratory laparotomy.
2. If the patient remains hemodynamically stable, open or endovascular revascularization.

Complications: Prolonged ischemia can result in bowel necrosis, perforation, peritonitis, sepsis, or death.

HYF: SMA is the most common location of obstruction. Pain is out of proportion to physical exam.

CHRONIC MESENTERIC ISCHEMIA

A 61-year-old F with PMH of STEMI s/p PCI with stent placement, HLD, HTN, and a significant smoking history presents with a 20-lb weight loss over the last 4 months. She reports having postprandial epigastric pain.

Management: Open or endovascular revascularization.

Complications: Weight loss is common because patients avoid eating to limit postprandial abdominal pain.

HYF: As with any vascular pathology, timing is key. Slow onset allows for development of collateral circulation.

ACUTE LIMB ISCHEMIA

A 65-year-old M with PMH of atrial fibrillation and a 40-pack-year smoking history p/w severe leg pain in his left leg. On exam, he is unable to move his toes, which are cyanotic.

Management:

1. Start IV heparin gtt.
2. Emergent revascularization.

Complications: Reperfusion syndrome, compartment syndrome (if ischemic for >6 hours).

HYF: Typically, motor dysfunction is preceded by sensory disturbances. If the patient has progressed to paralysis of the affected limb, immediate intervention is key. Watch out for the 6 P's: pale, pulseless, pain, paresthesia, poikilothermia, and paralysis.

PERIPHERAL ARTERY DISEASE

A 70-year-old M with PMH of CAD s/p CABG, HTN, T2DM, and a 50-pack-year smoking history presents with persistent cramping of his calves whenever he walks down his driveway to check his mailbox. He also has noticed some ulcers on his toes that have been present for <1 month. ABI is 0.3 on the left and 0.4 on the right, with a left toe pressure of 37 and a right toe pressure of 45.

Management:

1. ABI and other non-invasive imaging should be pursued to confirm the diagnosis.
2. Medical management with aspirin, statin, and cilostazol in conjugation with a supervised walking program.
3. Smoking cessation.
4. If symptoms persist or are significantly impacting quality of life, consider open (surgical bypass) or endovascular revascularization.

Complications: Patients with very low toe pressures (<40 mmHg) often have difficulty with wound healing on their feet. Proper shoes and stockings to help relieve pressure are extremely important to prevent wounds that can become infected.

HYF: Cramping with exercise is called claudication. It is a reproducible phenomenon and improves with rest. It can be confused with neurogenic claudication (eg, lumbar spinal stenosis), which is position-dependent. Look for someone who gets cramping any time they walk a certain distance.

LERICHE'S SYNDROME

A 60-year-old M with PMH of CAD, HTN, T2DM, and a 45-year smoking history presents with cramping of his hips, thighs, and calves. He also notes that he has erectile dysfunction.

Management:

1. If not debilitating, 1st-line treatment is non-surgical management with lifestyle changes (smoking cessation, exercise) and managing comorbidities (HTN, HLD, DM).
2. If persistent or severe disease, surgical revascularization (open or endovascular).

HYF: This is a special case of peripheral artery disease, specifically aortoiliac disease. Look for the classic triad of impotence, absent femoral pulses, and hip/buttock/calf claudication.

Venous Insufficiency: See p. 343.
Lower Extremity Ulceration: See p. 343.

(Continued)

18-2 Peripheral Vascular Disease

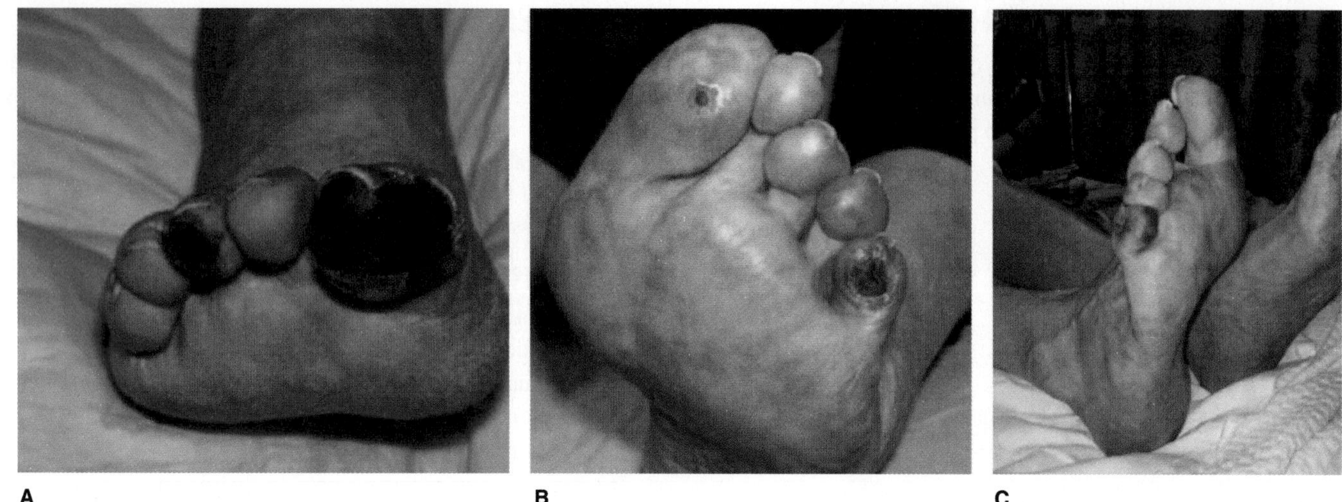
A
B
C

Acute ischemia of distal lower extremities.

19
Surgery: Breast

19-1 Malignant Breast Masses

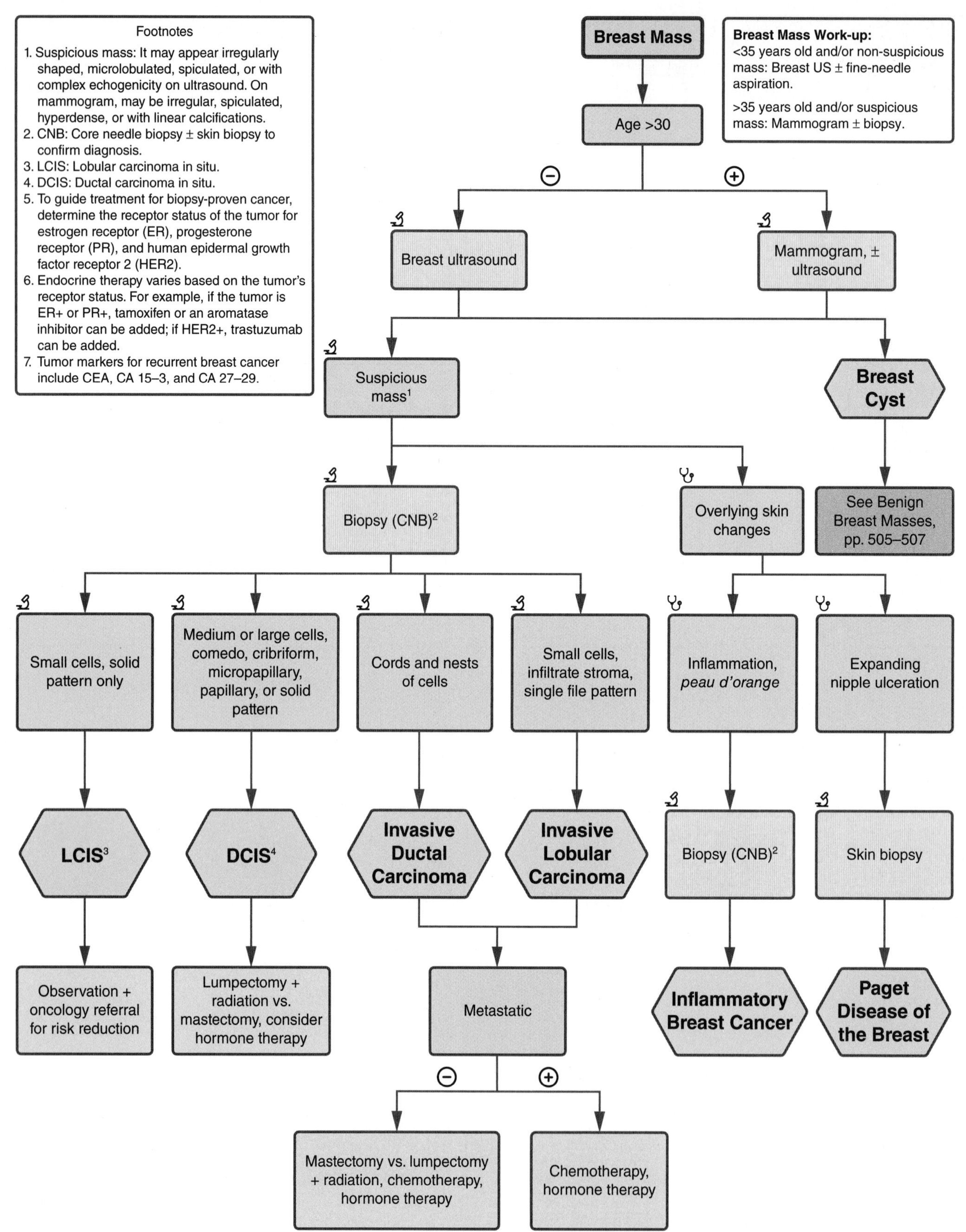
Footnotes
1. Suspicious mass: It may appear irregularly shaped, microlobulated, spiculated, or with complex echogenicity on ultrasound. On mammogram, may be irregular, spiculated, hyperdense, or with linear calcifications.
2. CNB: Core needle biopsy ± skin biopsy to confirm diagnosis.
3. LCIS: Lobular carcinoma in situ.
4. DCIS: Ductal carcinoma in situ.
5. To guide treatment for biopsy-proven cancer, determine the receptor status of the tumor for estrogen receptor (ER), progesterone receptor (PR), and human epidermal growth factor receptor 2 (HER2).
6. Endocrine therapy varies based on the tumor's receptor status. For example, if the tumor is ER+ or PR+, tamoxifen or an aromatase inhibitor can be added; if HER2+, trastuzumab can be added.
7. Tumor markers for recurrent breast cancer include CEA, CA 15–3, and CA 27–29.
Breast Mass
Breast Mass Work-up:
<35 years old and/or non-suspicious mass: Breast US ± fine-needle aspiration.
>35 years old and/or suspicious mass: Mammogram ± biopsy.
Age >30
Breast ultrasound
Mammogram, ± ultrasound
Suspicious mass[1]
Breast Cyst
Biopsy (CNB)[2]
Overlying skin changes
See Benign Breast Masses, pp. 505–507
Small cells, solid pattern only
Medium or large cells, comedo, cribriform, micropapillary, papillary, or solid pattern
Cords and nests of cells
Small cells, infiltrate stroma, single file pattern
Inflammation, peau d'orange
Expanding nipple ulceration
LCIS[3]
DCIS[4]
Invasive Ductal Carcinoma
Invasive Lobular Carcinoma
Biopsy (CNB)[2]
Skin biopsy
Observation + oncology referral for risk reduction
Lumpectomy + radiation vs. mastectomy, consider hormone therapy
Metastatic
Inflammatory Breast Cancer
Paget Disease of the Breast
Mastectomy vs. lumpectomy + radiation, chemotherapy, hormone therapy
Chemotherapy, hormone therapy

FIGURE 19.1

19-1 Malignant Breast Masses

LOBULAR CARCINOMA IN SITU (LCIS)

A 45-year-old F has a breast biopsy for a fibroadenoma that shows LCIS incidentally.

Management:

1. Clinical and imaging follow-up for classic LCIS.
2. Excision for non-classic LCIS.
3. Consider referral to oncology for risk-reduction strategies.

Complications: Increased risk in both breasts of developing breast cancer.

HYF: Classic pathology shows solid proliferation of small uniform cells with dyshesion.

DUCTAL CARCINOMA IN SITU (DCIS)

A 75-year-old F has a screening mammogram that shows linear branching microcalcifications in the left breast. Core biopsy shows DCIS.

Management:

1. Lumpectomy + radiation OR mastectomy with sentinel lymph node biopsy ± radiation.
2. Endocrine therapy used for chemoprevention.

Complications: Contralateral primary breast cancer possible after unilateral mastectomy or lumpectomy.

HYF: Non-invasive (premalignant) condition that does not usually present with a mass.

INFILTRATING DUCTAL CARCINOMA

A 40-year-old F with extensive family history of breast and ovarian cancer presents with a right breast mass. On **exam**, the mass is hard and immobile. On **imaging**, mammogram reveals a spiculated mass with microcalcifications. Breast US with biopsy confirms the diagnosis.

Management:

1. Staging with imaging.
2. Mastectomy vs. breast-conserving surgery + radiation.
3. Sentinel lymph node biopsy.
4. Adjuvant chemotherapy or endocrine therapy.
5. Refer for genetic counseling given this patient's family history (eg, *BRCA1/2* mutation).

Complications: Response to endocrine therapy dependent on hormone receptors.

HYF: Most common form of breast cancer. Pathology shows cords and nests of cells with varying gland formation.

INFILTRATING LOBULAR CARCINOMA

A 55-year-old F notices her nipple has become inverted on the right side. On **exam**, a palpable mass is felt underneath the areola.

Management:

1. Staging typically with MRI breast to evaluate extent of disease and contralateral disease.
2. Mastectomy vs. breast-conserving surgery + radiation.
3. Sentinel lymph node biopsy.
4. Adjuvant chemotherapy or endocrine therapy.

Complications: Response to endocrine therapy dependent on hormone receptors.

HYF: Pathology shows small cells infiltrating mammary stroma/adipose in a single line. Patients often have bilateral breast cancer.

INFLAMMATORY BREAST CANCER

A 40-year-old F was in clinic last week for progressive inflammation of her breast. She returns to clinic without improvement on antibiotics. On **exam**, the skin over her left breast is pink, thickened, and warm. On **imaging**, mammography shows a large area of calcification. Biopsy of the calcifications confirms invasive ductal carcinoma and punch biopsy of the skin confirms dermal involvement.

Management:

1. Neoadjuvant chemotherapy.
2. Mastectomy and radiation.

Complications:

- Pain, including bone and nerve pain.
- Poor prognosis.

HYF: Involves dermal lymphatic invasion leading to breast pain, erythema, edema, and prominent hair follicles; *peau d'orange* appearance of the breast is characteristic.

PAGET DISEASE OF THE BREAST

A 55-year-old F presents with a painful, itchy, ulcerated lesion on the right areola and nipple with palpable underlying mass. On **imaging**, mammogram reveals small microcalcifications suggestive of underlying DCIS. Skin biopsy confirms the diagnosis.

Management:

1. Treatment based on underlying cancer and stage.

Complications: Underlying invasive cancer is likely.

HYF: Paget cells are malignant, intraepithelial adenocarcinoma cells occurring in the epidermis of the nipple. Associated with DCIS or invasive carcinoma in majority of patients.

(Continued)

19-1 Malignant Breast Masses

BREAST CANCER IN PREGNANCY

A 35-year-old primigravida F in her 20th week of pregnancy presents with a new lump on self-examination.

Management:

1. Staging.
2. Mastectomy vs. breast-conserving surgery + radiation after delivery.
3. Sentinel lymph node biopsy with methylene blue only (no radiotracer during pregnancy).
4. Adjuvant chemotherapy possible after 1st trimester.

Complications: Radiation and chemotherapy during pregnancy are associated with fetal complications (highest risk during the 1st trimester).

HYF: Breastfeeding is safe and feasible after conclusion of treatment but not recommended from an irradiated breast.

MALE BREAST CANCER

A 60-year-old M with family history of breast cancer (*BRCA2* mutation) presents with **exam** findings of a painless, fixed subareolar mass in the left breast. On **imaging**, mammography results are suspicious for a malignant lesion. Core biopsy shows invasive ductal carcinoma.

Management:

1. Treat according to underlying cancer diagnosis.

HYF: Associated more with *BRCA2* mutation than *BRCA1*. Tamoxifen is preferred for adjuvant therapy. Men with breast cancer typically present at a more advanced stage and have overall worse prognosis.

Breast Cyst: See Benign Breast, pp. 505–507.

Common and Serious Side Effects of Breast Cancer Therapies

Chemotherapy (anthracyclines, taxanes, platinums, capecitabine)	General: Nausea, diarrhea, myelosuppression, alopecia, amenorrhea
	Anthracyclines: Cardiotoxicity, secondary leukemia
	Taxanes: Neuropathy, hypersensitivity reaction
	Platinums: Neuropathy, hypersensitivity reaction, ototoxicity, nephrotoxicity
	Capecitabine: Hand–foot syndrome, stomatitis
HER2-Targeted Therapy (trastuzumab, pertuzumab, T-DM1, neratinib)	General: Diarrhea, cardiotoxicity
	T-DM1: Thrombocytopenia, peripheral neuropathy, hyperbilirubinemia, transaminitis
Endocrine Therapy (SERMs, SERDs, aromatase inhibitors, ovarian suppression)	General: Hot flashes, arthralgia, myalgia, nausea, headache, vaginal dryness, mood swings, weight gain, hair thinning
	Tamoxifen: Endometrial cancer, venous thromboembolism, cataracts
	Aromatase inhibitors: ↓ bone mineral density

19-2 Benign Breast Masses

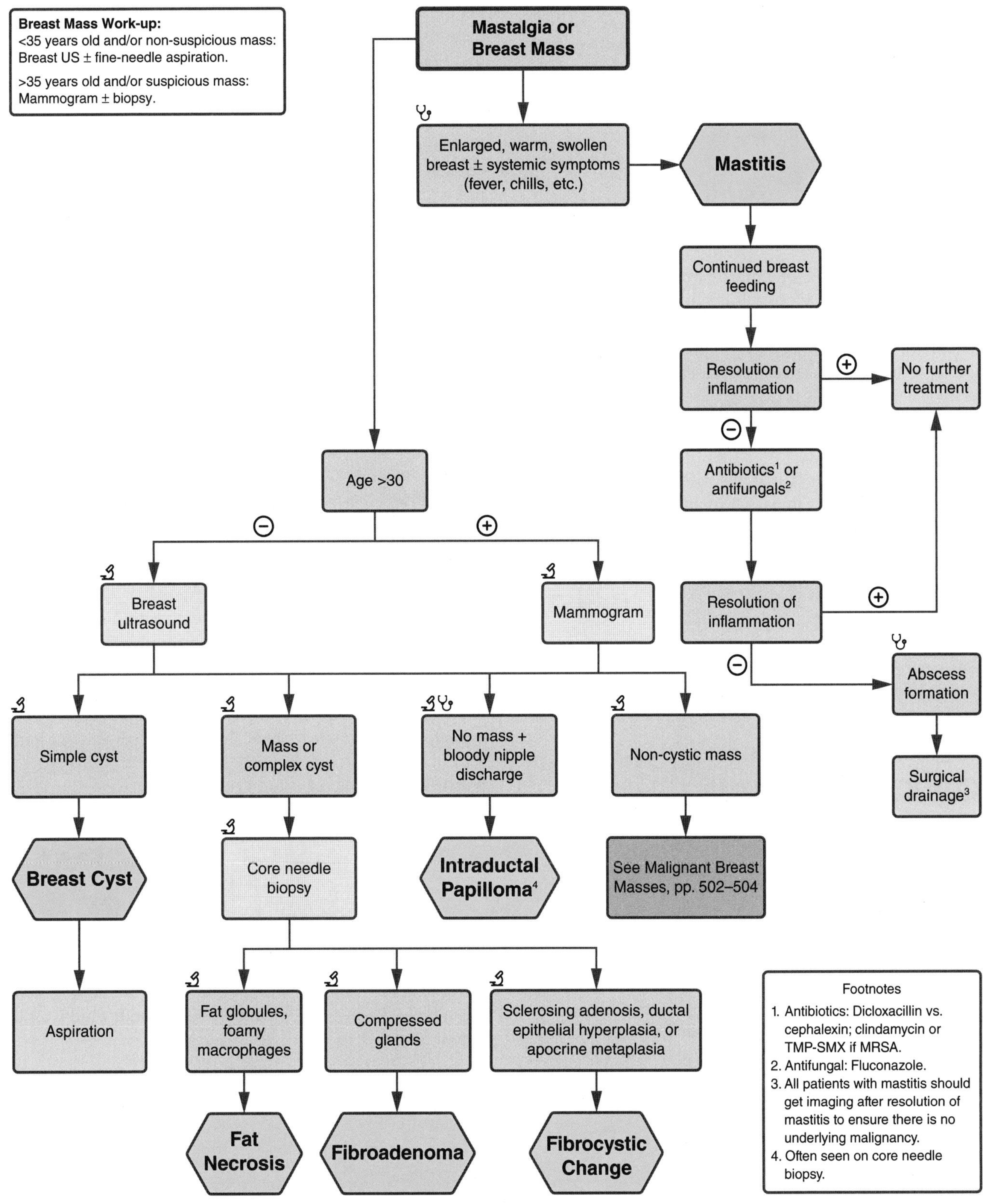

Breast Mass Work-up:
<35 years old and/or non-suspicious mass: Breast US ± fine-needle aspiration.
>35 years old and/or suspicious mass: Mammogram ± biopsy.
Mastalgia or Breast Mass
Enlarged, warm, swollen breast ± systemic symptoms (fever, chills, etc.)
Mastitis
Continued breast feeding
Resolution of inflammation
No further treatment
Antibiotics[1] or antifungals[2]
Resolution of inflammation
Abscess formation
Surgical drainage[3]
Age >30
Breast ultrasound
Mammogram
Simple cyst
Mass or complex cyst
No mass + bloody nipple discharge
Non-cystic mass
Breast Cyst
Core needle biopsy
Intraductal Papilloma[4]
See Malignant Breast Masses, pp. 502–504
Aspiration
Fat globules, foamy macrophages
Compressed glands
Sclerosing adenosis, ductal epithelial hyperplasia, or apocrine metaplasia
Fat Necrosis
Fibroadenoma
Fibrocystic Change
Footnotes
1. Antibiotics: Dicloxacillin vs. cephalexin; clindamycin or TMP-SMX if MRSA.
2. Antifungal: Fluconazole.
3. All patients with mastitis should get imaging after resolution of mastitis to ensure there is no underlying malignancy.
4. Often seen on core needle biopsy.

FIGURE 19.2

19-2 Benign Breast Masses

MASTITIS

A 25-year-old G1P1 F s/p spontaneous vaginal delivery 2 weeks ago who is currently breastfeeding presents with an enlarged, swollen, warm, and tender right breast. **Labs** show leukocytosis.

Management:

1. Continue breastfeeding.
2. Antibiotics (eg, nafcillin to cover MSSA).

Complications: Breast abscess.

HYF: Can be confused with inflammatory breast cancer; patients with inflammatory breast cancer will not respond to antibiotics. Evaluate with ultrasound if no improvement within 48–72 hours to rule out breast abscess. All patients with mastitis should undergo imaging after resolution of mastitis to ensure there is no underlying malignancy.

BREAST CYST

A 27-year-old F with no PMH presents with left breast pain. On **exam**, she has a small breast mass. On **imaging**, breast US shows well-defined, fluid-filled mass.

Management:

1. Breast US.
2. Drainage of breast cyst via needle aspiration.

HYF: For recurrent breast cysts, consider sending more extensive workup, including aspirate cultures, cell count, and a histologic sample. A breast cyst can also be excised if the cyst recurs or is bothersome to the patient.

INTRADUCTAL PAPILLOMA

A 37-year-old F presents with several months of bloody nipple discharge. On **exam**, she has no palpable breast masses. On **imaging**, mammography does not identify any lesions. Galactogram confirms the diagnosis.

Management:

1. Mammogram to rule out breast cancer.
2. Surgery to remove the affected duct.

HYF: Most common cause of bloody nipple discharge. Mammograms are indicated to rule out malignancy but will not show papillomas. Galactogram is diagnostic and guides surgical resection. Seen in young women age 20–40s. Associated with an increased risk of breast cancer.

FAT NECROSIS

A 37-year-old F s/p breast reduction surgery last month presents with a small breast mass on her post-op visit. On **exam**, she has a small breast mass in the right lower outer quadrant. On **imaging**, mammography shows a 2.5 × 2.8 cm calcified mass.

Management:

1. Biopsy to rule out breast cancer.
2. Reassurance.

HYF: Associated with breast trauma or breast surgery. Biopsy demonstrates fat globules. Fat necrosis is not associated with increased risk for breast cancer.

FIBROADENOMA

A 20-year-old F with no significant PMH presents with a breast mass in the upper outer quadrant of her left breast. On **exam**, she has a firm, well-circumscribed, mobile breast mass. On **imaging**, breast US or fine-needle aspiration confirms the diagnosis.

Management:

1. US shows a well-defined, solid mass.
2. Gold standard: Fine-needle aspiration is diagnostic and therapeutic.
3. Excisional biopsy if fine-needle aspiration is indeterminate.
4. Reassurance or removal.

HYF: Seen in young women (late teens, early 20s). Changes size over the course of a menstrual cycle. Not associated with increased risk for breast cancer. Surgical excision is optional for large, enlarging, or symptomatic fibroadenomas.

FIBROCYSTIC CHANGES

A 22-year-old F with no PMH presents with lumpy breasts. She reports bilateral breast tenderness and fluctuation in the size of the lumps related to her menstrual cycle (pain is worse in the last 2 weeks). On **exam**, she has small, cord-like, mobile breast masses bilaterally. On **imaging**, breast US shows simple cysts, which are aspirated, revealing clear fluid. The masses resolve after aspiration.

Management:

1. Breast US +/− fine-needle aspiration.
2. Start OCPs.
3. Follow-up reassurance only.

HYF: Similar to fibroadenoma, except with multiple lesions that change size over the course of the menstrual cycle. Some types of fibrocystic changes (eg, epithelial hyperplasia) are associated with increased risk of breast cancer while others are not (eg, apocrine metaplasia). Resolves with menopause. If bloody fluid is aspirated, send it for cytology.

PHYLLODES TUMOR

A 43-year-old F with no significant PMH presents with a painless and growing breast mass. On **imaging**, mammography shows smooth mass similar to a fibroadenoma, and biopsy confirms the diagnosis, revealing papillary projections of the stroma lined with epithelium, hyperplasia, and atypia.

Management:

1. Mammography.
2. Percutaneous biopsy (FNA or core needle) to confirm diagnosis.

19-2 Benign Breast Masses

3. Complete surgical excision.
4. Surveillance.

HYF: Presents similarly to a fibroadenoma but is larger and has associated risk of breast cancer. They can grow rapidly if not excised. Most are benign, but they have potential to become malignant sarcomas. Complete excision is required.

ATYPICAL HYPERPLASIA

A 70-year-old nulliparous F is found to have a lesion with microcalcifications on mammography. Core needle biopsy demonstrates hyperplasia of duct with atypia.

Management:

1. Mammography.
2. Core needle biopsy to confirm diagnosis.
3. Complete excision.
4. Surveillance +/– tamoxifen or aromatase inhibitors to reduce risk of breast cancer.

HYF: Can be ductal or lobular, filling part (but not the entirety) of a duct or lobule. Similar to a low-grade DCIS or LCIS, with an increased risk for breast cancer. Usually seen on mammogram and confirmed by tissue biopsy. Monitor with yearly mammograms and consider risk reduction with tamoxifen or aromatase inhibitor if postmenopausal.

20

Surgery: Ophthalmology

20-1 Adult Ophthalmology

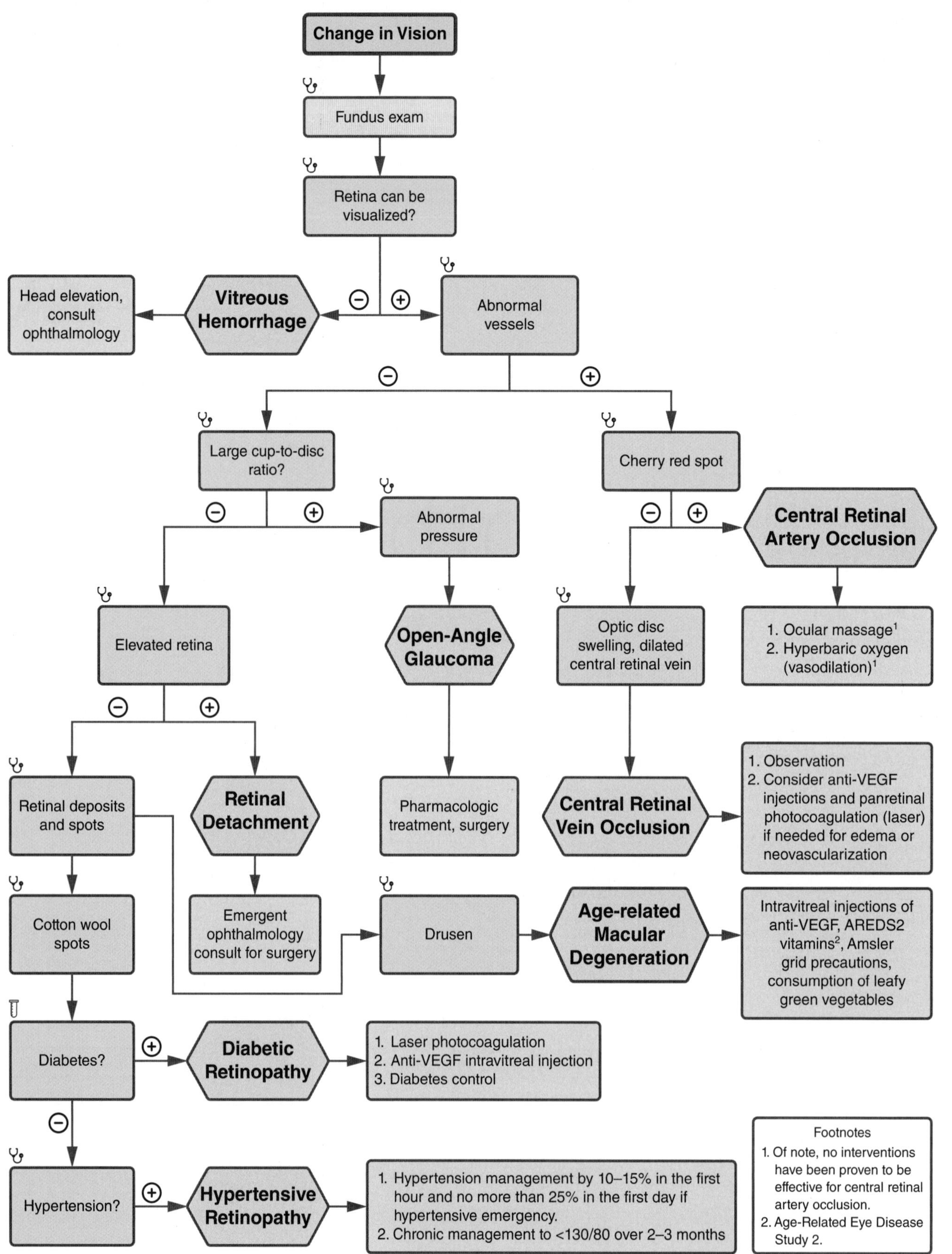
Change in Vision
Fundus exam
Retina can be visualized?
Vitreous Hemorrhage
Head elevation, consult ophthalmology
Abnormal vessels
Large cup-to-disc ratio?
Cherry red spot
Abnormal pressure
Central Retinal Artery Occlusion
Elevated retina
Open-Angle Glaucoma
Optic disc swelling, dilated central retinal vein
1. Ocular massage[1]
2. Hyperbaric oxygen (vasodilation)[1]
Retinal deposits and spots
Retinal Detachment
Pharmacologic treatment, surgery
Central Retinal Vein Occlusion
1. Observation
2. Consider anti-VEGF injections and panretinal photocoagulation (laser) if needed for edema or neovascularization
Cotton wool spots
Emergent ophthalmology consult for surgery
Drusen
Age-related Macular Degeneration
Intravitreal injections of anti-VEGF, AREDS2 vitamins[2], Amsler grid precautions, consumption of leafy green vegetables
Diabetes?
Diabetic Retinopathy
1. Laser photocoagulation
2. Anti-VEGF intravitreal injection
3. Diabetes control
Hypertension?
Hypertensive Retinopathy
1. Hypertension management by 10–15% in the first hour and no more than 25% in the first day if hypertensive emergency.
2. Chronic management to <130/80 over 2–3 months
Footnotes
1. Of note, no interventions have been proven to be effective for central retinal artery occlusion.
2. Age-Related Eye Disease Study 2.

FIGURE 20.1

20-1 Adult Ophthalmology

CMV RETINITIS

A 40-year-old M with PMH of untreated HIV presents with blurry vision, floaters, and photopsias over the past few days. Yellow-white hemorrhagic lesions are present on the fundus exam.

Management:

1. Diagnostic procedures such as aqueous or vitreous tap to test for CMV and other viruses.
2. IV, oral, and intravitreal anti-viral medications.
3. HAART in HIV+ patients.

Complications:

- Retinal detachment.
- Retinal scarring.

HYF: Risk factors include HIV, CD4 <50, or severe immunosuppression. Differentiation from acute retinal necrosis (ARN) is important as treatment is different. While patients can present with decreased visual acuity, floaters, photopsias, or scotomas, >50% of patients can be asymptomatic.

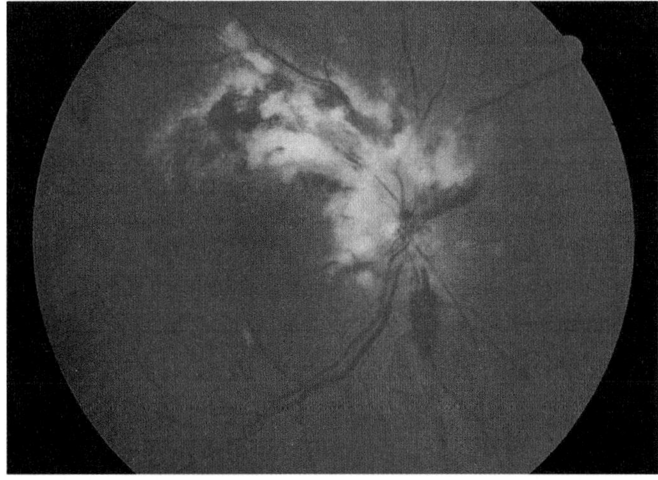

Hemorrhages and exudates ("cheese pizza" appearance) seen with CMV retinitis.

HERPES ZOSTER OPHTHALMICUS

An 82-year-old M presents with fever, malaise, burning and itching in the periorbital region, and eye pain. On exam, a vesicular rash is present in the area.

Management:

1. Corneal sensation, fluorescein staining, and dilated eye exam.
2. High-dose acyclovir (800 mg PO 5 times daily) for 7–10 days. Alternatively, famciclovir or valacyclovir.
3. Erythromycin ointment over skin rash to prevent bacterial superinfection.

Complications:

- Ptosis, lid scarring, ectropion/entropion.
- Permanent vision loss.

HYF: Hutchinson's sign (skin lesions at the tip of the nose) is a strong predictor of HZO as the nasociliary nerve is involved. Tzanck smear might reveal multinucleated giant cells. Age >60 and immunocompromise are the main risk factors.

ENDOPHTHALMITIS

A 65-year-old M with PMH of bilateral cataract surgery presents with pain, blurry vision, and floaters in the right eye. On exam, he has a swollen eyelid, hypopyon, and chemosis. B-scan (US) confirms the diagnosis.

Management:

1. Vitreous tap for culture (Gram stain, bacterial, and fungal) and injection of antibiotics/antifungals.
2. Vitrectomy if no improvement after injections or if vision is light perception.

Complications: Permanent vision loss.

HYF: Suspicion for endophthalmitis should be high after surgery, injections, globe rupture, or with bacteremia/fungemia.

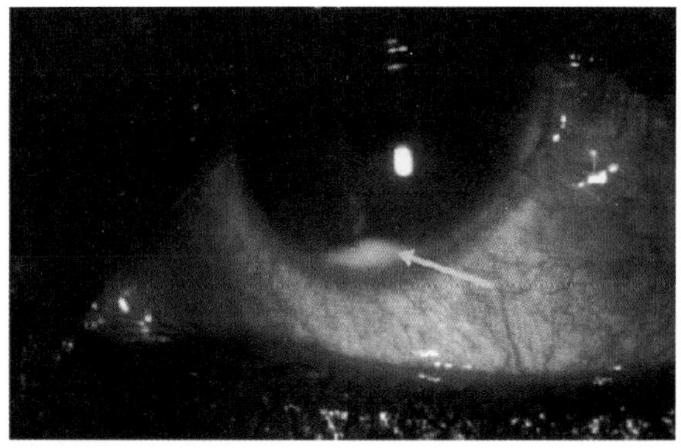

Hypopyon.

BLEPHARITIS

A 26-year-old F with PMH of atopy presents with foreign body sensation, burning, and crusting at both eyelid margins. On exam, there is meibomian gland inspissation and erythema of the eyelids.

Management:

1. Warm compresses and eyelid massage.
2. Eyelid hygiene with baby shampoo.

Complications: Rare, but can cause eye dryness, corneal neovascularization and ulceration.

(Continued)

20-1 Adult Ophthalmology

HYF: With blepharitis, erythema is localized to the eyelids, as opposed to conjunctival involvement in conjunctivitis.

SCLERITIS

A 45-year-old F with PMH of lupus presents with severe, boring pain in the left eye that wakes her from sleep. On exam, her sclera is diffusely red; uvea looks normal.

Management:

1. NSAIDs in mild to moderate cases.
2. Systemic steroids in severe cases and then immunosuppressive therapy (azathioprine, methotrexate).
3. Perform B-scan (US) to check for posterior scleritis.
4. Evaluate for the underlying cause.

Complications: Scleral thinning, cataract, glaucoma, vision loss.

HYF: Most often there is an underlying systemic disease. Scleritis should be differentiated from episcleritis, which is usually idiopathic, non-vision threatening, and blanches with phenylephrine.

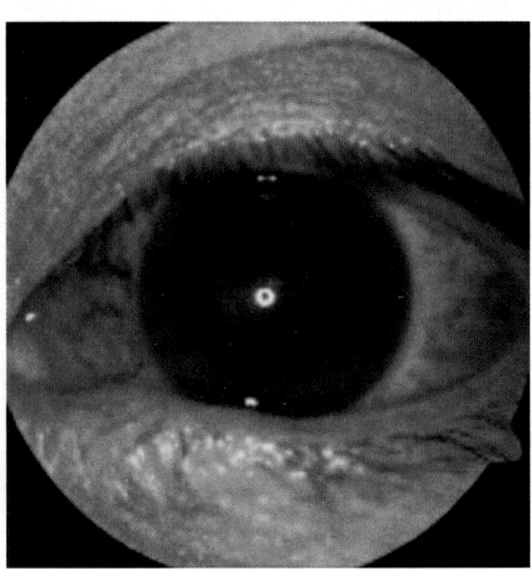

Diffuse anterior scleritis. Note the deep, dark vessels.

BACTERIAL CONJUNCTIVITIS

A 32-year-old M presents with left-sided eye pain and foreign body sensation that began 2 days ago. In the morning, it is difficult for him to open his eyes. On exam, he has conjunctival edema and injection. Purulent discharge appears after wiping; no follicles are present on the conjunctiva.

Management:

1. Copious irrigation.
2. Proper hygiene and hand washing instructions.
3. Topical erythromycin/azithromycin or polymyxin-trimethoprim and systemic antibiotics if concern for *N. gonorrhoeae* or *C. trachomatis.*

Complications: Blindness if untreated. Patients with *N. gonorrhoeae* or *C. trachomatis* are at increased risk of corneal involvement and perforation.

HYF: Continuous purulent discharge is suggestive. Can be hyperacute when infected by *N. gonorrhoeae* and can be transmitted from the genitals to the hands and then the eyes. Other common causes: *S. aureus*, *S. pneumoniae*, *Moraxella*.

VIRAL CONJUNCTIVITIS

A 25-year-old F with PMH of a recent URI presents with gritting and burning sensation in the right eye for the past week. Exam shows diffuse conjunctival edema and follicular reaction, as well as watery discharge.

Management:

1. Cold compresses and artificial tears for comfort.
2. Proper hygiene and hand washing instructions.

Complications: Corneal inflammation, pseudomembrane formation, conjunctival scarring, symblepharon formation.

HYF: Most common cause of conjunctivitis. Most common etiology is adenovirus. Other viruses: HSV, VZV, picornavirus, HIV. May see preauricular lymphadenopathy. Commonly presents with prodromal symptoms after a viral infection.

ALLERGIC CONJUNCTIVITIS

An 18-year-old M with PMH of eczema presents with bilateral watery eye discharge and itchiness since yesterday. On exam, he has diffuse conjunctival edema and papillary reaction.

Management:

1. Over-the-counter antihistamines and/or decongestants for symptom control.
2. Mast cell stabilizer if recurrent.

Complications: Conjunctival and corneal scarring.

HYF: Presents bilaterally. Pruritus and history of atopy are suggestive.

UVEITIS

A 32-year-old M presents with blurry vision and photophobia. On exam, there is anterior chamber reaction (hypopyon).

Management:

1. Topical steroids and cycloplegics.
2. Workup for cause of uveitis (eg, autoimmune or infectious causes).

20-1 Adult Ophthalmology

Complications:

- Cataract.
- Band keratopathy.
- Intraocular hypertension.

HYF: Involves inflammation of the uveal tract (iris, choroid, ciliary body). HLA-B27 mutation is a risk factor.

PHOTOKERATITIS

A 26-year-old F presents with severe eye pain and light sensitivity in both eyes. On exam, she has excessive tearing and chemosis. She recently came back from a ski trip in Colorado and did not wear ski goggles during the trip.

Management:

1. Supportive care with topical antibiotic ointment, artificial tears, and oral analgesics.

Complications: Self-resolves within days.

HYF: Due to corneal epithelial damage. UV-protective eyewear can help prevent it. Common after travel to high altitudes and areas with high UV reflection (snow, water, sand) and can be seen in welders and those who use tanning beds.

CAVERNOUS SINUS THROMBOSIS

A 30-year-old F presents with diplopia, nausea/vomiting, and a new headache. She has an unremarkable history and started taking oral contraceptives 3 months ago. On exam, she has proptosis and ophthalmoplegia.

Management:

1. MRI of brain and orbit and MRV (if contraindicated or unavailable, consider CT with and without contrast).
2. Broad-spectrum IV antibiotics if concern for infectious cause.
3. Anticoagulation (controversial but should be considered).
4. Treat underlying cause (infection, tumor, inflammation, etc.).

Complications:

- Visual loss.
- Death.

HYF: Requires urgent evaluation as it can be life and vision threatening.

DIABETIC RETINOPATHY

A 75-year-old F with PMH of diabetes presents with decreased vision. Fundus exam shows microaneurysms, exudates, and cotton wool spots. Recent A1c is 8.2 on labs.

Management:

1. Anti-VEGF intravitreal injections for macular edema.
2. Panretinal photocoagulation.
3. Blood sugar and blood pressure control.

Complications: Vitreous hemorrhage, tractional retinal detachment, permanent vision loss.

HYF: This is the leading cause of blindness in the US and is based on severity of stages from mild, moderate, to severe non-proliferative retinopathy and proliferative retinopathy. Patients with diabetes should be screened yearly and more frequently if they have signs of retinopathy.

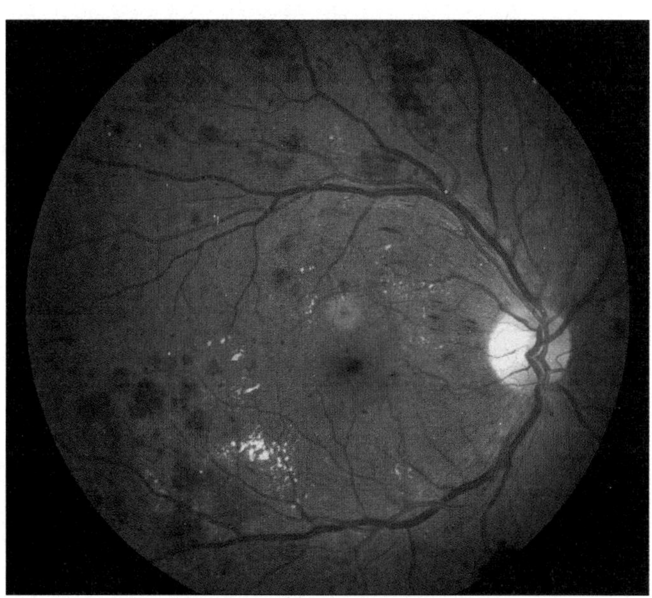

Scattered flame hemorrhages and macular exudates in non-proliferative diabetic retinopathy.

HYPERTENSIVE RETINOPATHY

A 75-year-old M with PMH of HTN presents for an annual checkup. His visual acuity has decreased by one line since his last exam 2 years ago. On exam, his retinal vessels appear narrow and nicked. He also has small areas with exudates and cotton wool spots on fundus exam.

Management:

1. Hypertension management by 10–15% in the first hour and no more than 25% in the first day if hypertensive emergency.
2. Chronic management to BP <130/80 over 2–3 months.

Complications: Retinal vascular diseases (eg, arterial and vein occlusions), neovascularization of the retina.

HYF: Can be acute and/or chronic.

(Continued)

20-1 Adult Ophthalmology

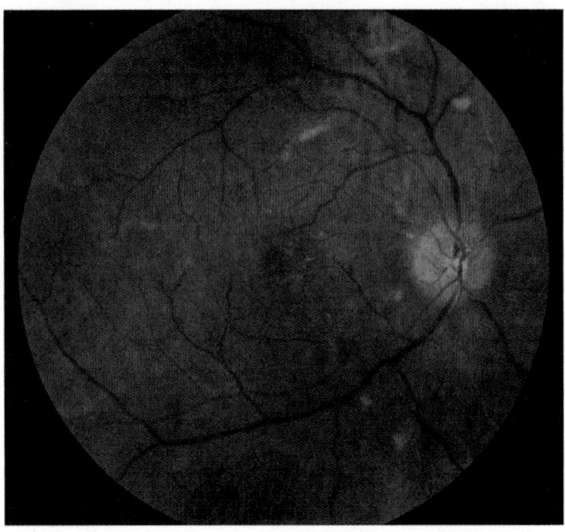

Blurred optic disc, scattered hemorrhages, cotton-wool spots, and foveal exudate can be seen in hypertensive retinopathy.

OPEN-ANGLE GLAUCOMA

A 50-year-old M with family history of glaucoma presents for routine checkup. His IOP is 21 and 23 mmHg in right and left eyes, respectively. On the fundus exam, the cup-to-disc ratio is 0.6 bilaterally.

Management:

1. Baseline visual field testing.
2. Pharmacologic (eye drops):
   a. 1st-line: Prostaglandin analogs (latanoprost, bimatoprost).
   b. β-blockers (timolol), carbonic anhydrase inhibitors (dorzolamide), α-2 agonists (brimonidine).
3. Surgery.

Complications: Visual field deficits.

HYF: Often asymptomatic. Most common in African Americans and Europeans. Be cautious about using β-blockers in those with asthma or bradycardia.

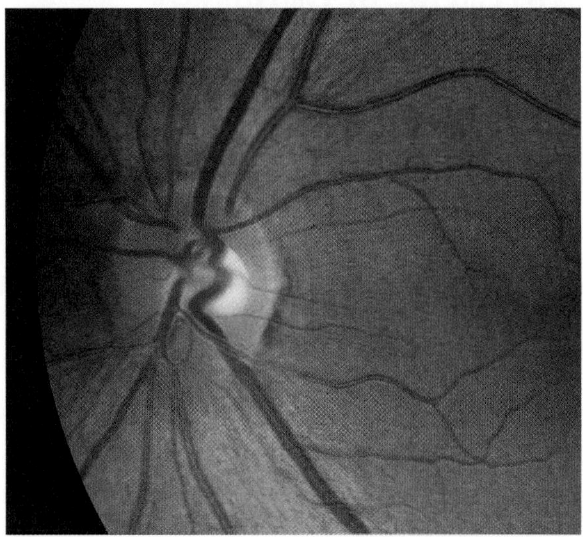

Glaucoma results in destruction of the neural rim and an enlarged, excavated cup, leading to "cupping."

ACUTE ANGLE CLOSURE GLAUCOMA

A 40-year-old M who just came from a movie theater presents with headache, nausea, blurry vision, halos, and right eye pain. On exam, his pupil is fixed, cornea is edematous, and conjunctiva is injected on the affected side.

Management:

1. Measure intraocular pressure.
2. Topical eye drops to lower intraocular pressure: β-blockers, carbonic anhydrase inhibitors, alpha-2 agonists.
3. Systemic acetazolamide if no contraindications.
4. Laser peripheral iridotomy is definitive treatment.

Complications: Permanent vision loss.

HYF: Pupillary dilation should be avoided until patients receive laser peripheral iridotomy.

CHRONIC DRY EYE SYNDROME

A 40-year-old F presents with blurry vision and foreign body sensation. She works as an executive at a local startup and noticed this recently gets worse toward the end of the day after using the computer all day.

Management:

1. Conservative management with artificial tears.
2. Lifestyle modifications.

Complications: Corneal neovascularization and scarring in severe cases.

HYF: Due to dryness secondary to windy weather and decreased frequency of blinking (reading, computer use). Also associated with Sjögren's syndrome.

PTERYGIUM

A 50-year-old M with unremarkable eye history presents with blurry vision. On exam, there is a wedge-shaped tissue between his conjunctiva and cornea, obscuring part of his visual axis.

Management:

1. Conservative management with artificial tears.
2. Surgical removal if visually significant.
3. UV protection.

Complications: Blurry vision.

HYF: Commonly seen in occupations with high level of UV exposure.

20-1 Adult Ophthalmology

AGED-RELATED MACULAR DEGENERATION

A 75-year-old F presents with bilateral loss of vision. Over the past year, she reports having difficulty driving at night. Peripheral vision is intact, but she endorses having blind spots in her central visual field. On fundus exam, drusen deposits are present near the macula.

Management:

1. AREDS2 vitamins
2. Avoid smoking. Eat leafy greens.
3. Amsler grid precautions.
4. Anti-VEGF injections if wet/neovascular AMD.

Complications: Permanent vision loss.

HYF: There are 2 subtypes: Wet (neovascular) with visual distortion and wavy lines, and dry (atrophic) with progressive blind spots. Smoking and age are risk factors.

RHEGMATOGENOUS RETINAL DETACHMENT

A 60-year-old F with a history of a motor vehicle accident 4 months ago presents with acute decline in vision. Patient reports seeing floaters, flashes, and a black curtain in part of his vision. Fundus exam shows an elevated gray-colored retina with a tear in the periphery.

Management:

1. Emergent ophthalmology consult for management (eg, pneumopexy, pars plana vitrectomy, scleral buckle).

Complications: Permanent loss of vision.

HYF: Retinal detachment is a vision-threatening condition and emergent medical care is necessary. It can present months after the trauma itself. Other risk factors include myopia more than 6.0D, previous retinal detachment, lattice degeneration, and family history.

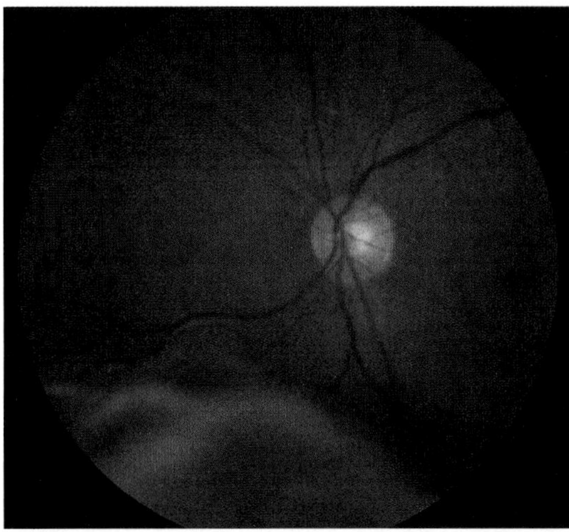

An elevated sheet of retinal tissue with folds can be seen in retinal detachment.

VITREOUS HEMORRHAGE

A 60-year-old M with diabetic retinopathy presents with acute decline in vision. Patient reports seeing red floaters. On exam, the fundus cannot be visualized.

Management:

1. Head elevation (30–45°) to settle the clot.
2. Ophthalmology consult to determine cause of vitreous hemorrhage.

Complications: Permanent loss of vision.

HYF: Vitreous hemorrhage has many different causes, including but not limited to posterior vitreous detachment, retinal tear, and proliferative diabetic retinopathy.

CENTRAL RETINAL ARTERY OCCLUSION

A 50-year-old M presents with sudden painless loss of vision in the right eye upon waking up in the morning. On exam, the fundus appears pale, fovea is cherry red color, and arterioles are attenuated ("box-carring"). On imaging, fundus fluorescein angiography shows occlusion of the central retinal artery.

Management:

1. Management of central retinal artery occlusion is controversial. Some options that have been proposed include ocular massage, hyperbaric oxygen, and anterior chamber paracentesis to lower intraocular pressure.
2. Full stroke workup.
3. Blood pressure, lipid, and blood sugar control.

Complications: Permanent vision loss, neovascularization of the retina.

HYF: Often encountered upon waking up and due to cholesterol emboli from carotid arteries or other regions. Stroke workup is imperative.

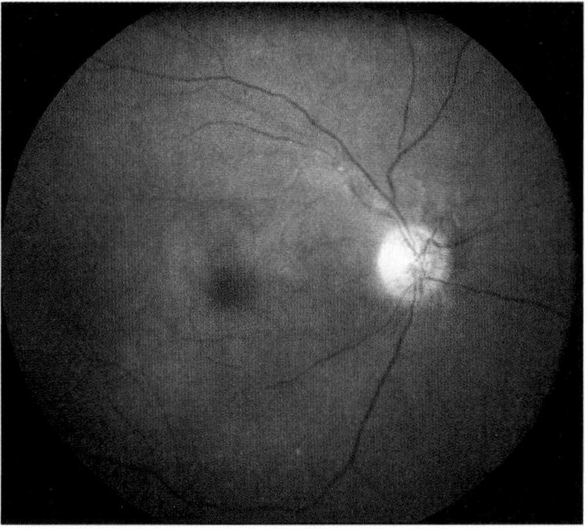

A central cherry red spot, Hollenhorst plaques, diffuse macular edema, and thready residual arterial flow can be visualized in this patient with central retinal artery occlusion.

(Continued)

20-1 Adult Ophthalmology

CENTRAL RETINAL VEIN OCCLUSION

A 50-year-old F with PMH of breast cancer presents with sudden, painless loss of vision in the right eye upon waking up in the morning. On fundus exam, there are diffuse retinal hemorrhages.

Management:

1. Monitoring of potential complications, such as neovascularization of the retina and macular edema, which can be managed with panretinal photocoagulation (laser) or anti-VEGF injections.
2. Blood pressure and blood sugar control.

Complications: Permanent vision loss, macular edema, neovascularization of the retina, neovascular glaucoma.

HYF: Characteristic fundus exam is known as the "blood and thunder" appearance. Risk factors: Hypertension, glaucoma, hyperviscosity.

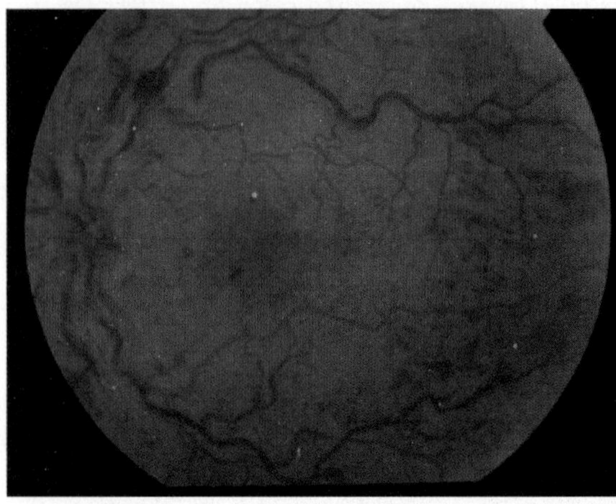

Disc swelling, retinal hemorrhages, and suffusion of the veins can be seen in central retinal vein occlusion.

OPTIC NEURITIS

A 40-year-old F with PMH of multiple sclerosis presents with left-sided eye pain that is exacerbated by eye movements and blurry vision. On exam, there is relative afferent pupillary defect and decreased color vision in the affected eye.

Management:

1. IV steroids.
2. MRI brain and orbit with and without contrast.
3. Consider plasmapheresis or IV immunoglobulin based on systemic causes.

Complications: Permanent loss of vision.

HYF: MRI will show optic nerve sheath enhancement. While optic neuritis can be an isolated occurrence, it is important to evaluate for multiple sclerosis. Other causes to consider are anti-MOG and neuromyelitis optica (NMO).

GRAVES OPHTHALMOPATHY

A 33-year-old F presents with double vision, proptosis, and eyelid retraction. Over the past few months, she has lost 10 lbs and reports insomnia as well as fatigue.

Management:

1. Hyperthyroidism/hypothyroidism workup and treatment.
2. Surgical management if necessary and only when thyroid disease is well-controlled.

Complications: Double vision from extraocular muscle enlargement and restriction, eyelid retraction, compressive optic neuropathy.

HYF: Risk factors are female sex, age, and smoking. Thyroid eye disease can present in hyperthyroid, hypothyroid, and euthyroid patients.

BACTERIAL KERATITIS/CORNEAL ULCER

A 25-year-old M presents with eye pain and redness. He is a contact lens wearer and sleeps in his contacts. On exam, mucopurulent discharge is present. There is a central round opacity on his cornea with fluorescein staining and hypopyon.

Management:

1. Gram stain, bacterial and fungal culture.
2. Topical broad-spectrum antibiotics.
3. Proper contact lens hygiene instructions.

Complications: Corneal scarring, corneal perforation, permanent vision loss.

HYF: *Pseudomonas*, *S. aureus*, and *Serratia* are the most common causes. Risk factors include contact lens wear and trauma.

VIRAL KERATITIS

A 25-year-old M presents with eye pain, redness, and tearing in 1 eye. On exam, corneal sensation in that eye is decreased. There are branched, tree-like dendritic erosions on fluorescein staining of the affected eye.

Management:

1. Topical trifluridine.
2. Oral antivirals (acyclovir).
3. Consider topical corticosteroids after several days of initiation with antivirals to minimize scarring.
4. Dilated eye exam to rule out retinal involvement.

Complications: Corneal scarring, neurotrophic keratopathy, permanent vision loss.

HYF: HSV and VZV are common causes. Risk factors: HIV, immunocompromise.

20-1 Adult Ophthalmology

FUNGAL KERATITIS

A 25-year-old M with PMH of HIV presents with progressively worsening eye pain, redness, and tearing over the past 2 months. On exam, there is a white stromal infiltrate with feathery borders.

Management:

1. Gram stain, bacterial and fungal culture.
2. Topical antifungal (eg, natamycin, amphotericin B).

Complications: Corneal scarring, corneal perforation, permanent vision loss.

HYF: Mostly seen in immunocompromised states, especially after trauma involving soil.

DACRYOCYSTITIS

A 46-year-old F presents with redness, swelling, and pain under the right eye. On exam, there is a fluctuant, warm mass at the medial canthus with purulent discharge from the punctum when compressed. She is febrile, and labs show leukocytosis.

Management:

1. Systemic antibiotics.
2. Surgical management when quiet after antibiotics.

Complications: Formation of fistulas and abscesses.

HYF: Mostly common causes are *S. aureus* or GBS.

PRESBYOPIA

A 55-year-old F presents with declining vision over the past several years, particularly at near distance. She has difficulty reading fine print.

Management:

1. Refraction and new prescription for reading glasses.

Complications: None.

HYF: Age-related loss of accommodation thought to be due to loss of lens elasticity.

20-2 Eye Trauma

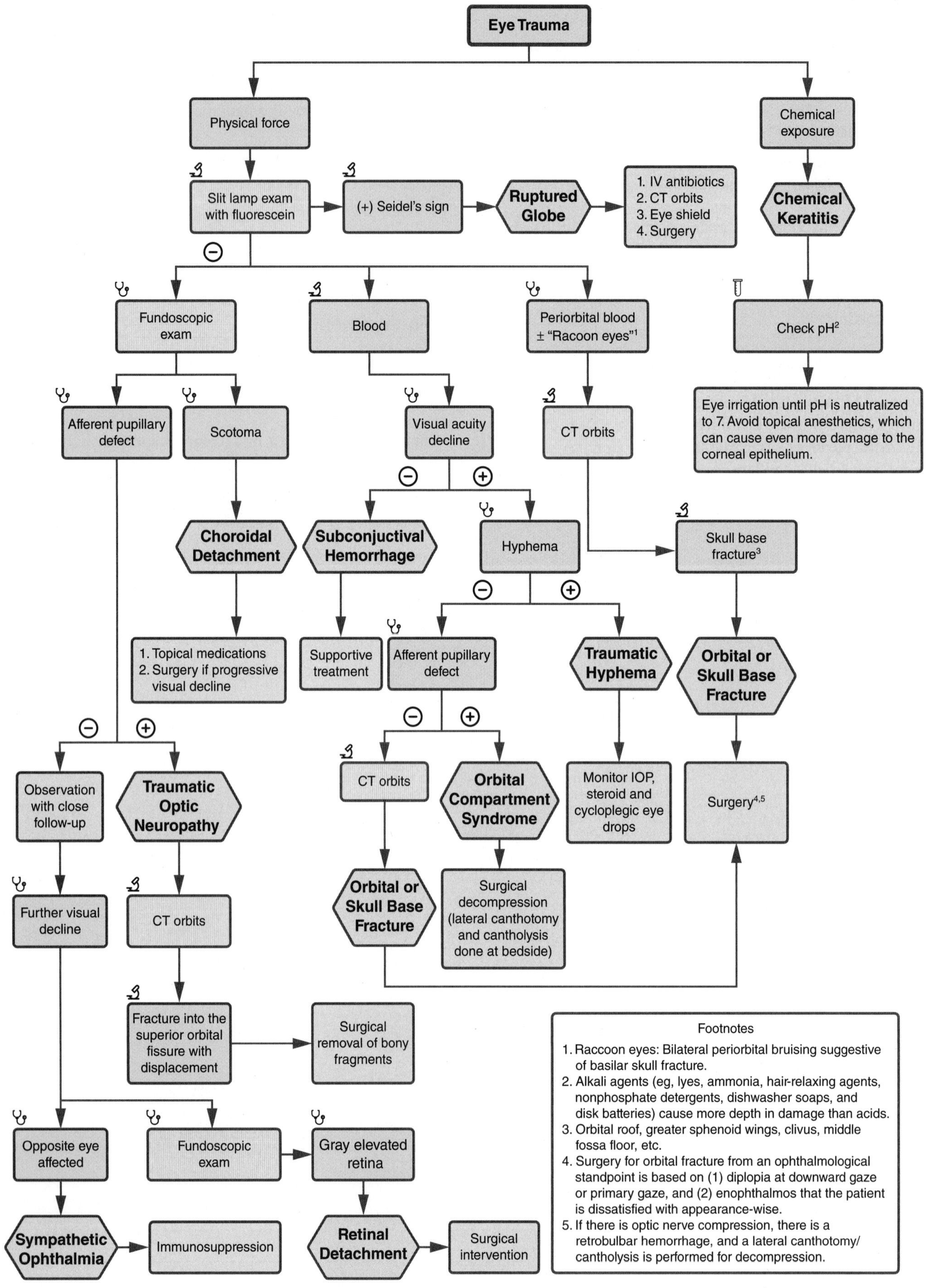
Eye Trauma
Physical force
Chemical exposure
Slit lamp exam with fluorescein
(+) Seidel's sign
Ruptured Globe
1. IV antibiotics
2. CT orbits
3. Eye shield
4. Surgery
Chemical Keratitis
Fundoscopic exam
Blood
Periorbital blood ± "Racoon eyes"[1]
Check pH[2]
Afferent pupillary defect
Scotoma
Visual acuity decline
CT orbits
Eye irrigation until pH is neutralized to 7. Avoid topical anesthetics, which can cause even more damage to the corneal epithelium.
Choroidal Detachment
Subconjuctival Hemorrhage
Hyphema
Skull base fracture[3]
1. Topical medications
2. Surgery if progressive visual decline
Supportive treatment
Afferent pupillary defect
Traumatic Hyphema
Orbital or Skull Base Fracture
Observation with close follow-up
Traumatic Optic Neuropathy
CT orbits
Orbital Compartment Syndrome
Monitor IOP, steroid and cycloplegic eye drops
Surgery[4,5]
Further visual decline
CT orbits
Orbital or Skull Base Fracture
Surgical decompression (lateral canthotomy and cantholysis done at bedside)
Fracture into the superior orbital fissure with displacement
Surgical removal of bony fragments
Opposite eye affected
Fundoscopic exam
Gray elevated retina
Sympathetic Ophthalmia
Immunosuppression
Retinal Detachment
Surgical intervention
Footnotes
1. Raccoon eyes: Bilateral periorbital bruising suggestive of basilar skull fracture.
2. Alkali agents (eg, lyes, ammonia, hair-relaxing agents, nonphosphate detergents, dishwasher soaps, and disk batteries) cause more depth in damage than acids.
3. Orbital roof, greater sphenoid wings, clivus, middle fossa floor, etc.
4. Surgery for orbital fracture from an ophthalmological standpoint is based on (1) diplopia at downward gaze or primary gaze, and (2) enophthalmos that the patient is dissatisfied with appearance-wise.
5. If there is optic nerve compression, there is a retrobulbar hemorrhage, and a lateral canthotomy/cantholysis is performed for decompression.

FIGURE 20.2

20-2 Eye Trauma

SUBCONJUNCTIVAL HEMORRHAGE

A 30-year-old M with PMH of COPD presents with red eye. **Exam** reveals a well-demarcated red patch under the conjunctiva.

Management:

1. Reassurance; self-resolves within 2 weeks.
2. BP management if due to HTN.
3. Coagulopathy workup if recurrent.

Complications: None, as it is a benign condition.

HYF: Can present after physical trauma such as excessive rubbing or Valsalva maneuver (eg, coughing). Patients with coagulopathies are at higher risk and need to be evaluated further if there is recurrence.

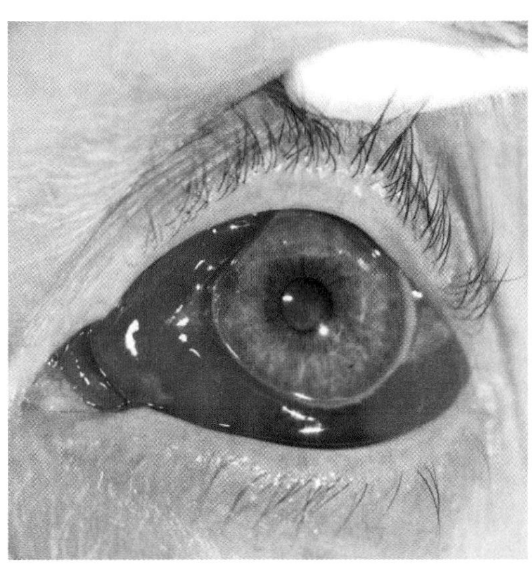

Subconjunctival hemorrhage that completely surrounds the eye.

SYMPATHETIC OPHTHALMIA

A 35-year-old M with PMH of globe rupture in right eye presents with blurry vision, eye pain, and photophobia in the left eye. **Exam** shows conjunctival injection, anterior chamber reaction, and keratic precipitates on the cornea.

Management:

1. Workup to rule out infectious causes.
2. Oral or IV corticosteroids for acute management.
3. Immunomodulators (eg, cyclosporine or azathioprine).

Complications: Vision-threatening disease with 1/2 of patients with 20/40 or worse vision and 1/3 of patients becoming legally blind.

HYF: This is a form of bilateral, granulomatous uveitis from prior uveal antigen exposure. Presentation includes classic findings of uveitis and should be differentiated from Vogt-Koyanagi-Harada syndrome (an autoimmune disease with similar presentation). History of trauma or surgery is key to correct diagnosis, and aggressive treatment is needed.

CHOROIDAL DETACHMENT

A 24-year-old F boxer presents with blurry vision after being hit multiple times in the face. Fundus **exam** shows retinal edema and sub-retinal hemorrhage. On **imaging**, US confirms fluid accumulation in the suprachoroidal space.

Management:

1. Corticosteroids and cycloplegics.
2. Surgical drainage if large; otherwise self-absorbs.

Complications: Poor visual outcome if large and untreated.

HYF: Two types (hemorrhagic vs. serous) exist. Serous is associated with low intraocular pressure, usually from overfiltration after surgery or retinal detachment. Hemorrhagic is most often seen after trauma. Other causes include cancer, certain medications, and inflammation.

TRAUMATIC HYPHEMA

A 17-year-old M presents with pain and blurry vision after a direct hit to the face in a paintball game. On **exam**, blood is present in his anterior chamber, and his pupils are unequal.

Management:

1. Monitor IOP.
2. Steroid and cycloplegic eye drops.
3. Keep head of bed elevated and avoid strenuous activities.

Complications: Increased intraocular pressure, re-bleeding, corneal blood staining, angle recession glaucoma (long-term).

HYF: Hyphema can cause an increase in intraocular pressure due to blockage of aqueous humor drainage. If intraocular pressures are elevated, patients are at higher risk of glaucomatous damage and corneal blood staining. Patients with sickle cell disease require lower intraocular pressure. Consider CT to rule out orbital fracture based on the nature of trauma.

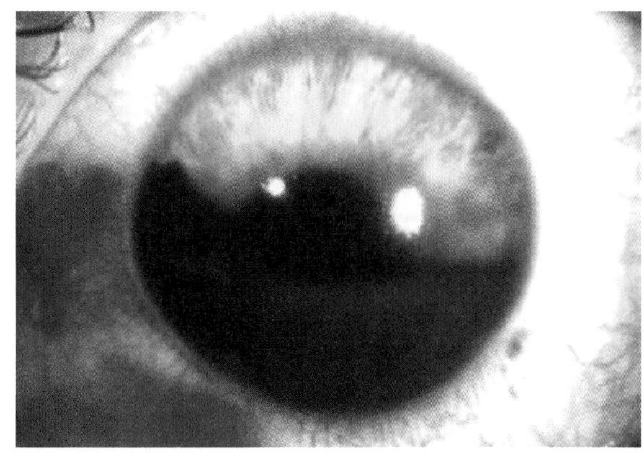

Traumatic hyphema with associated subconjunctival hemorrhage.

(Continued)

20-2 Eye Trauma

GLOBE RUPTURE

A 40-year-old F firefighter presents with decreased vision after she was blasted by an explosion. On exam, there is iris peaking and (+) Seidel's sign on her cornea.

Management:

1. Emergent ophthalmology consult and surgical repair.
2. CT orbit with and without contrast (thin cut) to rule out intraocular foreign body.
3. Prophylactic IV antibiotics.
4. Anti-nausea and pain medications.
5. Tetanus prophylaxis.

Complications:

- Traumatic cataract
- Endophthalmitis
- Retinal detachment and choroidal detachment.

HYF: Signs of globe rupture include 360° bullous subconjunctival hemorrhage, peaked iris, and positive Seidel's sign. Delay in surgical care can increase risk of infection and sympathetic ophthalmia.

ORBITAL/SKULL FRACTURE

A 50-year-old F presents with pain and double vision after a biking accident. On exam, she has significant bruising around the eyes ("raccoon eyes") with crepitus but full eye movements.

Management:

1. CT scan.
2. IOP monitoring for increased intraocular pressure secondary to compression from retrobulbar hemorrhage.
3. Corticosteroids and ice to reduce inflammation.
4. Consult (Ophthalmology, OMFS, or Neurosurgery) for surgical management.

Complications: Persistent double vision and enophthalmos.

HYF: It is important to evaluate extraocular movements to assess for entrapment, which more commonly occurs in children due to greenstick fractures. Crepitus is highly suggestive of this condition. Can simultaneously present with other conditions such as hyphema and optic nerve injury. Full ophthalmic evaluation is recommended. Avoid any actions that increase intra-nasal pressure (eg, nose blowing).

TRAUMATIC OPTIC NEUROPATHY

A 50-year-old M construction worker presents with loss of color vision in the right eye after a fall and direct trauma to the head. On exam, he has an afferent pupillary defect. Fundus exam is normal.

Management:

1. Rule out other causes.
2. CT orbit to rule out bony fragment impingement.
3. Observation.
4. Some studies suggest high-dose steroids (controversial).

Complications: Vision loss.

HYF: Optic nerve atrophy and pallor can take weeks to appear on imaging and exam. Acutely, diagnosis is made clinically. CT orbit is important to rule out bony fragment impingement, which can be reversible with surgery. Otherwise, interventions such as steroids are not proven to be effective.

CHEMICAL KERATITIS

A 21-year-old M presents with eye pain and foreign body sensation after a chemical incident at a research lab. On exam, his conjunctiva appears abnormally white.

Management:

1. Copious irrigation with Morgan lens.
2. pH strip to ensure pH is around 7. If not at 7, continue irrigation.
3. Sweep fornices and flip eyelids to ensure no material left in eye.
4. Topical antibiotic ointment, artificial tears, cycloplegics, and possible steroid eye drops.
5. Emergent ophthalmology consult for follow-up.

Complications:

- Conjunctival ischemia
- Corneal damage/ulcer
- Globe perforation.

HYF: Never use neutralizing agents as they can result in exothermic chemical reactions and exacerbate the injury. Injury with alkali agents penetrates further relative to those with acidic agents. Whitening of the conjunctiva is a worrisome sign as it means there is ischemia and higher risk of poor healing.

Retinal Detachment: See p. 515.

21
Surgery: Transplant

21-1 Transplant Rejection

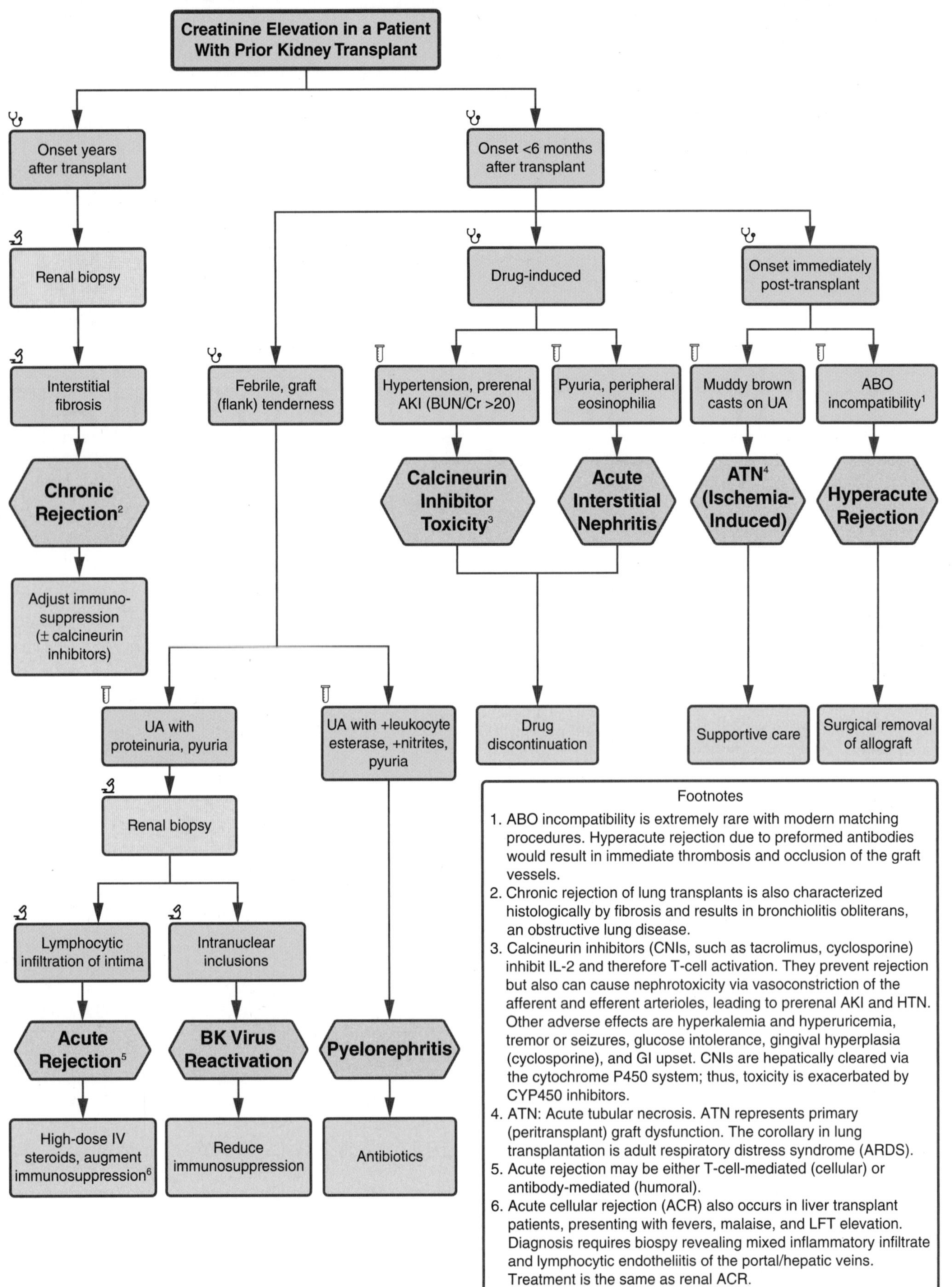
Creatinine Elevation in a Patient With Prior Kidney Transplant
Onset years after transplant
Renal biopsy
Interstitial fibrosis
Chronic Rejection[2]
Adjust immuno-suppression (± calcineurin inhibitors)
Onset <6 months after transplant
Febrile, graft (flank) tenderness
Drug-induced
Onset immediately post-transplant
Hypertension, prerenal AKI (BUN/Cr >20)
Pyuria, peripheral eosinophilia
Muddy brown casts on UA
ABO incompatibility[1]
Calcineurin Inhibitor Toxicity[3]
Acute Interstitial Nephritis
ATN[4] (Ischemia-Induced)
Hyperacute Rejection
UA with proteinuria, pyuria
UA with +leukocyte esterase, +nitrites, pyuria
Drug discontinuation
Supportive care
Surgical removal of allograft
Renal biopsy
Lymphocytic infiltration of intima
Intranuclear inclusions
Acute Rejection[5]
BK Virus Reactivation
Pyelonephritis
High-dose IV steroids, augment immunosuppression[6]
Reduce immunosuppression
Antibiotics

Footnotes

1. ABO incompatibility is extremely rare with modern matching procedures. Hyperacute rejection due to preformed antibodies would result in immediate thrombosis and occlusion of the graft vessels.
2. Chronic rejection of lung transplants is also characterized histologically by fibrosis and results in bronchiolitis obliterans, an obstructive lung disease.
3. Calcineurin inhibitors (CNIs, such as tacrolimus, cyclosporine) inhibit IL-2 and therefore T-cell activation. They prevent rejection but also can cause nephrotoxicity via vasoconstriction of the afferent and efferent arterioles, leading to prerenal AKI and HTN. Other adverse effects are hyperkalemia and hyperuricemia, tremor or seizures, glucose intolerance, gingival hyperplasia (cyclosporine), and GI upset. CNIs are hepatically cleared via the cytochrome P450 system; thus, toxicity is exacerbated by CYP450 inhibitors.
4. ATN: Acute tubular necrosis. ATN represents primary (peritransplant) graft dysfunction. The corollary in lung transplantation is adult respiratory distress syndrome (ARDS).
5. Acute rejection may be either T-cell-mediated (cellular) or antibody-mediated (humoral).
6. Acute cellular rejection (ACR) also occurs in liver transplant patients, presenting with fevers, malaise, and LFT elevation. Diagnosis requires biospy revealing mixed inflammatory infiltrate and lymphocytic endotheliitis of the portal/hepatic veins. Treatment is the same as renal ACR.

FIGURE 21.1

21-1 Transplant Rejection

INFECTION PROPHYLAXIS

A 41-year-old F with PMH of ESRD due to lupus nephritis on dialysis presents for evaluation for possible renal transplant.

Management:

1. Pre-transplant testing: UA, CXR, serologies (CMV, HSV, VZV, EBV, HIV, HBV, HCV, *Treponema pallidum*, measles, mumps, rubella), TB test.
2. Treat all active infections.
3. Vaccines: PCV13 and PPSV23 (pneumococcal), annual influenza, HBV (plus any vaccines not up-to-date).
4. Post-transplant prophylaxis: TMP-SMX for *Pneumocystis jirovecii*, valganciclovir/ganciclovir for CMV and routine CMV viral load monitoring.

Complications: Side effects from antibiotics used for infection prophylaxis (eg, nausea, diarrhea, allergic reactions).

HYF: Live vaccines should be avoided in immunocompromised hosts. Prophylactic regimen will need to be tailored to each patient based on exposures, comorbidities, and the organ being transplanted.

IMMUNOSUPPRESSION IN SOLID ORGAN TRANSPLANTS

A 41-year-old F with PMH of ESRD due to lupus nephritis on dialysis is admitted for renal transplantation.

Management:

1. Induction immunosuppression: Rabbit anti-thymocyte globulin (adverse effects include infusion reactions, serum sickness, and cytopenias) or basiliximab (IL-2 receptor antagonist).
2. Maintenance immunosuppression (regimen varies based on patient/donor risk stratification): Prednisone, calcineurin inhibitor (tacrolimus or cyclosporine), antimetabolite (azathioprine or mycophenolate).
3. Regular laboratory monitoring for infection, drug toxicity, and graft dysfunction or rejection.

Complications:

- Opportunistic infections (eg, *Pneumocystis carinii* pneumonia; viral infections such as CMV, EBV, BK polyomavirus, JC polyomavirus; fungal infections such as aspergillosis, histoplasmosis, cryptococcal meningitis, blastomycosis, coccidioidomycosis).
- Post-transplant malignancy (eg, non-Hodgkin lymphoma, squamous cell carcinoma of the skin, Kaposi sarcoma, anal or vulval carcinoma, hepatocellular carcinoma).

HYF: In the early post-transplant period (3–6 months), intense immunosuppression is required. Induction therapy involves anti-T-lymphocyte antibodies, both lymphocyte-depleting antibodies (thymoglobulin) and non-depleting antibodies (basiliximab). Maintenance therapy often involves a 3-drug regimen consisting of systemic steroids, a calcineurin inhibitor (eg, tacrolimus, cyclosporine), and antiproliferative agents (eg, sirolimus, mycophenolate mofetil, azathioprine). Long-term management of solid organ transplants includes monitoring for the adverse effects of immunosuppressive therapy.

ACUTE RENAL TRANSPLANT REJECTION

A 58-year-old M with PMH of ESRD s/p deceased donor kidney transplantation 5 months ago presents to clinic with Cr 1.8 (baseline ~1.0). Renal biopsy reveals lymphocytic infiltrate.

Management:

1. Pulse-dose IV glucocorticoids.
2. Rabbit anti-thymocyte globulin for T-cell-mediated rejection.
3. Plasmapheresis, IVIG, and/or rituximab for antibody-mediated rejection.

Complications:

- Recurrent rejection.
- Graft loss.
- Long-term allograft dysfunction.

HYF: Acute transplant rejection can be asymptomatic and may present with only elevated Cr/LFTs. Biopsy is required to confirm the diagnosis and distinguish from BK virus reactivation. Repeated episodes of acute rejection (weeks to months) can lead to chronic graft dysfunction (months to years).

CHRONIC RENAL TRANSPLANT REJECTION

A 58-year-old M with PMH of ESRD s/p deceased donor kidney transplantation 2 years ago presents to clinic with Cr 1.8 (baseline ~1.0) and hypertension. Renal biopsy reveals interstitial fibrosis with intimal thickening and tubular atrophy.

Management:

1. Optimize immunosuppression.
2. Reduce dose of calcineurin inhibitor.
3. Repeat transplant for ESRD.

Complications: Progression to ESRD, hypertension, proteinuria.

HYF: Type II and IV hypersensitivity reaction due to CD4+ T cells attacking host antigen-presenting cells. Differentiate chronic and acute rejection via time course and biopsy findings.

PNEUMOCYSTIS PNEUMONIA (PCP)

A 61-year-old F with PMH of alcoholic cirrhosis s/p liver transplant 8 months ago, who has been poorly compliant with her TMP-SMX prophylaxis, presents with 2 weeks of dry cough and fever. On **imaging**, CXR shows bilateral diffuse interstitial infiltrates. Sputum microscopy shows *Pneumocystis jirovecii.*

Management:

1. TMP-SMX (recommend sensitization if allergic).
2. Supportive care and prevent ventilator barotrauma.
3. Corticosteroids for moderate-severe ARDS (PaO_2 <70, A-a gradient ≥35 mmHg, or SpO_2 <92%).

21-1 Transplant Rejection

Solid Organ Transplant Rejection

Type	Onset	Mechanism	Treatment
Hyperacute	Immediate	Preformed antibodies react to donor tissue due to ABO incompatibility and activate the complement system. Presents during surgery with thrombosis of graft vessels and tissue ischemia. Type II hypersensitivity.	Graft removal.
Acute (most common)	Weeks to months (usually <6 months)	Cellular and humoral response against donor MHC (class I or II), leading to leukocyte infiltration of graft vessels and graft destruction. Type IV hypersensitivity.	Cytotoxic agents, corticosteroids.
Chronic	Months to years	Chronic cellular and humoral immune response, leading to intimal thickening, interstitial fibrosis, parenchymal atrophy, and gradual loss of graft function. Refractory to immunosuppressants. Types II and IV hypersensitivity.	Minimize episodes of acute rejection. Consider new organ transplant.

Complications: Fulminant hypoxic respiratory failure.

HYF: *Pneumocystis jirovecii* cannot be cultured, and so it must be visualized on direct microscopy of sputum or bronchoalveolar lavage. For PCP prophylaxis, TMP-SMX (or dapsone and atovaquone if sulfa allergy) is recommended lifelong for lung transplant recipients and 6–12 months after other solid organ transplants.

CMV PNEUMONITIS

A 21-year-old M with PMH of cystic fibrosis s/p lung transplant 2 months ago presents with 2 days of dyspnea and dry cough. On **imaging**, CXR shows patchy opacities. **Labs** show elevated CMV viral load on plasma PCR. Transbronchial biopsy reveals CMV inclusion bodies.

Management:

1. Oral valganciclovir (or IV ganciclovir if severe).
2. Consider reducing immunosuppression.
3. Monitor CMV viral load.

Complications:

- Other tissue-invasive diseases (eg, pancytopenia from bone marrow involvement, bloody diarrhea with shallow ulcers on colonoscopy in CMV colitis).
- Long-term allograft dysfunction and early mortality.

HYF: Lung biopsy is required to distinguish CMV pneumonitis and acute allograft rejection. CMV pneumonitis may be distinguished from other opportunistic pulmonary infections by the lack of hemoptysis (vs. *Aspergillosis*) and the acute onset (vs. the more indolent PCP).

CALCINEURIN INHIBITOR TOXICITY

A 54-year-old F with PMH of ESRD s/p renal transplant 6 months ago presents with decreased urine output and dental changes. On **exam**, she has gingival hyperplasia and costovertebral angle tenderness. **Labs** show BUN of 38 and a Cr of 6.5 (baseline of 2.8).

Management:

1. Discontinue cyclosporine.
2. Try a different calcineurin inhibitor.

Complications:

- Nephrotoxicity leading to graft failure.
- Diabetes mellitus.
- Neurotoxicity.

HYF: The probability of having neurotoxic and nephrotoxic effects increases if you take multiple calcineurin inhibitors simultaneously.

HYPERACUTE REJECTION 2/2 ABO INCOMPATIBILITY

A 29-year-old F with PMH of lupus nephritis complicated by ESRD is admitted for renal transplant. In the operating room, she becomes tachycardic and hypotensive within minutes of anastomosing the donor kidney to the patient's renal vessels. Dark red urine is seen draining from the Foley catheter.

Management:

1. Remove the graft.
2. Supportive care.

Complications:

- Graft failure.
- Hypotension.
- Shock.
- Death.

HYF: Can be prevented with a preoperative blood type and cross. ABO incompatibility results from type 2 hypersensitivity reaction (preformed host antibodies against donor RBCs), causing small vessel thrombi that lead to graft failure.

22
Surgery: Anesthesia

22-1 Anesthesia

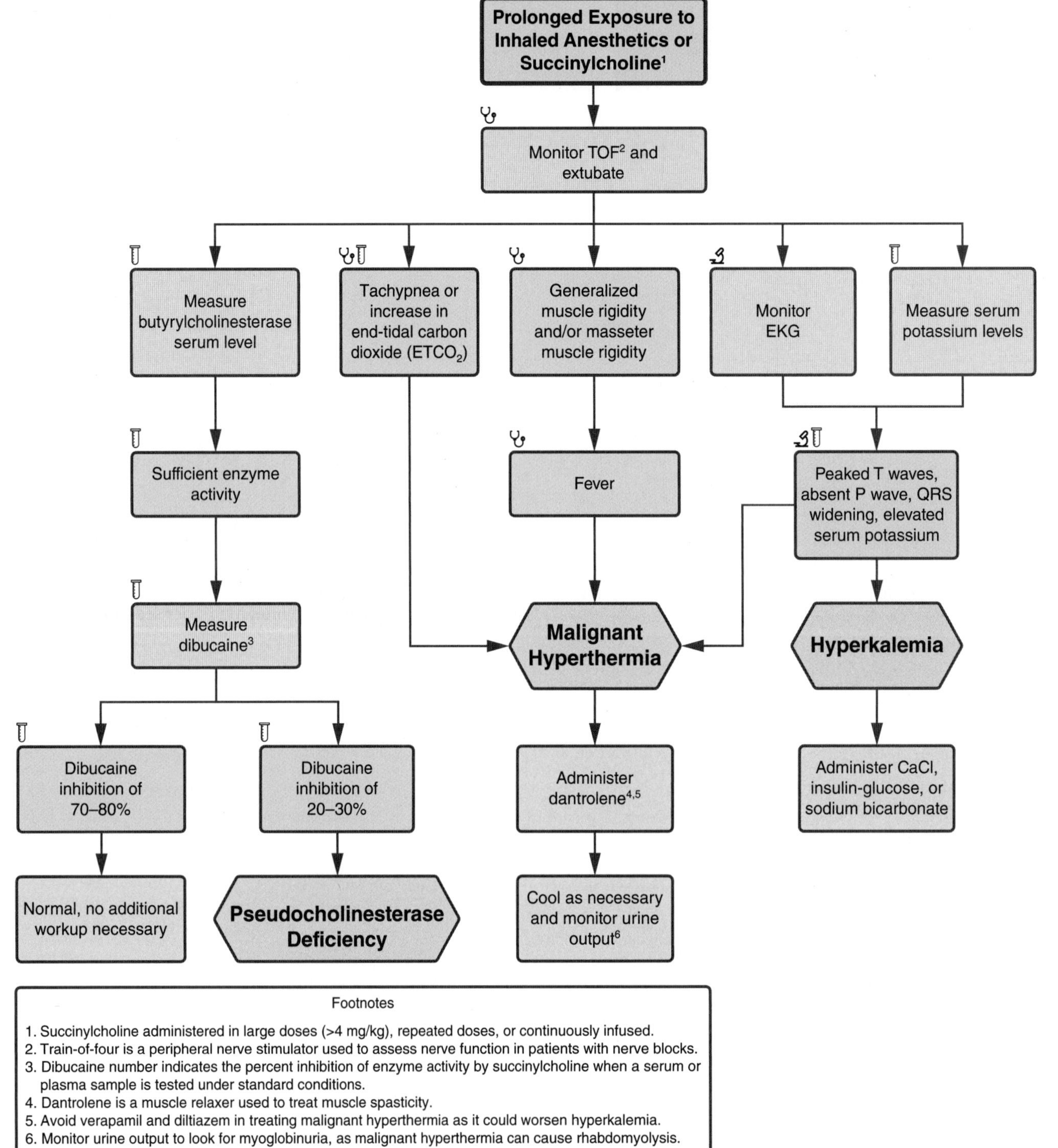
Prolonged Exposure to Inhaled Anesthetics or Succinylcholine[1]
Monitor TOF[2] and extubate
Measure butyrylcholinesterase serum level
Tachypnea or increase in end-tidal carbon dioxide ($ETCO_2$)
Generalized muscle rigidity and/or masseter muscle rigidity
Monitor EKG
Measure serum potassium levels
Sufficient enzyme activity
Fever
Peaked T waves, absent P wave, QRS widening, elevated serum potassium
Measure dibucaine[3]
Malignant Hyperthermia
Hyperkalemia
Dibucaine inhibition of 70–80%
Dibucaine inhibition of 20–30%
Administer dantrolene[4,5]
Administer CaCl, insulin-glucose, or sodium bicarbonate
Normal, no additional workup necessary
Pseudocholinesterase Deficiency
Cool as necessary and monitor urine output[6]

Footnotes

1. Succinylcholine administered in large doses (>4 mg/kg), repeated doses, or continuously infused.
2. Train-of-four is a peripheral nerve stimulator used to assess nerve function in patients with nerve blocks.
3. Dibucaine number indicates the percent inhibition of enzyme activity by succinylcholine when a serum or plasma sample is tested under standard conditions.
4. Dantrolene is a muscle relaxer used to treat muscle spasticity.
5. Avoid verapamil and diltiazem in treating malignant hyperthermia as it could worsen hyperkalemia.
6. Monitor urine output to look for myoglobinuria, as malignant hyperthermia can cause rhabdomyolysis.

FIGURE 22.1

22-1 Anesthesia

OPIOID OVERDOSE

A 27-year-old F presents to the ED with decreased HR, BP, and respiratory depression on exam. She is non-responsive to questions, and she has pinpoint pupils. After looking in the emergency medical record, she has recently sought treatment at the local crisis center for unspecified substance use disorder.

Management:

1. Administer naloxone (0.4–0.8 mg). Depending on symptom recovery, administer additional doses. After 10 mg total, consider other reasons for respiratory depression.
2. Obtain serum glucose, EKG, and CXR to rule out hypoglycemia, methadone or loperamide toxicity, and/or acute lung injury.
3. Monitor respiration with bedside end-tidal CO_2 monitor.

Complications: Common side effects of naloxone include nausea, diarrhea, fever, and body aches. More severe side effects include cardiac arrhythmias, dyspnea, pulmonary edema, and seizures.

HYF:

- When treating an opioid overdose, administer naloxone in increasing doses or frequency until symptoms reverse.
- In patients with opioid dependence, use initial dose of 0.1–0.2 mg to avoid acute withdrawal or if there are concerns with concurrent stimulant overdose.

MALIGNANT HYPERTHERMIA

A 51-year-old M presents for a laparoscopic cholecystectomy. His medical history includes HTN, GERD, and osteoarthritis. Previous surgery for a foot repair was uneventful. The patient denies any personal or family history of anesthetic complications. After premedication, anesthesia is induced with 100 μg fentanyl, 50 mg lidocaine, 200 mg propofol, and 160 mg succinylcholine at 7:30 a.m. A rapid intubation is performed. The operation is successful with no complications, and the patient is admitted in stable condition to the ward. There was no dysuria, but the patient begins to complain of muscle aches and stiffness in the jaw, neck, and lower back at approximately 9:20 a.m.

Management:

1. Administer dantrolene for muscle spasticity, and monitor HR.
2. Initiate cooling measures.
3. Contact local malignant hyperthermia hotline and begin workup, including creatine kinase, basic metabolic panel, and urinalysis.

Complications: If not treated promptly, malignant hyperthermia can cause rhabdomyolysis, kidney failure, and death.

HYF: Generalized muscle rigidity and especially masseter rigidity following administration of succinylcholine is a red flag for malignant hyperthermia.

PSEUDOCHOLINESTERASE (PCHE) DEFICIENCY

A 72-year-old F presents for a parotidectomy. Endotracheal intubation is facilitated with succinylcholine. General anesthesia is induced with 200 mg propofol and 100 mg lidocaine IV. Muscle paralysis is confirmed with a peripheral nerve stimulator via a train-of-four (TOF) technique without any twitch. The serum PChE during surgery was deficient at 1000 IU/L. After 6 hours of general anesthesia, an acceptable TOF was obtained. Propofol infusion was terminated and endotracheal tube removed.

Management:

1. Maintain mechanical ventilation under sedation while paralytic is cleared.
2. If paralytic reversal is necessary, fresh frozen plasma or exogenous RBC can be administered.
3. If pseudocholinesterase deficiency is uncertain, continue with dibucaine number and genetic testing.

Complications: Anticholinesterase agents inhibit PChE activity and can lead to worsening of paralysis.

HYF:

- In cases of prolonged paralysis, measure PChE during surgery and post-op. Confirm PChE deficiency with dibucaine number and genetic testing.
- If reversal is necessary, transfuse the patient with plasma or RBC.

23 Pediatrics

23-1 Early Childhood Well-Child Check

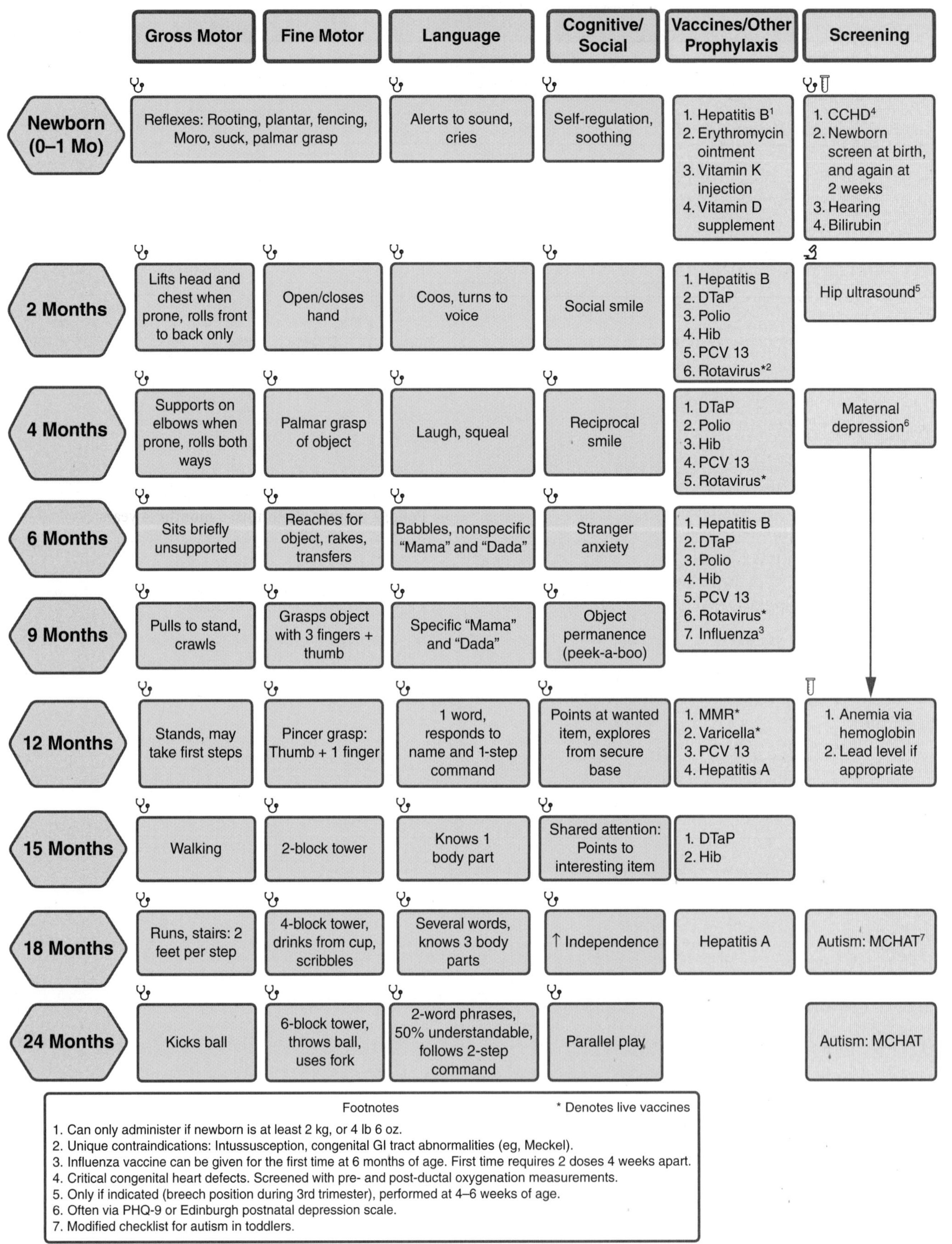
Well-Child Check 0–24 Months
Developmental Milestones
Gross Motor
Fine Motor
Language
Cognitive/ Social
Vaccines/Other Prophylaxis
Screening
Newborn (0–1 Mo)
Reflexes: Rooting, plantar, fencing, Moro, suck, palmar grasp
Alerts to sound, cries
Self-regulation, soothing
1. Hepatitis B1 2. Erythromycin ointment 3. Vitamin K injection 4. Vitamin D supplement
1. CCHD4 2. Newborn screen at birth, and again at 2 weeks 3. Hearing 4. Bilirubin
2 Months
Lifts head and chest when prone, rolls front to back only
Open/closes hand
Coos, turns to voice
Social smile
1. Hepatitis B 2. DTaP 3. Polio 4. Hib 5. PCV 13 6. Rotavirus*2
Hip ultrasound5
4 Months
Supports on elbows when prone, rolls both ways
Palmar grasp of object
Laugh, squeal
Reciprocal smile
1. DTaP 2. Polio 3. Hib 4. PCV 13 5. Rotavirus*
Maternal depression6
6 Months
Sits briefly unsupported
Reaches for object, rakes, transfers
Babbles, nonspecific "Mama" and "Dada"
Stranger anxiety
1. Hepatitis B 2. DTaP 3. Polio 4. Hib 5. PCV 13 6. Rotavirus* 7. Influenza3
9 Months
Pulls to stand, crawls
Grasps object with 3 fingers + thumb
Specific "Mama" and "Dada"
Object permanence (peek-a-boo)
12 Months
Stands, may take first steps
Pincer grasp: Thumb + 1 finger
1 word, responds to name and 1-step command
Points at wanted item, explores from secure base
1. MMR* 2. Varicella* 3. PCV 13 4. Hepatitis A
1. Anemia via hemoglobin 2. Lead level if appropriate
15 Months
Walking
2-block tower
Knows 1 body part
Shared attention: Points to interesting item
1. DTaP 2. Hib
18 Months
Runs, stairs: 2 feet per step
4-block tower, drinks from cup, scribbles
Several words, knows 3 body parts
↑ Independence
Hepatitis A
Autism: MCHAT7
24 Months
Kicks ball
6-block tower, throws ball, uses fork
2-word phrases, 50% understandable, follows 2-step command
Parallel play
Autism: MCHAT
Footnotes
* Denotes live vaccines
1. Can only administer if newborn is at least 2 kg, or 4 lb 6 oz.
2. Unique contraindications: Intussusception, congenital GI tract abnormalities (eg, Meckel).
3. Influenza vaccine can be given for the first time at 6 months of age. First time requires 2 doses 4 weeks apart.
4. Critical congenital heart defects. Screened with pre- and post-ductal oxygenation measurements.
5. Only if indicated (breech position during 3rd trimester), performed at 4–6 weeks of age.
6. Often via PHQ-9 or Edinburgh postnatal depression scale.
7. Modified checklist for autism in toddlers.

FIGURE 23.1

23-1 Early Childhood Well-Child Check

EARLY CHILDHOOD WELL-CHILD CHECK (1 MONTH–2 YEARS)

Screening:

1. Anemia screen: Once between 9–15 months, higher risk if child drinks >24 oz of cow's milk per day. Usually, anemia is due to iron deficiency → treat with iron supplementation.
2. Lead screen: If home was built before 1978, there is risk of lead-based paint, which can cause developmental delay. Can also present with constipation, abdominal pain, petechiae (thrombocytopenia), anemia, and lead lines on gingiva. Treatment for lead poisoning: Succimer, dimercaprol, EDTA.
3. Tuberculosis screening if any of the following risk factors: Immunosuppression, clinical suspicion, recent immigration from endemic area, or contact with individuals who are HIV+, homeless, or have active TB.
4. Autism screen: At 18 and 24 months. If screen is positive, refer to early intervention services.

Normal Developmental Screening: Screen at every well-child visit and/or if any concerns arise.

- 2 months: Social smile.
- 4 months: Reciprocal smile, recognizes voices.
- 6 months: Can sit up, roll over, stranger anxiety.
- 9 months: Pull to stand, crawl, object permanence.
- 1 year old: Walks, points to objects.
- 2 years old: **"rule of 2's"** - **200** words, **2**-word sentences, **50%** understandable by a stranger, parallel play.

Anticipatory Guidance:

- Teething: Starts between 4–6 months, can offer teething rings or toys, fluoride varnish at each well-child check, brush or wipe gums 2 times daily.
- Toilet training: Usually starts at >18 months of age.
- Tantrums: Start at age 2 years, regular routines can help, ignore behaviors unless dangerous to self or others, positive reinforcement of good behaviors.
- Nutrition: Wean off the bottle by 12 months of age for dental health, transition from breastmilk or formula to whole milk by 12 months, introduce common allergens (tree nuts, peanuts, egg) around 4–6 months.
- Physical activity: Safe play, taking turns.
- Safety: Windows, water safety, chemicals/medications in locked storage, firearm storage safety, and proper car seat use.

Vaccines:

- Hepatitis B: Newborn, 2 months, 4 months, 6 months.
- Hepatitis A: 12 months, 18 months.
- DTaP (Diphtheria, Tetanus, and acellular Pertussis): 2 months, 4 months, 6 months, 4 years, and 11 years.
- Hib (*Haemophilus influenzae* B): 2 months, 4 months, 6 months, 15 months.
- PCV13 (pneumococcal): 2 months, 4 months, 6 months, 12 months.
- MMR* (measles, mumps, rubella): 12 months, 4 years.
- Varicella*: 12 months, 4 years.
- Flu: Give annually, first dose requires 2 shots 4 weeks apart and can be given starting at age 6 months.
- Polio: 2 months, 4 months, 6 months, 4 years.
- Rotavirus*: 2 months, 4 months, 6 months.
- *Live vaccines:
  - Unique contraindications include severe immunodeficiency and pregnancy.
  - Household contacts of pregnant persons can still obtain a live vaccine.
- General contraindications for vaccines:
  - Anaphylaxis to that vaccine previously.
  - Current fever.
  - Egg allergy is not a contraindication.

23-2 Middle Childhood and Adolescent Well-Child Check

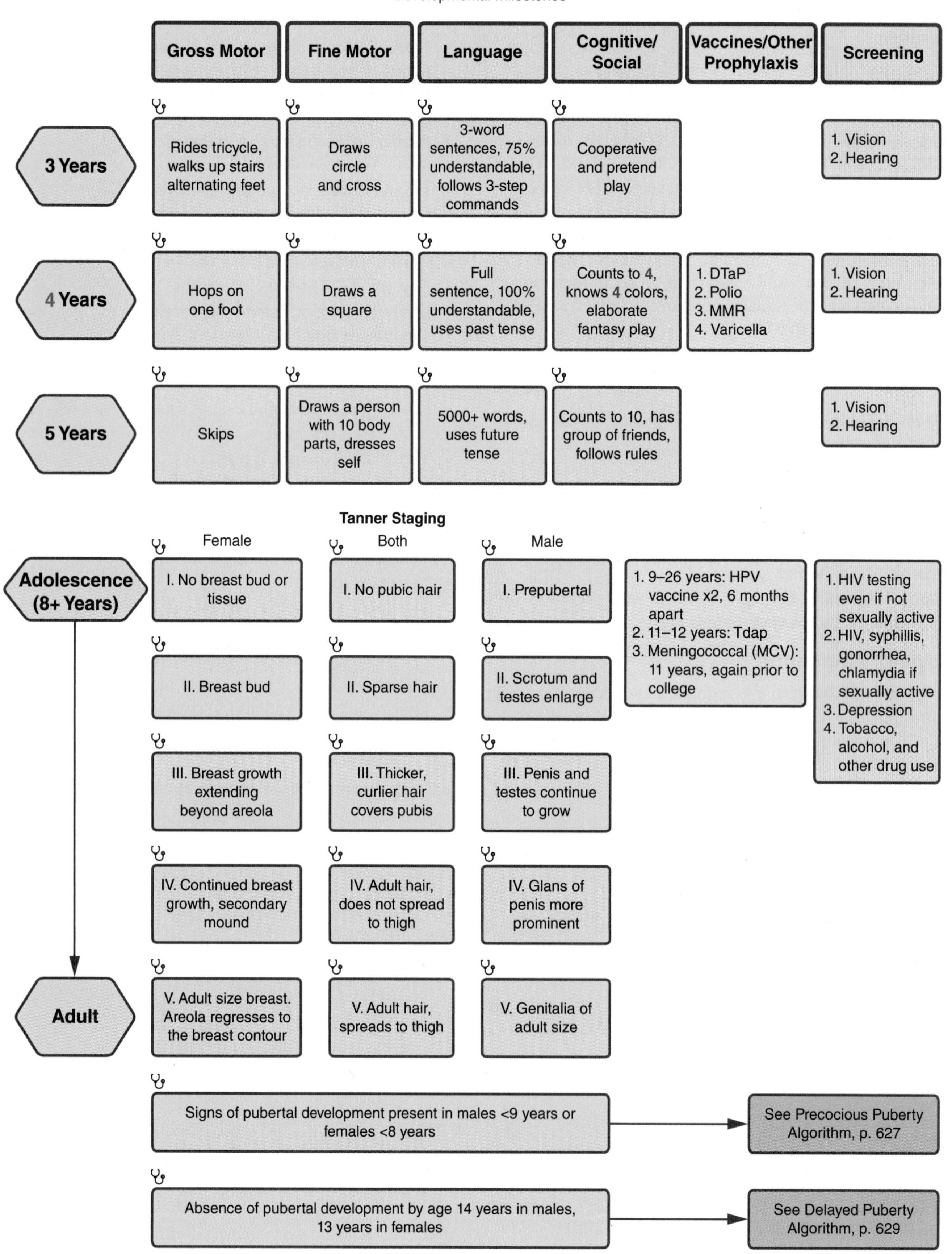
Well-Child Check: 3+ Years
Developmental Milestones
Gross Motor
Fine Motor
Language
Cognitive/ Social
Vaccines/Other Prophylaxis
Screening
3 Years
Rides tricycle, walks up stairs alternating feet
Draws circle and cross
3-word sentences, 75% understandable, follows 3-step commands
Cooperative and pretend play
1. Vision
2. Hearing
4 Years
Hops on one foot
Draws a square
Full sentence, 100% understandable, uses past tense
Counts to 4, knows 4 colors, elaborate fantasy play
1. DTaP
2. Polio
3. MMR
4. Varicella
1. Vision
2. Hearing
5 Years
Skips
Draws a person with 10 body parts, dresses self
5000+ words, uses future tense
Counts to 10, has group of friends, follows rules
1. Vision
2. Hearing
Tanner Staging
Female
Both
Male
Adolescence (8+ Years)
I. No breast bud or tissue
I. No pubic hair
I. Prepubertal
1. 9–26 years: HPV vaccine x2, 6 months apart
2. 11–12 years: Tdap
3. Meningococcal (MCV): 11 years, again prior to college
1. HIV testing even if not sexually active
2. HIV, syphillis, gonorrhea, chlamydia if sexually active
3. Depression
4. Tobacco, alcohol, and other drug use
II. Breast bud
II. Sparse hair
II. Scrotum and testes enlarge
III. Breast growth extending beyond areola
III. Thicker, curlier hair covers pubis
III. Penis and testes continue to grow
IV. Continued breast growth, secondary mound
IV. Adult hair, does not spread to thigh
IV. Glans of penis more prominent
Adult
V. Adult size breast. Areola regresses to the breast contour
V. Adult hair, spreads to thigh
V. Genitalia of adult size
Signs of pubertal development present in males <9 years or females <8 years
See Precocious Puberty Algorithm, p. 627
Absence of pubertal development by age 14 years in males, 13 years in females
See Delayed Puberty Algorithm, p. 629

FIGURE 23.2

23-2 Middle Childhood and Adolescent Well-Child Check

MIDDLE CHILDHOOD WELL-CHILD CHECK (3–10 YEARS OLD)

Screening:

1. Blood pressure: If elevated, repeat ambulatory monitoring.
2. Vision and hearing at 3-year and 4-year visits: Refer to ophthalmology or audiology as needed.
3. BMI: If elevated, refer to nutritionist, keep food diary, address physical activity, and consider screening labs: Hemoglobin A1C (type II diabetes), ALT (NAFLD), fasting lipid panel (dyslipidemia).

Developmental/Psychosocial Screening:

- 3 years old **"rule of 3's"**: **1000** words, 3-word sentences, cooperative play, ride tricycle, 75% understandable by a stranger.
- 4 years old: Hop on 1 foot, draw circle or line, cooperative play, use full sentences.
- Autism: Refer for formal evaluation if concerns on initial screening.
- Attention deficit hyperactivity disorder: Difficulty in **2 settings** (ie, school and home), inattention, impulsivity, hyperactivity.
  - Rule out vision and hearing issues, inadequate sleep (eg, OSA), and absence seizures first.

Anticipatory Guidance:

- Seat belt and helmet use.
- Limit fast food.
- Encourage fruits and veggies.
- Physical activity.
- Limit screen time.
- Sleep hygiene.
- Water safety (swim lessons early).
- Start of sexual development as early as age 8–9.

Vaccines:

- Annual influenza vaccine.
- COVID-19 vaccine (ages 5+).

ADOLESCENT WELL-CHILD CHECK (11–18 YEARS OLD)

Screening:

1. HIV (other STIs):
   a. All patients get a **one-time HIV screen** if not sexually active.
   b. **If sexually active, screen for gonorrhea, chlamydia, HIV, and syphilis, and consider herpes (if history positive and lesions).**
2. BMI: If elevated, refer to nutritionist, keep food diary, address physical activity, and consider screening labs: Hemoglobin A1C (type II diabetes), ALT (NAFLD), fasting lipid panel (dyslipidemia).
3. Blood pressure: If elevated, repeat ambulatory monitoring.
4. Vision/hearing: Refer to ophthalmology or audiology as needed.
5. Tobacco, alcohol, substance use: CRAFFT questionnaire (Car, Relax, Alone, Forget, Friends, Trouble).
6. Depression (ages 12+ or if concerned): PHQ-9 (patient health questionnaire), GAD-7 (generalized anxiety disorder).
7. Hepatitis C: **All patients age 18+ get a one-time screening** unless they have additional risk factors.
8. Dyslipidemia via fasting lipid panel.

Developmental Screening: Tanner staging.

Anticipatory Guidance:

- Puberty (in order): Thelarche, pubarche, menarche.
  - Precocious puberty: Age 8 years or younger in females, age 9 years or younger in males.
- Safe sex/contraception: Barrier use AND additional contraception with each intercourse. STI testing after each new partner or if concerns. Use shared decision-making when choosing contraception method. Options from most to least effective: etonogestrel implant, copper or levonorgestrel IUD, permanent sterilization, progesterone injection, and combined or progestin only oral contraceptives. IUDs can also provide emergency contraception.
- Physical activity.
- Limiting screen time.
- Limit fast food, increase fruits and veggies.
- Sleep hygiene.
- Gun safety.

Vaccines:

- Annual influenza vaccine.
- COVID 19 vaccine.
- HPV: 2 doses.
- Tdap booster at age 11 years.
- Meningococcal.

23-2 Middle Childhood and Adolescent Well-Child Check

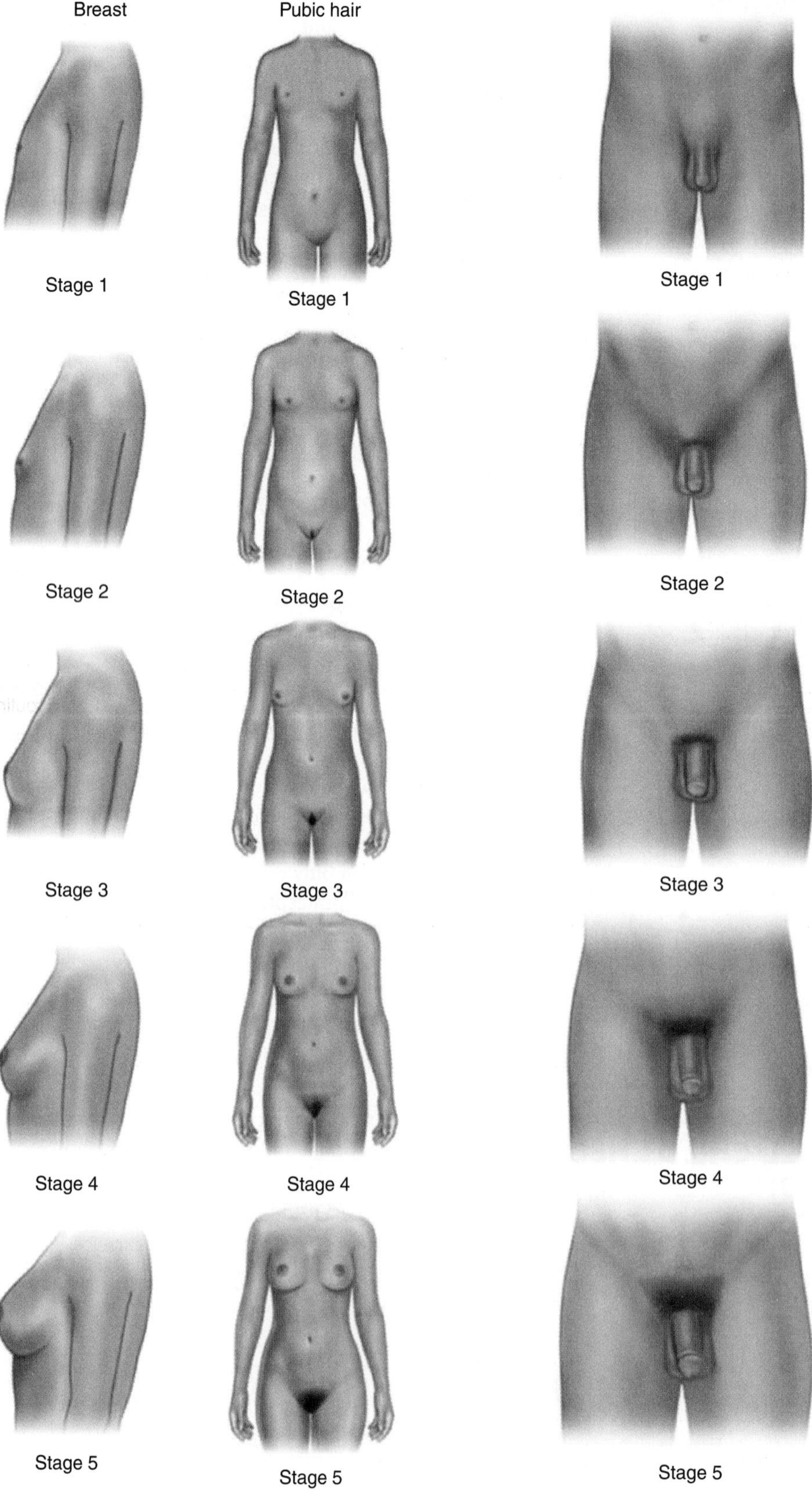
Breast
Pubic hair
Stage 1
Stage 1
Stage 1
Stage 2
Stage 2
Stage 2
Stage 3
Stage 3
Stage 3
Stage 4
Stage 4
Stage 4
Stage 5
Stage 5
Stage 5

Tanner staging of pubertal development.

23-3 Term and Preterm Infant Care

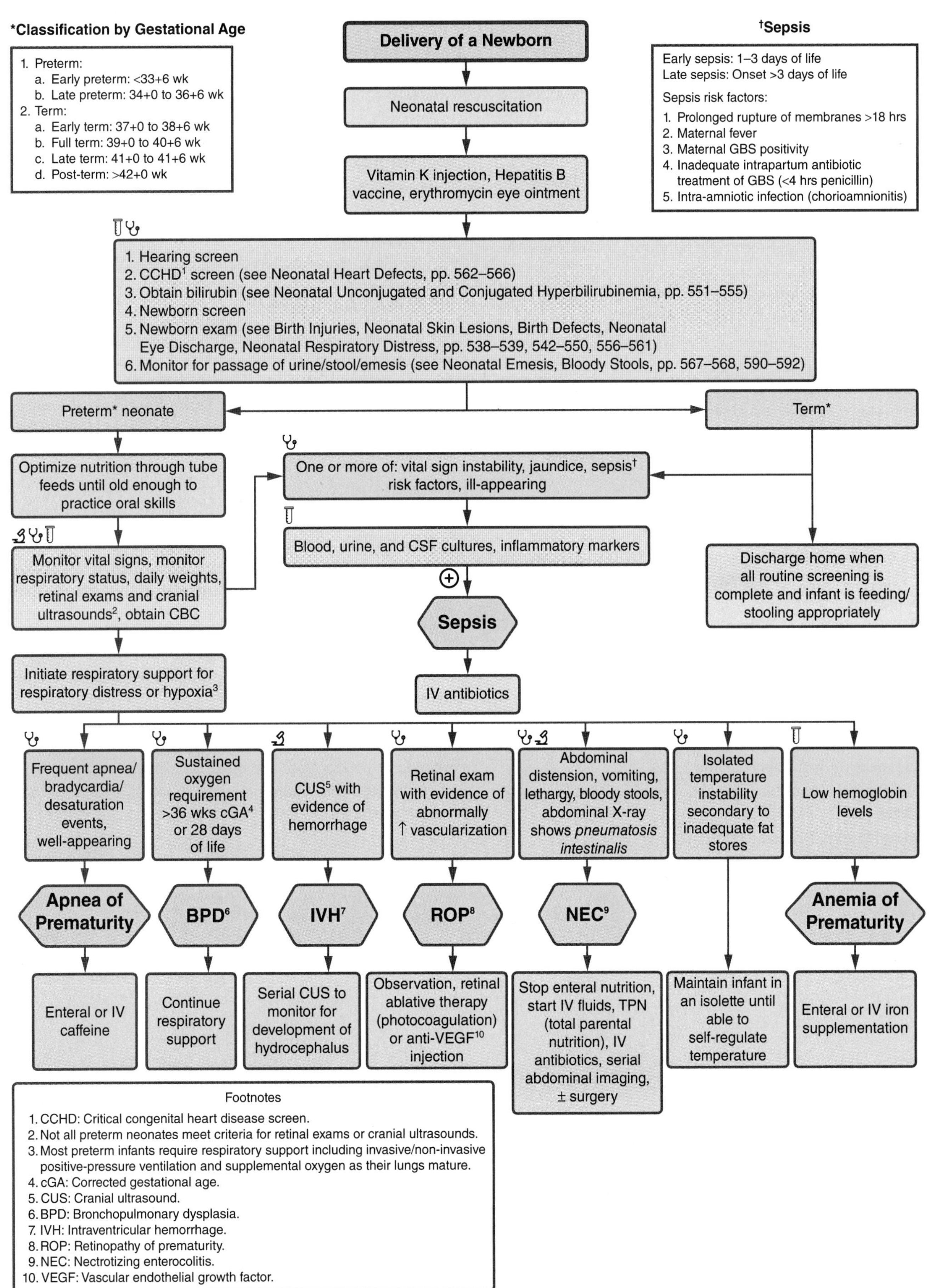

*Classification by Gestational Age
1. Preterm:
a. Early preterm: <33+6 wk
b. Late preterm: 34+0 to 36+6 wk
2. Term:
a. Early term: 37+0 to 38+6 wk
b. Full term: 39+0 to 40+6 wk
c. Late term: 41+0 to 41+6 wk
d. Post-term: >42+0 wk
Delivery of a Newborn
Neonatal rescuscitation
Vitamin K injection, Hepatitis B vaccine, erythromycin eye ointment
†Sepsis
Early sepsis: 1–3 days of life
Late sepsis: Onset >3 days of life
Sepsis risk factors:
1. Prolonged rupture of membranes >18 hrs
2. Maternal fever
3. Maternal GBS positivity
4. Inadequate intrapartum antibiotic treatment of GBS (<4 hrs penicillin)
5. Intra-amniotic infection (chorioamnionitis)
1. Hearing screen
2. CCHD[1] screen (see Neonatal Heart Defects, pp. 562–566)
3. Obtain bilirubin (see Neonatal Unconjugated and Conjugated Hyperbilirubinemia, pp. 551–555)
4. Newborn screen
5. Newborn exam (see Birth Injuries, Neonatal Skin Lesions, Birth Defects, Neonatal Eye Discharge, Neonatal Respiratory Distress, pp. 538–539, 542–550, 556–561)
6. Monitor for passage of urine/stool/emesis (see Neonatal Emesis, Bloody Stools, pp. 567–568, 590–592)
Preterm* neonate
Term*
Optimize nutrition through tube feeds until old enough to practice oral skills
One or more of: vital sign instability, jaundice, sepsis† risk factors, ill-appearing
Blood, urine, and CSF cultures, inflammatory markers
Monitor vital signs, monitor respiratory status, daily weights, retinal exams and cranial ultrasounds[2], obtain CBC
Discharge home when all routine screening is complete and infant is feeding/stooling appropriately
Sepsis
IV antibiotics
Initiate respiratory support for respiratory distress or hypoxia[3]
Frequent apnea/bradycardia/desaturation events, well-appearing
Sustained oxygen requirement >36 wks cGA[4] or 28 days of life
CUS[5] with evidence of hemorrhage
Retinal exam with evidence of abnormally ↑ vascularization
Abdominal distension, vomiting, lethargy, bloody stools, abdominal X-ray shows pneumatosis intestinalis
Isolated temperature instability secondary to inadequate fat stores
Low hemoglobin levels
Apnea of Prematurity
BPD[6]
IVH[7]
ROP[8]
NEC[9]
Anemia of Prematurity
Enteral or IV caffeine
Continue respiratory support
Serial CUS to monitor for development of hydrocephalus
Observation, retinal ablative therapy (photocoagulation) or anti-VEGF[10] injection
Stop enteral nutrition, start IV fluids, TPN (total parental nutrition), IV antibiotics, serial abdominal imaging, ± surgery
Maintain infant in an isolette until able to self-regulate temperature
Enteral or IV iron supplementation
Footnotes
1. CCHD: Critical congenital heart disease screen.
2. Not all preterm neonates meet criteria for retinal exams or cranial ultrasounds.
3. Most preterm infants require respiratory support including invasive/non-invasive positive-pressure ventilation and supplemental oxygen as their lungs mature.
4. cGA: Corrected gestational age.
5. CUS: Cranial ultrasound.
6. BPD: Bronchopulmonary dysplasia.
7. IVH: Intraventricular hemorrhage.
8. ROP: Retinopathy of prematurity.
9. NEC: Nectrotizing enterocolitis.
10. VEGF: Vascular endothelial growth factor.

FIGURE 23.3

23-3 Term and Preterm Infant Care

TERM NEWBORN CARE

Screening:

1. Hearing screen: Refer to audiology if infant does not pass screen bilaterally.
2. Critical congenital heart disease screen: Screening is performed by placing a pulse oximeter on the infant's right upper extremity and either lower extremity. Difference in oxygen saturations between both extremities is then interpreted.
   a. Failed screening if SpO_2 <90% in any extremity or if FiO2 difference is >3% between right hand (preductal) and either foot (postductal).
   b. Critical cyanotic lesions typically caught on prenatal echo (see Pediatric Cardiology, pp. 562–566).
3. Hyperbilirubinemia: Bilirubin is measured within first day of life with overall goal to avoid kernicterus (see Neonatal Jaundice algorithm, p. 551)
   a. Physiologic jaundice usually peaks by 3–4 days old.
   b. Risk factors: ABO or Rh incompatibility, low birth weight, prematurity, sibling with hyperbilirubinemia, cephalohematoma.
4. State newborn screen: Screen for various illnesses, including genetic illnesses. Content differs by state.
5. Check red reflex to ensure no cataracts or retinoblastoma.
6. Start vitamin D supplement, especially if exclusively breastfeeding.
7. Hip US: Obtain at 4–6 weeks of life to screen for hip dysplasia if infant were ever in breech position during the 3rd trimester.

Anticipatory Guidance:

- Should be feeding every 2–3 hours to avoid hypoglycemia, as newborns have low liver glycogen stores.
- Should make 6+ wet diapers a day.
- May lose up to 10% of birth weight, should regain birth weight by 2 weeks old.
- Avoid sudden infant death syndrome (SIDS):
  - Put infant on back to sleep in crib/bassinet with nothing around them.
  - Fully immunize the child.
  - Avoid secondhand smoke exposure.
- If febrile or hypothermic, see a doctor immediately to rule out sepsis.

Vaccines/Prophylaxis: "Eyes and Thighs" (Thighs Refers to Location of Shots)

- Hepatitis B.
- Erythromycin: Prophylaxis for gonococcal neonatal conjunctivitis.
- Vitamin K: Prevents hemorrhagic disease of the newborn.

NEONATAL SEPSIS

A 3-day-old, full-term infant presents to the emergency room with 1 day of poor feeding, fevers, and mild increased work of breathing. On exam, the infant is inconsolable, fussy, and febrile with moderate subcostal retractions. Labs show normal white count and elevated CRP. Urine, blood, and CSF cultures are obtained and pending.

Management:

1. Hospital admission and initiation of antibiotics.
2. IV antibiotics should cover for group B *Streptococcus*, *E. coli*, and *Listeria*. Ampicillin + gentamicin or ampicillin + cefotaxime/ceftazidime are good choices (ceftriaxone should not be used in infants <1 month old due to risk of kernicterus).
3. Supportive care.

Complications: Meningitis leading to poor neurodevelopmental outcomes.

HYF: Neonates are at high risk for invasive bacterial infections secondary to GBS from the birth canal or *E. coli* from urine. All fevers in neonates should be taken seriously, even if the infant is well-appearing.

23-3 Term and Preterm Infant Care

PRETERM NEWBORN COMPLICATIONS

APNEA OF PREMATURITY

A 2-day old F born at 32 weeks GA has frequent desaturation events accompanied by bradycardia, which resolve when her nurse stimulates her by touch.

Management:

1. Apnea resolves usually by 36–40 weeks corrected gestation.
2. Some desaturation events can resolve on their own, but some require stimulation and/or supplemental oxygen.
3. Consider use of caffeine.

Complications: No substantial evidence for long-term consequences.

HYF: All premature infants are at risk of apnea (15–20 second pauses in breathing) due to immature respiratory drive. Think of it as a normal physiologic condition in premature infants rather than truly pathological.

INTRAVENTRICULAR HEMORRHAGE

A 3-day-old F born at 29 weeks GA is found to have hemorrhage in her ventricles on screening cranial ultrasound.

Management:

1. Routine prevention for babies <30 weeks or <1500 grams:
   a. Elevate head to decrease ICP.
   b. Limit care times for the baby to minimize movement.
   c. Keep head midline to prevent compression of the jugular vein and improve cerebral perfusion pressure.
2. For known IVH, follow-up assessments via cranial ultrasounds or MRI are performed to assess for evolving bleed. Refer to a neurodevelopmental pediatrician.

Complications:

- Post-hemorrhagic hydrocephalus requiring shunt placement.
- Parenchymal bleed.
- Cerebral palsy.

HYF: Intraventricular hemorrhages originate in the fragile germinal matrix and are graded I–IV depending on the extent of the bleed. Not prevented by vitamin K.

RETINOPATHY OF PREMATURITY

A 3-week-old infant born at 27 weeks GA is found to have retinal neovascularization on fundus exam.

Management:

1. Laser photocoagulation.
2. Intravitreal anti-VEGF injection.

Complications:

- Retinal detachment.
- Blindness.

HYF: Retinopathy of prematurity occurs when there is neovascularization of the retina. Supplemental oxygen after birth, low birth weight, premature birth, and gestational age of <28 weeks are risk factors.

Necrotizing Enterocolitis: See Bloody Stools, p. 590.

*Other complications include bronchopulmonary dysplasia (BPD), anemia of prematurity, and hypoxic ischemic encephalopathy (HIE), which are not usually tested on USMLE Step 2.

23-4 Birth Injuries

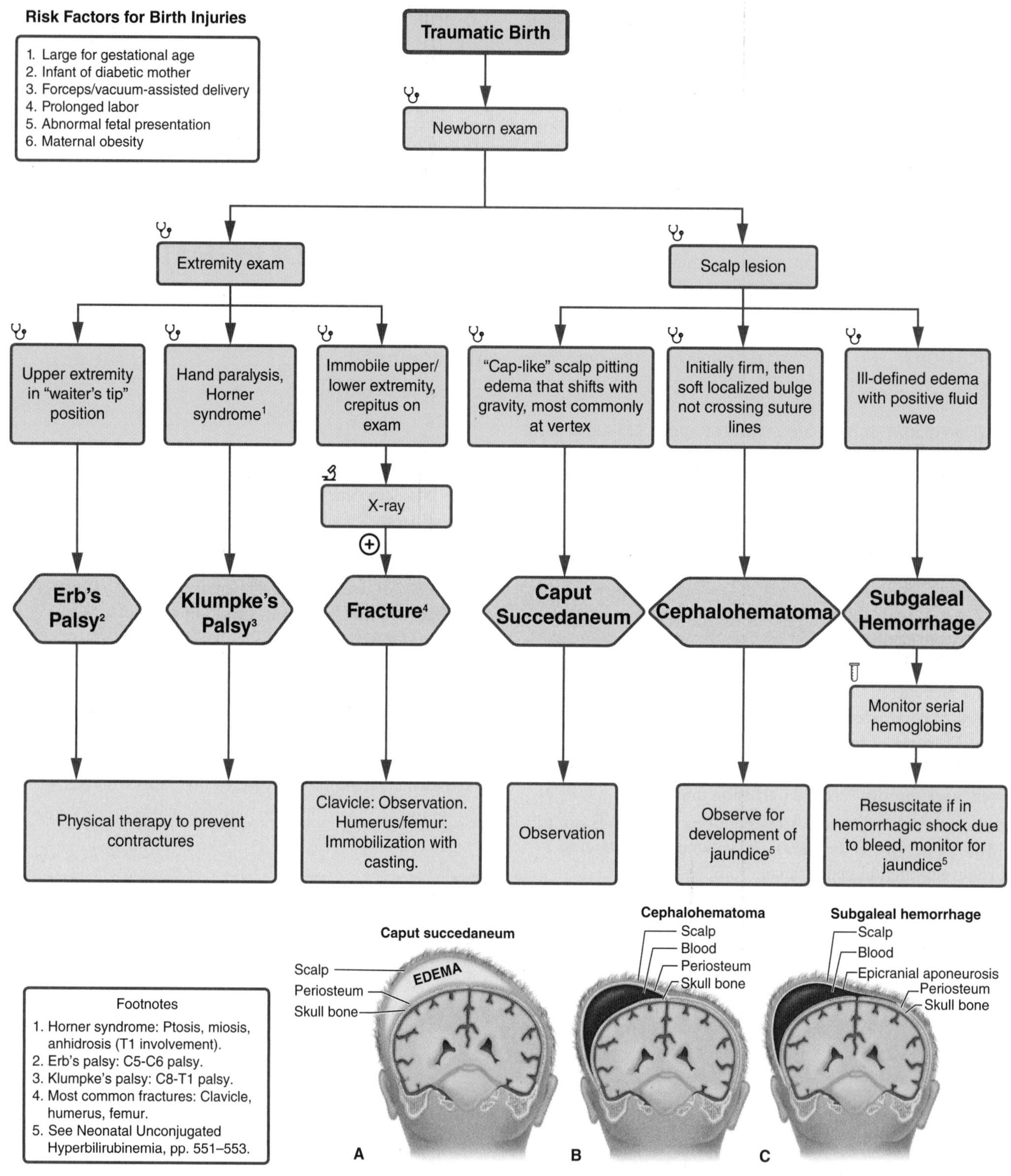
Risk Factors for Birth Injuries
1. Large for gestational age
2. Infant of diabetic mother
3. Forceps/vacuum-assisted delivery
4. Prolonged labor
5. Abnormal fetal presentation
6. Maternal obesity
Traumatic Birth
Newborn exam
Extremity exam
Scalp lesion
Upper extremity in "waiter's tip" position
Hand paralysis, Horner syndrome[1]
Immobile upper/ lower extremity, crepitus on exam
X-ray
"Cap-like" scalp pitting edema that shifts with gravity, most commonly at vertex
Initially firm, then soft localized bulge not crossing suture lines
Ill-defined edema with positive fluid wave
Erb's Palsy[2]
Klumpke's Palsy[3]
Fracture[4]
Caput Succedaneum
Cephalohematoma
Subgaleal Hemorrhage
Monitor serial hemoglobins
Physical therapy to prevent contractures
Clavicle: Observation. Humerus/femur: Immobilization with casting.
Observation
Observe for development of jaundice[5]
Resuscitate if in hemorrhagic shock due to bleed, monitor for jaundice[5]
Caput succedaneum
Scalp
Periosteum
Skull bone
EDEMA
Cephalohematoma
Scalp
Blood
Periosteum
Skull bone
Subgaleal hemorrhage
Scalp
Blood
Epicranial aponeurosis
Periosteum
Skull bone
A
B
C

Figure 23.4.1

Footnotes
1. Horner syndrome: Ptosis, miosis, anhidrosis (T1 involvement).
2. Erb's palsy: C5-C6 palsy.
3. Klumpke's palsy: C8-T1 palsy.
4. Most common fractures: Clavicle, humerus, femur.
5. See Neonatal Unconjugated Hyperbilirubinemia, pp. 551–553.

FIGURE 23.4

23-4 Birth Injuries

INFANT OF DIABETIC MOTHER

A 1-hour-old, full-term, large for gestational age (LGA) F born to a 32-year-old G1P1 mom with pregnancy complicated by poorly controlled gestational diabetes presents with vaginal delivery complicated by shoulder dystocia. On **exam**, she has crepitus on palpation of the right clavicle, decreased Moro reflex on the right side, and a cone-shaped head with cap-like edema crossing suture lines. **Labs** show hypoglycemia.

Management:

1. Obtain extremity X-ray to evaluate for clavicular fracture; no intervention required.
2. No intervention required for the "cone head." This is a normal finding due to cephalic molding when the infant passes through the birth canal.
3. No intervention for the normal superficial edema above the periosteum, called *caput succedaneum*.
4. Serial glucose checks with glucose gel/feeds administration when hypoglycemic.

Complications:

- LGA, organomegaly, shoulder dystocia: Poorly controlled maternal diabetes leads to *in utero* fetal hyperglycemia because glucose passes freely through the placenta, unlike insulin. Fetal hyperglycemia during the 3rd trimester causes macrosomia and organomegaly, increasing risk for shoulder dystocia and difficult extraction.
- Hypoglycemia: Fetal hyperglycemia leads to fetal hyperinsulinemia, which in turn leads to neonatal hypoglycemia, as the infant is no longer exposed to excess maternal glucose.

HYF: Clavicular fracture is the most common fracture in neonates and rarely requires intervention. Hypoglycemia is the most common complication for infants of diabetic mothers.

ERB'S PALSY

A 4-hour-old LGA infant with delivery complicated by shoulder dystocia presents with unilateral immobile upper extremity with arm adducted and internally rotated and forearm extended. **Exam** shows decreased Moro and biceps reflex on the affected side, but grasp reflex remains intact.

Management:

1. Referral to PT/OT to prevent contractures.
2. Majority have spontaneous recovery if the damage resulted from mild nerve compression/stretching.

Complications:

- Contractures due to prolonged immobility.
- Lasting deficits may develop if there was nerve rupture or avulsion.

HYF: Most common brachial plexus injury. Involves C5–C6 ± C7 nerve roots with classic **waiter's tip** position due to weakness of the deltoid and infraspinatus muscles (C5), biceps (C6), and wrist/finger extensors (C7).

KLUMPKE'S PALSY

A 3-hour-old LGA M with delivery complicated by shoulder dystocia presents with unilateral hand paralysis, ptosis, and pupillary constriction. On **exam**, he has intact Moro and biceps reflexes and a **claw hand**, but grasp reflex is absent.

Management:

1. Referral to PT/OT to prevent finger contractures using finger splints.

Complications:

- Contractures due to prolonged immobility.
- Lasting deficits may develop if there was nerve rupture or avulsion.

HYF: Lower brachial plexus injury involving C8–T1 nerve roots causes weakness of muscles innervated by the ulnar nerve (eg, intrinsic hand muscles). Associated with Horner syndrome: Miosis, ptosis, anhidrosis.

CEPHALOHEMATOMA

A 2-day-old F is born to a 24-year-old G3P3 mother whose pregnancy was complicated by gestational diabetes. Forceps were required during delivery due to large size for gestational age. On **exam**, the baby is crying vigorously and has a large area of soft, purple/red swelling that does not cross suture lines. On **labs**, indirect bilirubin measures 8.0 mg/dL.

Management:

1. Observation. Most resolve spontaneously without complications.
2. Serial bilirubin checks to evaluate the need for phototherapy for hyperbilirubinemia.

Complications: Hyperbilirubinemia and jaundice as the hematoma is resorbed.

HYF: Cephalohematomas are subperiosteal hemorrhages that cannot cross suture lines and predispose to neonatal jaundice. They are slow bleeds that may take 1–2 days to appear. Risk factors include instrument-assisted delivery (eg, forceps, vacuum).

SUBGALEAL HEMORRHAGE

A 5-day-old, full-term, LGA M with history of vacuum-assisted delivery presents with tachycardia, pallor, hypotension, and shock. On **exam**, he has shifting scalp edema with positive fluid wave most notable at the base of the neck.

Management:

1. Close monitoring of vital signs. Obtain serial head circumference measurements and hemoglobin/hematocrit checks to monitor progression of bleed.
2. Volume resuscitation with blood products/fluids.

Complications: Development of hemorrhagic shock in infants with subgaleal bleeds is associated with high infant mortality.

HYF: Subgaleal hemorrhage is a serious, rare bleed between the galeal aponeurosis and periosteum that can lead to significant blood loss and hemorrhagic shock. Vacuum-assisted delivery predisposes newborns to this birth injury, as traction during instrumented delivery causes shearing of emissary veins between scalp and dural sinuses.

23-5 Abnormal Newborn Screen

CONGENITAL ADRENAL HYPERPLASIA (CAH)

A 10-day-old infant with a history of home birth and no prenatal care presents to the emergency room for poor feeding and lethargy. **Exam** shows an ill-appearing infant, poor capillary refill, non-palpable pulses, and ambiguous genitalia. **Labs** are notable for hyponatremia to 124 and elevated 17-hydroxyprogesterone levels.

Management:

1. Hydrocortisone for glucocorticoid replacement.
2. Fludrocortisone for mineralocorticoid replacement.
3. Intensive care support if infant presents in adrenal crisis.

Complications:

- Adrenal crisis and shock.
- Poor growth and development.
- Infertility and reproductive problems.

HYF: The most common cause of CAH is 21-hydroxylase deficiency leading to classic CAH, which is characterized by salt-wasting due to lack of mineralocorticoids and hemodynamic instability caused by lack of glucocorticoids. Shunting of mineralocorticoid/glucocorticoid precursors to sex hormone synthesis leads to genital virilization. In females, virilization leads to ambiguous genitalia, while in males, virilization leads to hyperpigmented scrotum with excessive rugae. Other enzyme deficiencies that can lead to less

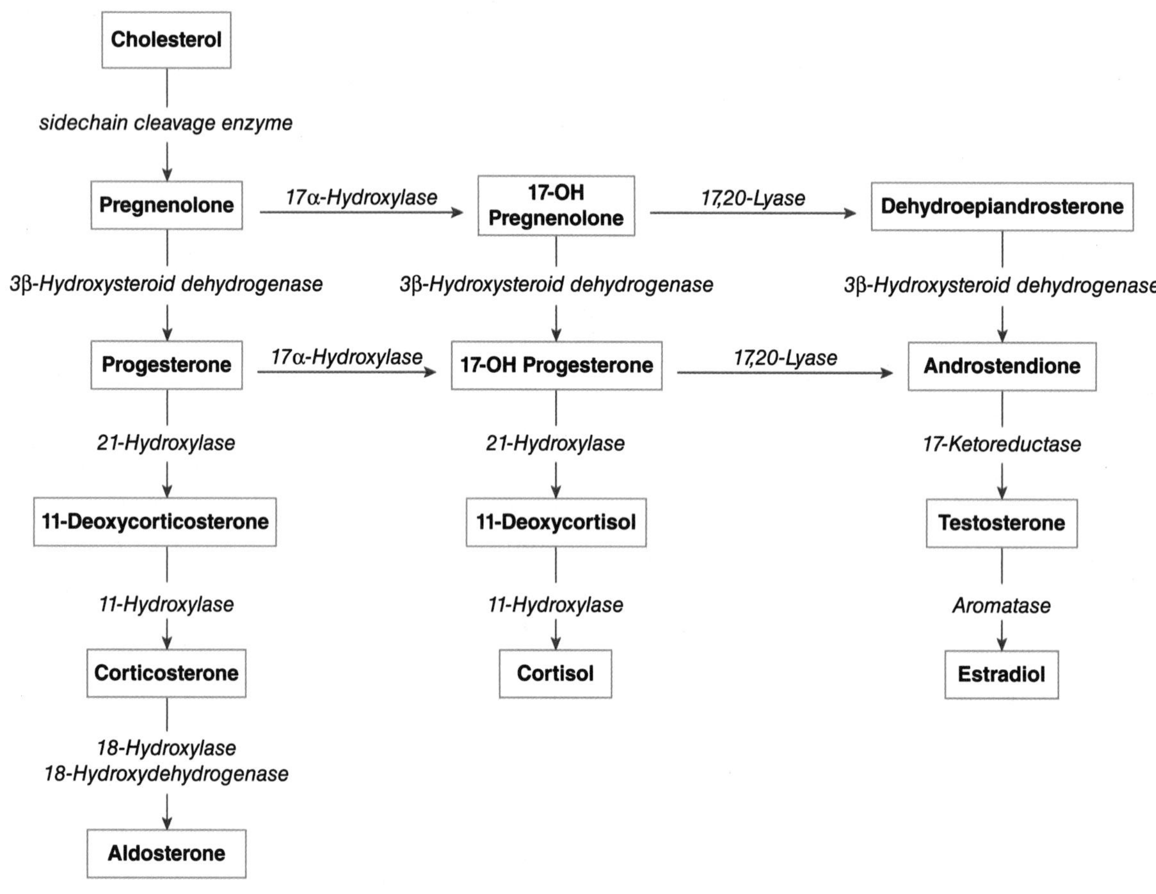
Cholesterol
sidechain cleavage enzyme
Pregnenolone
17α-Hydroxylase
17-OH Pregnenolone
17,20-Lyase
Dehydroepiandrosterone
3β-Hydroxysteroid dehydrogenase
3β-Hydroxysteroid dehydrogenase
3β-Hydroxysteroid dehydrogenase
Progesterone
17α-Hydroxylase
17-OH Progesterone
17,20-Lyase
Androstendione
21-Hydroxylase
21-Hydroxylase
17-Ketoreductase
11-Deoxycorticosterone
11-Deoxycortisol
Testosterone
11-Hydroxylase
11-Hydroxylase
Aromatase
Corticosterone
Cortisol
Estradiol
18-Hydroxylase
18-Hydroxydehydrogenase
Aldosterone

Steroidogenesis pathway.

23-5 Abnormal Newborn Screen

Forms of Congenital Adrenal Hyperplasia and Their Characteristics

Enzyme Deficiency	21-Hydroxylase	11β-Hydroxylase	17α-Hydroxylase
Presentation	Ambiguous genitalia in females. Most commonly presents in infancy with salt wasting or childhood with precocious puberty. Hypotension.	Ambiguous genitalia in females. Postnatal virilization in males and females. Hypertension.	Ambiguous genitalia (undescended testes) in males. Hypertension.
Adrenal crisis	Yes	Rare	No
Glucocorticoids	↓	↓	↓
Mineralocorticoids	↓	↓ Aldosterone, ↑ 11-DOC	↑
Androgens	↑	↑	↓
[Na^+]	↓	↑	↑
[K^+]	↑	↓	↓
Lab tests	↓ Cortisol ↑ ACTH, ↑ plasma renin ↑ 17-OHP	↓ Cortisol ↑ ACTH, ↓ plasma renin ↑ 11-deoxycortisol, ↑ DOC	↓ Cortisol ↑ ACTH, ↓ plasma renin ↑ DOC, ↑ corticosterone ↓ androstenedione
Treatment	Glucocorticoid (hydrocortisone) replacement. Mineralocorticoid (fludrocortisone) replacement. Sodium chloride supplementation.	Hydrocortisone.	Hydrocortisone. XY: orchiopexy or removal of intra-abdominal testes. Sex hormone replacement consistent with the individual's gender identity.

DHEA: dehydroepiandrosterone, DOC: deoxycorticosterone, 17-OHP: 17-hydroxyprogesterone.

severe, non–salt-wasting phenotypes include 11-beta-hydroxylase and 17-alpha-hydroxylase deficiency.

CYSTIC FIBROSIS (CF)

A 2-month-old F with history of meconium ileus, abnormal newborn screen, and familial history of cystic fibrosis presents with positive sweat chloride and genetic testing for cystic fibrosis.

Management:

1. Serial PFTs for monitoring disease progression.
2. Hospital admission and IV antibiotic therapy for CF exacerbations secondary to infection, which are heralded by shortness of breath, fever, and worsening PFTs.
3. CFTR modulator therapy.

Complications:

- Exocrine pancreatic insufficiency.
- Bronchiectasis secondary to recurrent sinopulmonary infections, especially with pseudomonas.
- Shortened life expectancy.

HYF: Caused by a mutation in the cystic fibrosis transmembrane conductance regulator (*CFTR*) gene, the most common mutation being ΔF508.

23-6 Neonatal Skin Lesions

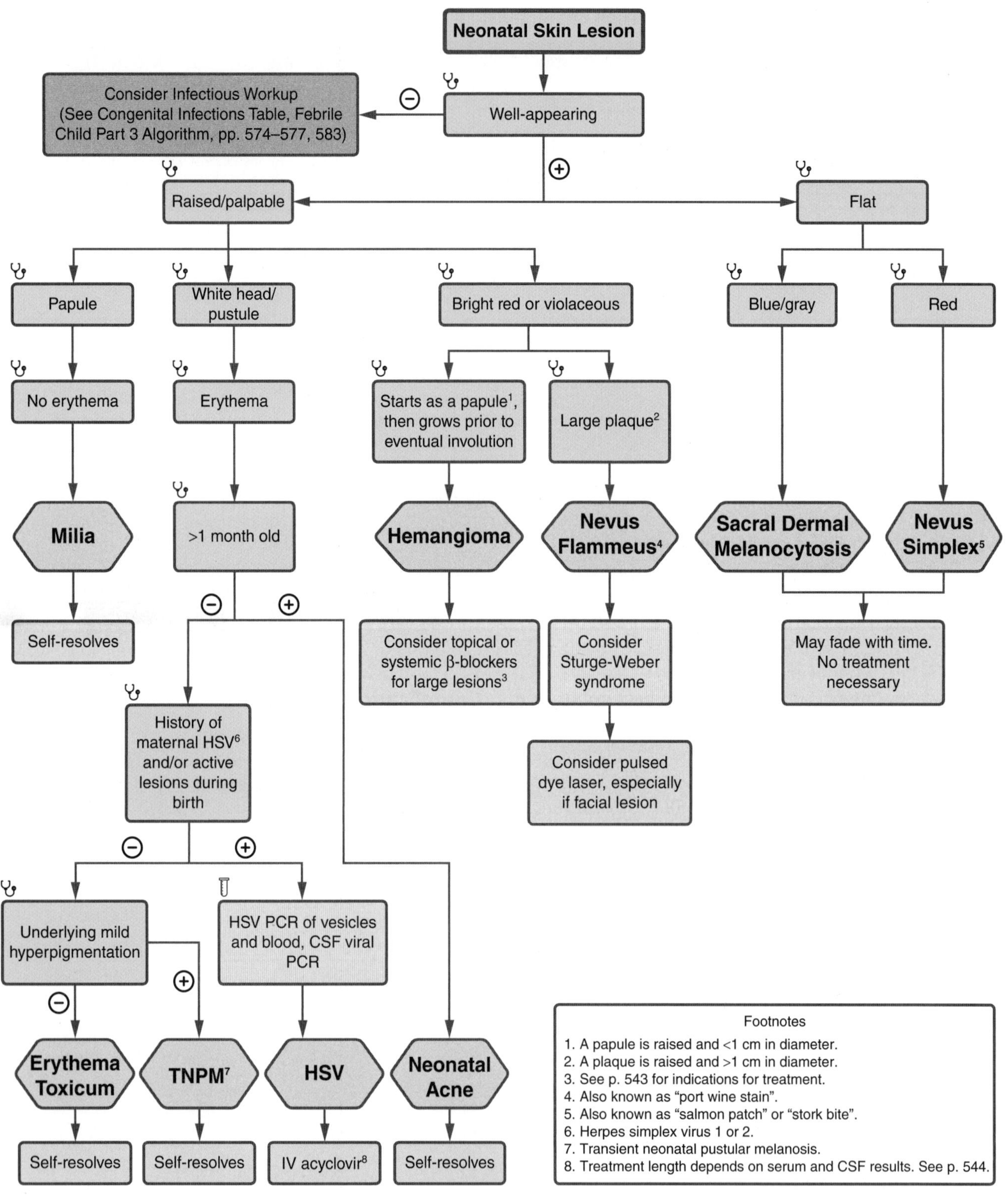
Neonatal Skin Lesion
Well-appearing
Consider Infectious Workup (See Congenital Infections Table, Febrile Child Part 3 Algorithm, pp. 574–577, 583)
Raised/palpable
Flat
Papule
White head/ pustule
Bright red or violaceous
Blue/gray
Red
No erythema
Erythema
Starts as a papule[1], then grows prior to eventual involution
Large plaque[2]
Milia
>1 month old
Hemangioma
Nevus Flammeus[4]
Sacral Dermal Melanocytosis
Nevus Simplex[5]
Self-resolves
Consider topical or systemic β-blockers for large lesions[3]
Consider Sturge-Weber syndrome
May fade with time. No treatment necessary
History of maternal HSV[6] and/or active lesions during birth
Consider pulsed dye laser, especially if facial lesion
Underlying mild hyperpigmentation
HSV PCR of vesicles and blood, CSF viral PCR
Erythema Toxicum
TNPM[7]
HSV
Neonatal Acne
Self-resolves
Self-resolves
IV acyclovir[8]
Self-resolves

Footnotes

1. A papule is raised and <1 cm in diameter.
2. A plaque is raised and >1 cm in diameter.
3. See p. 543 for indications for treatment.
4. Also known as "port wine stain".
5. Also known as "salmon patch" or "stork bite".
6. Herpes simplex virus 1 or 2.
7. Transient neonatal pustular melanosis.
8. Treatment length depends on serum and CSF results. See p. 544.

FIGURE 23.6

23-6 Neonatal Skin Lesions

STRAWBERRY (INFANTILE) HEMANGIOMA

A 4-month-old M is brought to his pediatrician for a well-child check. He is growing well along the 30th percentile for weight. His mom noted that he has 2 red spots on his chest that seem bigger than they were 3 months ago. Exam shows a 3-cm red, sharply demarcated raised plaque on the his chest.

Management:

1. Benign: No treatment.
2. Consider treating with topical or oral β-blockers if the lesion is located in cosmetically important areas, may interfere with function (eg, eyelid), large, or symptomatic.
3. If lesion is located on the neck in the "beard distribution," consider ENT consult to evaluate for airway hemangiomas.

Complications:

- Near the eye: Disrupted development of vision.
- Bleeding/ulceration, especially if on lip or neck.
- Disfigurement if on nose, ears.
- Airway hemangiomas can cause airway obstruction.

HYF: Infantile hemangiomas are benign vascular tumors that are usually not obvious at birth. They appear in the first few weeks of life as a red or purple, blanching macule and grow rapidly to a larger papule or larger mass until age ~1 year, after which they usually start regressing. Large segmental infantile hemangiomas can be associated with other developmental anomalies and can be part of PHACES and LUMBAR syndrome requiring further workup.

NEVUS FLAMMEUS (PORT WINE STAIN)

A 2-month-old M presents with blanchable dark red/violaceous plaques and scattered papules on the left side of his face. Parents say it started out as a lighter pink color at birth and has become more purple over time. It does not seem to bother him and doesn't bleed. He has had no fevers. Because of the location of the lesions, his pediatrician decides to get a head MRI.

Management:

1. Benign: No treatment is absolutely necessary.
2. Consider treating with laser therapy to prevent disfigurement, especially if the lesion is located on the face.

Complications: Disfigurement.

HYF: Port wine stains (nevus flammeus) occur most frequently on the face but can be present on any body part. They can be distinguished from a *nevus simplex* ("stork bite"), which are usually midline and fade with time. Port wine stains can be associated with a variety of syndromes, including Sturge-Weber syndrome (due to a mutation in the *GNAQ* gene), which usually presents with a port wine stain in the trigeminal nerve distribution and leptomeningeal capillary-venous malformation.

CONGENITAL DERMAL MELANOCYTOSIS

A 10-day-old term M is at his pediatrician's office for a weight check. His weight is now above his birth weight. On exam, he appears vigorous. He has a small sacral dimple with visible base and flat, gray-blue patches of discoloration on his back and buttocks.

Management:

1. Benign: No treatment.

Complications: None.

HYF: Congenital dermal melanocytosis (Mongolian spots, slate-gray patch) presents as gray-blue, flat patches on the lower back and self-resolves within the first decade of life. Due to improper migration or clearance of melanocytes from the fetal dermal layer. More prevalent in Asian, Black, and Hispanic populations. It is important not to confuse it with bruising or non-accidental trauma.

ERYTHEMA TOXICUM NEONATORUM

A 3-day-old term F is at her first visit with the pediatrician. She is down 6% from birth weight. Her mom is having some difficulty with breastfeeding. Exam shows jaundice and the following skin finding:

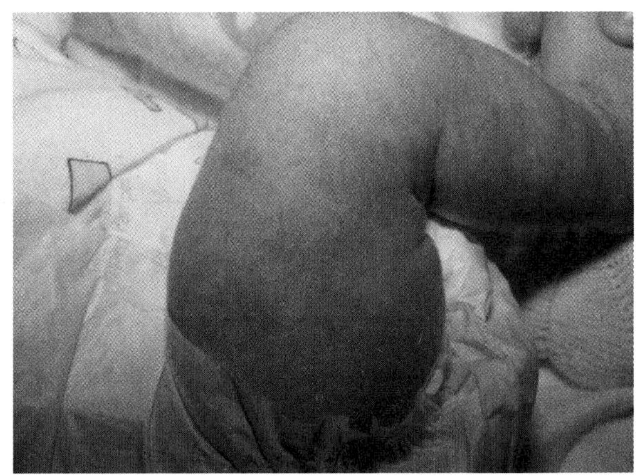

Neonatal extremity with classic erythema toxicum.

Management:

1. Benign: No treatment.

Complications: None.

HYF: Erythema toxicum is a benign, asymptomatic newborn rash that presents in the first 72 hours of life and self-resolves. It presents as scattered white/yellow pustules on an erythematous base, so it is important to distinguish it from varicella or herpes simplex infections.

TRANSIENT NEONATAL PUSTULAR MELANOSIS

A 7-day-old M presents with new white/yellow pustules and darker brown macules on his neck, as shown below. He doesn't have any fevers and has been feeding normally.

Management:

1. Benign: No treatment.

Complications: None.

23-6 Neonatal Skin Lesions

HYF: Transient neonatal pustular melanosis is thought to be a variant of erythema toxicum and usually occurs in neonates with darker skin. It can leave hyperpigmentation that fades with time.

HERPES SIMPLEX VIRUS (HSV)

A 12-day-old M presents with a rash. On exam, he is well-appearing and afebrile. He has an area of erythema on his arm with an overlying vesicle and a blister on his hard palate. His mom says he was feeding well initially by bottle but now he doesn't seem to want it at all. Labs show low platelet count and elevated AST and ALT. HSV PCR swabs of the vesicle and oral mucosa and HSV PCR of the blood and CSF are obtained and still pending.

Management:

1. Start IV acyclovir immediately when suspected – do not wait for PCR results.
2. If only skin and mucous membrane involvement: 14 days of acyclovir.
3. If blood or CNS involvement: 21 days of acyclovir.

Complications: SEM (skin, eye, mucosa) disease may progress to disseminated or CNS disease if not treated early.

HYF: HSV skin and mucosal infections can occur by intrapartum transmission to baby if mom has active lesions during delivery (horizontal transmission). This is distinct from vertical transmission of HSV during pregnancy, where teratogenic effects can occur. Newborns with suspected HSV must get blood and CSF tested for HSV to determine the appropriate treatment duration.

INFANTILE ACNE

A 3-month-old F presents with a rash that appeared on her face in the past week. It doesn't seem to be bothering her too much, and she has had no fevers. Exam shows open and closed comedones, as well as inflammatory papules, pustules, and nodules.

Management:

1. Benign: No treatment.

Complications: None. Usually self-resolves.

HYF: Infantile acne is thought to be caused by exposure to maternal hormones and can present anywhere from 6 weeks to 12 months of age.

Milia: See p. 320.

Nevus Simplex: See p. 315.

23-7 Birth Defects: Part 1

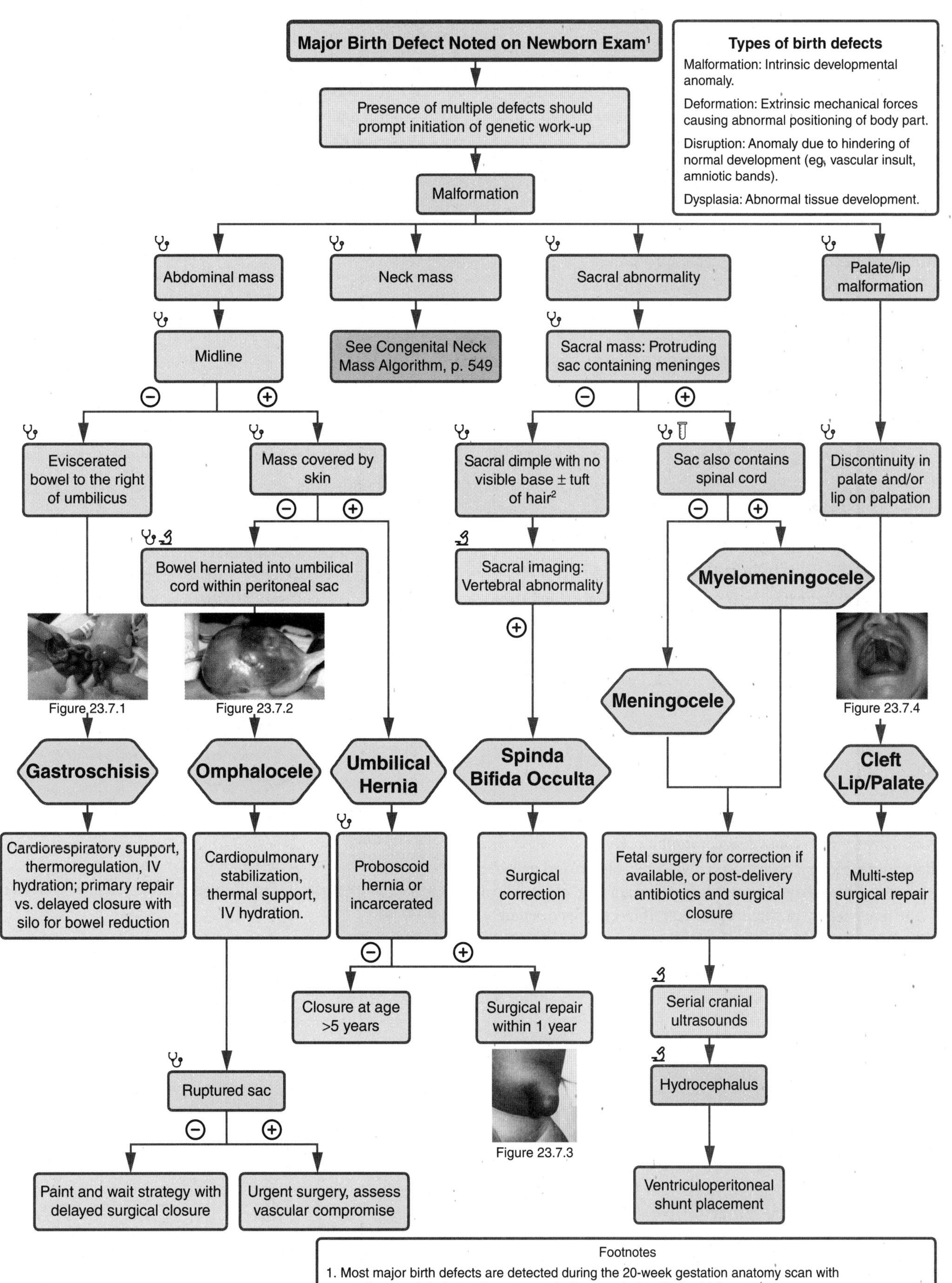

Major Birth Defect Noted on Newborn Exam[1]
Types of birth defects
Malformation: Intrinsic developmental anomaly.
Deformation: Extrinsic mechanical forces causing abnormal positioning of body part.
Disruption: Anomaly due to hindering of normal development (eg, vascular insult, amniotic bands).
Dysplasia: Abnormal tissue development.
Presence of multiple defects should prompt initiation of genetic work-up
Malformation
Abdominal mass
Neck mass
Sacral abnormality
Palate/lip malformation
Midline
See Congenital Neck Mass Algorithm, p. 549
Sacral mass: Protruding sac containing meninges
Eviscerated bowel to the right of umbilicus
Mass covered by skin
Sacral dimple with no visible base ± tuft of hair[2]
Sac also contains spinal cord
Discontinuity in palate and/or lip on palpation
Bowel herniated into umbilical cord within peritoneal sac
Sacral imaging: Vertebral abnormality
Myelomeningocele
Figure 23.7.1
Figure 23.7.2
Meningocele
Figure 23.7.4
Gastroschisis
Omphalocele
Umbilical Hernia
Spinda Bifida Occulta
Cleft Lip/Palate
Cardiorespiratory support, thermoregulation, IV hydration; primary repair vs. delayed closure with silo for bowel reduction
Cardiopulmonary stabilization, thermal support, IV hydration.
Proboscoid hernia or incarcerated
Surgical correction
Fetal surgery for correction if available, or post-delivery antibiotics and surgical closure
Multi-step surgical repair
Closure at age >5 years
Surgical repair within 1 year
Serial cranial ultrasounds
Figure 23.7.3
Hydrocephalus
Ruptured sac
Paint and wait strategy with delayed surgical closure
Urgent surgery, assess vascular compromise
Ventriculoperitoneal shunt placement
Footnotes
1. Most major birth defects are detected during the 20-week gestation anatomy scan with an ultrasound, but, very few are surgically corrected until after birth.
2. If a sacral dimple has a visible base, no need to perform sacral ultrasound or be concerned for defect.

FIGURE 23.7

23-7 Birth Defects: Part 1

GASTROSCHISIS

A girl born at 36 weeks GA has a defect in her abdominal wall and protrusion of her bowels to the right of this defect. **Labs/Imaging**: On a 20-week prenatal ultrasound, free-floating bowel loops were visualized, and maternal AFP levels were high.

Management:

1. Vaginal delivery is not contraindicated.
2. Cardiorespiratory support is often needed.
3. OG tube placement for stomach decompression.
4. Maintenance IV fluids due to increased evaporative losses.
5. Plastic bag covering the lower half of the baby and bowels to prevent fluid loss.
6. If small, primary repair in single operation. If large, staged repair with silo for bowel reduction.

Complications:

- Bowel wall thickening and rind formation from exposure to amniotic fluid.
- Preterm birth.
- C-section delivery.

HYF: Gastroschisis results from incomplete closure of the abdominal wall during gestation and is more common in pregnancies with young maternal age.

OMPHALOCELE

A baby girl infant born at 37 weeks GA with pregnancy complicated by limited prenatal care is delivered with a protruding sac containing abdominal contents. On **exam**, she is also noted to have bilateral ear pits and a large tongue.

Management

1. Vaginal delivery is possible if small omphalocele.
2. Paint and wait: Keep the sac covered with petroleum and gauze to promote epithelialization prior to delayed surgical closure. If small, primary repair in single operation. If large, staged repair.
3. Cardiorespiratory support is often needed.

Complications:

- Rupture of the omphalocele; if the liver is involved, liver injury can result. Requires urgent surgery.
- C-section delivery.
- Preterm birth.
- Complications related to surgical repair.

HYF: Normal fetal development involves mid-gut bowel herniation around 6 weeks gestation, but omphalocele occurs when the gut fails to rotate and return to the abdominal cavity. It is associated with advanced maternal age, Beckwith-Wiedemann syndrome (as in the case above), and trisomies 13, 21, and 18.

SPINA BIFIDA

A 2-day-old M is born at 36 weeks GA to a G1P1 mom whose pregnancy was complicated by poor prenatal care and epilepsy on valproic acid. On **exam**, he is noted to have a tuft of hair at the midline of his sacrum. On **imaging**, sacral ultrasound shows a spinal cord defect.

Management:

1. Prevention: Folic acid supplementation during pregnancy.
2. Early surgical repair, often with shunt placement.

Complications:

- Neurogenic bowel and bladder.
- Motor delays, weakness, spasticity, contractures.

HYF: Spina bifida is a failure of neural tube closure during embryogenesis. Risk factors include folate deficiency during pregnancy, maternal diabetes, and certain teratogens like valproic acid. There are varying degrees of disease:

- No deformity visible, but there is a tuft of hair or dimple covering the defect.
- *Meningocele*: The meninges and CSF protrude.
- *Myelomeningocele*: The meninges, CSF, and spinal cord elements protrude.

23-8 Birth Defects: Part 2

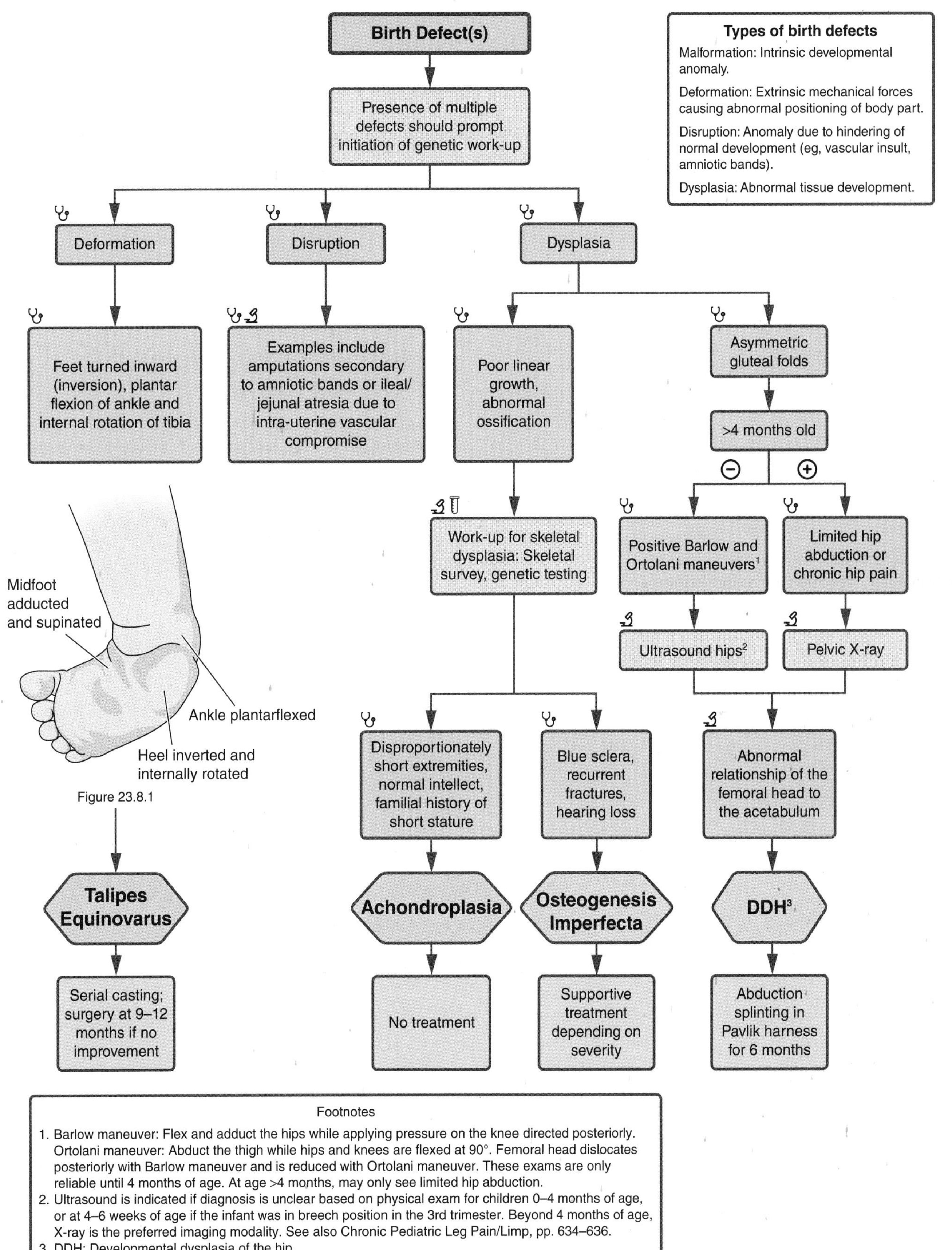

Birth Defect(s)
Presence of multiple defects should prompt initiation of genetic work-up
Types of birth defects
Malformation: Intrinsic developmental anomaly.
Deformation: Extrinsic mechanical forces causing abnormal positioning of body part.
Disruption: Anomaly due to hindering of normal development (eg, vascular insult, amniotic bands).
Dysplasia: Abnormal tissue development.
Deformation
Disruption
Dysplasia
Feet turned inward (inversion), plantar flexion of ankle and internal rotation of tibia
Examples include amputations secondary to amniotic bands or ileal/jejunal atresia due to intra-uterine vascular compromise
Poor linear growth, abnormal ossification
Asymmetric gluteal folds
>4 months old
Work-up for skeletal dysplasia: Skeletal survey, genetic testing
Positive Barlow and Ortolani maneuvers[1]
Limited hip abduction or chronic hip pain
Ultrasound hips[2]
Pelvic X-ray
Midfoot adducted and supinated
Ankle plantarflexed
Heel inverted and internally rotated
Figure 23.8.1
Disproportionately short extremities, normal intellect, familial history of short stature
Blue sclera, recurrent fractures, hearing loss
Abnormal relationship of the femoral head to the acetabulum
Talipes Equinovarus
Achondroplasia
Osteogenesis Imperfecta
DDH[3]
Serial casting; surgery at 9–12 months if no improvement
No treatment
Supportive treatment depending on severity
Abduction splinting in Pavlik harness for 6 months

Footnotes

1. Barlow maneuver: Flex and adduct the hips while applying pressure on the knee directed posteriorly. Ortolani maneuver: Abduct the thigh while hips and knees are flexed at 90°. Femoral head dislocates posteriorly with Barlow maneuver and is reduced with Ortolani maneuver. These exams are only reliable until 4 months of age. At age >4 months, may only see limited hip abduction.
2. Ultrasound is indicated if diagnosis is unclear based on physical exam for children 0–4 months of age, or at 4–6 weeks of age if the infant was in breech position in the 3rd trimester. Beyond 4 months of age, X-ray is the preferred imaging modality. See also Chronic Pediatric Leg Pain/Limp, pp. 634–636.
3. DDH: Developmental dysplasia of the hip.

FIGURE 23.8

23-8 Birth Defects: Part 2

TALIPES EQUINOVARUS (CLUBFOOT)

A gravid mother presents to the clinic for a routine exam and fetal ultrasound. On **imaging**, ultrasound shows that the fetus has a foot turned inward, on its side, and downward.

Management:

1. Manual repositioning and serial casting post-birth.
2. If repositioning fails, surgical release of contractures.

Complications: Permanent deformity leading to difficulty with ambulation.

HYF: CAVE: **C**avus, **A**dduction, **V**arus, **E**quinus.

ACHONDROPLASIA

A 5-year-old F presents to the clinic for a well-child check. On **exam**, she has macrocephaly, frontal bossing, rhizomelic limb shortening, bowed legs, and is <5%-ile for height.

Management:

1. Molecular genetic testing for fibroblast growth factor receptor 3 (*FGFR3*).
2. Physical therapy.
3. Orthopedic interventions when indicated.

Complications:

- Recurrent otitis media and/or hearing loss.
- Hydrocephalus from foramen magnum stenosis.

HYF: Autosomal dominant condition caused by gain-of-function mutations in *FGFR3*.

OSTEOGENESIS IMPERFECTA

A 7-year-old F with PMH of hearing loss presents to the clinic for a routine visit. Routine vitals show that she is <5%ile for height. On **exam**, she has blue sclera, scoliosis, and multiple bruises. On **imaging**, a radiographic survey shows multiple fractures in various locations and generalized lower bone density. She is unable to detail the mechanism of injury for fractures. There is a positive family history of osteogenesis imperfecta.

Management:

1. Physical therapy.
2. Bisphosphonates.
3. Regular surveillance.

Complications:

- Sometimes associated with malignant hyperthermia.
- Bony tumors such as osteogenic sarcoma.

HYF: Connective tissue disorder commonly caused by mutations in type 1 collagen (*Col1A*). Non-accidental trauma must be investigated and ruled out due to the presence of multiple fractures and easy bruising.

DEVELOPMENTAL DYSPLASIA OF THE HIP (DDH)

A 6-year-old F presents with 2 months of right hip pain and 3 days of limping. On **exam**, her right leg is 1 cm shorter than the left. She has asymmetric inguinal skin folds and pain on external rotation of the right hip. On **imaging**, X-ray shows a poorly formed femoral head.

Management:

1. 1–6 months: Abduction device (eg, Pavlik Harness).
2. 6–18 months: Closed reduction with hip spica cast.
3. 18+ months: Open reduction with orthopedic surgery.

Complications:

- Avascular necrosis of the femoral head.
- Accelerated osteoarthritis.
- Leg length discrepancy (eg, Galeazzi test).
- Recurrence.

HYF: All babies who were in breech position in the 3rd trimester are screened for DDH with bilateral hip ultrasonography at age 4–6 weeks. After age 4 months, X-ray is preferred to assess acetabular development and positioning. Serial hip exams with the Barlow and Ortolani maneuvers from birth to age 1 year to assess joint stability help catch this diagnosis early. If not caught, it can cause hip pain and limp in later childhood.

23-9 Birth Defects: Part 3

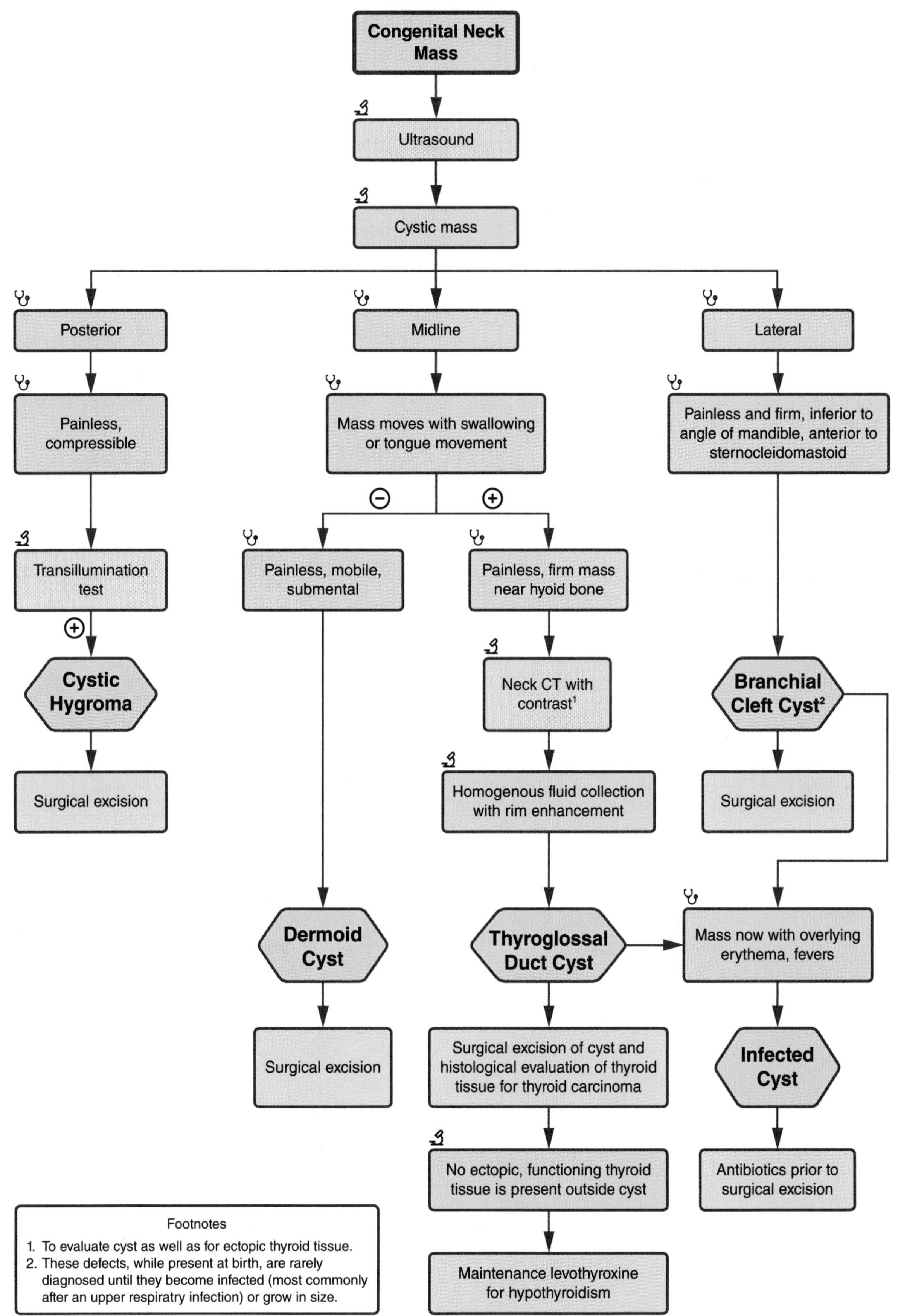
Congenital Neck Mass
Ultrasound
Cystic mass
Posterior
Midline
Lateral
Painless, compressible
Mass moves with swallowing or tongue movement
Painless and firm, inferior to angle of mandible, anterior to sternocleidomastoid
Transillumination test
Painless, mobile, submental
Painless, firm mass near hyoid bone
Cystic Hygroma
Neck CT with contrast[1]
Branchial Cleft Cyst[2]
Surgical excision
Homogenous fluid collection with rim enhancement
Surgical excision
Dermoid Cyst
Thyroglossal Duct Cyst
Mass now with overlying erythema, fevers
Surgical excision
Surgical excision of cyst and histological evaluation of thyroid tissue for thyroid carcinoma
Infected Cyst
No ectopic, functioning thyroid tissue is present outside cyst
Antibiotics prior to surgical excision
Maintenance levothyroxine for hypothyroidism

Footnotes

1. To evaluate cyst as well as for ectopic thyroid tissue.
2. These defects, while present at birth, are rarely diagnosed until they become infected (most commonly after an upper respiratory infection) or grow in size.

FIGURE 23.9

23-9 Birth Defects: Part 3

CYSTIC HYGROMA

A 1-month-old F born to a mother with inconsistent prenatal care/screenings presents for evaluation of neck swelling. **Exam** reveals a compressible, fluctuant mass in the posterior neck region with (+) transillumination test.

Management:

1. US for diagnosis.
2. If planning to surgically excise, perform CT or MRI.
3. They can spontaneously regress. Excise if compressing surrounding structures.

Complications:

- Hygromas can recur after excision.
- Depending on location, cystic hygromas can eventually block the airway or compromise swallowing.
- Associated with heart defects.

HYF: Cystic hygromas are malformations of the lymphatic system commonly associated with Turner syndrome and can be identified *in utero.*

BRANCHIAL CLEFT CYST

An 11-year-old F with PMH of asthma presents with cough and sore throat. **Exam** shows a painless, firm mass anterior to the sternocleidomastoid that does not move when she swallows. On **imaging**, US shows a mass with homogeneous low echogenicity.

Management:

1. Ultrasound.
2. If planning excision, perform CT or MRI.
3. Excision of mass and rest of tract.

Complications:

- May have fistula with external fluid drainage.
- Recurrent infections.
- Abscess formation.

HYF: Arises due to incomplete involution of branchial clefts. Anatomic position is key to diagnosis. Infections can lead to enlargement and associated dysphagia/airway obstruction.

DERMOID CYST

An 11-year-old M with no significant PMH presents with dysphagia. **Exam** shows a nontender, midline, submental growth that does not move when he swallows. On **imaging**, US reveals a cystic mass.

Management:

1. Ultrasound.
2. Surgical excision.
3. Evaluate histology of excised sample for possible malignancy.

Complications:

- Cysts can also be intracranial or intra-abdominal.
- Compression of adjacent structures.
- Aspiration/biopsy can cause infection.

HYF: Arises from trapped epithelial debris in deep tissue.

THYROGLOSSAL DUCT CYST (INFECTED CYST)

A 7-year-old F with PMH of tonsillitis presents with throat pain. **Exam** shows a non-tender, mid-line mass that elevates when she swallows. **Labs** reveal high TSH and low free T4 levels.

Management:

1. CT neck with contrast.
2. Fine needle aspiration with stain and culture.
3. Antibiotics and surgical excision.

Complications:

- Infection ± abscess.
- Draining sinus tract formation.
- Cancer associated with ectopic thyroid tissue in cyst.
- Hypothyroidism.

HYF: Arises due to incomplete closure of the thyroglossal duct. Radiation therapy for head and neck cancers can lead to enlargement of thyroglossal duct cyst.

23-10 Neonatal Unconjugated Hyperbilirubinemia

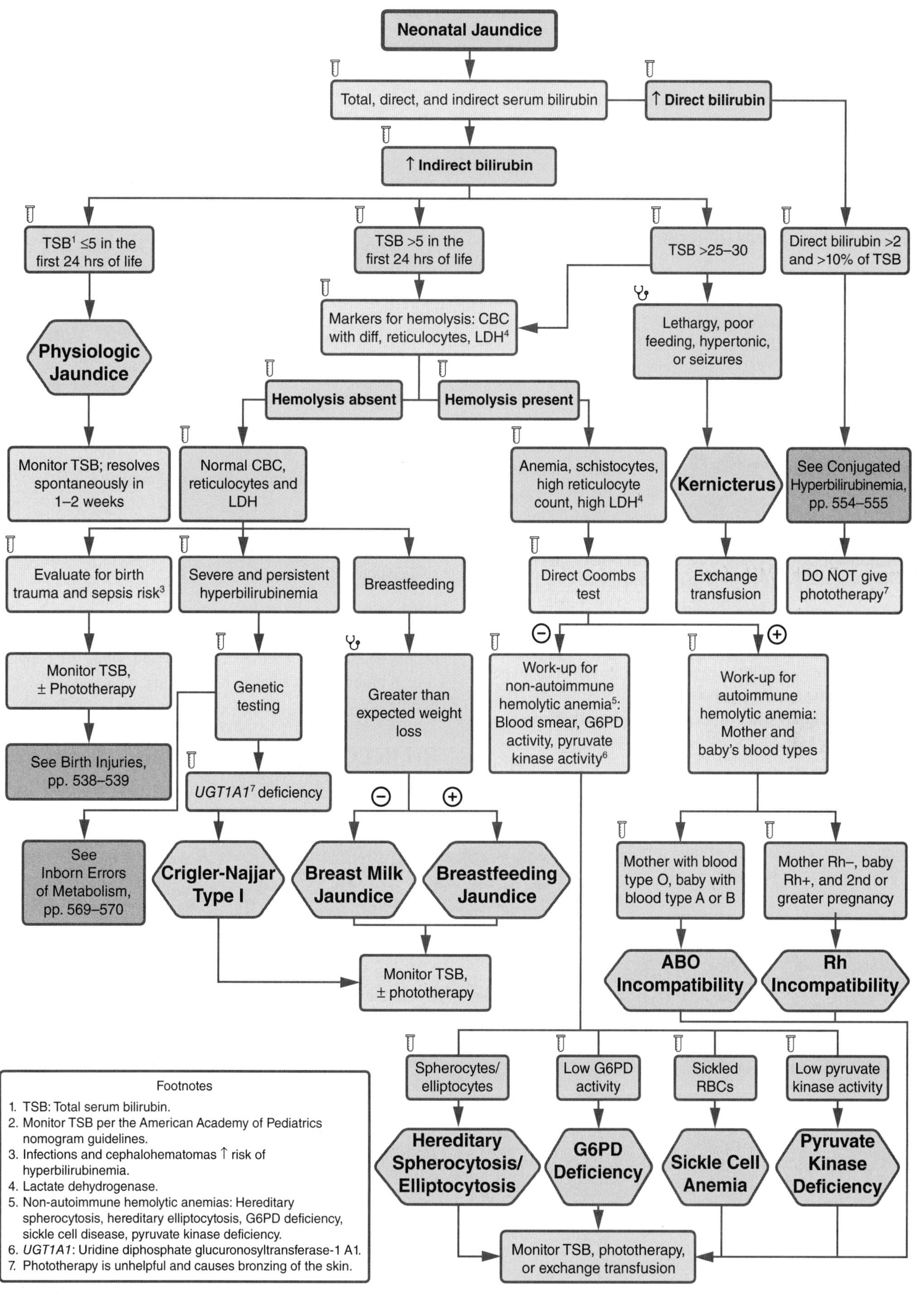

Neonatal Jaundice
Total, direct, and indirect serum bilirubin
↑ Direct bilirubin
↑ Indirect bilirubin
TSB¹ ≤5 in the first 24 hrs of life
TSB >5 in the first 24 hrs of life
TSB >25–30
Direct bilirubin >2 and >10% of TSB
Physiologic Jaundice
Markers for hemolysis: CBC with diff, reticulocytes, LDH⁴
Lethargy, poor feeding, hypertonic, or seizures
Hemolysis absent
Hemolysis present
Monitor TSB; resolves spontaneously in 1–2 weeks
Normal CBC, reticulocytes and LDH
Anemia, schistocytes, high reticulocyte count, high LDH⁴
Kernicterus
See Conjugated Hyperbilirubinemia, pp. 554–555
Evaluate for birth trauma and sepsis risk³
Severe and persistent hyperbilirubinemia
Breastfeeding
Direct Coombs test
Exchange transfusion
DO NOT give phototherapy⁷
Monitor TSB, ± Phototherapy
Genetic testing
Greater than expected weight loss
Work-up for non-autoimmune hemolytic anemia⁵: Blood smear, G6PD activity, pyruvate kinase activity⁶
Work-up for autoimmune hemolytic anemia: Mother and baby's blood types
See Birth Injuries, pp. 538–539
UGT1A1⁷ deficiency
See Inborn Errors of Metabolism, pp. 569–570
Crigler-Najjar Type I
Breast Milk Jaundice
Breastfeeding Jaundice
Mother with blood type O, baby with blood type A or B
Mother Rh–, baby Rh+, and 2nd or greater pregnancy
Monitor TSB, ± phototherapy
ABO Incompatibility
Rh Incompatibility
Spherocytes/ elliptocytes
Low G6PD activity
Sickled RBCs
Low pyruvate kinase activity
Hereditary Spherocytosis/ Elliptocytosis
G6PD Deficiency
Sickle Cell Anemia
Pyruvate Kinase Deficiency
Monitor TSB, phototherapy, or exchange transfusion

Footnotes

1. TSB: Total serum bilirubin.
2. Monitor TSB per the American Academy of Pediatrics nomogram guidelines.
3. Infections and cephalohematomas ↑ risk of hyperbilirubinemia.
4. Lactate dehydrogenase.
5. Non-autoimmune hemolytic anemias: Hereditary spherocytosis, hereditary elliptocytosis, G6PD deficiency, sickle cell disease, pyruvate kinase deficiency.
6. *UGT1A1*: Uridine diphosphate glucuronosyltransferase-1 A1.
7. Phototherapy is unhelpful and causes bronzing of the skin.

FIGURE 23.10

23-10 Neonatal Unconjugated Hyperbilirubinemia

PHYSIOLOGIC JAUNDICE

A 24-hour old F born full-term has a total serum bilirubin of 4.0 mg/dL. Direct bilirubin is 0.1 mg/dL. On exam, she is vigorous and pink. She has started feeding some colostrum. On labs, the mother's blood type is A+, the baby's is A–, and the Coombs test is negative.

Management:

1. Continue to encourage breastfeeding.
2. Clinical follow-up. Usually self-resolves by age 1–2 weeks.

HYF: Jaundice in term, healthy babies with no risk factors for hyperbilirubinemia is a relatively benign finding. Physiologic jaundice is due to *unconjugated* hyperbilirubinemia. The underlying cause is multifactorial (eg, high RBC turnover, ↓ uridine diphosphogluconurate glucuronosyltransferase [UGT] activity in the immature liver).

BREASTFEEDING JAUNDICE

A 2-day-old M born at 39w5d to a 28-year-old G1P1 mom with pregnancy complicated by gestational hypertension presents with an indirect bilirubin of 7.0 mg/dL. On exam, his weight is down 10% from birth. He is jaundiced and appears dehydrated with a sunken fontanelle. Breastfeeding has been suboptimal. He is making 1 dark brown stool daily. On labs, the mother's blood type is A+, the baby's is A–, and Coombs test is negative.

Management:

1. Consider phototherapy or exchange transfusion based on guidelines that take gestational age, age in hours of life, and risk factors for neurotoxicity (eg, kernicterus).
2. Consider lactation consult or formula supplementation.
3. IV fluids as needed.
4. Close clinical follow-up.

HYF: Breastfeeding jaundice occurs when there is inadequate intake of breast milk and is reflected by a higher degree of weight loss, dehydration, and lack of yellow, soft, seedy stools. Presents earlier than breast milk jaundice.

BREAST MILK JAUNDICE

A 5-day-old M born at 39w5d to a 28-year-old G3P3 mom presents with an indirect bilirubin of 8.0 mg/dL. On exam, his weight is down 3% from birth. He is well-appearing, vigorous, and jaundiced. Breastfeeding has been going well, and he is making 2–3 yellow, seedy stools daily. On labs, the mother's blood type is A+, the baby's is A–, and Coombs test is negative.

Management:

1. Continue to encourage breastfeeding.
2. Consider phototherapy or exchange transfusion based on guidelines that take gestational age, age in hours of life, and risk factors for neurotoxicity (eg, kernicterus).
3. Clinical follow-up.

HYF: Breast milk jaundice, as opposed to breastfeeding jaundice (lack of milk), is due to high levels of β-glucuronidase in breast milk, which deconjugate intestinal bilirubin and increase enterohepatic circulation. It starts at age 3–5 days and peaks at 2 weeks. Babies usually have a normal degree of weight loss after birth and plenty of yellow, soft, seedy stools.

ABO INCOMPATIBILITY (HEMOLYTIC DISEASE OF THE NEWBORN)

A 1-day-old M born at 39w5d to a 28-year-old G1P1 mom with an uncomplicated pregnancy presents with an indirect bilirubin of 6.0 mg/dL. On exam, his weight is down 5% from birth. He is well-appearing but jaundiced. On labs, the mother's blood type is O-, baby's blood is type B-, and the Coombs test is positive. The baby has been breastfeeding well and passed meconium.

Management:

1. Consider phototherapy or exchange transfusion.
2. Close follow-up of bilirubin.
3. Obtain CBC to monitor degree of anemia.

Complications:

- Significant anemia due to hemolysis.
- Kernicterus.

HYF: ABO incompatibility presents with indirect hyperbilirubinemia as a result of IgG-mediated autoimmune hemolysis. It occurs when the mother has type O blood, while the baby has type A or B blood and is actively hemolyzing. This can occur in the 1st pregnancy.

RH INCOMPATIBILITY

A 1-day-old M born at 39w5d to a 28-year-old G2P2 mom with uncomplicated pregnancy presents with an indirect bilirubin of 6.0mg/dL. On exam, his weight is down 5% from birth. He is well-appearing but jaundiced. On labs, the mother's blood type is O-, the baby's blood type O+, and the direct Coombs test is positive. The baby has been breastfeeding well and passed meconium.

Management:

1. Consider phototherapy or exchange transfusion.
2. Obtain CBC.
3. Close follow-up of bilirubin.

Complications:

- Significant anemia due to hemolysis.
- Kernicterus.

HYF: Rhesus (Rh) incompatibility presents with indirect hyperbilirubinemia as a result of autoimmune hemolysis. The D antigen (ie, Rh[D]) is the most immunogenic in the Rh complex. Rh(D) antigen alloimmunization occurs when a Rh(D)-negative female's bloodstream is exposed to Rh(D)-positive fetal RBCs during an index pregnancy (ie, during delivery, procedures such as

23-10 Neonatal Unconjugated Hyperbilirubinemia

amniocentesis, or abortion). Anti-D immunoglobulin (RhoGAM) injections are given at 28 weeks' gestation during pregnancy and at high-risk times (eg, within 72 hours of delivery) to prevent the mother's development of anti-D antibodies. The Kleihauer-Betke test is used to determine the dose of RhoGAM beyond the initial dose (usually 300 mcg) at 28 weeks' gestation.

G6PD DEFICIENCY

A 3-week-old M born full-term presents with jaundice and dark urine. He was recently hospitalized for febrile UTI. **Labs** show ↓ hemoglobin, ↑ bilirubin and LDH, and ↓ haptoglobin. Direct Coombs test is negative. Blood smear shows bite cells with Heinz bodies.

Management:

1. Avoid oxidative stressors: Fava beans, sulfa drugs (Bactrim), dapsone, antimalarials (quinines), isoniazid, infections/illness.
2. Supportive care.
3. If this is the first episode, conduct G6PD activity testing to make the genetic diagnosis after recovery.

HYF: G6PD deficiency is an X-linked recessive defect that causes hemolytic anemia and indirect hyperbilirubinemia. G6PD deficiency leads to impaired glutathione synthesis. G6PD activity testing has low sensitivity in acute hemolytic episodes; if negative, perform repeat testing 3 months afterwards.

Crigler-Najjar Type I: Hereditary unconjugated hyperbilirubinemia leading to reduced (Type II) or absent (Type I) UDP-glucoronosyltransferase (UGT) activity. Type I often has serum bilirubin in the 20-50 mg/dL range.
Pyruvate Kinase Deficiency: Autosomal recessive hemolytic anemia causing RBC hemolysis. Commonly presents with neonatal jaundice, gallstones and iron overload.
Hereditary Spherocytosis/Elliptocytosis: See p. 98.
Sickle Cell Anemia: See p. 97.

23-11 Neonatal Conjugated Hyperbilirubinemia

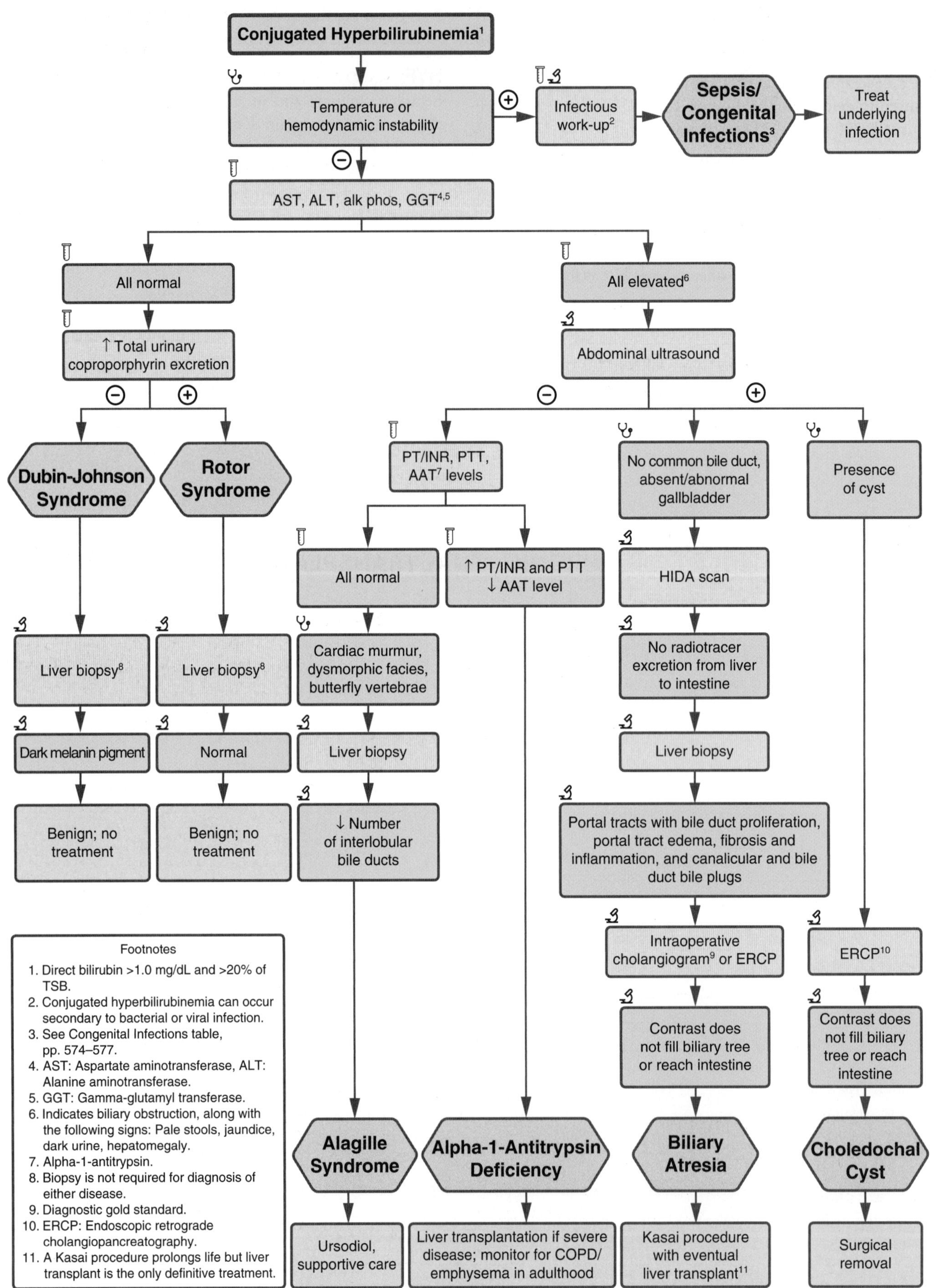
Conjugated Hyperbilirubinemia[1]
Temperature or hemodynamic instability
Infectious work-up[2]
Sepsis/ Congenital Infections[3]
Treat underlying infection
AST, ALT, alk phos, GGT[4,5]
All normal
↑ Total urinary coproporphyrin excretion
Dubin-Johnson Syndrome
Rotor Syndrome
Liver biopsy[8]
Liver biopsy[8]
Dark melanin pigment
Normal
Benign; no treatment
Benign; no treatment
All elevated[6]
Abdominal ultrasound
PT/INR, PTT, AAT[7] levels
All normal
↑ PT/INR and PTT ↓ AAT level
Cardiac murmur, dysmorphic facies, butterfly vertebrae
Liver biopsy
↓ Number of interlobular bile ducts
Alagille Syndrome
Ursodiol, supportive care
Alpha-1-Antitrypsin Deficiency
Liver transplantation if severe disease; monitor for COPD/ emphysema in adulthood
No common bile duct, absent/abnormal gallbladder
HIDA scan
No radiotracer excretion from liver to intestine
Liver biopsy
Portal tracts with bile duct proliferation, portal tract edema, fibrosis and inflammation, and canalicular and bile duct bile plugs
Intraoperative cholangiogram[9] or ERCP
Contrast does not fill biliary tree or reach intestine
Biliary Atresia
Kasai procedure with eventual liver transplant[11]
Presence of cyst
ERCP[10]
Contrast does not fill biliary tree or reach intestine
Choledochal Cyst
Surgical removal

Footnotes

1. Direct bilirubin >1.0 mg/dL and >20% of TSB.
2. Conjugated hyperbilirubinemia can occur secondary to bacterial or viral infection.
3. See Congenital Infections table, pp. 574–577.
4. AST: Aspartate aminotransferase, ALT: Alanine aminotransferase.
5. GGT: Gamma-glutamyl transferase.
6. Indicates biliary obstruction, along with the following signs: Pale stools, jaundice, dark urine, hepatomegaly.
7. Alpha-1-antitrypsin.
8. Biopsy is not required for diagnosis of either disease.
9. Diagnostic gold standard.
10. ERCP: Endoscopic retrograde cholangiopancreatography.
11. A Kasai procedure prolongs life but liver transplant is the only definitive treatment.

FIGURE 23.11

23-11 Neonatal Conjugated Hyperbilirubinemia

DUBIN-JOHNSON SYNDROME (DJS)

A 13-year-old F presents with jaundice, fatigue, and abdominal pain. Her mother says that this has happened multiple times and usually self-resolves. **Labs** show total bilirubin of 16 mg/dL and direct bilirubin of 12.0 mg/dL. Urine bilirubin assay is positive. Liver biopsy shows dark pigmentation of hepatic cells.

Management:

1. Benign – no treatment necessary.

HYF: DJS is a rare autosomal-recessive condition that is benign. Symptoms can present in times of illness or other stressors (eg, puberty, pregnancy). It is caused by a defective liver transport system, leading to decreased excretion of conjugated bilirubin into the hepatic bile canaliculi.

ROTOR SYNDROME

A 2-month-old F is brought in by her parents for a well-child visit. Her mother mentions that her jaundice never resolved after birth. **Labs** show total bilirubin of 6.0 mg/dL with direct bilirubin of 4.0 mg/dL, but AST and ALT are normal. Testing reveals elevated urinary coproporphyrin excretion.

Management:

1. Benign – no treatment necessary.

HYF: This is another relatively benign condition that presents in infancy and early childhood. It is caused by impaired storage of conjugated bilirubin in hepatocytes.

ALAGILLE SYNDROME

A 2-year-old F with a history of developmental delay, faltering growth, and VSD presents with severe jaundice. On **exam**, she is found to have a broad forehead and nasal bridge, triangular face with pointed chin, and prominent ears. **Labs** show conjugated hyperbilirubinemia, elevated LFTs, high cholesterol, and triglycerides. Liver biopsy reveals bile duct paucity. On **imaging**, X-rays reveal butterfly vertebrae.

Management:

1. Supportive symptomatic treatment for cholestasis, pruritus (eg, ursodeoxycholic acid).
2. Liver transplantation.
3. Subspecialty management of cardiac and renal anomalies.
4. No intervention usually required for vertebral or ophthalmologic differences.
5. Nutrition management, often including supplementation of fat-soluble vitamins.

HYF: Alagille Syndrome is an autosomal dominant disorder caused by a pathogenic variant in *JAG1* or *NOTCH2* genes, and usually results in hepatic cholestasis and growth difficulties. The major clinical features include cardiac defects, hepatic issues, renal abnormalities, skeletal abnormalities (including pathologic fracture), ophthalmologic changes, dysmorphic facies, and vascular anomalies (eg, aneurysms, Moyamoya syndrome).

BILIARY ATRESIA

A 3-week-old M born full-term presents with jaundice, dark urine, pale stools, and abdominal distention. **Exam** shows hepatomegaly and scleral icterus. **Labs** show total bilirubin of 6.0 mg/dL with direct bilirubin of 5.0 mg/dL. On **imaging**, US shows enlarged liver, small gallbladder, and absent common bile duct. Liver biopsy shows intrahepatic duct proliferation, fibrosis, and portal tract edema. Cholangiography shows biliary obstruction.

Management:

1. Surgical hepatoportoenterostomy (Kasai procedure).
2. Fat-soluble vitamin supplementation.
3. Ursodeoxycholic acid.
4. Liver transplant is the definitive treatment.

Complications:

- Extrahepatic bile duct fibrosis → cirrhosis → liver failure → hepatosplenomegaly.
- Neurodevelopmental delays from hyperbilirubinemia.

HYF: Progressive destruction of the extrahepatic biliary ducts results in direct hyperbilirubinemia because conjugated bilirubin cannot be excreted from the liver into the small intestine. Symptoms present within the first 2 months of life, classically with acholic stools.

BILIARY CYST

A 2-year-old M presents with abdominal pain and jaundice. **Labs** show a total bilirubin of 6.0 mg/dL with conjugated bilirubin of 5.0 mg/dL and lipase of 1533. **Exam** reveals a palpable mass in the RUQ. On **imaging**, US reveals a cyst of the common bile duct.

Management:

1. Surgical removal of the cyst.

Complications:

- Biliary fibrosis → cirrhosis → liver failure.
- Neurodevelopmental delays from hyperbilirubinemia.
- Pancreatitis.
- Cholangiocarcinoma in adulthood.

HYF: The majority of biliary cysts (ie, choledochal cysts) present at age <10 years. Cysts can cause pancreatitis in later childhood or may only present later in adulthood. Biliary cysts can present similarly to biliary atresia in infancy with elevated LFTs in a cholestatic pattern, as they are both obstructive biliary pathologies.

23-12 Neonatal Eye Discharge

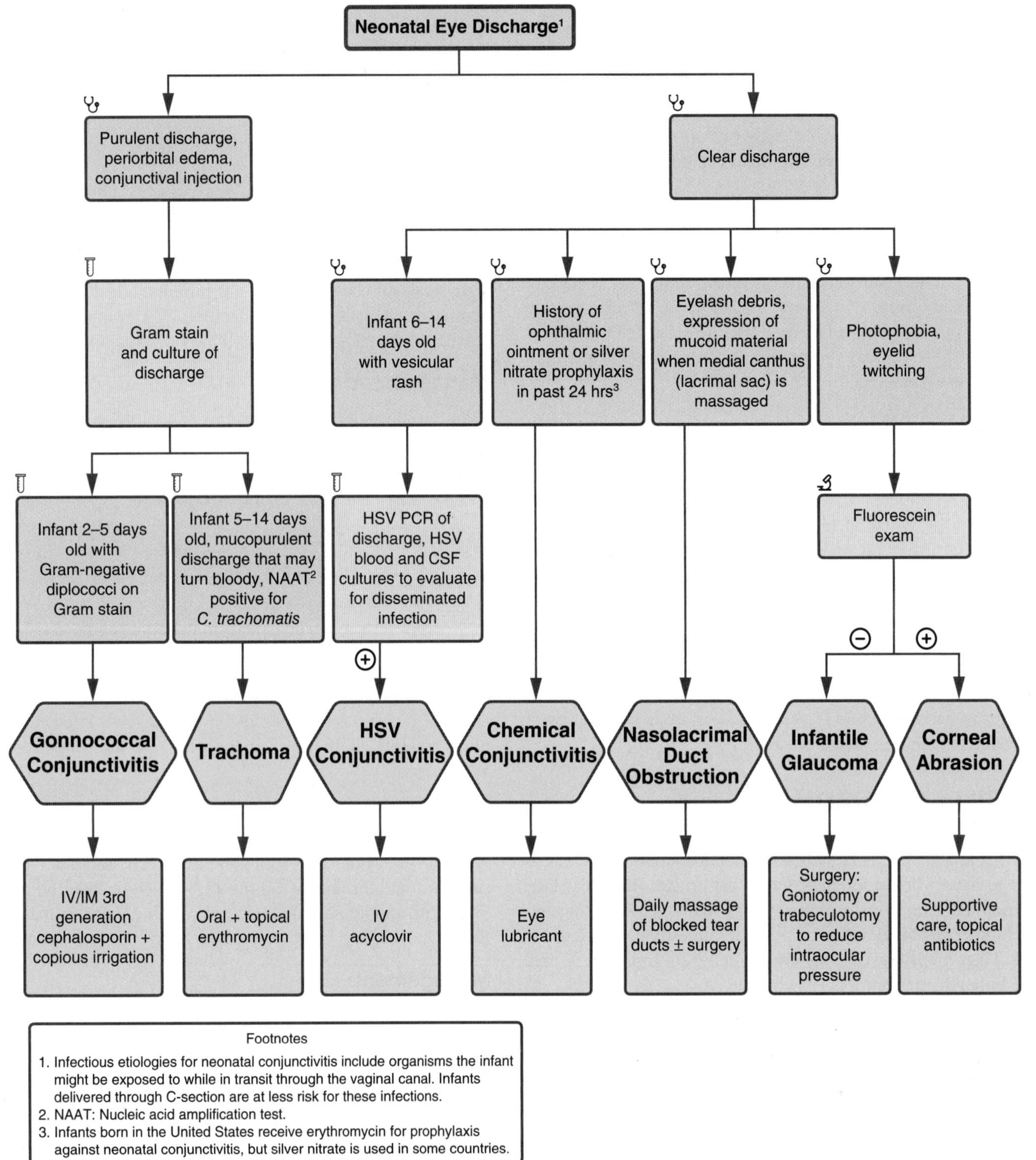

Neonatal Eye Discharge[1]
Purulent discharge, periorbital edema, conjunctival injection
Clear discharge
Gram stain and culture of discharge
Infant 6–14 days old with vesicular rash
History of ophthalmic ointment or silver nitrate prophylaxis in past 24 hrs[3]
Eyelash debris, expression of mucoid material when medial canthus (lacrimal sac) is massaged
Photophobia, eyelid twitching
Infant 2–5 days old with Gram-negative diplococci on Gram stain
Infant 5–14 days old, mucopurulent discharge that may turn bloody, NAAT[2] positive for C. trachomatis
HSV PCR of discharge, HSV blood and CSF cultures to evaluate for disseminated infection
Fluorescein exam
⊖
⊕
Gonnococcal Conjunctivitis
Trachoma
HSV Conjunctivitis
Chemical Conjunctivitis
Nasolacrimal Duct Obstruction
Infantile Glaucoma
Corneal Abrasion
IV/IM 3rd generation cephalosporin + copious irrigation
Oral + topical erythromycin
IV acyclovir
Eye lubricant
Daily massage of blocked tear ducts ± surgery
Surgery: Goniotomy or trabeculotomy to reduce intraocular pressure
Supportive care, topical antibiotics

Footnotes

1. Infectious etiologies for neonatal conjunctivitis include organisms the infant might be exposed to while in transit through the vaginal canal. Infants delivered through C-section are at less risk for these infections.
2. NAAT: Nucleic acid amplification test.
3. Infants born in the United States receive erythromycin for prophylaxis against neonatal conjunctivitis, but silver nitrate is used in some countries.

FIGURE 23.12

23-12 Neonatal Eye Discharge

NEONATAL GONOCOCCAL CONJUNCTIVITIS

A 3-day-old baby born without prenatal care presents with profuse purulent right-eye discharge. On exam, he has severe eyelid swelling, chemosis, and mucopurulent discharge.

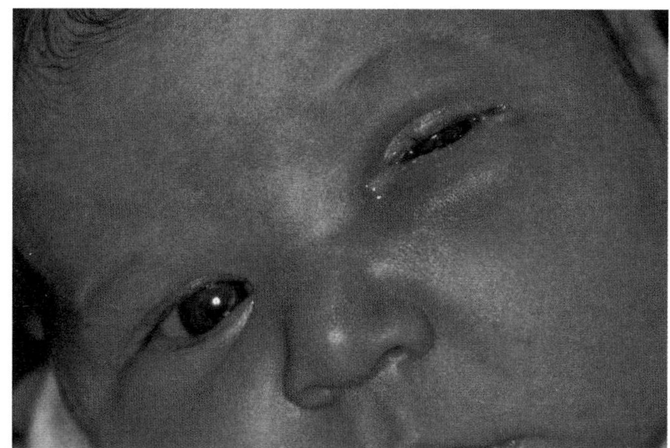

Unilateral purulent discharge with associated periorbital edema and erythema.

Management:

1. Gram stain and culture on chocolate agar (Thayer-Martin media may also be used).
2. Copious topical irrigation of normal saline to remove mucopurulent discharge.
3. Work-up of systemic disease, treatment is required for 7–14 days. If isolated to eye, one dose of IM 3rd generation cephalosporin.

Complications:

- Corneal ulceration, perforation, scarring.
- Endophthalmitis.
- Blindness if left untreated.

HYF: Preventative care includes maternal screening for gonorrhea prior to delivery. Symptoms are hyperacute, usually within 3–5 days of life. Timing of symptom onset is characteristic and helpful to distinguish from chlamydial conjunctivitis. Can effectively be prevented by prophylactic erythromycin ointment.

NEONATAL CHLAMYDIAL CONJUNCTIVITIS (TRACHOMA)

A 2-week-old F presents with serosanguinous eye discharge. Exam shows mild eyelid swelling. On labs, NAAT is positive for *C. trachomatis*.

Management:

1. Erythromycin drops QID.
2. Oral erythromycin for 2–3 weeks.
3. Work-up of systemic disease.

Complications:

- Corneal ulceration, perforation, scarring.
- Endophthalmitis.
- Blindness if left untreated.

HYF: Discharge can be watery to mucopurulent and usually not as copious as gonococcal infection. Symptoms usually present later around 5–14 days. Cannot be prevented by routine prophylaxis with erythromycin ointment.

NEONATAL CHEMICAL CONJUNCTIVITIS

A newborn presents with tearing within hours of birth after prophylactic treatment for gonococcal infection with silver nitrate.

Management:

1. Lubrication.

Complications: None.

HYF: Appears soon after birth and spontaneously resolves within 2–4 days. Application of silver nitrate is no longer a routine practice.

NASOLACRIMAL DUCT OBSTRUCTION (DACRYOSTENOSIS)

A term 5-week-old M presents with increased tearing from the right eye. On exam, he has lid crusting and a clear bluish mass overlying the lacrimal sac. Conjunctival injection is absent. Upon palpation over the lacrimal sac, there is reflux of mucoid material from the punctum.

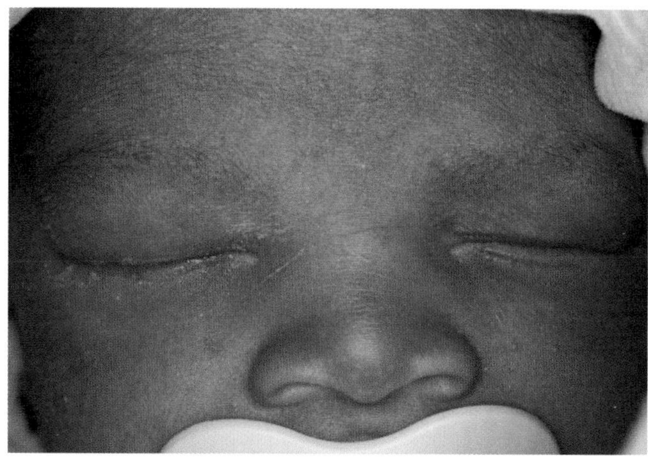

Mild crusting noted along lashline.

Management:

1. Observation with lacrimal massage.
2. Probing if no resolution by age 6 months.

Complications:

- Dacryocystitis.

HYF: Distinguish this from other newborn ophthalmic conditions (eg, infection) by lack of conjunctival injection. Purulence, tenderness, and swelling are more concerning for dacryocystitis.

HSV Conjunctivitis: See pp. 512, 611.

23-13 Neonatal Respiratory Distress

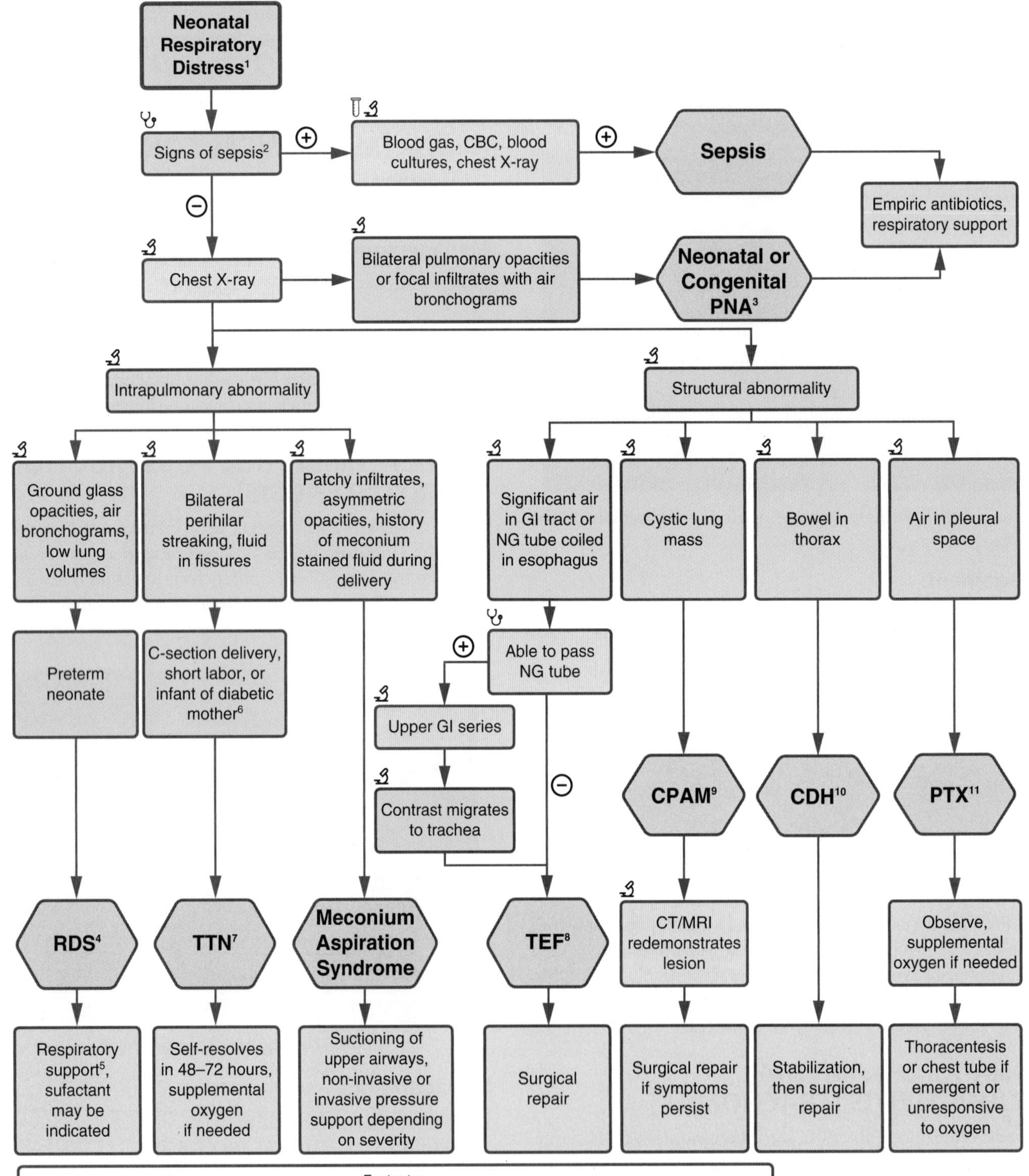
Neonatal Respiratory Distress[1]
Signs of sepsis[2]
+
Blood gas, CBC, blood cultures, chest X-ray
+
Sepsis
Empiric antibiotics, respiratory support
−
Chest X-ray
Bilateral pulmonary opacities or focal infiltrates with air bronchograms
Neonatal or Congenital PNA[3]
Intrapulmonary abnormality
Structural abnormality
Ground glass opacities, air bronchograms, low lung volumes
Bilateral perihilar streaking, fluid in fissures
Patchy infiltrates, asymmetric opacities, history of meconium stained fluid during delivery
Significant air in GI tract or NG tube coiled in esophagus
Cystic lung mass
Bowel in thorax
Air in pleural space
Preterm neonate
C-section delivery, short labor, or infant of diabetic mother[6]
Able to pass NG tube
+
Upper GI series
Contrast migrates to trachea
−
CPAM[9]
CDH[10]
PTX[11]
RDS[4]
TTN[7]
Meconium Aspiration Syndrome
TEF[8]
CT/MRI redemonstrates lesion
Observe, supplemental oxygen if needed
Respiratory support[5], sufactant may be indicated
Self-resolves in 48–72 hours, supplemental oxygen if needed
Suctioning of upper airways, non-invasive or invasive pressure support depending on severity
Surgical repair
Surgical repair if symptoms persist
Stabilization, then surgical repair
Thoracentesis or chest tube if emergent or unresponsive to oxygen

Footnotes

1. Tachypnea, intercostal/subcostal retractions, nasal flaring, head bobbing, hypoxia.
2. Signs of sepsis: Ill-appearing, temperature instability, maternal chorioamnionitis or untreated GBS. Obtain sepsis work-up as described. No lab findings are required to start empiric antibiotic treatment if the infant is ill-appearing.
3. Pneumonia.
4. Respiratory distress syndrome.
5. May include supplemental oxygen and/or pressure support.
6. These are only risk factors for TTN, not required clinical criteria.
7. Transient tachypnea of the newborn; caused by amniotic fluid in the lungs.
8. Tracheoesophageal fistula.
9. Congenital pulmonary airway malformation.
10. Congenital diaphragmatic hernia.
11. Pneumothorax.

FIGURE 23.13

23-13 Neonatal Respiratory Distress

NEONATAL OR CONGENITAL PNEUMONIA

A 2-day-old-infant born at 35 weeks GA develops increased work of breathing, tachycardia, and lethargy. On **imaging**, CXR shows bilateral pulmonary opacities.

Management:

1. Sepsis workup.
2. Supportive care in the NICU.
3. Empiric antibiotics, typically ampicillin and gentamicin.

Complications: Typically good outcomes, though preterm infants are at increased risk.

HYF: May be early onset (acquired from mother, diagnosed ≤7 days old) or late onset (community- or hospital-acquired, diagnosed ≥8 days old). Premature infants are at higher risk of pneumonia.

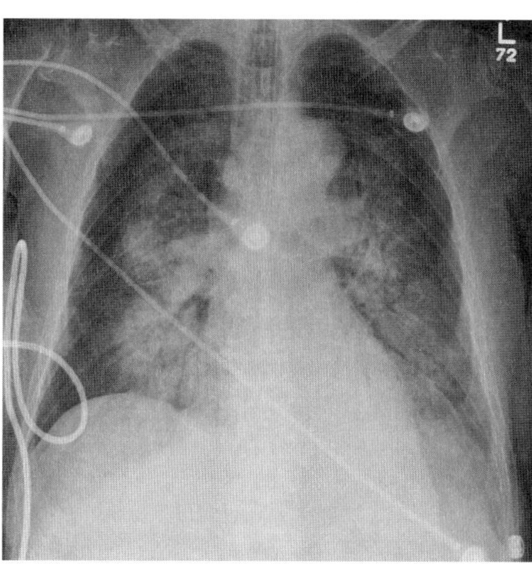
L
72

Congenital pneumonia.

RESPIRATORY DISTRESS SYNDROME (RDS)

A F born at 28 weeks GA presents with respiratory distress in the delivery room with tachypnea, grunting, and retractions. Symptoms improve with supportive care per neonatal resuscitation program (NRP). On **imaging**, CXR shows diffuse reticulogranular ground glass appearance with air bronchograms.

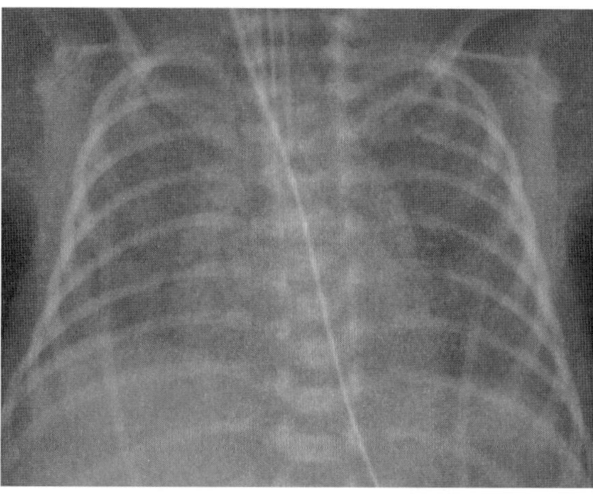

Respiratory distress syndrome.

Management:

1. Antenatal steroids for gestational age <34 weeks.
2. Supportive care, likely in the NICU.
3. Ventilatory and oxygenation support.
4. Consider surfactant administration if hypoxic despite positive pressure ventilation.

Complications:

- Respiratory failure.
- Bronchopulmonary dysplasia.
- Complications of intubation/ventilation (retinopathy of prematurity, subglottic stenosis, pneumothorax).

HYF: Incidence is highest in preterm infants due to decreased production and secretion of surfactant secondary to prematurity.

TRANSIENT TACHYPNEA OF THE NEWBORN (TTN)

A 1-hour-old infant born at 36 weeks GA via C-section develops tachypnea and retractions at 1 hour of life. On **exam**, lung sounds are clear. Work of breathing is improved by supplemental oxygen, and symptoms resolve within 24 hours. On **imaging**, CXR shows streaky interstitial markings.

Management:

1. Supportive care, nutrition optimization.
2. Supplemental oxygen.
3. Fluid restriction during the first day of life.

Complications: None.

HYF: Due to retained fetal lung fluid, leading to decreased lung compliance. Most commonly seen after cesarean delivery due to absent thoracic squeeze by the vaginal canal or in short/absent labor and in late-preterm infants (34–37 weeks) due to lower maternal stress hormone exposure. Usually occurs within 2 hours of delivery. A diagnosis of exclusion.

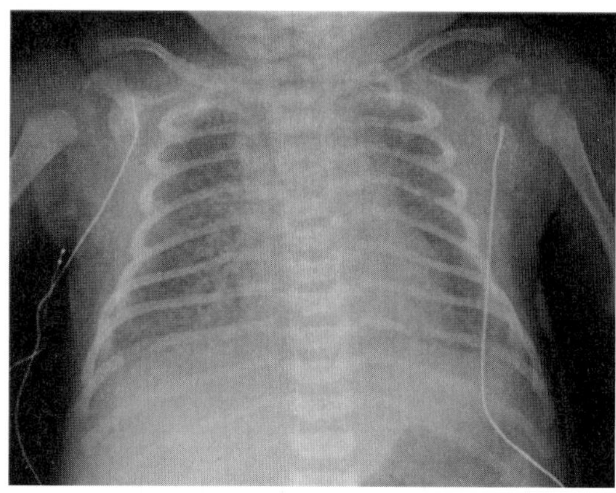

Transient tachypnea of the newborn.

23-13 Neonatal Respiratory Distress

MECONIUM ASPIRATION SYNDROME

A 2-hour-old infant born at 41 weeks GA with meconium-stained amniotic fluid at delivery has respiratory distress, tachypnea, and cyanosis during resuscitation that improves with supplemental oxygen. On **imaging**, subsequent CXR shows bilateral patchy infiltrates and flattened diaphragm.

Management:

1. Supportive care and standard management per neonatal resuscitation program (NRP).
2. ~30% require intubation due to respiratory failure.
3. Surfactant and iNO administration are not routine but may be considered in severely ill patients with refractory symptoms.

Complications:

- ECMO rarely required due to severe disease.
- Can be associated with pneumothorax (10–30%).
- May see long-term reactive airway disease.

HYF: Meconium aspiration results in surfactant deactivation and pneumonitis. No longer recommend routine intubation for infants with MAS. More common in post-term infants and infants born to mothers with symptoms of chorioamnionitis.

TRACHEOESOPHAGEAL FISTULA (TEF)

A 4-hour-old term newborn with respiratory distress has an unusually high secretion burden and difficulty feeding. On **imaging**, chest and abdominal X-rays are significant for large amounts of air in the intestines.

Management:

1. Diagnosed by failure to pass an NG tube and CXR showing NG tube coiled in the esophagus and gas-filled GI tract.
2. Surgical correction typically has excellent prognosis, although TEF with associated esophageal atresia has higher mortality and higher risk of complications.

Complications: Gastroesophageal reflux due to impaired esophageal motility.

HYF: May be associated with **VACTERL** anomalies (**V**ertebral, **A**nal, **C**ardiac, **T**racheal, **E**sophageal, **R**enal, **L**imb). Polyhydramnios can be seen *in utero*.

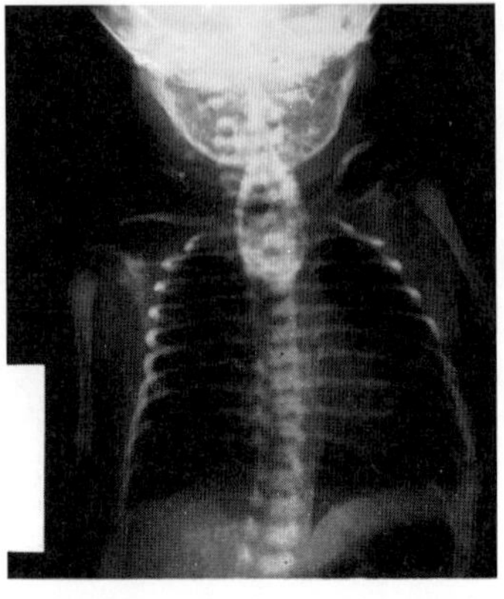

Tracheoesophageal fistula. A coiled NG tube can be visualized in the esophagus.

CONGENITAL PULMONARY AIRWAY MALFORMATION (CPAM)

A 2-hour-old M born at 38 weeks GA is in respiratory distress with increased work of breathing. The infant's mother recalls "an abnormality" on the 2nd trimester prenatal ultrasound. On **imaging**, CXR shows a cystic mass in the left lung base.

Management:

1. Supportive care.
2. Fetal echo to rule out congenital cardiac anomalies.
3. If symptomatic, immediate further imaging and surgical repair.
4. Asymptomatic patients can have imaging at 6 months old.

Complications:

- Mediastinal shift with large lesions, with possible compression of IVC and heart leading to hydrops.
- Compression of esophagus leading to small stomach and polyhydramnios.
- May be associated with malignancy.
- Can see pneumothorax due to air leak.
- Infection of the malformation.

HYF: Consists of hamartomatous or dysplastic lung tissue mixed with normal lung. May be associated with congenital abnormalities (10–20%). Usually diagnosed on prenatal ultrasound. Large or rapidly growing lesions may cause mediastinal shift and compression of intra-thoracic organs.

CONGENITAL DIAPHRAGMATIC HERNIA (CDH)

A full term neonate with a prenatal history of polyhydramnios has respiratory distress. On **imaging**, CXR demonstrates presence of bowel in the left hemithorax.

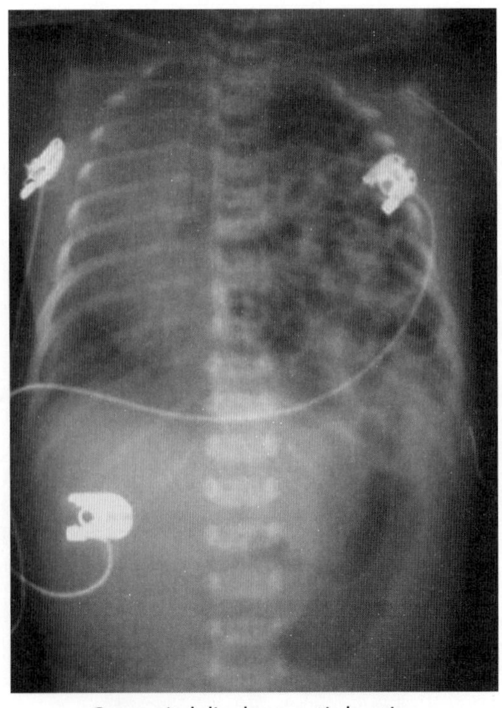

Congenital diaphragmatic hernia.

23-13 Neonatal Respiratory Distress

Management:

1. Stabilization and medical management preoperatively with ventilator support.
2. Surgical correction.

Complications:

- Pulmonary hypertension.
- Chronic lung disease due to pulmonary hypoplasia.

HYF: Most commonly see herniation into posterior left hemithorax. Typically diagnosed on prenatal ultrasound and confirmed with postnatal CXR.

PNEUMOTHORAX

A neonate born at 34 weeks GA develops sudden onset respiratory distress with tachypnea. Exam shows decreased breath sounds on the right side.

Management:

1. Can diagnose with CXR, ultrasound, or transillumination.
2. Infants not requiring O_2 supplementation may be closely observed.
3. Provide supplemental O_2 as needed to maintain O_2 saturations.
4. Thoracentesis is indicated for emergent treatment for infants not responding to resuscitation with bradycardia and cyanosis.

Complications: Complications due to thoracentesis or chest tube.

HYF: Chest tubes are not routinely placed in the delivery room, but they may be indicated for patients who develop a pneumothorax following initiation of mechanical ventilation.

23-14 Neonatal Heart Defects

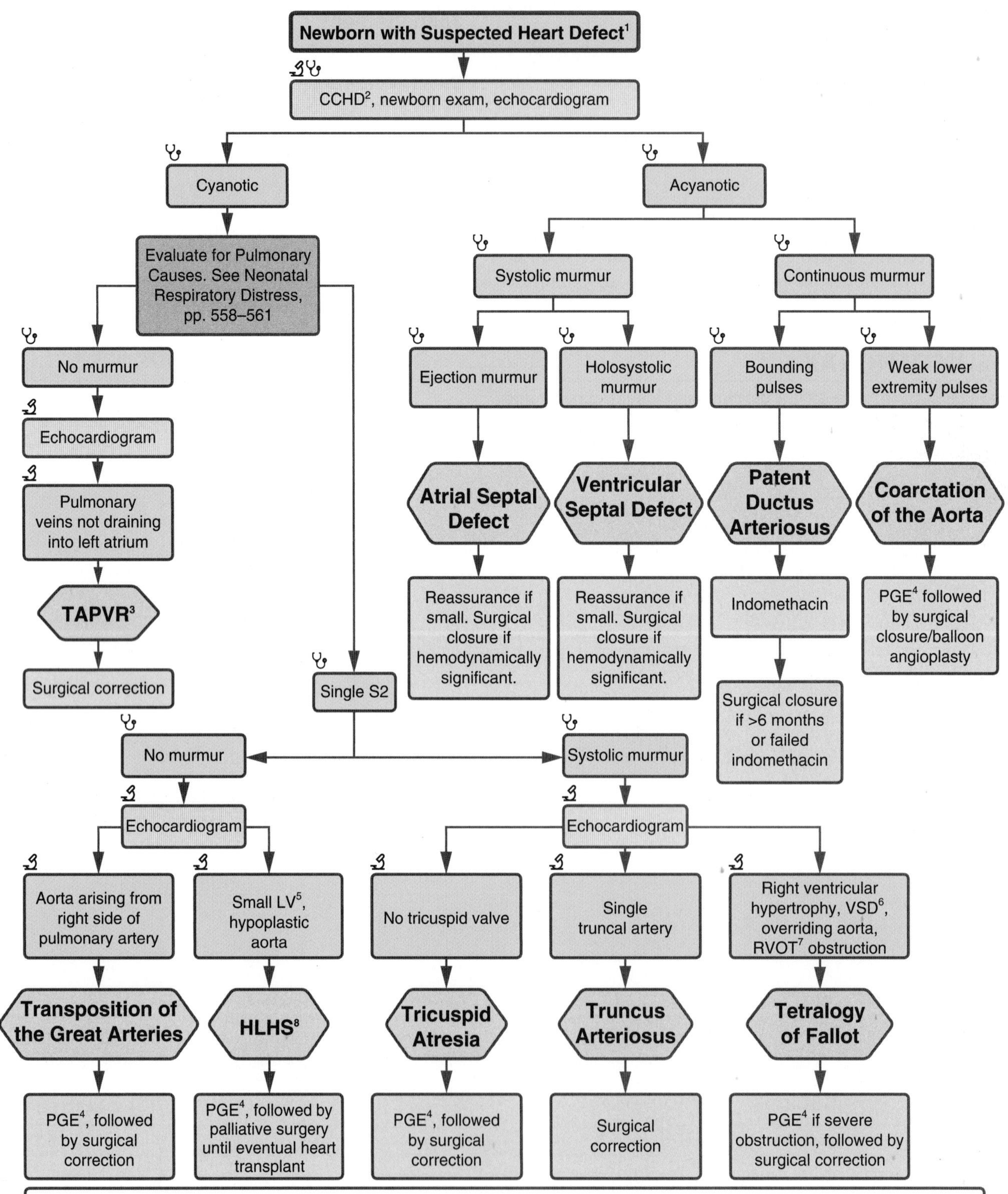

Newborn with Suspected Heart Defect[1]
CCHD[2], newborn exam, echocardiogram
Cyanotic
Acyanotic
Evaluate for Pulmonary Causes. See Neonatal Respiratory Distress, pp. 558–561
No murmur
Echocardiogram
Pulmonary veins not draining into left atrium
TAPVR[3]
Surgical correction
Single S2
No murmur
Systolic murmur
Echocardiogram
Aorta arising from right side of pulmonary artery
Transposition of the Great Arteries
PGE[4], followed by surgical correction
Small LV[5], hypoplastic aorta
HLHS[8]
PGE[4], followed by palliative surgery until eventual heart transplant
No tricuspid valve
Tricuspid Atresia
PGE[4], followed by surgical correction
Single truncal artery
Truncus Arteriosus
Surgical correction
Right ventricular hypertrophy, VSD[6], overriding aorta, RVOT[7] obstruction
Tetralogy of Fallot
PGE[4] if severe obstruction, followed by surgical correction
Systolic murmur
Ejection murmur
Atrial Septal Defect
Reassurance if small. Surgical closure if hemodynamically significant.
Holosystolic murmur
Ventricular Septal Defect
Reassurance if small. Surgical closure if hemodynamically significant.
Continuous murmur
Bounding pulses
Patent Ductus Arteriosus
Indomethacin
Surgical closure if >6 months or failed indomethacin
Weak lower extremity pulses
Coarctation of the Aorta
PGE[4] followed by surgical closure/balloon angioplasty

Footnotes

1. A majority of infants with heart defects are prenatally diagnosed during the 20-week gestation anatomy scan. However, many infants present primarily with faltering growth, cyanosis, or fatigue and diaphoresis with feeding, which can be signs of developing heart failure. Additionally, any infant with a diastolic or continuous murmur should obtain an echocardiogram to screen for CCHD.
2. CCHD: Critical congenital heart disease screen. Pulse oximetry of the right hand and either foot is performed. Presence of a cyanotic heart defect is considered if any reading is <89% or if lower extremity reading is significantly lower than upper extremity reading.
3. TAPVR: Total anomalous pulmonary venous return.
4. PGE: Prostaglandin E. Maintains the ductus arteriosus patent. Used in ductal-dependant lesions.
5. LV: Left ventricle.
6. VSD: Ventricular septal defect.
7. RVOT: Right ventricular outflow tract.
8. HLHS: Hypoplastic left heart syndrome.

FIGURE 23.14

23-14 Neonatal Heart Defects

NON-CYANOTIC HEART DEFECTS

ATRIAL SEPTAL DEFECT

A newborn presents with a midsystolic ejection murmur best heard over the 2nd intercostal space and fixed split S2. Echocardiogram confirms the defect's size and location.

Management:

1. Reassurance: Small defects are most likely to close spontaneously.
2. Surgical closure for severe L → R shunting or evidence of right heart enlargement.

Complications:

- Other AV canal defects.
- Arrhythmias.
- Volume overload/heart failure.
- Pulmonary hypertension.

HYF: Murmur is usually from flow across the pulmonary valve, not flow across the ASD. EKG may show right ventricular hypertrophy. CXR may show cardiomegaly and increased pulmonary vascularity. Associated with trisomy 21 and Holt-Oram (heart-hand) syndrome. Secundum defects are the most common.

VENTRICULAR SEPTAL DEFECT

A 2-week-old with poor weight gain presents with a harsh holosystolic murmur heard best at the left lower sternal border. Echocardiogram confirms the defect's size and location.

Management:

1. Small defects close spontaneously by age 2 years.
2. Medical management for mild to moderate heart failure.
3. Surgical repair for hemodynamically significant VSD resulting in pulmonary overcirculation and severe heart failure.

Complications:

- Pulmonary hypertension.
- Eisenmenger syndrome.
- Aortic regurgitation.
- Endocarditis.

HYF: Most common CHD. Can develop displaced apical impulse and palpable thrill. The intensity of the murmur is inversely related to size of defect. Associated with trisomy 21 and CHARGE syndrome (mutation in *CHD7*).

PATENT DUCTUS ARTERIOSUS

A newborn M presents with feeding difficulty and poor weight gain. On exam, he has a continuous murmur best heard at the left subclavicular region and bounding pulses.

Management:

1. NSAID (indomethacin or ibuprofen) in preterm infants.
2. Observation in term asymptomatic infants <6 kg and infants with severe pulmonary hypertension.
3. Ligation/occlusion in term infants >6 kg with moderate to severe PDA, small audible PDA, or history of endocarditis.

Complications:

- Left-sided cardiac overload.
- Pulmonary hypertension.

HYF: EKG may show left ventricular hypertrophy. CXR may show cardiomegaly. Associated with congenital rubella syndrome.

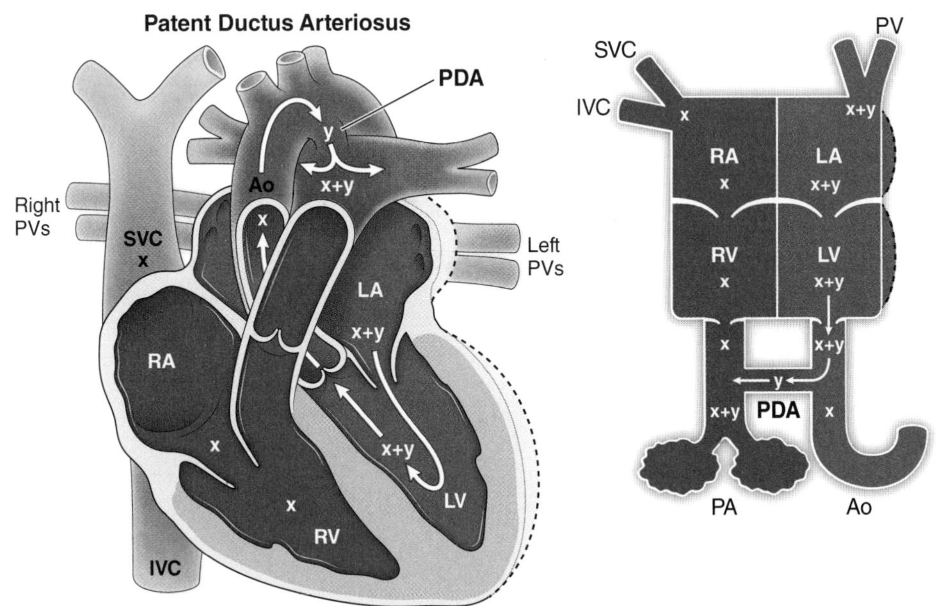
Patent Ductus Arteriosus
PDA
y
Ao
x+y
x
Right PVs
SVC
x
Left PVs
LA
x+y
RA
x
x+y
x
LV
RV
IVC
SVC
PV
IVC
x
x+y
RA
x
LA
x+y
RV
x
LV
x+y
x
x+y
y
x+y
PDA
x
PA
Ao

Diagram illustrating a left-to-right shunt from the descending aorta to the main pulmonary artery via the patent ductus arteriosus.

23-14 Neonatal Heart Defects

COARCTATION OF THE AORTA

A newborn F presents with asymptomatic hypertension and cyanosis in the lower extremities. On exam, she has a continuous murmur, diminished and delayed femoral pulses, and upper and lower extremity blood pressure differential. Echocardiogram confirms the defect.

Management:

1. Prostaglandin E1 (PGE) to keep ductus arteriosus open.
2. Surgical closure/balloon angioplasty if large gradient, hypertension, collateral flow, or symptoms of heart failure.

Complications:

- Recoarctation.
- Heart failure.
- Systemic hypertension.
- Aneurysms.

HYF: Occurs distal to left subclavian in most patients due to thickening of the tunica media at the junction of ductus arteriosus and aortic arch. EKG may show LVH. CXR may show cardiomegaly, pulmonary congestion, and rib notching. If severe, coarctation of the aorta may be dependent on a patent ductus arteriosus; when it closes on day 3 of life, infants can go into heart failure. Associated with Turner syndrome. 2/3rds of patients have a bicuspid aortic valve.

EISENMENGER SYNDROME

An 18-year-old M with a history of unrepaired VSD presents with syncope. On exam, he has cyanosis, edema, and hepatomegaly.

Management:

1. Medical management of heart failure.
2. Cardiac transplant.

Complications:

- Heart failure.
- Iron-deficiency anemia.
- Pulmonary artery thrombosis.

HYF: Most commonly caused by VSD (33%), ASD (30%), and PDA (14%). EKG may show right ventricular hypertrophy or biventricular hypertrophy. CXR shows RV enlargement and pulmonary artery dilation.

CYANOTIC HEART DEFECTS

TRUNCUS ARTERIOSUS

A term newborn M fails his CCHD screen at 3 days of life. On exam, he has mild intercostal retractions and a systolic murmur with ejection click. Femoral pulses are bounding. On imaging, CXR shows an enlarged cardiac silhouette ("boot-shaped heart") and increased pulmonary vascular markings. EKG shows right-axis deviation. Echocardiogram shows a VSD and a single truncal valve with a common ventricular outflow tract.

Management:

1. Administer PGE to sustain the PDA.
2. Diuretics to improve pulmonary congestion.
3. Respiratory support via positive pressure if needed.
4. Urgent surgical correction.

Complications:

- Heart failure.
- Iron deficiency anemia.
- Pulmonary artery thrombosis.
- Death within 2 months if no surgical repair.

HYF: Truncus arteriosus occurs when the single truncal root does not divide into aortic and pulmonic arteries during embryogenesis. It is frequently associated with DiGeorge syndrome (22q11 gene deletion).

TETRALOGY OF FALLOT

A 2-day-old M develops cyanosis and respiratory distress. He has a grade II crescendo-decrescendo systolic ejection murmur best heard at the LUSB with radiation to the back. On imaging, echocardiogram reveals pulmonary artery stenosis, right ventricular hypertrophy, an overriding aorta, and a VSD.

Management:

1. Administer PGE to sustain the PDA.
2. Surgical correction.

23-14 Neonatal Heart Defects

Complications:

- Heart failure.
- Arrhythmia from surgical repair.

HYF: PROVe: Pulmonary stenosis, RVH, Overriding Aorta, VSD. Tetralogy of Fallot can also present later in toddlerhood and result in "tet spells," cyanotic episodes due to decreased systemic vascular resistance and leading to a right-to-left shunt across the VSD.

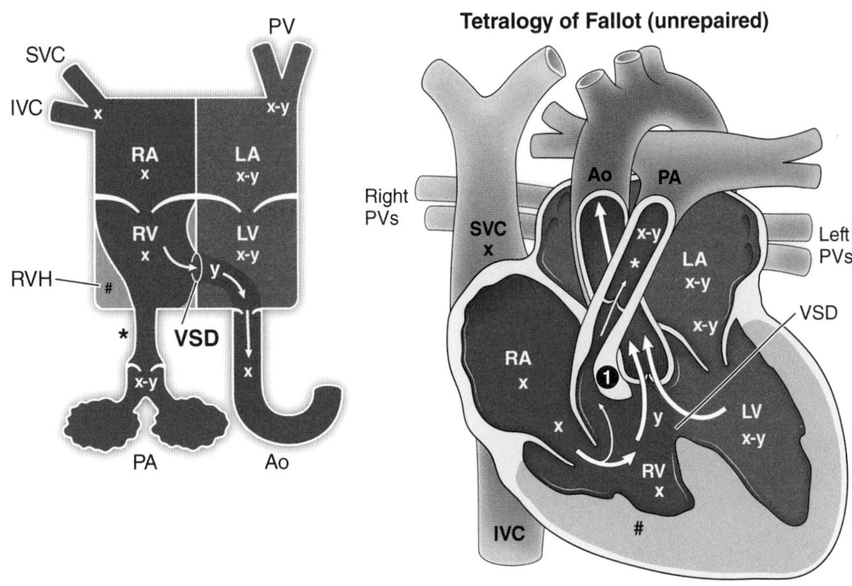
SVC
IVC
PV
RA
x
LA
x-y
RV
x
LV
x-y
RVH
VSD
PA
Ao
Tetralogy of Fallot (unrepaired)
Right PVs
Left PVs
SVC
IVC
Ao
PA
LA
RA
RV
LV

Right ventricular outflow tract obstruction leads to a right-to-left shunt via the ventricular septal defect (VSD).

TOTAL ANOMALOUS PULMONARY VENOUS RETURN (TAPVR)

A 10-hour-old M develops respiratory distress, hypoxia, and cyanosis. **Exam** shows tachycardia with a grade III systolic heart murmur. On **imaging**, echocardiogram reveals an enlarged right atrium and right ventricle, as well as pulmonary veins entering the right atrium rather than the left. Right-to-left shunting is seen across an ASD.

Management:

1. Supportive care, including respiratory support if needed.
2. Surgical correction.

Complications: Death if not surgically corrected.

HYF: TAPVR is a cyanotic defect often accompanied by an ASD, resulting in a systolic heart murmur and mixing of blood, allowing oxygenated blood to enter the systemic vascular system.

TRANSPOSITION OF THE GREAT ARTERIES

A 5-day-old F develops tachypnea and hypoxia with cyanosis. **Exam** shows regular rate and rhythm without murmur. EKG is normal. On **imaging**, echocardiogram reveals that the aorta originates at the RV, and the pulmonary artery originates at the LV.

Transposition of the great arteries

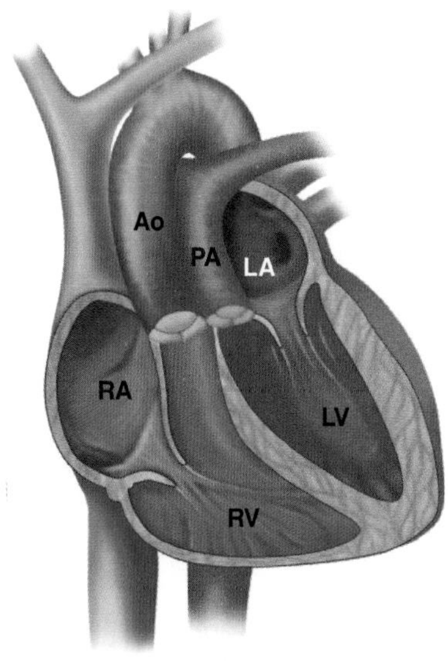
Ao
PA
LA
RA
LV
RV

23-14 Neonatal Heart Defects

Management:

1. Administer PGE to sustain the PDA.
2. Surgical correction.

Complications: Death if not surgically repaired.

HYF: EKG may show right axis deviation and RVH as it pumps against systemic pressures. This cyanotic heart defect is often accompanied by other defects, such as VSD or ASD, which allow mixing of blood for less severe presentation.

HYPOPLASTIC LEFT HEART SYNDROME (HLHS)

A 3-day-old F with limited prenatal care develops tachycardia, hypotension, and cyanosis. On **exam**, her femoral pulses are weak, and she has a grade III systolic murmur over the RUSB. On **imaging**, echocardiogram shows a small left ventricle, very small ascending aorta, aortic stenosis, and dilated right atrium and right ventricle.

Management:

1. Administer PGE to sustain the PDA.
2. Avoid supplemental oxygen to prevent decreasing pulmonary vascular resistance. Keeping a greater pulmonary vascular resistance relative to systemic vascular resistance aids the shunting of blood to systemic circulation.
3. Three-stage surgical palliation around 7–10 days of life, 6–9 months old, and lastly at 2 years old.
4. Eventual heart transplantation.

Complications:

- Death in the first week of life if not surgically corrected.
- Pulmonary hypertension.

HYF: HLHS is usually diagnosed prenatally and results from underdevelopment of the left side of the heart, resulting in single-ventricle physiology. Surgical palliation was developed relatively recently in the last 3 decades.

23-15 Neonatal Emesis

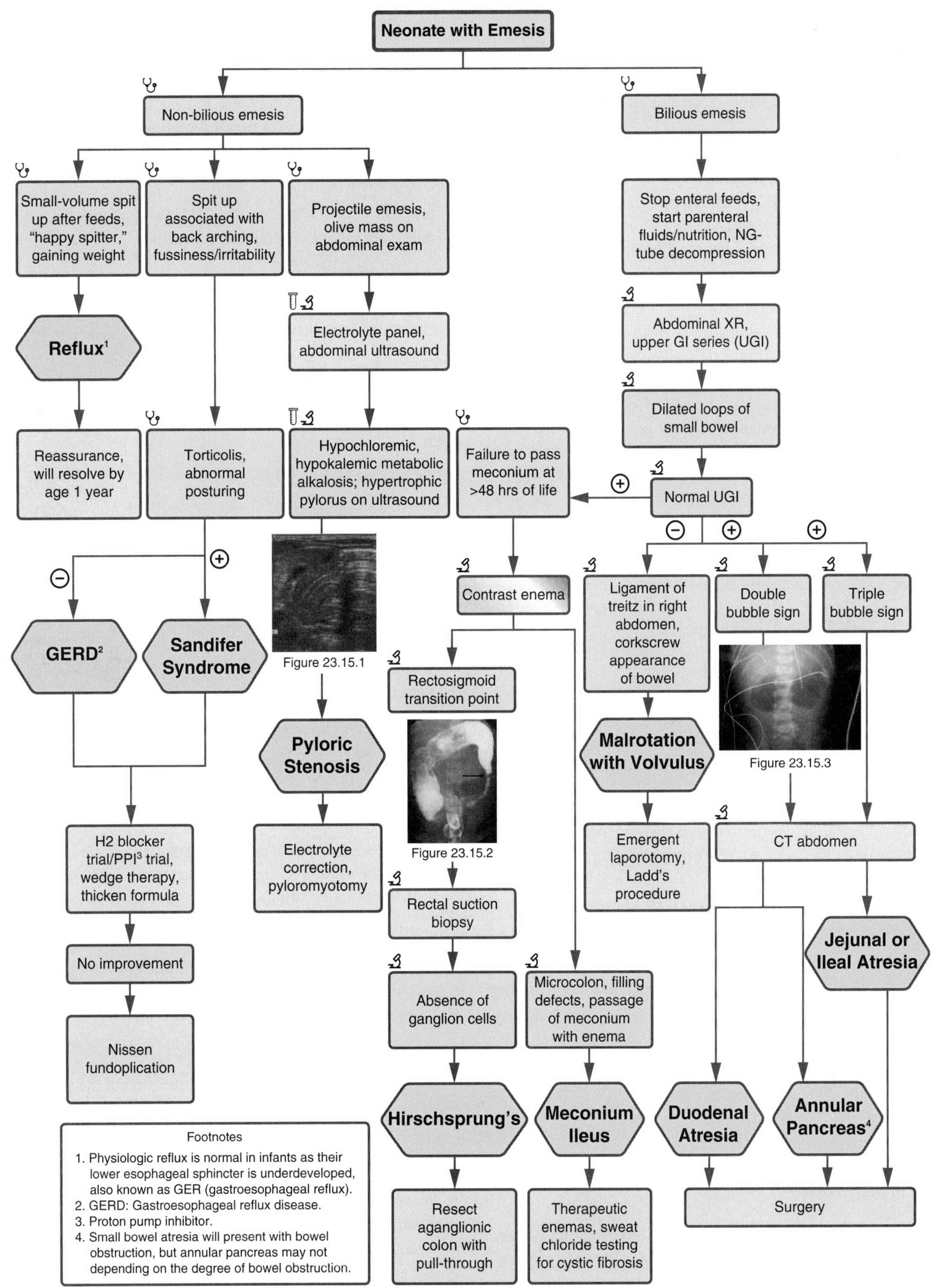

Neonate with Emesis
Non-bilious emesis
Bilious emesis
Small-volume spit up after feeds, "happy spitter," gaining weight
Spit up associated with back arching, fussiness/irritability
Projectile emesis, olive mass on abdominal exam
Stop enteral feeds, start parenteral fluids/nutrition, NG-tube decompression
Reflux[1]
Electrolyte panel, abdominal ultrasound
Abdominal XR, upper GI series (UGI)
Dilated loops of small bowel
Reassurance, will resolve by age 1 year
Torticolis, abnormal posturing
Hypochloremic, hypokalemic metabolic alkalosis; hypertrophic pylorus on ultrasound
Failure to pass meconium at >48 hrs of life
Normal UGI
Contrast enema
Ligament of treitz in right abdomen, corkscrew appearance of bowel
Double bubble sign
Triple bubble sign
GERD[2]
Sandifer Syndrome
Figure 23.15.1
Rectosigmoid transition point
Pyloric Stenosis
Malrotation with Volvulus
Figure 23.15.3
Figure 23.15.2
H2 blocker trial/PPI[3] trial, wedge therapy, thicken formula
Electrolyte correction, pyloromyotomy
Emergent laporotomy, Ladd's procedure
CT abdomen
Rectal suction biopsy
No improvement
Jejunal or Ileal Atresia
Absence of ganglion cells
Microcolon, filling defects, passage of meconium with enema
Nissen fundoplication
Hirschsprung's
Meconium Ileus
Duodenal Atresia
Annular Pancreas[4]
Resect aganglionic colon with pull-through
Therapeutic enemas, sweat chloride testing for cystic fibrosis
Surgery
Footnotes
1. Physiologic reflux is normal in infants as their lower esophageal sphincter is underdeveloped, also known as GER (gastroesophageal reflux).
2. GERD: Gastroesophageal reflux disease.
3. Proton pump inhibitor.
4. Small bowel atresia will present with bowel obstruction, but annular pancreas may not depending on the degree of bowel obstruction.

FIGURE 23.15

23-15 Neonatal Emesis

GASTROESOPHAGEAL REFLUX DISEASE (GERD)

A 2-month-old previously healthy term F presents with persistent spit-up after feeds leading to inadequate weight gain.

Management:

1. Positional interventions: Keeping infant upright after meals.
2. H2 blockers (famotidine), which can be escalated to proton pump inhibitors (omeprazole).
3. Nissen fundoplication if very severe with continued failure to gain weight.

Complications:

- Discomfort.
- Poor weight gain.

HYF: All infants will have spit-ups after feeds. As long as the infant is gaining adequate weight, this is not pathological. Intervention is only indicated if there are concerns for slower weight gain and ascending aspiration.

HYPERTROPHIC PYLORIC STENOSIS

A 5-week-old M presents with 2 days of projectile vomiting after every feed. On **exam**, an olive-shaped mass in the epigastrium is palpable. **Labs** show a metabolic alkalosis with hypokalemia. On **imaging**, US shows a hypertrophic pylorus.

Management:

1. IV fluids, correct electrolyte imbalances.
2. Surgical correction with pyloromyotomy.

Complications:

- Faltering growth.

HYF: Most commonly seen in first born male infants between 3–6 weeks of age when the pylorus starts to hypertrophy.

MALROTATION WITH OR WITHOUT VOLVULUS

A 3-day-old M born at 40 weeks GA presents with bilious emesis. On **imaging**, abdominal X-ray shows proximal bowel obstruction and distal gas. Upper GI series shows malpositioned ligament of Treitz.

Management:

1. Stabilization and decompression.
2. Ladd's procedure.

Complications: Midgut volvulus (emergency!): Vascular compromise or perforation.

HYF: It is possible to have malrotation without volvulus. In these cases, Ladd's procedure can be performed as an elective procedure. However, these children are at risk for volvulizing at any moment.

HIRSCHSPRUNG'S DISEASE

A 1-week-old F born at 39 weeks GA presents with bilious emesis and abdominal distension. When she was in the nursery, she did not pass meconium until day 3 of life. On **imaging**, abdominal X-ray shows dilated small bowel loops. Anorectal manometry is abnormal. Rectal suction biopsy shows absence of ganglion cells.

Management:

1. Surgical resection of distal bowel that is aganglionic.
2. Assess for other congenital abnormalities.

Complications:

- Enterocolitis (emergency!)
- Constipation, incontinence.

HYF: Occurs due to failed migration of neural crest cells to the distal colon and rectum. Delayed passage of meconium (past 45 hours of life) is a frequent part of the history. Associated with trisomy 21.

MECONIUM ILEUS

A 2-day-old M born at 37 weeks GA with a family history of cystic fibrosis presents with abdominal distension and failure to pass meconium. On **imaging**, contrast radiograph shows dilated small bowel and dense opacities suggestive of inspissated meconium in the terminal ileum.

Management:

1. Stabilization.
2. Therapeutic enemas.
3. Surgery if needed.

Complications:

- GI complications, perforation.
- Cholestasis.

HYF: Meconium ileus is highly suggestive of an underlying diagnosis of cystic fibrosis (CF). Refer infants for CF testing, as this may be the presenting symptom.

INTESTINAL ATRESIA

A 1-day-old F with trisomy 21 born at 34 weeks GA presents with bilious emesis. On **imaging**, abdominal X-ray shows a double bubble sign (dilated stomach and duodenum).

Management:

1. NG/OG tube placement for decompression of the stomach.
2. Hydration, correction of electrolyte abnormalities.
3. Surgical correction.

Complications:

- Short gut syndrome.
- Associated chromosomal/cardiac abnormalities.
- Anastomotic dysfunction, stricture, adhesions.

HYF: Duodenal atresia is more common than jejunal atresia and is associated with trisomy 21.

23-16 Genetic Disorders: Inborn Errors of Metabolism

PHENYLKETONURIA (PKU)

A 6-month-old F born full-term presents with developmental regression (loss of sitting), lethargy, and new seizures. On **exam**, she has a musty body odor, and **labs** show elevated plasma phenylalanine and elevated phenylalanine to tyrosine ratio. Sequencing of *PAH* reveals a pathogenic variant.

Management:

1. Conversion to low-phenylalanine diet.
2. Referral to neurodevelopmental specialist.

HYF: PKU is tested on the newborn screen and is asymptomatic if managed on low-phenylalanine diet since infancy. Developmental delay and regression are progressive over time if not on a restricted diet.

FABRY DISEASE

A 5-year-old M with PMH of anhidrosis presents with acroparesthesias with burning pain in extremities after exercise. On **exam**, he has angiokeratomas on the hips, back, and thighs. Echocardiogram shows left ventricular hypertrophy similar to hypertrophic cardiomyopathy, as well as mitral valve insufficiency. **Labs** show decreased alpha-galactosidase A activity, and sequencing of *GLA* shows pathogenic mutation.

Management:

1. EKG and echocardiogram if not already available.
2. Urinalysis and renal function studies (Cr, BUN) to assess for proteinuria and CKD.
3. Referral for consideration of enzyme replacement therapy.

Complications:

- Cerebrovascular accident.
- CKD progressing to ESRD.

HYF: Fabry is X-linked–recessive and typically appears in mid- to late childhood with multisystem involvement, typically a combination of vascular and neurologic problems with fulminant onset. It is not included on most states' newborn screens due to limited treatment options.

KRABBE SYNDROME

A 6-month-old F with a history of poor perinatal care presents with feeding difficulties and loss of milestones such as cooing and head control. On **exam**, she has lower extremity spasticity, axial hypotonia, and fisting. **Labs** show decreased *GALC* activity, and targeted sequencing confirms pathogenic variant in *GALC*.

Management:

1. Referral to neurodevelopmental specialist.
2. Audiology assessment for hearing loss.
3. Brain MRI to determine degree of progression: namely, risk of apneas and temperature instability.
4. Nerve conduction testing for peripheral motor neuropathy.
5. Consider bone marrow transplant.

HYF: Krabbe is a leukodystrophy, meaning it generally affects the CNS and PNS but in a global fashion. Think leukodystrophy if only the nervous system is involved.

GAUCHER SYNDROME

An 18-year-old M presents with bone pain in the upper extremities. On **exam**, he has hepatosplenomegaly. **Labs** show low bone mineral density and pancytopenia. On **imaging**, x-ray reveals osteolytic lesions. Targeted sequencing shows pathogenic mutation in *GBA*.

Management:

1. Enzyme replacement therapy.
2. CBC monitoring for transfusion needs.
3. Skeletal assessment.

HYF: Gaucher is a lysosomal storage disorder and is associated with the Ashkenazi Jewish founder effect. The most common subtype affects adolescents and adults (type 1) and can be a cancer mimic.

NIEMANN-PICK SYNDROME

A 1-year-old M has jaundice, hepatosplenomegaly, hypotonia, and cherry red macular spots bilaterally. On **imaging**, CXR shows pulmonary infiltrates bilaterally. Targeted sequencing shows a pathogenic variant in *NPC1*.

Management:

1. Brain MRI to determine extent of disease.
2. EEG for seizure assessment.
3. Referral to neurodevelopmental specialist.

HYF: Niemann-Pick is progressive and currently has no treatment aside from supportive therapy. Both Neimann-Pick and Tay-Sachs are lysosomal storage disorders and exhibit cherry red macula, but the former is more visceral and the latter more neurologic.

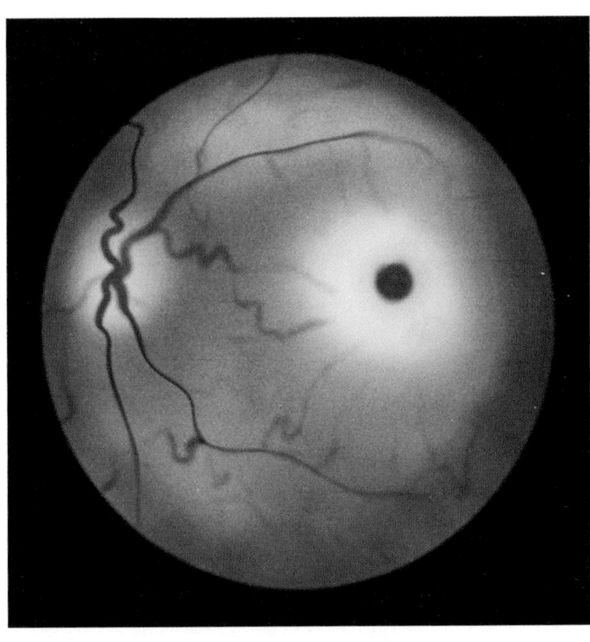

Cherry red spot on macula.

23-16 Genetic Disorders: Inborn Errors of Metabolism

TAY-SACHS SYNDROME (TSS)

A 4-month-old term M presents with extremity weakness, regression of motor skills, and exaggerated startle response. On **exam**, he has hypotonia and a cherry red spot on the macula with normal liver and spleen. Targeted sequencing shows a pathogenic variant in *HEXA*.

Management:

1. Neuro-evaluation with MRI and EEG.
2. Nutritional support.
3. Referral to neurodevelopmental specialist.

HYF: TSS is a progressive neurologic disorder with no direct treatment aside from supportive therapy. It is distinguished from NPS by lack of liver or spleen abnormalities. Higher incidence in the Ashkenazi Jewish population.

METACHROMATIC LEUKODYSTROPHY

A 2-year-old F presents with frequent falls, dysarthria, and gross motor developmental regression. On **exam**, she has lower extremity spasticity. On **imaging**, brain MRI shows diffuse symmetric hyperintensities suggestive of leukodystrophy. Targeted sequencing shows a pathogenic variant in *ARSA*.

Management:

1. Bone marrow transplant.
2. EEG and neurology referral for seizure management.

HYF: Metachromatic leukodystrophy is very similar in presentation to Krabbe syndrome and requires MRI and genetic testing to differentiate. MRI is the most sensitive modality for detecting leukodystrophies.

HURLER SYNDROME

An 18-month-old M has corneal clouding, an umbilical hernia, coarse facial features, hepatosplenomegaly, global developmental delay, and limited joint range of motion on **exam**. Targeted sequencing reveals a pathogenic variant in *IDUA*.

Management:

1. Bone marrow transplant.
2. Referral to neurodevelopmental specialist.
3. Ophthalmologic evaluation for cataracts and glaucoma.
4. Echocardiogram for progressive valvular dysfunction risk.

HYF: Hurler syndrome is the most severe of the mucopolysaccharidoses and is characteristically associated with corneal clouding.

HUNTER SYNDROME

A 30-month-old F with a history of poor perinatal care presents with loss of motor and speech milestones. On **exam**, she has short stature, coarse facial features, and hepatosplenomegaly, with no corneal clouding. Targeted sequencing reveals a pathogenic variant in *IDS*.

Management:

1. Echocardiogram for valvular dysfunction.
2. Brain MRI to evaluate for common abnormalitis, including hydrocephalus, ventriculomegaly, and enlarged subarachnoid spaces.
3. Referral to neurodevelopmental specialist.

HYF: Hunter is generally similar to but milder in presentation than Hurler with no ophthalmologic involvement. **Hunters need their eyes to hunt** (no corneal clouding).

HOMOCYSTINURIA

An 8-year-old F presents with a stroke to the ED. On **exam**, she has tall stature, severe myopia with glasses, and pectus excavatum. On **imaging**, CXR shows scoliosis. **Labs** show elevated plasma homocysteine levels, and targeted sequencing reveals a pathogenic variant in *CBS*.

Management:

1. Trial of pyridoxine therapy (can reduce homocysteine levels).
2. Methionine-restricted diet.
3. Ophthalmology referral for ectopia lentis surveillance.
4. DEXA scan every 3–5 years.

Complications: High risk of future thromboembolism.

HYF: Stroke is the major cause of morbidity and mortality in this population.

FRIEDRICH'S ATAXIA

A 12-year-old M presents with gradually progressive lower extremity weakness, and on **exam** has gait and limb ataxia with dysarthria. Echocardiogram shows hypertrophic cardiomyopathy. **Labs** reveal hyperglycemia with elevated HbA1c. Targeted sequencing shows a pathogenic variant in *FXN*.

Management:

1. Neurology referral.
2. Physical and occupational therapy.

HYF: Friedrich's ataxia is a trinucleotide repeat disorder (GAA) in the *FXN* gene and is autosomal recessive. Thus, it does not undergo anticipation, unlike many other trinucleotide repeat disorders.

PRADER-WILLI SYNDROME

An 8-year-old M with a history of perinatal feeding difficulty presents with hyperphagia, obesity, and global developmental delay. On **exam**, he has a thin vermilion border, hypogonadism, and hypotonia. Combined DNA methylation studies and sequencing reveal imprinting failure on the paternal allele of chromosome 15q11.2–q13.

Management:

1. Prevention of obesity complications (diabetes, cholesterol screening, sleep apnea testing).
2. Referral to endocrinology for management of GH replacement for short stature.
3. Prevention of food hoarding.

HYF: Prader-Willi syndrome is believed to affect hypothalamic detection of satiety, leading to characteristic hyperphagia with primarily central obesity.

23-17 Genetic Disorders: Aneuploidy

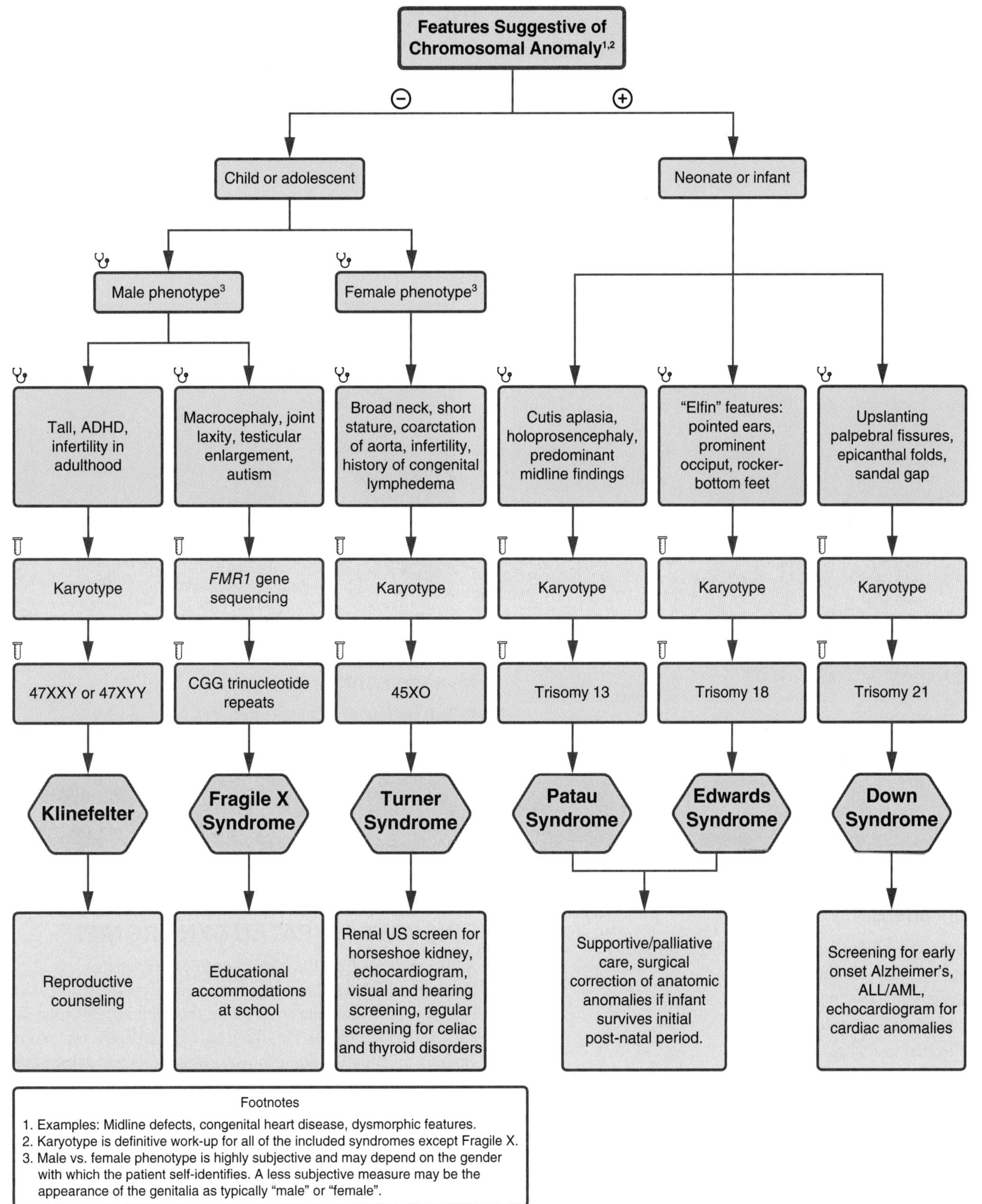
Features Suggestive of Chromosomal Anomaly[1,2]
⊖
⊕
Child or adolescent
Neonate or infant
Male phenotype[3]
Female phenotype[3]
Tall, ADHD, infertility in adulthood
Macrocephaly, joint laxity, testicular enlargement, autism
Broad neck, short stature, coarctation of aorta, infertility, history of congenital lymphedema
Cutis aplasia, holoprosencephaly, predominant midline findings
"Elfin" features: pointed ears, prominent occiput, rocker-bottom feet
Upslanting palpebral fissures, epicanthal folds, sandal gap
Karyotype
FMR1 gene sequencing
Karyotype
Karyotype
Karyotype
Karyotype
47XXY or 47XYY
CGG trinucleotide repeats
45XO
Trisomy 13
Trisomy 18
Trisomy 21
Klinefelter
Fragile X Syndrome
Turner Syndrome
Patau Syndrome
Edwards Syndrome
Down Syndrome
Reproductive counseling
Educational accommodations at school
Renal US screen for horseshoe kidney, echocardiogram, visual and hearing screening, regular screening for celiac and thyroid disorders
Supportive/palliative care, surgical correction of anatomic anomalies if infant survives initial post-natal period.
Screening for early onset Alzheimer's, ALL/AML, echocardiogram for cardiac anomalies
Footnotes
1. Examples: Midline defects, congenital heart disease, dysmorphic features.
2. Karyotype is definitive work-up for all of the included syndromes except Fragile X.
3. Male vs. female phenotype is highly subjective and may depend on the gender with which the patient self-identifies. A less subjective measure may be the appearance of the genitalia as typically "male" or "female".

FIGURE 23.17

23-17 Genetic Disorders: Aneuploidy

TRISOMY 21 (DOWN SYNDROME)

A term M with a history of limited prenatal care presents with poor feeding. On **exam**, he has hypotonia, up-slanting palpebral fissures, a protruding tongue, Brushfield spots in the eyes, and a single palmar crease. Echocardiogram shows complete AV septal defect. On **labs**, karyotype reveals trisomy 21.

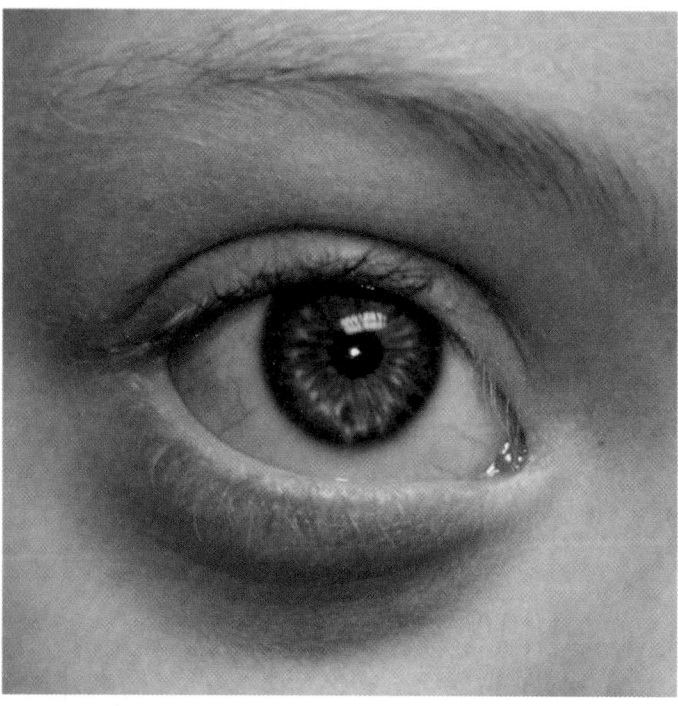

Upslanting palpebral fissures and Brushfield spots.

Management:

1. Hearing screen.
2. Referral to neurodevelopmental specialist.
3. Thyroid screening.

Complications:

- Transient myeloproliferative disorder (neonatal).
- Acute lymphocytic leukemia.
- Obesity.
- Obstructive sleep apnea.
- Intellectual disability.
- Atlantoaxial instability: Misalignment of C1 and C2.
- Hirschsprung disease and bowel obstruction/constipation.
- Dementia (adulthood, 50% by 6th decade).

HYF: Though trisomy 21 is associated with potential medical problems, patients often live fulfilling, rich lives. Trisomy 21 is not usually genetically inherited but can be if a parent has a balanced translocation of chromosome 21 that they pass on to their child.

TRISOMY 18 (EDWARDS SYNDROME)

A late-preterm F with a history of poor prenatal care presents with feeding difficulties. On **exam**, she has low tone, "rocker bottom" feet, microcephaly, and hand contractures (clenched hands with overlapping digits). **Labs/imaging**: echocardiogram shows large VSD. Karyotype shows trisomy 18.

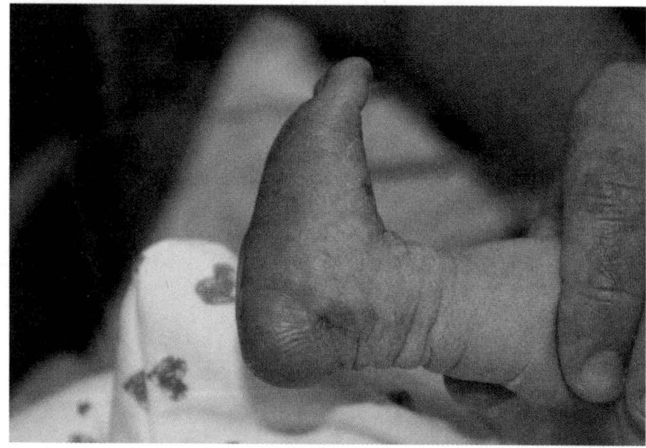

Rocker bottom feet.

Management:

1. Full cardiac evaluation (leading cause of death).
2. Swallow evaluation for aspiration risk.
3. Sleep study for apnea concern.

HYF: Most cases do not survive to birth, with only around 10% of patients surviving until 1 year of life. Shared decision-making with families is essential to discuss goals of care and risks/benefits of major surgery (eg, heart surgery).

TRISOMY 13 (PATAU SYNDROME)

A late-preterm F with a history of poor prenatal care is born with omphalocele and a congenital open wound on scalp. On **exam**, she has cutis aplasia of the scalp along the midline, low tone, low-set ears, and a cleft palate. On **imaging**, brain MRI shows holoprosencephaly. Echocardiogram shows a large VSD. On **labs**, karyotype shows trisomy 13.

23-17 Genetic Disorders: Aneuploidy

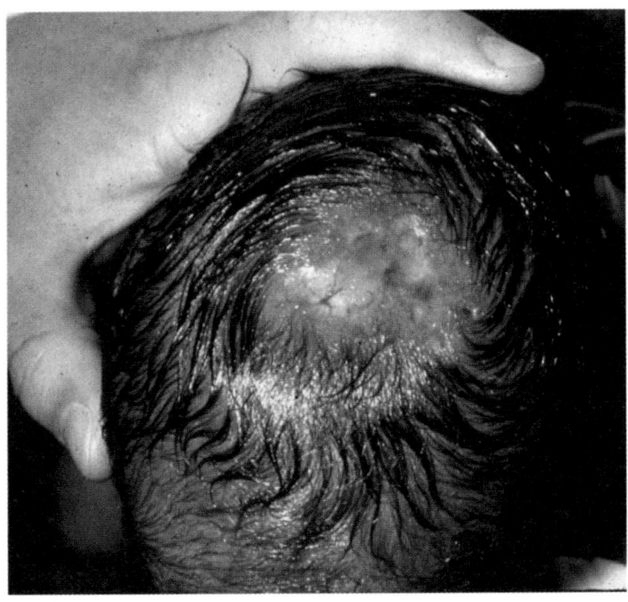

Cutis aplasia of the neonatal scalp.

HYF: Trisomy 13 has the worst prognosis of the trisomies with >90% mortality in the perinatal period. Phenotype is highly variable, but midline defects such as cutis aplasia, holoprosencephaly, and myelomeningocele are highly suggestive.

TURNER SYNDROME (45X,O)

A 15-year-old F with PMH of short stature and coarctation of the aorta s/p repair in infancy presents with delayed puberty. On **exam**, she has a wide-webbed neck, shield chest, and bilateral ptosis. **Labs** show elevated FSH. On **imaging**, pelvic ultrasound shows streak ovaries. Karyotype shows presence of only 1 X chromosome.

Management:

1. Consider growth hormone supplementation if height <5th percentile.
2. Renal ultrasound to assess for VUR and other collecting system malformations.
3. Cardiac evaluation with EKG to assess QT prolongation and echocardiogram if not already performed.
4. Estrogen supplementation in adolescence.
5. Monitoring of blood pressure.

HYF: Turner syndrome is associated with conditions associated with estrogen deficiency seen in postmenopausal women, such as osteopenia/osteoporosis and endometrial hyperplasia.

KLINEFELTER SYNDROME (47,XXY/47,XYY)

An 18-year-old M with PMH of cryptorchidism s/p repair in infancy, tall stature, and ADHD presents with gynecomastia. He has small testicles on **exam**. On **labs**, karyotype shows 47,XXY.

Management:

1. Referral to endocrinology to discuss testosterone therapy.
2. Fertility counseling if desired.
3. Screening for dyslipidemia and type 2 diabetes in older age.

HYF: Klinefelter is the most common full trisomy, affecting 1:500–1:000 men with wide phenotypic variability. It is most commonly discovered during work-up for male infertility.

OTHER CHROMOSOMAL ABNORMALITIES

FRAGILE X SYNDROME

A 5-year-old M with PMH of recurrent otitis media, moderate global developmental delay, and autism presents with anger and behavioral outbursts. On **exam**, he has hypotonia, macroorchidism, large ears, and joint laxity. On **labs**, PCR of *FMR1* gene shows 250 trinucleotide repeats of CGG.

Management:

1. Echocardiogram monitoring for development of aortic root dilation.
2. Neurobehavioral support.
3. Speech, language, and occupational therapy.

HYF: Fragile X is a trinucleotide repeat expansion disorder affecting *FMR1* that is most reliably detectable with targeted testing. SNP array will not capture this disorder. Severity of phenotype is correlated with number of trinucleotide repeats. Males are more affected than females.

23-18 TORCH Infections

Congenital infections

Infection	Source	Signs/Symptoms		Prevention
Toxoplasma gondii	Oocytes in cat feces, undercooked meat	"Classic triad"[1]: • Hydrocephalus • Chorioretinitis[2] • *Intracranial* calcifications (especially in the basal ganglia) Others: thrombocytopenia (petechiae/purpura), anemia, fever, hepatosplenomegaly, jaundice, lymphadenopathy, seizures, rash, microcephaly	Intracranial calcifications.	Pregnant persons should avoid undercooked meat and changing the cat litter
Rubella	Human droplets	Most tested: • Patent ductus arteriosus • Sensorineural hearing loss • Cataracts • "Blueberry muffin" rash[3] Others: Other congenital heart defects (eg, ASD and VSD), anemia, thrombocytopenia (petechiae/purpura), hepatosplenomegaly, jaundice, microcephaly, cerebral calcifications, radiolucent bone disease[4], IUGR	"Blueberry muffin" rash.	Maternal vaccination **prior** to pregnancy[5]

23-18 TORCH Infections

Cytomegalovirus	Bodily fluids, most commonly urine or saliva of young children	Most tested: • Thrombocytopenia: petechiae • Jaundice at birth • Sensorineural hearing loss • Chorioretinitis • Hypotonia and poor suck • *Periventricular* calcifications • IUGR Others: Hepatosplenomegaly, microcephaly, anemia	Periventricular calcifications	Avoiding high-risk exposure
HSV	Maternal genital lesions present during birth	Symptoms present between birth and 6 weeks of life: • Vesicles of the skin, eyes, or oral mucosa • Fever or hypothermia • Meningitis • Seizure • Viral hepatitis, liver failure • Thrombocytopenia	Vesicular lesions.	Acyclovir at 36 weeks for pregnant women with recurrent genital HSV

(*Continued*)

23-18 TORCH Infections

Congenital infections (Continued)

Infection	Source	Signs/Symptoms		Prevention
Syphilis	Sexual transmission of the *Treponema pallidum* spirochete	Early findings: • Hepatomegaly • Jaundice • Rhinitis; white discharge • Maculopapular rash • Lymphadenopathy • Localized bone demineralization Late findings: • Frontal bossing, saddle nose • Saber shins: Anterior bowing of the tibias • Hutchinson teeth[6] • Sensorineural hearing loss • Eye findings: Keratitis, glaucoma, corneal scarring	Skin peeling rash. 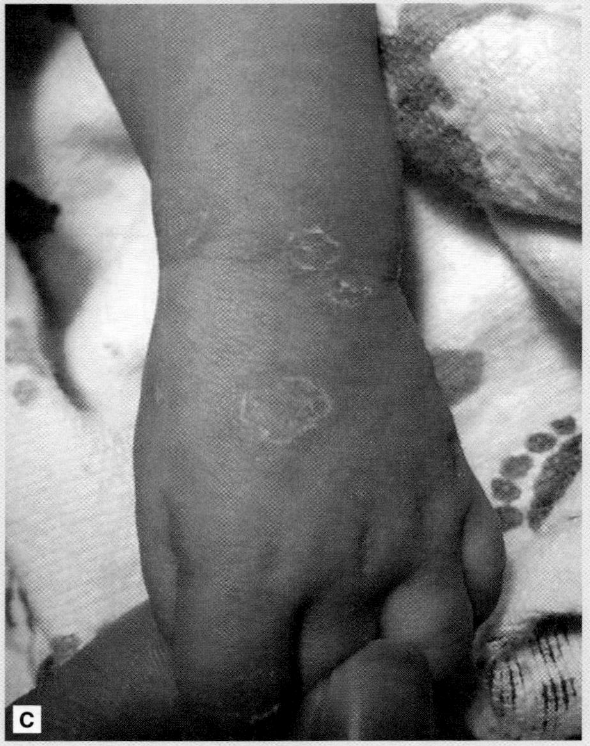 C Hutchinson teeth. 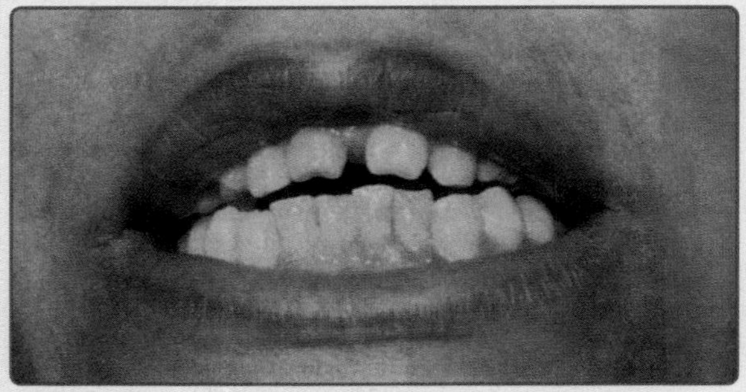	Avoid high-risk exposure

23-18 TORCH Infections

Parvovirus B19	Respiratory droplets	• Severe aplastic anemia • Hydrops fetalis[7] • Fetal death	Hydrops fetalis. 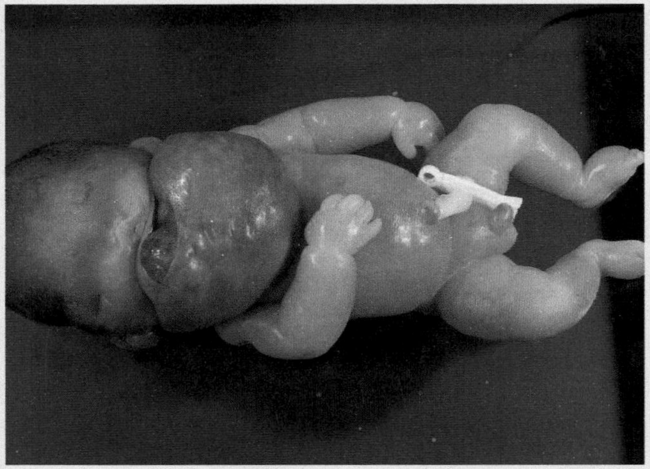	Avoid high-risk exposure
Zika	Sexual transmission by infected person, or *Aedes* mosquito bite	• Severe microcephaly with partially collapsed skull • Cerebellar or parenchymal calcifications • Ventriculomegaly • Eye findings: Chorioretinal atrophy, coloboma, optic nerve hypoplasia • IUGR		Avoid endemic areas (eg, South America) and high-risk exposure, practice protected sex

[1]True triad is actually only seen in 10% of patients.
[2]Leading to vision loss, cataracts, glaucoma, retinal detachment.
[3]Name for dermal erythropoiesis.
[4]Rubella inhibits mitosis in bones, causing focal lesions of osteoporosis and leading to radiolucent bands in the metaphyses.
[5]The MMR (measles, mumps, rubella) vaccine is live and therefore should not be given to pregnant women.
[6]Hypoplastic, notched permanent teeth.
[7]Excess amniotic fluid and fluid build-up in the fetus, including ascites, skin edema, pericardial effusion, pleural effusion.

23-19 Childhood Presentations

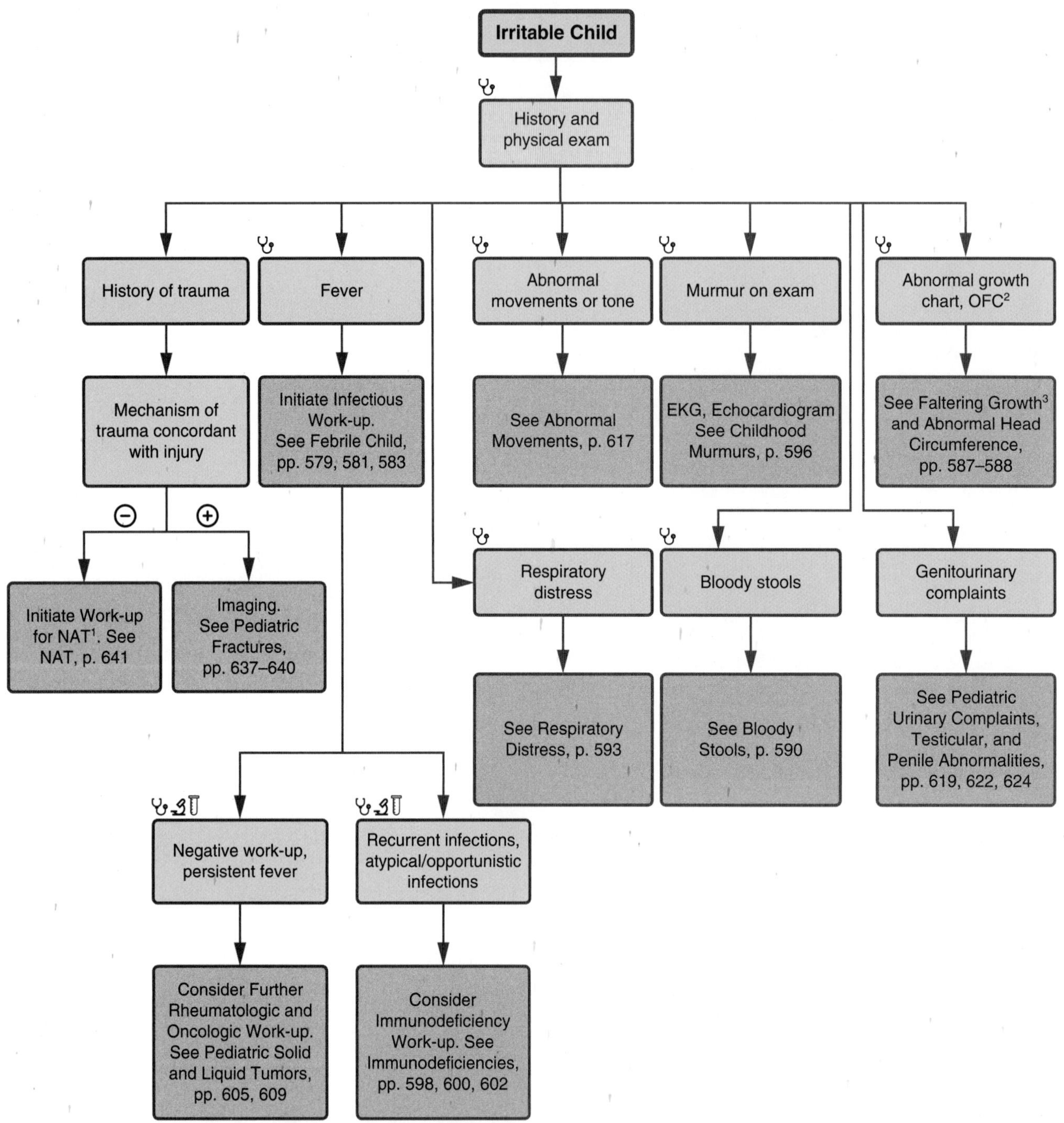
Irritable Child
History and physical exam
History of trauma
Fever
Abnormal movements or tone
Murmur on exam
Abnormal growth chart, OFC[2]
Mechanism of trauma concordant with injury
Initiate Infectious Work-up. See Febrile Child, pp. 579, 581, 583
See Abnormal Movements, p. 617
EKG, Echocardiogram See Childhood Murmurs, p. 596
See Faltering Growth[3] and Abnormal Head Circumference, pp. 587–588
⊖
⊕
Initiate Work-up for NAT[1]. See NAT, p. 641
Imaging. See Pediatric Fractures, pp. 637–640
Respiratory distress
Bloody stools
Genitourinary complaints
See Respiratory Distress, p. 593
See Bloody Stools, p. 590
See Pediatric Urinary Complaints, Testicular, and Penile Abnormalities, pp. 619, 622, 624
Negative work-up, persistent fever
Recurrent infections, atypical/opportunistic infections
Consider Further Rheumatologic and Oncologic Work-up. See Pediatric Solid and Liquid Tumors, pp. 605, 609
Consider Immunodeficiency Work-up. See Immunodeficiencies, pp. 598, 600, 602

When evaluating a child that is irritable or fussy, it is important to obtain a detailed history from the caregivers and perform a thorough physical exam prior to deciding what work-up is appropriate. Children are unique in that they may not be the best historians, which makes us rely heavily on the physical exam. Moreover, the list of differential diagnoses under consideration can change significantly based on the age of the child presenting to care. Keep this core concept in mind when evaluating a child that presents to you for evaluation.
The next section of this chapter will go through the most common chief complaints that children present with, either in the primary care setting or in the emergency room.

Footnotes

1. Non-accidental trauma.
2. Occipito-frontal circumference.
3. Faltering growth is also referred to as failure to gain weight and was previously known as failure to thrive.

FIGURE 23.19

23-20 Febrile Child: Part 1

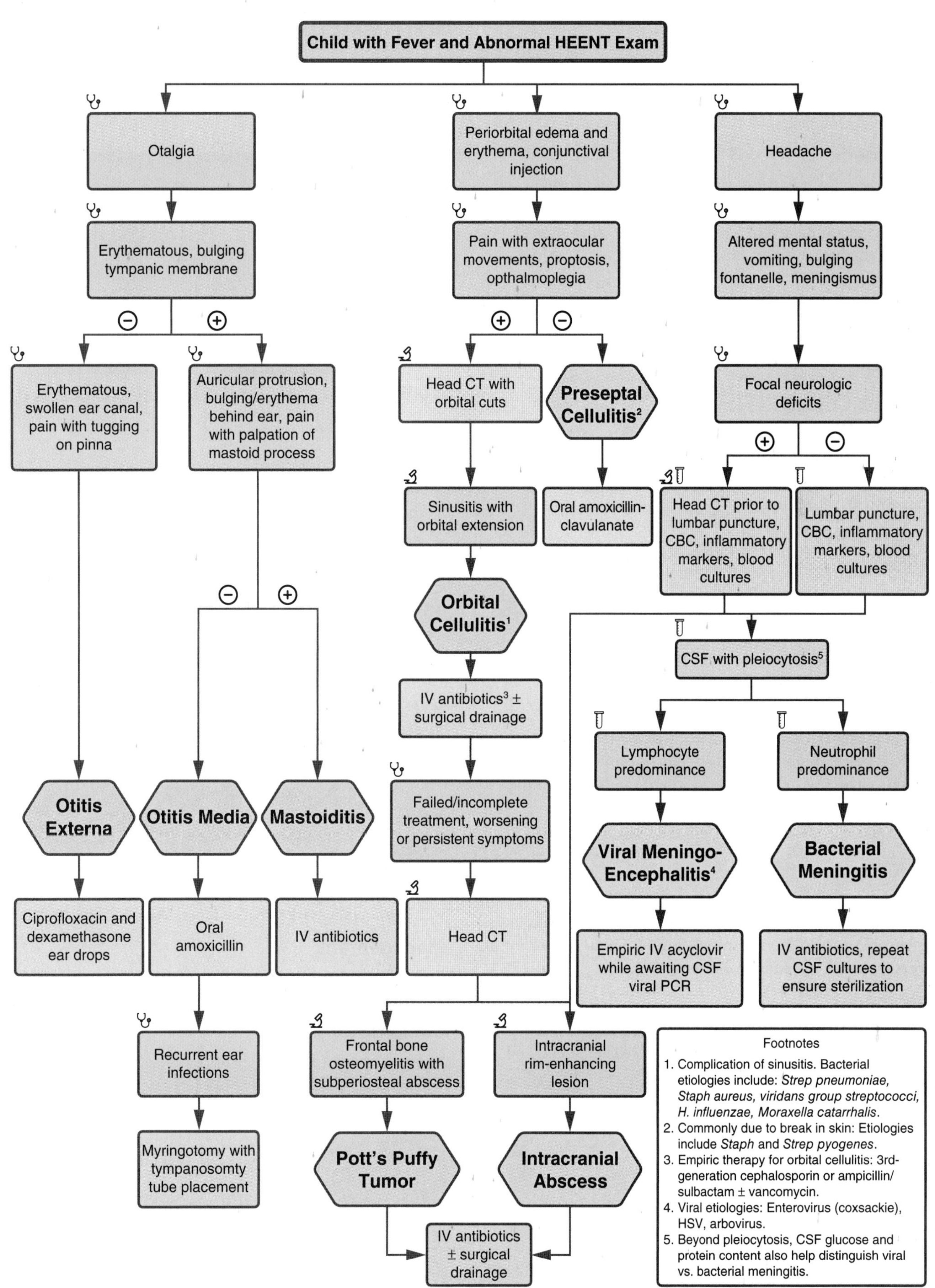
Child with Fever and Abnormal HEENT Exam
Otalgia
Periorbital edema and erythema, conjunctival injection
Headache
Erythematous, bulging tympanic membrane
Pain with extraocular movements, proptosis, opthalmoplegia
Altered mental status, vomiting, bulging fontanelle, meningismus
Erythematous, swollen ear canal, pain with tugging on pinna
Auricular protrusion, bulging/erythema behind ear, pain with palpation of mastoid process
Head CT with orbital cuts
Preseptal Cellulitis2
Focal neurologic deficits
Sinusitis with orbital extension
Oral amoxicillin-clavulanate
Head CT prior to lumbar puncture, CBC, inflammatory markers, blood cultures
Lumbar puncture, CBC, inflammatory markers, blood cultures
Orbital Cellulitis1
CSF with pleiocytosis5
IV antibiotics3 ± surgical drainage
Lymphocyte predominance
Neutrophil predominance
Otitis Externa
Otitis Media
Mastoiditis
Failed/incomplete treatment, worsening or persistent symptoms
Viral Meningo-Encephalitis4
Bacterial Meningitis
Ciprofloxacin and dexamethasone ear drops
Oral amoxicillin
IV antibiotics
Head CT
Empiric IV acyclovir while awaiting CSF viral PCR
IV antibiotics, repeat CSF cultures to ensure sterilization
Recurrent ear infections
Frontal bone osteomyelitis with subperiosteal abscess
Intracranial rim-enhancing lesion
Myringotomy with tympanosomty tube placement
Pott's Puffy Tumor
Intracranial Abscess
IV antibiotics ± surgical drainage

Footnotes

1. Complication of sinusitis. Bacterial etiologies include: *Strep pneumoniae, Staph aureus, viridans group streptococci, H. influenzae, Moraxella catarrhalis*.
2. Commonly due to break in skin: Etiologies include *Staph* and *Strep pyogenes*.
3. Empiric therapy for orbital cellulitis: 3rd-generation cephalosporin or ampicillin/sulbactam ± vancomycin.
4. Viral etiologies: Enterovirus (coxsackie), HSV, arbovirus.
5. Beyond pleiocytosis, CSF glucose and protein content also help distinguish viral vs. bacterial meningitis.

FIGURE 23.20

23-20 Febrile Child: Part 1

PRESEPTAL CELLULITIS

A 3-year-old F presents with 4 days of left periorbital edema and erythema after falling down from a trampoline and hitting the corner of her left eye on a sharp end. On exam, she has no proptosis or pain with eye movements.

Management:

1. Oral amoxicillin-clavulanic acid to cover for *Staph*, *Strep*, and anaerobes.
2. Consider including MRSA coverage if no response after 48 hours of therapy or if purulence is present.

Complications: Progression to orbital cellulitis.

HYF: Fever may or may not be present. Most often, there is a preceding history of an upper respiratory infection or trauma to the periorbital area.

ORBITAL CELLULITIS

A 3-year-old M presents with 3 days of fever and right swollen eye. On exam, he has proptosis as well as painful and limited extraocular movement. On imaging, CT shows inflammation of extraocular muscles with fat stranding.

Management:

1. IV antibiotics.
2. Drainage of abscesses.

Complications:

- Necrotizing fasciitis.
- Loss of vision.
- Intracranial extension.

HYF: Trauma and local infection such as paranasal sinusitis are highly suggestive. Important to distinguish from preseptal cellulitis, which is a less serious condition where infection is limited to the anterior segment of the orbital septum.

OTITIS EXTERNA

A 10-year-old M presents with 2 days of right-sided ear pain, fever, and discharge a few days after restarting swim lessons. Exam shows erythema of external auditory canal, copious discharge from the right ear, pain on manipulation of pinna, and an intact, non-erythematous tympanic membrane.

Management:

1. Antibiotic ear drops containing steroids (eg, ciprofloxacin and dexamethasone). Antibiotics should cover *Staph aureus* and *Pseudomonas*.
2. Ibuprofen and/or acetaminophen for pain control.
3. Prevention: Vinegar or hydrogen peroxide ear drops after swimming.

Complications:

- Mastoiditis.
- Malignant otitis externa.

HYF: Commonly called "swimmer's ear." Treatment with antibiotic drops avoids progression to mastoiditis and spread of infection to mastoid bone and air cells requiring surgical intervention.

OTITIS MEDIA

A 5-month-old previously healthy F presents with 3 days of fever, increased fussiness, and grabbing at her left ear. On exam, otoscopic evaluation reveals erythematous, bulging tympanic membrane with purulence.

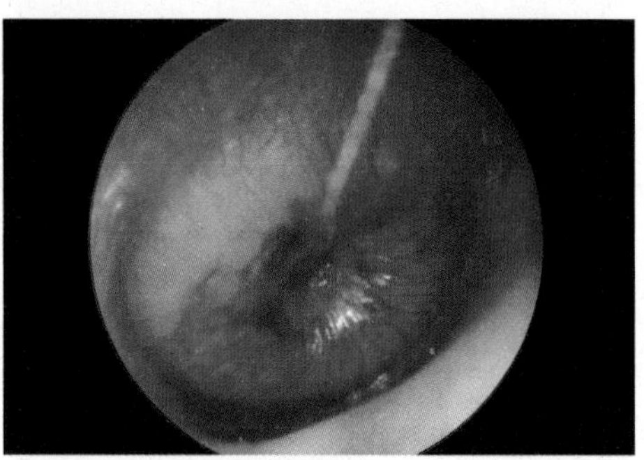

Notable erythema of tympanic membrance with visible meniscus of effusion.

Management:

1. High dose of oral amoxicillin in order to cover *H. influenzae*, *Moraxella*, *Strep. pneumo*, Group A *Strep*, and *Staph. aureus*.
2. Ibuprofen or acetaminophen for ear pain.

Complications:

- Cholesteatoma
- Hearing loss
- Perforation of tympanic membrane.
- Mastoiditis.
- Recurrent otitis media.

HYF: Otitis media is more common in children, given their shorter, more horizontally positioned eustachian tubes. Ear tubes are placed to facilitate drainage of purulent effusion in children with recurrent otitis media.

BACTERIAL MENINGITIS

A 10-year-old previously healthy M presents with 5 days of high fevers, neck stiffness, fatigue, and confusion. On exam, he has no focal neurologic deficits but (+) Kernig and Brudzinski signs. LP shows pleocytosis with neutrophilic predominance, low glucose, and high protein on labs.

Management:

1. Hospital admission with IV antibiotics while awaiting CSF cultures to speciate.

Complications:

- Septic shock.
- Intracranial abscess.
- Long-term neurodevelopmental abnormalities.

HYF: *Strep. pneumo* is the most common etiology for bacterial meningitis in all age groups (excluding infants).

Pathogen	Patient population affected
Group B Strep, *E. coli*, Listeria	Infant <3 m.o
Neisseria meningitidis	Adolescents
Strep. pneumo	All ages
Haemophilus influenzae type B	Unvaccinated

23-21 Febrile Child: Part 2

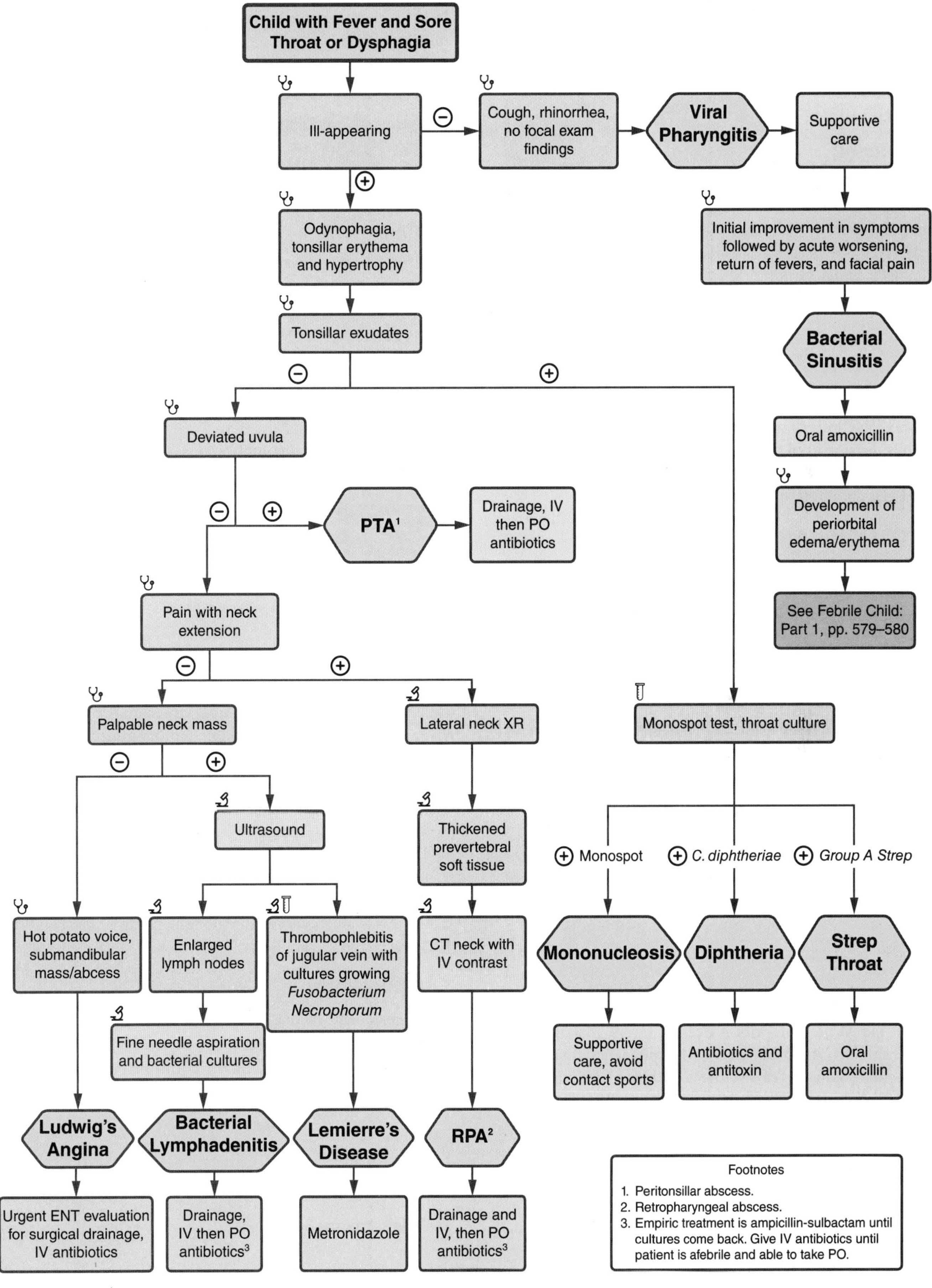
Child with Fever and Sore Throat or Dysphagia
Ill-appearing
Cough, rhinorrhea, no focal exam findings
Viral Pharyngitis
Supportive care
Initial improvement in symptoms followed by acute worsening, return of fevers, and facial pain
Bacterial Sinusitis
Oral amoxicillin
Development of periorbital edema/erythema
See Febrile Child: Part 1, pp. 579–580
Odynophagia, tonsillar erythema and hypertrophy
Tonsillar exudates
Deviated uvula
PTA[1]
Drainage, IV then PO antibiotics
Pain with neck extension
Palpable neck mass
Lateral neck XR
Monospot test, throat culture
Ultrasound
Thickened prevertebral soft tissue
Monospot
C. diphtheriae
Group A Strep
Hot potato voice, submandibular mass/abcess
Enlarged lymph nodes
Thrombophlebitis of jugular vein with cultures growing Fusobacterium Necrophorum
CT neck with IV contrast
Mononucleosis
Diphtheria
Strep Throat
Fine needle aspiration and bacterial cultures
Supportive care, avoid contact sports
Antibiotics and antitoxin
Oral amoxicillin
Ludwig's Angina
Bacterial Lymphadenitis
Lemierre's Disease
RPA[2]
Urgent ENT evaluation for surgical drainage, IV antibiotics
Drainage, IV then PO antibiotics[3]
Metronidazole
Drainage and IV, then PO antibiotics[3]
Footnotes
1. Peritonsillar abscess.
2. Retropharyngeal abscess.
3. Empiric treatment is ampicillin-sulbactam until cultures come back. Give IV antibiotics until patient is afebrile and able to take PO.

FIGURE 23.21

23-21 Febrile Child: Part 2

SINUSITIS

A 13-year-old M presents to the clinic 10 days after an initial visit for viral pharyngitis. He notes that, as of 2 days ago, his fevers have returned and he now has facial pain. On **exam**, transillumination of his sinuses reveals unilateral dullness.

Management:

1. Sinus irrigation.
2. Decongestant. Humidification.
3. Empiric treatment with amoxicillin or amoxicillin-clavulanate to cover for *Streptococcus pneumoniae*, *H. influenzae*, *Moraxella*, *Staph*, Group A *Strep*, and oral anaerobes.

Complications:

- Orbital cellulitis.
- Intracranial extension (meningitis, abscess).
- Pott's puffy tumor.

HYF: Maxillary and ethmoid sinuses are present at birth but do not completely develop until the first years of life. Frontal and sphenoid sinuses do not fully develop until age ~10 years. True sinusitis is therefore less common in very young children.

PERITONSILLAR ABSCESS

A 6-year-old presents with 4 days of high fevers, sore throat, poor appetite, odynophagia, and drooling with a "hot potato voice." Oropharyngeal **exam** reveals lateral deviation of uvula with a medially displaced, fluctuant tonsil.

Management:

1. Hospitalization for IV fluids and IV antibiotics.
2. IV ampicillin-sulbactam or PO amoxicillin-clavulanic acid are both good choices that cover oral flora, including oral anaerobes.
3. Airway evaluation to ensure no impending airway compromise.
4. Surgical drainage.

Complications:

- Extension into parapharyngeal/prevertebral space.
- Laryngeal edema.
- Sepsis.

HYF: These infections are usually polymicrobial.

MONONUCLEOSIS

A 17-year-old M presents with a week of fevers, malaise, fatigue, and sore throat. On **exam**, he has lymphadenopathy, tonsillar enlargement, oropharyngeal erythema with exudates, and hepatosplenomegaly. On **labs**, heterophile antibody testing is (+). Blood smear shows atypical lymphocytes.

Management:

1. Supportive care with IV fluids, pain control, and antipyretics.
2. Abstinence from contact sports to avoid splenic rupture.

Complications:

- Splenic rupture.
- Characteristic rash when treated with amoxicillin.

HYF: Caused by EBV, although CMV infection can mimic mononucleosis.

STREPTOCOCCAL PHARYNGITIS

A 7-year-old F presents with multiple days of fevers, sore throat, and malaise. On **exam**, she has tonsillar enlargement with exudates, palatal petechiae, and cervical lymphadenopathy. On **labs**, rapid strep antigen test and throat culture both are (+) for Group A *Strep*.

Management:

1. Strep throat will resolve spontaneously without antibiotics. Treatment with penicillin or amoxicillin is to prevent rheumatic fever.
2. Supportive care.

Complications:

- Suppurative complications: Oropharyngeal abscess, and infection spread.
- Immune mediated complications: Post-streptococcal glomerulonephritis, acute rheumatic fever.
- Toxin-mediated complication: Scarlet fever.

HYF: The Centor criteria includes 4 components: fever, tonsillar exudate, anterior cervical lymphadenopathy, and absence of cough. Having >3 components increases the likelihood of strep throat. Lab testing is needed for definitive diagnosis.

RETROPHARYNGEAL ABSCESS

A 3-year-old M presented with 3 days of high fevers, neck pain, and dysphagia. On **exam**, he has an erythematous posterior oropharynx and pain with neck extension. On **imaging**, lateral neck X-ray shows prevertebral space thickening.

Management:

1. Hospitalization for IV fluids and IV antibiotics.
2. IV ampillicin-sulbactam or oral amoxicillin-clavulanic acid are both good choices that cover oral flora, including oral anaerobes.
3. Airway evaluation to ensure no impending airway compromise.
4. Surgical drainage.

Complications:

- Extension into mediastinal (danger) space leading to mediastinitis.
- Airway obstruction.
- Lemierre's disease (suppurative thrombophlebitis of internal jugular vein).
- Sepsis.

HYF: Retropharyngeal lymph nodes involute by age 3–5 years; thus, RPAs are mostly seen in children age <5 years.

Ludwig's Angina: See p. 456.

23-22 Febrile Child: Part 3

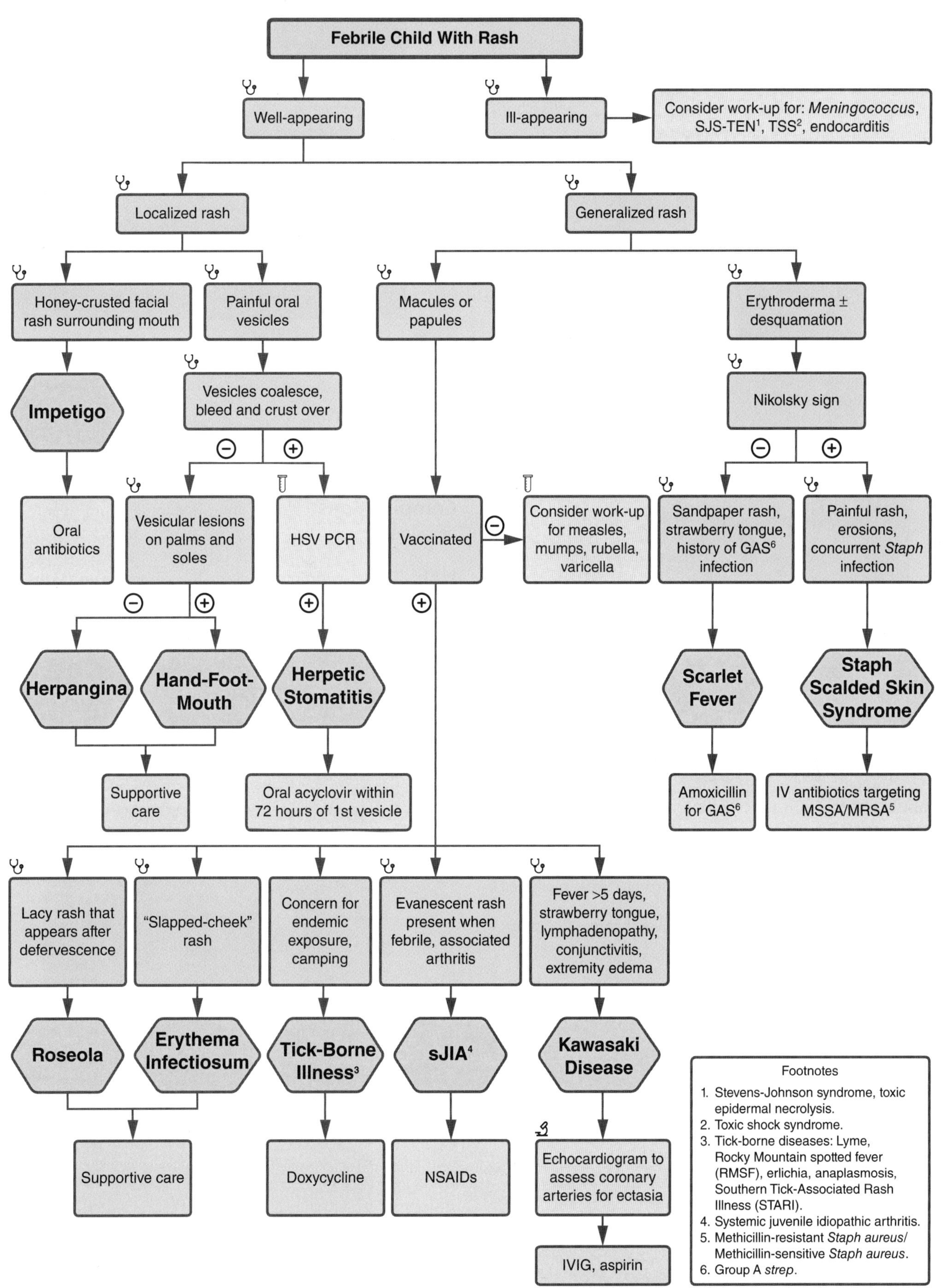
Febrile Child With Rash
Well-appearing
Ill-appearing
Consider work-up for: *Meningococcus*, SJS-TEN[1], TSS[2], endocarditis
Localized rash
Generalized rash
Honey-crusted facial rash surrounding mouth
Painful oral vesicles
Macules or papules
Erythroderma ± desquamation
Impetigo
Vesicles coalesce, bleed and crust over
Nikolsky sign
Oral antibiotics
Vesicular lesions on palms and soles
HSV PCR
Vaccinated
Consider work-up for measles, mumps, rubella, varicella
Sandpaper rash, strawberry tongue, history of GAS[6] infection
Painful rash, erosions, concurrent *Staph* infection
Herpangina
Hand-Foot-Mouth
Herpetic Stomatitis
Scarlet Fever
Staph Scalded Skin Syndrome
Supportive care
Oral acyclovir within 72 hours of 1st vesicle
Amoxicillin for GAS[6]
IV antibiotics targeting MSSA/MRSA[5]
Lacy rash that appears after defervescence
"Slapped-cheek" rash
Concern for endemic exposure, camping
Evanescent rash present when febrile, associated arthritis
Fever >5 days, strawberry tongue, lymphadenopathy, conjunctivitis, extremity edema
Roseola
Erythema Infectiosum
Tick-Borne Illness[3]
sJIA[4]
Kawasaki Disease
Supportive care
Doxycycline
NSAIDs
Echocardiogram to assess coronary arteries for ectasia
IVIG, aspirin
Footnotes
1. Stevens-Johnson syndrome, toxic epidermal necrolysis.
2. Toxic shock syndrome.
3. Tick-borne diseases: Lyme, Rocky Mountain spotted fever (RMSF), erlichia, anaplasmosis, Southern Tick-Associated Rash Illness (STARI).
4. Systemic juvenile idiopathic arthritis.
5. Methicillin-resistant *Staph aureus*/ Methicillin-sensitive *Staph aureus*.
6. Group A *strep*.

FIGURE 23.22

23-22 Febrile Child: Part 3

IMPETIGO

A 2-year-old previously healthy M presents with 3 days of rash around his mouth. His mom says she's been putting ointment on it every day, but it doesn't seem to help. On exam, he has honey-crusted perioral lesions in an erythematous base.

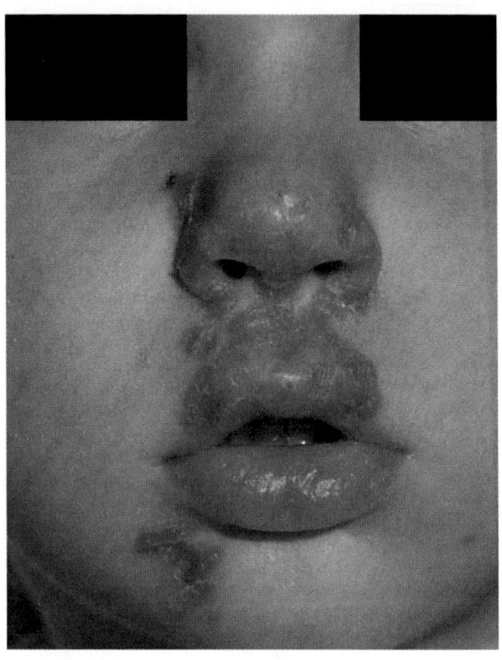

Honey crusted lesions seen in impetigo.

Management:

1. Keep skin clean with soap and water.
2. Topical antibiotic ointment covering skin flora, including *Staph* and Group A *Strep* (eg, mupirocin).

Complications:

- If GAS: Scarlet fever (toxin-mediated), Post-strep glomerulonephritis (immune-mediated), but NOT acute rheumatic fever.
- If *Staph. aureus*: Staph scalded skin syndrome (toxin-mediated).

HYF: Most skin and soft tissue infections are either due to Group A *Strep* or *Staph aureus.*

HAND-FOOT-MOUTH DISEASE

A 15-month-old, previously healthy F presents with multiple days of poor oral intake, pain with swallowing, refusal to eat, and 1 day of rash on her hands and soles of her feet. Exam reveals painful oral lesions in the posterior pharynx.

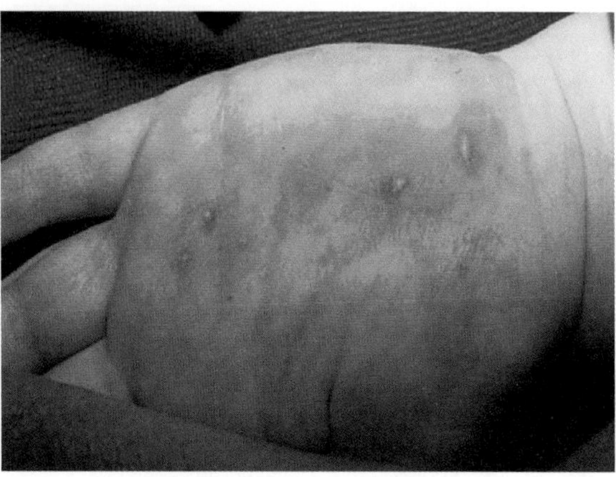

Erythematous papules on palms characteristic of hand-foot-mouth disease.

Management:

1. Supportive care: oral anesthetic, NSAIDs, acetaminophen, hydration, cold popsicles.

Complications: Poor oral intake due to pain causing dehydration.

HYF: Viral syndrome caused by coxsackie A virus. When lesions are limited to the posterior oropharynx, it is referred to as "herpangina."

SCARLET FEVER

A 5-year-old previously healthy M presents with 3 days of sore throat and fevers, and 1 day of papular, erythematous, sandpaper rash. Exam reveals a negative Nikolsky sign.

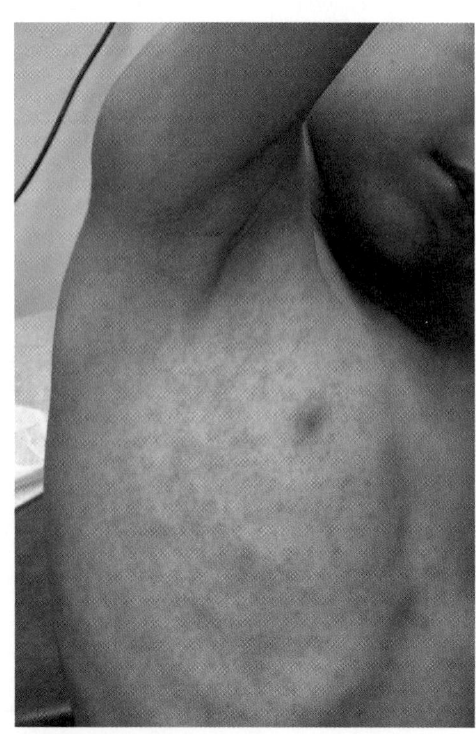

Classic sandpaper rash in scarlet fever.

23-22 Febrile Child: Part 3

Management:

1. Oral antibiotics to treat Group A *Strep* (eg, penicillin/amoxicillin).

Complications: Complications are dependant on original site of GAS infection. See streptococcal pharyngitis and impetigo sections.

HYF: Scarlet fever is a toxin-mediated process following a localized GAS infection, most commonly pharyngitis but can also be impetigo. This condition can also present with a "strawberry tongue" and should be distinguished from Kawasaki disease.

STAPH SCALDED SKIN SYNDROME

A 3-year-old presents with multiple days of fever, perioral impetiginous rash, and now progressive diffuse and painful erythroderma. There is a positive Nikolsky sign on exam.

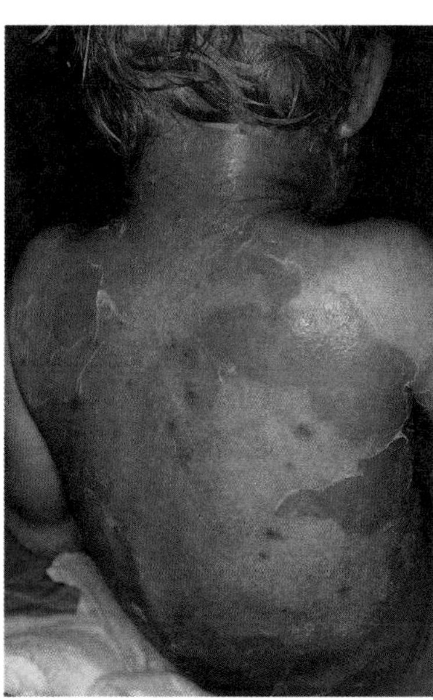

Staphylococcal scalded skin syndrome. Flaccid blisters have sloughed, leaving denuded areas of "scalded skin".

Management:

1. Antibiotics to cover MSSA (eg, nafcillin, amoxicillin).
2. Supportive care mainly via IV hydration and wound care.

Complications:

- Dehydration due to increased insensible losses secondary to loss of skin integrity. This is similar to the pathophysiology of dehydration due to severe burns.
- Sepsis.

HYF: A painful rash that classically starts in the bodily creases, including the armpits and groin. Staph scalded skin can look similar to SJS-TEN, however staph scalded skin does not affect mucosa and there is ususally a clear nidus of infection (eg, impetigo).

ROSEOLA

An 18-month-old M presents with 4 days of high fevers to 104.9 °F (40.5 °C). Today, he no longer has fevers but has developed a lacy rash. His dad says it started on his face and has been spreading down to his legs.

Management:

1. Antipyretics and supportive care.

Complications: Dehydration.

HYF: Also known as "sixth disease," roseola is caused by human herpesvirus-6 (HHV-6). Rash characteristically appears after defervescence.

PARVOVIRUS B-19 (ERYTHEMA INFECTIOSUM)

A daycare teacher presents with her 2-year-old M for a febrile illness. Both she and her son have a history of sickle cell disease. His mother has symptoms of headache and joint pain, and he has a cough and rhinorrhea. On labs, his CBC shows anemia with a low reticulocyte count. Exam shows a "slapped-cheek" rash.

Management:

1. Antipyretics and supportive care.

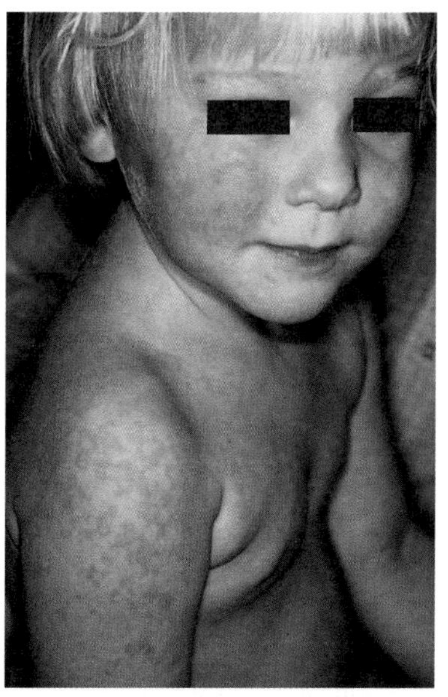

"Slapped-cheek" rash of face along with rash on torso.

23-22 Febrile Child: Part 3

Complications:

- Aplastic anemia.
- Hydrops fetalis due to vertical transmission in pregnant mothers. See TORCH infection section.

HYF: Parvovirus is also known as fifth disease. Classically, it does not require any treatment. Can induce apalstic crisis through marrow suppression in individuals with risk factors.

KAWASAKI DISEASE

A 5-year-old F presents with 6 days of fever, fatigue, swollen hands, and a rash. On **exam**, she has marked generalized lymphadenopathy, conjunctivitis, and peripheral edema with desquamation of her feet. **Labs** show leukocytosis and thrombocytosis, elevated ESR and CRP, elevated AST and ALT, and low albumin.

Management:

1. IVIG.
2. Aspirin.
3. Obtain echocardiogram to evaluate for coronary artery aneurysm.

Complications

- Coronary aneurysm.
- Corornary artery thrombosis, myocardial infarction.
- Myocarditis.
- Coronary artery aneurysm
- Heart failure.

HYF: Kawasaki disease is a multisystemic acute vasculitis. Diagnostic criteria: CRASH Diagnostic criteria: CRASH and BURN. **C**onjunctivitis, **R**ash, **A**denopathy, **S**trawberry tongue, **H**ands and **F**eet (extremity changes), BURN: fever >5 days. Kawasaki disease is one of the only pediatric indications for aspirin therapy. Aspirin is generally avoided in children due to risk of Reye syndrome.

23-23 Faltering Growth

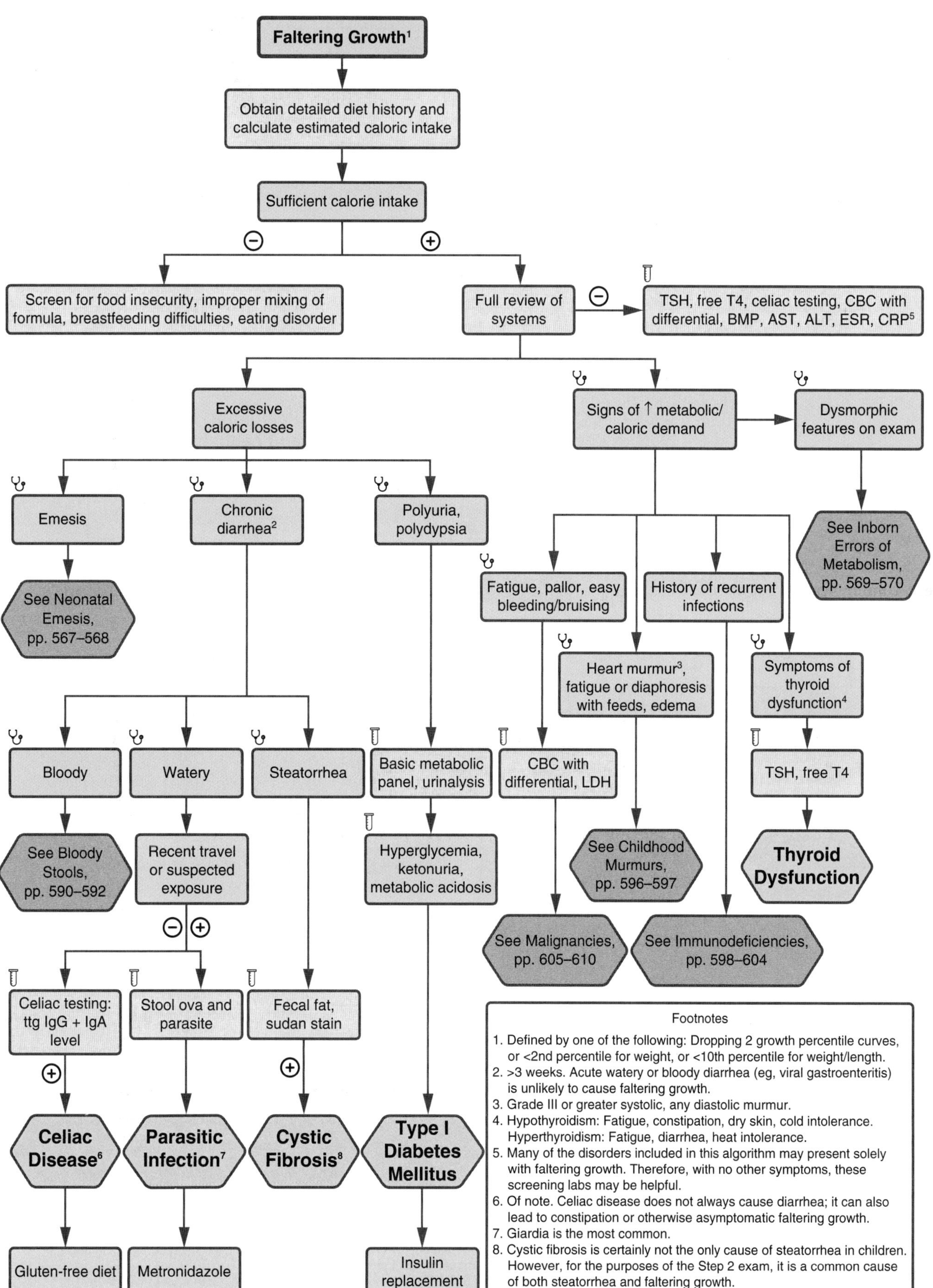
Faltering Growth[1]
Obtain detailed diet history and calculate estimated caloric intake
Sufficient calorie intake
Screen for food insecurity, improper mixing of formula, breastfeeding difficulties, eating disorder
Full review of systems
TSH, free T4, celiac testing, CBC with differential, BMP, AST, ALT, ESR, CRP[5]
Excessive caloric losses
Signs of ↑ metabolic/ caloric demand
Dysmorphic features on exam
See Inborn Errors of Metabolism, pp. 569–570
Emesis
Chronic diarrhea[2]
Polyuria, polydypsia
See Neonatal Emesis, pp. 567–568
Fatigue, pallor, easy bleeding/bruising
History of recurrent infections
Heart murmur[3], fatigue or diaphoresis with feeds, edema
Symptoms of thyroid dysfunction[4]
Bloody
Watery
Steatorrhea
Basic metabolic panel, urinalysis
CBC with differential, LDH
TSH, free T4
See Bloody Stools, pp. 590–592
Recent travel or suspected exposure
Hyperglycemia, ketonuria, metabolic acidosis
See Childhood Murmurs, pp. 596–597
Thyroid Dysfunction
See Malignancies, pp. 605–610
See Immunodeficiencies, pp. 598–604
Celiac testing: ttg IgG + IgA level
Stool ova and parasite
Fecal fat, sudan stain
Celiac Disease[6]
Parasitic Infection[7]
Cystic Fibrosis[8]
Type I Diabetes Mellitus
Gluten-free diet
Metronidazole
Insulin replacement
Footnotes
1. Defined by one of the following: Dropping 2 growth percentile curves, or <2nd percentile for weight, or <10th percentile for weight/length.
2. >3 weeks. Acute watery or bloody diarrhea (eg, viral gastroenteritis) is unlikely to cause faltering growth.
3. Grade III or greater systolic, any diastolic murmur.
4. Hypothyroidism: Fatigue, constipation, dry skin, cold intolerance. Hyperthyroidism: Fatigue, diarrhea, heat intolerance.
5. Many of the disorders included in this algorithm may present solely with faltering growth. Therefore, with no other symptoms, these screening labs may be helpful.
6. Of note. Celiac disease does not always cause diarrhea; it can also lead to constipation or otherwise asymptomatic faltering growth.
7. Giardia is the most common.
8. Cystic fibrosis is certainly not the only cause of steatorrhea in children. However, for the purposes of the Step 2 exam, it is a common cause of both steatorrhea and faltering growth.

FIGURE 23.23

23-24 Abnormal Head Circumference

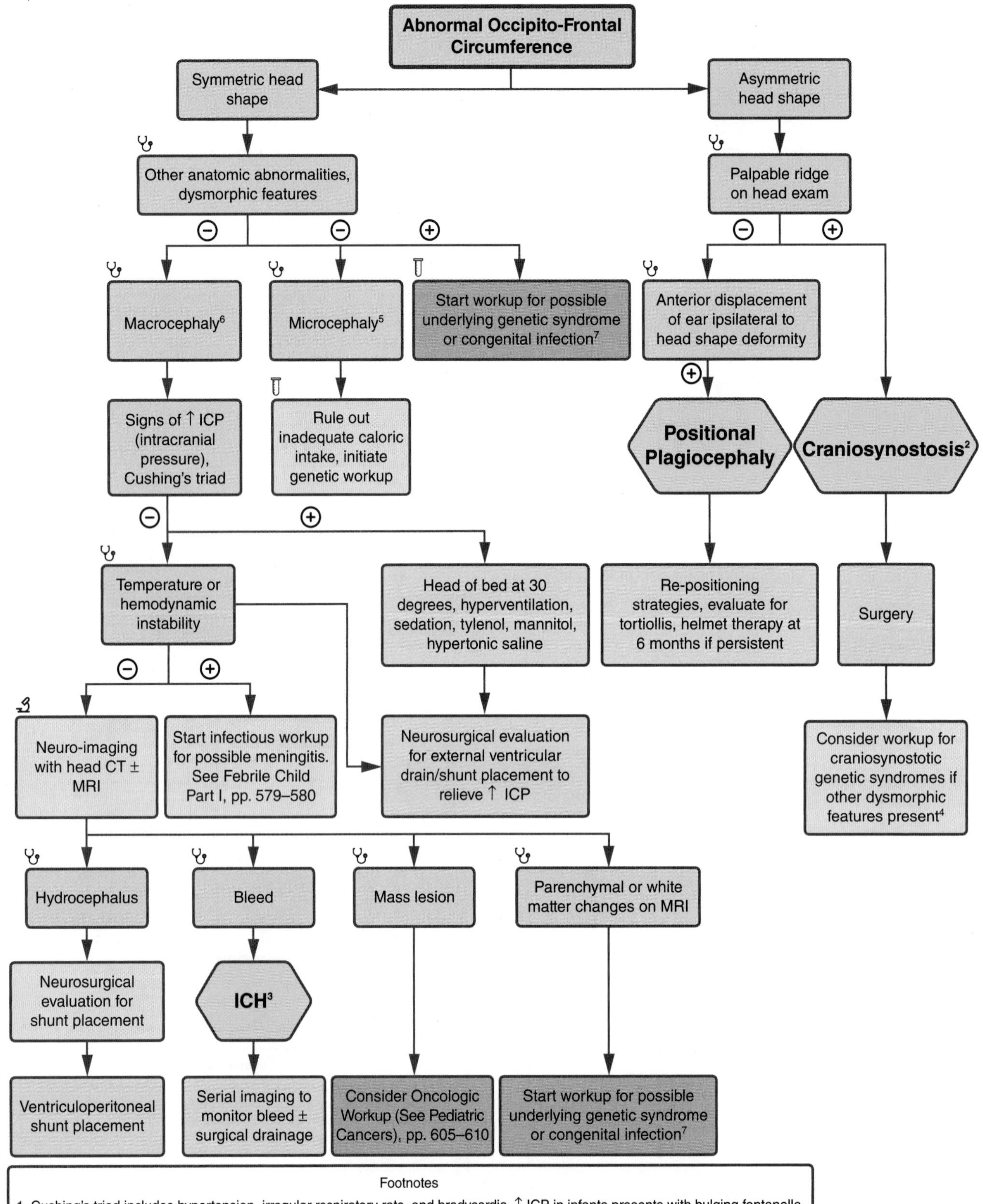

Abnormal Occipito-Frontal Circumference
Symmetric head shape
Asymmetric head shape
Other anatomic abnormalities, dysmorphic features
Palpable ridge on head exam
Macrocephaly6
Microcephaly5
Start workup for possible underlying genetic syndrome or congenital infection7
Anterior displacement of ear ipsilateral to head shape deformity
Signs of ↑ ICP (intracranial pressure), Cushing's triad
Rule out inadequate caloric intake, initiate genetic workup
Positional Plagiocephaly
Craniosynostosis2
Temperature or hemodynamic instability
Head of bed at 30 degrees, hyperventilation, sedation, tylenol, mannitol, hypertonic saline
Re-positioning strategies, evaluate for tortiollis, helmet therapy at 6 months if persistent
Surgery
Neuro-imaging with head CT ± MRI
Start infectious workup for possible meningitis. See Febrile Child Part I, pp. 579–580
Neurosurgical evaluation for external ventricular drain/shunt placement to relieve ↑ ICP
Consider workup for craniosynostotic genetic syndromes if other dysmorphic features present4
Hydrocephalus
Bleed
Mass lesion
Parenchymal or white matter changes on MRI
Neurosurgical evaluation for shunt placement
ICH3
Ventriculoperitoneal shunt placement
Serial imaging to monitor bleed ± surgical drainage
Consider Oncologic Workup (See Pediatric Cancers), pp. 605–610
Start workup for possible underlying genetic syndrome or congenital infection7

Footnotes

1. Cushing's triad includes hypertension, irregular respiratory rate, and bradycardia. ↑ ICP in infants presents with bulging fontanelle, fussiness, irritability and inconsolability. They may or may not have nausea and vomiting given presence of fontanelle as pop-off valve. Cushing's triad would be a very late sign.
2. Craniosynostoses: Metopic suture- trigonocephaly, Coronal suture- brachycephaly, Saggital suture-dolichocephaly/scaphocephaly.
3. Intracranial hemorrhage.
4. Craniosynostosis syndromes include Apert syndrome, Crouzon syndrome, Seathre-Chotzen syndrome, Pfeiffer syndrome.
5. Defined by head circumferance less than 3 to 5 standard deviations below the mean.
6. Defined by head circumferance greater than 2 standard deviations from the mean or >97th percentile.
7. See Congenital Infections table and Genetic Syndromes algorithms, see pp. 569–577.

FIGURE 23.24

23-24 Abnormal Head Circumference

POSITIONAL PLAGIOCEPHALY

The mom of a 2-month-old M says he always likes to turn his head to the left. She is concerned that his head is becoming flatter on that side. On **exam**, he has an asymmetric head, open anterior and posterior fontanelles with no overlying sutures, and some frictional alopecia on the left side are noted.

Management:

1. Evaluate for torticollis, which can make it difficult for infants to move their heads in the direction opposite of their tightened sternocleidomastoid.
2. More "tummy time" to relieve pressure off the head.
3. Tricks to change head positioning, including placing interesting visuals on the side opposite the preferred side.
4. Helmet therapy if still present and significant at age 6 months.

Complications: Persistent asymmetric head shape.

HYF: Positional plagiocephaly is a common benign head asymmetry in infants, and no fused sutures should be palpable as ridge.

CRANIOSYNOSTOSIS

A 6-month-old M presents to his pediatrician's office for a wellness visit. On **exam**, He is noted to have frontal bossing and a palpable vertical ridge on his forehead. On **imaging**, head CT scan shows premature fusion of the metopic suture.

Management:

1. Surgical correction.

Complications: Restricted brain development, resulting in neurodevelopmental delays.

HYF: Craniosynostosis occurs when there is premature closure of cranial sutures. It can be associated with certain genetic syndromes but is most often sporadic.

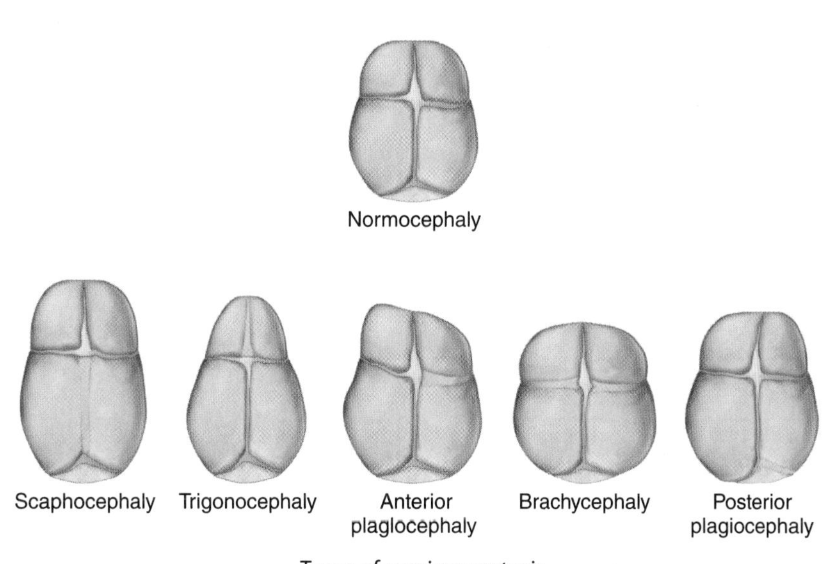
Normocephaly
Scaphocephaly
Trigonocephaly
Anterior plaglocephaly
Brachycephaly
Posterior plagiocephaly

Types of craniosynostosis.

23-25 Bloody Stools

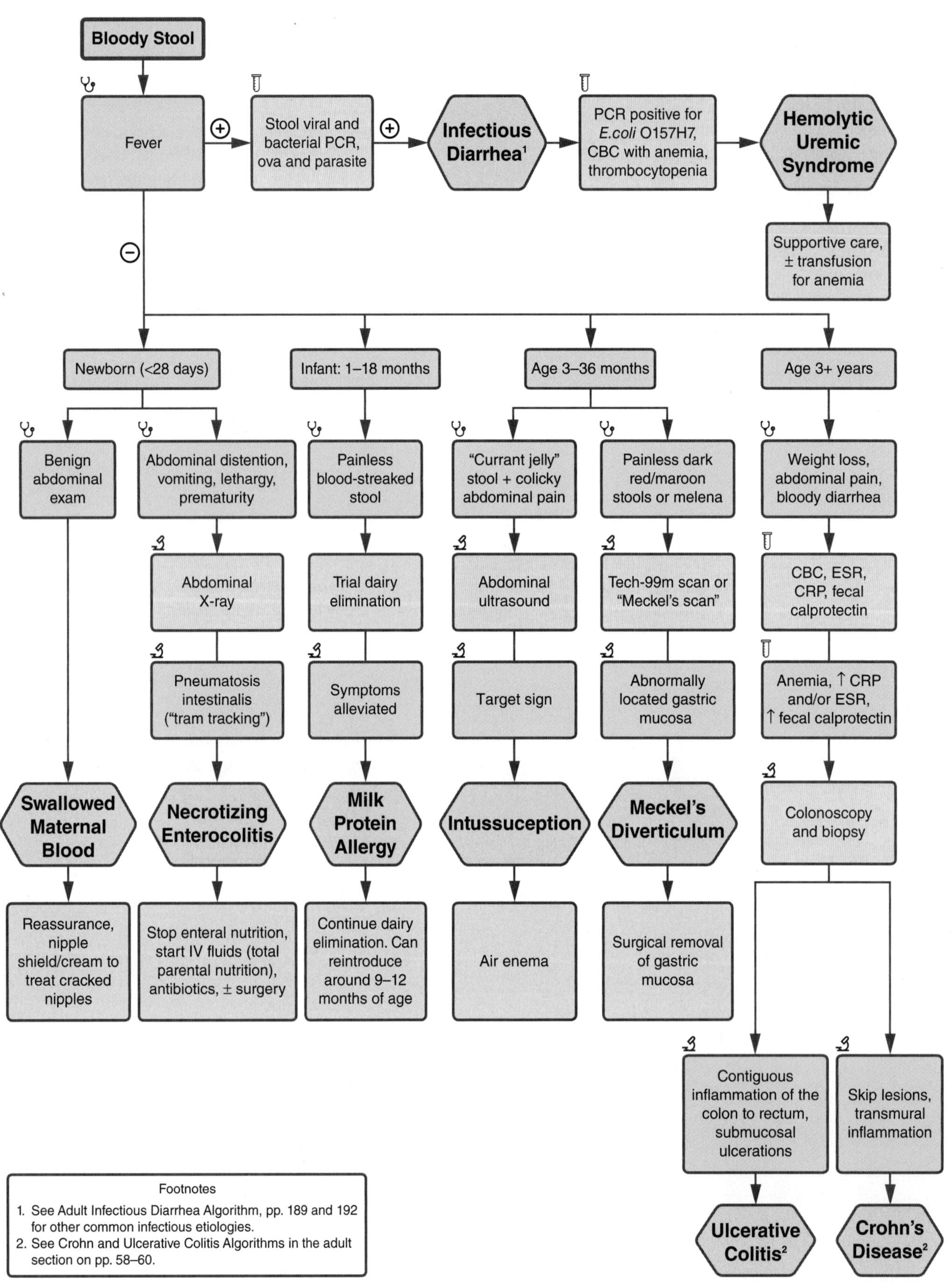

Bloody Stool
Fever
+
Stool viral and bacterial PCR, ova and parasite
+
Infectious Diarrhea[1]
PCR positive for E.coli O157H7, CBC with anemia, thrombocytopenia
Hemolytic Uremic Syndrome
Supportive care, ± transfusion for anemia
−
Newborn (<28 days)
Infant: 1–18 months
Age 3–36 months
Age 3+ years
Benign abdominal exam
Abdominal distention, vomiting, lethargy, prematurity
Painless blood-streaked stool
"Currant jelly" stool + colicky abdominal pain
Painless dark red/maroon stools or melena
Weight loss, abdominal pain, bloody diarrhea
Abdominal X-ray
Trial dairy elimination
Abdominal ultrasound
Tech-99m scan or "Meckel's scan"
CBC, ESR, CRP, fecal calprotectin
Pneumatosis intestinalis ("tram tracking")
Symptoms alleviated
Target sign
Abnormally located gastric mucosa
Anemia, ↑ CRP and/or ESR, ↑ fecal calprotectin
Swallowed Maternal Blood
Necrotizing Enterocolitis
Milk Protein Allergy
Intussuception
Meckel's Diverticulum
Colonoscopy and biopsy
Reassurance, nipple shield/cream to treat cracked nipples
Stop enteral nutrition, start IV fluids (total parental nutrition), antibiotics, ± surgery
Continue dairy elimination. Can reintroduce around 9–12 months of age
Air enema
Surgical removal of gastric mucosa
Contiguous inflammation of the colon to rectum, submucosal ulcerations
Skip lesions, transmural inflammation
Ulcerative Colitis[2]
Crohn's Disease[2]
Footnotes
1. See Adult Infectious Diarrhea Algorithm, pp. 189 and 192 for other common infectious etiologies.
2. See Crohn and Ulcerative Colitis Algorithms in the adult section on pp. 58–60.

FIGURE 23.25

23-25 Bloody Stools

HEMOLYTIC UREMIC SYNDROME (HUS)

A 3-year-old F presents with 3 days of diarrhea that has become bloody in the last 24 hours, abdominal pain, fever, and vomiting. Her mom says they had a neighborhood barbecue and is worried that her hamburger was not fully cooked. **Labs** show mild anemia and thrombocytopenia, creatinine of 1.2, and elevated indirect bilirubin. UA shows 2+ proteins and 21-100 RBCs. Peripheral smear reveals schistocytes. Coombs test is negative.

Management:

1. Supportive care, especially fluid resuscitation.
2. Dialysis if severe renal failure or electrolyte derangements (eg, hyperkalemia).
3. Blood transfusion for significant anemia.
4. Avoid platelet transfusion, as they will be consumed.
5. Avoid antibiotics, as they increase the risk of complications.

Complications:

- Chronic kidney disease or end-stage renal disease.
- Diabetes mellitus.
- Seizures.
- Stroke.

HYF: HUS is a thrombotic microangiopathy that occurs secondary to bacterial infection, most often due to Shiga-like toxin (verotoxin) from *E. coli (O157: H7)* or by Shiga toxin from *Shigella dystenteriae.* Atypical HUS can occur from other bacteria (eg, *Strep pneumoniae*) or drugs. Most common in children age <5 years. Risk factors include recent antibiotics or antimotility agents (eg, loperamide) to treat the diarrhea.

NECROTIZING ENTEROCOLITIS (NEC)

A 5-day-old F born at 31 weeks GA presents with hypothermia, bloody stools, and significant abdominal distention. On **imaging**, abdominal X-ray shows dilated bowel loops and *pneumatosis intestinalis* as below. On **labs**, CBC shows leukocytosis and anemia.

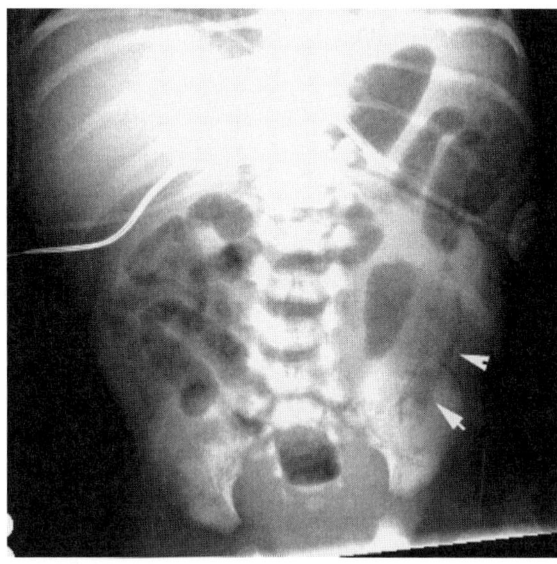

Tram-tracking along bowel wall indicative of pneumatosis intestinalis.

Management:

1. Bowel rest: no enteral feeds, TPN.
2. Nasogastric tube for decompression.
3. Broad-spectrum IV antibiotics.
4. Serial X-rays.
5. Surgery if perforation or worsening serial X-rays.

Complications:

- Intestinal perforation.
- Sepsis.
- Anemia.
- Shock secondary to blood loss or sepsis.

HYF: NEC is most likely to occur in preterm neonates with low birth weight in the first days or weeks of life. Enteral feeding with formula is a risk factor. *Pneumatosis intestinalis* is the pathognomonic finding on X-ray thought to be secondary to bacterial translocation to bowel wall in premature intestines. In addition, portal venous gas can also be seen on imaging.

MILK PROTEIN ALLERGY

A 2-month-old, previously healthy term F presents with 1 week of blood-streaked stools. She has been growing and developing well and feeding ~32 oz of formula daily. Her mom thinks she has been more fussy lately but has had no fevers or vomiting.

Management:

1. Trial dairy elimination: switch to hydrolyzed formula and eliminate dairy for breastfeeding mom.

HYF: Painless, blood-streaked stools in an otherwise healthy infant can sometimes be due to food protein–induced allergic proctocolitis from milk or soy. It is diagnosed based on clinical history alone and usually self-resolves by age 1 year.

INTUSSUSCEPTION

A 2-year-old M presents with severe intermittent abdominal pain. His mom says he develops bouts of crying and bending of his knees. During the most recent episode, he also vomited and developed mucousy stools that look like currant jelly. On **exam**, there is a RUQ sausage-shaped mass and abdominal tenderness. On **imaging**, abdominal US shows a "target" sign:

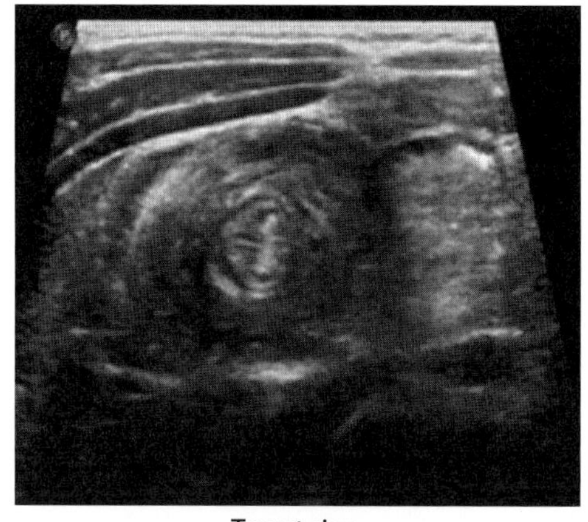

Target sign.

23-25 Bloody Stools

Management:

1. US-guided air insufflation or saline enema: Diagnostic and therapeutic.
2. Surgery if peritoneal signs or if air enema is unsuccessful.

Complications:

- Small bowel obstruction.
- Intestinal perforation.
- Anemia.
- Electrolyte abnormalities.

HYF: Intussusception usually occurs in children aged 6–36 months and is due to telescoping of the large intestine or small intestine into the large intestine most commonly at "the" ileocecal junction. Small bowel into small bowel intusseception is benign requiring no intervention and is usually an incidental finding. It can also result from a pathologic lead point such as Meckel's diverticulum or inflammation from prior gastroenteritis. Associated with Henoch-Schonlein Purpura (usually ileoileal involvement), Celiac disease, intestinal tumor, and the rotavirus vaccine. A history of intussusception is a contraindication to the rotavirus vaccine.

MECKEL'S DIVERTICULUM

A 1-year-old previously healthy M presents with 1 week of painless hematochezia. His mom says he has been acting like his normal self with a regular appetite. On **imaging**, a Technetium-99m scan shows ectopic gastric tissue. On **labs**, CBC shows a hemoglobin of 10.5.

Management:

1. Definitive treatment: Surgical excision of diverticulum.

Complications:

- Anemia.
- Intestinal perforation.
- Abdominal obstruction.
- Intussusception: Diverticulum acts as a lead point.

HYF: Meckel's diverticulum is caused by a failure of the vitelline duct to obliterate during fetal development, resulting in gastric tissue within the small intestine that secretes HCl and causes painless ulceration and bleeding. Rule of 2s: 2% prevalence; presentation by age 2; 2:1 M:F ratio; located within 2 feet of ileocecal valve; 2 types of ectopic tissue: gastric/pancreatic; 2 inches long.

INFLAMMATORY BOWEL DISEASE (ULCERATIVE COLITIS)

A 12-year-old, previously healthy F presents with a 10-lb weight loss in the last 3 months, as well as intermittent bloody diarrhea. She feels fatigued and complains of daily abdominal pain. **Exam** shows abdominal tenderness, pale conjunctiva, mouth ulcerations, and erythematous nodules on her shins. **Labs** show hemoglobin of 7.8, WBC of 25,000, and CRP of 9.0. On **imaging**, colonoscopy shows shallow ulcerations, pseudopolyps, and inflammation throughout her colon. Pathology shows chronic inflammation of the mucosa leading to crypt abscess formation.

Management:

1. Steroids.
2. 5-ASA agents (eg, mesalamine, sulfasalazine).
3. ± biologic agents (eg, infliximab).

Complications:

- Anemia.
- Treatment-related complications: Immunosuppression, osteopenia (steroids).
- Toxic megacolon.
- Colorectal cancer.

HYF: IBD usually presents in teenagers and young adults rather than infancy. Anemia is common due to chronic inflammation and intestinal losses. Extraintestinal manifestations can include arthritis, uveitis, erythema nodosum, and pyoderma gangrenosum. Symptoms can worsen with pregnancy; most UC medications are considered safe throughout pregnancy.

Infectious Diarrhea: See pp. 189–193.
Ulcerative Colitis: See p. 60.
Crohn's Disease: See p. 60.

23-26 Childhood Respiratory Distress

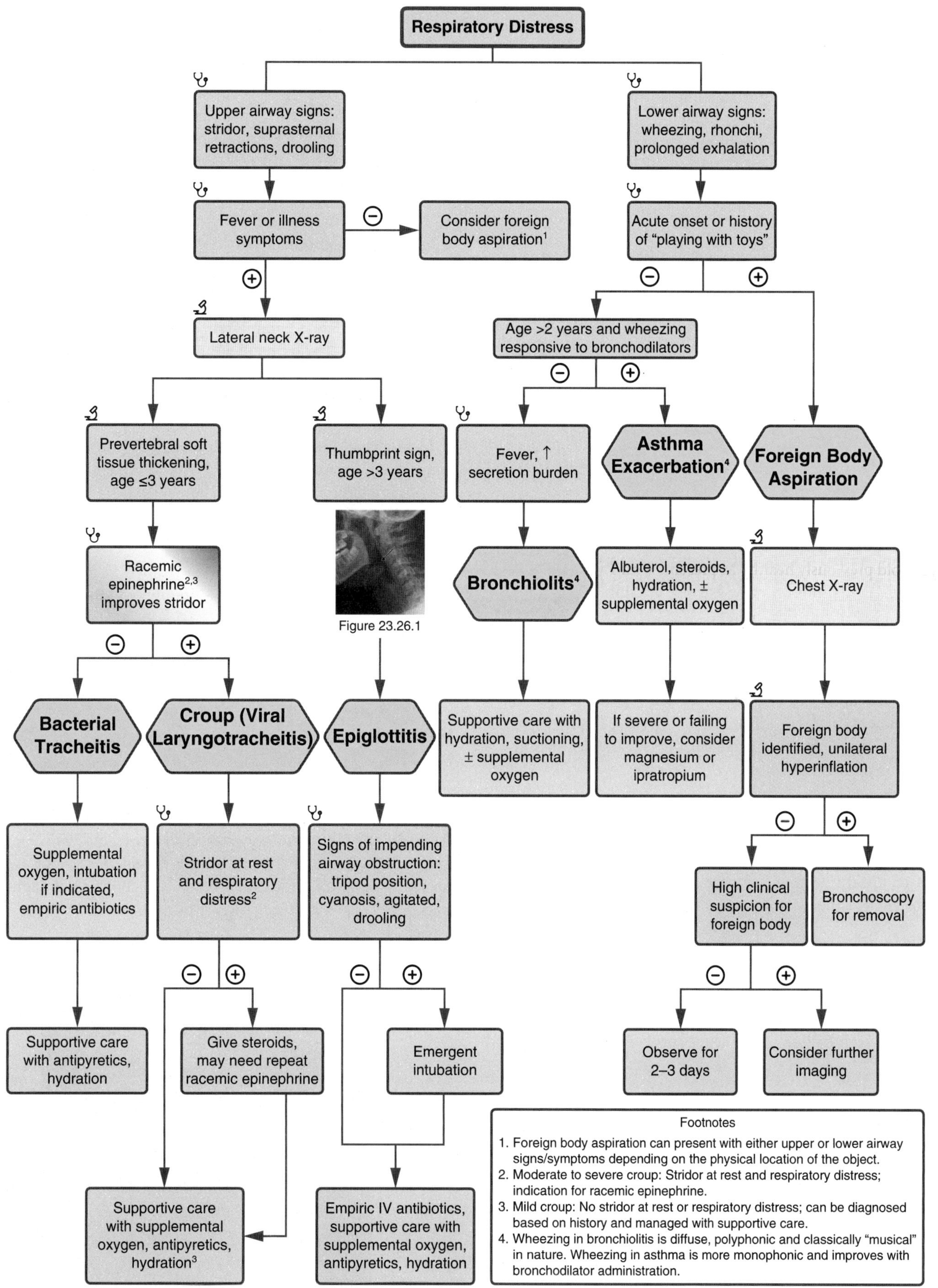
Respiratory Distress
Upper airway signs: stridor, suprasternal retractions, drooling
Lower airway signs: wheezing, rhonchi, prolonged exhalation
Fever or illness symptoms
Consider foreign body aspiration[1]
Acute onset or history of "playing with toys"
Lateral neck X-ray
Age >2 years and wheezing responsive to bronchodilators
Prevertebral soft tissue thickening, age ≤3 years
Thumbprint sign, age >3 years
Fever, ↑ secretion burden
Asthma Exacerbation[4]
Foreign Body Aspiration
Racemic epinephrine[2,3] improves stridor
Figure 23.26.1
Bronchiolits[4]
Albuterol, steroids, hydration, ± supplemental oxygen
Chest X-ray
Bacterial Tracheitis
Croup (Viral Laryngotracheitis)
Epiglottitis
Supportive care with hydration, suctioning, ± supplemental oxygen
If severe or failing to improve, consider magnesium or ipratropium
Foreign body identified, unilateral hyperinflation
Supplemental oxygen, intubation if indicated, empiric antibiotics
Stridor at rest and respiratory distress[2]
Signs of impending airway obstruction: tripod position, cyanosis, agitated, drooling
High clinical suspicion for foreign body
Bronchoscopy for removal
Supportive care with antipyretics, hydration
Give steroids, may need repeat racemic epinephrine
Emergent intubation
Observe for 2–3 days
Consider further imaging
Supportive care with supplemental oxygen, antipyretics, hydration[3]
Empiric IV antibiotics, supportive care with supplemental oxygen, antipyretics, hydration
Footnotes
1. Foreign body aspiration can present with either upper or lower airway signs/symptoms depending on the physical location of the object.
2. Moderate to severe croup: Stridor at rest and respiratory distress; indication for racemic epinephrine.
3. Mild croup: No stridor at rest or respiratory distress; can be diagnosed based on history and managed with supportive care.
4. Wheezing in bronchiolitis is diffuse, polyphonic and classically "musical" in nature. Wheezing in asthma is more monophonic and improves with bronchodilator administration.

FIGURE 23.26

23-26 Childhood Respiratory Distress

ASTHMA EXACERBATION

A 7-year-old M with PMH of asthma, eczema, and seasonal allergies presents to the emergency room for fevers and increased work of breathing. His younger brother came down with a viral upper respiratory infection last week, and now he has similar symptoms. He admits to intermittently forgetting to take his inhaler every day and has missed multiple doses. On **exam**, he has suprasternal and subcostal retractions with diffuse biphasic wheezing.

Management:

1. See pp. 258, 272 for management of acute asthma exacerbation and maintenance therapy.

Complications: Respiratory failure.

HYF: Asthma is more common in children with other atopic conditions, including eczema and allergies (atopic triad). Exacerbations are commonly triggered by viral respiratory infections, tobacco smoke, and exercise.

FOREIGN BODY ASPIRATION

A 22-month-old M presents with sudden-onset respiratory distress. His parents report that he was playing with some toys when he suddenly started crying and coughing. **Exam** reveals stridor, decreased breath sounds in the right lower lung field, and right-sided wheezing. On **imaging**, CXR shows hyperinflation of the right lower lobe and left mediastinal shift.

Management:

1. Auscultation is key to identifying unilateral pulmonary discrepancy.
2. Airway management for unstable patients; CPR, ventilation, and intubation as indicated.
3. Supplemental oxygen if indicated.
4. Bronchoscopy is always necessary if degree of suspicion is high.

Complications: Delayed diagnosis can lead to airway inflammation or distal infection, which can result in bronchiectasis or post-obstructive pneumonia.

HYF: History concerning for aspiration episode may be absent. Chest X-ray may identify a foreign body, but its absence is not exclusionary. Another key presentation is pneumonia that improves with treatment but recurs. Bronchoscopy is always necessary with moderate to high degree of suspicion and is both diagnostic and therapeutic.

BRONCHIOLITIS

A 13-month-old previously healthy F presents with a 3-day history of fever, cough, nasal congestion, and increased work of breathing. **Exam** reveals tachypnea, intercostal retractions, belly push, nasal flaring, and diffuse crackles and wheezing. After suctioning her nose, you note that her work of breathing improves.

Management:

1. Diagnosis is clinical; no labs or imaging indicated.
2. Treatment is supportive: hydration (IV fluids), suctioning, supplemental oxygen if needed.
3. Admit patients who require IV fluid hydration or supplemental oxygen. Patients with good oral intake and oxygen saturations may be observed at home.
4. Recent studies have shown minimal to no benefit of bronchodilators for wheezing in these cases.

Complications:

- Apnea (infants <2 months).
- Respiratory failure.
- Recurrent wheezing in childhood.

HYF: Most commonly caused by RSV in the winter season, though it may also be due to parainfluenza, influenza, or metapneumovirus. Certain high-risk populations may qualify for palivizumab, a monoclonal antibody against RSV as prophylaxis.

BACTERIAL TRACHEITIS

A 15-month-old M presents with several days of fever, cough, and congestion. **Exam** is notable for stridor, cough, and intercostal retractions. On **imaging**, AP and lateral neck X-rays show narrowing of the trachea.

Management:

1. Airway management.
2. Supportive respiratory care.
3. Empiric antibiotics (ceftriaxone + vancomycin).

Complications: Complications occur in a minority of patients, most often due to consequences of airway obstruction.

HYF: Most commonly caused by *S. aureus* and *H. influenzae* type b (Hib) and usually presents with fever.

CROUP (LARYNGOTRACHEITIS)

An 8-month-old, previously healthy M presents with 2 days of fever, congestion, and cough. **Exam** is notable for stridor at rest, a hoarse, barking cough, and intercostal retractions. On **imaging**, AP neck X-ray shows a "steeple sign" from subglottic edema.

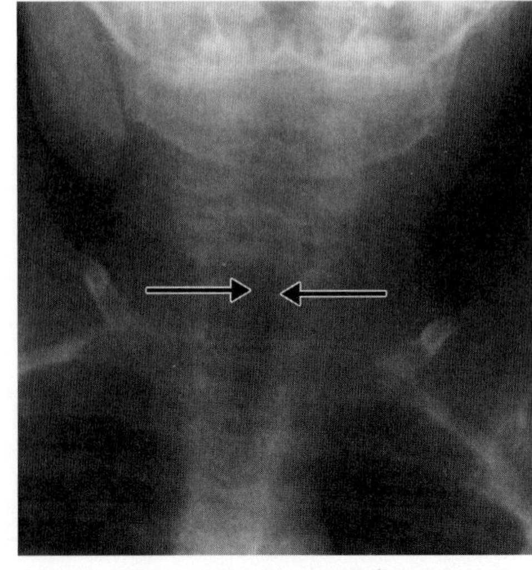

Steeple sign.

23-26 Childhood Respiratory Distress

Management:

1. Steroids (eg, dexamethasone) for mild croup.
2. Racemic epinephrine for moderate to severe croup.
3. Supportive care: Oxygen, antipyretics, hydration.

Complications:

- Respiratory failure.
- Secondary bacterial infection, causing progression to bacterial tracheitis.
- Patient may develop recurrent croup.

HYF: Acute viral inflammatory disease of the larynx most commonly caused by parainfluenza and found in children age 3 months to 3 years.

EPIGLOTTITIS

A 5-year-old incompletely vaccinated F presents with a fever of 102.2 °F (39 °C), pain with swallowing, and increased oral secretions. **Exam** is notable for tripod positioning, muffled voice, drooling, inspiratory retractions, and laryngotracheal tenderness. On **imaging**, lateral neck X-ray shows a "thumbprint sign."

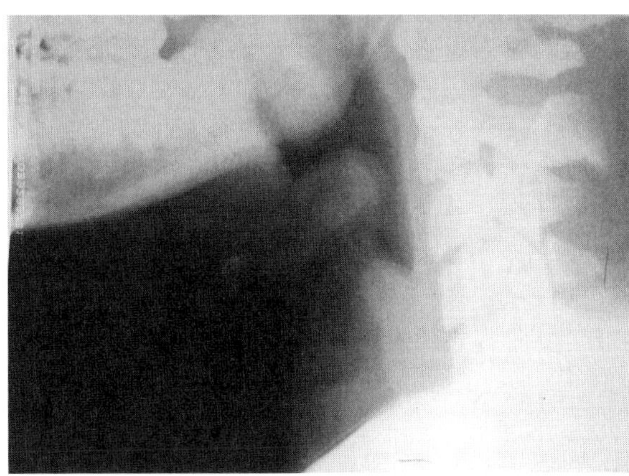

Epiglottic edema (thumbprint sign) in epiglottitis.

Management:

1. Airway management: Due to potential laryngospasm, perform endotracheal intubation with ENT surgeon or anesthesiologist present.
2. Start IV antibiotics (ceftriaxone + vancomycin).

Complications:

- Airway obstruction or death.
- Epiglottic abscess or secondary infection.

HYF: Diagnosis is clinical; imaging is not required. Commonly caused by *H. influenzae* type b (Hib), especially if unvaccinated, but can also be caused by *S. pneumoniae* or *S. aureus.* Patients may sit in the "tripod" position (neck hyperextended, leaning forward) to maximize air entry.

23-27 Childhood Murmurs

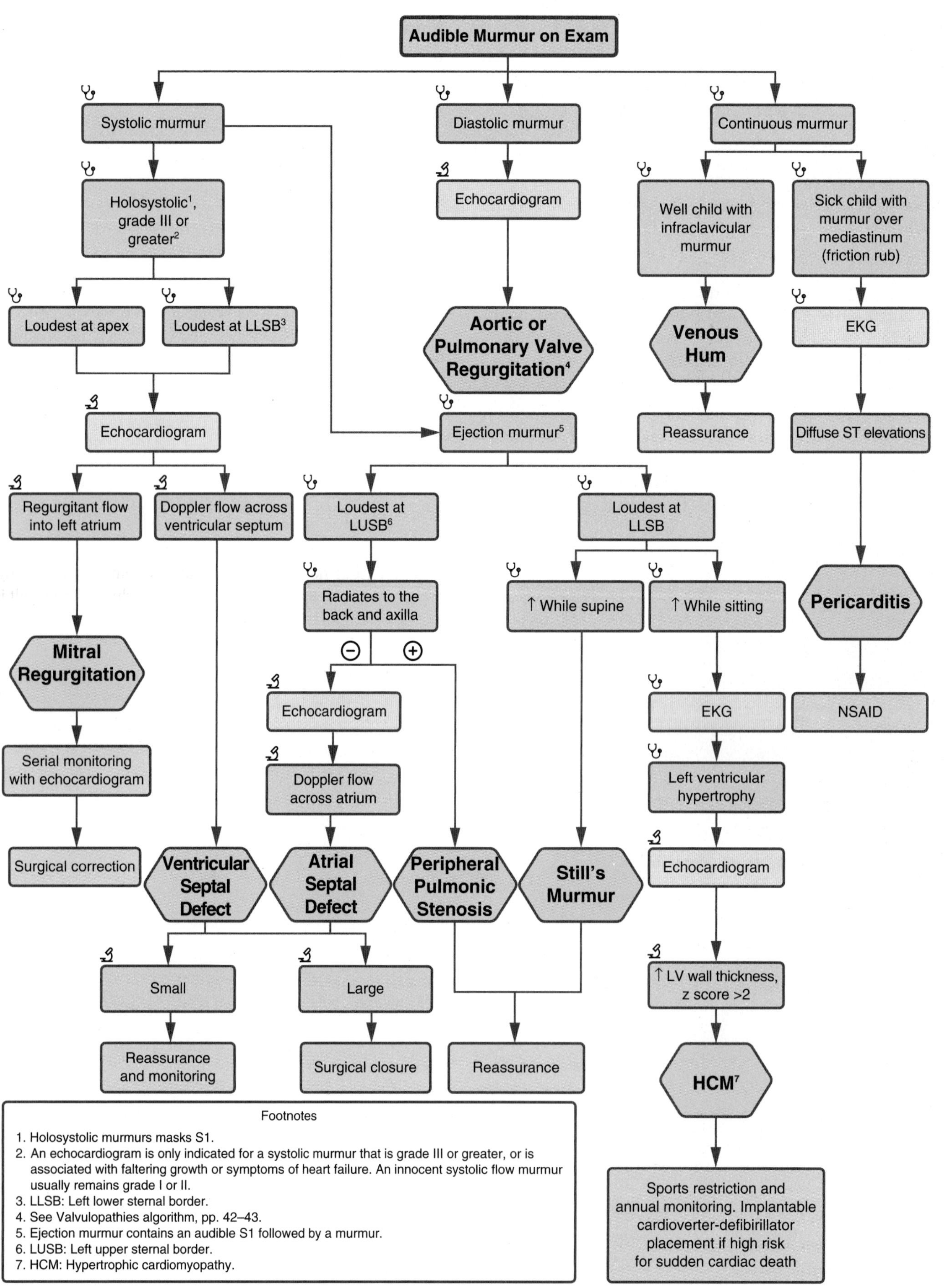
Audible Murmur on Exam
Systolic murmur
Diastolic murmur
Continuous murmur
Holosystolic[1], grade III or greater[2]
Echocardiogram
Well child with infraclavicular murmur
Sick child with murmur over mediastinum (friction rub)
Loudest at apex
Loudest at LLSB[3]
Aortic or Pulmonary Valve Regurgitation[4]
Venous Hum
EKG
Echocardiogram
Ejection murmur[5]
Reassurance
Diffuse ST elevations
Regurgitant flow into left atrium
Doppler flow across ventricular septum
Loudest at LUSB[6]
Loudest at LLSB
Radiates to the back and axilla
↑ While supine
↑ While sitting
Pericarditis
Mitral Regurgitation
⊖
⊕
Echocardiogram
EKG
NSAID
Serial monitoring with echocardiogram
Doppler flow across atrium
Left ventricular hypertrophy
Surgical correction
Ventricular Septal Defect
Atrial Septal Defect
Peripheral Pulmonic Stenosis
Still's Murmur
Echocardiogram
Small
Large
↑ LV wall thickness, z score >2
Reassurance and monitoring
Surgical closure
Reassurance
HCM[7]
Sports restriction and annual monitoring. Implantable cardioverter-defibirillator placement if high risk for sudden cardiac death
Footnotes
1. Holosystolic murmurs masks S1.
2. An echocardiogram is only indicated for a systolic murmur that is grade III or greater, or is associated with faltering growth or symptoms of heart failure. An innocent systolic flow murmur usually remains grade I or II.
3. LLSB: Left lower sternal border.
4. See Valvulopathies algorithm, pp. 42–43.
5. Ejection murmur contains an audible S1 followed by a murmur.
6. LUSB: Left upper sternal border.
7. HCM: Hypertrophic cardiomyopathy.

FIGURE 23.27

23-27 Childhood Murmurs

SYSTOLIC MURMURS

PERIPHERAL PULMONIC STENOSIS (PPS)

A 3-day-old F born at 36 weeks gestation has a grade I mid-systolic ejection murmur best heard over the LUSB that also radiates to the axilla and back.

Management:

1. Reassurance and monitoring.

Complications: None.

HYF: A PPS murmur is most likely in a premature neonate and occurs because the pulmonary arteries are not fully developed at birth. It usually resolves over time as the pulmonary arteries dilate.

STILL'S MURMUR

A 2-year-old healthy F with normal growth and development presents with a musical, soft, vibratory systolic ejection murmur best heard over the left lower sternal border. It increases in intensity when she is supine.

Management:

1. Reassurance; usually resolves by adulthood.

Complications: None.

HYF: Still's murmurs are the most common benign murmurs of childhood and do not require further workup or treatment. In general, if a child's growth trend is reassuring, a significant heart anomaly is unlikely. You can distinguish this murmur from the murmur of HCM because Still's murmurs increase in intensity when the patient is supine.

HYPERTROPHIC CARDIOMYOPATHY (HCM)

A previously healthy 15-year-old M presents to his pediatrician's office after experiencing chest pain, dizziness, and dyspnea during a basketball game. **Exam** reveals an S4 heart sound and systolic ejection murmur that decreases in intensity when supine. The murmur gets louder with Valsalva maneuvers and standing. On **imaging**, EKG reveals left axis deviation and increased QRS amplitudes in the precordial leads (V1–V6). Echocardiogram shows impaired diastolic function and asymmetrical thickening of the anterior interventricular septum.

Management:

1. Avoid strenuous exercise.
2. If symptomatic, β-blockers.
3. Surgical intervention via alcohol septal ablation or septal myectomy only if resistant to lifestyle modifications and medical management.

Complications:

- Sudden death, most often with exercise.
- Ventricular arrhythmias.
- Congestive heart failure.
- Atrial fibrillation.

HYF: Hypertrophic cardiomyopathy is an autosomal dominant disorder in genes that encode sarcomere proteins (eg, myosin, troponin, acting, and titin) and can be either obstructive or non-obstructive. Valsalva maneuvers and standing decrease ventricular volume (decreased preload), which increases the LV outflow gradient and the murmur intensity. β-blockers, handgrip, and supine positioning, on the other hand, increase preload and therefore decrease the murmur intensity.

CONTINUOUS MURMURS

VENOUS HUM

A 3-year-old, previously healthy M presents with a soft, continuous murmur best heard right under the clavicles. The murmur disappears when he lies down or extends his neck and turns his head to the right.

Management:

1. Reassurance.

Complications: None.

HYF: A venous hum is a continuous murmur that results from normal venous flow through the jugular veins. By extending and turning the neck, the jugular vein can be occluded and result in the disappearance of the murmur.

VIRAL PERICARDITIS

A previously healthy 4-year-old F presents with 1 week of rhinorrhea, cough, and 3 days of fever. Her dad brings her to the ED because she is complaining of chest pain. On **exam**, she is tachycardic with a continuous murmur and friction rub. EKG reveals diffuse ST elevations. On **imaging**, an echocardiogram shows a small pericardial effusion. On **labs**, ESR, CRP, and troponin are elevated. CXR reveals an enlarged cardiac silhouette.

Management:

1. Course of NSAIDs (eg, ibuprofen, indomethacin, or naproxen) varying between 3 days and 2 weeks.
2. Steroids if NSAIDs are contraindicated.

Complications:

- Pericardial effusion.
- Cardiac tamponade.
- Obstructive heart failure.

HYF: Pericarditis in children is often viral in etiology but can also be idiopathic, autoimmune (eg, secondary to JIA, SLE) or caused by malignancy. In all cases, a course of NSAIDs is necessary to reduce pericardial inflammation. Treatment of the underlying cause or of a significant pericardial effusion via pericardiocentesis (if present) is also necessary.

*See also the Neonatal Heart Defects algorithm on pp. 562-566 for murmurs found in ASD, VSD, and other heart anomalies.

23-28 Immunologic Disorders: Part 1

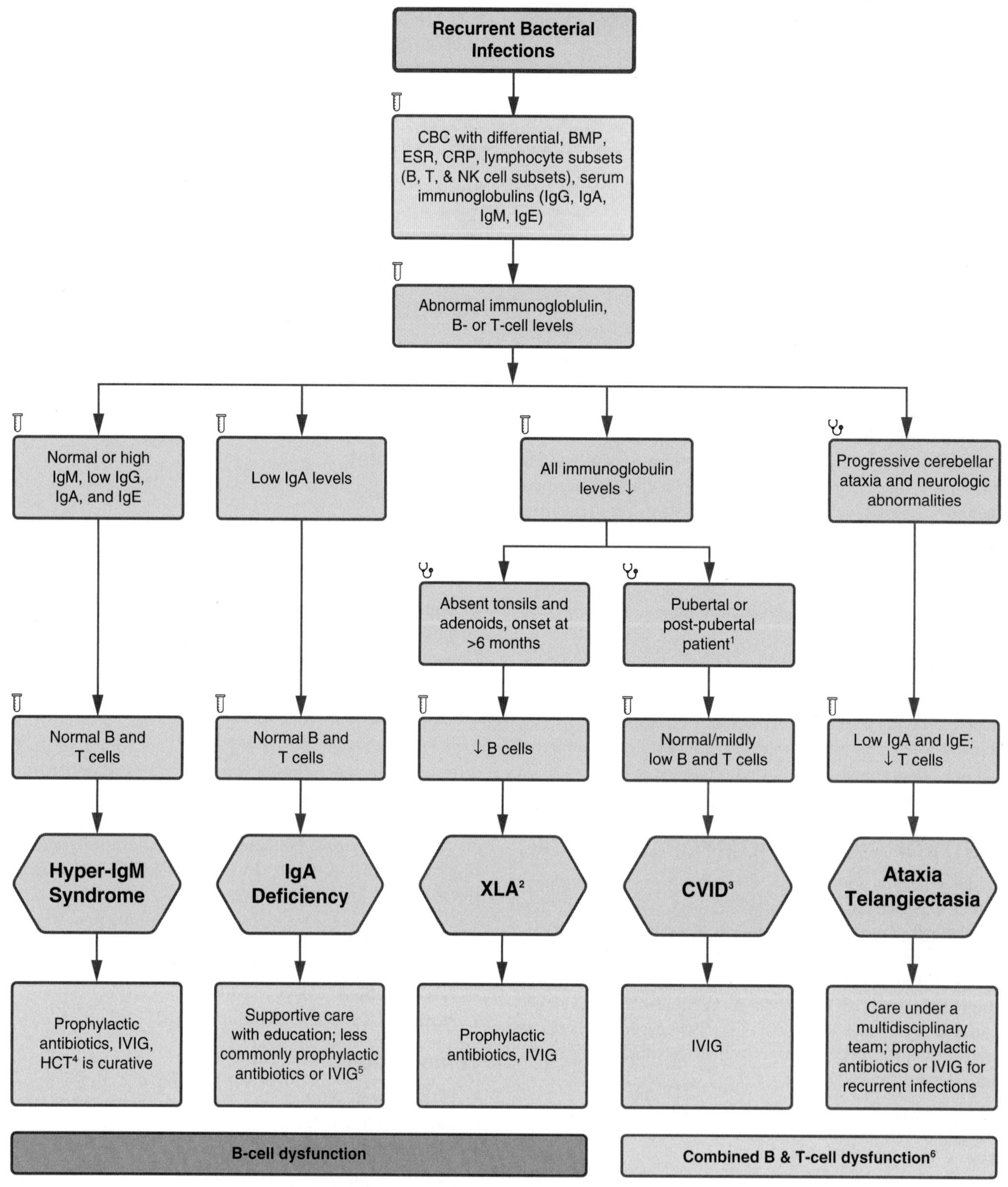
Recurrent Bacterial Infections
CBC with differential, BMP, ESR, CRP, lymphocyte subsets (B, T, & NK cell subsets), serum immunoglobulins (IgG, IgA, IgM, IgE)
Abnormal immunogloblulin, B- or T-cell levels
Normal or high IgM, low IgG, IgA, and IgE
Low IgA levels
All immunoglobulin levels ↓
Progressive cerebellar ataxia and neurologic abnormalities
Absent tonsils and adenoids, onset at >6 months
Pubertal or post-pubertal patient[1]
Normal B and T cells
Normal B and T cells
↓ B cells
Normal/mildly low B and T cells
Low IgA and IgE; ↓ T cells
Hyper-IgM Syndrome
IgA Deficiency
XLA[2]
CVID[3]
Ataxia Telangiectasia
Prophylactic antibiotics, IVIG, HCT[4] is curative
Supportive care with education; less commonly prophylactic antibiotics or IVIG[5]
Prophylactic antibiotics, IVIG
IVIG
Care under a multidisciplinary team; prophylactic antibiotics or IVIG for recurrent infections
B-cell dysfunction
Combined B & T-cell dysfunction[6]

Footnotes

1. Older age of onset can often differentiate CVID from XLA.
2. X-linked agammaglobulinemia.
3. Combined variable immunodeficiency.
4. Hematopoietic stem cell transplant.
5. With IgA deficiency, most individuals are asymptomatic and about 30% have recurrent sinopulmonary disorders, *Giardia* infections, and anaphylactic transfusion reactions.
6. Because much of the specific antibody production by B cells requires intact T-cell function, most T-cell defects lead to combined immunodeficiency.

FIGURE 23.28

23-28 Immunologic Disorders: Part 1

B-CELL DISORDERS

HYPER-IGM SYNDROME

A 6-month-old presents with with severe and recurrent sinus infections and pneumonia. **Exam** notable for LLL crackles. **Labs** reveal normal lymphocyte number, elevated IgM, and low levels of all other immunoglobulins.

Management:

1. Treat active infection.
2. Antibiotic prophylaxis.
3. IVIG.

Complications: Severe sinopulmonary infections due to impaired immunoglobulins.

HYF: Due to absence of CD40 ligand that typically allows class-switching from IgM to other immunoglobulin classes.

IGA DEFICIENCY

A 6-year-old M with PMH of celiac disease presents with his third episode of *Giardia* infection. **Labs** reveal low IgA levels.

Management:

1. Supportive care.

Complications:

- Anaphylactic reaction to transfusions.
- Associated with a celiac-like syndrome.
- Recurrent respiratory or GI infections due to lack of IgA.
- Associated with recurrent giardiasis.

HYF: Most common form of immunodeficiency and can be completely asymptomatic. Can see allergic reaction with blood transfusions. IVIG is not usually indicated.

X-LINKED AGAMMAGLOBULINEMIA

A 7-month-old M presents with recurrent episodes of otitis media and pneumonia. **Exam** is notable for absence of tonsils. **Labs** demonstrate absent immunoglobulins and absent B cells.

Management:

1. Treat active infections.
2. Start prophylactic antibiotics.
3. IVIG.

Complications:

- Life-threatening.
- Classically see infections with encapsulated organisms (*Pseudomonas, S. pneumoniae, Haemophilus*).

HYF: Absence of tonsils and other lymphoid tissue. X-linked recessive disorder due to a defect in bruton tyrosine kinase (Btk). Symptoms are classically seen after 6 months old, as this is the age when transplacentally transferred maternal immunoglobulins are no longer active.

COMBINED B- AND T-CELL DISORDERS

COMMON VARIABLE IMMUNODEFICIENCY (CVID)

A 15-year-old F who is small for her age presents with history of recurrent episodes of otitis media, pneumonia, and chronic sinusitis. **Exam** reveals diffuse wheezing and splenomegaly. **Labs** reveal low IgG, IgA, and IgM levels.

Management:

1. IVIG.

Complications: Complications due to years of recurrent infections leading to chronic pulmonary disease.

HYF: Typically a combined B- and T-cell defect. B cells cannot differentiate into plasma cells, which are responsible for secreting immunoglobulins. Absence of immunoglobulins leads to recurrent infections.

ATAXIA TELANGIECTASIA

A 15-month-old with a history of delayed walking presents with recurrent respiratory tract infections. **Exam** reveals several cafe-au-lait macules and diffuse coarse breath sounds. **Labs** reveal elevated AFP and low IgA; subsequent studies demonstrate pathogenic *ATM* gene variant.

Management:

1. Supportive care with a multidisciplinary team, management of disease complications.
2. Management of acute infections.

Complications:

- Eye movement abnormalities develop in elementary-age children.
- Cognitive and speech deficits.
- Peripheral neuropathy.
- May see oculocutaneous telangiectasias in toddlers or older; may see other skin abnormalities such as cafe au lait macules or cutaneous granulomatous lesions.
- Bronchiectasis or interstitial lung disease.
- Increased risk of malignancy.

HYF: Due to autosomal recessive defect in *ATM* gene, which is responsible for dsDNA repair mechanisms. Characterized by progressive cerebellar degeneration, oculocutaneous telangiectasias, immunodeficiency, and increased risk of malignancy. Immunodeficiency is due to low levels of T cells and immunoglobulins. May result in abnormal newborn screen.

23-29 Immunologic Disorders: Part 2

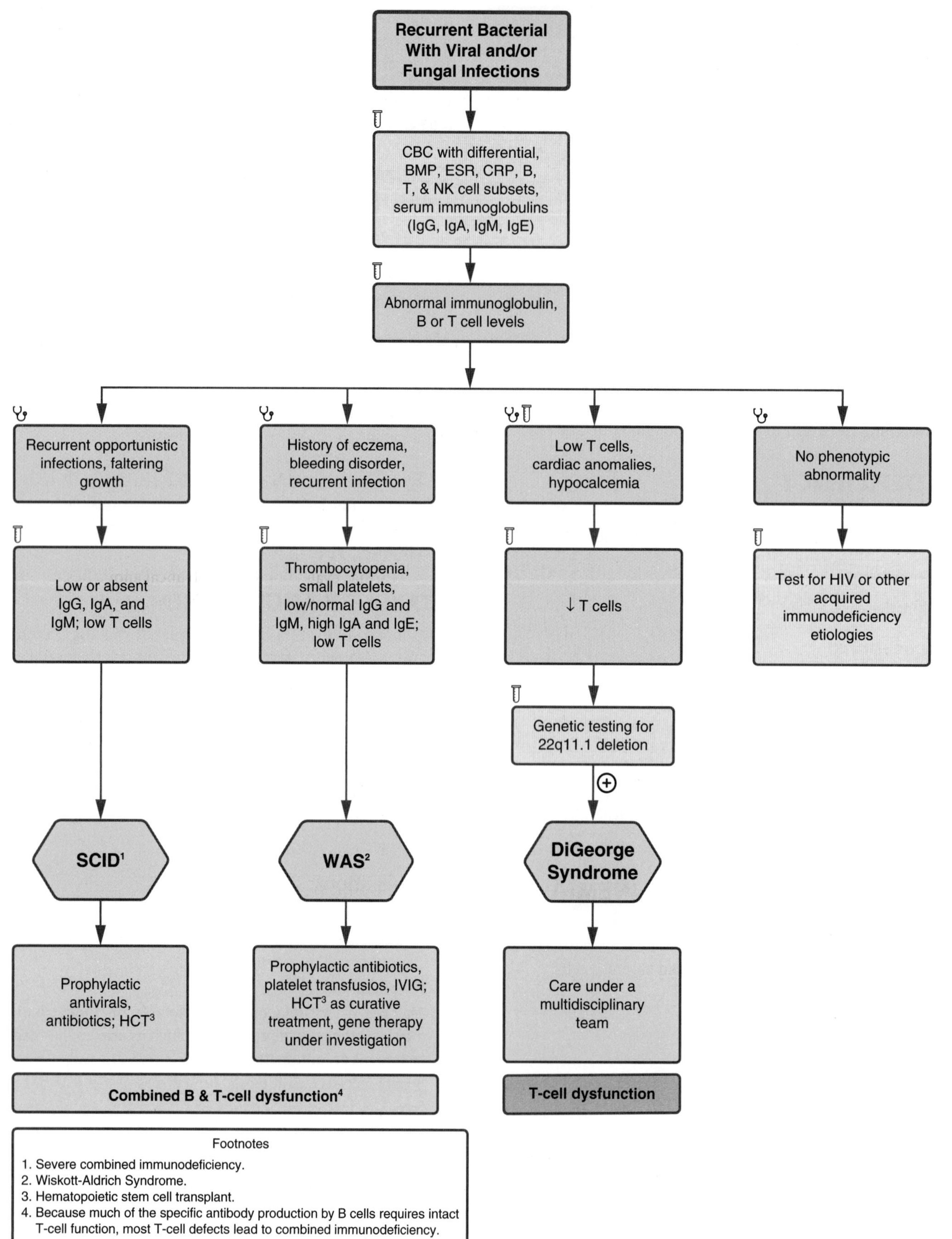
Recurrent Bacterial With Viral and/or Fungal Infections
CBC with differential, BMP, ESR, CRP, B, T, & NK cell subsets, serum immunoglobulins (IgG, IgA, IgM, IgE)
Abnormal immunoglobulin, B or T cell levels
Recurrent opportunistic infections, faltering growth
History of eczema, bleeding disorder, recurrent infection
Low T cells, cardiac anomalies, hypocalcemia
No phenotypic abnormality
Low or absent IgG, IgA, and IgM; low T cells
Thrombocytopenia, small platelets, low/normal IgG and IgM, high IgA and IgE; low T cells
↓ T cells
Test for HIV or other acquired immunodeficiency etiologies
Genetic testing for 22q11.1 deletion
+
SCID[1]
WAS[2]
DiGeorge Syndrome
Prophylactic antivirals, antibiotics; HCT[3]
Prophylactic antibiotics, platelet transfusios, IVIG; HCT[3] as curative treatment, gene therapy under investigation
Care under a multidisciplinary team
Combined B & T-cell dysfunction[4]
T-cell dysfunction
Footnotes
1. Severe combined immunodeficiency.
2. Wiskott-Aldrich Syndrome.
3. Hematopoietic stem cell transplant.
4. Because much of the specific antibody production by B cells requires intact T-cell function, most T-cell defects lead to combined immunodeficiency.

FIGURE 23.29

23-29 Immunologic Disorders: Part 2

COMBINED B- AND T-CELL DISORDERS

SEVERE-COMBINED IMMUNODEFICIENCY (SCID)

A 6-month-old M who recently moved to the United States has a history of recurrent infections, including pneumonia and chronic diarrhea. He presents with faltering growth. **Exam** reveals a small-for-his-age infant with diffuse coarse crackles on lung exam, oral thrush, and absent lymphoid tissue. **Labs** are notable for low T- and B-cell levels.

Management:

1. Protective measures.
2. Antibiotic and antiviral prophylaxis, including TMP-SMX for PJP prophylaxis.
3. Hematopoietic stem cell transplant.

Complications:

- If untreated, it is often fatal in the first year.
- Severe recurrent infections with bacterial, viruses, fungi, *Pneumocystis jiroveci.*

HYF: Typically presents with abnormal newborn screen. Usually X-linked recessive due to a defect in both B and T cells, which is caused by a defect in stem cell maturation and low adenosine deaminase.

WISKOTT-ALDRICH SYNDROME

An 8-month-old M with a history of severe eczema and recurrent infections presents with a new petechial rash and bloody stools. **Labs** are significant for thrombocytopenia and a deleterious mutation in the *WAS* gene.

Management:

1. Prophylactic antibiotics.
2. Platelet transfusions.
3. Sometimes IVIG or hematopoietic cell transplant.

Complications:

- May see early signs of prolonged bleeding, such as from the umbilical stump or with circumcision.
- Most common infections are of encapsulated organisms: *Streptococcus pneumoniae*, *Neisseria meningitidis*, and *Haemophilus influenzae.*
- Increased risk of malignancy.

HYF: X-linked recessive disorder. **WATER** triad: **W**iskott-**A**ldrich, **T**hrombocytopenia, **E**czema, **R**ecurrent infections.

22Q11 DELETION SPECTRUM (DIGEORGE SYNDROME)

A 1-month-old M with a history of global developmental delay and recurrent bacterial infections presents with intermittent muscle spasms and convulsions with concern for seizure. On **exam**, he has positive Chvostek sign, hyperreflexia, submucosal cleft palate, and prominent ears. On **imaging**, echocardiogram shows a small VSD. EKG shows QT prolongation. **Labs** show severe hypocalcemia with hypoparathyroidism. SNP array is positive for deletion in 22q11.2.

Management:

1. Calcium supplementation if needed.
2. Full cardiac evaluation for conotruncal anomalies.
3. Palate correction to assist with feeding, respiration, and prevention of aspiration.
4. Neurodevelopmental support if needed.

HYF: Previously called DiGeorge or velocardiofacial syndrome, this disorder has wide phenotypic variability depending on the size of the deletion. Calcium homeostasis typically improves after the neonatal period. **CATCH22**: **C**ardiac defects, **A**bnormal facial features, **T**hymic hypoplasia, **C**left palate, and **H**ypocalcemia/**H**ypoparathyroidism.

23-30 Immunologic Disorders: Part 3

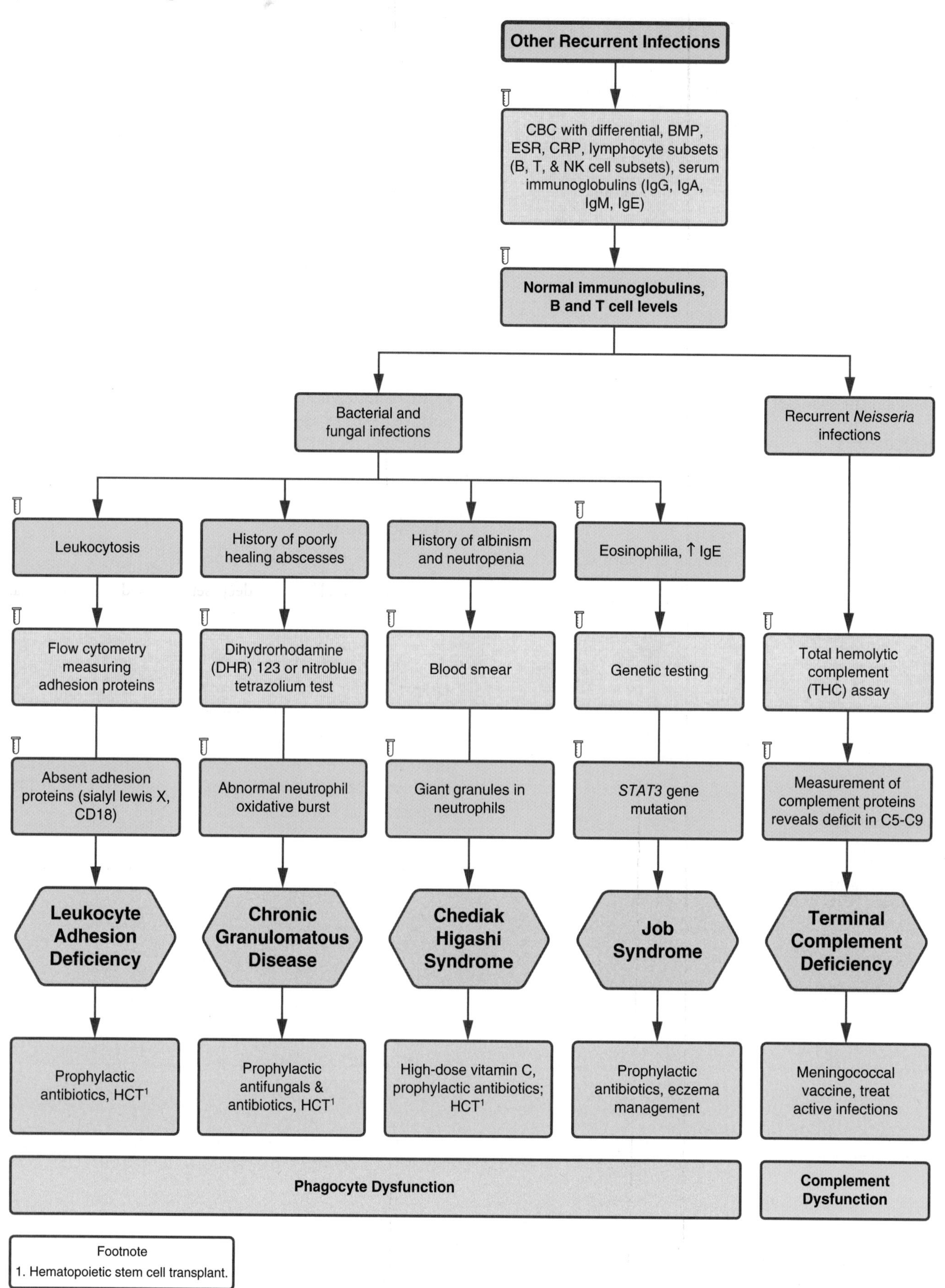
Other Recurrent Infections
CBC with differential, BMP, ESR, CRP, lymphocyte subsets (B, T, & NK cell subsets), serum immunoglobulins (IgG, IgA, IgM, IgE)
Normal immunoglobulins, B and T cell levels
Bacterial and fungal infections
Recurrent *Neisseria* infections
Leukocytosis
History of poorly healing abscesses
History of albinism and neutropenia
Eosinophilia, ↑ IgE
Flow cytometry measuring adhesion proteins
Dihydrorhodamine (DHR) 123 or nitroblue tetrazolium test
Blood smear
Genetic testing
Total hemolytic complement (THC) assay
Absent adhesion proteins (sialyl lewis X, CD18)
Abnormal neutrophil oxidative burst
Giant granules in neutrophils
STAT3 gene mutation
Measurement of complement proteins reveals deficit in C5-C9
Leukocyte Adhesion Deficiency
Chronic Granulomatous Disease
Chediak Higashi Syndrome
Job Syndrome
Terminal Complement Deficiency
Prophylactic antibiotics, HCT[1]
Prophylactic antifungals & antibiotics, HCT[1]
High-dose vitamin C, prophylactic antibiotics; HCT[1]
Prophylactic antibiotics, eczema management
Meningococcal vaccine, treat active infections
Phagocyte Dysfunction
Complement Dysfunction
Footnote
1. Hematopoietic stem cell transplant.

FIGURE 23.30

23-30 Immunologic Disorders: Part 3

PHAGOCYTE DISORDERS

LEUKOCYTE ADHESION DEFICIENCY

A 5-week-old F presents with omphalitis with delayed separation of the umbilical cord stump. **Exam** is notable for absence of purulent material at the infection site. **Labs** reveal leukocytosis of 68K WBCs, and flow cytometry reveals deficiency of CD18.

Management:

1. Supportive care.
2. Prophylactic antibiotics.
3. Severe cases may require hematopoietic or bone marrow transplant.

Complications:

- Recurrent bacterial infections, primarily affecting skin and mucosal surfaces.
- Infections are typically due to *Staph aureus* and gram-negative organisms, as well as *Candida* and *Aspergillus*.

HYF: Classically, delayed separation of the umbilical cord is seen. Absence of CD18 results in defective leukocyte migration and chemotaxis. Can see significant leukocytosis due to margination and inability to migrate extravascularly. Inability of leukocytes to arrive at site of injury/infection leads to absence of pus formation.

CHRONIC GRANULOMATOUS DISEASE (CGD)

A 3-year-old M with a history of poor wound healing and recurrent fungal infections presents with *Staph aureus* pneumonia. On **labs**, dihydrorhodamine oxidation test reveals defective neutrophil superoxide production.

Management:

1. Prophylactic antifungals.
2. Daily prophylactic antibiotics (TMP-SMX).
3. May benefit from IFN-gamma or, more rarely, hematopoietic cell transplantation.

Complications:

- Recurrent infections by catalase positive organisms.
  SPACE-Kitty is CATalase positive: *Staph aureus*, **P**seudomonas, Aspergillus, Candida, *E. coli*, **K**lebsiella.
- Severe occult infection, as infections may be relatively asymptomatic early on.
- Most common infectious sites are lungs, skin, and GI tract.

HYF: Most commonly diagnosed in toddlers ages 2–4 years. Classically, recurrent poorly healing abscesses are seen.

CHEDIAK HIGASHI SYNDROME

A 13-month-old M with very fair skin and light-colored hair and eyes presents with recurrent pyogenic infections and easy bruising. **Labs** demonstrate neutropenia, and blood smear reveals large inclusions in all nucleated blood cells.

Management:

1. High-dose vitamin C.
2. Bone marrow transplant is curative.
3. Hematopoietic cell transplantation.

Complications:

- Recurrent infections involving mucosal membranes, skin, and respiratory tract.
- Most common infectious organisms are gram-positive (*Staph aureus*) and gram-negative bacteria and fungi.
- Progressive peripheral neuropathy.
- Most common life-threatening complication is genetic form of hemophagocytic lymphohistiocytosis.

HYF: Autosomal recessive disease characterized by defective degranulation of neutrophils, easy bleeding, partial oculocutaneous albinism, light skin, and silvery hair. Most patients do not survive beyond 7 years if they do not undergo bone marrow transplantation.

JOB SYNDROME

A 9-year-old M with a history of severe eczema and recurrent bacterial and candidal infections presents with *Staph aureus* pneumonia. **Labs** reveal high levels of IgE and peripheral eosinophilia. **Exam** is notable for frontal bossing, deep-set eyes, and severe eczema.

Management:

1. Management of eczema symptoms.
2. Prophylactic antibiotics.
3. Aggressive treatment of infections.
4. Treatment of any accompanying syndromic features.

Complications:

- Chronic lung disease due to recurrent infections.
- Patients are at increased risk of lymphoma.
- Recurrent skin and pulmonary infections usually with *Staph aureus* or *Candida*.

HYF: Due to a defect in neutrophil chemotaxis and significantly decreased or absent CD4+ T cells. **FATED**: coarse **F**acies, **A**bscesses, retained primary **T**eeth, hyper-Ig**E**/**E**osinophilia, **D**ermatologic issues (severe eczema). Can also see scoliosis, osteoporosis, frequent fractures, and neurologic and vascular abnormalities.

COMPLEMENT DISORDERS

HEREDITARY ANGIOEDEMA

A 5-year-old M with a history of colicky abdominal pain presents with facial swelling after a fall. **Exam** is notable for diffuse facial edema without urticaria. **Labs** reveal low C4 and low levels of C1-inhibitor protein.

Management:

1. Treat acute attacks with C1-inhibitor protein.
2. Early intubation if signs of laryngeal involvement.
3. Avoidance of triggers.

23-30 Immunologic Disorders: Part 3

Complications:

- Attacks involving the upper airway can result in laryngeal edema and airway obstruction.
- Gastrointestinal attacks present with nausea, vomiting, and diarrhea due to bowel wall edema.

HYF: Classically due to C1 esterase deficiency; lack of C1 inhibitor results in excessive activation of the cytokine cascade and overproduction of bradykinin, leading to vasodilation and angioedema. Symptoms are not responsive to antihistamines. Attacks typically last 2–3 days, usually provoked by stress or trauma.

TERMINAL COMPLEMENT DEFICIENCY

A 5-year-old presents with recurrent *Neisseria* infections. **Labs** are significant for low CH50 levels, and specific complement levels reveal inadequate amounts of terminal complement.

Management:

1. Meningococcal vaccine.
2. Antibiotic treatment of bacterial infections.

Complications: Recurrent *Neisseria* infections.

HYF: Loss of terminal complement leads to lack of formation of membrane attack complex. Can rarely see lupus or glomerulonephritis.

23-31 Pediatric Solid Tumors

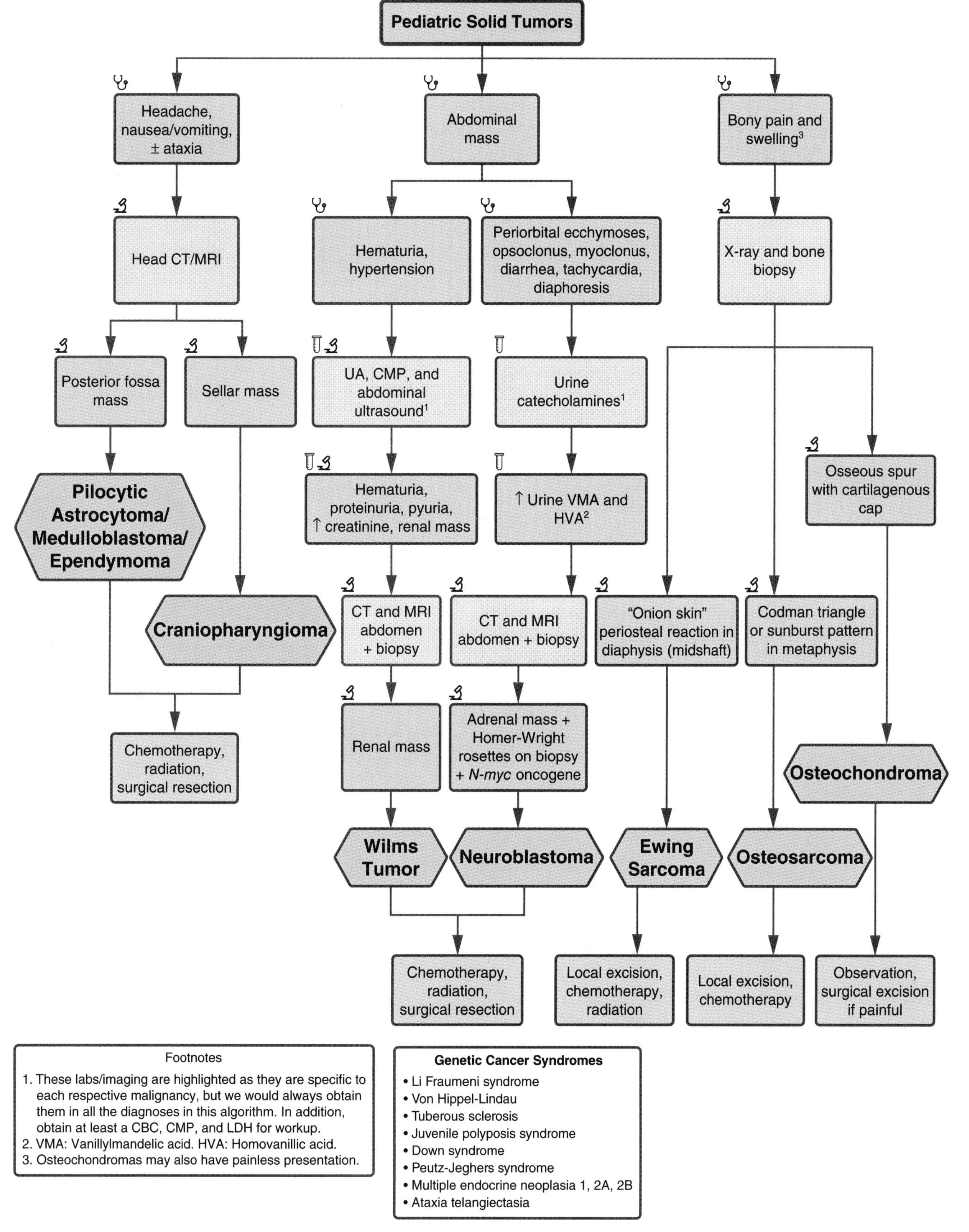

Pediatric Solid Tumors
Headache, nausea/vomiting, ± ataxia
Abdominal mass
Bony pain and swelling[3]
Head CT/MRI
Hematuria, hypertension
Periorbital ecchymoses, opsoclonus, myoclonus, diarrhea, tachycardia, diaphoresis
X-ray and bone biopsy
Posterior fossa mass
Sellar mass
UA, CMP, and abdominal ultrasound[1]
Urine catecholamines[1]
Osseous spur with cartilagenous cap
Pilocytic Astrocytoma/ Medulloblastoma/ Ependymoma
Hematuria, proteinuria, pyuria, ↑ creatinine, renal mass
↑ Urine VMA and HVA[2]
Craniopharyngioma
CT and MRI abdomen + biopsy
CT and MRI abdomen + biopsy
"Onion skin" periosteal reaction in diaphysis (midshaft)
Codman triangle or sunburst pattern in metaphysis
Chemotherapy, radiation, surgical resection
Renal mass
Adrenal mass + Homer-Wright rosettes on biopsy + N-myc oncogene
Osteochondroma
Wilms Tumor
Neuroblastoma
Ewing Sarcoma
Osteosarcoma
Chemotherapy, radiation, surgical resection
Local excision, chemotherapy, radiation
Local excision, chemotherapy
Observation, surgical excision if painful
Footnotes
1. These labs/imaging are highlighted as they are specific to each respective malignancy, but we would always obtain them in all the diagnoses in this algorithm. In addition, obtain at least a CBC, CMP, and LDH for workup.
2. VMA: Vanillylmandelic acid. HVA: Homovanillic acid.
3. Osteochondromas may also have painless presentation.
Genetic Cancer Syndromes
• Li Fraumeni syndrome
• Von Hippel-Lindau
• Tuberous sclerosis
• Juvenile polyposis syndrome
• Down syndrome
• Peutz-Jeghers syndrome
• Multiple endocrine neoplasia 1, 2A, 2B
• Ataxia telangiectasia

FIGURE 23.31

23-31 Pediatric Solid Tumors

ABDOMINAL TUMORS

WILMS TUMOR (NEPHROBLASTOMA)

A 3-year-old previously healthy M presents with bloody urine and abdominal pain. On **exam**, he has elevated BP of 122/84 and a smooth, right-sided abdominal mass. On **labs**, CBC shows mild anemia and leukocytosis, and UA has 3+ RBCs and 3+ WBCs. On **imaging**, abdominal ultrasound reveals a right renal mass, and CT abdomen is able to better characterize the tumor.

Management:

1. CT chest/abdomen/pelvis to characterize the tumor and evaluate for metastasis.
2. ± Biopsy.
3. Surgical resection first, followed by chemotherapy ± radiation.

HYF: Wilms tumor does not cross midline, while neuroblastoma can. Associated syndromes include **WAGR** (**W**ilms tumor, **A**niridia, **G**enitourinary anomalies, mental **R**etardation) and Beckwith-Wiedemann Syndrome.

NEUROBLASTOMA

A 15-month-old previously healthy F presents with fatigue, frequent fevers, and distended abdomen. **Exam** shows pallor and a palpable abdominal mass that crosses the midline. **Labs** reveal leukocytosis, anemia, and elevated LDH. On **imaging**, CT scan of the abdomen shows a mass of the adrenal medulla. Homer-Wright pseudorosettes are seen on biopsy of the mass. On **labs**, urine studies show elevated levels of homovanillic acid (HVA) and vanillylmandelic acid (VMA).

Management:

1. CT chest, abdomen, and pelvis to investigate for metastases.
2. Surgical resection, chemotherapy, ± radiation.

Complications:

- Horner syndrome (ptosis, miosis, anhidrosis) if involvement of the cervical sympathetic chain or thoracic region.
- Paralysis or neurologic changes if involvement of the spinal cord.
- Bone metastasis and pathologic fractures.

HYF: Neuroblastoma is a tumor of neural crest origin. The most common presentation is an abdominal mass from a tumor of the adrenal medulla. *N-myc* gene amplification is associated with poor prognosis.

BONE TUMORS

OSTEOID OSTEOMA

A 16-year-old M develops progressively worsening nocturnal thigh pain that improves after he takes ibuprofen. On **exam**, there is point tenderness and swelling of the proximal femur, and he walks with a limp. On **imaging**, X-ray shows a 1-cm round lucency at the proximal femur.

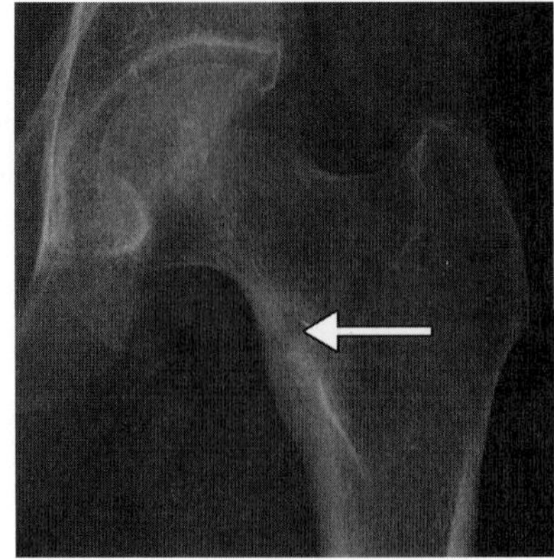

Round lucent lesion of osteoid osteoma.

Management:

1. Clinical features and imaging (X-ray, CT) are sufficient for diagnosis.
2. NSAIDs for symptom management.
3. Surveillance X-rays every 6 months.
4. Frequently self-resolve. For refractory symptoms, consider surgery, ablation, or cryotherapy.

Complications:

- Scoliosis.
- Muscular atrophy.
- Leg-length discrepancy.

HYF: Look for nocturnal pain that improves with NSAIDS. Benign **b**one tumors that start with **o** are more common in **bo**ys.

OSTEOCHONDROMA

A 14-year-old M presents with 2 months of left thigh pain following a minor fall. **Exam** reveals a non-tender, firm mass at the distal femur. On **imaging**, X-ray of the left thigh shows an osseous spur with a cartilaginous cap, continuous with the cortex.

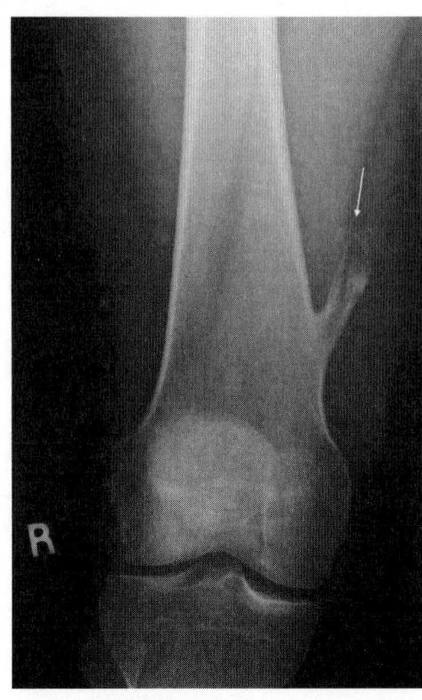
R

Arrow showing pedunculated lesion of distal femur.

23-31 Pediatric Solid Tumors

Management:

1. Often no intervention, as these stop growing when the growth plates close.
2. MRI ± surgical resection if there is tumors concern for tissue impingement, spinal cord encroachment, or new or worsening pain.

Complications:

- Rarely transforms into chondrosarcoma.
- If multiple, rule out hereditary multiple osteochondroma.
- Possible local irritation, arthritis of the hip if at proximal femur.

HYF: Mostly commonly found in the distal femur or proximal humerus. May be painless.

EWING SARCOMA

A 13-year-old F presents with 3 weeks of progressive pain in her right arm. The pain seems to be worse at night. On **imaging**, X-ray reveals an "onion skin" periosteal reaction of the right humerus. **Labs** show elevated LDH.

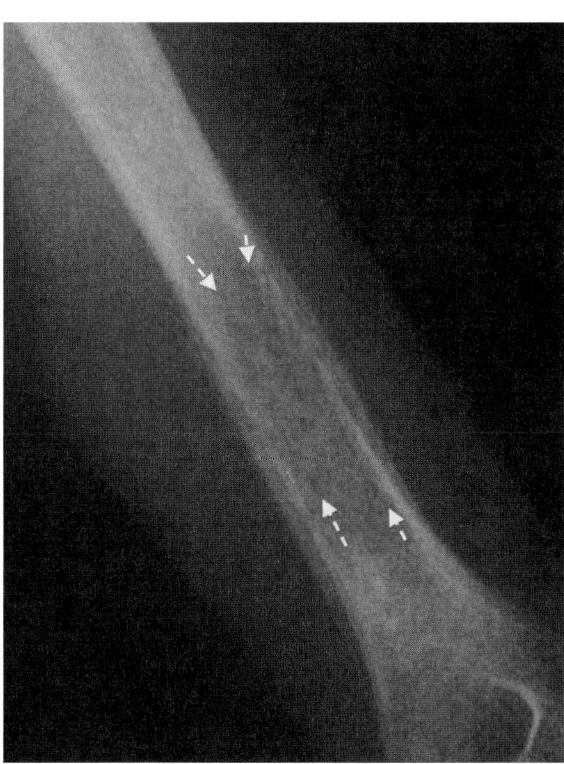

Ewing sarcoma.

Management:

1. Bone scan, CT scan, and MRI to look for metastasis.
2. Chemotherapy, surgical resection ± radiation.

Complications:

- Pathologic fractures.
- Aggressive tumor with early metastasis.

HYF: The most common bone malignancy in teenagers, and most commonly found in the diaphysis of long bones and the pelvis. Associated with t(11:22) translocation.

OSTEOSARCOMA

A 13-year-old previously healthy M presents with progressive left leg pain that worsens with activity. His mother notes that he has lost some weight. On **labs**, CBC shows leukocytosis and anemia. On **imaging**, X-ray shows a sunburst pattern with Codman's triangle.

Management:

1. Biopsy.
2. Chemotherapy, surgical resection ± radiation.

Complications:

- Horner syndrome (ptosis, miosis, anhidrosis) if involvement of the cervical sympathetic chain or thoracic region.
- Paralysis or neurologic changes if involvement of the spinal cord.
- Bone metastasis and pathologic fractures.

HYF: Bimodal age distribution: Peak in ages 10–14 and then around age 65. Codman triangle or sunburst pattern can sometimes be seen on X-ray in metaphysis of long bones. Associated with familial retinoblastoma.

INTRACRANIAL TUMORS

MEDULLOBLASTOMA

A 5-year-old F presents with morning headaches and vomiting, ataxia, and blurry vision. On **imaging**, head MRI reveals a mass occupying the fourth ventricle. Biopsy of the mass shows Homer-Wright rosettes.

Management:

1. Chemotherapy, surgical resection ± radiation.

Complications:

- Compression of the 4th ventricle causing communicating hydrocephalus and symptoms of increased intracranial pressure, including papilledema and blurry vision.
- Herniation.
- Cranial nerve palsies if spread into the brainstem.

HYF: Medulloblastomas are highly malignant posterior fossa tumors originating from the cerebellum that grow into the 4th ventricle.

23-31 Pediatric Solid Tumors

CRANIOPHARYNGIOMA

A 10-year-old previously healthy M presents with worsening headaches, and his mom says he is always "running into things." On exam, he has bitemporal hemianopsia and is not growing in height as expected. On imaging, hand X-ray shows delayed bone age. Labs show low IGF-1 and low T4 with inappropriately normal TSH. Head MRI reveals a sellar mass.

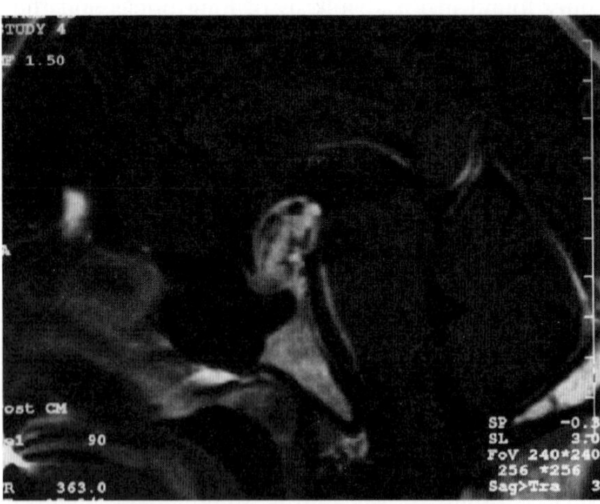

Craniopharyngioma as seen on MRI.

Management:

1. Endocrine work-up, including X-ray for bone age and levels of IGF-1 (for growth deficiency), free T4 and TSH, morning FSH and LH (for delayed puberty workup), and morning cortisol (to investigate for ACTH deficiency). Children are often followed by endocrinology.
2. Full evaluation by neuro-ophthalmology for eye exam and visual field testing.
3. Chemotherapy, surgical resection ± radiation.

Complications:

- Compression of the optic chiasm causing bitemporal hemianopsia.
- Pituitary and hypothalamic dysfunction: obesity, growth hormone deficiency leading to short stature, delayed puberty from low gonadotropin secretion, central hypothyroidism, ACTH deficiency, vasopressin deficiency (diluted urine).

HYF: Craniopharyngiomas are derived from the craniopharyngeal duct connected to Rathke pouch, a structure that develops into the anterior pituitary gland during embryogenesis.

23-32 Pediatric Liquid Tumors

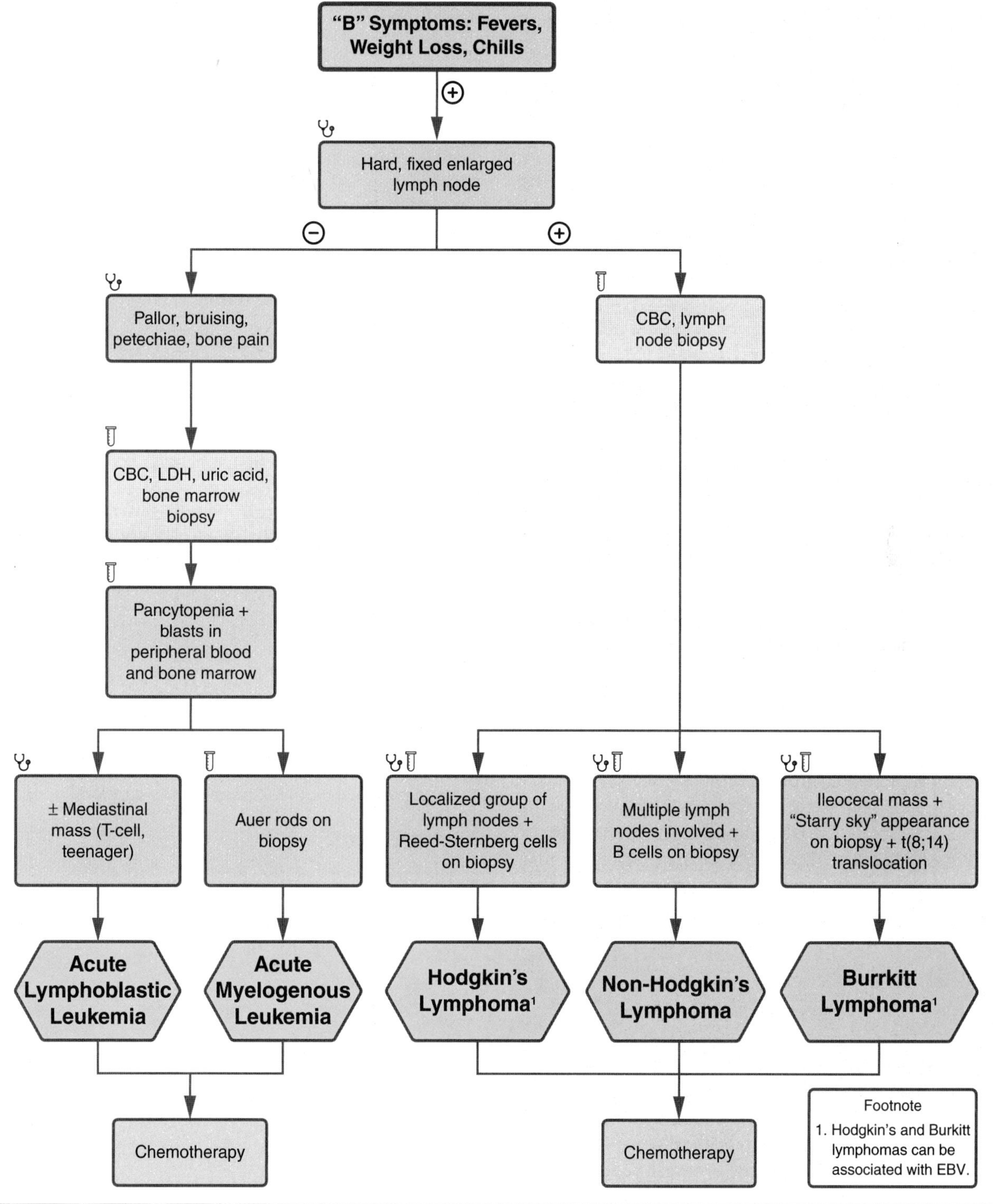
"B" Symptoms: Fevers, Weight Loss, Chills
+
Hard, fixed enlarged lymph node
−
+
Pallor, bruising, petechiae, bone pain
CBC, lymph node biopsy
CBC, LDH, uric acid, bone marrow biopsy
Pancytopenia + blasts in peripheral blood and bone marrow
± Mediastinal mass (T-cell, teenager)
Auer rods on biopsy
Localized group of lymph nodes + Reed-Sternberg cells on biopsy
Multiple lymph nodes involved + B cells on biopsy
Ileocecal mass + "Starry sky" appearance on biopsy + t(8;14) translocation
Acute Lymphoblastic Leukemia
Acute Myelogenous Leukemia
Hodgkin's Lymphoma1
Non-Hodgkin's Lymphoma
Burrkitt Lymphoma1
Chemotherapy
Chemotherapy
Footnote
1. Hodgkin's and Burkitt lymphomas can be associated with EBV.

FIGURE 23.32

23-32 Pediatric Liquid Tumors

HODGKIN'S LYMPHOMA

A 17-year-old previously healthy F presents with low-grade fevers, night sweats, weight loss, and localized supraclavicular lymphadenopathy on exam. Lymph node biopsy shows Reed-Sternberg cells.

Management:

1. CT chest/abdomen/pelvis for staging.
2. Chemotherapy, immunotherapy, ± radiation.

HYF: Hodgkin's lymphoma is a B-cell lymphoma and has an overall good prognosis. Reed-Sternberg cells arise from germinal center B cells and have an "owl eye" appearance.

BURKITT LYMPHOMA

A 5-year-old previously healthy F presents with weight loss, abdominal pain, and bloody stools. On labs, CBC is notable for anemia and leukocytosis, LDH and uric acid levels are elevated, and BMP shows elevated potassium and phosphorus. On imaging, abdominal CT scan shows an ileocecal mass. Biopsy of the mass shows a "starry sky" appearance.

Management:

1. CT chest/abdomen/pelvis + bone marrow biopsy to help with staging.
2. Chemotherapy ± radiation.

Complications:

- Tumor lysis syndrome: Usually seen after administration of chemotherapy or in rapidly growing tumors with high cell turnover. Occurs due to release of intracellular contents of dying cancer cells into the bloodstream, causing electrolyte abnormalities. These include hyperphosphatemia, hyperkalemia, hyperuricemia (DNA turnover), and hypocalcemia. These electrolyte abnormalities in turn can lead to fatal arrhythmias and/or renal failure.
- Burkitt lymphoma carries a higher risk of tumor lysis syndrome due to its rapid growth.

HYF: Burkitt lymphoma is a type of non-Hodgkin lymphoma that often presents with a submandibular or ileocecal mass. The most commonly associated translocation, t(8;14)(q24;q32), causes overexpression of the *c-MYC* oncogene. Patients with EBV or HIV infection are at increased risk of developing the disease. The "starry sky" appearance on histopathology is due to clearing of the cellular debris by macrophages.

ACUTE LYMPHOBLASTIC LEUKEMIA (ALL)

A 7-year-old M presents with 4 weeks of fatigue, frequent fevers, and a new "rash." On exam, he has conjunctival pallor, petechiae on his abdomen, and hepatosplenomegaly. On labs, CBC reveals significant leukocytosis, anemia, and thrombocytopenia. LDH is elevated. Bone marrow biopsy shows 30% lymphoblasts.

Management:

1. Obtain lumbar puncture to evaluate for CNS involvement.
2. Obtain chest X-ray to evaluate for mediastinal mass.
3. Chemotherapy, immunotherapy, and/or hematopoietic stem cell transplant.
4. Stem cell transplant.

Complications:

- T-cell ALL can present with a mediastinal mass causing SVC-like syndrome.
- Higher risk of infection during chemotherapy treatment due to neutropenia.
- Tumor lysis syndrome.
- Hyperleukocytosis (WBC >100,000), causing viscous blood that can lead to end-organ damage in the lungs and brain due to tissue hypoxia.
- Bleeding due to thrombocytopenia.

HYF: ALL can be B- or T-cell derived and most commonly occurs in children. Patients with trisomy 21 are at higher risk for this malignancy. B-cell ALL associated with the Philadelphia chromosome t(9;22) has a less favorable prognosis but can be targeted with imatinib.

LANGERHANS CELL HISTIOCYTOSIS

A 10-year-old M with PMH of refractory otitis media presents with a red papular rash on his face and 2 months of polyuria and polydipsia. Exam shows mastoid swelling. On imaging, X-ray shows a punched-out lytic lesion of the temporal bone.

Management:

1. Diagnostic FNA or core biopsy.
2. Skeletal survey ± CT head and spine.
3. Surgical resection of skull lesions.
4. Chemotherapy ± radiation if multifocal.
5. Evaluation for diabetes insipidus.

Complications:

- Loose teeth and jaw pain.
- Proptosis.
- Refractory otitis media.
- Hearing loss.
- Diabetes insipidus due to involvement of the pituitary gland.

HYF: Characterized by diabetes insipidus, skin rash, and refractory otitis media. Skin and bone lesions are the most common.

23-33 Pediatric Ophthalmology

TRACHOMA

A 6-year-old M whose family recently moved from Ethiopia presents with eye redness, discomfort, and tearing. On exam, pale follicles are present on the conjunctiva, and there is tarsal inflammation. On labs, PCR swab of the eyelid is positive for *Chlamydia trachomatis*.

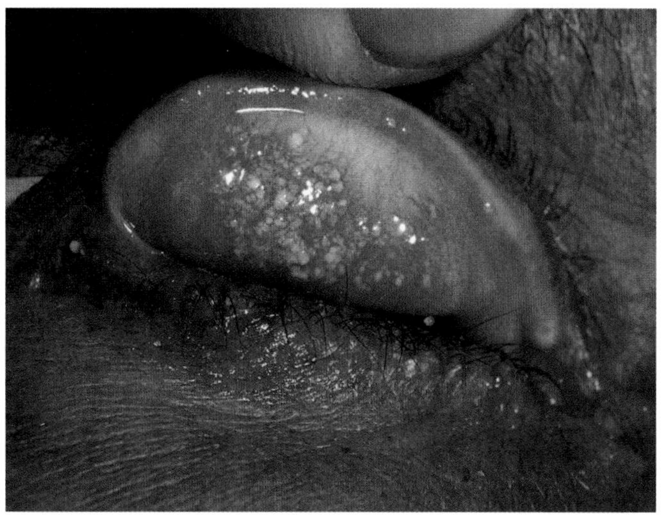

Prominent follicles under the upper eyelid seen in trachoma.

Management:

1. Oral azithromycin.
2. Fluorescein exam to assess corneal damage.
3. Surgical management (reserved for late and advanced cases) for those with misdirected eyelashes or eyelid margins.

Complications:

- Conjunctival scarring.
- Cicatricial entropion and trichiasis.
- Corneal opacification and vascularization.

HYF: One of the leading causes of preventable blindness globally, especially in endemic regions. Active disease presents with follicular conjunctivitis. Repeat infection and inflammation leads to scarring and cicatricial changes.

BACTERIAL CONJUNCTIVITIS

A 10-year-old M presents with right eye pain, redness, and discharge for the past 10 days. On exam, he has conjunctival edema and injection with mucopurulent discharge. He does not have any blurry vision or pain with eye movements.

Management:

1. Proper hygiene and hand washing as it is a contagious condition.
2. Supportive therapy with cool compresses and preservative free artificial tears.
3. Topical antibiotics (eg, neomycin/polymyxin B/bacitracin).

Complications:

Low risk for complications except in the cases of *Chlamydia* and *Neisseria gonorrhea*, which have increased risk of corneal involvement.

HYF: Most cases are acute, self-limited, and contagious.

VIRAL CONJUNCTIVITIS

An 8-year-old F recovering from a recent URI presents with a gritty and burning sensation in the right eye for the past week. On exam, she has bilateral conjunctivitis and clear discharge.

Management:

1. Proper hygiene and hand washing, as it is a contagious condition.
2. Supportive therapy with cool compresses and preservative-free artificial tears.

Complications: Rare, but some patients can have pseudomembrane formation and corneal infiltrates.

HYF: Most common cause is adenovirus. Commonly presents with prodromal symptoms after a viral infection. It is very infectious, and patients should be counseled on avoiding personal care objects and frequent hand washing.

ALLERGIC CONJUNCTIVITIS

A 13-year-old F with PMH of eczema presents with bilateral eye discharge and itchiness since yesterday. Exam shows bilateral conjunctivitis, edematous nasal turbinates, and a transverse nasal crease ("allergic salute").

Management:

1. Antihistamines (eg, cetirizine, diphenhydramine, or loratadine) for symptom control. Patients with accompanying allergic rhinitis can also use intranasal steroids (eg, fluticasone).
2. Mast cell stabilizer if recurrent.

Complications: None.

HYF: Always presents bilaterally and is much shorter in duration compared to other causes of conjunctivitis. Pruritus and history of atopy is suggestive. Usually presents in older children, as seasonal allergies are uncommon <5 years of age.

UVEITIS

A 7-year-old F with PMH of juvenile idiopathic arthritis presents for a routine eye exam. On exam, she has anterior chamber cell reaction.

Management:

1. Topical steroids.
2. Systemic immunosuppression.

Complications:

- Cataract.
- Band keratopathy.
- Glaucoma.

23-33 Pediatric Ophthalmology

HYF: Uveitis in children is associated with juvenile idiopathic arthritis (JIA). Unlike presentation in adults, children rarely have symptoms of photophobia or eye pain. All patients with JIA should be screened for uveitis.

MYOPIA

A 8-year-old M presents with progressive decline in vision requiring him to squint when in class. He has not been prescribed glasses before. Slit lamp exam is unremarkable.

Management:

1. Glasses prescription.
2. Low dose atropine.

Complications:

- Retinal detachment (if more than 6D of myopia).

HYF: Those of Asian ancestry or with family history of myopia are at a higher risk.

STRABISMUS

A 4-year-old M is brought in by parents after his eyes were noted to be misaligned. On exam, his left eye moves to the center when covering the right ("cover-uncover test") and has a more pronounced red reflex.

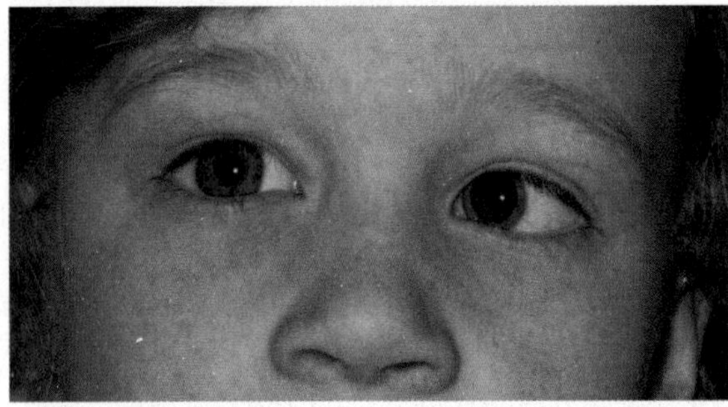

Esotropia of left eye in comparison to right eye that is midline.

Management:

1. Patching of the unaffected eye or using cycloplegic drops to blur the unaffected eye to strengthen the affected eye and prevent amblyopia.
2. Refractive correction of the affected eye.
3. Strabismus surgery.

Complications:

- Amblyopia.

HYF: Head tilt and intermittently deviated eyes for >4 months are suggestive of strabismus. It can be congenital or due to secondary causes of visual deprivation, such as cataracts. If age <5 years, there is a high risk of developing amblyopia. Strabismus is a leading cause of amblyopia in children. They need to be addressed by a pediatric ophthalmologist to prevent irreversible vision loss in the amblyopic eye.

AMBLYOPIA

A 5-year-old M with congenital uncorrected ptosis of the right eye is found to have 20/60 vision in the right eye on exam. Vision in the left eye is 20/20.

Management:

1. Surgical correction of ptosis.
2. Patching of the unaffected eye.

Complications:

- Treat underlying cause of amblyopia.
- Difficult to reverse as patients become older.

HYF: Strabismus, asymmetric refractive error of eyes, ptosis, or any other causes of visual deprivation can cause amblyopia. Amblyopia concerns visual acuity, while strabismus is ocular misalignment.

ECTOPIA LENTIS

A 14-year-old M presents with right-sided decline in vision. On exam, he is in the 98th percentile for height, has pectus excavatum and long fingers, and his lens is dislocated superiorly.

Management:

1. Surgical correction.
2. Workup for genetic causes, such as Marfan syndrome.

Complications: Blurry vision.

HYF: Superior dislocation is associated with Marfan syndrome (as seen in this patient), while inferior dislocation is associated with homocystinuria. In Alport syndrome, dislocation is variable. Can also happen after forceful blunt trauma without genetic predisposition.

RETINOBLASTOMA

A 1-year-old F with misaligned eyes is found to have an absent right red reflex and leukocoria. On fundus exam, a mass is found in the retina.

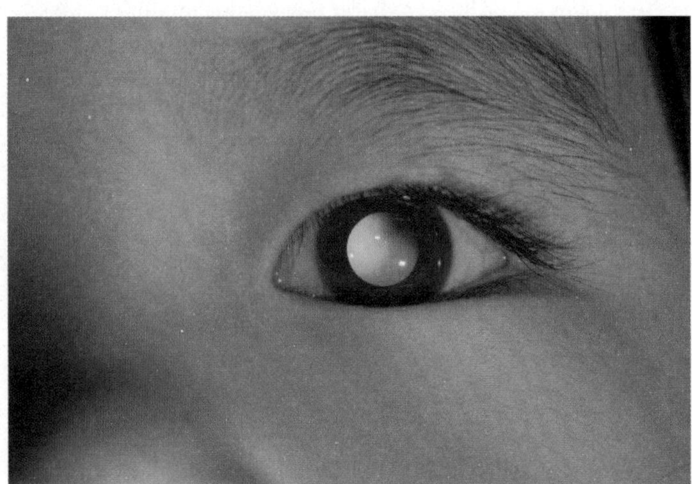

Leukocoria (white pupil) is seen in retinoblastoma.

Management:

1. Imaging studies, including ocular ultrasound, CT scan, and/or MRI brain and orbit.
2. Surgical and oncologic evaluation.

23-33 Pediatric Ophthalmology

Complications:

- Vision loss.
- Metastasis and death, if untreated.

HYF: >95% survival rate. *RB1* mutation is a risk factor. Need to distinguish from other causes of leukocoria, such as congenital cataracts.

NEUROFIBROMATOSIS TYPE 1

An 8-year-old M presents with blurry vision. On exam, multiple café au lait spots and axillary freckling are present. Slit lamp exam reveals Lisch nodules.

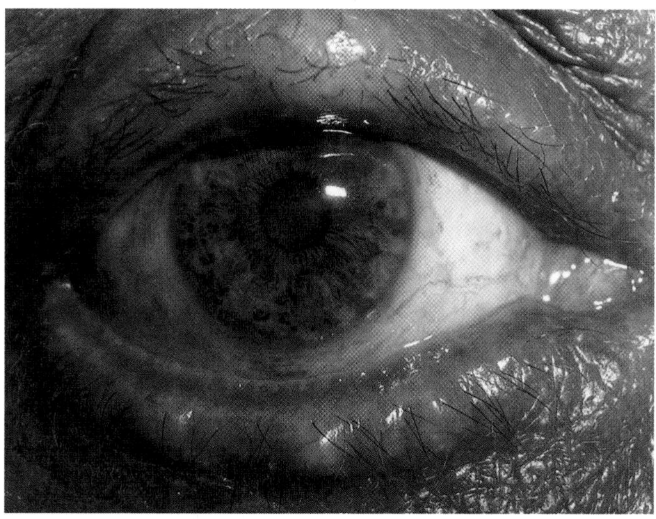

Lisch nodules.

Management:

1. Genetic testing for *NF1* mutation.

Complications:

- Color vision change.
- Optic nerve atrophy.
- Vision loss.

HYF:

NF1 is a neurocutaneous disorder associated with café au lait macules, axillary freckling, and neurofibromas.

23-34 Abnormal Tone

HYPERTONIA

CEREBRAL PALSY (CP)

A 4-year-old F with a history of preterm birth at 32 weeks gestation, seizures, and delayed milestones presents with tight muscles that are impeding daily care. On **exam**, she has hyperreflexia and hypertonia in the lower extremities. On **imaging**, review of prior MRI after birth shows periventricular leukomalacia.

Management:

1. Symptomatic management: Botox injections, anti-spastic medications (eg, baclofen).
2. Nutritional support.
3. Physical and occupational therapy.

Complications:

- Gross and fine motor delay.
- Muscle contractures.
- Increased oral secretions.

HYF: CP is a term describing a group of permanent, non-progressive motor disorders attributed to a intrauterine or perinatal insult (perinatal asphyxia, neonatal stroke, IVH, chorioamnionitis). The greatest risk factor for CP is prematurity (<37 weeks gestation).

NEONATAL TETANUS

A 7-day-old F born at 39 weeks GA via home-birth presents with progressive inability to breastfeed starting at day 5 of life and now has stopped breastfeeding completely. Father says he cut the cord with kitchen scissors at birth. On **exam**, baby has clenched fists, high muscle tone, trismus and is arching her back (opisthotonus).

Management:

1. Treatment of acute tetanus is mainly supportive in the intensive care unit with ventilatory support to prevent respiratory failure from spastic paralysis.
2. Use of antispasmodics can be helpful.
3. Prognosis is poor despite administration of antibiotics and tetanus toxoid immunoglobulin.
4. Given poor prognosis of tetanus, prophylaxis is key.

Complications:

- Rigors and muscle spasms.
- Lockjaw, trismus.
- Death can occur if not properly treated.

HYF: Spastic paralysis in tetanus is exotoxin-mediated (tetanospasmin).

HYPOTONIA

SPINAL MUSCULAR ATROPHY (WERDNIG-HOFFMANN DISEASE)

A 4-month-old M born full-term presents with head control. On **exam**, he has proximal muscle weakness (lower >> upper extremities), absent DTRs, and tongue fasciculations. Genetic testing shows deletion in *SMN1* gene.

Management:

1. Symptomatic management.
2. Physical and occupational therapy.
3. Nusinursen.

Complications:

- The most common cause of death is respiratory insufficiency and aspiration pneumonia due to ineffective airway clearance.

HYF: If the patient presents with more acute-onset hypotonia, consider other diagnoses, such as polio (unvaccinated or from underdeveloped country) or botulism (honey ingestion).

BOTULISM

A 4-month-old healthy F presents with difficulty with feeds, decreased movement, constipation, and inability to open her eyes. On **exam**, she has ptosis and generalized weakness.

Management:

1. Supportive care.
2. IV human-derived botulism IgG.
3. Stool testing for botulism spores and/or toxin.

Complications: Respiratory compromise.

HYF: Botulism can be caused by eating foods contaminated with *Clostridium botulinum* spores, which colonize the GI tract and produce toxin that leads to impairment of presynaptic acetylcholine release into the neuromuscular junction. It can also be caused by ingestion of inhaled environmental dust contaminated with botulism spores (eg, construction sites). It usually causes GI upset, then acute onset of bilateral cranial nerve abnormalities, followed by descending flaccid paralysis. Counsel families to avoid giving babies honey prior to 1 year of age.

23-35 Progressive Muscle Weakness

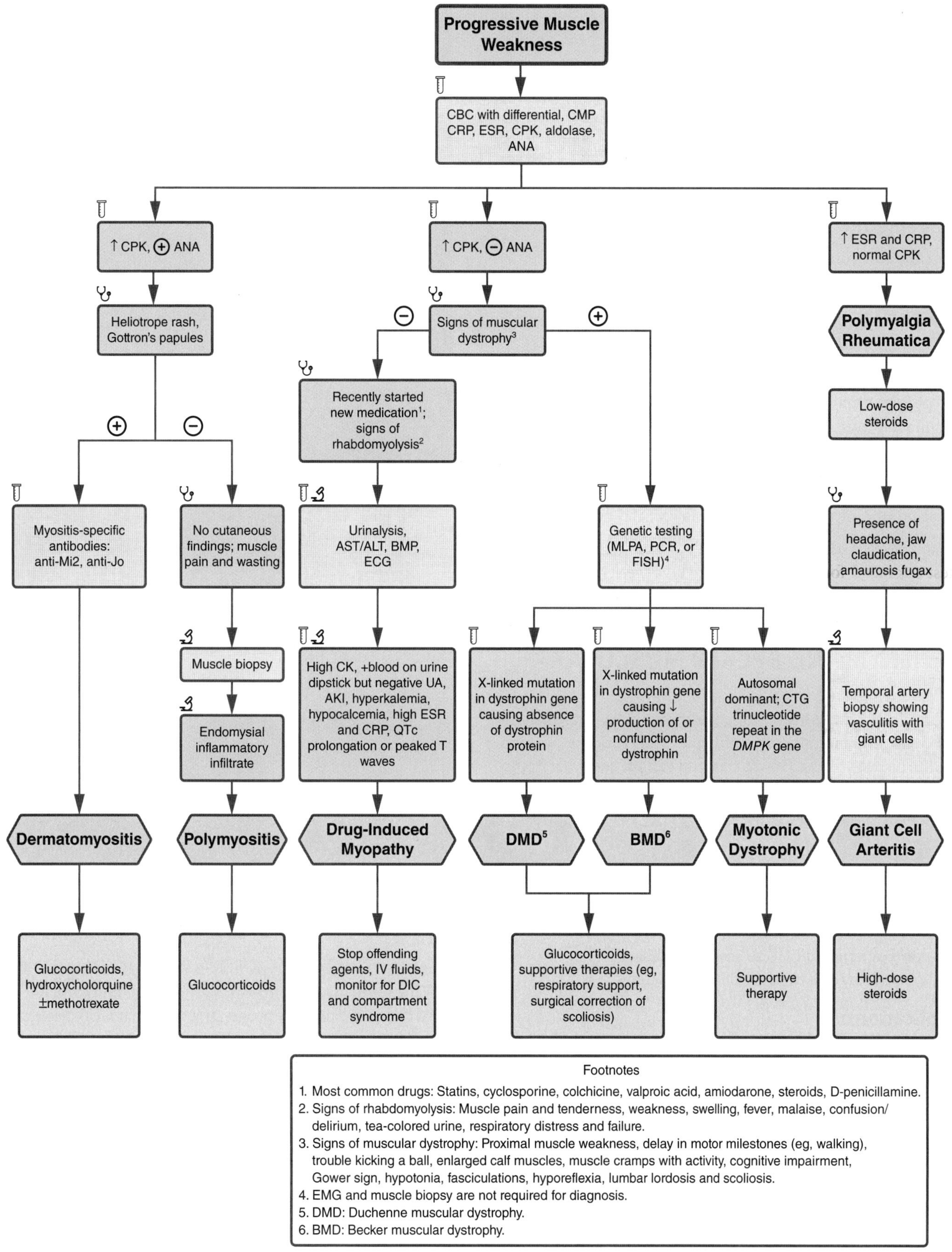
Progressive Muscle Weakness
CBC with differential, CMP CRP, ESR, CPK, aldolase, ANA
↑ CPK, ⊕ ANA
↑ CPK, ⊖ ANA
↑ ESR and CRP, normal CPK
Heliotrope rash, Gottron's papules
⊕
⊖
Signs of muscular dystrophy[3]
⊖
⊕
Polymyalgia Rheumatica
Recently started new medication[1]; signs of rhabdomyolysis[2]
Low-dose steroids
Myositis-specific antibodies: anti-Mi2, anti-Jo
No cutaneous findings; muscle pain and wasting
Urinalysis, AST/ALT, BMP, ECG
Genetic testing (MLPA, PCR, or FISH)[4]
Presence of headache, jaw claudication, amaurosis fugax
Muscle biopsy
Endomysial inflammatory infiltrate
High CK, +blood on urine dipstick but negative UA, AKI, hyperkalemia, hypocalcemia, high ESR and CRP, QTc prolongation or peaked T waves
X-linked mutation in dystrophin gene causing absence of dystrophin protein
X-linked mutation in dystrophin gene causing ↓ production of or nonfunctional dystrophin
Autosomal dominant; CTG trinucleotide repeat in the DMPK gene
Temporal artery biopsy showing vasculitis with giant cells
Dermatomyositis
Polymyositis
Drug-Induced Myopathy
DMD[5]
BMD[6]
Myotonic Dystrophy
Giant Cell Arteritis
Glucocorticoids, hydroxycholorquine ±methotrexate
Glucocorticoids
Stop offending agents, IV fluids, monitor for DIC and compartment syndrome
Glucocorticoids, supportive therapies (eg, respiratory support, surgical correction of scoliosis)
Supportive therapy
High-dose steroids
Footnotes
1. Most common drugs: Statins, cyclosporine, colchicine, valproic acid, amiodarone, steroids, D-penicillamine.
2. Signs of rhabdomyolysis: Muscle pain and tenderness, weakness, swelling, fever, malaise, confusion/delirium, tea-colored urine, respiratory distress and failure.
3. Signs of muscular dystrophy: Proximal muscle weakness, delay in motor milestones (eg, walking), trouble kicking a ball, enlarged calf muscles, muscle cramps with activity, cognitive impairment, Gower sign, hypotonia, fasciculations, hyporeflexia, lumbar lordosis and scoliosis.
4. EMG and muscle biopsy are not required for diagnosis.
5. DMD: Duchenne muscular dystrophy.
6. BMD: Becker muscular dystrophy.

FIGURE 23.35

23-35 Progressive Muscle Weakness

JUVENILE POLYMYOSITIS/ DERMATOMYOSITIS

A 7-year-old F with a history of Raynaud comes to the clinic for evaluation of progressive difficulty climbing stairs and brushing her hair, amongst other daily activities. Her mother notes that she has some discoloration of her skin around the eyes, upper neck, and on her knuckles. **Labs** show elevated creatine kinase and ESR. Muscle biopsy shows perivascular, mononuclear infiltrate.

Management:

1. Systemic corticosteroids.
2. Methotrexate or hydroxychloroquine is often used in dermatomyositis.
3. Sun protection for dermatomyositis.

Complications:

- Dysphagia secondary to esophageal muscle weakness.
- Respiratory muscle weakness leading to respiratory difficulties.
- Calcinosis.

HYF: Patients also present with characteristic dermatologic findings, including Gottron's papules, shawl sign, and heliotrope rash. Anti-Jo-1 antibodies may be positive. Polymyositis presents similarly but without the dermatologic findings, and it usually has more severe muscle weakness. Muscle biopsy shows endomysial, mononuclear infiltrate.

DUCHENNE AND BECKER MUSCULAR DYSTROPHIES

A 4-year-old M with a history of gross motor delay presents with muscle weakness and difficulty getting up from a sitting position. On **exam**, he has positive Gower sign and calf pseudohypertrophy, and he walks on his toes. **Labs** show elevated CK and aldolase. Genetic testing shows a deletion in the dystrophin gene. Muscle biopsy shows muscle degeneration and fibrosis.

Management:

1. Glucocorticoids.
2. Physical and occupational therapy.
3. Echocardiogram and ECG to screen for dilated cardiomyopathy and conduction abnormalities.

Complications:

- Scoliosis.
- Restrictive lung disease.
- Dilated cardiomyopathy.
- Cardiac or respiratory failure is usually cause of death.

HYF: Duchenne muscular dystrophy presents early in life (age 2–3 years), whereas Becker muscular dystrophy presents later (age 5–15) with less severe symptoms. The Gower sign occurs when a child stands via tripod positioning due to calf weakness. Both are X-linked recessive disorders.

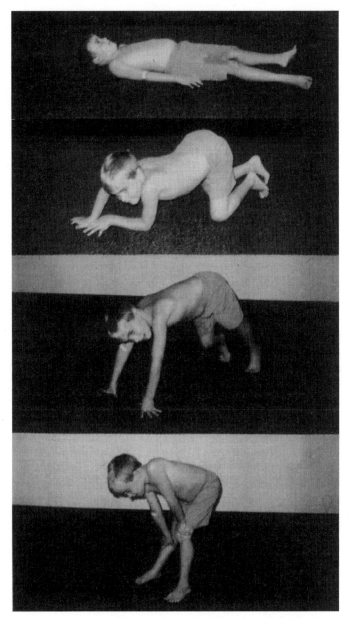

Positive Gower sign seen in Duchenne and Becker muscular dystrophies.

Myotonic Dystrophy: Type 1 is a trinucleotide repeat disorder (CTG) caused by an autosomal dominant mutation in *DMPK* (chr. 19) and heralded by progressive muscular weakness and myotonia (impaired muscle relaxation). Associated with frontal balding, cataracts, and cardiac arrhythmias. Most commonly presents in adulthood but can present in infancy as hypotonia. Treatment is supportive, as there are currently no disease-modifying agents.

Polymyalgia Rheumatica: See p. 307.
Drug-Induced Myopathy: See p. 307.
Giant Cell Arteritis: See p. 768.

23-36 Abnormal Movements: Seizures

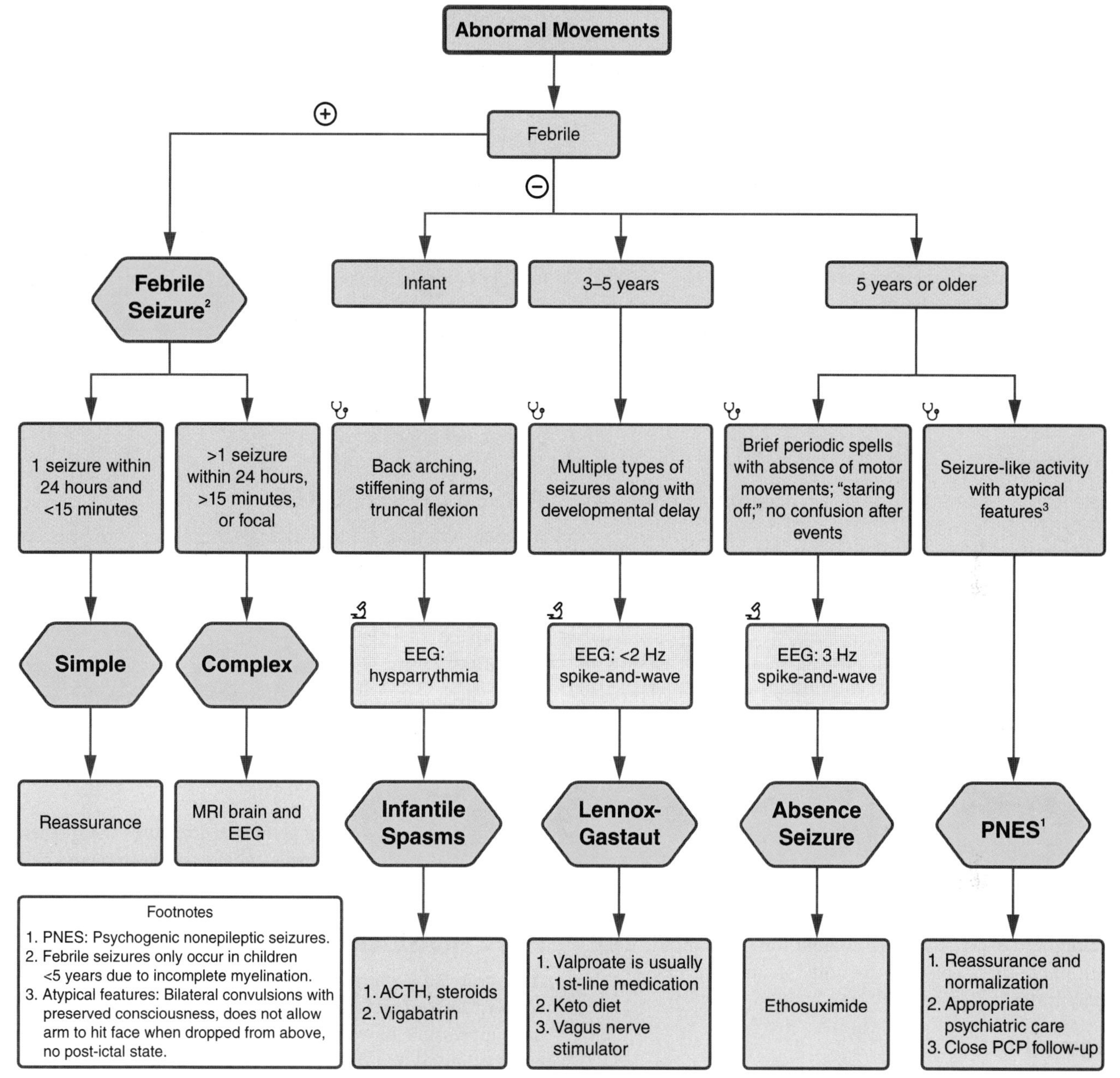
Abnormal Movements
Febrile
⊕
⊖
Febrile Seizure[2]
Infant
3–5 years
5 years or older
1 seizure within 24 hours and <15 minutes
>1 seizure within 24 hours, >15 minutes, or focal
Back arching, stiffening of arms, truncal flexion
Multiple types of seizures along with developmental delay
Brief periodic spells with absence of motor movements; "staring off;" no confusion after events
Seizure-like activity with atypical features[3]
Simple
Complex
EEG: hysparrythmia
EEG: <2 Hz spike-and-wave
EEG: 3 Hz spike-and-wave
Reassurance
MRI brain and EEG
Infantile Spasms
Lennox-Gastaut
Absence Seizure
PNES[1]
Footnotes
1. PNES: Psychogenic nonepileptic seizures.
2. Febrile seizures only occur in children <5 years due to incomplete myelination.
3. Atypical features: Bilateral convulsions with preserved consciousness, does not allow arm to hit face when dropped from above, no post-ictal state.
1. ACTH, steroids
2. Vigabatrin
1. Valproate is usually 1st-line medication
2. Keto diet
3. Vagus nerve stimulator
Ethosuximide
1. Reassurance and normalization
2. Appropriate psychiatric care
3. Close PCP follow-up

FIGURE 23.36

23-36 Abnormal Movements: Seizures

FEBRILE SEIZURES

A 13-month-old F with home temperature of 103.5 °F (39.7 °C) presents with 30-second generalized tonic-clonic seizure. On **exam**, she has notable rhinorrhea and cough. On **labs**, nasal swab is positive for rhinovirus.

Management:

1. For simple febrile seizures (>1 seizure within 24 hours <15 minutes in duration), no further workup. Give symptomatic care and reassurance.
2. For complex febrile seizures (>1 seizure within 24 hours, >15 minutes, or focal), consider further workup such as EEG or brain MRI.
3. If meningitis is suspected or infant <12 months, follow the appropriate work-up.

Complications:

- Simple febrile seizures have a good prognosis, and usually no neurologic sequelae occur.
- Complex febrile seizures that develop into status epilepticus should be rescued with benzodiazepines (see Neurology section).

HYF: Febrile seizures occur between 6 months and 5 years of age. They are associated with recent immunization but are NOT a contraindication to future vaccination. Overall risk of developing epilepsy is low. Antipyretics do not reduce risk of future febrile seizures.

INFANTILE SPASMS

A 9-month-old M born term without complications presents with new onset of brief episodes of forward flexion of the head accompanied by either flexion or extension of both arms, brief eye-rolling, and a cry. **Exam** is notable for gross motor delay, and multiple of these episodes are noted in an hour. EEG shows hypsarrhythmia.

Management:

1. ACTH.
2. Vigabatrin if spasms are refractory to ACTH.

Complications:

- Generally poor neurologic prognosis.
- May develop into Lennox-Gastaut syndrome.

HYF: When the 3 components of spasms, neurodevelopmental regression, and hypsarrhythmia are present, the eponym "West Syndrome" is commonly used.

LENNOX-GASTAUT SYNDROME

A 4-year-old M with PMH of infantile spasms presents with absence, atonic and generalized clonic seizures, and developmental delay. Interictal EEG shows a slow (<2.5 Hz), generalized spike-and-wave pattern.

Management:

1. Valproate is 1st-line therapy.
2. Keto diet.
3. Vagus nerve stimulator.

Complications: Developmental delay.

HYF: Lennox-Gastaut syndrome is generally diagnosed with the triad of multiple seizure types, cognitive delay, and the typical EEG pattern mentioned above.

ABSENCE SEIZURES

A 7-year-old M with PMH of ADHD presents with brief episodes of staring off in class. On **exam**, he has a 15-second staring spell when asked to hyperventilate. EEG shows 3 Hz spike-and-wave form.

Management:

1. Ethosuximide or valproate.

Complications:

- Possible developmental delay.

HYF: Absence seizures are generalized seizures that present with 10–20 seconds of staring spells, which can be triggered by hyperventilation. There is no post-ictal period. Presents age 4–10.

PSYCHOGENIC NONEPILEPTIC SEIZURES

A 16-year-old F whose parents are recently divorced presents with concern for seizures. She has no post-ictal period. On **exam**, she has suppressible movement of upper extremities and resistance to eye opening. When the MD performs an arm-drop test, she avoids hitting her face.

Management:

1. Reassurance.
2. Appropriate psychiatric care.

HYF: True seizures are non-suppressible movements. Screen patient for underlying stressors or psychiatric pathologies and treat accordingly. Psychogenic seizures can co-occur with true seizures or be seen in family members of those with true seizures.

23-37 Pediatric Urinary Complaints

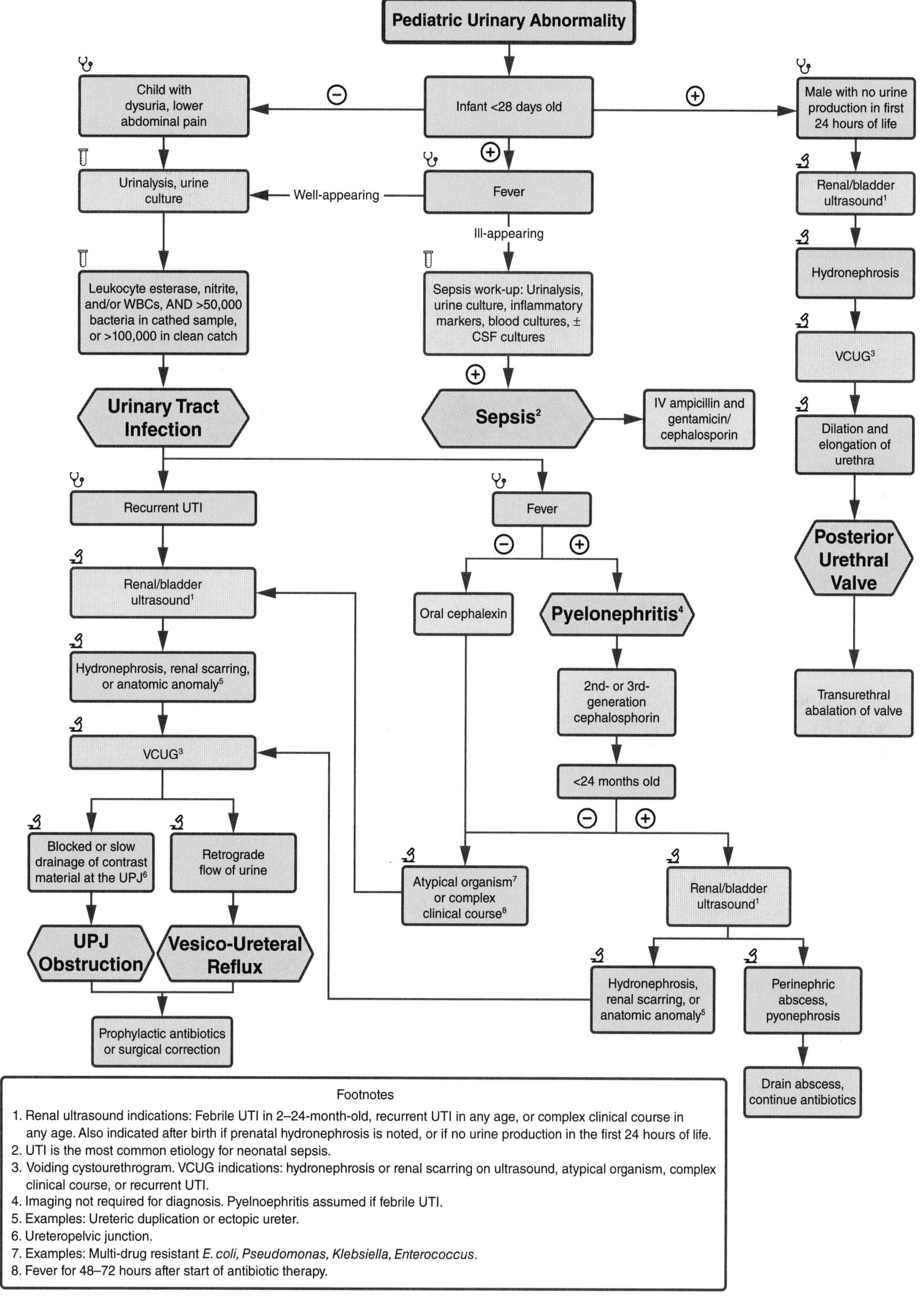
Pediatric Urinary Abnormality
Infant <28 days old
Child with dysuria, lower abdominal pain
Male with no urine production in first 24 hours of life
Fever
Well-appearing
Ill-appearing
Urinalysis, urine culture
Renal/bladder ultrasound[1]
Hydronephrosis
Leukocyte esterase, nitrite, and/or WBCs, AND >50,000 bacteria in cathed sample, or >100,000 in clean catch
Sepsis work-up: Urinalysis, urine culture, inflammatory markers, blood cultures, ± CSF cultures
VCUG[3]
Urinary Tract Infection
Sepsis[2]
IV ampicillin and gentamicin/ cephalosporin
Dilation and elongation of urethra
Recurrent UTI
Fever
Posterior Urethral Valve
Renal/bladder ultrasound[1]
Oral cephalexin
Pyelonephritis[4]
Hydronephrosis, renal scarring, or anatomic anomaly[5]
2nd- or 3rd-generation cephalosphorin
Transurethral abalation of valve
VCUG[3]
<24 months old
Blocked or slow drainage of contrast material at the UPJ[6]
Retrograde flow of urine
Atypical organism[7] or complex clinical course[8]
Renal/bladder ultrasound[1]
UPJ Obstruction
Vesico-Ureteral Reflux
Hydronephrosis, renal scarring, or anatomic anomaly[5]
Perinephric abscess, pyonephrosis
Prophylactic antibiotics or surgical correction
Drain abscess, continue antibiotics

Footnotes

1. Renal ultrasound indications: Febrile UTI in 2–24-month-old, recurrent UTI in any age, or complex clinical course in any age. Also indicated after birth if prenatal hydronephrosis is noted, or if no urine production in the first 24 hours of life.
2. UTI is the most common etiology for neonatal sepsis.
3. Voiding cystourethrogram. VCUG indications: hydronephrosis or renal scarring on ultrasound, atypical organism, complex clinical course, or recurrent UTI.
4. Imaging not required for diagnosis. Pyelnoephritis assumed if febrile UTI.
5. Examples: Ureteric duplication or ectopic ureter.
6. Ureteropelvic junction.
7. Examples: Multi-drug resistant *E. coli, Pseudomonas, Klebsiella, Enterococcus*.
8. Fever for 48–72 hours after start of antibiotic therapy.

FIGURE 23.37

23-37 Pediatric Urinary Complaints

URINARY TRACT INFECTION

A 4-year-old F presents with 2 days of fever, abdominal pain, and burning sensation when she urinates. On **labs**, UA shows positive leukocyte esterase and nitrites, 50+ WBC/hpf, and moderate bacteria. Urine culture grows >100,000 colony forming units of *E. coli*.

Management:

1. 7 days of oral 1st-generation cephalosporin (eg, cephalexin), TMP-SMX, or nitrofurantoin.
2. Obtain renal bladder ultrasound if persistent or worsening fevers despite antibiotic therapy.
3. Consider VCUG to rule out VUR if: ≥2 febrile UTIs, fever ≥102.2 °F (39 °C) with bacteria other than *E. coli*, abnormal renal US, or chronic kidney disease.

Complications:

- Pyelonephritis, leading to renal abscess or sepsis.

HYF: Diagnosis of UTI requires a urinalysis with:

- Nitrites, leukocyte esterase, and/or WBCs.
  AND
- >50,000 colonies in a cathed urine sample, or >100,000 colonies in a clean catch.

Not all bacteria form nitrites (eg, *Enterococci*), so the presence of leukocyte esterase is more sensitive for UTI diagnosis. *E. coli* is the most common etiology.

PYELONEPHRITIS

A 20-month-old previously healthy F presents with 2 days of fever and poor feeding. **Exam** shows suprapubic and costovertebral angle tenderness. On **labs**, UA shows positive leukocyte esterase and nitrites, 50+ WBC/hpf, and moderate bacteria. Urine culture grows >100,000 colony forming units of *E. coli*.

Management:

1. 7–10 days of a 2nd-generation cephalosporin or fluoroquinolone. Use IV antibiotics until fever resolves if age <2 months or does not tolerate PO.
2. Renal and bladder ultrasound (RBUS) if indicated (see algorithm).
3. Voiding cystourethrogram if indicated (see algorithm).

Complications:

- Renal abscess or sepsis.

HYF: A UTI accompanied by fever is considered pyelonephritis – diagnostic criteria does not include imaging. Children <2 years should get RBUS. Risk factors include female sex, anatomical abnormalities, constipation, and bowel/bladder dysfunction.

POSTERIOR URETHRAL VALVES

A 36-hour-old M in the nursery has passed meconium but has not yet urinated. On **exam**, he has suprapubic fullness. **Labs** show normal electrolytes and creatinine. On **imaging**, RBUS show a distended bladder with a thickened bladder wall and bilateral hydronephrosis.

Management:

1. Bladder decompression with catheterization.
2. VCUG to rule out vesicoureteral reflux.
3. Cystoscopy to confirm diagnosis.
4. PUV ablation and/or surgical correction (ie, urinary diversion).

Complications:

- Oligohydramnios and Potter sequence *in utero*.
- Recurrent UTI: renal scarring, CKD, HTN.
- Vesicoureteral reflux.
- Hydronephrosis.
- Renal scarring, chronic kidney disease, hypertension as a result of either recurrent UTI or hydronephrosis.

HYF: Most common cause of urinary tract obstruction in newborn boys. PUV most commonly presents *in utero* with hydronephrosis on prenatal screening US and sometimes oligohydramnios leading to pulmonary hypoplasia and Potter sequence. Patients with PUV often do not have increased creatinine, as the mother's kidneys clear it when *in utero*.

URETEROPELVIC JUNCTION (UPJ) OBSTRUCTION

A 16-year-old M with PMH of pyelonephritis presents with left flank pain after drinking beer with his friends. **Exam** reveals mild left CVA tenderness. He is afebrile. On **labs**, CBC is normal. BMP is remarkable for creatinine of 1.5.

Management:

1. Evaluate for hydronephrosis via RBUS.
2. Evaluate for UPJ obstruction via diuretic renography.
3. Consider antibiotic prophylaxis.
4. Consider surgical correction for symptomatic patients or those with impaired renal function.

Complications:

- Recurrent UTIs.
- Hydronephrosis.
- Nephrolithiasis.
- Hematuria.
- Renal scarring, chronic kidney disease, hypertension as a result of either recurrent UTI or hydronephrosis.

HYF: Commonly presents after activity causing diuresis (ie, drinking caffeine or alcohol). Diagnosis is made by diuretic renography showing impaired drainage of kidney. Associated with horseshoe kidney.

VESICOURETERAL REFLUX (VUR)

A 6-year-old F with a prior history of UTI at age 4 presents for dysuria. On **labs**, UA and urine culture confirm UTI. On **imaging**, RBUS shows moderate left hydronephrosis. VCUG shows reflux of contrast into the left ureter.

23-37 Pediatric Urinary Complaints

Management:

1. Treat recurrent UTI.
2. Consider antibiotic prophylaxis.
3. Monitor hydronephrosis with routine US.
4. Consider definitive correction with surgery (ie, ureteral reimplantation) for breakthrough UTI or worsening hydronephrosis.

Complications:

- Recurrent UTI.
- Hydronephrosis.
- Renal scarring, chronic kidney disease, hypertension as a result of either recurrent UTI or hydronephrosis.

HYF: VUR is 2× as common in females as males and greatly increases the risk of pyelonephritis and urosepsis. VCUG is the imaging modality of choice to diagnose VUR.

ECTOPIC URETER

A 4-year-old F with a history of several UTIs in infancy presents with persistent urinary incontinence. On **labs**, CBC and BMP are normal. On **imaging**, RBUS shows a dilated right ureter implanting low on the bladder.

Management:

1. CT or MRI for further evaluation as needed.
2. Surgical removal of affected ureter segment, possible removal of kidney.

Complications:

- Recurrent UTI.
- Hydronephrosis.
- Incontinence if implanting below urinary sphincter.
- Renal scarring, chronic kidney disease, hypertension as a result of either recurrent UTI or hydronephrosis.

HYF: Ectopic ureters are 6× more common in females than males. Presentation is usually a UTI but may include persistent incontinence in females if the ureter implants below the external urinary sphincter.

23-38 Penile Abnormality

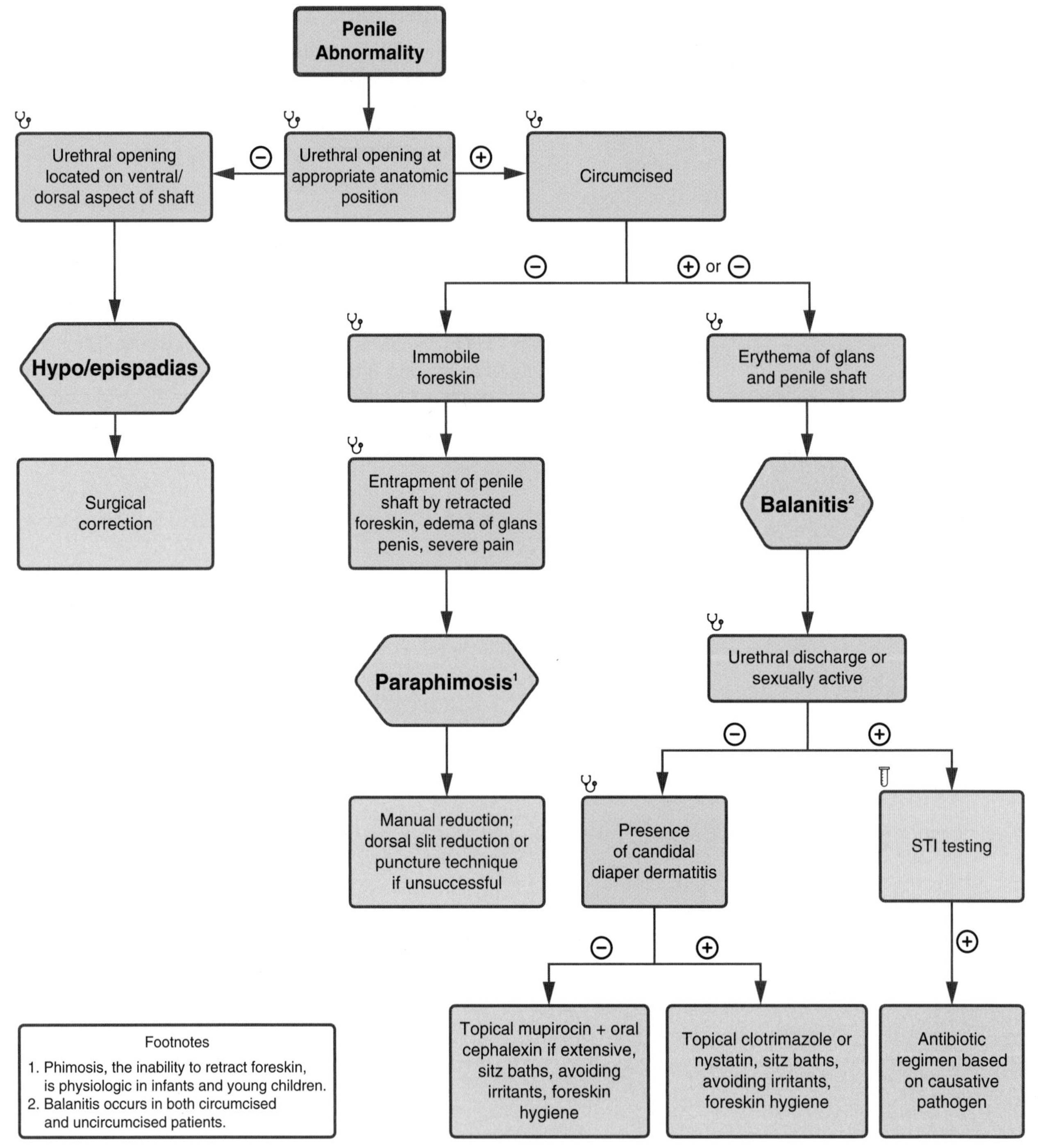
Penile Abnormality
Urethral opening located on ventral/ dorsal aspect of shaft
Urethral opening at appropriate anatomic position
Circumcised
⊕ or ⊖
Hypo/epispadias
Surgical correction
Immobile foreskin
Entrapment of penile shaft by retracted foreskin, edema of glans penis, severe pain
Paraphimosis[1]
Manual reduction; dorsal slit reduction or puncture technique if unsuccessful
Erythema of glans and penile shaft
Balanitis[2]
Urethral discharge or sexually active
Presence of candidal diaper dermatitis
STI testing
Topical mupirocin + oral cephalexin if extensive, sitz baths, avoiding irritants, foreskin hygiene
Topical clotrimazole or nystatin, sitz baths, avoiding irritants, foreskin hygiene
Antibiotic regimen based on causative pathogen
Footnotes
1. Phimosis, the inability to retract foreskin, is physiologic in infants and young children.
2. Balanitis occurs in both circumcised and uncircumcised patients.

FIGURE 23.38

23-38 Penile Abnormality

HYPOSPADIAS

A 1-day-old term M has 2 meatal openings on the ventral side of his penis.

Management:

1. Do not circumcise.
2. Surgical correction if the meatus is significantly displaced or the patient has problems with urination.

Complications: Possible complications of surgery include urethral fistulas, strictures, and diverticula.

HYF: Circumcision is never performed in these patients, as the foreskin is used for subsequent urethroplasty. Severe hypospadias can be indicative of a disorder of sex development, like androgen insensitivity.

EPISPADIAS

A 3-day-old M presents with findings of urethral exposure on the dorsal side of his penis.

Management:

1. Do not circumcise.
2. Surgical correction of urethral opening and any associated anatomic abnormalities.

Complications:

- Surgical complications such as urethral strictures.
- Bladder exstrophy.

HYF: Circumcision is never performed in these patients, as the foreskin is used for subsequent urethroplasty. Epispadias is often associated with bladder exstrophy, a defect in which the bladder and urethra herniate through the ventral abdominal wall.

PARAPHIMOSIS

A 15-year-old uncircumcised M presents with severe penile pain and dysuria. On exam, it is difficult to retract the foreskin around the glans, and the visible glans appears swollen and cyanotic.

Management:

1. Manual reduction, or
2. Surgical correction.
3. Later elective circumcision to prevent recurrence.

Complications: Penile glans ischemia and necrosis.

HYF: Paraphimosis is a urologic emergency, occurs in uncircumcised boys, and is most common in the teenage years. It is distinct from phimosis, which usually occurs in younger children (2–4 years old) and involves only difficulty with retracting the foreskin due to scarring and stenosis.

BALANITIS

A 10-month-old M presents to his pediatrician for a diaper rash. On exam, he has a swollen, red penile glans and diaper dermatitis with surrounding satellite lesions.

Management:

1. Topical mupirocin.
2. If severe, oral antibiotics (eg, cephalexin).
3. Topical antifungals if candidal dermatitis is present.
4. If secondary to a STI in a teenager, treat with the appropriate antibiotics.

Complications: In uncircumcised boys, balanitis can lead to phimosis or paraphimosis.

HYF: Balanitis is inflammation of the penile glans and most common in uncircumcised boys due to poor hygiene and accumulation of smegma (dead epithelium and oily secretions) under the foreskin, which increases the risk for bacterial or fungal growth. *Candida albicans* is often responsible for balanitis in infants. In teenagers, however, STIs can result in balanitis and cause painful urination and foul-smelling discharge.

23-39 Testicular Abnormality

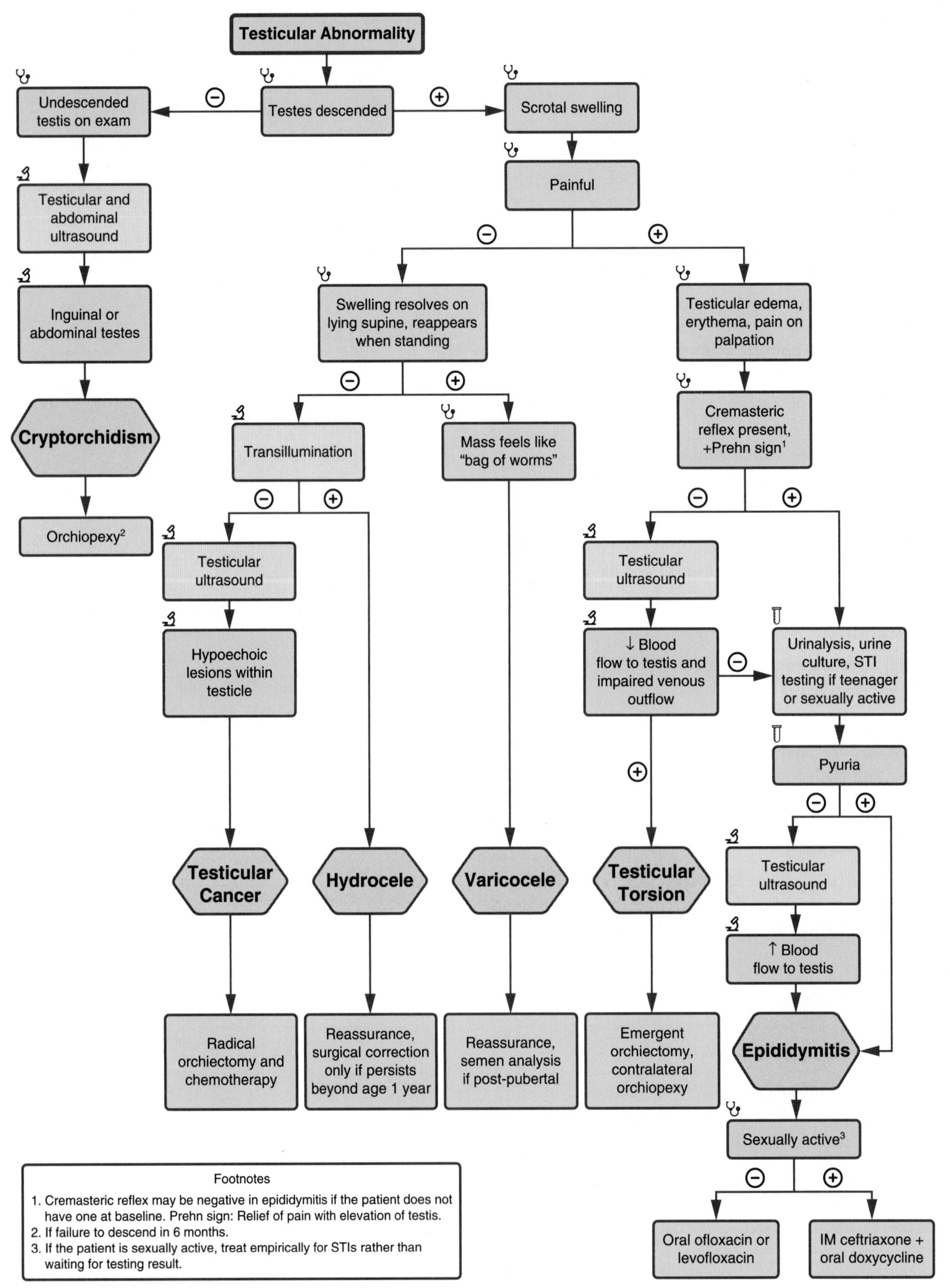
Testicular Abnormality
Testes descended
Undescended testis on exam
Scrotal swelling
Testicular and abdominal ultrasound
Painful
Inguinal or abdominal testes
Swelling resolves on lying supine, reappears when standing
Testicular edema, erythema, pain on palpation
Cryptorchidism
Transillumination
Mass feels like "bag of worms"
Cremasteric reflex present, +Prehn sign1
Orchiopexy2
Testicular ultrasound
Testicular ultrasound
Hypoechoic lesions within testicle
↓ Blood flow to testis and impaired venous outflow
Urinalysis, urine culture, STI testing if teenager or sexually active
Pyuria
Testicular ultrasound
Testicular Cancer
Hydrocele
Varicocele
Testicular Torsion
↑ Blood flow to testis
Radical orchiectomy and chemotherapy
Reassurance, surgical correction only if persists beyond age 1 year
Reassurance, semen analysis if post-pubertal
Emergent orchiectomy, contralateral orchiopexy
Epididymitis
Sexually active3
Oral ofloxacin or levofloxacin
IM ceftriaxone + oral doxycycline
Footnotes
1. Cremasteric reflex may be negative in epididymitis if the patient does not have one at baseline. Prehn sign: Relief of pain with elevation of testis.
2. If failure to descend in 6 months.
3. If the patient is sexually active, treat empirically for STIs rather than waiting for testing result.

FIGURE 23.39

23-39 Testicular Abnormality

CRYPTORCHIDISM

A 3-week-old M presents at his pediatrician's office. On **exam**, his right testis is not palpable in his scrotum. On **imaging**, abdominal US reveals a testis in the abdominal cavity.

Management:

1. Surgical correction via orchiopexy.

Complications:

- Testicular cancer.
- Infertility.

HYF: Testes usually descend into the scrotum while *in utero*. If they fail to do so, they may remain in the abdominal cavity or inguinal canal, higher-temperature environments that increase the risk of testicular cancer and infertility. Early intervention is crucial to prevent these complications.

TESTICULAR CANCER

A 17-year-old M presents with a painless right scrotal mass he noticed while showering. On **exam**, he has a firm, non-tender testicular nodule that does not transilluminate. **Labs** reveal elevated hCG. On **imaging**, US shows a well-defined, hypoechoic lesion in the right testicle.

Management:

1. Sperm cryopreservation.
2. Radical orchiectomy.
3. Possible adjuvant chemotherapy.

Complications:

- Metastasis.
- Reactive hydrocele.
- Infertility secondary to surgery.

HYF: Do NOT biopsy testicular masses due to risk of tumor seeding.

HYDROCELE

An 8-month-old M presents with painless scrotal swelling present since birth. On **exam**, he has a non-tender, fluctuant, transilluminating fluid collection in his right hemi-scrotum. The collection is not reducible.

Management:

1. Monitor for resolution. Most congenital hydroceles will resolve by age 1.
2. Surgery if concerns for infertility or unresolved by age 1.

Complications:

- Incarcerated inguinal hernia.
- Large hydroceles may be bothersome.

HYF: Spermatoceles can also transilluminate. Inguinal hernia may mimic hydrocele on exam but will be reducible. Hydroceles may also be reactive to trauma, torsion, tumor, or infection.

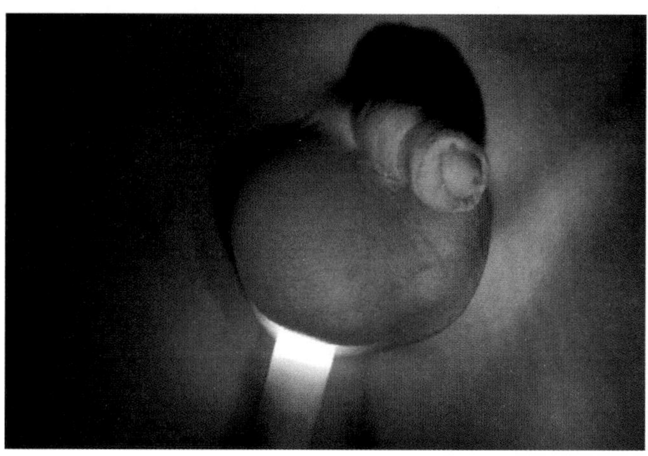

Transillumination of hydrocele.

VARICOCELE

A 13-year-old previously healthy M presents with a feeling of fullness in his left hemi-scrotum upon standing. On **exam**, he has a "bag of worms"-like mass that resolves upon lying supine. On **imaging**, scrotal US shows dilated vessels that reflux on Doppler with Valsalva.

Management:

1. Supportive care.
2. Surgery is indicated for pain or infertility concerns.

Complications: Infertility.

HYF: "Bag of worms" finding is due to dilation of the pampiniform plexus. Varicoceles can be secondary to compression of the spermatic vein by a retroperitoneal mass.

TESTICULAR TORSION

A 12-year-old M presents to the emergency department with severe sudden abdominal pain and vomiting. On **exam**, his right testis is red and swollen, and he has exquisite tenderness to palpation. He also has a (–) Prehn sign and absent right cremasteric reflex. On **labs**, UA is normal. On **imaging**, testicular Doppler US shows impaired venous blood flow.

Management:

1. Emergent surgical correction with orchiectomy and contralateral orchiopexy.

Complications:

- Loss of the testis.
- Infertility.
- Infection.

HYF: This is a urologic emergency due to the high risk of testicular loss by ischemia. Unlike epididymitis, pain in testicular torsion worsens with elevation of the scrotum (negative Prehn sign).

23-39 Testicular Abnormality

EPIDIDYMITIS

A 15-year-old M presents with gradual onset of scrotal pain and swelling, dysuria, urinary frequency, and intermittent penile discharge. On **exam**, there is tenderness to palpation of the scrotum with (+) Prehn sign, as well as significant inguinal lymphadenopathy. He is sexually active. On **labs**, urine chlamydia PCR is positive. UA shows hematuria and pyuria. On **imaging**, testicular Doppler US reveals inflammation of the epididymis and testis with intact venous blood flow.

Management:

1. If STI present, administer appropriate antibiotic treatment (ceftriaxone and doxycycline).
2. If *E. coli* more likely, fluoroquinolones.
3. If due to activity, rest and anti-inflammatory medications.

Complications:

- Epididymal abscess.
- Infertility due to fibrosis.

HYF: Epididymitis can be distinguished from testicular torsion by its more gradual rather than acute onset. It is most commonly due to gonorrhea or chlamydia but can also be caused by *E. coli*, mumps virus, or activities with repetitive movement, like running. It is important to obtain a testicular US in any case with scrotal pain to rule out testicular torsion.

23-40 Precocious Puberty

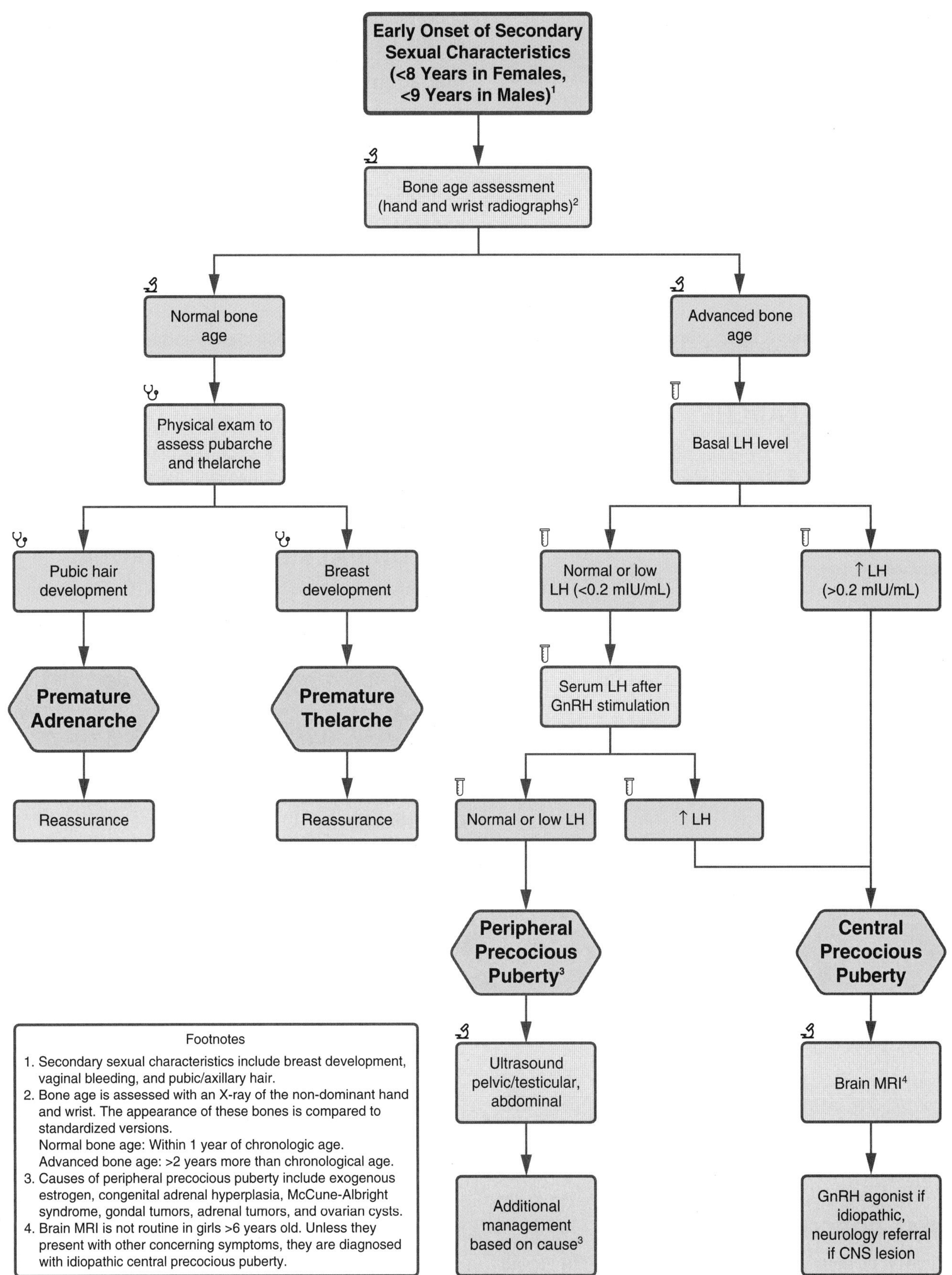
Early Onset of Secondary Sexual Characteristics (<8 Years in Females, <9 Years in Males)[1]
Bone age assessment (hand and wrist radiographs)[2]
Normal bone age
Advanced bone age
Physical exam to assess pubarche and thelarche
Basal LH level
Pubic hair development
Breast development
Normal or low LH (<0.2 mIU/mL)
↑ LH (>0.2 mIU/mL)
Premature Adrenarche
Premature Thelarche
Serum LH after GnRH stimulation
Reassurance
Reassurance
Normal or low LH
↑ LH
Peripheral Precocious Puberty[3]
Central Precocious Puberty
Ultrasound pelvic/testicular, abdominal
Brain MRI[4]
Additional management based on cause[3]
GnRH agonist if idiopathic, neurology referral if CNS lesion

Footnotes

1. Secondary sexual characteristics include breast development, vaginal bleeding, and pubic/axillary hair.
2. Bone age is assessed with an X-ray of the non-dominant hand and wrist. The appearance of these bones is compared to standardized versions.
   Normal bone age: Within 1 year of chronologic age.
   Advanced bone age: >2 years more than chronological age.
3. Causes of peripheral precocious puberty include exogenous estrogen, congenital adrenal hyperplasia, McCune-Albright syndrome, gondal tumors, adrenal tumors, and ovarian cysts.
4. Brain MRI is not routine in girls >6 years old. Unless they present with other concerning symptoms, they are diagnosed with idiopathic central precocious puberty.

FIGURE 23.40

23-40 Precocious Puberty

PREMATURE ADRENARCHE

A 6-year-old F with a history of obesity presents for concerns of pubic and underarm hair. On **exam**, she has dark, coarse hair on the pubis and under the axillae with no other abnormal findings. **Imaging** shows normal radiographic bone age.

Management:

1. Reassurance.

Complications:

- In obese children: PCOS, type 2 diabetes or other metabolic syndrome.

HYF: Premature adrenarche is more common in obese children. With normal bone age, it does not require additional management.

PREMATURE THELARCHE

A 4-year-old F presents with a mildly tender breast mass. On **exam**, she has bilateral, firm 1-cm masses posterior to the nipple. **Imaging** shows normal radiographic bone age.

Management:

1. Reassurance.

Complications: None.

HYF: Premature thelarche with normal bone age does not require further management.

PERIPHERAL PRECOCIOUS PUBERTY

A 6-year-old F has an episode of vaginal bleeding. On **exam**, she has breast buds bilaterally. **Imaging** shows advanced bone age. **Labs** show low basal LH.

Management:

1. Pelvic US.
2. Reassurance.

Complications:

- Poor self-esteem in adolescents.
- Premature fusion of growth plates that may cause reduced adult height potential.

HYF: Ovarian cysts are the most common cause of peripheral precocious puberty in females. Additional causes of peripheral precocious puberty include exogenous estrogen, congenital adrenal hyperplasia, McCune-Albright syndrome, gonadal tumors, and adrenal tumors.

CENTRAL PRECOCIOUS PUBERTY

A 5-year-old M presents with axillary and pubic hair. His growth chart shows that his height has increased from the 30th to the 55th percentile. On **exam**, he has coarse, dark hair over the pubis and under the axillae. **Labs/Imaging** show advanced bone age and very elevated LH.

Management:

1. GnRH agonist: Leuprolide.
2. Brain MRI.
3. Treatment varies based on size, age, and other features if CNS tumor is identified.

Complications:

- Poor self-esteem in adolescents.
- Premature fusion of growth plates that may cause reduced adult height potential.
- Complications of CNS tumors include gelastic seizures (seizures with laughing and giggling), behavior and cognitive disturbances.

HYF: CNS tumors can cause precocious puberty with advanced bone age and elevated LH. The most common CNS tumor to cause precocious puberty is a benign hypothalamic hamartoma. Central precocious puberty may also be idiopathic.

MCCUNE-ALBRIGHT SYNDROME

A 5-year-old F with a history of multiple fractures presents with growth of pubic and axillary hair, as well as breast development. On **exam**, she has coarse, dark hair across the pubis and under her axillae, as well as breast buds and multiple large macules on her right torso. **Labs/Imaging** show advanced bone age, low serum LH, and ovarian cysts on US.

Management:

1. Aromatase inhibitor (eg, letrozole).

Complications:

- Recurrent fracture.
- Recurrent ovarian cysts.
- Thyrotoxicosis.
- Acromegaly.
- Cushing's syndrome.

HYF: McCune-Albright syndrome is the triad of irregular café au lait macules, polyostotic fibrous dysplasia (presents as recurrent fractures), and peripheral precocious puberty. It occurs much more often in girls than in boys. Due to mutation in *GNAS*, which encodes a subunit of the Gs protein that activates adenylyl cyclase, leading to excess stimulation of endocrine function.

23-41 Delayed Puberty

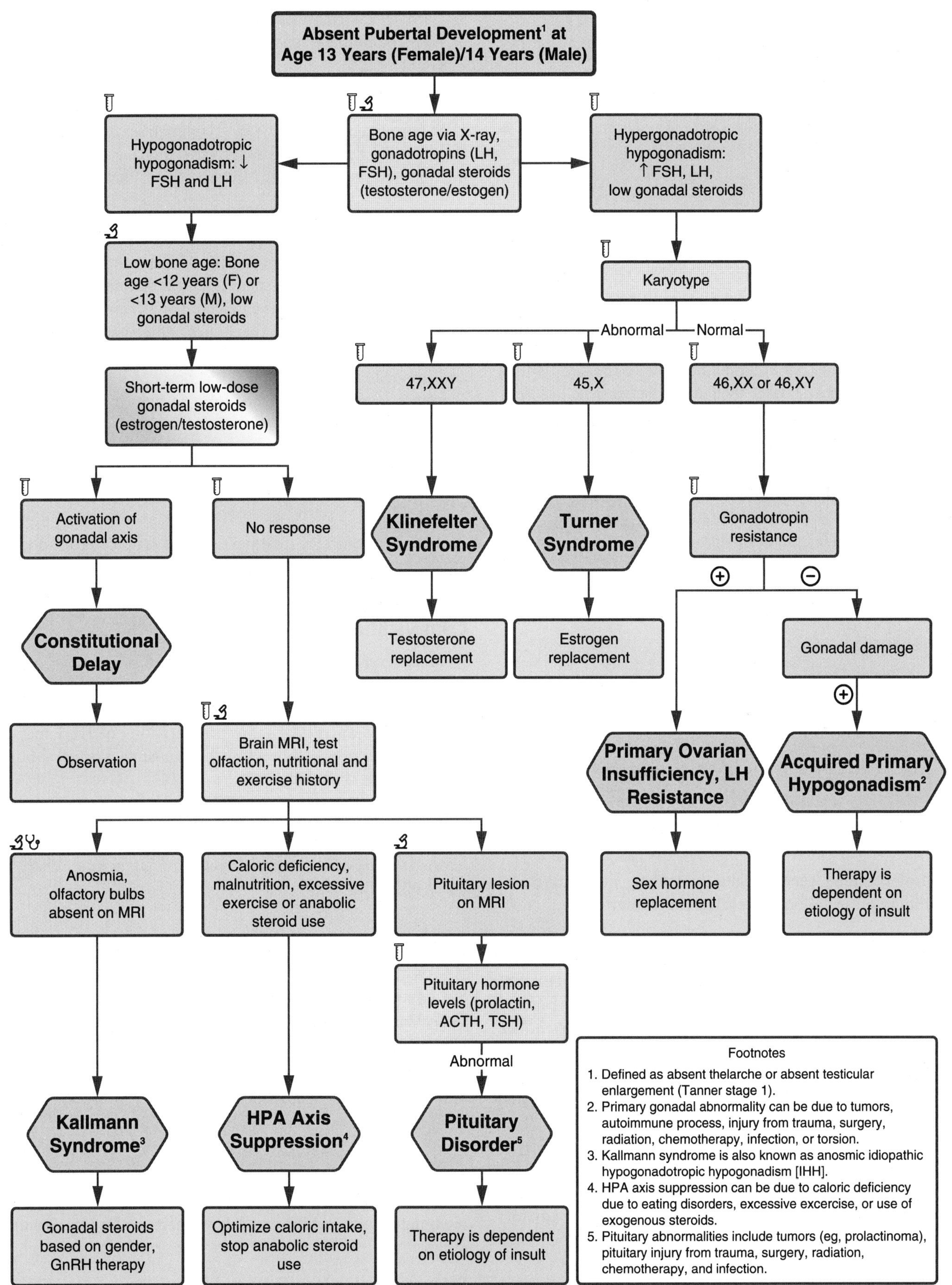

Absent Pubertal Development[1] at Age 13 Years (Female)/14 Years (Male)
Bone age via X-ray, gonadotropins (LH, FSH), gonadal steroids (testosterone/estogen)
Hypogonadotropic hypogonadism: ↓ FSH and LH
Hypergonadotropic hypogonadism: ↑ FSH, LH, low gonadal steroids
Low bone age: Bone age <12 years (F) or <13 years (M), low gonadal steroids
Short-term low-dose gonadal steroids (estrogen/testosterone)
Karyotype
Abnormal
Normal
47,XXY
45,X
46,XX or 46,XY
Activation of gonadal axis
No response
Klinefelter Syndrome
Turner Syndrome
Gonadotropin resistance
Constitutional Delay
Testosterone replacement
Estrogen replacement
Gonadal damage
Observation
Brain MRI, test olfaction, nutritional and exercise history
Primary Ovarian Insufficiency, LH Resistance
Acquired Primary Hypogonadism[2]
Anosmia, olfactory bulbs absent on MRI
Caloric deficiency, malnutrition, excessive exercise or anabolic steroid use
Pituitary lesion on MRI
Sex hormone replacement
Therapy is dependent on etiology of insult
Pituitary hormone levels (prolactin, ACTH, TSH)
Abnormal
Kallmann Syndrome[3]
HPA Axis Suppression[4]
Pituitary Disorder[5]
Gonadal steroids based on gender, GnRH therapy
Optimize caloric intake, stop anabolic steroid use
Therapy is dependent on etiology of insult
Footnotes
1. Defined as absent thelarche or absent testicular enlargement (Tanner stage 1).
2. Primary gonadal abnormality can be due to tumors, autoimmune process, injury from trauma, surgery, radiation, chemotherapy, infection, or torsion.
3. Kallmann syndrome is also known as anosmic idiopathic hypogonadotropic hypogonadism [IHH].
4. HPA axis suppression can be due to caloric deficiency due to eating disorders, excessive excercise, or use of exogenous steroids.
5. Pituitary abnormalities include tumors (eg, prolactinoma), pituitary injury from trauma, surgery, radiation, chemotherapy, and infection.

FIGURE 23.41

23-41 Delayed Puberty

CONSTITUTIONAL DEVELOPMENTAL GROWTH DELAY

A 13-year-old previously healthy F presents with absent pubertal development. On **exam**, she has Tanner stage 1 breast buds and pubic hair. **Labs/Imaging** show low LH/FSH and bone age less than chronological age.

Management:

1. Reassurance and observation.
2. Severe CDGD may be difficult to differentiate from central hypogonadotropic hypogonadism, and the latter may be ruled out with pubertal priming with a trial of low-dose sex steroids.

Complications: May cause low self-esteem in adolescence.

HYF: This is a diagnosis of exclusion and due to transient GnRH deficiency. It has a genetic basis, though no marker gene has been identified. Inheritance pattern is closest to autosomal dominant with incomplete penetration. Take a focused familial pubertal history.

KLINEFELTER SYNDROME

A previously healthy 16-year-old M presents with concerns for lack of pubertal development. On **exam**, his testicles are small and firm, leg length is disproportionately large for height, and he has gynecomastia. **Lab** evaluation shows elevated LH/FSH, and karyotype is performed, revealing 47,XXY.

Management:

1. Testosterone replacement is the mainstay of treatment for virilization and improvement of bone density.

Complications:

- Infertility is the most commonly observed complication due to progressive testicular fibrosis.
- Gynecomastia, higher risk of breast cancer.
- Osteoporosis.

HYF: Most common genotype due to meiotic nondisjunction. Most common presentation is in evaluation of infertility.

TURNER SYNDROME

An 11-year-old F with no remote history of cardiac surgery presents to establish care with a new PCP and has height that is approximately 2 standard deviations below the average for females in her age. **Exam** reveals a young woman with a broad chest, wide-spaced nipples, cubitus valgus, and genu valgum. **Labs** reveal elevated FSH/LH and karyotype of 45,X.

Management:

1. Recombinant human growth hormone (despite normal growth hormone levels) and exogenous estrogen at 11–12 years of age.
2. Screening for cardiac and renal anomalies at time of diagnosis.
3. Screening for metabolic syndrome, hypertension, and autoimmune complications.

Complications:

- Infertility and growth delay.
- Cardiac abnormalities (bicuspid aortic valve, coarctation of the aorta, pulmonary venous abnormalities).
- Higher risk for autoimmune conditions, liver disease, hypertension, and bony abnormalities.

HYF: Turner syndrome is the most common sex chromosome abnormality in females. Bicuspid aortic valve and coarctation of the aorta are commonly tested cardiac complications of Turner syndrome.

KALLMANN SYNDROME

A 15-year-old M with a remote history of cryptorchidism s/p repair presents with concern for small testicular size and lack of pubertal development. **Exam** reveals eunuchoid body habitus, testicular volume of 3 mL, and sparse axillary and pubic hair. Neurologic exam reveals deficit in cranial nerve I. **Labs** reveal low serum testosterone and low FSH/LH. Presumptive diagnosis of Kallmann syndrome (anosmic idiopathic hypogonadotropic hypogonadism [IHH]) is made.

Management:

1. Pubertal induction: Testosterone for males; exogenous estrogen for females.
2. Fertility-promoting treatment. In males, testosterone doesn't restore spermatogenesis; instead, administer exogenous hCG or pulsatile GnRH therapy.

Complications:

- More severe cases in males may present with microphallus and/or cryptorchidism. Newborn girls with IHH have no obvious reproductive findings.
- While not universal, some presentations of IHH may have non-reproductive findings, such as anosmia, skeletal abnormalities, or cleft lip/palate.

HYF: Isolated GnRH deficiencies are difficult to distinguish from constitutional growth delay. However, adrenarche may occur in isolated GnRH deficiencies, whereas adrenarche and pubarche are delayed in CDHD.

HPA AXIS SUPPRESSION

A 15-year-old F tells her doctor that she has not had her period yet. She started developing breast buds around 12 years of age and has pubic hair but no axillary hair. She likes to run track for her school. On **exam**, BMI is in the 7th percentile.

Management

1. Reassurance.

Complications: None.

HYF: Excessive exercise has been shown to suppress the HPA axis in young athletes, which can delay puberty or lead to anovulatory cycles.

Primary Ovarian Insufficiency, LH Resistance: See p. 699.
Acquired Primary Hypogonadism: See p. 702.
Pituitary Disorder: See pp. 488-490.

23-42 Acute Leg Pain/Limp

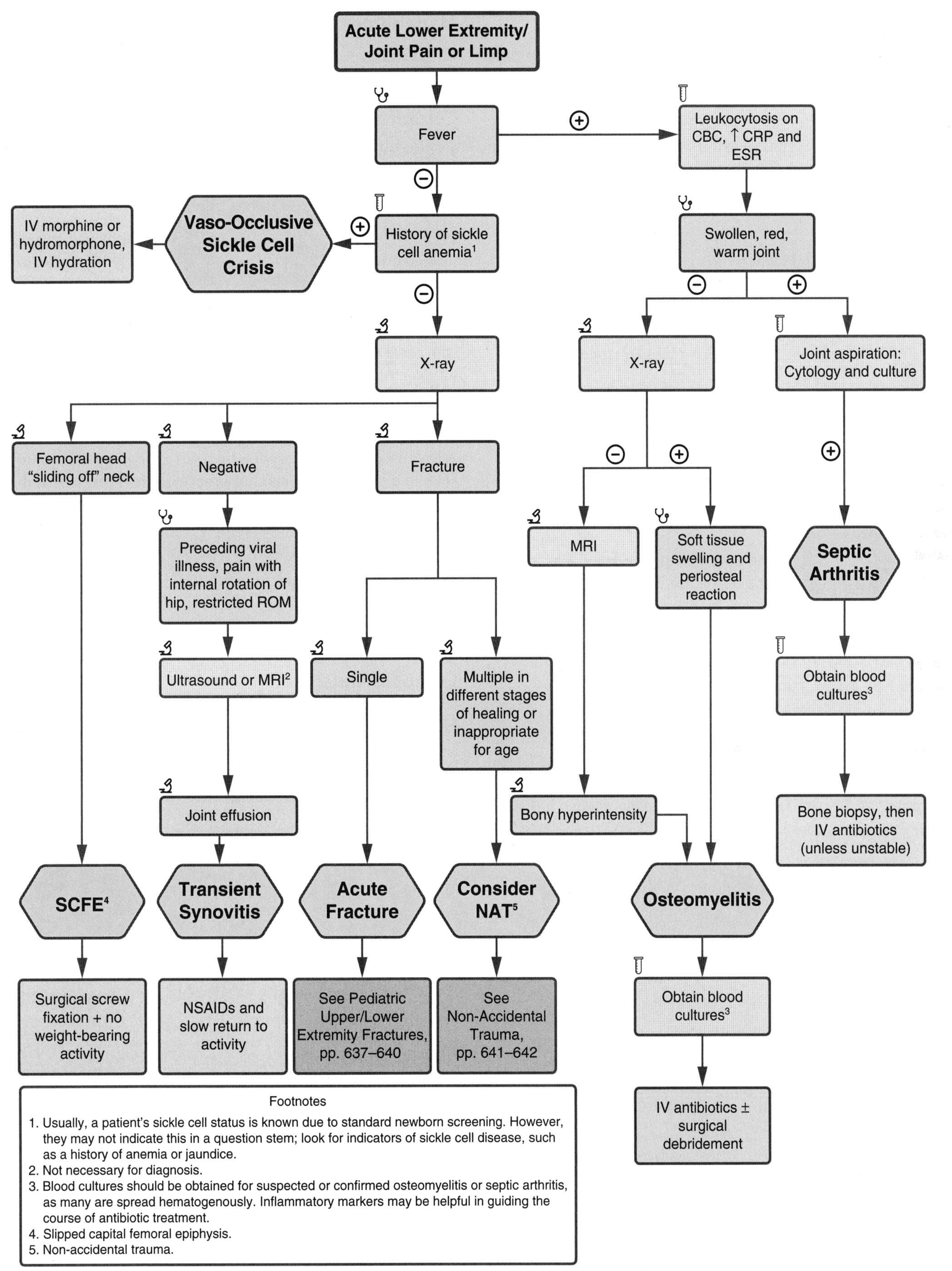
Acute Lower Extremity/ Joint Pain or Limp
Fever
⊕
Leukocytosis on CBC, ↑ CRP and ESR
⊖
History of sickle cell anemia[1]
⊕
Vaso-Occlusive Sickle Cell Crisis
IV morphine or hydromorphone, IV hydration
⊖
X-ray
Femoral head "sliding off" neck
Negative
Fracture
Preceding viral illness, pain with internal rotation of hip, restricted ROM
Ultrasound or MRI[2]
Joint effusion
Single
Multiple in different stages of healing or inappropriate for age
SCFE[4]
Transient Synovitis
Acute Fracture
Consider NAT[5]
Surgical screw fixation + no weight-bearing activity
NSAIDs and slow return to activity
See Pediatric Upper/Lower Extremity Fractures, pp. 637–640
See Non-Accidental Trauma, pp. 641–642
Swollen, red, warm joint
⊖
⊕
X-ray
Joint aspiration: Cytology and culture
⊖
⊕
MRI
Soft tissue swelling and periosteal reaction
Bony hyperintensity
Osteomyelitis
Obtain blood cultures[3]
IV antibiotics ± surgical debridement
⊕
Septic Arthritis
Obtain blood cultures[3]
Bone biopsy, then IV antibiotics (unless unstable)

Footnotes

1. Usually, a patient's sickle cell status is known due to standard newborn screening. However, they may not indicate this in a question stem; look for indicators of sickle cell disease, such as a history of anemia or jaundice.
2. Not necessary for diagnosis.
3. Blood cultures should be obtained for suspected or confirmed osteomyelitis or septic arthritis, as many are spread hematogenously. Inflammatory markers may be helpful in guiding the course of antibiotic treatment.
4. Slipped capital femoral epiphysis.
5. Non-accidental trauma.

FIGURE 23.42

23-42 Acute Leg Pain/Limp

SEPTIC ARTHRITIS

A 7-year-old F presents with fever and left knee pain for the past 2 days. **Exam** shows a swollen and red knee with palpable effusion. Passive knee extension and flexion are limited. On **imaging**, X-rays show soft tissue swelling. On **labs**, CBC shows leukocytosis and elevated ESR/CRP. US-guided arthrocentesis is performed with aspiration of cloudy fluid. Cytology shows elevated WBCs >80,000 per mm^3. Initial cultures grow Gram-positive cocci.

Management:

1. Initiate therapy with IV antibiotics and trend serial inflammatory markers (CRP). Once CRP is nearly normalized, convert to oral antibiotics. Empiric treatment is usually IV ceftriaxone + vancomycin or piperacillin-tazobactam.
2. Obtain blood cultures, as many cases are hematogenously spread.

Complications:

- Joint degeneration and early arthritis.
- In septic arthritis of the hip: Femoral head necrosis.
- Bacteremia and sepsis.
- Joint loosening or dislocation.

HYF: Septic arthritis is most common in the knee, hip, shoulder, and ankle. Septic arthritis of the hip usually presents in kids <2 years old.

SLIPPED CAPITAL FEMORAL EPIPHYSIS (SCFE)

A 13-year-old M presents with 1 month of progressive right hip pain. He doesn't remember injuring himself. His height is in the 20th percentile for age and weight in the 99th percentile. **Exam** reveals altered gait with right foot pointed laterally, limited internal hip rotation, and external thigh rotation during passive hip flexion. On **imaging**, X-rays reveal:

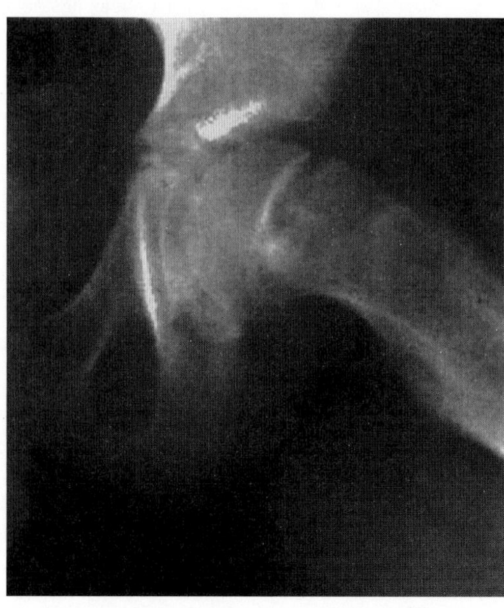

Displaced femoral epiphysis in SCFE.

Management:

1. Make non-weight bearing.
2. Immediate surgical fixation of the physis with screws.

Complications:

- Avascular necrosis of the femoral head.
- Accelerated osteoarthritis.
- Leg length discrepancy.

HYF: SCFE is characterized by anterosuperior displacement of the proximal femur relative to the femoral head. X-ray shows posteriorly displaced femoral epiphysis ("Ice cream slipping off a cone"). May present with referred knee or thigh pain rather than hip pain. Most common in obese adolescents (age 10–16), but hypothyroidism, renal disease, and radiation history are also risk factors. Both hips can often be affected, leading to a classic waddling gait.

TRANSIENT SYNOVITIS

A 6-year-old M presents with 2 days of right hip pain and limping. He had a URI 2 weeks ago but otherwise has been well and hasn't fallen recently. **Exam** reveals a limping gait and decreased ROM of the hip, though he is able to bear weight. **Labs** are normal. On **imaging**, X-rays are normal. Hip US shows bilateral hip effusions.

Management:

1. NSAIDs.
2. Self-resolution within 1–4 weeks.

Complications: None.

HYF: Transient synovitis (ie, toxic synovitis or reactive arthritis) occurs most commonly in children ages 3-8 years after a viral infection (eg, GI, respiratory). X-rays are usually normal. Hip US may show unilateral or bilateral effusions (even with only 1 affected hip).

OSTEOMYELITIS

A 4-year-old M presents with 3 days of a limp and fever. He complains of pain in his right leg. On **exam**, he has TTP of the tibia and overlying erythema. On **imaging**, X-rays of the right lower leg are negative for bony changes, but there is soft tissue swelling. MRI shows bony hyperintensity of the tibia. **Labs** reveal leukocytosis and elevated ESR/CRP.

Management:

1. IV antibiotics for a variable amount of time (pending clinical improvement and downtrending inflammatory markers), then transition to PO antibiotics; empiric treatment is usually IV ceftriaxone + vancomycin or piperacillin-tazobactam.
2. Obtain blood cultures, as many cases are hematogenously spread.
3. Surgical drainage if abscess.
4. Surgical debridement if no improvement on antibiotics (persistent fevers, persistently elevated inflammatory markers).

23-42 Acute Leg Pain/Limp

Complications:

- Septic arthritis.
- Pathologic fracture.
- Abscess.
- Bone deformity.
- Bacteremia and sepsis.

HYF: X-rays may be negative in the first 14 days of infection. Special considerations in osteomyelitis and septic arthritis: The most common pathogens are *Staph aureus*, MRSA, and *Strep* species. In sickle cell disease, *Salmonella* is more common than *Staph aureus*. *Kingella* is becoming more common in children <3 years old. In adolescents, consider *Neisseria gonorrhoeae*.

Vaso-Occlusive Sickle Cell Crisis: See Sickle Cell Anemia on p. 97.

23-43 Chronic Leg Pain/Limp

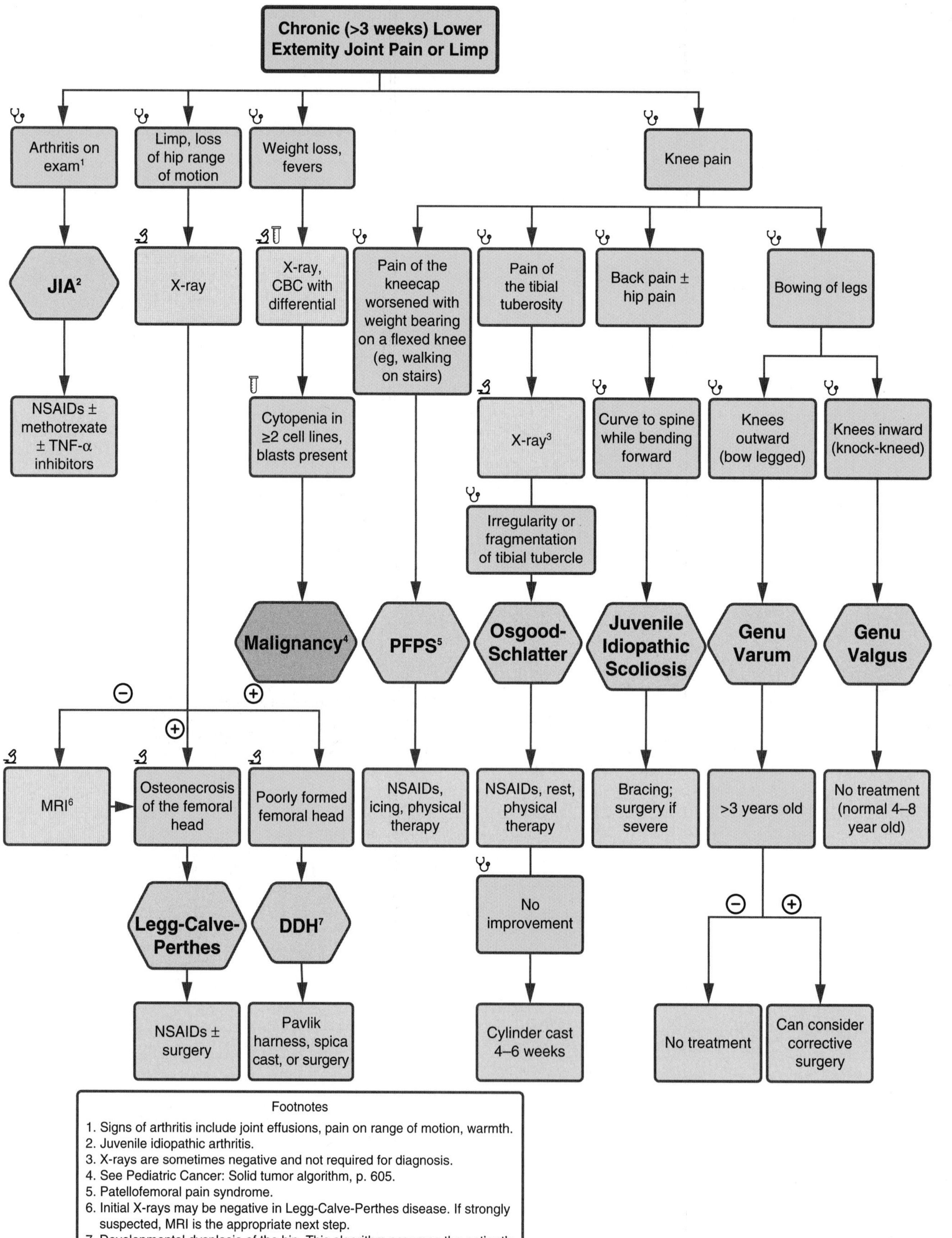

Chronic (>3 weeks) Lower Extemity Joint Pain or Limp
Arthritis on exam[1]
Limp, loss of hip range of motion
Weight loss, fevers
Knee pain
JIA[2]
X-ray
X-ray, CBC with differential
Pain of the kneecap worsened with weight bearing on a flexed knee (eg, walking on stairs)
Pain of the tibial tuberosity
Back pain ± hip pain
Bowing of legs
NSAIDs ± methotrexate ± TNF-α inhibitors
Cytopenia in ≥2 cell lines, blasts present
X-ray[3]
Curve to spine while bending forward
Knees outward (bow legged)
Knees inward (knock-kneed)
Irregularity or fragmentation of tibial tubercle
Malignancy[4]
PFPS[5]
Osgood-Schlatter
Juvenile Idiopathic Scoliosis
Genu Varum
Genu Valgus
⊖
⊕
⊕
MRI[6]
Osteonecrosis of the femoral head
Poorly formed femoral head
NSAIDs, icing, physical therapy
NSAIDs, rest, physical therapy
Bracing; surgery if severe
>3 years old
No treatment (normal 4–8 year old)
Legg-Calve-Perthes
DDH[7]
No improvement
⊖
⊕
NSAIDs ± surgery
Pavlik harness, spica cast, or surgery
Cylinder cast 4–6 weeks
No treatment
Can consider corrective surgery

Footnotes

1. Signs of arthritis include joint effusions, pain on range of motion, warmth.
2. Juvenile idiopathic arthritis.
3. X-rays are sometimes negative and not required for diagnosis.
4. See Pediatric Cancer: Solid tumor algorithm, p. 605.
5. Patellofemoral pain syndrome.
6. Initial X-rays may be negative in Legg-Calve-Perthes disease. If strongly suspected, MRI is the appropriate next step.
7. Developmental dysplasia of the hip. This algorithm assumes the patient's age is at least >4 months; see Birth Defects: Dysplasias and Deformations algorithm for DDH in 0–4 months of age, p. 547.

FIGURE 23.43

23-43 Chronic Leg Pain/Limp

JUVENILE IDIOPATHIC ARTHRITIS (JIA)

A 10-year-old F presents for 6 weeks of joint pain in her right knee, left wrist, and both ankles. It is worse in the mornings, as she feels more stiff at that time. Her symptoms improve throughout the day. Ibuprofen helps. **Exam** reveals joint effusions and warmth in her bilateral ankles, wrists, and knees. There is no overlying erythema. **Labs** show mild anemia, leukocytosis, elevated ESR and CRP, and mildly positive ANA. Slit lamp examination is positive for uveitis.

Management:

1. 1st-line: NSAIDs (ibuprofen, naproxen, meloxicam).
2. 2nd-line: Methotrexate.
3. 3rd-line: TNF-α inhibitors (infliximab, etanercept).
4. 4th-line: Intra-articular steroid injections.

Complications:

- Chronic arthritis.
- Leg length discrepancy.
- Anemia of chronic disease.

HYF: JIA includes multiple subsets (eg, oligoarticular, polyarticular, systemic) that all present with chronic joint pain and stiffness that is worse in the mornings. Hip pain is rare. It is a clinical diagnosis that does not require imaging, though MRI would show inflammatory changes.

Major types of juvenile idiopathic arthritis

Subtype	Oligoarticular (50%)	Polyarticular (40%)	Systemic (10%)
Clinical Features	- Age 2–3 years (F > M) - Arthritis in <4 large joints (except hips) - Uveitis and iridocyclitis are common	- Age 2–5, 10–14 years (F > M) - Arthritis in 5+ joints - Spine and hand involvement (hand deformities, dactylitis) - Fever, rare uveitis or irdocyclitis, growth retardation	- Age <18 years (F = M) - Any number of joints involved >6 weeks - Quotidian fever, maculopapular rash, hepatosplenomegaly, lymphadenopathy, pericarditis, growth retardation
Labs	Weakly ANA (+)	- Weakly ANA (+) in younger ages, RF (+) in older ages - ↑ ESR - Anemia	- ANA (–), RF (–) - ↑ ESR - Leukocytosis, anemia

PATELLOFEMORAL PAIN SYNDROME (PFPS)

A 15-year-old F is seen for 2 months of right knee pain and a sensation of knee buckling. It is worse when she walks upstairs, squats, or sits for prolonged periods. She has recently been running on the school track team. On **exam**, she has pain on palpation of the patella. There is no redness or joint swelling.

Management:

1. Activity modification.
2. NSAIDs.
3. Physical therapy with emphasis on quadriceps and hip abductors.

Complications: Patellofemoral osteoarthritis.

HYF: Patients complain of generalized anterior knee pain that is worsened when bearing weight on a flexed knee. It is a clinical diagnosis only; no imaging is required.

OSGOOD-SCHLATTER DISEASE

A 15-year-old M presents with 1 month of left knee pain. It is worse when he plays basketball. On **exam**, he has TTP of the tibial tuberosity. There is no swelling or joint erythema. On **imaging**, knee X-ray shows the following:

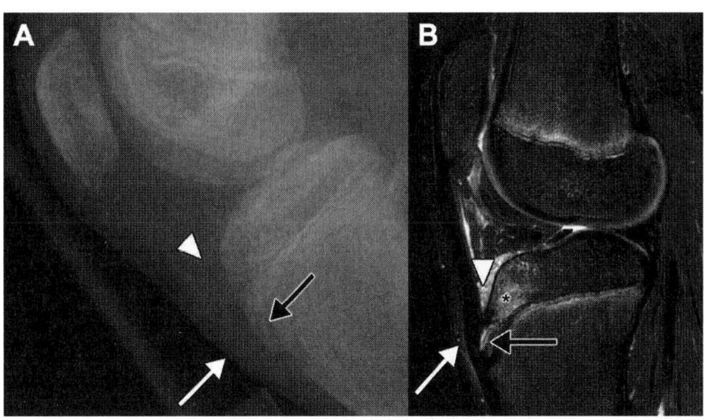
A
B

Fragmentation of the tibial tubercle in Osgood-Schlatter Disease.

Management:

1. NSAIDs.
2. Rest.
3. Physical therapy.

Complications: Bony prominence of the tibial tubercle.

HYF: Most common in adolescent boys during periods of rapid growth and athletes with repetitive activity, especially jumping and kneeling. X-rays are not required for diagnosis but may show lifting, irregularity, or fragmentation of the tibial tubercle.

23-43 Chronic Leg Pain/Limp

SCOLIOSIS

A 14-year-old M presents with right convex thoracic curvature that has been discovered incidentally.

Management:

1. Physical exam: Evaluation of spinal shape, Adam forward bend test demonstrates C- or S-shaped deviation of spinous processes. Can see "rib hump" or "lumbar hump."
2. Obtain X-ray to determine cobb angle if there is more than 7° deviation on scoliometer measurements.
3. Treatment:
   a. Cobb angle 10–19°: Monitoring.
   b. 20–29°: Monitoring or bracing.
   c. 30–39°: Bracing.
   d. >40°: Surgery.

Complications:

- Progression of scoliosis, in severe cases, can cause respiratory and cardiopulmonary impairment.
- Regardless of treatment, chronic back pain is possible, although functional impairment in treated patients is low.

HYF: Infant form <4 years old, juvenile form 4–9 years old, adolescent form >10 years old. Infant and juvenile forms often present with left curvature, adolescent with right curvature. Diagnosis is made on exam. X-ray is for determining prognosis and treatment.

GENU VARUM/VALGUS

A 4-year-old presents with bowing in of knees.

Management:

1. Observation and reassurance: Primary genu valgus is only considered pathological if persistence continues after 10 years. Primary genus varus is only considered pathological if persistence continues after 3 years.
2. Surgical correction in persistent cases.

Complications: Gait abnormalities.

HYF: Almost always presents as a sign of underlying pathology. Likely pathologies include rickets, skeletal dysplasia, and neoplasms, and workup should include these.

LEGG-CALVE-PERTHES (LCP) DISEASE

A 6-year-old M presents with progressively worsening left hip pain over the last month and a limp in the last week. On **exam**, his left hip has limited ROM on abduction and internal rotation and proximal thigh atrophy. (+) Trendelenburg sign. On **imaging**, X-rays of his pelvis and lower extremities are negative. MRI shows avascular osteonecrosis of the left femoral head. On **labs**, CBC, CRP, and ESR are normal.

Management:

1. NSAIDs.
2. Avoid weight bearing.
3. Splinting, possible surgical repair (if >8 years old).

HYF: Affects boys between ages 3–12 (peaks at age 6). It may present with direct hip pain or referred groin or knee pain. X-rays may show sclerosis and fragmentation of the femoral head in later disease, but they may be negative in early disease.

Developmental Dysplasia of the Hip: See p. 548.

23-44 Pediatric Upper Extremity Fractures

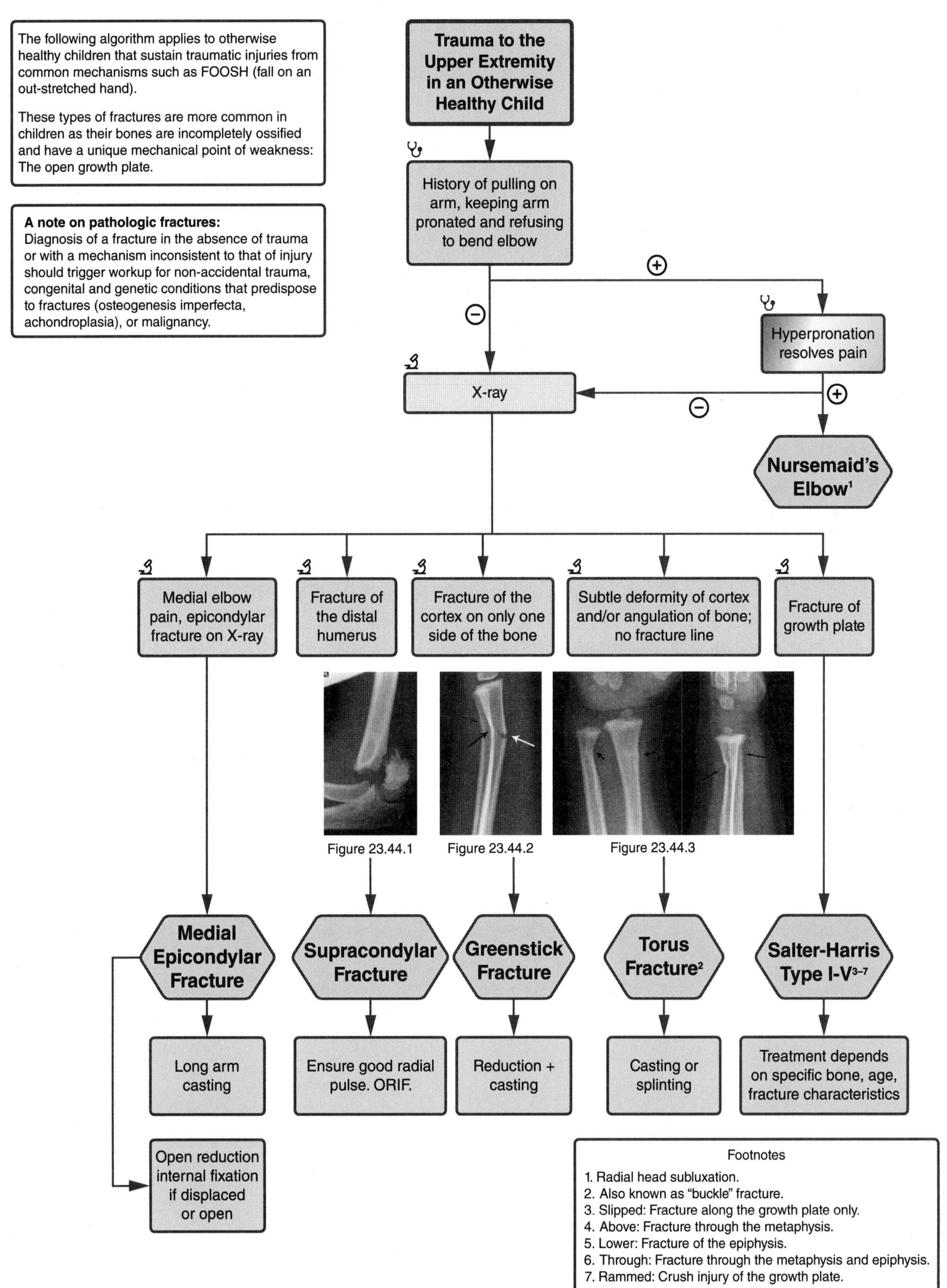

The following algorithm applies to otherwise healthy children that sustain traumatic injuries from common mechanisms such as FOOSH (fall on an out-stretched hand).
These types of fractures are more common in children as their bones are incompletely ossified and have a unique mechanical point of weakness: The open growth plate.
A note on pathologic fractures:
Diagnosis of a fracture in the absence of trauma or with a mechanism inconsistent to that of injury should trigger workup for non-accidental trauma, congenital and genetic conditions that predispose to fractures (osteogenesis imperfecta, achondroplasia), or malignancy.
Trauma to the Upper Extremity in an Otherwise Healthy Child
History of pulling on arm, keeping arm pronated and refusing to bend elbow
Hyperpronation resolves pain
X-ray
Nursemaid's Elbow1
Medial elbow pain, epicondylar fracture on X-ray
Fracture of the distal humerus
Fracture of the cortex on only one side of the bone
Subtle deformity of cortex and/or angulation of bone; no fracture line
Fracture of growth plate
Figure 23.44.1
Figure 23.44.2
Figure 23.44.3
Medial Epicondylar Fracture
Supracondylar Fracture
Greenstick Fracture
Torus Fracture2
Salter-Harris Type I-V3-7
Long arm casting
Ensure good radial pulse. ORIF.
Reduction + casting
Casting or splinting
Treatment depends on specific bone, age, fracture characteristics
Open reduction internal fixation if displaced or open
Footnotes
1. Radial head subluxation.
2. Also known as "buckle" fracture.
3. Slipped: Fracture along the growth plate only.
4. Above: Fracture through the metaphysis.
5. Lower: Fracture of the epiphysis.
6. Through: Fracture through the metaphysis and epiphysis.
7. Rammed: Crush injury of the growth plate.

FIGURE 23.44

23-44 Pediatric Upper Extremity Fractures

RADIAL HEAD SUBLUXATION (NURSEMAID'S ELBOW)

A 3-year-old F presents with elbow pain after her mom suddenly pulled her away from an incoming car while crossing the street. On **exam**, she is holding her forearm extended and pronated and refuses to bend her elbow. Hyperpronation of the forearm results in a pop, after which she recovers full range of motion.

Management:

1. Manual reduction by hyperpronation, or supination of the forearm at 90° of flexion.
2. No X-rays are indicated unless there is an atypical mechanism of injury or edema of the elbow.

Complications: Recurrence in about one-third of patients.

HYF: Nursemaid's elbow is a subluxation of the radial head under the annular ligament and occurs typically in ages 1–4 years.

SUPRACONDYLAR FRACTURE

A 7-year-old M presents with elbow pain and swelling after falling on an outstretched hand while playing basketball. On **imaging**, X-ray shows a fracture of the distal humerus.

Management:

1. Thorough neurovascular examination. Ensure good radial pulse to monitor for brachial artery injury.
2. Splint vs. cast immobilization depending on operative plan.
3. ± closed or open reduction.

Complications:

- Nerve injury: Median, ulnar, or radial nerve palsy.
- Brachial artery injury, which can lead to compartment syndrome.
- Volkmann ischemic contracture secondary to compartment syndrome/brachial artery injury.

HYF: Supracondylar fractures are common pediatric fractures often caused by a fall on an outstretched hand. A supracondylar fracture often results in posterior displacement of the distal humerus fragment; the anteriorly displaced proximal fragment can entrap the median nerve and brachial artery located anteriorly to the humerus. X-ray often shows a fracture line and posterior fat pad (ie, sail sign). Operative urgency depends on displacement and neurovascular status.

GREENSTICK FRACTURE

A 6-year-old F fell off the monkey bars onto her right side. She got up and immediately felt pain in her right lateral forearm. On **imaging**, X-rays show a fracture of the ulnar periosteum and cortex that does not extend to the other side of the bone.

Management:

1. Closed reduction under sedation.
2. Cast immobilization (bivalved long arm cast).
3. Repeat X-rays at 10-14 days.

Complications: Refracture.

HYF: Greenstick fractures often occur from a FOOSH. On X-ray, the cortex is fractured on the opposite side from which a compressive force was applied, rather than extending through the width of the bone.

TORUS FRACTURE (BUCKLE FRACTURE)

An 8-year-old M trips while playing soccer and complains of wrist pain. **Exam** shows swelling of the distal forearm. On **imaging**, X-rays show a subtle angulation of the bones and no fracture line.

Management:

1. Cast vs. splint immobilization.

Complications: Generally favorable outcomes.

HYF: Torus fractures (ie, "buckle" fractures) also commonly occur from a FOOSH. They are essentially "kinks" in the softer, more malleable pediatric bone.

Salter-Harris Fractures, Type I-V: See p. 640.

23-45 Pediatric Lower Extremity Fractures

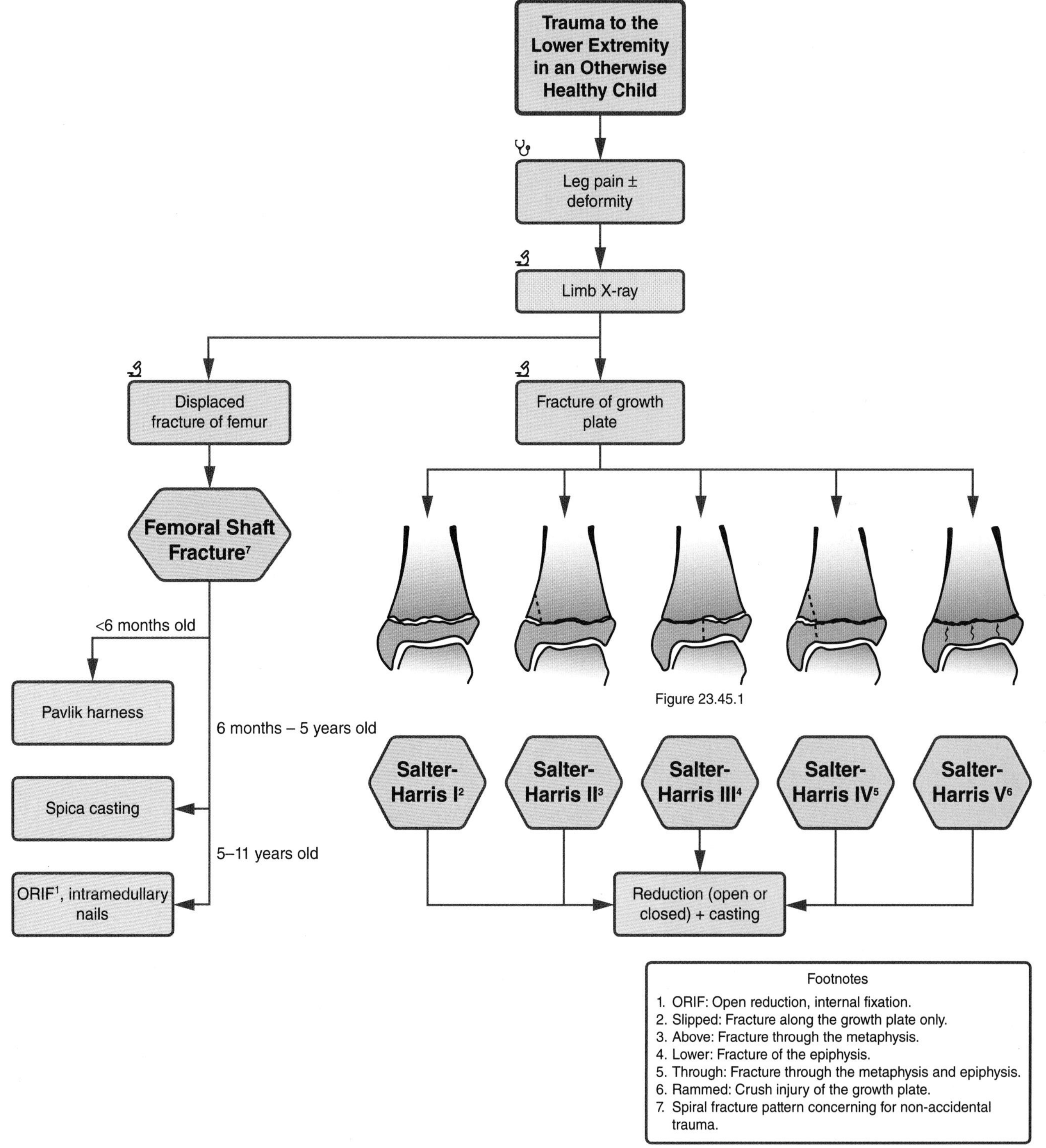
Trauma to the Lower Extremity in an Otherwise Healthy Child
Leg pain ± deformity
Limb X-ray
Displaced fracture of femur
Fracture of growth plate
Femoral Shaft Fracture7
<6 months old
Pavlik harness
6 months – 5 years old
Spica casting
5–11 years old
ORIF1, intramedullary nails
Figure 23.45.1
Salter-Harris I2
Salter-Harris II3
Salter-Harris III4
Salter-Harris IV5
Salter-Harris V6
Reduction (open or closed) + casting

Footnotes

1. ORIF: Open reduction, internal fixation.
2. Slipped: Fracture along the growth plate only.
3. Above: Fracture through the metaphysis.
4. Lower: Fracture of the epiphysis.
5. Through: Fracture through the metaphysis and epiphysis.
6. Rammed: Crush injury of the growth plate.
7. Spiral fracture pattern concerning for non-accidental trauma.

FIGURE 23.45

23-45 Pediatric Lower Extremity Fractures

FEMORAL SHAFT FRACTURE

A 17-year-old M presents after driving his ATV over a cliff. He was discovered unconscious on the scene with a visible deformity of his quadricep. On exam, he can move his foot, but it is noticeably dusky with a thready posterior tibial pulse.

Management:

1. If stable, Pavlik harness for age <6 months old; spica casting for age 0–5 years; intramedullary nailing for >5 yo.
2. If there are more serious injuries preventing surgical intervention, can temporize with external fixation or traction.

Complications:

- Leg-length discrepancy.
- Osteonecrosis of femoral head.
- Nonunion/malunion.
- Refracture.

HYF: This is the 2nd most common pediatric fracture. Fall is the most common mechanism, followed by motor vehicle accident. Neurovascular status determines urgency as well as open fixation (ORIF, urgent if any neurovascular compromise). High rate of fracture union.

SALTER-HARRIS FRACTURES

A 12-year-old F presents with pain, swelling, and loss of range of motion in her ankle after she jumped off a tall boulder during a family hike. On imaging, X-rays show the following:

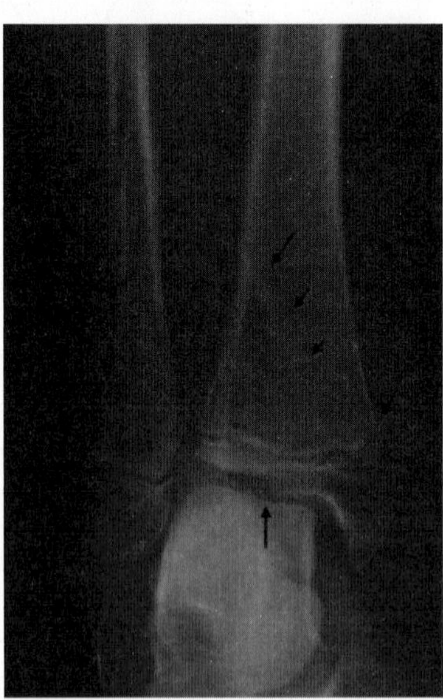

Arrows pointing to type 4 Salter-Harris fracture of the distal tibia.

Management:

1. Management of Salter-Harris fractures depends on many factors including the affected bone, displacement, neurovascular status, and age of patient.

Complications:

- Limb length discrepancy or deformity due to growth arrest.
- Decreased ROM.
- Premature osteoarthritis.
- Formation of physeal bars.

HYF: Salter-Harris fractures are fractures that include any growth plate and usually occur during a child's growth spurt. SALTER – Slipped (I): Fracture along the growth plate. Above (II): Fracture through the metaphysis. Lower (III): Fracture of the epiphysis. Through (IV, pictured above): Fracture through the metaphysis and epiphysis. Rammed (V): Crush injury of the growth plate.

DISTAL FEMORAL PHYSEAL FRACTURE

A 7-year-old M was playing football when he was hit in the knee with a helmet during a tackle. Since then, he has been complaining of pain around his knee and developed a limp. On exam, his leg is warm and well-perfused without weakness or numbness.

Management:

1. Limb X-ray may detect physeal widening or other evidence of growth plate injury.
2. MRI can confirm diagnosis.
3. Casting 4–6 weeks for non-displaced fractures.
4. Closed reduction percutaneous pinning (CRPP) vs. ORIF for displacement or articular involvement.

Complications:

- Non-union.
- Limb length discrepancy.
- Angular deformity (most common).
- Popliteal injury.

HYF: These fractures occur with direct trauma and only occur in children with open growth plates. These fractures are high risk for growth arrest. CRPP is the preferred treatment option. Can be confused with collateral ligament injury.

23-46 Non-Accidental Trauma

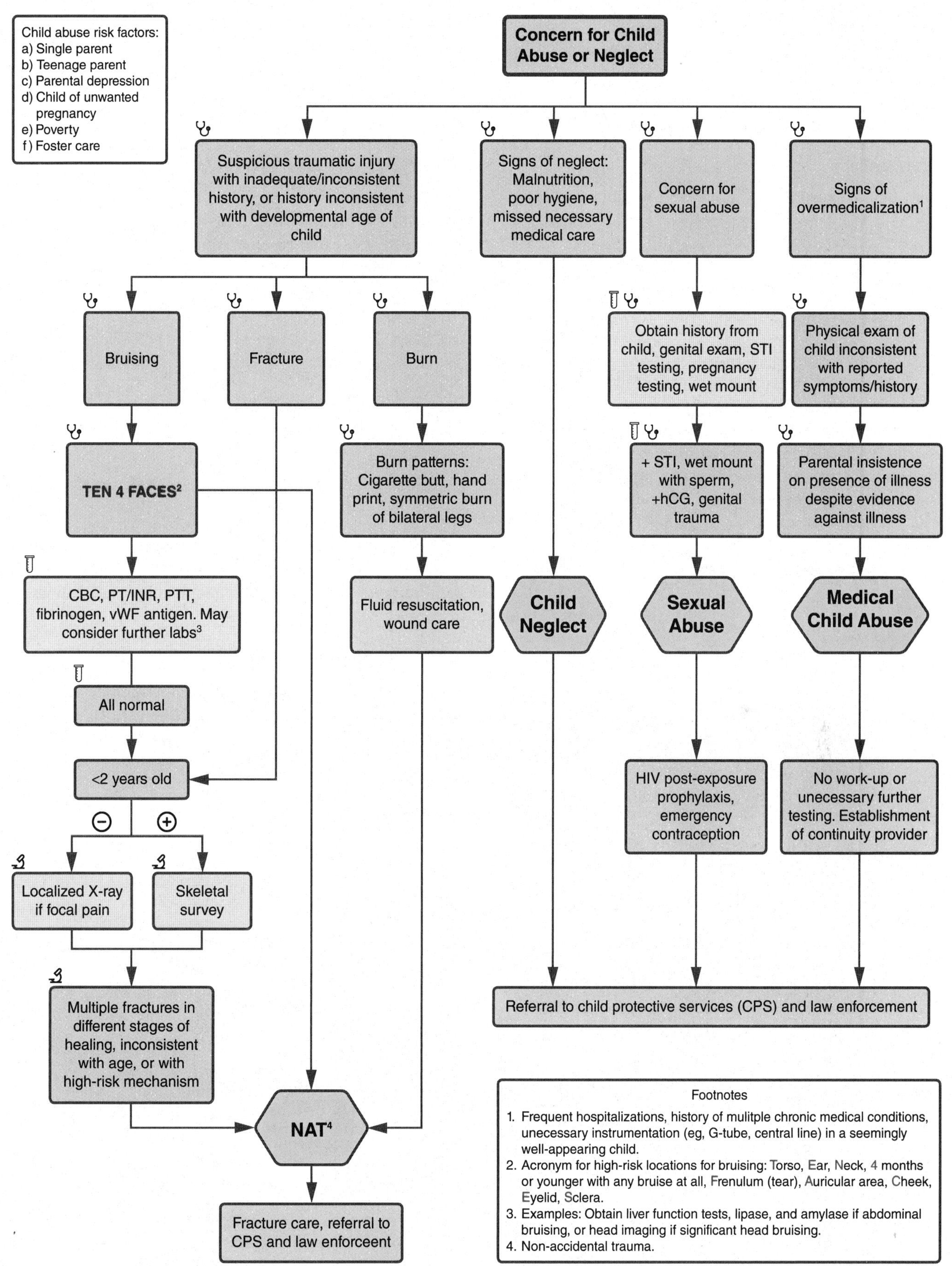

Child abuse risk factors:
a) Single parent
b) Teenage parent
c) Parental depression
d) Child of unwanted pregnancy
e) Poverty
f) Foster care
Concern for Child Abuse or Neglect
Suspicious traumatic injury with inadequate/inconsistent history, or history inconsistent with developmental age of child
Signs of neglect: Malnutrition, poor hygiene, missed necessary medical care
Concern for sexual abuse
Signs of overmedicalization1
Bruising
Fracture
Burn
Obtain history from child, genital exam, STI testing, pregnancy testing, wet mount
Physical exam of child inconsistent with reported symptoms/history
TEN 4 FACES2
Burn patterns: Cigarette butt, hand print, symmetric burn of bilateral legs
+ STI, wet mount with sperm, +hCG, genital trauma
Parental insistence on presence of illness despite evidence against illness
CBC, PT/INR, PTT, fibrinogen, vWF antigen. May consider further labs3
Fluid resuscitation, wound care
Child Neglect
Sexual Abuse
Medical Child Abuse
All normal
<2 years old
HIV post-exposure prophylaxis, emergency contraception
No work-up or unecessary further testing. Establishment of continuity provider
Localized X-ray if focal pain
Skeletal survey
Multiple fractures in different stages of healing, inconsistent with age, or with high-risk mechanism
Referral to child protective services (CPS) and law enforcement
NAT4
Fracture care, referral to CPS and law enforceent
Footnotes
1. Frequent hospitalizations, history of mulitple chronic medical conditions, unecessary instrumentation (eg, G-tube, central line) in a seemingly well-appearing child.
2. Acronym for high-risk locations for bruising: Torso, Ear, Neck, 4 months or younger with any bruise at all, Frenulum (tear), Auricular area, Cheek, Eyelid, Sclera.
3. Examples: Obtain liver function tests, lipase, and amylase if abdominal bruising, or head imaging if significant head bruising.
4. Non-accidental trauma.

FIGURE 23.46

23-46 Non-Accidental Trauma

HIGH-RISK BRUISING: LOCATION

An 18-month-old M is taken to the ED by his mom because she noticed some redness in his left eye. She says she's not sure how he got it. On exam, you also note a torn upper anterior frenulum and bruising of the left ear.

Management:

1. Obtain CBC, coagulation profile, and von Willebrand testing.
2. Obtain AST, ALT, and amylase to evaluate for abdominal trauma.
3. Retinal exam by ophthalmology.
4. Skeletal survey.
5. Notify Child Protective Services.

HYF: TEN 4 FACES. Suspect "high-risk" bruising or bruising that might indicate non-accidental trauma in the following places if <4 years old: Torso, Ear, Neck, 4 months or younger with any bruise at all (as they are non-mobile), Frenulum (tear), Auricular area, Cheek, Eyelid, Sclera. Obtain the labs above to screen for blood clotting disorders and a retinal exam to assess for retinal hemorrhages. A skeletal survey to evaluate for fractures is indicated because the child is <2 years old and cannot localize pain effectively.

HIGH-RISK BRUISING: PATTERNED

A 1-month-old F is brought to her pediatrician because the mom says she's been fussier in the last 2 days. On exam, she has a patterned bruise on the left side of her face as pictured below

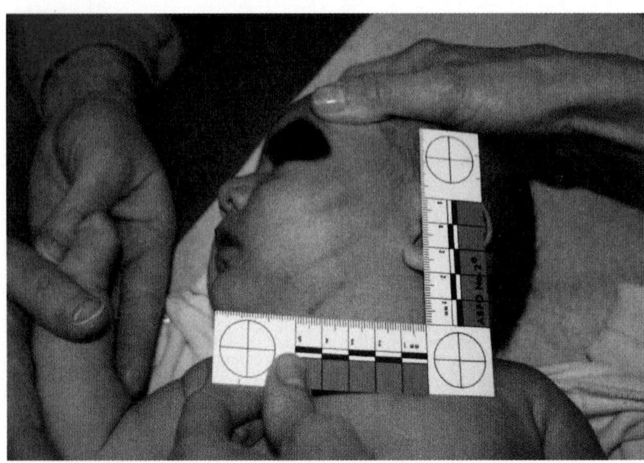

Patterned bruising of cheek in the impression of a handprint.

Management:

1. Obtain CBC, coagulation profile, and von Willebrand testing.
2. Obtain AST, ALT, and amylase to evaluate for abdominal trauma.
3. Obtain a head CT to rule out intracranial bleed.
4. Skeletal survey.
5. Retinal exam by ophthalmology.
6. Notify CPS.

HYF: Any patterned bruise on a child of any age is highly concerning for non-accidental trauma, though exceptions include traditions of coining or cupping. In this case, the bruise has a handprint pattern. Other common patterns include cord loops, small, round cigarette burns, or bite marks. In a child <1 year of age, evidence of head trauma warrants a head CT scan to rule out intracranial bleed, even in the absence of neurologic changes.

ABUSIVE HEAD TRAUMA

A 6-week-old M is brought to the ED because he has been extra fussy and not breastfeeding well. On exam, he is lethargic and tachycardic. Eye exam reveals retinal hemorrhages bilaterally. On imaging, head CT shows a right frontal subdural hematoma.

Management:

1. Obtain CBC, coagulation profile, and von Willebrand testing.
2. Obtain AST, ALT, and amylase to evaluate for abdominal trauma.
3. Obtain head CT. If positive for bleed, obtain head MRI.
4. Skeletal survey.
5. Retinal exam by ophthalmology.
6. Notify CPS.

HYF: Previously known as "shaken baby syndrome," abusive head trauma in infants most commonly results in subdural hematomas from rupture of the bridging veins. Spinal injuries, encephalopathy, skull fractures, and extensive retinal hemorrhages can also result from this type of injury.

HIGH-RISK FRACTURES

A 10-month-old F presents to the ED because her mom noticed she doesn't want to crawl as much as she used to. On exam, she seems to be moving her left leg more than her right. On imaging, X-ray of the hip reveals a classic metaphyseal lesion of the proximal humerus.

Management:

1. Obtain AST, ALT, and amylase to evaluate for abdominal trauma.
2. Skeletal survey.
3. Notify CPS.

HYF: Classic metaphyseal lesions are bucket handle fractures in infants (<1 year old) that are highly concerning for NAT. The mechanism is usually a torsional force near the growth plate. The following fracture locations are high-risk and require further investigation for NAT:

- Any fracture in a non-mobile infant.
- Ribs.
- Sternum.
- Spinous process.
- Scapula.
- Pelvis.
- Multiple fractures at different stages of healing.

24
Obstetrics

24-1 Vaginal Bleeding in Pregnancy

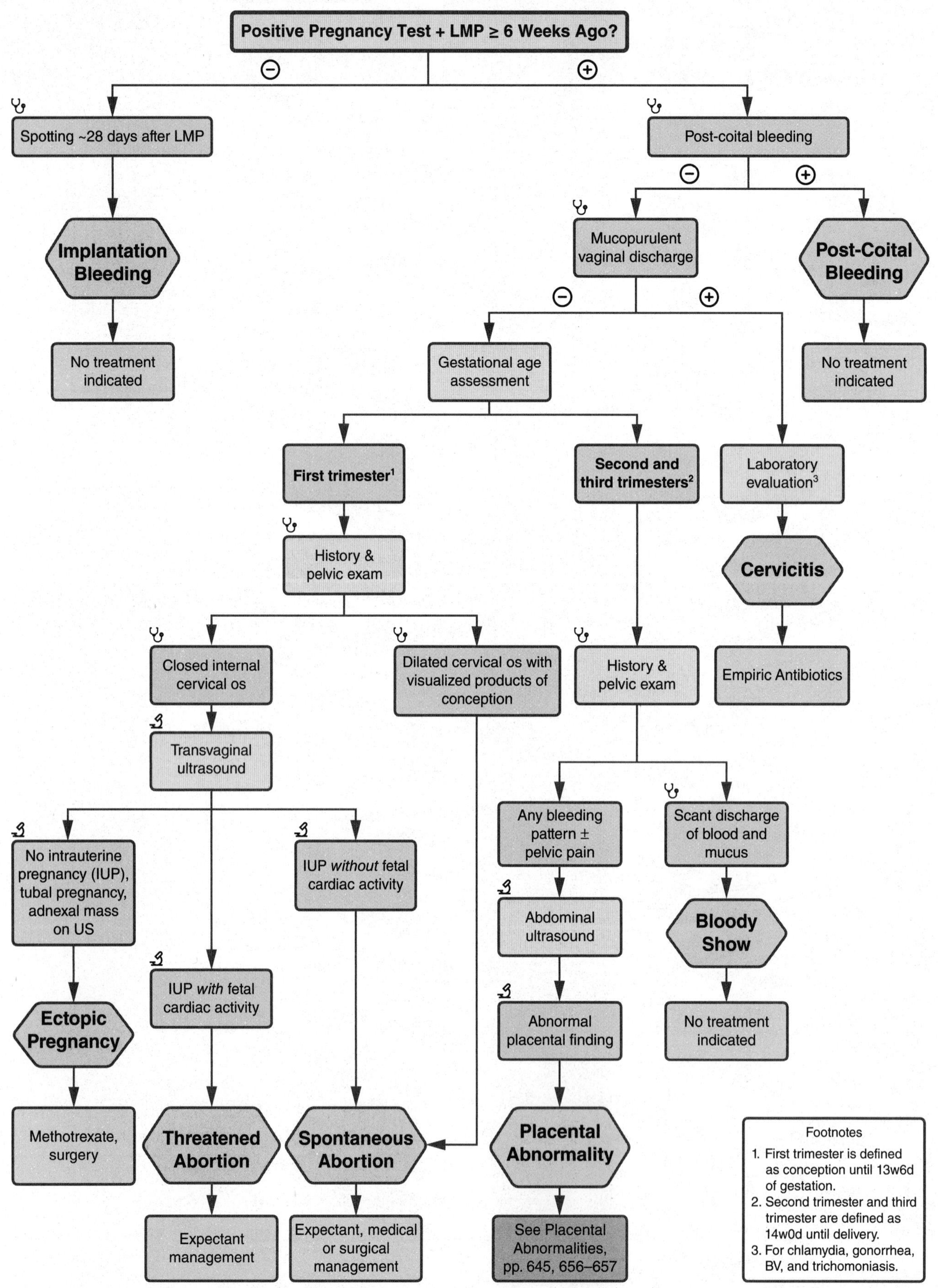
Positive Pregnancy Test + LMP ≥ 6 Weeks Ago?
Spotting ~28 days after LMP
Implantation Bleeding
No treatment indicated
Post-coital bleeding
Mucopurulent vaginal discharge
Post-Coital Bleeding
No treatment indicated
Gestational age assessment
First trimester[1]
Second and third trimesters[2]
Laboratory evaluation[3]
History & pelvic exam
Cervicitis
Closed internal cervical os
Dilated cervical os with visualized products of conception
History & pelvic exam
Empiric Antibiotics
Transvaginal ultrasound
No intrauterine pregnancy (IUP), tubal pregnancy, adnexal mass on US
IUP *without* fetal cardiac activity
Any bleeding pattern ± pelvic pain
Scant discharge of blood and mucus
Abdominal ultrasound
Bloody Show
IUP *with* fetal cardiac activity
Ectopic Pregnancy
Abnormal placental finding
No treatment indicated
Methotrexate, surgery
Threatened Abortion
Spontaneous Abortion
Placental Abnormality
Expectant management
Expectant, medical or surgical management
See Placental Abnormalities, pp. 645, 656–657
Footnotes
1. First trimester is defined as conception until 13w6d of gestation.
2. Second trimester and third trimester are defined as 14w0d until delivery.
3. For chlamydia, gonorrhea, BV, and trichomoniasis.

FIGURE 24.1

24-1 Vaginal Bleeding in Pregnancy

IMPLANTATION BLEEDING

A 27-year-old F with unremarkable PMH and LMP 4 weeks ago presents with 1 day of spotting. **Exam** and **labs** are normal.

Management: No management necessary.

Complications: None.

HYF: Implantation bleeding is a diagnosis of exclusion.

POST-COITAL BLEEDING

A 24-year-old F G1P0 at 24w5d presents with spotting after sexual intercourse. **Exam** and **imaging** are unremarkable.

Management: No management necessary.

Complications: None.

HYF: Post-coital bleeding is much more common in pregnancy due to the presence of cervical ectropion and increased blood flow to the genital tract.

CERVICITIS

A 22-year-old F G1P0 at 15w2d presents with thick, yellow vaginal discharge and occasional light bleeding. **Exam** shows friable cervix with mucopurulent discharge at the cervical os.

Management:

1. Test for chlamydia, gonorrhea, BV, and trichomoniasis.
2. Treat empirically to cover chlamydia and gonorrhea.

Complications: Endometritis, pelvic inflammatory disease.

HYF: The primary risk factor for infectious cervicitis is sexual activity because of increased risk for STIs.

ECTOPIC PREGNANCY

A 30-year-old F with a positive home pregnancy test and LMP 6 weeks ago presents with 1 day of light vaginal bleeding. **Exam** shows unilateral adnexal tenderness. **Labs** show β-hCG of 3000 mIU/mL. On **imaging**, transvaginal ultrasound (TVUS) shows a thin endometrial stripe and no intrauterine gestation.

Management:

1. IM methotrexate. Monitor hCG levels until undetectable.
2. Salpingectomy or salpingostomy in the case of hemodynamic instability, rupture, or failed medical therapy.

Complications:

- Tubal rupture and hemorrhage (potentially fatal).
- Tubal abortion.

HYF: Any patient presenting with bleeding and pain in early pregnancy is assumed to have an ectopic pregnancy until definitively excluded with imaging and labs.

THREATENED ABORTION

A 32-year-old F G2P1 at 10w3d presents with 2 days of vaginal bleeding and cramping. **Exam** shows closed internal cervical os. On **imaging**, transvaginal ultrasound (TVUS) shows intrauterine pregnancy with fetal cardiac activity.

Management: No management necessary.

Complications: Spontaneous abortion.

HYF: In up to 90–96% of pregnancies at 7–11 weeks' gestation that present with vaginal bleeding with fetal cardiac activity, bleeding resolves and the pregnancy is not lost.

SPONTANEOUS ABORTION

A 26-year-old F G1P0 at 7w4d presents with 1 day of heavy vaginal bleeding and cramping. **Exam** shows dilated internal cervical os with blood in the vaginal vault. On **imaging**, TVUS shows intrauterine pregnancy with no fetal cardiac activity.

Management:

1. Expectant management – available to hemodynamically stable patients in the 1st trimester.
2. Medical management – with mifepristone-misoprostol combined regimen.
3. Surgical management – with vacuum aspiration of uterus.

Complications:

- Incomplete emptying of the uterus.
- Infection, hemorrhage.

HYF: Risk factors include extremes of age, previous pregnancy loss, medical conditions (infection, obesity, diabetes), and medications/substance use.

PLACENTAL ABNORMALITY

A 37-year-old F G2P1 at 28w5d presents with 3 days of painless vaginal bleeding. **Exam** is unremarkable. On **imaging**, TVUS shows placental tissue covering the cervix (placenta previa).

Management: Dependent on type of placental abnormality.

Complications: Dependent on type of placental abnormality.

HYF: See Placental Abnormalities on pp. 656–657.

BLOODY SHOW

A 35-year-old F G2P1 at 39w1d presents with scant discharge of bloody mucus and contractions. **Exam** shows cervix is 2 cm dilated. On **imaging**, transvaginal ultrasound shows vertex fetus.

Management: No management necessary.

Complications: None.

HYF: Bloody show signifies the impending onset of labor and may precede it by ≤72 hours.

24-2 Recurrent Pregnancy Loss

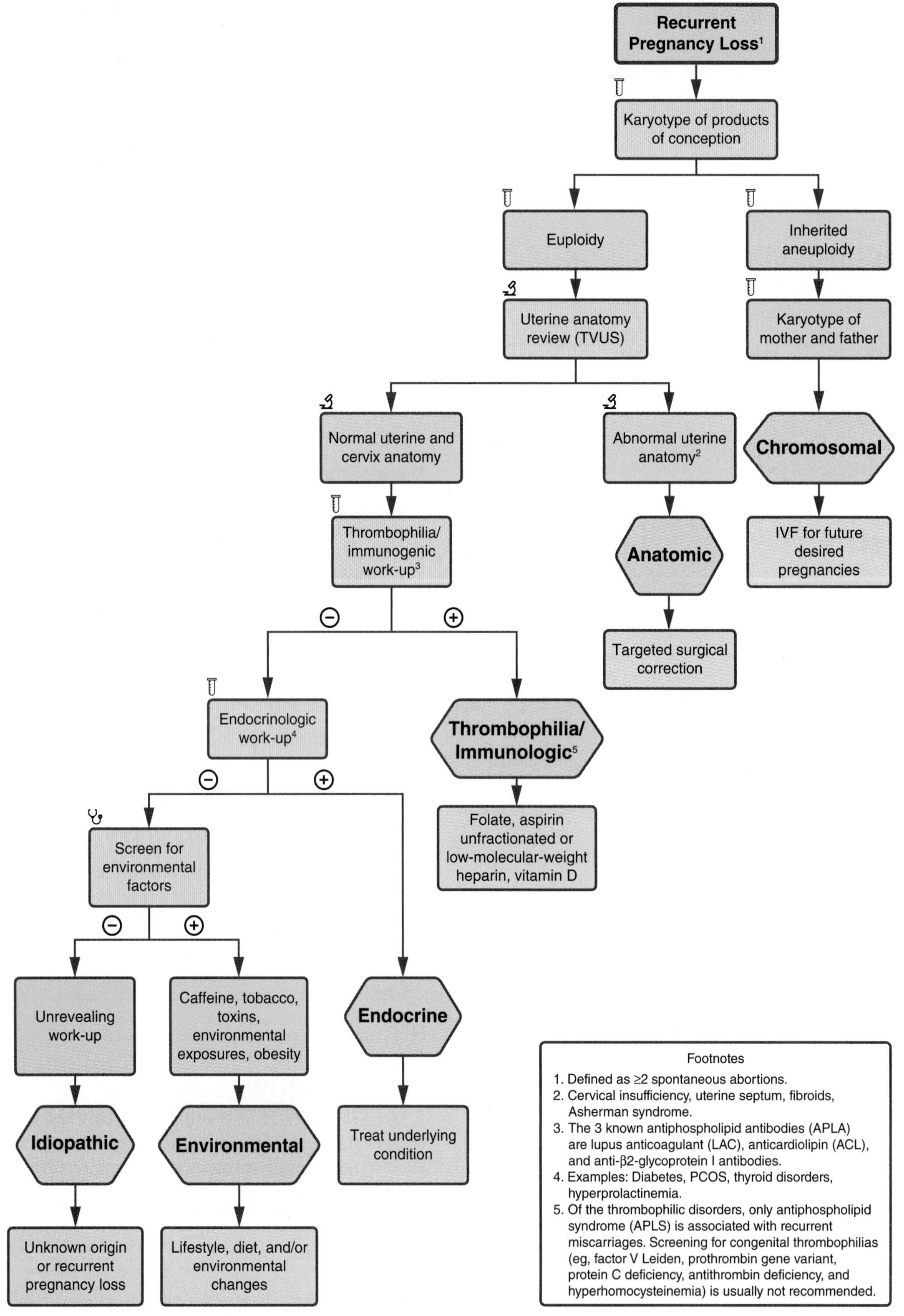

Recurrent Pregnancy Loss[1]
Karyotype of products of conception
Euploidy
Inherited aneuploidy
Uterine anatomy review (TVUS)
Karyotype of mother and father
Normal uterine and cervix anatomy
Abnormal uterine anatomy[2]
Chromosomal
Thrombophilia/ immunogenic work-up[3]
Anatomic
IVF for future desired pregnancies
Targeted surgical correction
Endocrinologic work-up[4]
Thrombophilia/ Immunologic[5]
Folate, aspirin unfractionated or low-molecular-weight heparin, vitamin D
Screen for environmental factors
Unrevealing work-up
Caffeine, tobacco, toxins, environmental exposures, obesity
Endocrine
Idiopathic
Environmental
Treat underlying condition
Unknown origin or recurrent pregnancy loss
Lifestyle, diet, and/or environmental changes
Footnotes
1. Defined as ≥2 spontaneous abortions.
2. Cervical insufficiency, uterine septum, fibroids, Asherman syndrome.
3. The 3 known antiphospholipid antibodies (APLA) are lupus anticoagulant (LAC), anticardiolipin (ACL), and anti-β2-glycoprotein I antibodies.
4. Examples: Diabetes, PCOS, thyroid disorders, hyperprolactinemia.
5. Of the thrombophilic disorders, only antiphospholipid syndrome (APLS) is associated with recurrent miscarriages. Screening for congenital thrombophilias (eg, factor V Leiden, prothrombin gene variant, protein C deficiency, antithrombin deficiency, and hyperhomocysteinemia) is usually not recommended.

FIGURE 24.2

24-2 Recurrent Pregnancy Loss

RECURRENT PREGNANCY LOSS

Defined as having ≥2 miscarriages. After 3 repeated miscarriages, assessment with physical exam and appropriate testing are recommended.

CHROMOSOMAL

A 39-year-old F G1P0 with no PMH presents with 1st-trimester vaginal bleeding. **Exam** shows products of conception in the vaginal vault. On **imaging**, US shows missed abortion.

Management:

1. Management of spontaneous abortion (uterine evacuation, medical management, expectant management; RhoGAM if Rh-negative).
2. Karyotype of products of conception.
3. Consider IVF for future pregnancies, depending on chromosomal abnormality.

Complications: High risk of subsequent pregnancy with chromosomal abnormality with maternal age >35.

HYF: Contributes to ~50% of SABs in 1st trimester, 20–30% of 2nd-trimester losses, and 5–10% of 3rd-trimester losses.

ANATOMIC

A 28-year-old F G1P0 at 10 weeks GA with PMH of uterine surgery presents with vaginal bleeding. On **imaging**, she is found to have a complete spontaneous abortion and a uterine septum.

Management:

1. Management of spontaneous abortion (see above).
2. Targeted surgical correction of anatomic abnormality.

Complications: Recurrent spontaneous abortion.

HYF: Uterine abnormalities include Asherman syndrome, adhesions, submucosal fibroids, retrograde uterus, and uterine septum. Cervical abnormalities include cervical insufficiency or DES exposure. Of note, a history of cervical conization or loop electrosurgical excision procedure (LEEP) is NOT associated with recurrent miscarriages.

IMMUNOLOGIC/THROMBOPHILIA

A 30-year-old F G3P0020 with PMH of recurrent pregnancy loss presents with 1st-trimester bleeding. On **imaging**, US shows evidence of missed abortion. **Labs** reveal (+) lupus anticoagulant and anticardiolipin antibodies concerning for antiphospholipid syndrome.

Management:

1. Management of spontaneous abortion (see p. 645).
2. Subsequent pregnancies: Unfractionated heparin or low-molecular-weight heparin for thrombotic prophylaxis.

Complications: Pregnancy without thrombotic prophylaxis is at risk for fetal demise and thrombosis. Avoid vitamin K antagonists during pregnancy due to risk of teratogenicity and pregnancy loss.

HYF: If antiphospholipid antibodies are detected, false-positive VDRL and falsely prolonged PTT may be seen. Antiphospholipid syndrome effects can be remembered as "**CLOTS**" (**C**oagulation defect, **L**ivedo reticularis, **O**bstetric [recurrent spontaneous abortion], **T**hrombocytopenia [↓ platelets], **S**LE association).

ENDOCRINE

A 28-year-old F with PMH of polycystic ovary syndrome presents with 1st-trimester vaginal bleeding. On **imaging**, US reveals a complete spontaneous abortion.

Management:

1. Management of spontaneous abortion (see p. 645).
2. Treat underlying endocrine disorders.

Complications: Diabetes mellitus can contribute to adverse pregnancy in addition to recurrent pregnancy loss.

HYF: Endocrine disorders account for 8–12% of recurrent pregnancy loss. Examples include thyroid disorders, luteal phase defects, polycystic ovary syndrome, hyperprolactinemia, and diabetes.

ENVIRONMENTAL

A 25-year-old F with PMH of alcohol use disorder presents with 1st-trimester vaginal bleeding. On **imaging**, US shows a complete spontaneous abortion.

Management:

1. Management of spontaneous abortion (see p. 645).
2. For subsequent pregnancies, limit exposure to environmental teratogens.

Complications: Environmental teratogens can cause spontaneous abortion or congenital anomalies.

HYF: Confirmed teratogens: Heavy metals (lead and mercury), alcohol, and ionizing radiation. Suspected teratogens: Tobacco, excessive caffeine (>500 mg/day), and drugs.

24-3 Hypertension in Pregnancy

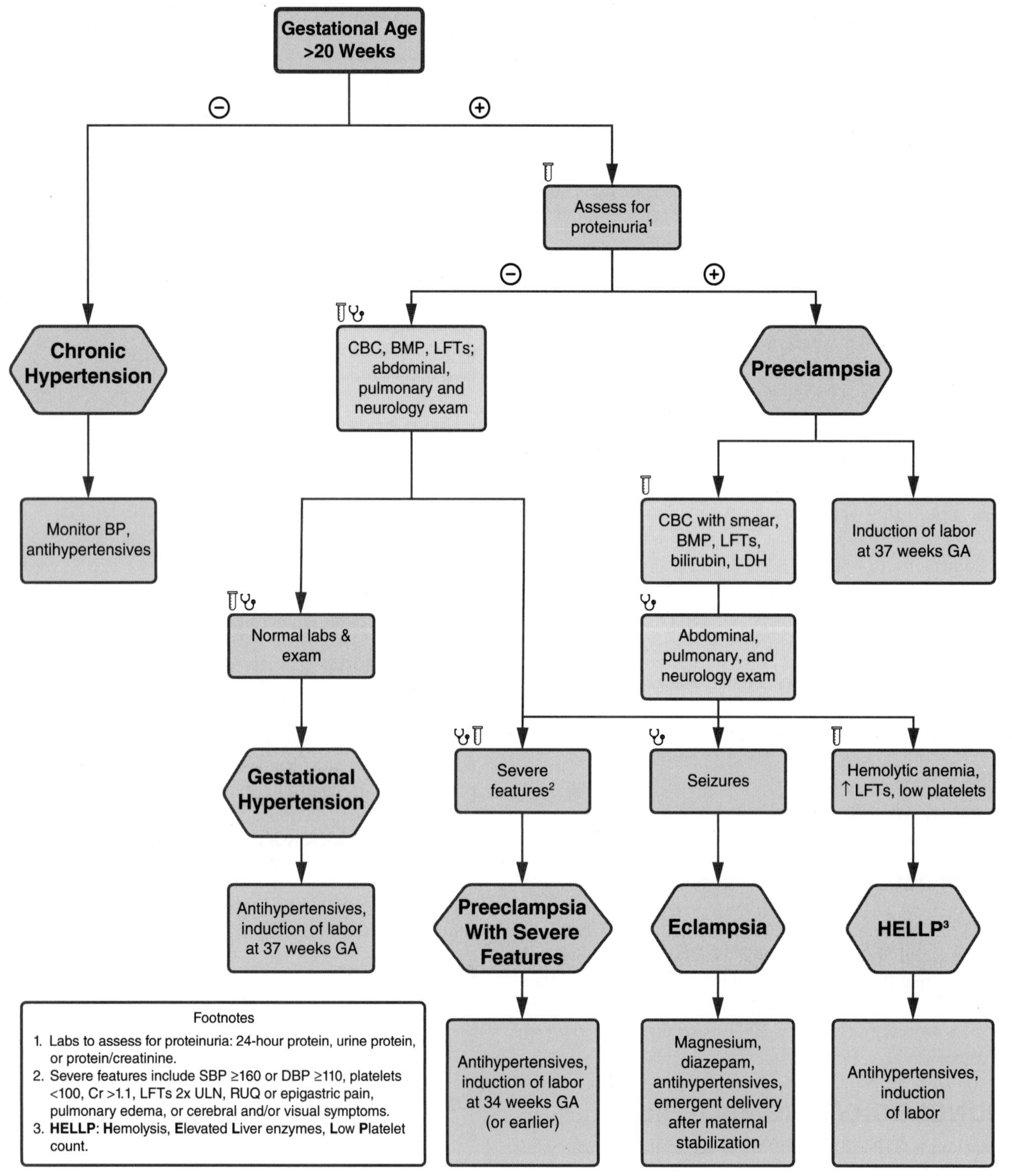
Gestational Age >20 Weeks
⊖
⊕
Assess for proteinuria[1]
⊖
⊕
Chronic Hypertension
CBC, BMP, LFTs; abdominal, pulmonary and neurology exam
Preeclampsia
Monitor BP, antihypertensives
CBC with smear, BMP, LFTs, bilirubin, LDH
Induction of labor at 37 weeks GA
Normal labs & exam
Abdominal, pulmonary, and neurology exam
Gestational Hypertension
Severe features[2]
Seizures
Hemolytic anemia, ↑ LFTs, low platelets
Antihypertensives, induction of labor at 37 weeks GA
Preeclampsia With Severe Features
Eclampsia
HELLP[3]
Antihypertensives, induction of labor at 34 weeks GA (or earlier)
Magnesium, diazepam, antihypertensives, emergent delivery after maternal stabilization
Antihypertensives, induction of labor
Footnotes
1. Labs to assess for proteinuria: 24-hour protein, urine protein, or protein/creatinine.
2. Severe features include SBP ≥160 or DBP ≥110, platelets <100, Cr >1.1, LFTs 2x ULN, RUQ or epigastric pain, pulmonary edema, or cerebral and/or visual symptoms.
3. HELLP: Hemolysis, Elevated Liver enzymes, Low Platelet count.

FIGURE 24.3

24-3 Hypertension in Pregnancy

CHRONIC HYPERTENSION

A 29-year-old F G1P0 at 10 weeks GA with PMH of HTN presents with blood pressure of 151/91 on exam at her first prenatal visit. Blood pressure taken at her preconception visit was 142/93.

Management:

1. Closely monitor BP. Start 81 mg ASA at 12 weeks for preeclampsia prevention.
2. Antihypertensives (methyldopa, labetalol, nifedipine).
3. If SBP >160 or DBP >110, treat with short-acting labetalol, hydralazine, or nifedipine (considered a hypertensive crisis).

Complications: Similar to preeclampsia complications (see below).

HYF: A diagnosis of chronic hypertension is made in pregnant patients at <20 weeks GA with elevated blood pressures and no proteinuria. The diagnosis may also be made if elevated BP persists for >12 weeks postpartum. Up to 1/3 of patients with chronic hypertension develop superimposed preeclampsia.

PREECLAMPSIA (WITH AND WITHOUT SEVERE FEATURES)

A 28-year-old F G1P0 at 31 weeks GA presents with blood pressure of 153/94 and lower-extremity edema on exam. Labs are notable for 24-hour urine protein of 389 mg.

Management:

1. Assess for severe features; closely monitor BP.
2. Delivery no later than 37 weeks GA.
3. Antihypertensives (methyldopa, labetalol, nifedipine).
4. If severe preeclampsia, control BPs with labetalol or hydralazine and proceed to induction of labor when stabilized.
5. Prevention of intrapartum seizures with magnesium sulfate drip (continue for 24 hours postpartum).

Complications:

- Prematurity, fetal distress, stillbirth.
- Placental abruption.
- Seizures, stroke.
- Fetal/maternal death.
- IUGR.

HYF: Preeclampsia can be diagnosed with either new-onset hypertension and proteinuria OR new-onset hypertension with any of the severe features (with or without proteinuria).

GESTATIONAL HYPERTENSION

A 31-year-old F G2P1 at 27 weeks GA presents with blood pressure of 149/82 and 144/91 on 2 subsequent readings. Labs demonstrate no significant proteinuria.

Management:

1. Closely monitor BP.
2. Antihypertensives (methyldopa, labetalol, nifedipine).
3. If SBP >160 or DBP >110, treat with short-acting labetalol, hydralazine, or nifedipine (hypertensive crisis).
4. Induction of labor at 37 weeks GA or sooner if medications are required to control severe-range BP elevations.

Complications: Similar to preeclampsia complications (see above).

HYF: A diagnosis of gestational hypertension is made in patients >20 weeks GA with elevated blood pressure and no proteinuria (blood pressure may not persist >12 weeks postpartum). Up to 25% of patients with gestational hypertension go on to develop preeclampsia.

ECLAMPSIA

A 27-year-old F G1P0 at 30 weeks GA and PMH of preeclampsia presents with headaches, blurry vision, and epigastric pain and develops a seizure while in OB triage. On exam, her vital signs are notable for blood pressure in the 160s/100s.

Management:

1. Stabilize the patient and prepare for immediate delivery.
2. Seizure control and prophylaxis with magnesium. Add IV diazepam for recurrent seizures.
3. Control BP with IV labetalol and/or hydralazine.

Complications:

- Placental abruption.
- DIC.
- Acute renal failure.
- Aspiration pneumonia, pulmonary edema.
- Hypoxic encephalopathy.
- Maternal/fetal death.

HYF: 1 in 4 eclamptic seizures occur during the postpartum period (most within 48 hours).

HELLP (HEMOLYSIS, ELEVATED LFTs, LOW PLATELETS)

A 26-year-old F G1P0 at 32 weeks GA presents with RUQ pain, headache, and blood pressure of 155/89 and 157/95. Labs show elevated LFTs, anemia, and thrombocytopenia.

Management:

1. Similar to preeclampsia with severe features (see above).

Complications:

- Bleeding, DIC.
- Placental abruption.
- Acute renal failure.
- Maternal/fetal death.

HYF: HELLP is a variant of preeclampsia, and the prognosis is poor.

***Identifying elevated blood pressure in pregnancy:**

- Elevated blood pressure: SBP >140 or DBP >90 on 2 readings (taken ≥4 hours apart).
- Severely elevated blood pressure: SBP >160 or DBP >110.
- Selecting an antihypertensive medication in pregnancy: Do not give ACE inhibitors or diuretics.

24-4 Diabetes in Pregnancy

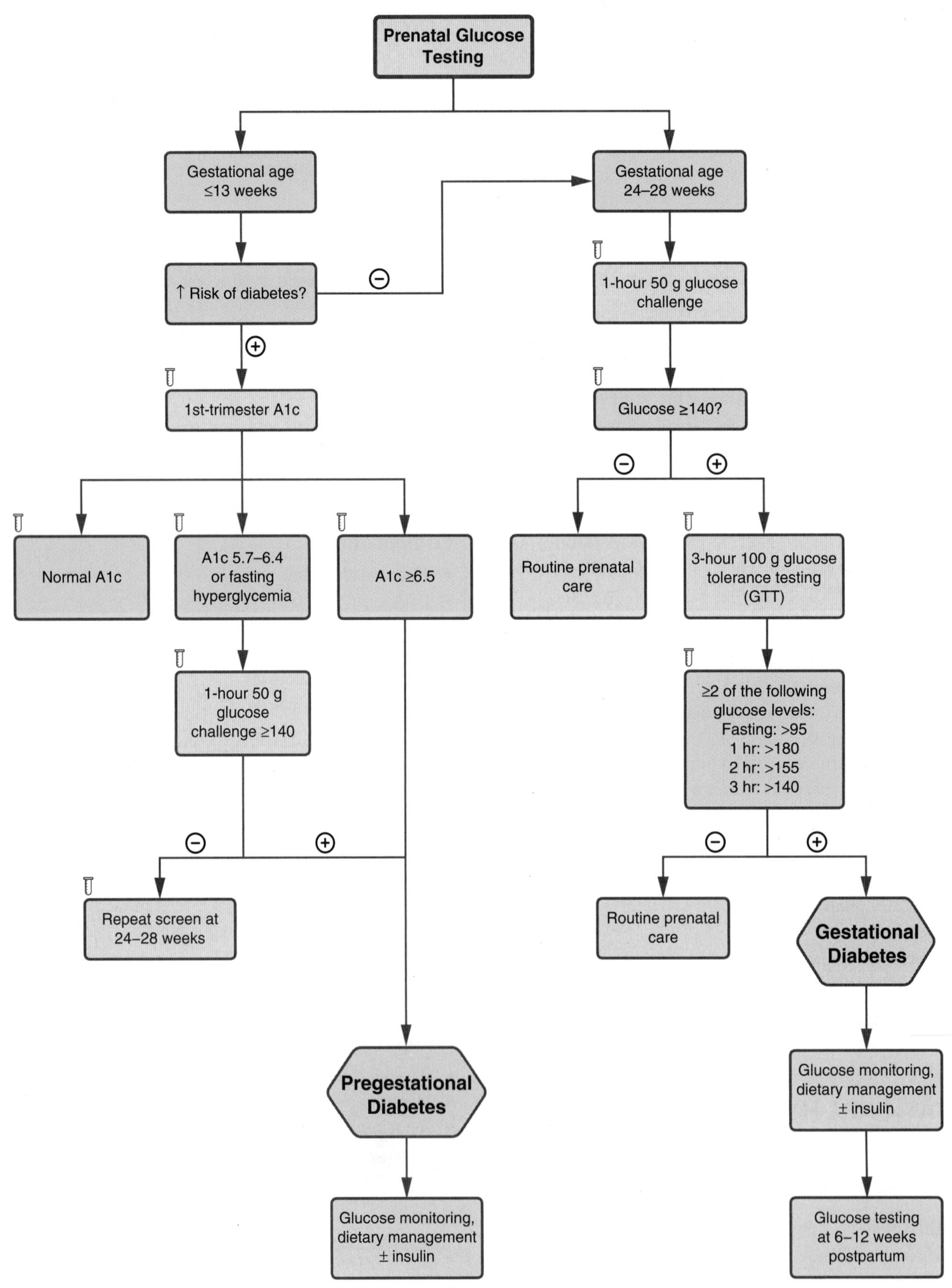
Prenatal Glucose Testing
Gestational age ≤13 weeks
↑ Risk of diabetes?
⊖
⊕
1st-trimester A1c
Normal A1c
A1c 5.7–6.4 or fasting hyperglycemia
A1c ≥6.5
1-hour 50 g glucose challenge ≥140
⊖
⊕
Repeat screen at 24–28 weeks
Pregestational Diabetes
Glucose monitoring, dietary management ± insulin
Gestational age 24–28 weeks
1-hour 50 g glucose challenge
Glucose ≥140?
⊖
⊕
Routine prenatal care
3-hour 100 g glucose tolerance testing (GTT)
≥2 of the following glucose levels:
Fasting: >95
1 hr: >180
2 hr: >155
3 hr: >140
⊖
⊕
Routine prenatal care
Gestational Diabetes
Glucose monitoring, dietary management ± insulin
Glucose testing at 6–12 weeks postpartum

FIGURE 24.4

24-4 Diabetes in Pregnancy

PREGESTATIONAL DIABETES

A 34-year-old F G2P1 at 6 weeks GA with family history of type 2 diabetes mellitus (T2DM) presents for establishment of prenatal care.

Management:

1. HbA1c for diagnosis.
2. Folate supplements.
3. Glucose control: Diet, exercise, oral agents, insulin.
4. Frequent follow-up.
5. Monitor fetal growth.
6. Regular antenatal testing.

Complications:

- Fetus/neonate: Congenital anomalies, polyhydramnios, fetal growth restriction, macrosomia, shoulder dystocia, birth injury, RDS, hypoglycemia, hyperbilirubinemia, childhood obesity (long-term).
- Gestational carrier: DKA (T1DM), HHS (T2DM), nephropathy, diabetic retinopathy, hypertension, preeclampsia.
- Birth: Miscarriage, preterm delivery, cesarean delivery.

HYF: Screen for T2DM during the 1st trimester in patients with increased risk of diabetes. Glucose control is crucial, especially during organogenesis (0–8 weeks GA).

GESTATIONAL DIABETES

A 38-year-old F G2P1 at 25 weeks GA with PMH of gestational diabetes in prior pregnancy presents for follow-up after she was found to have a serum glucose of 150 after 1-hour GTT at last visit.

Management:

1. 3-hour GTT for diagnosis.
2. Glucose control: Diet, exercise, oral agents (glyburide, metformin), insulin.
3. Frequent follow-up.
4. Monitor fetal growth.
5. Regular antenatal testing (if medications required).
6. T2DM screening 6 weeks postpartum.

Complications:

- Fetus/neonate: Polyhydramnios, risks of macrosomia (shoulder dystocia, birth injury), stillbirth, RDS, hypoglycemia, hyperbilirubinemia, childhood obesity (long-term).
- Gestational carrier: Hypertension, preeclampsia, progression to T2DM.
- Birth: Cesarean delivery.

HYF: GDM screening occurs at 24–28 weeks GA. Hormones released by the placenta cause/increase insulin resistance; prior history of GDM increases risk in future pregnancies.

Glucose Tolerance Test (GTT) for Gestational Diabetes Screening

	3-hour 100 g GTT	2-hour 75 g GTT
	≥2 of the following values diagnostic of GDM:	≥1 of the following values diagnostic of GDM:
Fasting	>95	>92
1 hour	>180	>180
2 hours	>155	>153
3 hours	>140	

24-5 Anemia in Pregnancy

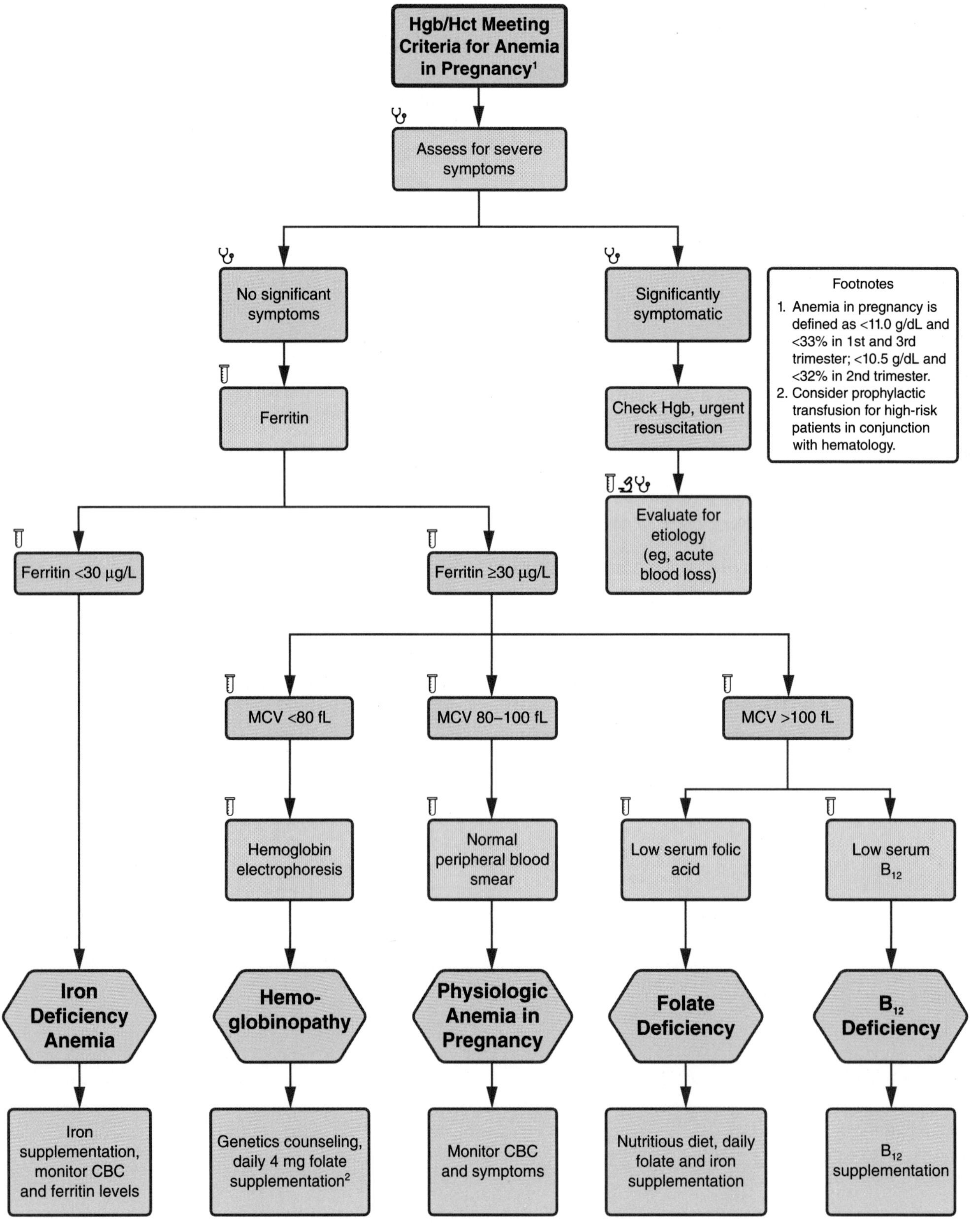
Hgb/Hct Meeting Criteria for Anemia in Pregnancy[1]
Assess for severe symptoms
No significant symptoms
Significantly symptomatic
Ferritin
Check Hgb, urgent resuscitation
Evaluate for etiology (eg, acute blood loss)
Ferritin <30 μg/L
Ferritin ≥30 μg/L
MCV <80 fL
MCV 80–100 fL
MCV >100 fL
Hemoglobin electrophoresis
Normal peripheral blood smear
Low serum folic acid
Low serum B12
Iron Deficiency Anemia
Hemo-globinopathy
Physiologic Anemia in Pregnancy
Folate Deficiency
B12 Deficiency
Iron supplementation, monitor CBC and ferritin levels
Genetics counseling, daily 4 mg folate supplementation[2]
Monitor CBC and symptoms
Nutritious diet, daily folate and iron supplementation
B12 supplementation
Footnotes
1. Anemia in pregnancy is defined as <11.0 g/dL and <33% in 1st and 3rd trimester; <10.5 g/dL and <32% in 2nd trimester.
2. Consider prophylactic transfusion for high-risk patients in conjunction with hematology.

FIGURE 24.5

24-5 Anemia in Pregnancy

IRON DEFICIENCY ANEMIA

A 20-year-old F G3P0 at 20 weeks GA presents with Hgb of 10 on prenatal screening **labs**. Follow-up ferritin level is 12 μg/L.

Management:

1. Iron supplementation (PO or IV). Continue postpartum if ferritin levels have not normalized.
2. Diet changes to incorporate iron-rich foods (eg, animal products, greens).

Complications:

- Mother: Lowered tolerance to blood loss and infection.
- Fetal: Low birth weight, IUGR, prematurity, perinatal mortality.

HYF: Most common cause of anemia in pregnancy.

HEMOGLOBINOPATHIES (EG, SICKLE CELL DISEASE, HB S-C DISEASE, BETA THALASSEMIA, ALPHA THALASSEMIA)

A 20-year-old F with PMH of sickle cell disease presents with acute vaso-occlusive crisis and 1 week of nausea and vomiting. **Exam** is significant for signs of dehydration. On **labs**, CBC shows microcytic anemia. Rapid pregnancy test is (+).

Management:

1. Genetic testing of partner to assess for fetal risk.
2. High-dose daily PO folate supplementation (4 mg/day).
3. Treat underlying disease.
4. Monitor CBC.

Complications:

- Sickle cell disease: Maternal infection, pregnancy-induced hypertension, heart failure, pulmonary infarction, fetal growth restriction, preterm delivery, low birth weight, increased pregnancy termination complications.
- Hb S-C disease: Pulmonary infarction.
- Alpha thalassemia: Hydrops fetalis.

HYF: Diagnosis of fetal hemoglobinopathy should not change obstetric management.

PHYSIOLOGIC ANEMIA IN PREGNANCY

A 28-year-old F G4P2 at 18 weeks GA presents with Hgb of 9 on prenatal screening **labs**. Follow-up ferritin level is 40 μg/L. Peripheral blood smear shows normal morphology.

Management:

1. Monitor CBC levels.

HYF: A diagnosis of exclusion. In pregnancy, plasma volume, RBC volume, and hemoglobin mass all expand, resulting in hemodilution and increased iron demand.

FOLATE DEFICIENCY

A 26-year-old F G2P0 at 10 weeks GA with PMH of epilepsy controlled with carbamazepine presents with oral ulcers. On **labs**, CBC is significant for macrocytic anemia, serum folic acid = 1.7 ng/mL, and serum vitamin B_{12} = 324 pg/mL.

Management:

1. Daily PO folate supplementation.
2. PO iron supplementation.
3. Nutritious diet.

Complications: Increased risk of neural tube defects.

HYF: Most common cause of macrocytic anemia in pregnancy. Very similar clinical presentation to B_{12} deficiency.

B_{12} DEFICIENCY

A 34-year-old F G1P0 with PMH of partial gastrectomy presents with palpitations and numbness in her fingers. On **exam**, she has an erythematous and swollen tongue. On **labs**, CBC is significant for macrocytic anemia, serum folic acid of 5.6 ng/mL, and serum vitamin B_{12} of 178 pg/mL.

Management:

1. Daily vitamin B_{12} supplementation (parenteral if malabsorption is present).

Complications:

- Increased risk of neural tube defects.
- Irreversible neurologic deficits.

HYF: Highly associated with a history of malabsorption (Crohn's disease, celiac disease), autoimmune conditions (thyroid disease, vitiligo), medications (PPIs, metformin, NO). Very similar clinical presentation to folate deficiency but with a more indolent course.

24-6 Abnormal LFTs in Pregnancy

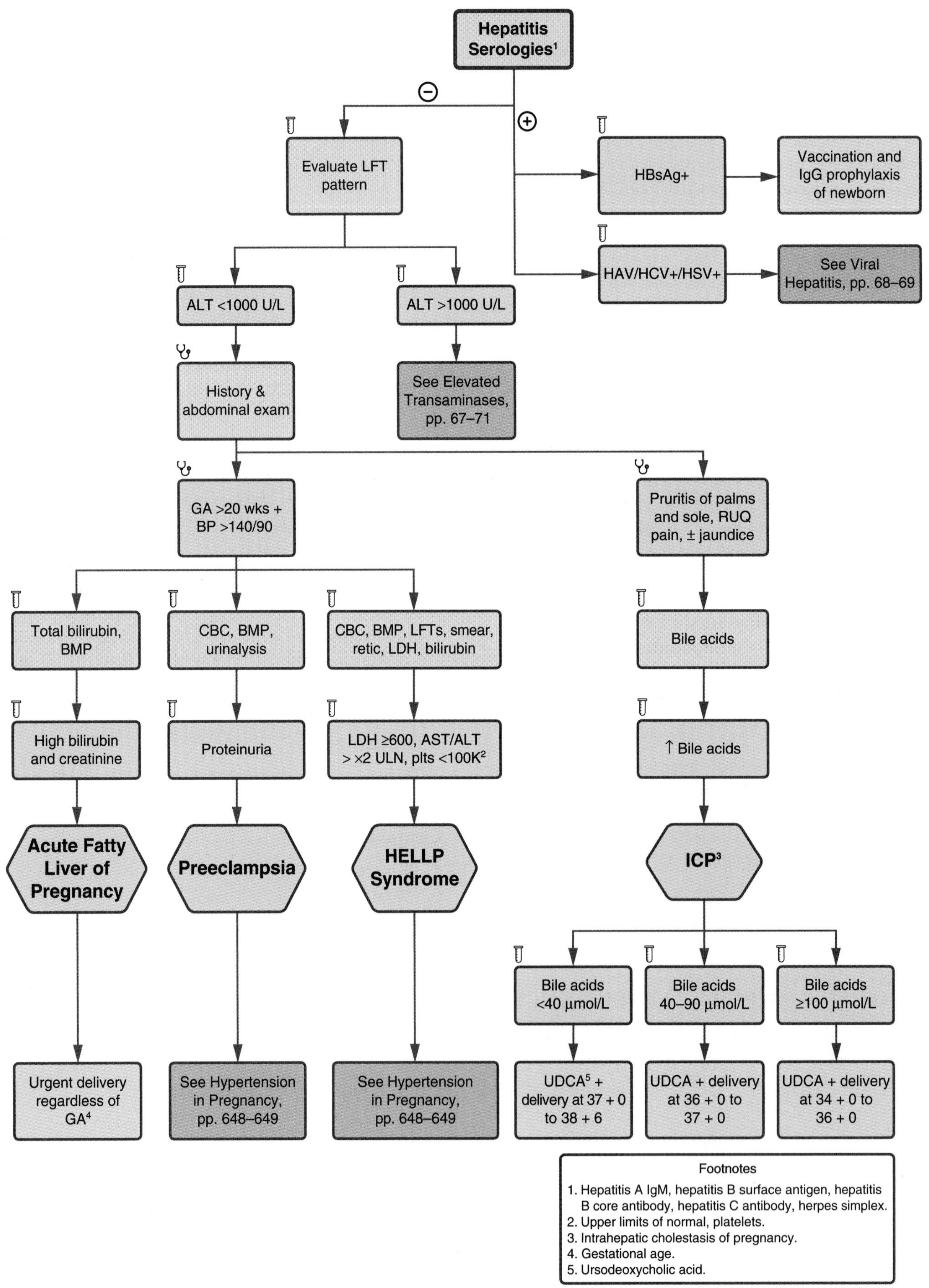

Hepatitis Serologies[1]
⊖
⊕
Evaluate LFT pattern
HBsAg+
Vaccination and IgG prophylaxis of newborn
HAV/HCV+/HSV+
See Viral Hepatitis, pp. 68–69
ALT <1000 U/L
ALT >1000 U/L
History & abdominal exam
See Elevated Transaminases, pp. 67–71
GA >20 wks + BP >140/90
Pruritis of palms and sole, RUQ pain, ± jaundice
Total bilirubin, BMP
CBC, BMP, urinalysis
CBC, BMP, LFTs, smear, retic, LDH, bilirubin
Bile acids
High bilirubin and creatinine
Proteinuria
LDH ≥600, AST/ALT > ×2 ULN, plts <100K[2]
↑ Bile acids
Acute Fatty Liver of Pregnancy
Preeclampsia
HELLP Syndrome
ICP[3]
Bile acids <40 µmol/L
Bile acids 40–90 µmol/L
Bile acids ≥100 µmol/L
Urgent delivery regardless of GA[4]
See Hypertension in Pregnancy, pp. 648–649
See Hypertension in Pregnancy, pp. 648–649
UDCA[5] + delivery at 37 + 0 to 38 + 6
UDCA + delivery at 36 + 0 to 37 + 0
UDCA + delivery at 34 + 0 to 36 + 0
Footnotes
1. Hepatitis A IgM, hepatitis B surface antigen, hepatitis B core antibody, hepatitis C antibody, herpes simplex.
2. Upper limits of normal, platelets.
3. Intrahepatic cholestasis of pregnancy.
4. Gestational age.
5. Ursodeoxycholic acid.

FIGURE 24.6

24-6 Abnormal LFTs in Pregnancy

ACUTE FATTY LIVER OF PREGNANCY

A 27-year-old F G1P0 at 34w0d GA presents with nausea, vomiting, RUQ abdominal pain, and anorexia. On **exam** and **labs**, she is hypertensive and hypoglycemic, with elevated creatinine, LFTs, and total bilirubin.

Management:

1. Prompt delivery of fetus.
2. Monitor chemistries, creatinine, and coagulation status.
3. Treat hypoglycemia, coagulopathy, liver failure, kidney injury as needed.

Complications:

- Hemorrhage.
- Acute kidney injury.
- Liver failure.

HYF: Typically presents between 30 and 38 weeks GA, but can be diagnosed at an earlier GA, or up to 4 days postpartum. 20–40% of patients are also diagnosed with preeclampsia. Approximately 20% of cases associated with long-chain 3-hydroxyacyl-CoA dehydrogenase (LCHAD) deficiency (genetic testing recommended).

INTRAHEPATIC CHOLESTASIS OF PREGNANCY

A 30-year-old F G2P0 at 3w5d presents with pruritis of palms and soles that is worse at night, RUQ abdominal pain, and nausea. On **exam** and **labs**, she is jaundiced with elevated LFTs and bile acids.

Management:

1. Ursodeoxycholic acid.
2. Time of delivery depends on level of bile acids (see algorithm).

Complications:

- Intrauterine demise.
- Meconium-stained amniotic fluid.
- Preterm delivery.
- Neonatal respiratory distress syndrome.
- Stillbirth.

HYF: Etiology likely involves a combination of genetic susceptibility (*MDR3* mutations), hormonal factors (more common in twin pregnancies and the 2nd half of pregnancy), and environmental factors. Fetal/neonatal complications are a result of bile acids crossing the placenta.

24-7 Placental Abnormalities

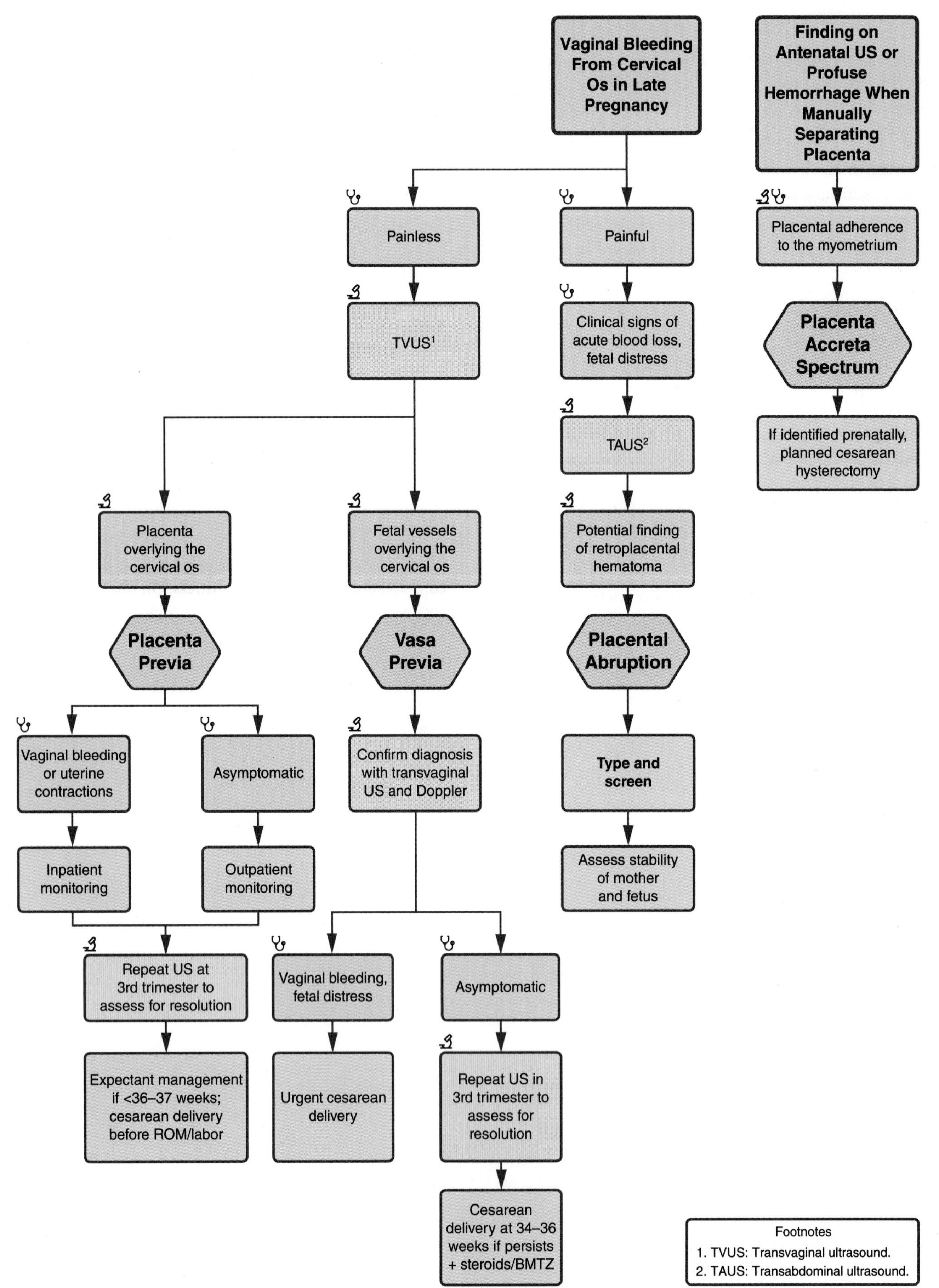
Vaginal Bleeding From Cervical Os in Late Pregnancy
Painless
TVUS[1]
Placenta overlying the cervical os
Placenta Previa
Vaginal bleeding or uterine contractions
Inpatient monitoring
Asymptomatic
Outpatient monitoring
Repeat US at 3rd trimester to assess for resolution
Expectant management if <36–37 weeks; cesarean delivery before ROM/labor
Fetal vessels overlying the cervical os
Vasa Previa
Confirm diagnosis with transvaginal US and Doppler
Vaginal bleeding, fetal distress
Urgent cesarean delivery
Asymptomatic
Repeat US in 3rd trimester to assess for resolution
Cesarean delivery at 34–36 weeks if persists + steroids/BMTZ
Painful
Clinical signs of acute blood loss, fetal distress
TAUS[2]
Potential finding of retroplacental hematoma
Placental Abruption
Type and screen
Assess stability of mother and fetus
Finding on Antenatal US or Profuse Hemorrhage When Manually Separating Placenta
Placental adherence to the myometrium
Placenta Accreta Spectrum
If identified prenatally, planned cesarean hysterectomy
Footnotes
1. TVUS: Transvaginal ultrasound.
2. TAUS: Transabdominal ultrasound.

FIGURE 24.7

24-7 Placental Abnormalities

PLACENTA ACCRETA SPECTRUM

A 39-year-old F G4P3 at 34 weeks GA with PMH of multiple cesarean deliveries presents with painless vaginal bleeding. On **imaging**, TVUS shows multiple irregular-shaped placental lacunae. Doppler shows turbulent blood flow through the lacunae.

Management:

1. Expectant management if <34 weeks.
2. Planned cesarean delivery prior to ROM/labor, immediately followed by total hysterectomy without placental removal.
3. Hemodynamic monitoring of pregnant person.

Complications:

- Severe antenatal hemorrhage in pregnant person.
- Coagulopathy (eg, DIC, VTE, renal failure) in pregnant person.
- Hysterectomy.
- Infection (eg, pneumonia, pyelonephritis, intra-abdominal or wound).
- Preterm birth.

HYF: Highly associated with a history of cesarean sections or other uterine surgeries.

- Placenta accreta: Placental attachment to myometrium without invasion.
- Placenta increta: Placental invasion of myometrial.
- Placenta percreta: Placental invasion beyond myometrium to surrounding structures (eg, bladder).

PLACENTA PREVIA

A 38-year-old F G4P3 at 30 weeks GA with a PMH of cesarean delivery and tobacco use disorder presents with painless, transient vaginal bleeding. On **imaging**, TVUS shows placenta overlying the internal cervical os.

Management:

1. Avoid digital and speculum exams.
2. Inpatient for symptomatic patients (vaginal bleeding or contractions), outpatient for asymptomatic patients.
3. Cesarean delivery prior to rupture of membranes or spontaneous labor; urgent cesarean delivery if fetal distress present.
4. Indications for delivery: Labor, uncontrolled bleeding, fetal distress, 36 weeks GA.

Complications:

- Antepartum hemorrhage in pregnant person.
- Preterm delivery.
- Perinatal mortality.

HYF: 90% of placenta previa cases that are low-lying placentas found at the anatomy US at 18–20 weeks GA will resolve. Resolution is defined as a placental edge >2 cm from the cervical os.

VASA PREVIA

A 28-year-old F G1P0 at 27 weeks GA presents with painless vaginal bleeding. On **imaging**, TVUS shows a low-lying placenta with a linear tubular echolucent body overlying the os. Color Doppler shows flow through this structure.

Management:

1. If vaginal bleeding or fetal distress is present, emergency cesarean delivery.
2. If asymptomatic: Repeat US in late 3rd trimester to assess for resolution, cesarean delivery prior to rupture of membranes/labor with delivery at 34–36 weeks GA.

Complications:

- Fetal hemorrhage, hypoxia, and mortality.
- Preterm delivery.

HYF: Acute vaginal bleeding in vasa previa is an emergency due to the risk of fetal hemorrhage.

PLACENTAL ABRUPTION

A 20-year-old F G1P0 with PMH of HTN presents with abrupt-onset vaginal bleeding and abdominal pain after a motor vehicle accident. **Exam** shows a rigid and tender uterus. Toco shows uterine contractions. FHR shows fetal distress. On **imaging**, US shows retroplacental hematoma.

Management:

1. Inpatient monitoring: IV fluids, IV access, continuous fetal monitoring, quantify blood loss, preparation for blood/blood product replacement (eg, type and screen).
2. Assess stability of birther and fetus.
3. Unstable patient: Urgent resuscitation.
   a. With fetal demise: The delivery method safest for pregnant person.
   b. With fetal viability: Urgent cesarean delivery.
4. Stable patient.
   a. With fetal distress: Urgent cesarean delivery.
   b. With reassuring fetal status: Close inpatient monitoring and expectant management until fetal maturity.
   c. With fetal demise: Vaginal delivery.

Complications:

- Hemorrhage in pregnant person.
- Coagulopathy (eg, DIC, renal failure) in pregnant person.
- Hysterectomy.
- Recurrent placental abruption.

HYF: Highly associated with previous history of abruption, HTN, tobacco use, cocaine use, and trauma to the abdomen.

24-8 Intrauterine Growth Restriction

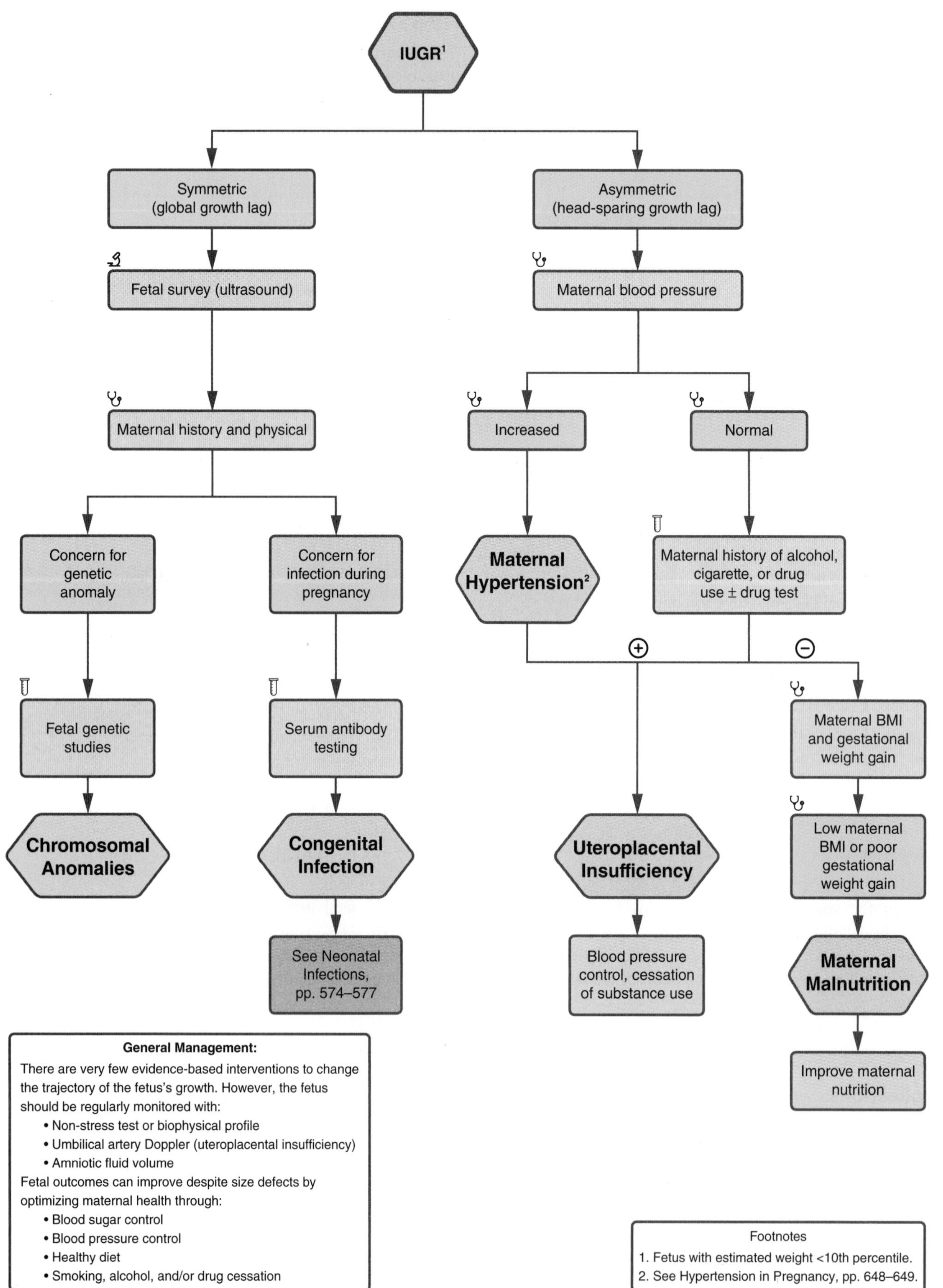
IUGR[1]
Symmetric (global growth lag)
Asymmetric (head-sparing growth lag)
Fetal survey (ultrasound)
Maternal blood pressure
Maternal history and physical
Increased
Normal
Concern for genetic anomaly
Concern for infection during pregnancy
Maternal Hypertension[2]
Maternal history of alcohol, cigarette, or drug use ± drug test
⊕
⊖
Fetal genetic studies
Serum antibody testing
Maternal BMI and gestational weight gain
Chromosomal Anomalies
Congenital Infection
Uteroplacental Insufficiency
Low maternal BMI or poor gestational weight gain
See Neonatal Infections, pp. 574–577
Blood pressure control, cessation of substance use
Maternal Malnutrition
Improve maternal nutrition

General Management:

There are very few evidence-based interventions to change the trajectory of the fetus's growth. However, the fetus should be regularly monitored with:

- Non-stress test or biophysical profile
- Umbilical artery Doppler (uteroplacental insufficiency)
- Amniotic fluid volume

Fetal outcomes can improve despite size defects by optimizing maternal health through:

- Blood sugar control
- Blood pressure control
- Healthy diet
- Smoking, alcohol, and/or drug cessation

Footnotes

1. Fetus with estimated weight <10th percentile.
2. See Hypertension in Pregnancy, pp. 648–649.

FIGURE 24.8

24-8 Intrauterine Growth Restriction

CHROMOSOMAL ABNORMALITIES (EG, TRISOMY 18)

A 27-year-old F G1P0 at 19 weeks GA with no PMH presents for her first prenatal exam. On **imaging**, US reveals estimated fetal weight and head circumference at 7th percentile, with clenched fists, overlapping fingers, and nuchal thickening.

Management:

1. Routine monitoring.

Complications:

- Death in utero.
- In those who survive birth, death within first 2 weeks of life.
- In those who survive to school age, profound intellectual disability.
- Rocker bottom feet.

HYF: Symmetric IUGR prior to 20 weeks suggests chromosomal abnormality.

The fetus in this vignette has Trisomy 18 (PRINCE Edward = **P**rominent occiput, **R**ocker bottom feet, **I**ntellectual disability, **N**ondisjunction, **C**lenched fists with overlapping fingers, low-set **E**ars).

Fetal observation should occur for at least 30 minutes. A normal score is 8 or 10 with normal amniotic fluid. A score of <8 or a score of ≤8 with abnormally low amniotic fluid requires further investigation.

The most common cause of a non-reactive stress test is a sleeping fetus. A nonreactive stress test requires follow-up with BPP.

CONGENITAL INFECTIONS

A 25-year-old F G1P0 at 20 weeks GA with no PMH presents for routine prenatal exam and reports having had a sore throat 3 weeks ago. On **exam**, she has a fundal height of 16 cm. **Imaging** shows an estimated fetal weight and head circumference in the 8th percentile.

Management:

1. Serum CMV IgG and IgM testing.
2. Regular monitoring of fetal growth.

Complications:

- Small-for-gestational-age infant.
- Preterm birth.
- See "Neonatal Infections" for other CMV complications.

HYF: Congenital infections and chromosomal anomalies are the most common causes of symmetric intrauterine growth restriction. TORCH (toxoplasmosis, other, rubella, CMV, HSV) infections can cause intrauterine growth restriction.

UTEROPLACENTAL INSUFFICIENCY

A 35-year-old F G1P0 at 32 weeks GA with PMH of HTN presents for routine prenatal visit. On **exam**, she has fundal height 28 cm. **Imaging** shows estimated fetal weight <10th percentile with head circumference consistent with 32 weeks.

Management:

1. Evaluate and treat any elevated blood pressure (see "Hypertensive Disorders in Pregnancy").
2. Assess for substance use. Counsel on smoking, alcohol, and drug cessation.
3. Routine monitoring with weekly BPP and umbilical artery Dopplers.

Complications:

- Small-for-gestational-age infant.
- Preterm birth.

HYF: Hypertension is a common cause of uteroplacental insufficiency, which is due to lack of sufficient spiral artery development and leads to "head-sparing" fetal growth restriction. Use of various substances in pregnancy may also lead to uteroplacental insufficiency.

Biophysical Profile (BPP)

Variable	2 points for:
Non-stress test	≥2 fetal heart rate (FHR) accelerations of at least 15 secs and 15 bmp
Fetal breathing movements	≥1 episodes of fetal breathing movements lasting 30 secs
Fetal movements	≥1 episodes of extension with return to flexion
Fetal tone	≥3 discrete body or limb movements
Amniotic fluid volume	Single deepest pocket ≥2 cm

MATERNAL MALNUTRITION

A 27-year-old F G2P1 at 29 weeks GA with PMH of anorexia presents for routine prenatal exam. On **exam**, she has normal blood pressure, and her fundal height is 25 cm. **Imaging** shows estimated fetal weight at 7th percentile with head circumference 30th percentile. There is no history of alcohol or drug use.

Management:

1. Measure BMI and assess for sufficient weight gain (see Fetal Size Defects: Macrosomia, pp. 660–661.)
2. Discuss dietary changes and improved nutrition.
3. Routine monitoring with umbilical Doppler.

Complications:

- Small-for-gestational-age infant.
- Preterm birth.

HYF: Low maternal BMI or poor gestational weight gain can lead to intrauterine growth restriction that is asymmetric (head-sparing).

Maternal Hypertension: See pp. 648–649.

24-9 Macrosomia

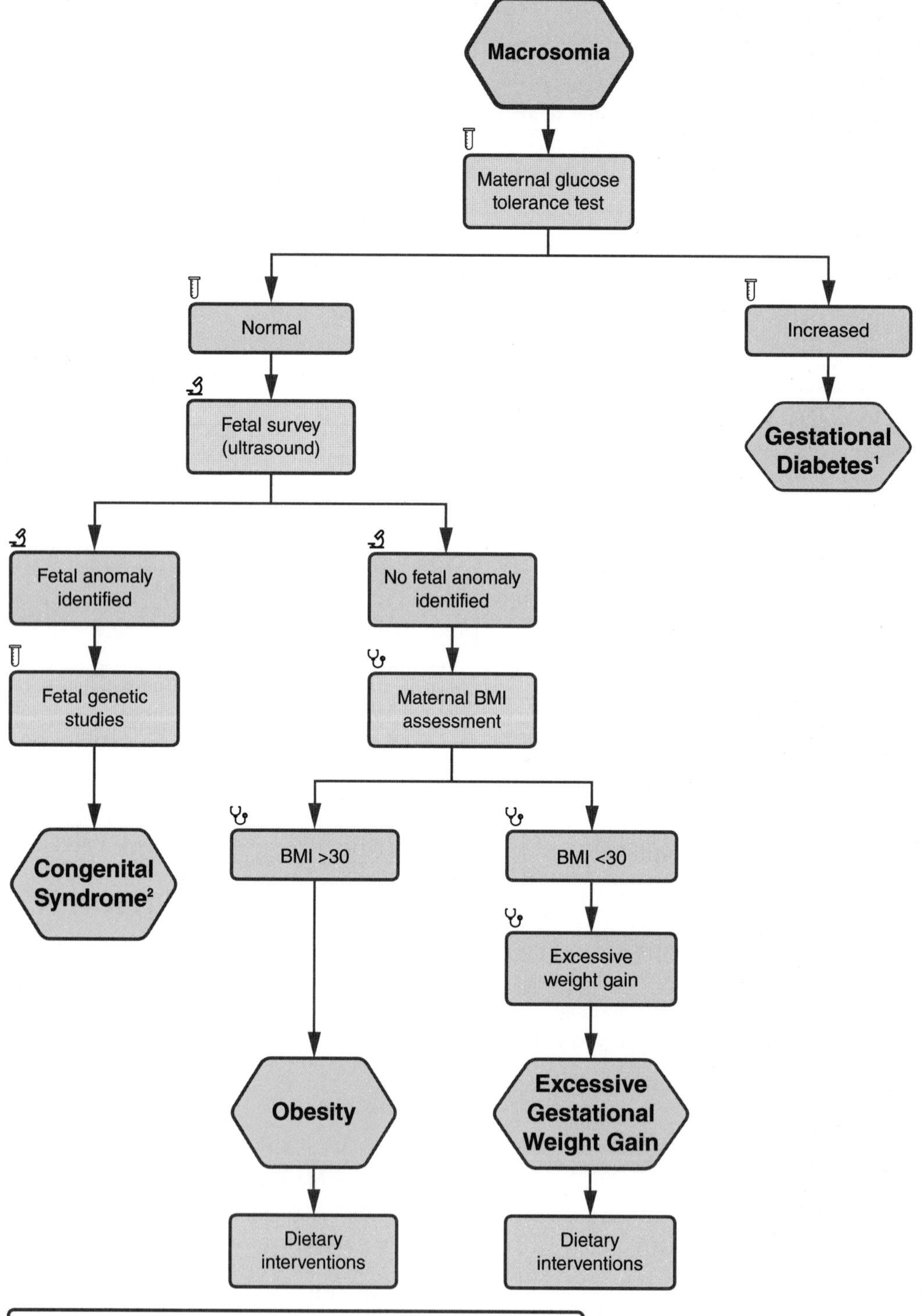
Macrosomia
Maternal glucose tolerance test
Normal
Increased
Gestational Diabetes[1]
Fetal survey (ultrasound)
Fetal anomaly identified
No fetal anomaly identified
Fetal genetic studies
Maternal BMI assessment
Congenital Syndrome[2]
BMI >30
BMI <30
Excessive weight gain
Obesity
Excessive Gestational Weight Gain
Dietary interventions
Dietary interventions

General Management:

There are very few evidence-based interventions to change the trajectory of the fetus's growth. However, the fetus should be regularly monitored with:

- Non-stress test or biophysical profile
- Umbilical artery Doppler (uteroplacental insufficiency)
- Amniotic fluid volume

Fetal outcomes can improve despite size defects by optimizing maternal health through:

- Blood sugar control
- Blood pressure control
- Healthy diet
- Smoking, alcohol, and/or drug cessation

Footnotes

1. See Diabetes in Pregnancy, pp. 650–651.
2. The most common congential syndrome causing macrosomia is Beckwith-Wiedemann.

FIGURE 24.9

24-9 Macrosomia

OBESITY

A 25-year-old F G3P2 at 32 weeks GA with no PMH presents for routine prenatal visit. On **exam**, she has a fundal height of 36 cm and BMI 37. **Imaging** shows estimated fetal weight at 97th percentile.

Management:

1. Dietary and lifestyle modifications.

Complications:

- Shoulder dystocia.
- Operative or cesarean delivery.
- Uterine rupture.
- Postpartum hemorrhage.
- Neonatal hypoglycemia.
- Neonatal polycythemia.
- Neonatal respiratory distress.

HYF: Obesity is a prominent risk factor for fetal macrosomia.

EXCESSIVE GESTATIONAL WEIGHT GAIN

A 23-year-old F G1P0 at 25 weeks GA with no PMH presents for routine prenatal visit. On **exam**, she has a fundal height of 28 cm and BMI 25. **Imaging** shows estimated fetal weight at 92nd percentile.

Management:

1. Assess gestational weight gain trajectory.
2. Dietary and lifestyle modification.

Complications: See Obesity above.

HYF: Excessive gestational weight gain is a risk factor for macrosomia irrespective of maternal BMI.

GESTATIONAL DIABETES

A 29-year-old F G2P1 at 26 weeks GA with no PMH presents for routine prenatal visit. On **exam**, she has a fundal height of 30 cm. **Imaging** shows estimated fetal weight at 98th percentile.

Management:

1. 1-hour glucose tolerance test.
2. If abnormal, 30-hour glucose tolerance test.
3. Lifestyle changes, blood sugar monitoring, and insulin if needed (see Diabetes in Pregnancy, pp. 650–651).
4. Continue monitoring fetal growth.

Complications: See Diabetes in Pregnancy.

HYF: See Diabetes in Pregnancy.

CONGENITAL SYNDROME (BECKWITH-WIEDEMANN)

A 32-year-old F G1P0 at 28 weeks GA with no PMH presents for routine prenatal visit. On **exam**, her fundal height is 32 cm and estimated fetal weight is 95th percentile. On **labs**, blood glucose testing is normal. On **imaging**, fetal US shows macroglossia.

Management:

1. Monitoring and treatment for hypoglycemia postnatally.
2. Management of any breathing or feeding difficulties arising from macroglossia.
3. Omphalocele repair.

Complications:

- Feeding and breathing difficulties.
- Wilms' tumor.
- Hepatoblastoma.
- Kidney abnormalities.
- Organ enlargement.
- Unusual ear creases and pits.

HYF: Beckwith-Wiedemann is the most common syndrome causing macrosomia.

Gestational Weight Gain

Pre-pregnancy BMI	Appropriate weight gain
< 18.5	28–40 lbs
18.5 to 24.9	25–35 lbs
25.0 to 29.9	15–25 lbs
≥ 30.0	11–20 lbs

24-10 Trophoblastic Disease

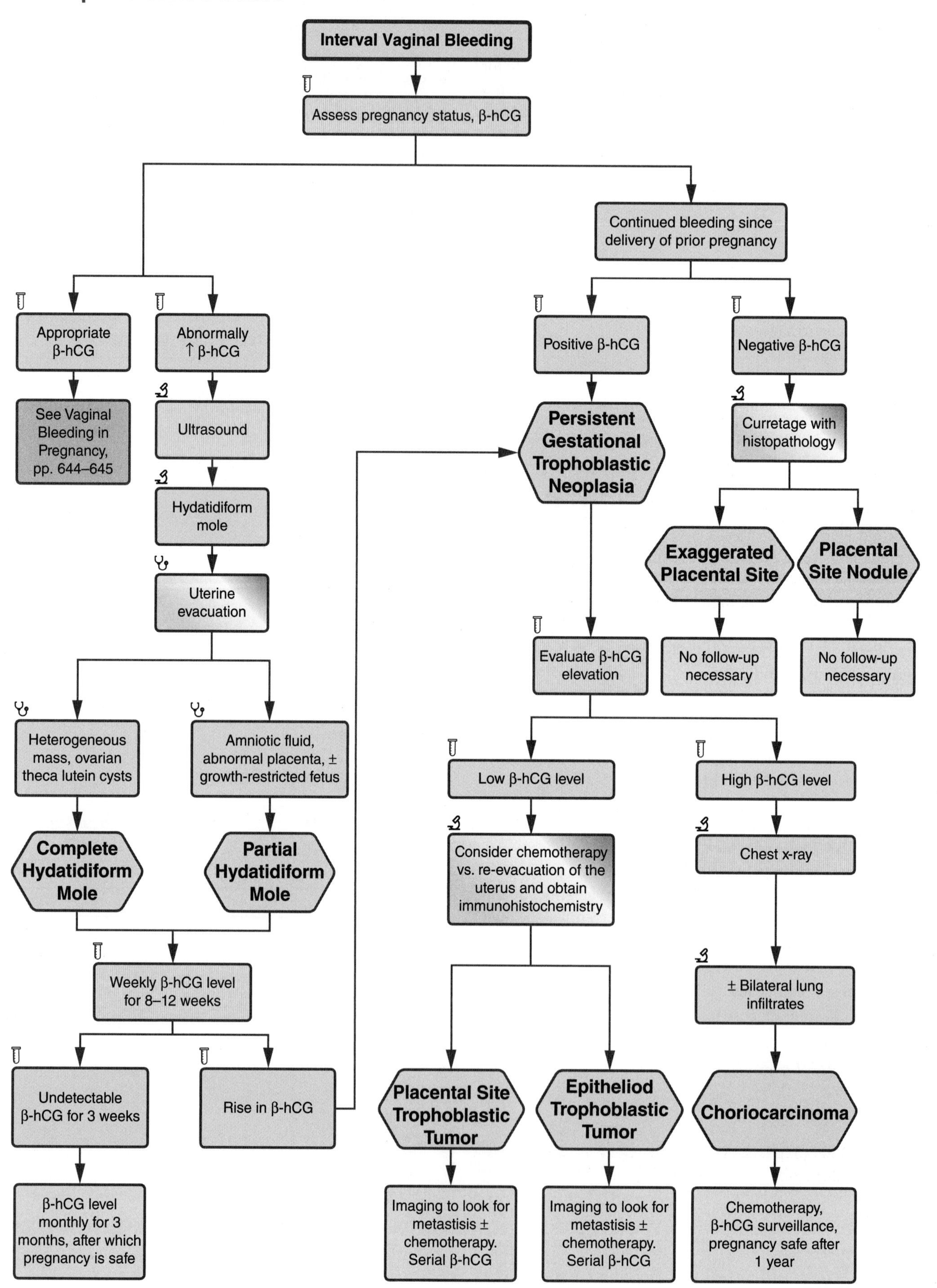
Interval Vaginal Bleeding
Assess pregnancy status, β-hCG
Continued bleeding since delivery of prior pregnancy
Appropriate β-hCG
Abnormally ↑ β-hCG
Positive β-hCG
Negative β-hCG
See Vaginal Bleeding in Pregnancy, pp. 644–645
Ultrasound
Persistent Gestational Trophoblastic Neoplasia
Curretage with histopathology
Hydatidiform mole
Exaggerated Placental Site
Placental Site Nodule
Uterine evacuation
Evaluate β-hCG elevation
No follow-up necessary
No follow-up necessary
Heterogeneous mass, ovarian theca lutein cysts
Amniotic fluid, abnormal placenta, ± growth-restricted fetus
Low β-hCG level
High β-hCG level
Complete Hydatidiform Mole
Partial Hydatidiform Mole
Consider chemotherapy vs. re-evacuation of the uterus and obtain immunohistochemistry
Chest x-ray
Weekly β-hCG level for 8–12 weeks
± Bilateral lung infiltrates
Undetectable β-hCG for 3 weeks
Rise in β-hCG
Placental Site Trophoblastic Tumor
Epitheliod Trophoblastic Tumor
Choriocarcinoma
β-hCG level monthly for 3 months, after which pregnancy is safe
Imaging to look for metastisis ± chemotherapy. Serial β-hCG
Imaging to look for metastisis ± chemotherapy. Serial β-hCG
Chemotherapy, β-hCG surveillance, pregnancy safe after 1 year

FIGURE 24.10

24-10 Trophoblastic Disease

EXAGGERATED PLACENTAL SITE

A 30-year-old F G1P0 with PMH of recent spontaneous abortion presents with postpartum bleeding. **Exam** shows a normal-size uterus. **Labs** reveal normal β-hCG level. On **imaging**, US shows echogenic lesions in the uterine cavity.

Management:

1. Curettage and pathologic review.
2. No further treatment or follow-up necessary.

Complications: Risk of postpartum hemorrhage.

HYF: Can occur following normal pregnancy, ectopic pregnancy, abortion, or hydatidiform mole. Excellent prognosis following curettage.

PLACENTAL SITE NODULE

A 29-year-old F G3P1 with PMH of dilation and curettage (D&C) 3 years ago presents with irregular menstrual bleeding. On **exam**, she has a normal-size uterus. **Labs** reveal normal β-hCG. On **imaging**, US shows thickened endometrium.

Management:

1. Removal by D&C and histopathology to confirm diagnosis.
2. No additional treatment or follow-up necessary.

Complications: Benign, without malignant potential.

HYF: An uncommon cause of abnormal bleeding post-pregnancy. Can present years after pregnancy.

COMPLETE HYDATIDIFORM MOLE

A 19-year-old F G1P0 at 12 weeks GA presents with vaginal bleeding, hyperemesis gravidarum, and nausea. **Exam** shows bloody discharge with clear vesicles in the vaginal vault. **Labs** show a β-hCG of >100,000.

Management:

1. D&C.
2. Regular β-hCG monitoring.

Complications:

- Persistent gestational trophoblastic neoplasia (15–20% continue to grow after D&C).
- Progression to choriocarcinoma (3%).
- Risk of future molar pregnancy (<1%).
- Sepsis.

HYF: 1–3 in 1000 pregnancies. More frequently at age extremes (<15 or >45). "Snowstorm uterus" on US. Diploid and no fetal parts.

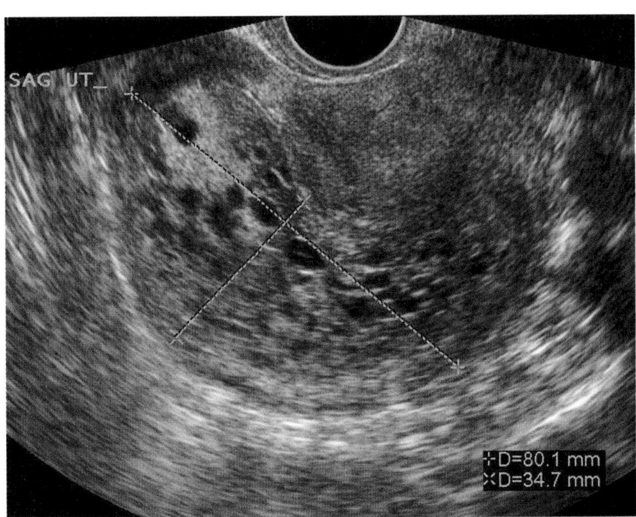
SAG UT
D=80.1 mm
D=34.7 mm

A complete hydatidiform mole with the characteristic "snowstorm" appearance on ultrasound.

PARTIAL HYDATIDIFORM MOLE

A 41-year-old F G1P0 at 10 weeks GA presents with vaginal bleeding. **Exam** shows a uterus greater than gravid date. **Labs** show abnormally elevated β-hCG. On **imaging**, cysts are seen in the uterus on US.

Management:

1. D&C.
2. Serial β-hCG monitoring.

Complications:

- Small risk of persistent gestational trophoblastic neoplasia or choriocarcinoma.
- Risk of future molar pregnancy (<1%).

HYF: Triploid and contains some fetal parts.

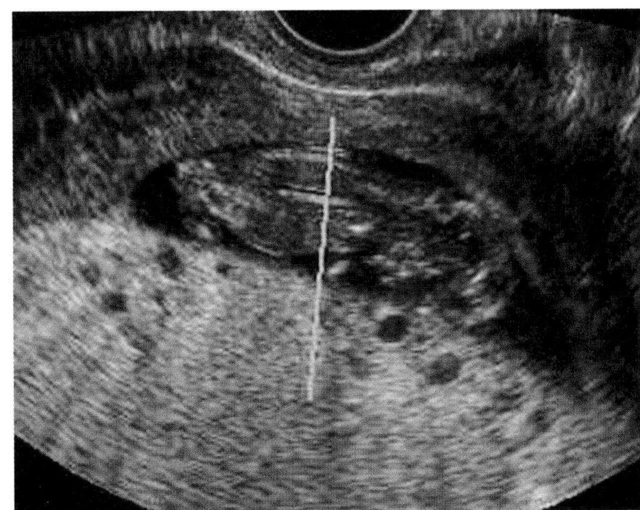

A partial hydatidiform mole on ultrasound.

(Continued)

24-10 Trophoblastic Disease

PLACENTAL SITE TROPHOBLASTIC TUMOR (PSTT)

A 32-year-old F with a full-term pregnancy 1 year ago presents with irregular vaginal bleeding, enlarged uterus, and a slightly elevated β-hCG.

Management:

1. US-guided D&C.
2. CXR or CT.
3. Hysterectomy with lymph node dissection.
4. ± chemotherapy depending on risk factors.

Complications:

- Metastasis to lungs and pelvic region.
- Less responsive to chemotherapy.

HYF: Extremely rare (1 in 100,000 pregnancies).

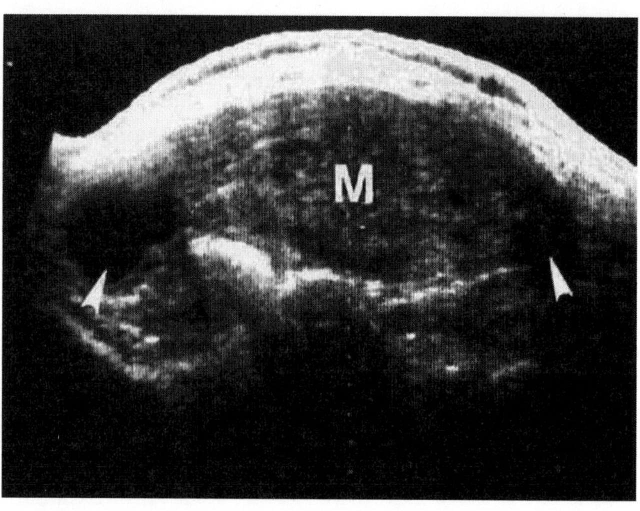
M

Trophoblastic disease. Transverse scan of the pelvis with a hydatidiform mole (M) and ovarian theca lutein cysts (*arrowheads*).

EPITHELIOID TROPHOBLASTIC TUMOR (ETT)

A 25-year-old F G1P1 presents with irregular vaginal bleeding. **Exam** shows enlarged uterus. **Labs** reveal a slightly elevated β-hCG.

Management:

1. Surgery.
2. Chemotherapy.

Complications:

- Relatively resistant to chemotherapy.
- Often misdiagnosed initially as choriocarcinoma, which can delay definitive surgical treatment.

HYF: ETT makes up 1% of all gestational trophoblastic neoplasias. Hysterectomy and surgical excision of metastases are the mainstays of treatment given chemoresistance.

CHORIOCARCINOMA

A 40-year-old F with PMH of spontaneous abortion 5 months ago presents with vaginal bleeding. On **exam**, she has an enlarged, soft uterus. **Labs** show elevated β-hCG.

Management:

1. D&C.
2. Chest x-ray, MRI, or CT to look for metastasis.
3. ± chemotherapy (methotrexate).
4. Serial β-hCG.

Complications:

- Metastasis (most commonly to the lungs, liver, brain).

HYF: Develops from a hydatidiform mole or following a spontaneous abortion. Choriocarcinoma has a 90–100% cure rate with chemotherapy.

24-11 Amniotic Fluid Abnormalities

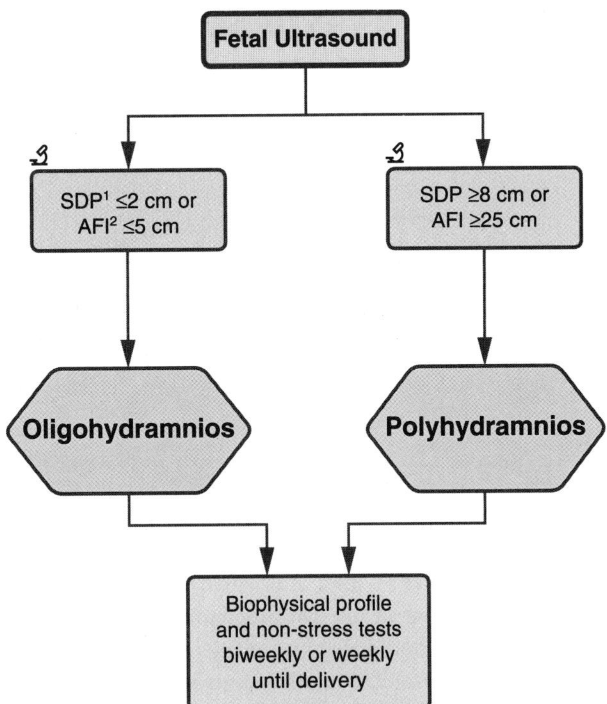
Fetal Ultrasound
SDP[1] ≤2 cm or AFI[2] ≤5 cm
SDP ≥8 cm or AFI ≥25 cm
Oligohydramnios
Polyhydramnios
Biophysical profile and non-stress tests biweekly or weekly until delivery

Common causes of oligohydramnios:

1. Fetal urinary tract abnormalities (renal agenesis, cystic renal disease, GU obstruction).
2. Uteroplacental insufficiency.
3. Rupture of membranes.
4. Postterm pregnancy (>41 weeks).
5. Placental abruption.
6. TORCH and other infections affecting the fetus.
7. Idiopathic.

Common causes of polyhydramnios:

1. GI tract abnormalities (tracheoesophageal fistula, anencephaly, duodenal atresia).
2. Pulmonary malformations.
3. Multiple gestation.
4. Maternal diabetes.
5. Aneuploidy.
6. Twin-twin transfusion syndrome.
7. High fetal cardiac output states (alloimmunization, parvovirus 19, fetomaternal hemorrhage, alpha thalessemia, G6PD deficiency).
8. Idiopathic.

Footnotes

1. SDP: Measurement of the single deepest fluid pocket.
2. AFI: Amniotic fluid index (sum of 4 largest pockets in specific areas around the fetus).

FIGURE 24.11

24-11 Amniotic Fluid Abnormalities

OLIGOHYDRAMNIOS

A 28-year-old F G1P0 at 35 weeks with PMH of uteroplacental insufficiency presents for routine prenatal visit. **Exam** shows uterine size less than expected for gestational age. On **imaging**, US shows amniotic fluid index of ≤5 cm.

Management:

1. Rule out inaccurate gestational dates.
2. Rule out PROM.
3. US evaluation of fetal and placental anatomy.
4. Plan delivery based on gestational age and fetal assessment.
5. Routine antenatal testing with BPP and non-stress tests.

Complications:

- Associated with 40-fold increase in prenatal mortality.
- Musculoskeletal abnormalities (clubfoot, facial distortion), pulmonary hypoplasia, umbilical cord compression, and intrauterine growth restriction.

HYF: Etiologies include fetal urinary tract abnormalities (renal agenesis, GU obstruction), chronic uteroplacental insufficiency, post-term pregnancy (>41 weeks), or rupture of membranes.

POLYHYDRAMNIOS

A 30-year-old F G1P0 with PMH of DM presents for prenatal visit. On **exam**, she has a fundal height greater than expected for gestational age. **Labs** are consistent with gestational diabetes. On **imaging**, US shows an amniotic fluid index of 30 cm.

Management:

1. US for fetal anomalies.
2. Rule out maternal diabetes.
3. Biophysical profile and nonstress tests weekly or biweekly until delivery, depending on severity of polyhydramnios.

Complications:

- Preterm birth.
- Placental abruption.
- Fetal anomalies.

HYF: 40% of polyhydramnios cases are idiopathic. May be present in normal pregnancies, but fetal chromosomal abnormalities should also be considered. Other etiologies include maternal DM, multiple gestation, isoimmunization, pulmonary abnormalities (cystic lung malformations), fetal GI tract abnormalities (duodenal atresia, tracheoesophageal fistula, anencephaly), and twin-twin transfusion syndrome.

24-12 Preterm Labor

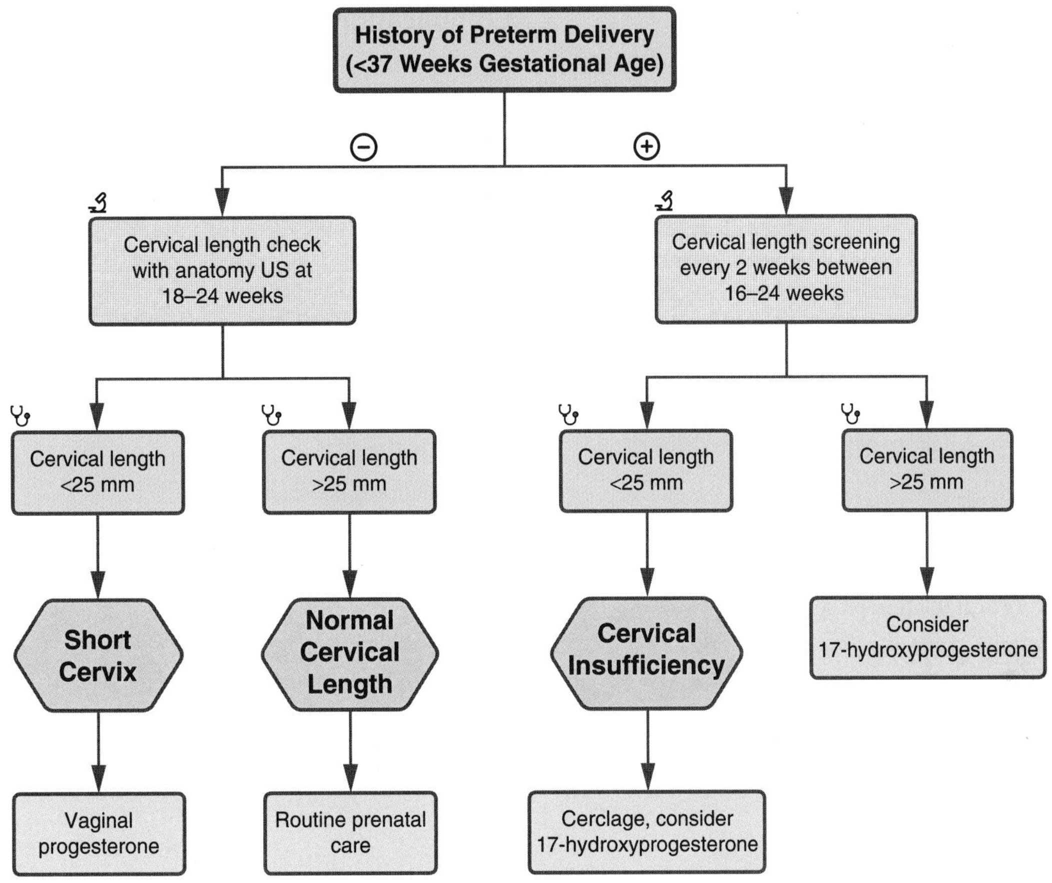
History of Preterm Delivery (<37 Weeks Gestational Age)
⊖
⊕
Cervical length check with anatomy US at 18–24 weeks
Cervical length screening every 2 weeks between 16–24 weeks
Cervical length <25 mm
Cervical length >25 mm
Cervical length <25 mm
Cervical length >25 mm
Short Cervix
Normal Cervical Length
Cervical Insufficiency
Consider 17-hydroxyprogesterone
Vaginal progesterone
Routine prenatal care
Cerclage, consider 17-hydroxyprogesterone

FIGURE 24.12

24-12 Preterm Labor

HISTORY OF PRETERM LABOR

A 34-year-old F G2P1 at 20 weeks GA with PMH of preterm labor presents for routine prenatal care. On exam, her cervical os is closed. On imaging, TVUS shows cervical length of 30 mm.

Management:

1. If cervical length <25 mm on TVUS, offer cerclage. If cervical >25 mm on TVUS, continue cervical length screening until 24 weeks and consider progesterone supplementation.

Complications: Preterm delivery.

HYF: Preterm labor is the #1 cause of adverse neonatal outcomes. The greatest risk factor is a history of prior preterm delivery.

CERVICAL INSUFFICIENCY

A 29-year-old F G3P0 at 10 weeks GA with PMH of 2 mid-trimester losses after painless cervical dilation presents with 1 mm of cervical dilation on exam.

Management:

1. Offer history-indicated cerclage at 12–14 weeks.

Complications: Preterm delivery.

HYF: Cervical insufficiency is suggested by the presence of both: 1) 1+ prior early preterm births and/or 2nd-trimester losses, and 2) TVUS cervical length <25 mm or cervical dilatation (eg, >1 cm) on digital exam (before 24 weeks GA).

SHORT CERVIX

A 36-year-old F G2P21 at 22 weeks GA with PMH of 1 prior full-term delivery presents with incidentally found short cervix on TVUS.

Management:

1. Vaginal progesterone.

Complications: Preterm delivery.

HYF: An incidentally found short cervix on routine TVUS increases the risk of a preterm delivery.

24-13 Fetal Heart Tracing

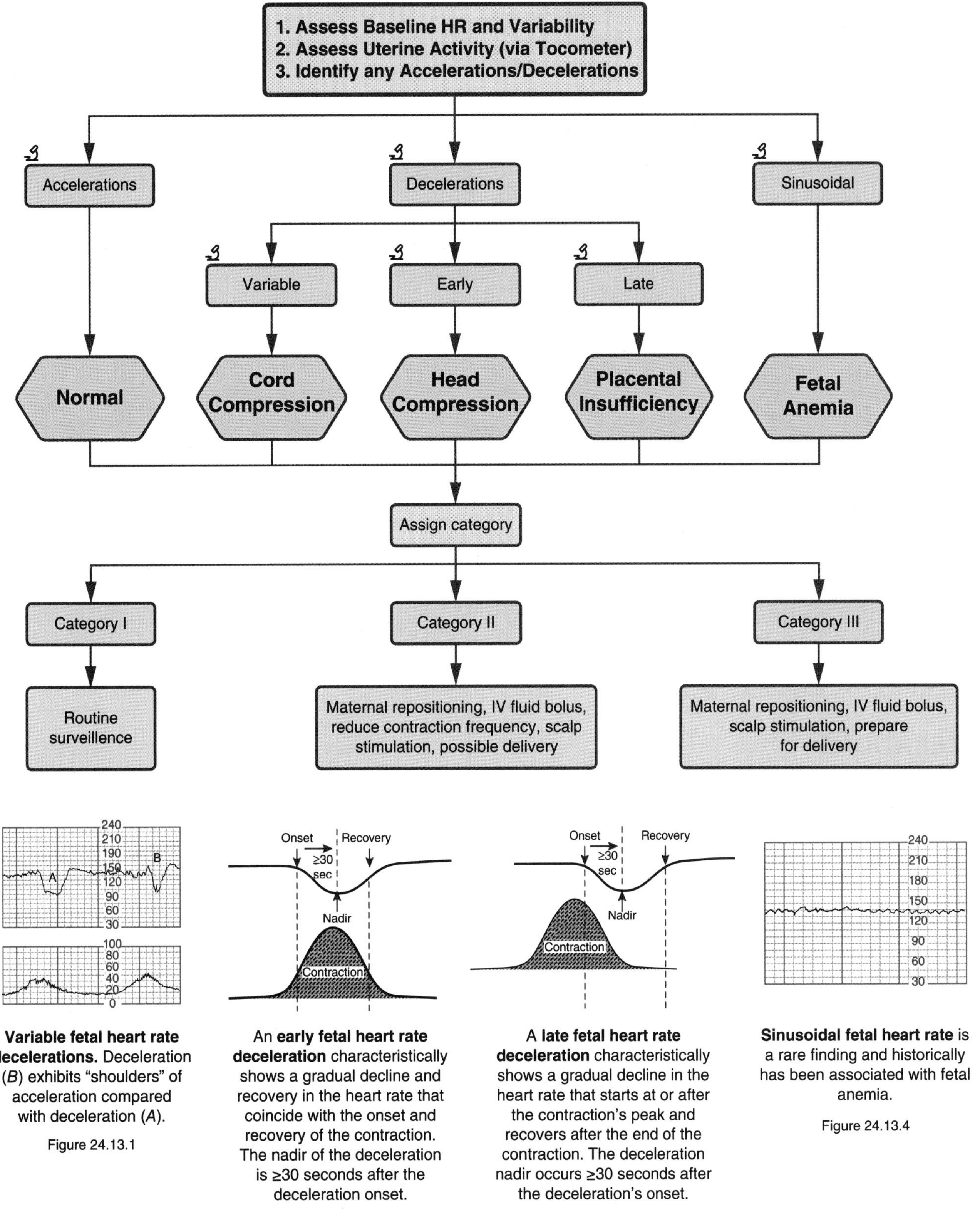
1. Assess Baseline HR and Variability
2. Assess Uterine Activity (via Tocometer)
3. Identify any Accelerations/Decelerations
Accelerations
Decelerations
Sinusoidal
Variable
Early
Late
Normal
Cord Compression
Head Compression
Placental Insufficiency
Fetal Anemia
Assign category
Category I
Category II
Category III
Routine surveillence
Maternal repositioning, IV fluid bolus, reduce contraction frequency, scalp stimulation, possible delivery
Maternal repositioning, IV fluid bolus, scalp stimulation, prepare for delivery
240
210
190
150
120
90
60
30
A
B
100
80
60
40
20
0
Onset
Recovery
≥30 sec
Nadir
Contraction
Onset
Recovery
≥30 sec
Nadir
Contraction
240
210
180
150
120
90
60
30

Variable fetal heart rate decelerations. Deceleration (*B*) exhibits "shoulders" of acceleration compared with deceleration (*A*).

Figure 24.13.1

An **early fetal heart rate deceleration** characteristically shows a gradual decline and recovery in the heart rate that coincide with the onset and recovery of the contraction. The nadir of the deceleration is ≥30 seconds after the deceleration onset.

Figure 24.13.2

A **late fetal heart rate deceleration** characteristically shows a gradual decline in the heart rate that starts at or after the contraction's peak and recovers after the end of the contraction. The deceleration nadir occurs ≥30 seconds after the deceleration's onset.

Figure 24.13.3

Sinusoidal fetal heart rate is a rare finding and historically has been associated with fetal anemia.

Figure 24.13.4

FIGURE 24.13

24-13 Fetal Heart Tracing

Fetal heart rate (FHR) monitoring is conducted either through external monitoring (Doppler ultrasound) or through an electrode attached to the fetal scalp. It is used to monitor fetal activity prenatally and during labor.

Components of a FHR evaluation include:

1. Baseline heart rate.
2. Variability.
3. Accelerations.
4. Decelerations.

BASELINE HEART RATES

- Normal: 110–160 beats per minute (bpm).
- Bradycardia: <110 bpm.
- Tachycardia: >160 bpm.

VARIABILITY

Variability is defined as fluctuations, irregular in amplitude and frequency, of the FHR around the baseline.

Absent	Indicates severe fetal acidemia
Minimal	<6 bpm; indicates fetal hypoxia, effects of opioids/ magnesium, fetal sleep cycle
Normal	6–25 bpm
Marked	>25 bpm; indicates fetal hypoxia, may portend a decrease in variability
Sinusoidal	A wave-link pattern with a cyclical frequency of 3–5 BPM

ACCELERATIONS

Accelerations are defined as a sudden FHR increase 15 of bpm above baseline. Duration of an acceleration must be <30 sec from onset to peak, with a duration of >15 sec and <2 min.

DECELERATIONS

Decelerations are defined as a decrease in FHR below baseline either associated (early/late) or unassociated (variable) with uterine contractions.

Early	Gradual decrease in FHR (onset to nadir >30 sec), nadir occurs at the same time as the peak of the contraction Cause: Head compression
Late	Gradual decrease in FHR (onset to nadir >30 sec), nadir occurs after the peak of the contraction Cause: Uteroplacental insufficiency
Variable	Abrupt decrease in FHR (onset to nadir <30 sec) of >15 bpm lasting ≥15 sec but <2 min Cause: Cord compression

VEaL CHoP: Variable decelerations = **C**ord compression, **E**arly decelerations = **H**ead compression, (**A**ccelerations = **O**kay), **L**ate decelerations = **P**lacental insufficiency.

CATEGORIZING FETAL HEART TRACINGS

Fetal heart tracings are assigned a category based on the appearance and features present. Category I tracings are normal, II are intermediate, and III are abnormal.

I	Normal baseline rate Moderate baseline variability No late/variable decelerations ± early decelerations
II	All tracings not categorized as I or III. Examples: Minimal/marked variability, prolonged decelerations, variable decelerations with prolonged return to baseline, recurrent late/variable decelerations with minimal/moderate variability
III	Absent variability and any of the following: 1. Recurrent late decelerations 2. Recurrent variable decelerations 3. Bradycardia 4. Sinusoidal pattern

Category II/III tracings require investigation into the cause of fetal distress. Repositioning, discontinuation of uterotonics, IV fluid bolus, correction of hypotension, modification of pushing efforts, scalp stimulation, and other interventions are often attempted. For persistently poor tracings, cesarean delivery is generally recommended.

24-14 Onset of Labor

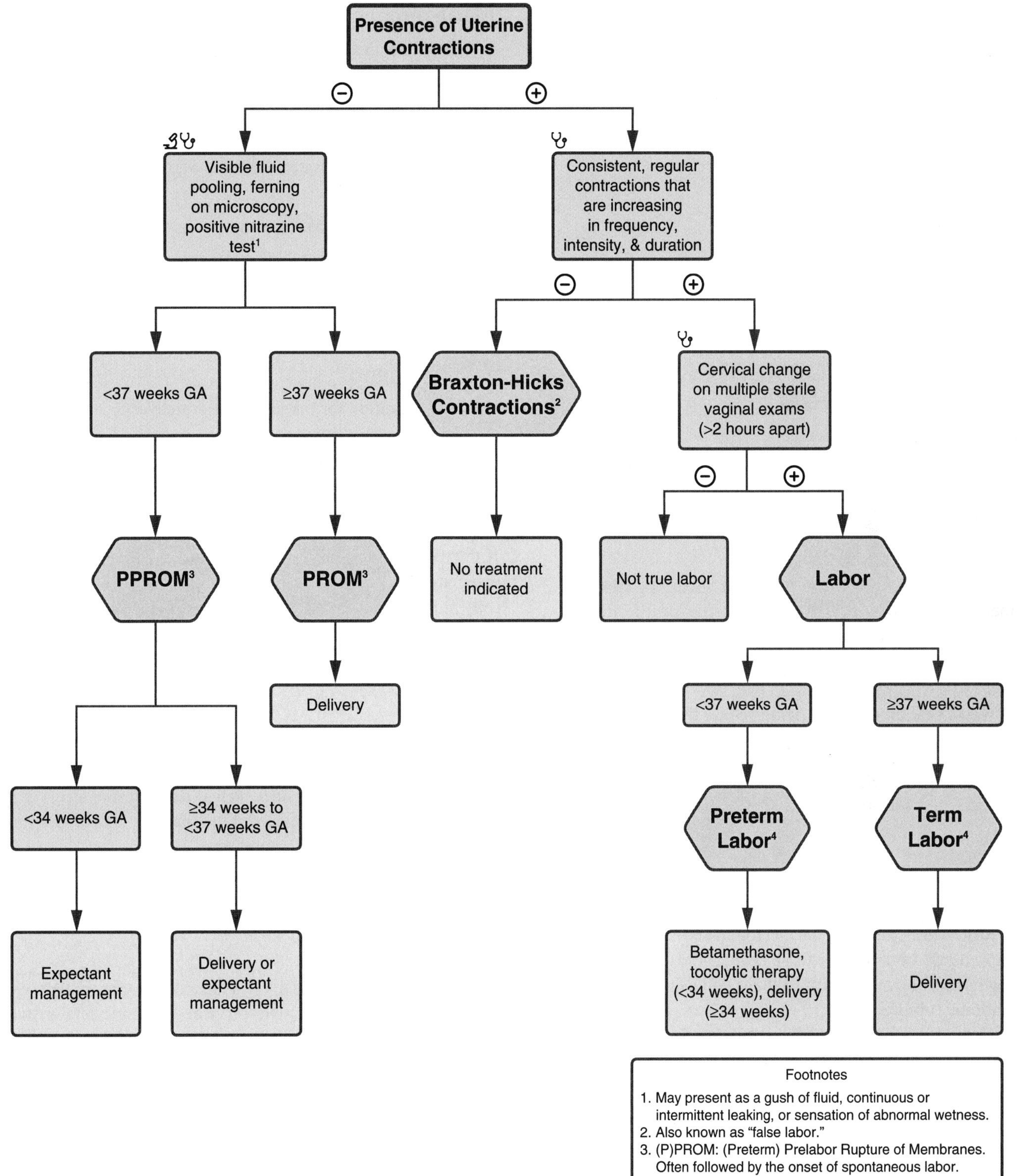
Presence of Uterine Contractions
⊖
⊕
Visible fluid pooling, ferning on microscopy, positive nitrazine test[1]
Consistent, regular contractions that are increasing in frequency, intensity, & duration
⊖
⊕
<37 weeks GA
≥37 weeks GA
Braxton-Hicks Contractions[2]
Cervical change on multiple sterile vaginal exams (>2 hours apart)
⊖
⊕
PPROM[3]
PROM[3]
No treatment indicated
Not true labor
Labor
Delivery
<37 weeks GA
≥37 weeks GA
<34 weeks GA
≥34 weeks to <37 weeks GA
Preterm Labor[4]
Term Labor[4]
Expectant management
Delivery or expectant management
Betamethasone, tocolytic therapy (<34 weeks), delivery (≥34 weeks)
Delivery
Footnotes
1. May present as a gush of fluid, continuous or intermittent leaking, or sensation of abnormal wetness.
2. Also known as "false labor."
3. (P)PROM: (Preterm) Prelabor Rupture of Membranes. Often followed by the onset of spontaneous labor.
4. Preterm: <37 weeks GA. Term: ≥37 weeks GA.

FIGURE 24.14

24-14 Onset of Labor

BRAXTON-HICKS CONTRACTIONS

A 28-year-old F G1P0 at 38w5d presents with 8 hours of irregular uterine cramping. **Exam** shows an undilated cervix. On **imaging**, transabdominal US reveals a cephalic fetal presentation with a normal amniotic fluid index.

Management: No treatment indicated.

Complications: None.

HYF: Braxton-Hicks contractions (also known as "false labor") may wane over time or may progress to the latent phase of true labor.

PRETERM PRELABOR RUPTURE OF MEMBRANES (PPROM)

A 30-year-old F G3P2 at 27 weeks presents with increased vaginal discharge. **Exam** reveals pooling of clear, nitrazine-positive fluid in the vagina with evidence of ferning. On **imaging**, transabdominal US shows an amniotic fluid index of 3 cm.

Management:

1. <34 weeks GA: Expectant management, including latency antibiotics, corticosteroids, and monitoring for infection.
2. ≥34 weeks to 37 weeks GA: Expectant management or immediate delivery, using shared decision-making with the patient to navigate the balance of benefits and risks.
3. ≥37 weeks GA: Immediate delivery, either by induction of labor or cesarean section.

Complications:

- Maternal: Intra- or postpartum infection (ie, chorioamnionitis), placental abruption, preterm delivery.
- Fetal: Complications of prematurity (respiratory distress, sepsis, necrotizing enterocolitis).

HYF: Risk factors for PPROM include history of prior PPROM, genital tract infection, antepartum bleeding, and cigarette smoking. Most patients who present with PPROM will deliver within 1 week of membrane rupture.

PRELABOR RUPTURE OF MEMBRANES (PROM)

A 30-year-old F G3P2 at 37 weeks presents after feeling a "gush of fluid." **Exam** shows pooling of clear, nitrazine-positive fluid in the vagina with evidence of ferning. On **imaging**, transabdominal US reveals a cephalic fetal presentation with an amniotic fluid index of 3 cm.

Management:

1. Immediate delivery, either by induction of labor or cesarean section.

Complications: Maternal and/or fetal infection.

HYF: PROM complicates about 8% of pregnancies.

PRETERM LABOR

A 17-year-old F G1P0 at 29w4d presents with regular, painful uterine contractions for the past 6 hours. Pelvic **exam** shows cervical dilation of 3 cm. On **imaging**, transvaginal ultrasound shows cervical length of 2.5 cm.

Management:

1. Hospitalization for management or delivery.
2. Betamethasone to reduce the risks associated with neonatal prematurity.
3. Tocolytic therapy (indomethacin) to delay delivery.
4. ≥34 weeks GA = delivery.

Complications: Preterm birth, neonatal complications of prematurity.

HYF: Preterm labor does not necessarily result in preterm birth. Preterm labor precedes about 50% of preterm births, and <10% of patients with diagnosed preterm labor will deliver within 7 days.

TERM LABOR

A 24-year-old F G2P1 at 39w1d presents with regular, painful contractions for the past 4 hours. Pelvic **exam** shows a cervix that is 4 cm dilated and 90% effaced. On **imaging**, transabdominal US reveals a cephalic fetal presentation.

Management: Admission for delivery.

Complications: None.

HYF: Labor consists of a 1st stage (onset to complete cervical dilation), 2nd stage (complete cervical dilation to fetal expulsion), and 3rd stage (fetal expulsion to placental expulsion). See Stages of Labor and Fetal Presentation, pp. 673–674.

24-15 Stages of Labor

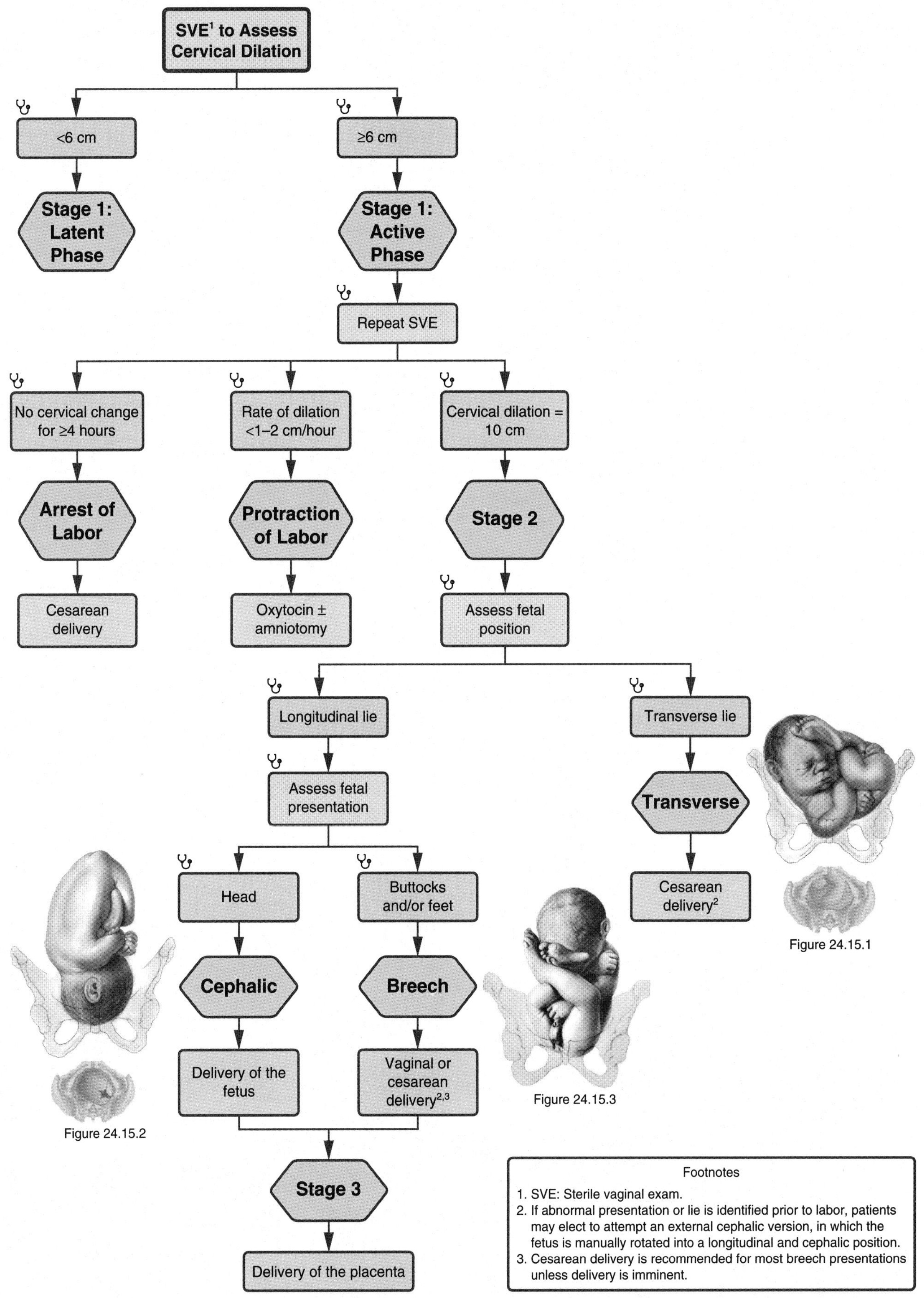
SVE[1] to Assess Cervical Dilation
<6 cm
≥6 cm
Stage 1: Latent Phase
Stage 1: Active Phase
Repeat SVE
No cervical change for ≥4 hours
Rate of dilation <1–2 cm/hour
Cervical dilation = 10 cm
Arrest of Labor
Protraction of Labor
Stage 2
Cesarean delivery
Oxytocin ± amniotomy
Assess fetal position
Longitudinal lie
Transverse lie
Assess fetal presentation
Transverse
Head
Buttocks and/or feet
Cesarean delivery[2]
Cephalic
Breech
Delivery of the fetus
Vaginal or cesarean delivery[2,3]
Stage 3
Delivery of the placenta
Figure 24.15.1
Figure 24.15.2
Figure 24.15.3
Footnotes
1. SVE: Sterile vaginal exam.
2. If abnormal presentation or lie is identified prior to labor, patients may elect to attempt an external cephalic version, in which the fetus is manually rotated into a longitudinal and cephalic position.
3. Cesarean delivery is recommended for most breech presentations unless delivery is imminent.

FIGURE 24.15

24-15 Stages of Labor

STAGES OF LABOR

Stage	Definition	Key Features
1 (Latent)	Onset of labor to 6-cm cervical dilation	Gradual cervical change
1 (Active)	6-cm to 10-cm (complete) cervical dilation	Rapid cervical change; protraction and/or arrest may occur (see below)
2	Complete cervical dilation to delivery of fetus	Course is dependent on fetal lie and presentation (see below)
3	Delivery of fetus to delivery of placenta	Duration is typically ≤30 minutes

Fetal Lie and Presentation

Fetal Lie	Fetal Presentation	Management	Complications
Longitudinal	Cephalic	Vaginal delivery	Arrest of descent[1]
Longitudinal	Breech	ECV[2] attempted before labor; TOL[3] if successful, cesarean delivery if unsuccessful	Fetal entrapment, hypoxic injury, umbilical cord prolapse, delivery-related trauma
Transverse	Shoulder, compound, funic[4]	ECV attempted before labor; TOL if successful, cesarean delivery if unsuccessful	Umbilical cord prolapse, delivery-related trauma, uterine rupture

1. Also known as "prolonged second stage"; can be reasonably diagnosed when a nulliparous patient has pushed for ≥3 hours (4 hours with epidural) or a multiparous patient has pushed for ≥2 hours (3 hours with epidural).
2. External cephalic version (ECV) is an elective procedure in which a fetus with an abnormal lie or presentation is manually rotated into a longitudinal and cephalic position through abdominal manipulation in order to increase the likelihood of vaginal cephalic birth. Ideally, abnormal lie/presentation is identified before the onset of labor, and ECV may be attempted as the first management step.
3. Trial of labor, with the goal of vaginal cephalic birth.
4. Umbilical cord is the presenting part.

PROTRACTION OF LABOR

A 31-year-old F G1P0 at 40 weeks presents with regular, painful uterine contractions for the past 6 hours. Exam shows cervical dilation of 6 cm. Three hours later, a repeat exam shows cervical dilation of 7 cm.

Management: Oxytocin for labor augmentation; amniotomy if adequate fetal descent (–2 station or lower).

Complications:

- Maternal: Operative vaginal delivery, cesarean delivery, 3rd/4th degree perineal lacerations, postpartum hemorrhage, intra-amniotic infection.
- Fetal: Fetal hypoxemia, respiratory distress syndrome, neonatal sepsis.

HYF: Protraction and/or arrest affect approximately 20% of all labors that end in a live birth. Risk factors include nulliparity, term or post-term pregnancy, maternal obesity, and cephalopelvic disproportion.

ARREST OF LABOR

A 40-year-old F G1P0 at 40 weeks presents with regular, painful uterine contractions for the past 6 hours. Exam shows cervical dilation of 7 cm. Two hours later, exam shows cervical dilation of 8 cm. Four hours later, cervical dilation is unchanged.

Management: Cesarean delivery.

Complications: Same as "Protraction of Labor."

HYF: In a patient whose membranes have ruptured and who has reached cervical dilation ≥6 cm, arrest of labor is diagnosed if there is no cervical change for ≥4 hours despite adequate contractions (>200 Montevideo units) *or* if there is no cervical change for ≥6 hours with inadequate contractions.

24-16 Postpartum Fever

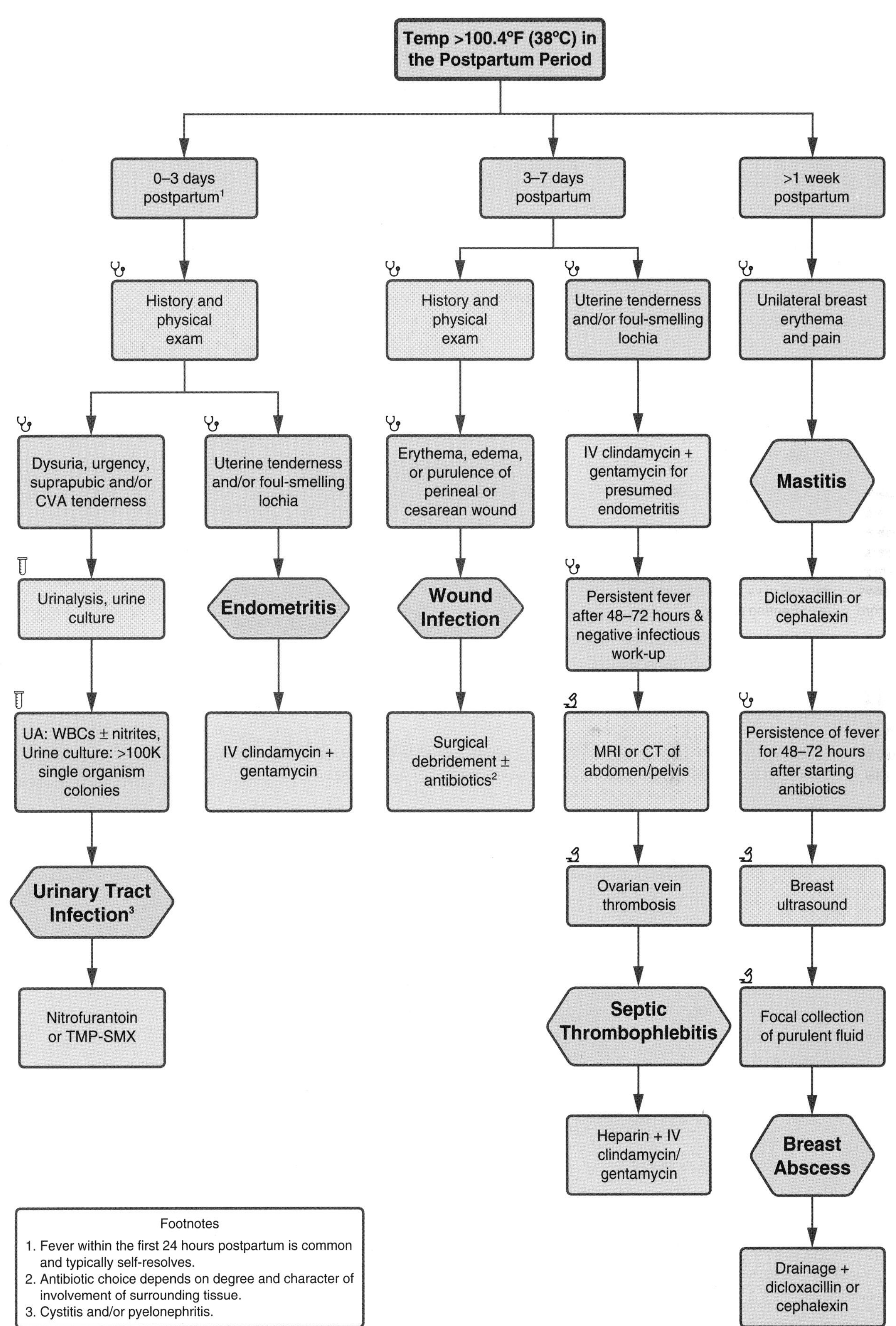
Temp >100.4°F (38°C) in the Postpartum Period
0–3 days postpartum1
3–7 days postpartum
>1 week postpartum
History and physical exam
History and physical exam
Uterine tenderness and/or foul-smelling lochia
Unilateral breast erythema and pain
Dysuria, urgency, suprapubic and/or CVA tenderness
Uterine tenderness and/or foul-smelling lochia
Erythema, edema, or purulence of perineal or cesarean wound
IV clindamycin + gentamycin for presumed endometritis
Mastitis
Urinalysis, urine culture
Endometritis
Wound Infection
Persistent fever after 48–72 hours & negative infectious work-up
Dicloxacillin or cephalexin
UA: WBCs ± nitrites, Urine culture: >100K single organism colonies
IV clindamycin + gentamycin
Surgical debridement ± antibiotics2
MRI or CT of abdomen/pelvis
Persistence of fever for 48–72 hours after starting antibiotics
Urinary Tract Infection3
Ovarian vein thrombosis
Breast ultrasound
Nitrofurantoin or TMP-SMX
Septic Thrombophlebitis
Focal collection of purulent fluid
Heparin + IV clindamycin/ gentamycin
Breast Abscess
Drainage + dicloxacillin or cephalexin

Footnotes

1. Fever within the first 24 hours postpartum is common and typically self-resolves.
2. Antibiotic choice depends on degree and character of involvement of surrounding tissue.
3. Cystitis and/or pyelonephritis.

FIGURE 24.16

24-16 Postpartum Fever

MASTITIS

A 21-year-old G1P1 postpartum day 2 presents with fever and localized pain/erythema of the right breast.

Management:

1. Dicloxacillin or cephalexin.
2. Complete emptying of breast.
3. NSAIDs, cold compresses.

Complications: Breast abscess.

HYF: If no clinical improvement within 48–72 hours of antibiotics, US is required to evaluate for breast abscess.

ENDOMETRITIS

A 27-year-old G2P2 postpartum day 2 with chorioamnionitis during labor presents with fever, uterine tenderness, and foul-smelling lochia.

Management:

1. IV clindamycin + gentamicin.

Complications: Septic pelvic thrombophlebitis.

HYF: Endometritis is a polymicrobial infection of the endometrium. Risk factors include cesarean delivery, prolonged rupture of membranes, and intrapartum infection.

WOUND INFECTION

A 36-year-old G3P2 postpartum day 3 s/p perineal laceration repair presents with fever and perineal pain, erythema, and edema.

Management:

1. Surgical debridement.
2. Antibiotics depending on extent of tissue involvement.

Complications:

- Cellulitis.
- Necrotizing fasciitis (rare).
- Sepsis.

HYF: Common causes of wound infections in the postpartum period include group A and group B *Streptococcus, Staphylococcus epidermidis, S. aureus, Escherichia coli, Proteus*, and cervicovaginal flora.

URINARY TRACT INFECTION

A 26-year-old G2P1 postpartum day 4 presents with fever and dysuria. Exam shows CVA tenderness. On **labs**, UA is (+) leukocyte esterase and nitrites.

Management:

1. UA, urine culture for diagnosis.
2. TMP-SMX or nitrofurantoin.
3. CT if no symptom improvement after 72 hours.

Complications:

- Bacteremia.
- Sepsis.
- Renal abscess.

HYF: Fever and CVA tenderness generally distinguish pyelonephritis from cystitis.

SEPTIC THROMBOPHLEBITIS

A 32-year-old G1P1 post-op day 5 s/p cesarean now presents with 4 days of persistent fever and lower abdominal pain with negative urinalysis. Currently on day 3 of broad-spectrum IV antibiotics.

Management:

1. Pelvic MRI or CT to confirm diagnosis.
2. Heparin.
3. IV clindamycin + gentamicin.

Complications: Pulmonary embolism.

HYF: Pelvic endothelial damage, venous stasis, and hypercoagulability contribute to the risk of septic pelvic thrombophlebitis. Risk factors include pelvic infection and cesarean delivery.

BREAST ABSCESS

A 29-year-old G3P3 on postpartum day 5 presents with persistent fever, erythema, and pain of the left breast on day 3 of antibiotics. She is found to have a fluctuant mass on exam.

Management:

1. Ultrasound to confirm diagnosis.
2. Incision and drainage or ultrasound-guided aspiration.
3. Dicloxacillin or cephalexin.

Complications:

- Recurrent infection.
- Mammary duct fistula.
- Milk fistula.

HYF: Milk drainage (continued breastfeeding, pumping) is important for clearing infection and pain relief.

24-17 Postpartum Hemorrhage

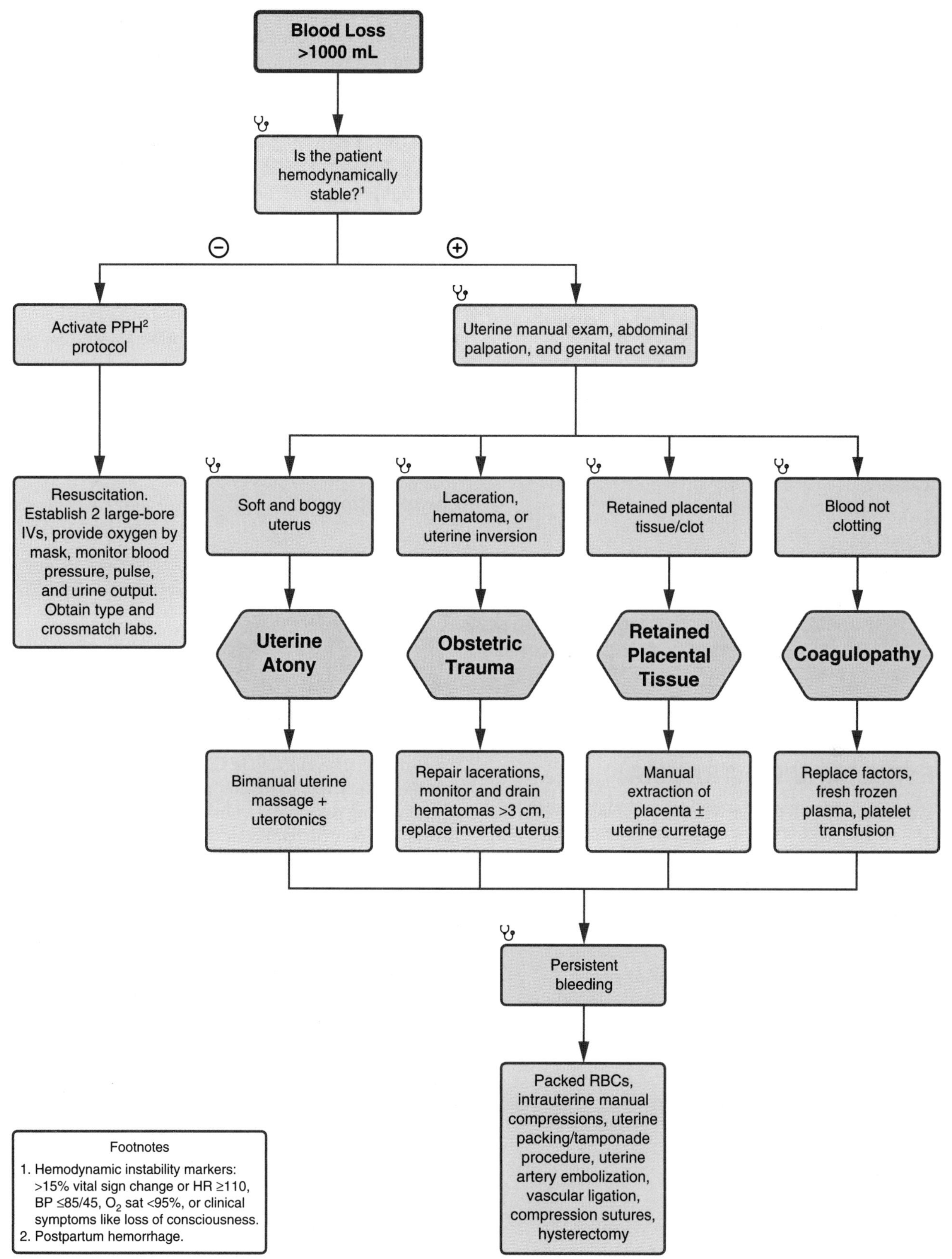
Blood Loss >1000 mL
Is the patient hemodynamically stable?1
⊖
⊕
Activate PPH2 protocol
Resuscitation. Establish 2 large-bore IVs, provide oxygen by mask, monitor blood pressure, pulse, and urine output. Obtain type and crossmatch labs.
Uterine manual exam, abdominal palpation, and genital tract exam
Soft and boggy uterus
Laceration, hematoma, or uterine inversion
Retained placental tissue/clot
Blood not clotting
Uterine Atony
Obstetric Trauma
Retained Placental Tissue
Coagulopathy
Bimanual uterine massage + uterotonics
Repair lacerations, monitor and drain hematomas >3 cm, replace inverted uterus
Manual extraction of placenta ± uterine curretage
Replace factors, fresh frozen plasma, platelet transfusion
Persistent bleeding
Packed RBCs, intrauterine manual compressions, uterine packing/tamponade procedure, uterine artery embolization, vascular ligation, compression sutures, hysterectomy
Footnotes
1. Hemodynamic instability markers: >15% vital sign change or HR ≥110, BP ≤85/45, O2 sat <95%, or clinical symptoms like loss of consciousness.
2. Postpartum hemorrhage.

FIGURE 24.17

24-17 Postpartum Hemorrhage

4Ts of Postpartum Hemorrhage: Tone, Trauma, Tissue, Thrombin.

UTERINE ATONY (TONE)

A 29-year-old G5P5 underwent a spontaneous vaginal birth of twin babies 30 minutes ago. Labor was complicated by chorioamnionitis. Placenta was delivered 30 minutes after birth. Cumulative blood loss was 1000 mL, and the patient continues to experience profuse vaginal bleeding. On exam, the uterus is soft and boggy on abdominal palpation.

Management:

1. Empty the bladder and conduct bimanual pelvic examination to remove any intrauterine clots.
2. Pitocin ± supplemental uterotonics (methergine, hemabate, misoprostol).
3. Uterine tamponade with intrauterine tamponade balloon or compression sutures (B-Lynch sutures) if bleeding persists.

Complications:

- Anemia.
- Hypovolemic shock.
- Sheehan syndrome.

HYF: The #1 cause of postpartum hemorrhage. Methergine is contraindicated in patients with a history of hypertension. Hemabate is contraindicated in patients with a history of asthma and can cause diarrhea. Misoprostol is contraindicated in patients with allergy to misoprostol and can cause transient hyperthermia.

OBSTETRIC TRAUMA (TRAUMA)

A 35-year-old G1P1 undergoes a forceps-assisted vaginal birth due to prolonged second stage of labor. Apgar scores were 7 and 9 at 1 and 5 minutes, respectively. Placenta was delivered 15 minutes after birth, and cumulative blood loss was 900 mL. On exam, uterine tone is firm. Patient continues to bleed.

Management:

1. Quick examination to identify source of bleeding.
2. Suture repair of open lacerations, drain hematomas >3 cm, replace inverted uterus.
3. Packing may be needed to establish hemostasis.

Complications: Genital tract hematoma.

HYF: Hemodynamic instability without obvious bleeding site should raise concern for intraperitoneal or retroperitoneal bleeding, requiring resuscitative measures and IR/surgical consult.

RETAINED PLACENTA (TISSUE)

A 37-year-old G3P2 underwent spontaneous vaginal birth 40 minutes ago. Patient has a history of one therapeutic abortion requiring D&C and prior vaginal birth with manual extraction of placenta. On exam, there is severe bleeding, but the placenta has not been delivered despite several attempts. Cumulative blood loss is >1200 mL.

Management:

1. Manual removal + prophylactic antibiotics with 1st-generation cephalosporins.
2. Uterine curettage or large oval forceps may be needed to remove retained tissue.
3. Uterine balloon tamponade or packing if severe bleeding persists.

Complications:

- Infection.
- Uterine perforation.
- Hysterectomy if placenta accreta spectrum. See p. 657.

HYF: Prior history of retained placenta is the most common risk factor for retained placenta.

COAGULOPATHY (THROMBIN)

A 33-year-old G2P2 undergoes emergent cesarean birth for nonreassuring fetal heart tracings. Cumulative blood loss was 1500 mL, and the patient was started on pitocin and IV fluid resuscitation while awaiting packed RBC. On exam, bleeding continues, and the patient is hemodynamically unstable.

Management:

1. Transfuse packed RBC, fresh frozen plasma, clotting factors, and platelets.
2. Support blood pressure with vasopressors.

Complications: Disseminated intravascular coagulation.

HYF: Excessive resuscitation with crystalloid fluid is associated with dilutional coagulopathy and can also contribute to pulmonary edema.

24-18 Postpartum Mood Changes

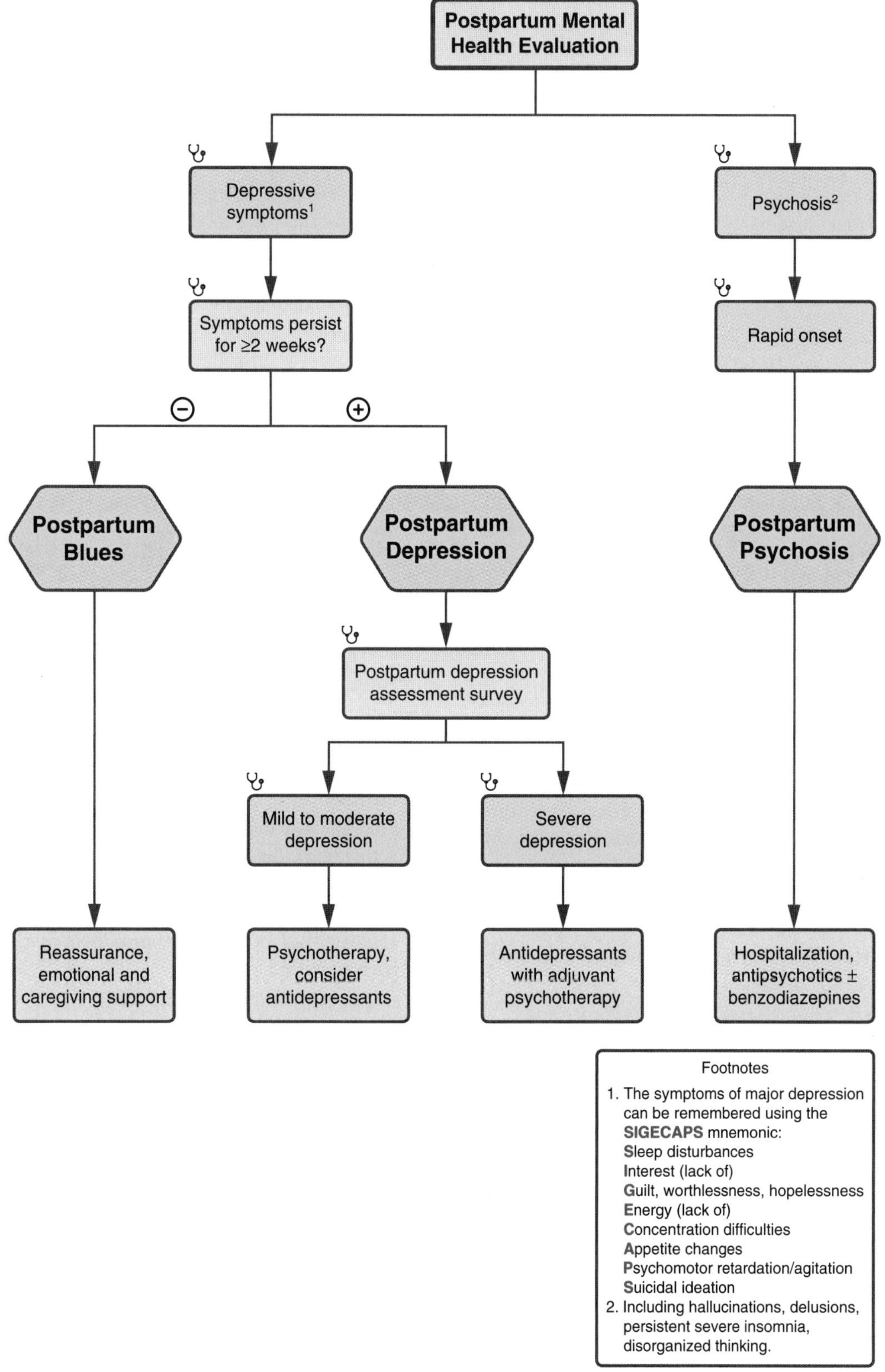
Postpartum Mental Health Evaluation
Depressive symptoms[1]
Psychosis[2]
Symptoms persist for ≥2 weeks?
Rapid onset
Postpartum Blues
Postpartum Depression
Postpartum Psychosis
Postpartum depression assessment survey
Mild to moderate depression
Severe depression
Reassurance, emotional and caregiving support
Psychotherapy, consider antidepressants
Antidepressants with adjuvant psychotherapy
Hospitalization, antipsychotics ± benzodiazepines

Footnotes

1. The symptoms of major depression can be remembered using the **SIGECAPS** mnemonic:
   Sleep disturbances
   Interest (lack of)
   Guilt, worthlessness, hopelessness
   Energy (lack of)
   Concentration difficulties
   Appetite changes
   Psychomotor retardation/agitation
   Suicidal ideation
2. Including hallucinations, delusions, persistent severe insomnia, disorganized thinking.

FIGURE 24.18

24-18 Postpartum Mood Changes

POSTPARTUM BLUES

A 27-year-old G1P1 comes to the office for a checkup 3 days after an uncomplicated vaginal delivery. The patient reports feeling sad and irritable and is tearful during the interview. **Exam** and **labs** are normal.

Management:

1. Inquire about suicidal ideation.
2. Screen for postpartum depression with a validated screening tool (eg, the Edinburgh Postnatal Depression Scale [EPDS] or PHQ-9).
3. Negative screen → offer reassurance and support.

Complications:

- Increased risk for subsequent depression and anxiety disorders.
- If symptoms persist >2 weeks or if suicidal ideation is present, the episode should be treated as postpartum depression.

HYF: Postpartum blues are common (occurring in 40–80% of postpartum patients) and are self-limited. Symptoms present within 2–3 days of delivery and resolve spontaneously within 2 weeks of onset.

POSTPARTUM DEPRESSION

A 27-year-old G1P1 presents for a checkup 6 weeks after an uncomplicated vaginal delivery. The patient has had difficulty sleeping over the past month and reports feeling fatigued and guilty about not wanting to spend more time with the baby. The patient admits to wondering if the baby would be better off alone. **Exam** and **labs** are normal.

Management:

1. Screen for postpartum depression with a validated screening tool (eg, EPDS or PHQ-9).
2. Positive screen → determine severity based on score and number of symptoms present.
3. Initiate treatment based on severity of depressive episode (psychotherapy is 1st-line for mild/moderate illness, antidepressants are 1st-line for severe illness); consider referring to a mental health specialist for ongoing care.

Complications:

- Recurrence of postpartum and/or non-postpartum depression (estimated to occur in 40–50% of patients).
- Impaired parental functioning, including difficulties with breast/chest-feeding, parental-infant bonding, and relationship with partner.
- Impaired infant/child development, including compromised health and safety, cognitive impairment, and psychopathology.

HYF: Postpartum depression occurs in 8–15% of postpartum patients and typically presents within 4–6 weeks of delivery (although it can present up to 1 year later). Note that postpartum blues and postpartum depression may present similarly. Postpartum depression is not a separate diagnosis in the DSM-5 and is diagnosed according to the same criteria as nonpuerperal major depression (≥5 symptoms persisting for ≥2 weeks). However, if symptoms persist for >2 weeks, *even if <5 symptoms are present*, it is recommended that the episode be treated as postpartum depression rather than postpartum blues. For this reason, a consideration of time course is prioritized over the number of symptoms present.

POSTPARTUM PSYCHOSIS

A 27-year-old G1P1 comes to the office for a checkup 1 week after an uncomplicated vaginal delivery. The patient appears disheveled and exhausted and expresses fears that the baby is "shrinking," despite appropriate weight gain. Their partner reports that the patient has barely slept for the past 3 days. **Exam** and **labs** are normal.

Management:

1. Hospitalize patient (usually necessary to ensure safety of patient and infant).
2. Initiate antipsychotic medication (older 2nd-generation antipsychotics are 1st-line, such as quetiapine, risperidone, and olanzapine).
3. For agitation and/or severe insomnia, consider adding a short-acting benzodiazepine (such as lorazepam).

Complications:

- Increased risk of recurrent episodes of psychosis outside of postpartum period.
- Impaired parental-infant bonding.
- Suicide, infanticide.

HYF: Postpartum psychosis is rare (occurring in 0.1–0.2% of postpartum patients) and presents within 2 weeks of delivery. It is strongly associated with bipolar disorder, and in patients with no previous psychiatric history, it has been shown to significantly predict a subsequent bipolar disorder diagnosis.

25

Gynecology

25-1 Acute Pelvic Pain

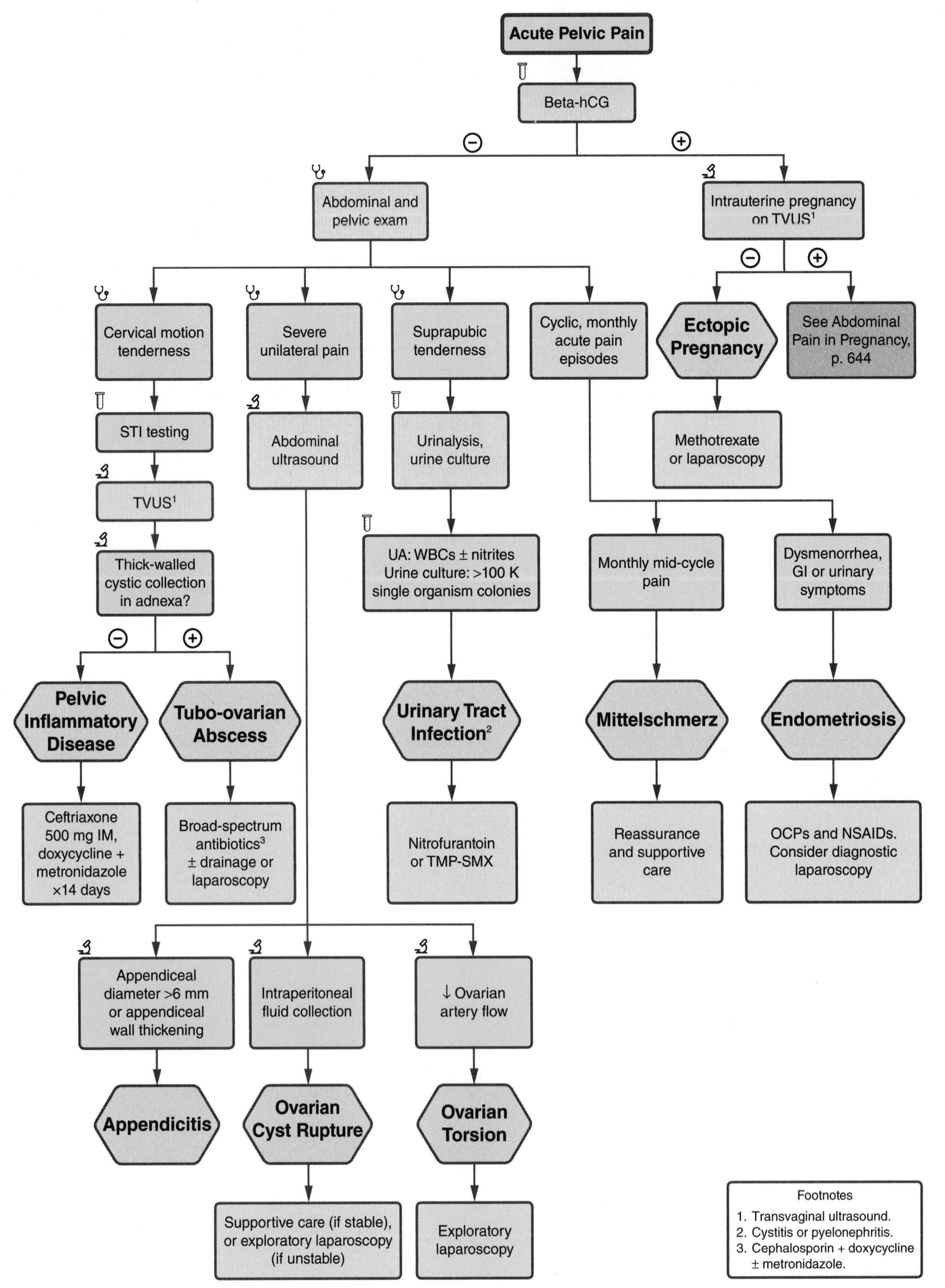
Acute Pelvic Pain
Beta-hCG
⊖
⊕
Abdominal and pelvic exam
Intrauterine pregnancy on TVUS[1]
⊖
⊕
Cervical motion tenderness
Severe unilateral pain
Suprapubic tenderness
Cyclic, monthly acute pain episodes
Ectopic Pregnancy
See Abdominal Pain in Pregnancy, p. 644
STI testing
Abdominal ultrasound
Urinalysis, urine culture
Methotrexate or laparoscopy
TVUS[1]
UA: WBCs ± nitrites
Urine culture: >100 K single organism colonies
Monthly mid-cycle pain
Dysmenorrhea, GI or urinary symptoms
Thick-walled cystic collection in adnexa?
⊖
⊕
Pelvic Inflammatory Disease
Tubo-ovarian Abscess
Urinary Tract Infection[2]
Mittelschmerz
Endometriosis
Ceftriaxone 500 mg IM, doxycycline + metronidazole ×14 days
Broad-spectrum antibiotics[3] ± drainage or laparoscopy
Nitrofurantoin or TMP-SMX
Reassurance and supportive care
OCPs and NSAIDs. Consider diagnostic laparoscopy
Appendiceal diameter >6 mm or appendiceal wall thickening
Intraperitoneal fluid collection
↓ Ovarian artery flow
Appendicitis
Ovarian Cyst Rupture
Ovarian Torsion
Supportive care (if stable), or exploratory laparoscopy (if unstable)
Exploratory laparoscopy
Footnotes
1. Transvaginal ultrasound.
2. Cystitis or pyelonephritis.
3. Cephalosporin + doxycycline ± metronidazole.

FIGURE 25.1

25-1 Acute Pelvic Pain

URINARY TRACT INFECTION

A 20-year-old F with no PMH presents with dysuria, urinary frequency, and suprapubic pain. On exam, she has suprapubic tenderness. On labs, urinalysis is positive for leukocyte esterase and nitrites.

Management:

1. Urinalysis, urine culture for diagnosis.
2. TMP-SMX or nitrofurantoin.

Complications:

- Progression of cystitis to pyelonephritis.
- Bacteremia.
- Sepsis.

HYF: Presence of pyuria is needed for diagnosis; fever and CVA tenderness generally distinguish pyelonephritis from cystitis.

MITTELSCHMERZ

A 16-year-old F with no PMH presents with bilateral lower abdominal pain occurring 2 weeks before menses each month for the past 6 months. No abnormalities on exam.

Management:

1. Reassurance.
2. Analgesics.
3. Consider OCPs for prevention.

Complications: None.

HYF: Mittelschmerz is caused by normal follicular enlargement prior to ovulation and/or normal follicular bleeding at the time of ovulation. Pain occurs approximately 14 days before menses each month.

OVARIAN CYST RUPTURE

A 26-year-old F with no PMH presents with sudden left lower abdominal pain, nausea, and vomiting. Pelvic exam reveals an adnexal mass. On imaging, abdominal US shows an intraperitoneal fluid collection.

Management:

1. Evaluate vital signs.
2. If hemodynamically stable: Supportive care.
3. If hemodynamically unstable: Exploratory laparoscopy.

Complications:

- Blood loss and associated sequelae.
- Ovarian torsion (prior to rupture).

HYF: Vital signs determine management due to risk of blood loss following cyst rupture.

OVARIAN TORSION

A 34-year-old F with PMH of ovarian cysts presents with severe, acute-onset left lower abdominal pain, nausea, and vomiting. Pelvic exam reveals an adnexal mass. On labs, abdominal US shows an enlarged left ovary with decreased arterial flow.

Management:

1. Exploratory laparoscopy (urgent).

Complications: Loss of affected ovary (and decreased fertility).

HYF: "Whirlpool sign" on US is pathognomonic for ovarian torsion. Risk factors include ovarian masses (commonly ovarian cysts or benign neoplasms).

Ectopic Pregnancy: See pp. 645, 709.

Endometriosis: See p. 685.

Pelvic Inflammatory Disease: See p. 704.

Tubo-Ovarian Abscess: See p. 709.

Appendicitis: See p. 80.

25-2 Dyspareunia

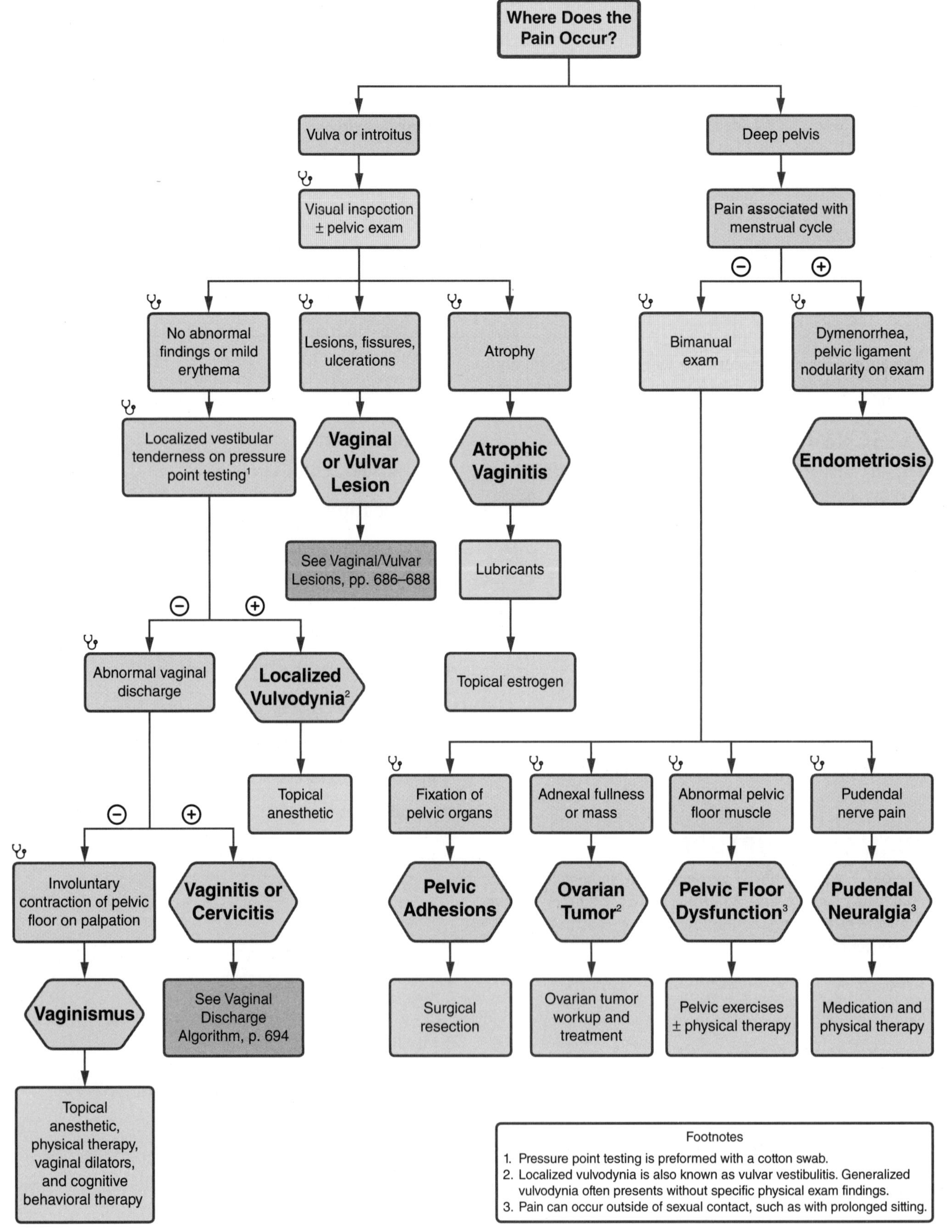
Where Does the Pain Occur?
Vulva or introitus
Deep pelvis
Visual inspection ± pelvic exam
Pain associated with menstrual cycle
No abnormal findings or mild erythema
Lesions, fissures, ulcerations
Atrophy
Bimanual exam
Dymenorrhea, pelvic ligament nodularity on exam
Localized vestibular tenderness on pressure point testing1
Vaginal or Vulvar Lesion
Atrophic Vaginitis
Endometriosis
See Vaginal/Vulvar Lesions, pp. 686–688
Lubricants
Abnormal vaginal discharge
Localized Vulvodynia2
Topical estrogen
Topical anesthetic
Fixation of pelvic organs
Adnexal fullness or mass
Abnormal pelvic floor muscle
Pudendal nerve pain
Involuntary contraction of pelvic floor on palpation
Vaginitis or Cervicitis
Pelvic Adhesions
Ovarian Tumor2
Pelvic Floor Dysfunction3
Pudendal Neuralgia3
Vaginismus
See Vaginal Discharge Algorithm, p. 694
Surgical resection
Ovarian tumor workup and treatment
Pelvic exercises ± physical therapy
Medication and physical therapy
Topical anesthetic, physical therapy, vaginal dilators, and cognitive behavioral therapy
Footnotes
1. Pressure point testing is preformed with a cotton swab.
2. Localized vulvodynia is also known as vulvar vestibulitis. Generalized vulvodynia often presents without specific physical exam findings.
3. Pain can occur outside of sexual contact, such as with prolonged sitting.

FIGURE 25.2

25-2 Dyspareunia

ATROPHIC VAGINITIS

A 66-year-old F with no PMH presents with painful sex. On exam, she has smooth and shiny vaginal epithelium with patchy erythema.

Management:

1. Increased use of lubricants.
2. Topical estrogen.

Complications: Increased risk of vaginal infection.

HYF: Atrophic vaginitis is common in postmenopausal women, as estrogen maintains vaginal lubrication.

ENDOMETRIOSIS

A 23-year-old F with no PMH presents with pelvic pain that worsens around the middle of each month. On exam, she has pelvic ligament nodularity. On imaging, US shows unilocular mass with homogeneous echoes.

Management:

1. NSAIDs.
2. Hormonal contraceptive.
3. Laparoscopic surgery for diagnosis and/or treatment.

Complications:

- Infertility.
- Abnormal uterine bleeding.
- Low back pain.

HYF: Definitive diagnosis of endometriosis can only be made with a biopsy, usually obtained through laparoscopic surgery.

VULVODYNIA

An 18-year-old F with no PMH presents with burning pain during sex. On exam, she has localized tenderness in the vestibule.

Management:

1. Assess relationship safety.
2. Assess anxiety with sexual contact.
3. Topical anesthetic.

Complications:

- Increased anxiety with sexual contact.
- Chronic dyspareunia.

HYF: Localized vulvodynia is a common cause of dyspareunia, particularly with introital burning pain.

VAGINISMUS

A 25-year-old F with no PMH presents with inability to engage in penetrative sex due to significant pain. On exam, she has spontaneous pelvic muscle contractions with palpation.

Management:

1. Physical therapy.
2. Topical anesthetic.
3. Consider cognitive behavioral therapy.

Complications:

- Inability to engage in penetrative sex.
- Chronic dyspareunia.

HYF: Vaginismus is due to pelvic muscle spasm. Some patients have preceding sexual trauma, and many have associated anxiety with sexual contact, which can develop before or after symptoms.

PELVIC ADHESIONS

A 32-year-old F with PMH of chlamydia and gonorrhea when she was 21 years old presents with pelvic pain, particularly during sex. On exam, she has reduced mobility of pelvic organs.

Management:

1. Laparoscopic lysis of adhesions (if symptomatic).
2. Hysterosalpingogram for fertility concerns.

Complications:

- Associated with pelvic inflammatory disease (PID) and co-occurs with: 1) perihepatitis or Fitz-Hugh-Curtis syndrome, 2) tubo-ovarian abscess.

HYF: Pelvic adhesions are commonly caused by PID but can also be caused by prior surgery or endometriosis.

PELVIC FLOOR DYSFUNCTION

A 55-year-old F with PMH of a car accident 3 months ago presents with pelvic pain during sex and difficulty voiding. On exam, she has increased tension in pelvic muscles.

Management:

1. Pelvic floor exercise and physical therapy.
2. Medication to maintain soft bowel movements.

Complications: Bowel and bladder dysfunction.

HYF: Pelvic floor dysfunction occurs most commonly after pregnancy or pelvic trauma and can also occur due to pelvic muscle overuse, advanced age, or obesity.

PUDENDAL NEURALGIA

A 28-year-old F who is 6 weeks postpartum presents with pain with sex and prolonged sitting. On exam, she has increased perineal tenderness.

Management:

1. Medication (steroids, local anesthetic, nerve block).
2. Physical therapy.
3. Consider surgery if resulting from surgery or nerve compression.

Complications:

- Bowel and bladder dysfunction.
- Altered sexual arousal (eg, persistent genital arousal disorder or erectile dysfunction in males).

HYF: Pudendal neuralgia most commonly occurs due to trauma, such as surgery or childbirth, or with repeated mechanical injury (eg, prolonged bike riding).

25-3 Vulvar/Vaginal Cancers

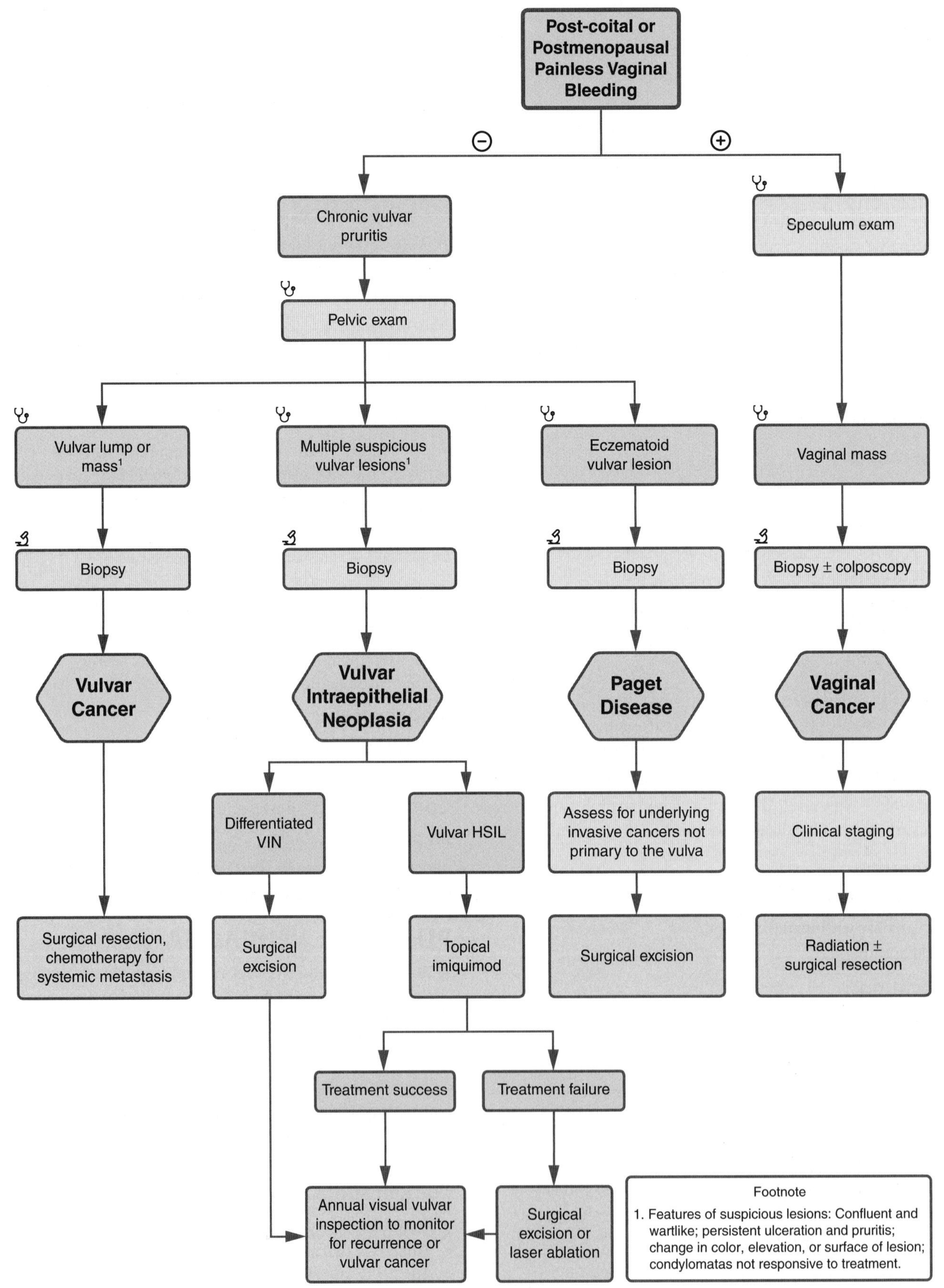
Post-coital or Postmenopausal Painless Vaginal Bleeding
⊖
⊕
Chronic vulvar pruritis
Speculum exam
Pelvic exam
Vulvar lump or mass[1]
Multiple suspicious vulvar lesions[1]
Eczematoid vulvar lesion
Vaginal mass
Biopsy
Biopsy
Biopsy
Biopsy ± colposcopy
Vulvar Cancer
Vulvar Intraepithelial Neoplasia
Paget Disease
Vaginal Cancer
Differentiated VIN
Vulvar HSIL
Assess for underlying invasive cancers not primary to the vulva
Clinical staging
Surgical resection, chemotherapy for systemic metastasis
Surgical excision
Topical imiquimod
Surgical excision
Radiation ± surgical resection
Treatment success
Treatment failure
Annual visual vulvar inspection to monitor for recurrence or vulvar cancer
Surgical excision or laser ablation
Footnote
1. Features of suspicious lesions: Confluent and wartlike; persistent ulceration and pruritis; change in color, elevation, or surface of lesion; condylomatas not responsive to treatment.

FIGURE 25.3

25-3 Vulvar/Vaginal Cancers

VULVAR CANCER

A 68-year-old postmenopausal F with PMH of lichen sclerosus presents with chronic vulvar pruritis. On exam, she has vulvar dystrophy concerning for lichen sclerosus; biopsy of the lesion shows vulvar SCC.

Management:

1. Extensive physical exam, including thorough pelvic/rectal exam and palpation of groin lymph nodes.
2. Biopsy all suspicious lesions.
3. Surgical excision with vulvoplasty and groin lymphadenectomy; neoadjuvant chemotherapy for advanced disease.

Complications: Complications related to surgical resection (eg, aesthetic changes to the vulva, wound seroma, genital prolapse).

HYF: High association with VIN (premalignant lesion); condyloma/HPV infection in younger patients; chronic vulvar dermatoses (eg, lichen sclerosis, squamous hyperplasia) in older patients.

VULVAR INTRAEPITHELIAL NEOPLASIA

A 27-year-old F with PMH of HIV presents with vulvar pain, irritation, and itching. Pelvic exam reveals multiple suspicious vulvar lesions; biopsy of the lesion shows vulvar HSIL.

Management:

1. Biopsy all suspicious lesions.
2. Treat all VIN cases due to malignancy potential.
   a. Vulvar HSIL (high grade squamous intraepithelial lesion): Medical management with topical imiquimod; surgical excision (cold-knife excision or LEEP) or LEEP if no resolution.
   b. Differentiated VIN (dVIN): Surgical excision (cold knife excision or LEEP).
3. Annual vulvar exams to assess for recurrence or possible progression to vulvar cancer.

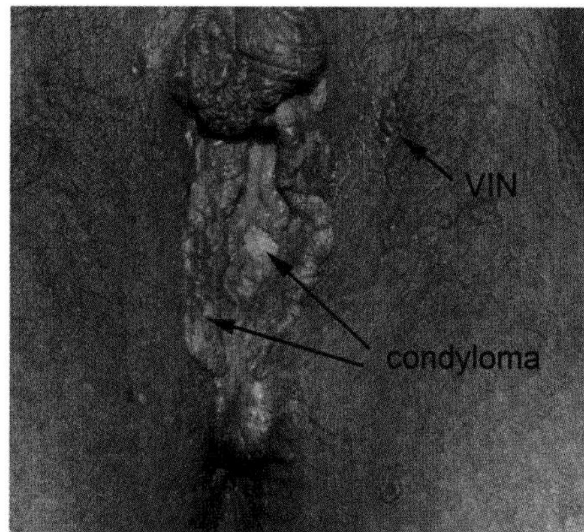
VIN
condyloma
A patient with stage 3 vulvar intraepithelial neoplasia and adjacent exophytic condyloma.

Complications: Vulvar cancer.

HYF: Premalignant lesion. Subtypes:

- vHSIL: Associated with carcinogenic genotypes of HPV, cigarette smoking, and immunosuppression. Typically presents in younger patients (<40 years old) with intermittent symptoms.
- dVIN: Associated with vulvar dermatoses (eg, lichen sclerosus). Typically presents in older patients (>60 years old) with chronic symptoms (especially vulvar pruritis).

PAGET DISEASE OF THE VULVA

A 62-year-old postmenopausal F presents with chronic vulvar pruritis, soreness, and oozing. Pelvic exam shows an eczematoid red macule on the vulva; biopsy of the lesion shows vacuolated Paget cells.

Management:

1. Biopsy all suspicious lesions.
2. Workup to look for presence of underlying primary invasive cancer of nearby structures (eg, cystoscopy).
3. Wide local excision.

Complications:

- Associated with underlying vulvar adenocarcinoma or primary invasive cancer in an extra-vulvar site (cervix, colon, bladder, gallbladder, breast).
- Multiple surgical excisions due to high recurrence rate.

HYF: Paget disease of the vulva is a skin cancer of the genital region arising from glandular epithelial cells.

VAGINAL CANCER

A 58-year-old postmenopausal F with PMH of total hysterectomy presents with painless postcoital bleeding, vaginal discharge, and constipation. Speculum exam reveals a nodular lesion on the upper posterior wall of the vagina. Histological assessment confirms the diagnosis of vaginal SCC.

Management:

1. Biopsy all suspicion lesions.
2. Clinical staging (cystoscopy, proctoscopy, chest radiography, CT, MRI, etc.).
3. Individualized treatment based on tumor characteristics: Radiation therapy ± surgical resection for operable tumors (for which resection will not compromise surrounding organs, eg, bladder or rectum).

Complications:

- Rectovaginal or vesicovaginal fistula in advanced disease.
- Complications related to radiation and surgery (consider patient preferences regarding sexual function).

HYF: Most tumors in the vagina are metastases of other cancers (especially cervical and vulvar). Primary vaginal cancers are highly associated with early hysterectomy and DES exposure in utero.

25-4 Vulvar/Vaginal Infections and Inflammation

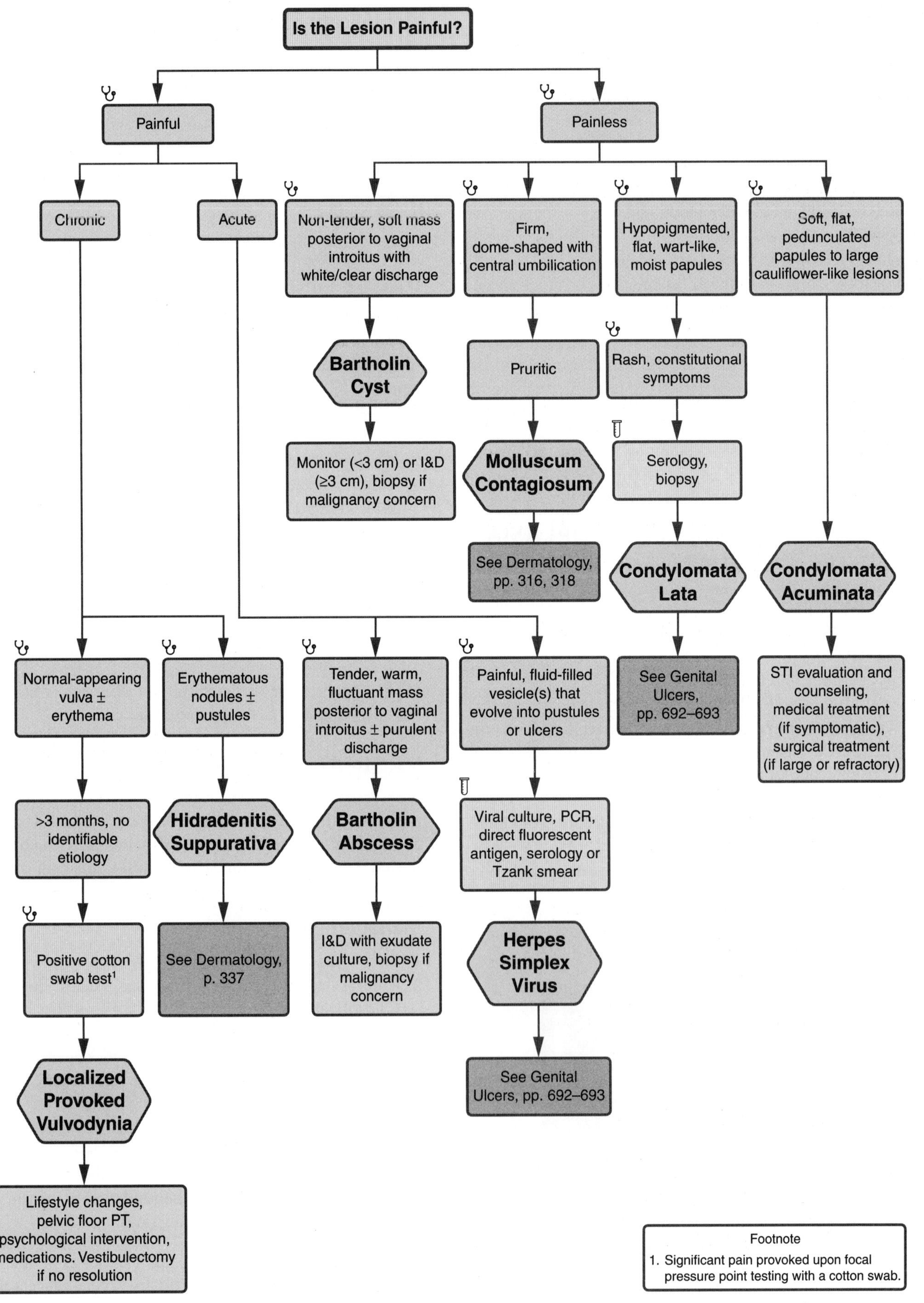

Is the Lesion Painful?
Painful
Painless
Chronic
Acute
Non-tender, soft mass posterior to vaginal introitus with white/clear discharge
Firm, dome-shaped with central umbilication
Hypopigmented, flat, wart-like, moist papules
Soft, flat, pedunculated papules to large cauliflower-like lesions
Bartholin Cyst
Pruritic
Rash, constitutional symptoms
Monitor (<3 cm) or I&D (≥3 cm), biopsy if malignancy concern
Molluscum Contagiosum
Serology, biopsy
See Dermatology, pp. 316, 318
Condylomata Lata
Condylomata Acuminata
Normal-appearing vulva ± erythema
Erythematous nodules ± pustules
Tender, warm, fluctuant mass posterior to vaginal introitus ± purulent discharge
Painful, fluid-filled vesicle(s) that evolve into pustules or ulcers
See Genital Ulcers, pp. 692–693
STI evaluation and counseling, medical treatment (if symptomatic), surgical treatment (if large or refractory)
>3 months, no identifiable etiology
Hidradenitis Suppurativa
Bartholin Abscess
Viral culture, PCR, direct fluorescent antigen, serology or Tzank smear
Positive cotton swab test[1]
See Dermatology, p. 337
I&D with exudate culture, biopsy if malignancy concern
Herpes Simplex Virus
Localized Provoked Vulvodynia
See Genital Ulcers, pp. 692–693
Lifestyle changes, pelvic floor PT, psychological intervention, medications. Vestibulectomy if no resolution
Footnote
1. Significant pain provoked upon focal pressure point testing with a cotton swab.

FIGURE 25.4

25-4 Vulvar/Vaginal Infections and Inflammation

BARTHOLIN CYST OR ABSCESS

A 23-year-old F presents with severe vulvar pain interfering with her ability to sit, walk, or have sex. Pelvic exam reveals a unilateral tender, warm, fluctuant mass in the lower medial labia majora with yellow-green discharge.

Management:

1. Cysts: Incision and drainage (I&D) if ≥3 cm. Abscesses: Culture exudate to exclude MRSA and I&D.
   a. I&D should include additional methods to keep the Bartholin tract open (eg, Word catheter).
2. Biopsy if signs of Bartholin gland carcinoma (eg, postmenopausal patient, solid component to mass, unresponsive to treatment).

Complications:

- Bartholin gland carcinoma.
- Bartholin gland excision (definitive treatment): Excessive bleeding, hematoma formation, infection, dyspareunia.

HYF: Diagnosis is clinical.

- Bartholin cysts are mostly asymptomatic, with occasional clear/white discharge, but if large, they can cause discomfort/pain during sex, sitting, or ambulating.
- Bartholin abscesses present with severe pain and purulent discharge (yellow/green).

GENITAL WARTS (CONDYLOMATA ACUMINATA)

A 28-year-old F presents with genital warts. Pelvic exam reveals multiple, soft, flesh-colored papillated plaques on the vulva.

Management:

1. Biopsy if diagnosis is unclear, lesion is refractory to treatment, or atypical features are present.
2. Assess for clinical features and need for STI testing; counsel and/or treat sexual partners.
3. Treat symptomatic or bothersome lesions: At-home topical imiquimod for non-pregnant patients who can comply with self-therapy; office-based trichloroacetic acid for pregnant patients or non-pregnant patients who cannot comply with self-therapy.
4. Surgical therapy for large or refractory lesions.

Complications: High recurrence rate regardless of treatment modality.

HYF: Associated with HPV infection, which resolves within 2 years for most immunocompetent patients.

LOCALIZED PROVOKED VULVODYNIA/ VESTIBULODYNIA

A 28-year-old F with no significant PMH presents with 4 months of persistent vulvar pain, especially during sex and with tight-fitting clothes. Pelvic exam is significant for normal-appearing vulva and significant pain elicited in the vulvar vestibule upon focal pressure point testing with a cotton swab.

Management:

1. Exclude other possible etiologies (eg, dermatoses, allergies, medications, menopause, infection, abuse).
2. Combination of the following modalities:
   a. Behavior modifications: Vulvar hygiene (eg, avoid products that cause dermatitis), loose clothes, ice the area, avoid activities that apply pressure to the vulva (eg, biking), Epsom salt or oatmeal baths, lubrication during sex, stress relief.
   b. Pelvic floor physical therapy.
   c. Psychological intervention (eg, CBT, sex therapy, couples therapy).
   d. Medication therapy: 1st-line is topical lidocaine or estradiol.
3. Surgery (vestibulectomy) if no resolution.

HYF: Formerly vulvar vestibulitis. Diagnosis of exclusion. Most common vulvodynia and most common cause of dyspareunia in premenopausal women.

*__Epidermal cyst:__ Usually asymptomatic but can occasionally get irritated, sore, or infected. Most arise from occlusion of pilosebaceous ducts. Diagnosis is clinical. Visual inspection of the vulva reveals a smooth, round, mobile, skin-colored nodule with central punctum. If stable and uninfected, no treatment needed. For inflamed cysts, triamcinolone injection. If fluctuant/infected, I&D.

Condylomata Lata (Syphilis): See p. 693.

***Molluscum Contagiosum*:** See pp. 316, 318.

Hidradenitis Suppurativa: See p. 337.

Herpes Simplex Virus: See p. 693.

25-5 Vulvar Dystrophies

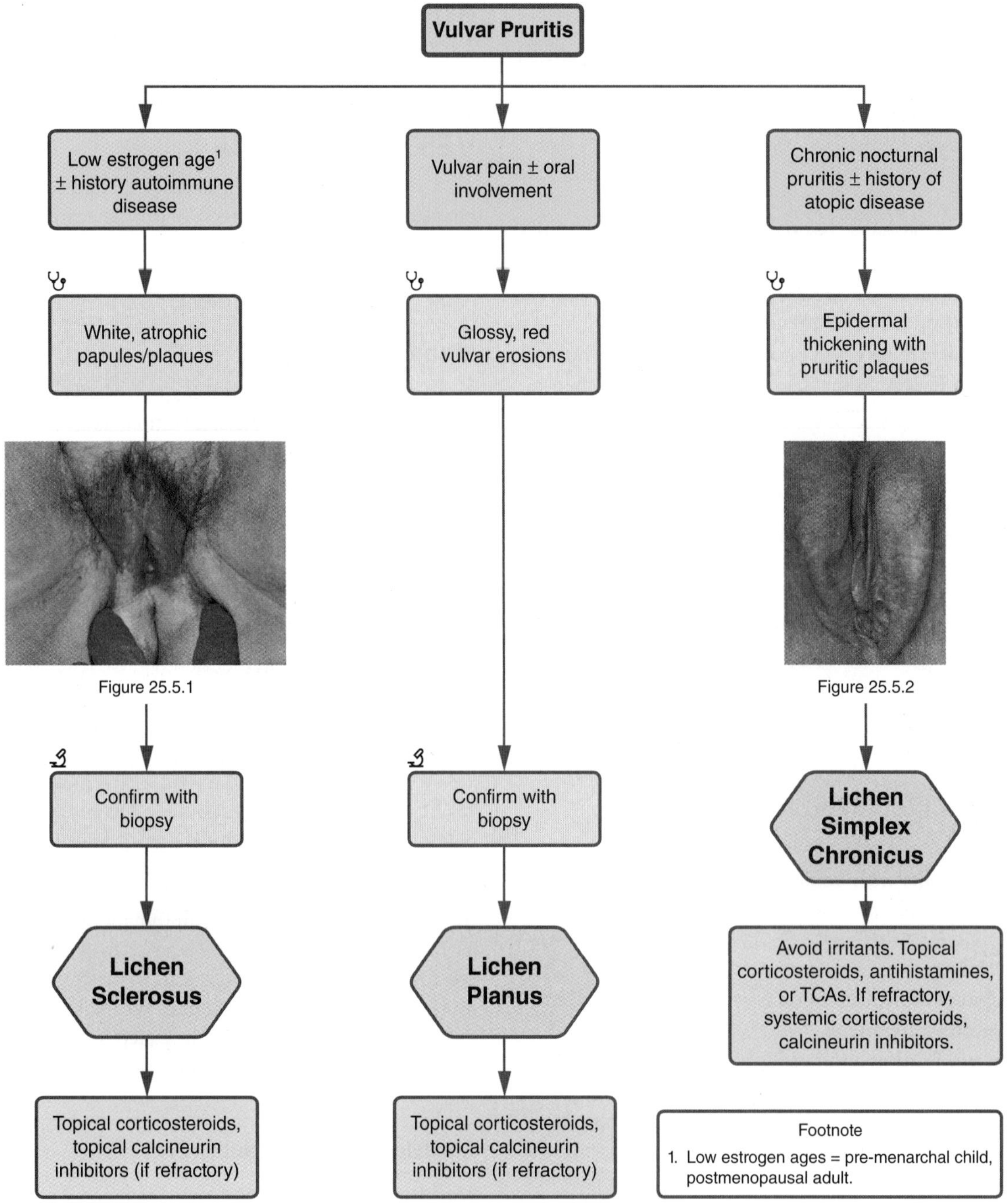
Vulvar Pruritis
Low estrogen age[1] ± history autoimmune disease
Vulvar pain ± oral involvement
Chronic nocturnal pruritis ± history of atopic disease
White, atrophic papules/plaques
Glossy, red vulvar erosions
Epidermal thickening with pruritic plaques
Figure 25.5.1
Figure 25.5.2
Confirm with biopsy
Confirm with biopsy
Lichen Simplex Chronicus
Lichen Sclerosus
Lichen Planus
Avoid irritants. Topical corticosteroids, antihistamines, or TCAs. If refractory, systemic corticosteroids, calcineurin inhibitors.
Topical corticosteroids, topical calcineurin inhibitors (if refractory)
Topical corticosteroids, topical calcineurin inhibitors (if refractory)
Footnote
1. Low estrogen ages = pre-menarchal child, postmenopausal adult.

FIGURE 25.5

25-5 Vulvar Dystrophies

LICHEN SCLEROSUS

A 62-year-old postmenopausal F with PMH of vitiligo presents with vulvar pruritis and dyspareunia. Pelvic exam shows flat, white, atrophic papules in a figure-eight distribution on the labia minora and perianal area, with noted erythema. Speculum exam shows a normal vagina and cervix, void of any lesions; punch biopsy of the lesion shows hyperkeratosis, epidermal atrophy (flattened rete ridges), and homogenization of collagen in the upper dermis overlying a lymphocytic infiltrate.

Management:

1. Punch biopsy to confirm diagnosis and exclude possible vulvar squamous cell carcinoma.
2. Topical high-potency corticosteroids (clobetasol), intralesional corticosteroid injection for thick hypertrophic plaques.
3. Topical calcineurin inhibitors for refractory cases.
4. Surveillance with regular vulvar examinations and biopsies if lesions worsen or change.

Complications:

- Progression to dVIN and vulvar SCC.
- Vulvar/vaginal adhesions and scarring, necessitating dilators or surgery.
- Loss of vulvar architecture.

HYF: Similar to lichen planus but does not involve the vagina or other mucosal surfaces. Associated with autoimmune disorders and low-estrogen states (premenarche and postmenopause).

LICHEN PLANUS

A 55-year-old F presents with vulvar pain and burning, dyspareunia, and dysuria. Pelvic exam reveals well-demarcated, bright-red vestibular patches with Wickham striae. Speculum exam shows vaginal inflammation; punch biopsy of the lesion shows pointed rete ridges and vacuolar change of the epidermal basal layer with upper-dermal lymphocytic infiltrate.

Management:

1. Punch biopsy to confirm diagnosis and exclude possible vulvar squamous cell carcinoma.
2. Topical high-potency corticosteroids (clobetasol).
3. Intravaginal corticosteroids (hydrocortisone) if vaginal involvement.
4. Topical calcineurin inhibitors for refractory cases.
5. Surveillance with regular vulvar examinations and biopsies if lesions worsen or change.

Complications:

- Progression to dVIN and vulvar SCC.
- Vulvar/vaginal adhesions and scarring, necessitating dilators or surgery.
- Loss of vulvar architecture.

HYF: Can involve mucosal surfaces, like the vagina and mouth (unlike lichen sclerosus). High recurrence rate that usually requires long-term maintenance therapy.

LICHEN SIMPLEX CHRONICUS

A 68-year-old F with PMH of atopic dermatitis presents with intensive vaginal pruritis that disturbs sleep. Pelvic exam shows thick, leathery vulvar skin (lichenification) with raised dark plaques and excoriations; punch biopsy of the lesion shows epidermal thickening, hyperkeratosis, spongiosis, and acanthosis.

Management:

1. Exclude underlying infection (eg, candidiasis) or disease (lichen sclerosus, lichen planus) that can cause vulvar pruritis.
2. Avoid irritants (eg, harsh soaps, rough clothing).
3. Topical moderate-potency corticosteroids (eg, triamcinolone).
4. Hydroxyzine or amitriptyline for nocturnal itching.
5. Systemic corticosteroids or topical calcineurin inhibitors for refractory cases.

HYF: Also known as squamous cell hyperplasia. This is a diagnosis of exclusion describing the non-neoplastic morphology of vulvar skin under chronic irritation/pruritis.

25-6 Genital Ulcers

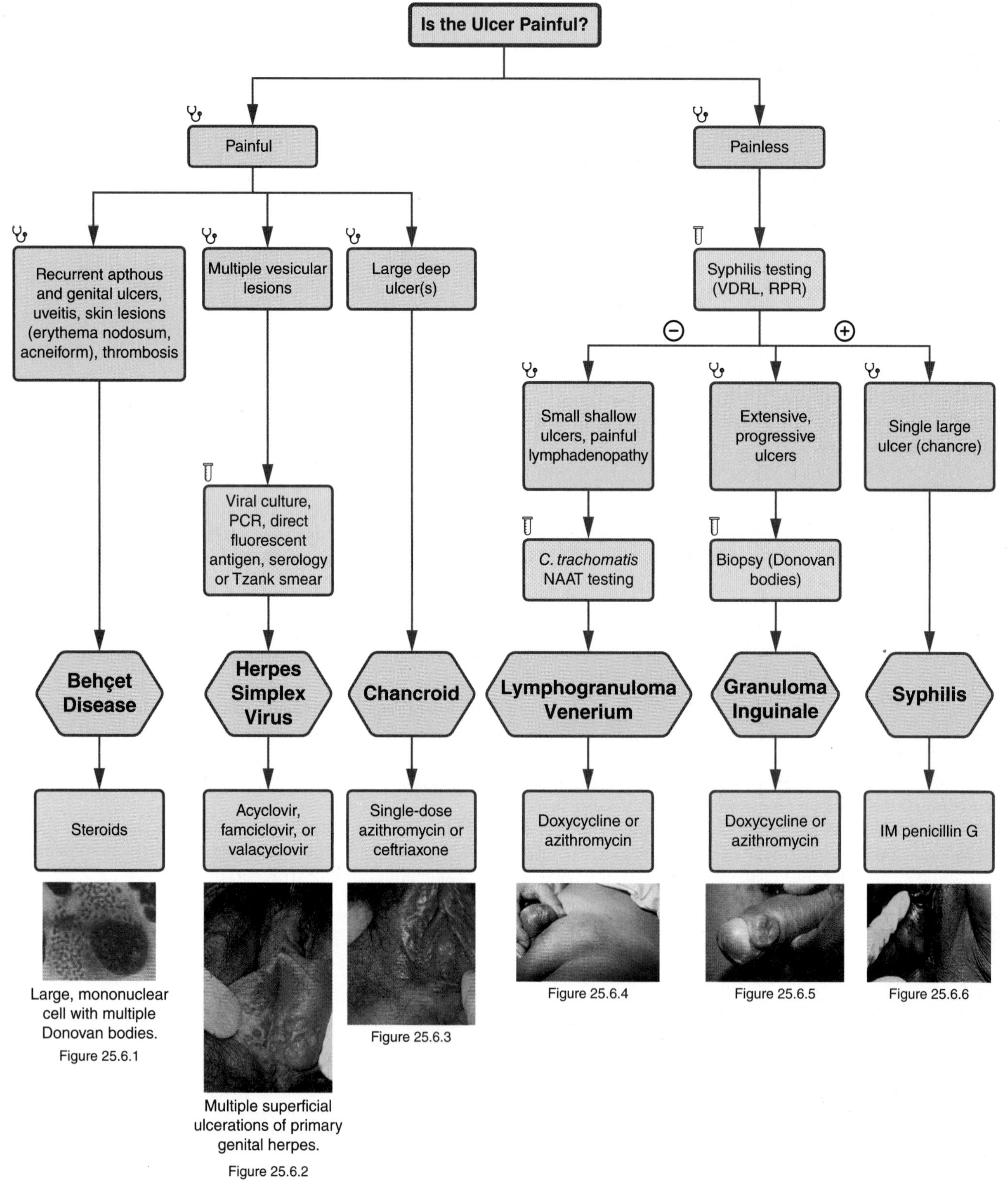
Is the Ulcer Painful?
Painful
Painless
Recurrent apthous and genital ulcers, uveitis, skin lesions (erythema nodosum, acneiform), thrombosis
Multiple vesicular lesions
Large deep ulcer(s)
Syphilis testing (VDRL, RPR)
⊖
⊕
Small shallow ulcers, painful lymphadenopathy
Extensive, progressive ulcers
Single large ulcer (chancre)
Viral culture, PCR, direct fluorescent antigen, serology or Tzank smear
C. trachomatis NAAT testing
Biopsy (Donovan bodies)
Behçet Disease
Herpes Simplex Virus
Chancroid
Lymphogranuloma Venerium
Granuloma Inguinale
Syphilis
Steroids
Acyclovir, famciclovir, or valacyclovir
Single-dose azithromycin or ceftriaxone
Doxycycline or azithromycin
Doxycycline or azithromycin
IM penicillin G

Large, mononuclear cell with multiple Donovan bodies.
Figure 25.6.1

Multiple superficial ulcerations of primary genital herpes.
Figure 25.6.2

Figure 25.6.3

Figure 25.6.4

Figure 25.6.5

Figure 25.6.6

FIGURE 25.6

25-6 Genital Ulcers

HERPES SIMPLEX VIRUS (HSV)

A 38-year-old F presents with vaginal burning and dysuria. On exam, she has red, shallow ulcers and vesicles. On **labs**, Tzanck smear shows multinucleated giant cells.

Management:

1. Confirm diagnosis with viral culture, PCR, direct fluorescent antibody test, serology, and/or Tzanck smear.
2. Acyclovir, famciclovir, or valacyclovir for primary infection.
3. If resistant to above treatment, foscarnet.

Complications:

- Recurrence of genital lesions.
- Aseptic meningitis.
- Sacral radiculitis (causing urinary retention).

HYF: HSV-2 is the most common cause of genital herpes, although HSV-1 is increasingly common.

CHANCROID (*HAEMOPHILUS DUCREYI*)

A 29-year-old F who recently immigrated to the United States presents with extreme vaginal pain. Exam reveals a single, well-demarcated, necrotic ulcer and inguinal lymphadenopathy.

Management:

1. Single-dose azithromycin or ceftriaxone.

Complications:

- Inguinal abscesses and buboes.
- Scarring and fibrosis.

HYF: Chancroid is rare in the US and starts as a papule before progressing to a pustule. The diagnosis is generally made on clinical grounds and is difficult to culture.

LYMPHOGRANULOMA VENEREUM (*CHLAMYDIA TRACHOMATIS*)

A 33-year-old F with PMH of *N. gonorrhoeae* presents with a painless, shallow vaginal ulcer and painful buboes on exam. On **labs**, NAAT testing for *Chlamydia trachomatis* is positive.

Management:

1. *Chlamydia trachomatis* NAAT testing.
2. Doxycycline or azithromycin.
3. Possible aspiration of buboes.

Complications:

- Anorectal symptoms.
- Scarring and fibrosis of the anogenital tract.

HYF: Lymphogranuloma venereum is caused by the L1, L2, and L3 *C. trachomatis* subtypes.

BEHÇET DISEASE

A 26-year-old F with PMH of aphthous ulcers and colitis presents with erythema nodosum and genital ulcers on exam.

Management:

1. Assessment for associated symptoms (see HYF below).
2. Steroids.

Complications: Thrombosis (a common cause of morbidity).

HYF: An autoimmune vasculitis characterized by recurrent aphthous ulcers and various systemic manifestations (including ocular involvement, skin lesions, gastrointestinal disease, neurologic symptoms, arthritis).

GRANULOMA INGUINALE (*KLEBSIELLA GRANULOMATIS*)

A 35-year-old F presents with a beefy-red, genital ulcer on exam. A biopsy of the ulcer demonstrates Donovan bodies.

Management:

1. Biopsy of lesion.
2. Doxycycline or azithromycin.

Complications:

- Lymphatic infections.
- Scarring and fibrosis.

HYF: A diagnosis of granuloma inguinale is confirmed with a biopsy with evidence of Donovan bodies.

SYPHILIS (*TREPONEMA PALLIDUM*)

A 31-year-old F presents with a new painless genital lesion. Exam is notable for an ulcer (chancre) and local lymphadenopathy. **Labs** are notable for a positive VDRL/RPR.

Management:

1. Confirmatory diagnostic testing.
2. Benzathine penicillin IM.
3. If allergic to penicillin, tetracycline or doxycycline.
4. If pregnant and allergic to penicillin, desensitization and treatment with penicillin.

Complications:

- Progression to secondary syphilis (4–8 weeks later: Fever, headache, diffuse maculopapular rash on the soles and palms, condyloma lata, possible meningitis, hepatitis, nephropathy, eye involvement).
- Progression to tertiary syphilis (1–20 years later: Granulomatous gummas, neurosyphilis with tabes dorsalis, Argyll Robertson pupils, aortic root disease).
- Congenital syphilis if infected during pregnancy.

HYF: Caused by the spirochete *T. pallidum*. Testing is often done with VDRL/RPR (rapid but many possible false positives) with confirmatory testing with treponemal tests (FTA-ABS).

25-7 Abnormal Vaginal Discharge

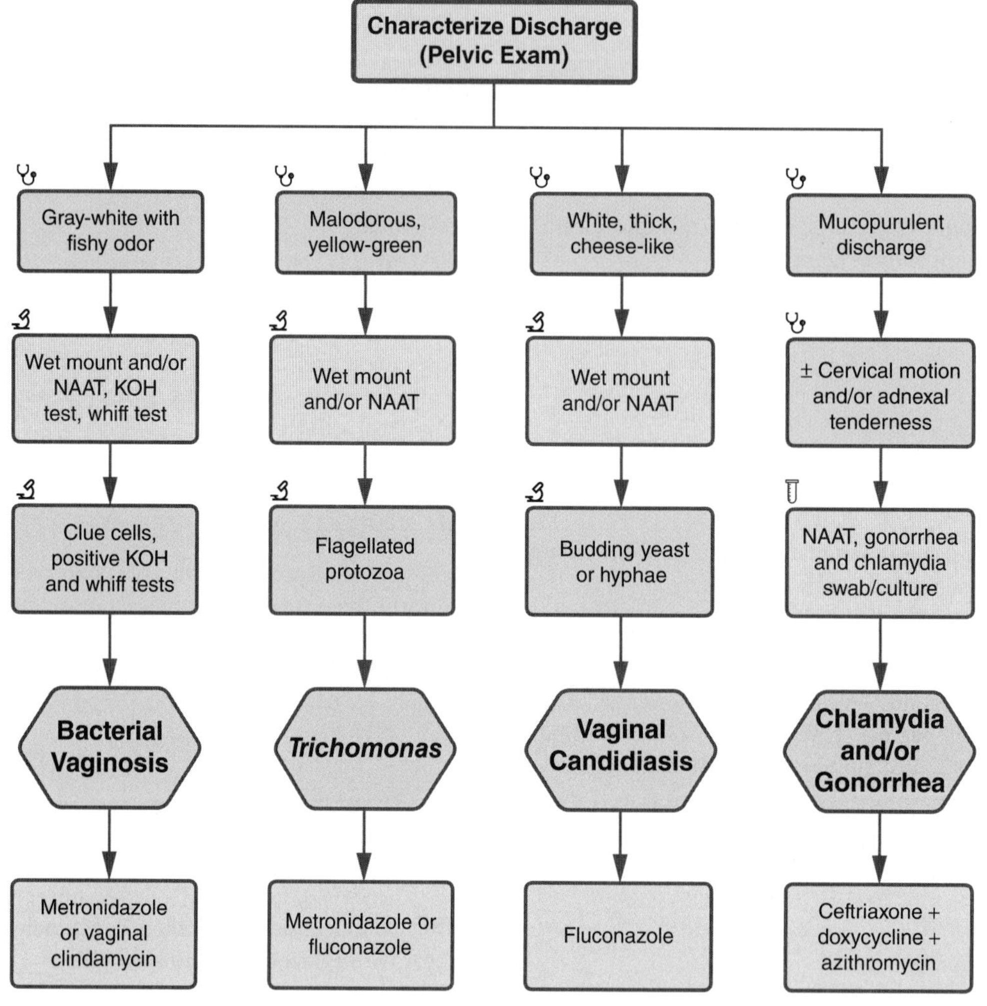
Characterize Discharge (Pelvic Exam)
Gray-white with fishy odor
Wet mount and/or NAAT, KOH test, whiff test
Clue cells, positive KOH and whiff tests
Bacterial Vaginosis
Metronidazole or vaginal clindamycin
Malodorous, yellow-green
Wet mount and/or NAAT
Flagellated protozoa
Trichomonas
Metronidazole or fluconazole
White, thick, cheese-like
Wet mount and/or NAAT
Budding yeast or hyphae
Vaginal Candidiasis
Fluconazole
Mucopurulent discharge
± Cervical motion and/or adnexal tenderness
NAAT, gonorrhea and chlamydia swab/culture
Chlamydia and/or Gonorrhea
Ceftriaxone + doxycycline + azithromycin

FIGURE 25.7

25-7 Abnormal Vaginal Discharge

BACTERIAL VAGINOSIS

A 30-year-old F presents with malaodorous discharge. **Exam** shows gray vaginal discharge. **Labs/Imaging:** Wet mount shows clue cells, and KOH preparation yields (+) whiff test.

Management:

1. Metronidazole (PO or vaginal) or vaginal clindamycin.

Complications:

- Pelvic inflammatory disease.
- If pregnant: Chorioamnionitis/endometritis, preterm delivery.

HYF: Caused by a change in vaginal flora (frequently due to increase in *Gardnerella vaginalis*); increased risk in pregnancy.

TRICHOMONAS

A 24-year-old F presents with dysuria, malodorous discharge, and pruritus. On **exam**, she has yellow-green vaginal discharge and petechiae on the cervix; wet mount shows motile trichomonads.

Management:

1. Single-dose PO metronidazole or fluconazole.
2. Treat partners.
3. Test for other STIs.

Complications:

- PID.
- If pregnant: Chorioamnionitis/endometritis, pre-term delivery.

HYF: Risk factors include unprotected sex.

VAGINAL CANDIDIASIS

A 35-year-old F presents with vulvar pruritus and increased vaginal discharge. **Exam** shows vulvar excoriations and thick, white vaginal discharge. KOH prep shows hyphae and budding yeasts.

Management:

1. Fluconazole (PO or topical).

Complications: None.

HYF: Risk factors include diabetes, pregnancy, and other immunocompromised states.

CHLAMYDIA

A 28-year-old F presents with vaginal discharge and dysuria. **Exam** shows mucopurulent discharge and cervical motion tenderness. On **labs**, urine culture is positive for *Chlamydia*.

Management:

1. Doxycycline x 7 days.
2. Single-dose azithromycin.
3. Single-dose IM ceftriaxone for presumptive coinfection with *Neisseria*.
4. Treat partners.

Complications:

- Pelvic inflammatory disease.
- Tubo-ovarian abscess.
- Infertility.

HYF: Treat for presumptive coinfection with *Neisseria* given high rates of co-occurrence.

GONORRHEA

A 19-year-old F presents with vaginal discharge and dysuria. **Exam** shows mucopurulent discharge and cervical motion tenderness. On **labs**, nucleic acid amplification test (NAAT) is (+) gonorrhea.

Management:

1. Single-dose IM ceftriaxone.
2. Treat for presumptive coinfection with *Chlamydia*: Doxycycline + azithromycin.
3. Treat partners.

Complications:

- Pelvic inflammatory disease.
- Tubo-ovarian abscess.
- Infertility.

HYF: Treat for presumptive coinfection with *Chlamydia* given high rates of co-occurrence.

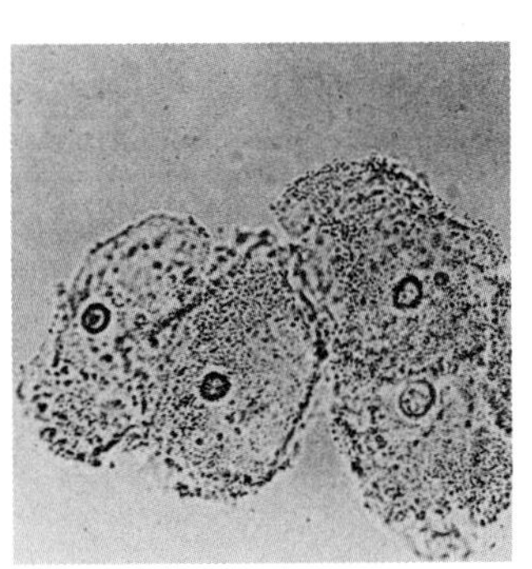

Clue cells.

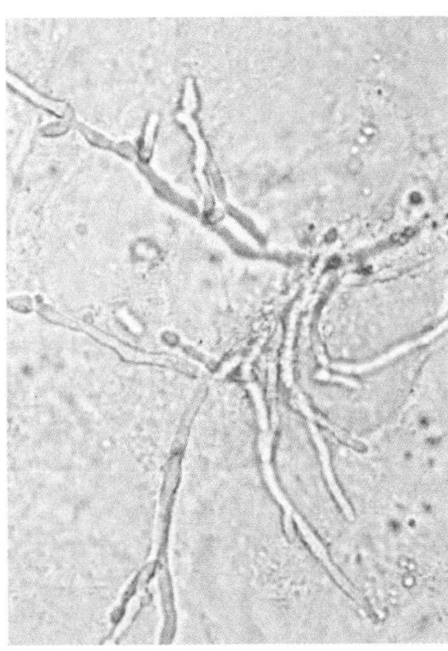

Candida albicans.

25-8 Incontinence

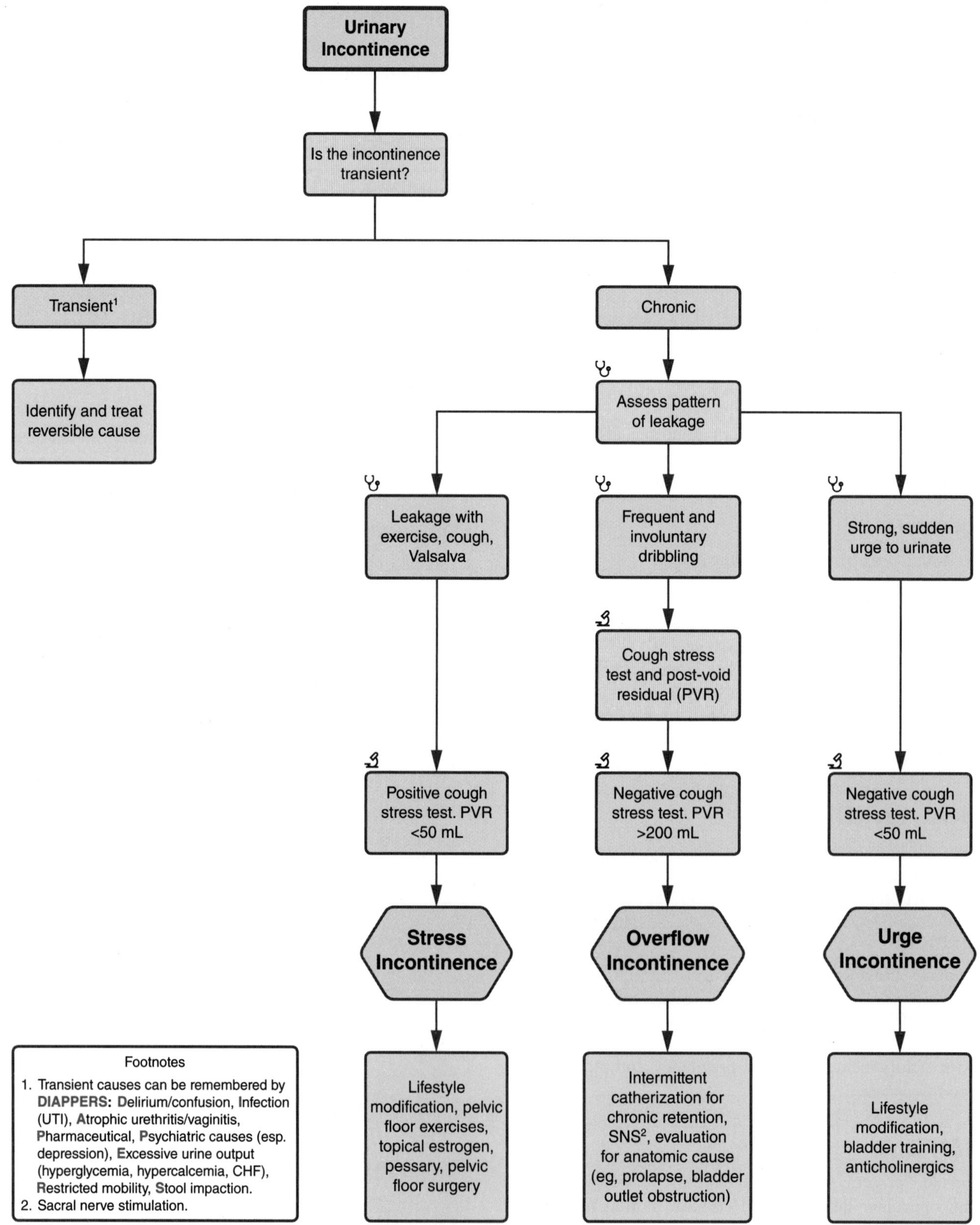
Urinary Incontinence
Is the incontinence transient?
Transient[1]
Chronic
Identify and treat reversible cause
Assess pattern of leakage
Leakage with exercise, cough, Valsalva
Frequent and involuntary dribbling
Strong, sudden urge to urinate
Cough stress test and post-void residual (PVR)
Positive cough stress test. PVR <50 mL
Negative cough stress test. PVR >200 mL
Negative cough stress test. PVR <50 mL
Stress Incontinence
Overflow Incontinence
Urge Incontinence
Lifestyle modification, pelvic floor exercises, topical estrogen, pessary, pelvic floor surgery
Intermittent catheterization for chronic retention, SNS[2], evaluation for anatomic cause (eg, prolapse, bladder outlet obstruction)
Lifestyle modification, bladder training, anticholinergics
Footnotes
1. Transient causes can be remembered by DIAPPERS: Delirium/confusion, Infection (UTI), Atrophic urethritis/vaginitis, Pharmaceutical, Psychiatric causes (esp. depression), Excessive urine output (hyperglycemia, hypercalcemia, CHF), Restricted mobility, Stool impaction.
2. Sacral nerve stimulation.

FIGURE 25.8

25-8 Incontinence

STRESS INCONTINENCE

A 64-year-old F G5P5 with PMH of HTN presents with leakage of urine when she laughs, coughs, or sneezes. She denies any fevers or difficulty or pain with urination. On **exam**, she has leakage with cough and Valsalva, and **labs** are significant for positive cough stress test and PVR <50 mL.

Management:

1. Lifestyle modification and pelvic floor exercises.
2. Topical estrogen for postmenopausal women.
3. Pessary.
4. Pelvic floor surgery or midurethral sling.

Complications:

- UTI.
- Emotional distress.
- Skin rashes and infections.

HYF: Stress incontinence is most commonly caused by weakened pelvic floor muscles, poor intrinsic sphincter function, or urethral hypermobility.

OVERFLOW INCONTINENCE

A 49-year-old F with PMH of DM2 and fibroids presents with urinary incontinence. The patient has frequent urinary accidents without warnings or triggers. She denies dysuria. On **exam**, she has a negative cough stress test and PVR >200 mL.

Management:

1. Cholinergic agonists.
2. Clean intermittent catheterization for chronic retention.
3. Sacral nerve stimulation.

Complications:

- UTI.
- Emotional distress.
- Skin rashes and infections.

HYF: Overflow incontinence is a problem of detrusor muscle underactivity or bladder outlet obstruction (eg, BPH).

URGE INCONTINENCE

A 37-year-old F G3P4 with no significant PMH presents with frequent, sudden urge to urinate. She is often unable to make it to the bathroom in time. She is s/p vaginal birth of twin babies 4 weeks ago via NSVD. On **exam**, she has a negative stress test and PVR <50 mL.

Management:

1. Lifestyle modification.
2. Bladder training.
3. Anticholinergics (oxybutynin).

Complications:

- UTI.
- Emotional distress.
- Skin rashes and infections.

HYF: This is a problem of detrusor muscle overstimulation. Often occurs at night and disrupts sleep.

25-9 Primary Amenorrhea

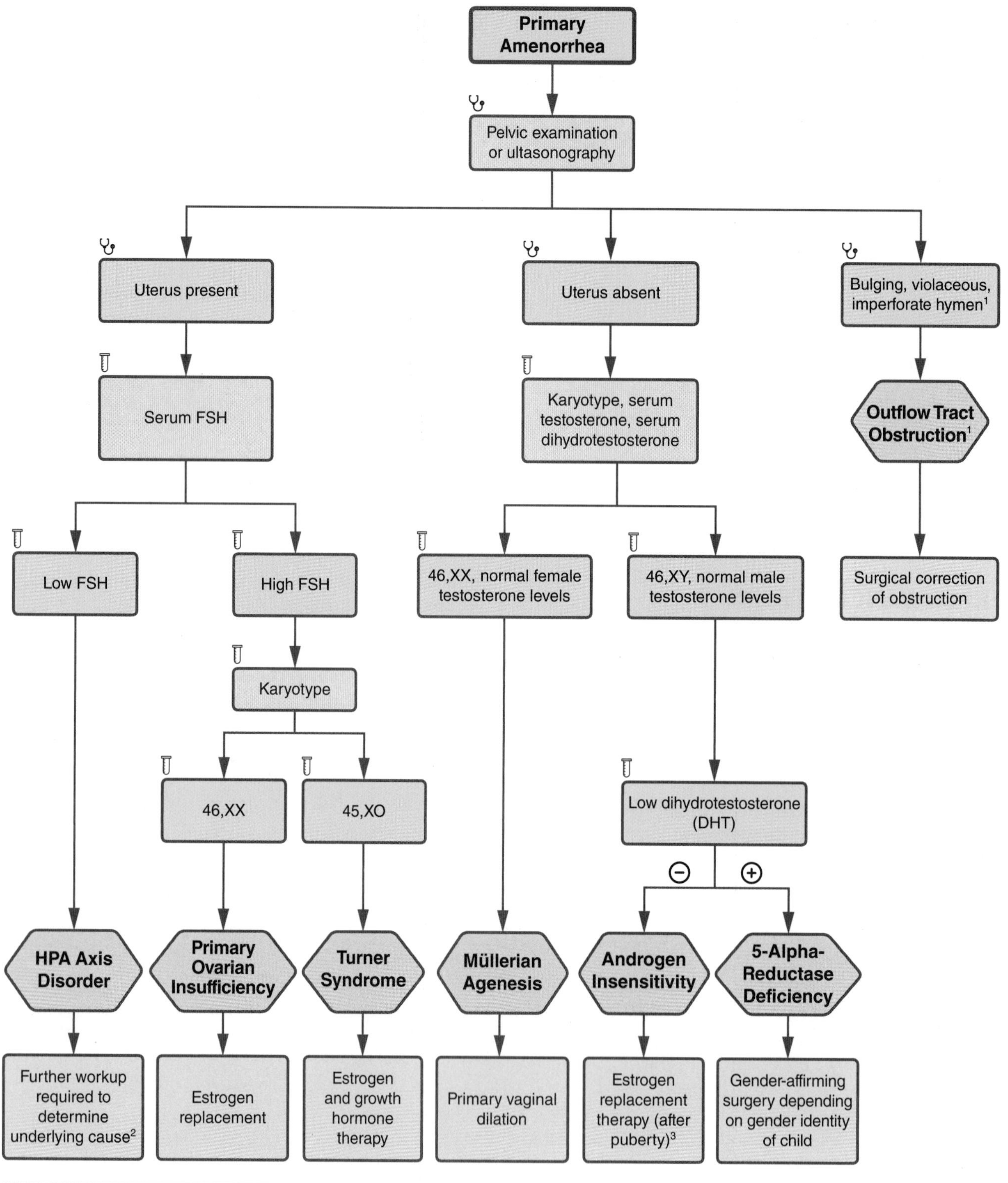
Primary Amenorrhea
Pelvic examination or ultasonography
Uterus present
Uterus absent
Bulging, violaceous, imperforate hymen[1]
Serum FSH
Karyotype, serum testosterone, serum dihydrotestosterone
Outflow Tract Obstruction[1]
Low FSH
High FSH
46,XX, normal female testosterone levels
46,XY, normal male testosterone levels
Surgical correction of obstruction
Karyotype
46,XX
45,XO
Low dihydrotestosterone (DHT)
⊖
⊕
HPA Axis Disorder
Primary Ovarian Insufficiency
Turner Syndrome
Müllerian Agenesis
Androgen Insensitivity
5-Alpha-Reductase Deficiency
Further workup required to determine underlying cause[2]
Estrogen replacement
Estrogen and growth hormone therapy
Primary vaginal dilation
Estrogen replacement therapy (after puberty)[3]
Gender-affirming surgery depending on gender identity of child

Footnotes

Primary amenorrhea is defined as the absence of menses at age 15 in the presence of secondary sexual characteristics and normal growth.

1. Examples of outflow tract obstructions include imperforate hymen (as described in the algorithm), transverse vaginal septum, and vaginal agenesis.
2. Possible HPA axis disorders include Kallman syndrome, consitutional delay, and functional hypothalamic amenorrhea.
3. Undescended testicles are removed due to cancer risk. Treatment is based on gender identity.

FIGURE 25.9

25-9 Primary Amenorrhea

HPA AXIS DISORDERS

A 15-year-old F presents with primary amenorrhea. On **exam**, she has short stature (constitutional delay), impaired sense of smell (Kallmann syndrome), and low BMI (functional hypothalamic amenorrhea).

Management:

1. Constitutional delay: Hormone replacement therapy.
2. Kallmann syndrome: Hormone replacement therapy.
3. Functional hypothalamic amenorrhea: Increase BMI and/or reduce stress.

Complications:

- Constitutional delay: Short stature.
- Kallmann syndrome: Urologic and neurologic abnormalities.
- Functional hypothalamic amenorrhea: Risk of cardiovascular disease and osteopenia.

HYF: Constitutional delay is more common in males than females.

OUTFLOW TRACT OBSTRUCTION

A 13-year-old F with PMH of cyclic abdominal pain presents with primary amenorrhea and a bulge in her vagina. **Exam** shows imperforate hymen. There are normal **labs** and **imaging** of the internal organs.

Management:

1. Identify types of obstruction (most common): Imperforate hymen, transverse vaginal septum, vaginal agenesis.
2. Surgical correction of obstruction.

Complications:

- Risk of endometriosis in long-standing cases.
- Risk of infertility and urinary retention if severe.

HYF: Transverse vaginal septum and imperforate hymen are the most common etiologies of primary amenorrhea in a patient with normal pubertal development and a uterus.

PRIMARY OVARIAN INSUFFICIENCY

A 13-year-old F presents with primary amenorrhea. On **exam**, she has no secondary sex characteristics. **Labs** show high FSH and low estrogen.

Management:

1. Hormone replacement therapy.
2. Psychological support.

Complications:

- Osteopenia.
- Cardiovascular disease.
- Hypothyroid or other endocrine disorders.

HYF: Varied etiology, all occurring before puberty: Chromosomal abnormalities, chemotherapy, radiation, premutation in FMR1 (fragile X), or endocrinopathy.

TURNER SYNDROME

A 15-year-old F presents with primary amenorrhea. On **exam**, she has short stature, shield chest, brachial > femoral pulse (coarctation of aorta), and high-arched palate. **Imaging** shows bicuspid aortic valve, horseshoe kidney, and streak ovaries. **Labs** show decreased estrogen and increased LH and FSH.

Management:

1. Short stature prevented by growth hormone therapy.

Complications: Common manifestations of Turner syndrome include:

- Coarctation of aorta.
- Hypertension.
- Hearing loss.
- Infertility (although pregnancy may be possible with IVF and exogenous estradiol + progesterone).

HYF: Turner syndrome is the most common cause of primary amenorrhea. Sex chromosome (usually X) loss often is due to nondisjunction during meiosis or mitosis.

MÜLLERIAN AGENESIS

A 15-year-old F with developmentally appropriate secondary sexual characteristics presents with primary amenorrhea. On **exam**, she has a vaginal dimple. On **imaging**, MRI shows rudimentary Müllerian structures.

Management:

1. Non-surgical vaginal elongation by dilation.
2. Psychological support.

Complications: Concomitant congenital malformations (especially of the urinary tract and skeleton) are present in up to 50% of patients with Müllerian agenesis.

HYF: Müllerian agenesis is caused by embryonic underdevelopment of the Müllerian duct with normal height, breast development, body hair, and external genitalia.

ANDROGEN INSENSITIVITY SYNDROME

A 15-year-old F presents with primary amenorrhea. **Exam** shows female external genitalia with scant axillary and pubic hair and rudimentary vagina. **Imaging** shows an absent uterus and fallopian tubes. **Labs** show increased testosterone, estrogen, and LH.

Management:

1. Treatment based on gender identity.
2. Hormone replacement therapy to prevent osteoporosis.

Complications: Normal functioning testes (often found in labia majora) are surgically removed to prevent malignancy.

HYF: Androgen insensitivity syndrome is caused by a defect in the androgen receptor, resulting in a normal-appearing female (46,XY DSD).

(Continued)

25-9 Primary Amenorrhea

5-ALPHA-REDUCTASE DEFICIENCY

A 15-year-old F assigned at birth individual presents with primary amenorrhea and virilization of genitals instead. **Labs** show normal male-range testosterone and disproportionately low dihydrotestosterone levels. On **imaging**, no uterus is present on US.

Management:

1. Gender-affirming care depending on child's gender identity.
2. Supplemental testosterone and fertility treatments per gender identity.

Complications:

- Infertility.
- Psychosexual, mental health challenges.

HYF: 5-alpha-reductase converts testosterone to DHT. Testosterone is responsible for development of internal genitalia (testicular), whereas DHT is responsible for development of external genitalia (scrotal and penile). Therefore, these children have ambiguous, female-appearing genitalia at birth and male gonads internally.

25-10 Secondary Amenorrhea

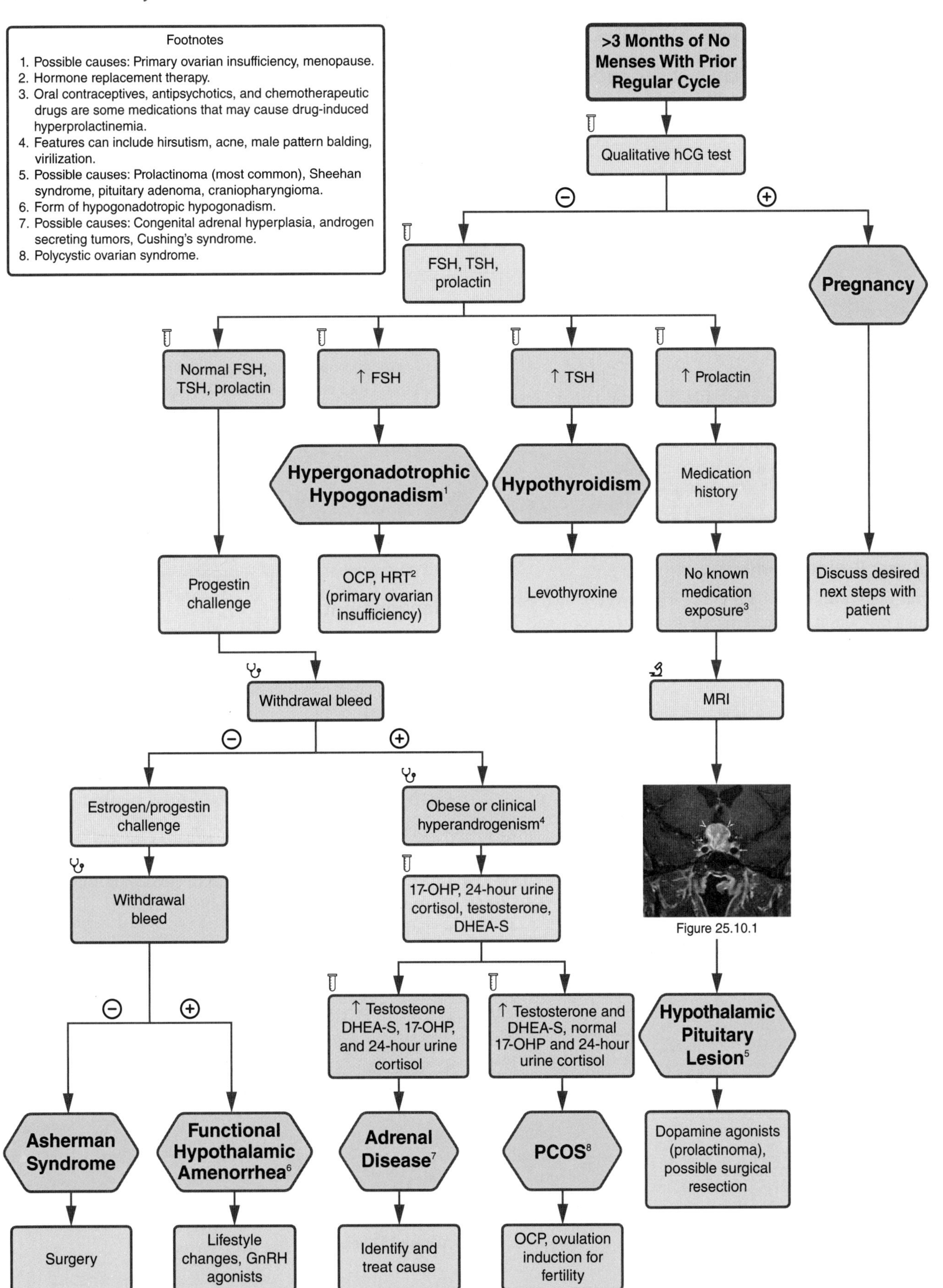
Footnotes
1. Possible causes: Primary ovarian insufficiency, menopause.
2. Hormone replacement therapy.
3. Oral contraceptives, antipsychotics, and chemotherapeutic drugs are some medications that may cause drug-induced hyperprolactinemia.
4. Features can include hirsutism, acne, male pattern balding, virilization.
5. Possible causes: Prolactinoma (most common), Sheehan syndrome, pituitary adenoma, craniopharyngioma.
6. Form of hypogonadotropic hypogonadism.
7. Possible causes: Congenital adrenal hyperplasia, androgen secreting tumors, Cushing's syndrome.
8. Polycystic ovarian syndrome.
>3 Months of No Menses With Prior Regular Cycle
Qualitative hCG test
⊖
⊕
FSH, TSH, prolactin
Pregnancy
Discuss desired next steps with patient
Normal FSH, TSH, prolactin
↑ FSH
↑ TSH
↑ Prolactin
Hypergonadotrophic Hypogonadism[1]
Hypothyroidism
Medication history
Progestin challenge
OCP, HRT[2] (primary ovarian insufficiency)
Levothyroxine
No known medication exposure[3]
Withdrawal bleed
MRI
⊖
⊕
Estrogen/progestin challenge
Obese or clinical hyperandrogenism[4]
Figure 25.10.1
Withdrawal bleed
17-OHP, 24-hour urine cortisol, testosterone, DHEA-S
⊖
⊕
↑ Testosterone DHEA-S, 17-OHP, and 24-hour urine cortisol
↑ Testosterone and DHEA-S, normal 17-OHP and 24-hour urine cortisol
Hypothalamic Pituitary Lesion[5]
Asherman Syndrome
Functional Hypothalamic Amenorrhea[6]
Adrenal Disease[7]
PCOS[8]
Dopamine agonists (prolactinoma), possible surgical resection
Surgery
Lifestyle changes, GnRH agonists
Identify and treat cause
OCP, ovulation induction for fertility

FIGURE 25.10

25-10 Secondary Amenorrhea

HYPERGONADOTROPIC HYPOGONADISM

Prototype: Primary Ovarian Insufficiency

A 39-year-old F presents with 1 year of hot flashes, night sweats, and increasing pain with sexual intercourse.

Management:

1. Estrogen replacement therapy (transdermal or vaginal).
2. Micronized progesterone.
3. Weight-bearing exercises, daily calcium.

Complications:

- Osteoporosis.
- Infertility.

HYF: Etiology varies, with 50% being idiopathic. Other causes of ovarian insufficiency: Chromosomal abnormalities (Turner syndrome and fragile X syndrome, galactosemia), ovarian damage (chemotherapy, radiation, surgery), autoimmune conditions.

HYPOTHALAMIC PITUITARY LESION

Prototype: Prolactinoma

A 37-year-old F with no PMH presents with 1 year of increasingly worsening new-onset headache, irregular menstruations, and difficulty getting pregnant. She also endorses 6 months of whitish nipple discharge.

Management:

1. Dopamine agonist.
2. Surgical resection.
3. Postoperative radiation therapy.

Complications: Infertility.

HYF: While most cases of hyperprolactinemia are due to an adenoma, some cases are idiopathic. It is important to rule out hypothyroidism and drug-induced hyperprolactinemia.

ASHERMAN SYNDROME

A 35-year-old F s/p 3 D&C therapeutic abortions presents with 1 year of no menses. She previously had regular periods. Three years ago, she started to have irregular periods, and last year, her menses stopped completely.

Management:

1. Hysteroscopic lysis of adhesions.

Complications:

- Chronic endometritis.
- Recurrent miscarriages.
- Infertility.

HYF: Hysteroscopy is both diagnostic and therapeutic.

FUNCTIONAL HYPOTHALAMIC AMENORRHEA

A 21-year-old F college cross-country runner presents with 2 years of amenorrhea. On **exam**, BMI is 18. On **labs**, FSH, TSH, and prolactin levels are normal.

Management:

1. Weight gain and decreased training/exercise.
2. Estrogen replacement therapy.

Complications: Osteoporosis.

HYF: Functional hypothalamic amenorrhea is a diagnosis of exclusion. While it is typically associated with the female-athlete triad (amenorrhea, osteoporosis, decreased caloric intake), it can be precipitated by a malabsorptive (celiac disease) or hypermetabolic state (high stress/cortisol) or as a result of an eating disorder.

POLYCYSTIC OVARIAN SYNDROME (PCOS)

A 27-year-old F G0P0 presents with 2 years of irregular menstrual periods, now having periods once per year. On **exam**, she has thick hair on the upper lips and chin, acne, and male-pattern balding.

Management:

1. Menstrual-dysfunction treatment (OCPs, progestin IUD, metformin).
2. Androgen-excess therapy (OCPs, spironolactone, GnRH agonists).
3. Infertility treatment (weight loss, letrozole, clomiphene, metformin).

Complications:

- Depression/anxiety.
- Infertility.
- Metabolic syndrome and CVD (screening for HTN, dyslipidemia, and diabetes is recommended).
- Endometrial carcinoma.

HYF: While diagnosis is suggested by meeting the Rotterdam criteria below, definitive diagnosis is based on exclusion of other mimics of PCOS (thyroid disease, non-classic congenital adrenal hyperplasia, hyperprolactinemia, and androgen-secreting tumors).

- Rotterdam criteria (2 out of 3 required for diagnosis):
  1. Oligo- and/or anovulation.
  2. Clinical and/or biochemical signs of hyperandrogenism.
  3. Polycystic ovaries on US.

Hypothyroidism: See pp. 137–139.

Adrenal Disease: See pp. 154–156.

25-11 Dysmenorrhea

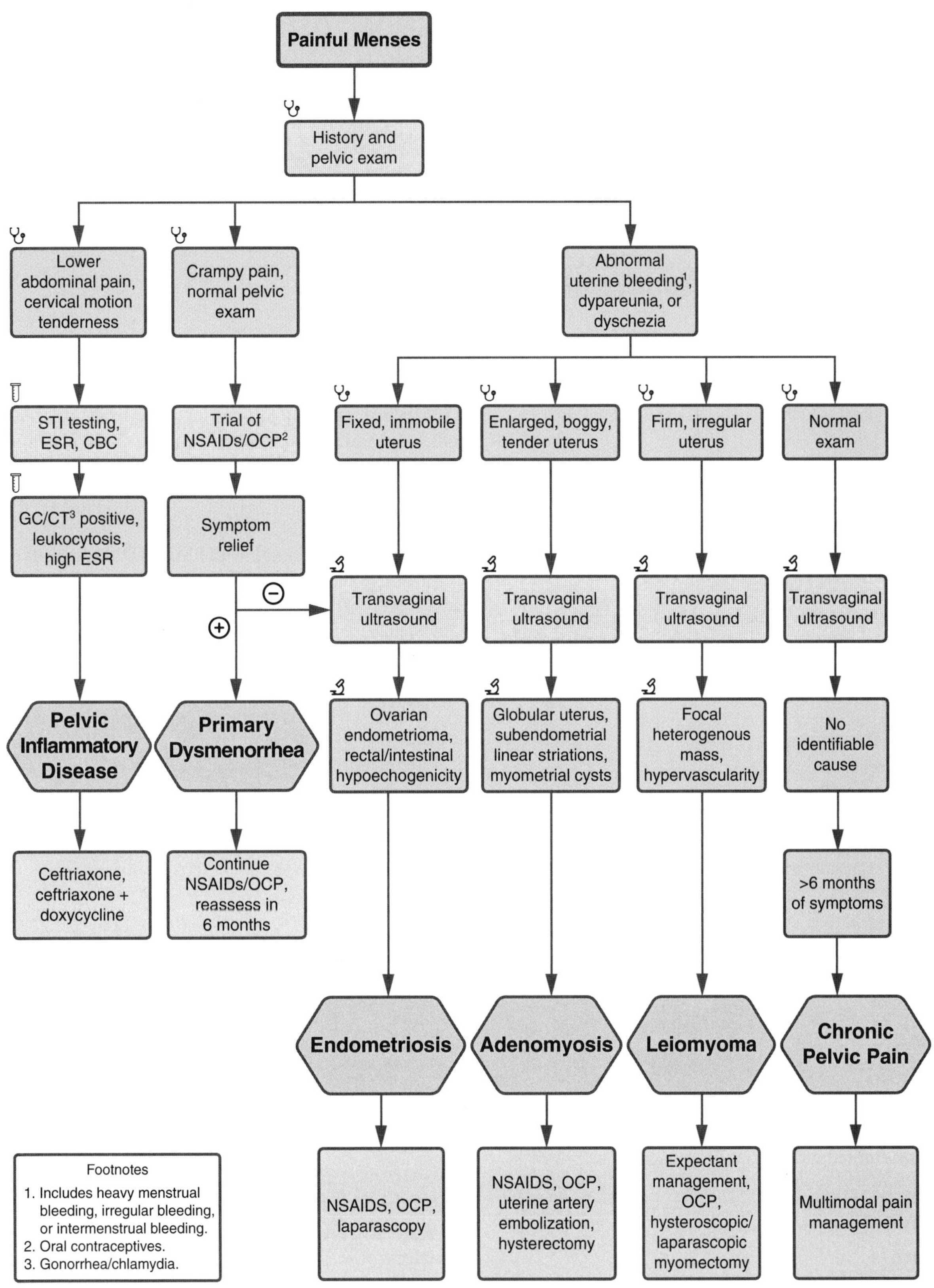
Painful Menses
History and pelvic exam
Lower abdominal pain, cervical motion tenderness
Crampy pain, normal pelvic exam
Abnormal uterine bleeding[1], dyspareunia, or dyschezia
STI testing, ESR, CBC
GC/CT[3] positive, leukocytosis, high ESR
Pelvic Inflammatory Disease
Ceftriaxone, ceftriaxone + doxycycline
Trial of NSAIDs/OCP[2]
Symptom relief
Primary Dysmenorrhea
Continue NSAIDs/OCP, reassess in 6 months
Fixed, immobile uterus
Enlarged, boggy, tender uterus
Firm, irregular uterus
Normal exam
Transvaginal ultrasound
Transvaginal ultrasound
Transvaginal ultrasound
Transvaginal ultrasound
Ovarian endometrioma, rectal/intestinal hypoechogenicity
Globular uterus, subendometrial linear striations, myometrial cysts
Focal heterogenous mass, hypervascularity
No identifiable cause
>6 months of symptoms
Endometriosis
Adenomyosis
Leiomyoma
Chronic Pelvic Pain
NSAIDS, OCP, laparascopy
NSAIDS, OCP, uterine artery embolization, hysterectomy
Expectant management, OCP, hysteroscopic/ laparascopic myomectomy
Multimodal pain management
Footnotes
1. Includes heavy menstrual bleeding, irregular bleeding, or intermenstrual bleeding.
2. Oral contraceptives.
3. Gonorrhea/chlamydia.

FIGURE 25.11

25-11 Dysmenorrhea

PELVIC INFLAMMATORY DISEASE

A 27-year-old F with multiple sexual partners presents with acute-onset lower abdominal pain and tenderness. She has cervical motion tenderness with mucopurulent endocervical discharge on pelvic exam.

Management:

1. Outpatient treatment: Ceftriaxone IM × 1 dose + doxycycline PO × 14 days + metronidazole × 14 days.
2. Inpatient treatment: Cefoxitin IV + doxycycline PO. 24 hours after clinical improvement: Stop cefoxitin, continue doxycycline, and add metronidazole × 14 days.

Complications:

- Tubo-ovarian abscess.
- Fitz-Hugh-Curtis syndrome.
- Infertility.

HYF: Presumptive clinical diagnosis is sufficient to initiate empiric antibiotic therapy in patients with suspicion for PID due to severity of reproductive repercussions (infertility).

PRIMARY DYSMENORRHEA

A 16-year-old F with no PMH presents with recurrent, crampy lower abdominal pain beginning several hours prior to onset of menses and lasting 1–3 days. She has a normal pelvic exam.

Management:

1. NSAIDs ± topical heat therapy.
2. Oral contraceptives (OCPs).

Complications: None.

HYF: Most common gynecological concern among adolescents. It is a diagnosis of exclusion when all possible pelvic pathologies have been ruled out.

ENDOMETRIOSIS

A 25-year-old F presents with painful menses, dyspareunia (pain with sexual intercourse), and dyschezia (pain with defecation). She and her partner have been actively trying to get pregnant for the past 4 years.

Management:

1. NSAIDs + OCPs.
2. GnRH agonists + norethindrone/GnRH antagonists.
3. Laparoscopy.

Complications:

- Endometrioma.
- Increased risk of epithelial ovarian cancer (clear-cell and endometroid).
- Infertility.

HYF: Leading cause of secondary dysmenorrhea. Laparoscopy can be diagnostic as well as therapeutic in patients with endometriosis. Patients present with the **3Ds – dysmenorrhea, dyschezia, dyspareunia.**

ADENOMYOSIS

A 45-year-old F presents with several years of worsening, heavy menstrual bleeding and painful menses. Pelvic exam reveals enlarged, boggy/tender uterus. On **imaging**, transvaginal US shows a globular uterus with subendometrial linear striations.

Management:

1. NSAIDs or OCPs.
2. Uterine artery embolization.
3. Hysterectomy.

Complications:

- Hysterectomy.
- Infertility.

HYF: While treatment is based on clinical diagnosis with imaging studies, a definitive diagnosis can only be made on pathology evaluation following a hysterectomy.

LEIOMYOMA

A 49-year-old nulliparous F with PMH of DM2 presents with 1 year of worsening heavy and prolonged menstrual bleeding, requiring pad changes every 2 hours. Menses began at age 10 and were previously regular. She also reports constipation and urinary frequency.

Management:

1. Medication management (OCPs, progestin IUDs).
2. Hysteroscopic/laparoscopic myomectomy.
3. Hysterectomy.

Complications:

- Placental abruption/fetal growth restriction.
- Infertility.
- Hysterectomy.

HYF: Most common pelvic tumor (benign). Management varies based on symptoms and whether the patient desires future fertility.

CHRONIC PELVIC PAIN

A 25-year-old F presents with 1 year of non-cyclic pelvic pain. She reports that her pain is worse with stress and during sexual intercourse. Pelvic exam and transvaginal US are normal.

Management:

1. NSAIDs/acetaminophen.
2. Oral contraceptive if cyclic exacerbation of pelvic pain.
3. Multimodal therapy (physical therapy, muscle relaxants, topical analgesics).

Complications:

- Depression.
- Hysterectomy.

HYF: This is a diagnosis of exclusion. For some, pelvic pain is due to central sensitization and is associated with somatic symptoms (eg, fatigue, poor sleep).

25-12 Abnormal Uterine Bleeding

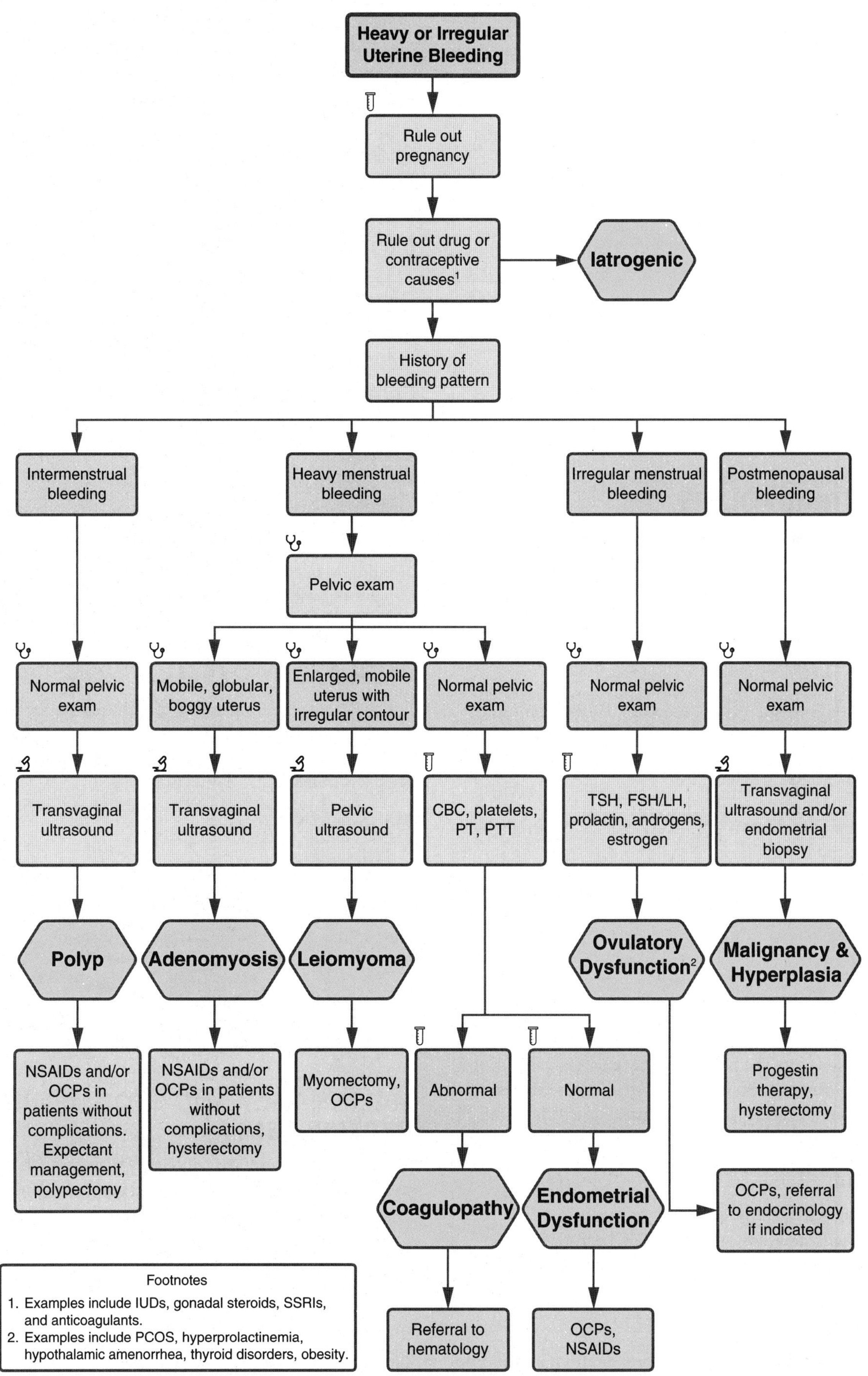
Heavy or Irregular Uterine Bleeding
Rule out pregnancy
Rule out drug or contraceptive causes[1]
Iatrogenic
History of bleeding pattern
Intermenstrual bleeding
Heavy menstrual bleeding
Irregular menstrual bleeding
Postmenopausal bleeding
Pelvic exam
Normal pelvic exam
Mobile, globular, boggy uterus
Enlarged, mobile uterus with irregular contour
Normal pelvic exam
Normal pelvic exam
Normal pelvic exam
Transvaginal ultrasound
Transvaginal ultrasound
Pelvic ultrasound
CBC, platelets, PT, PTT
TSH, FSH/LH, prolactin, androgens, estrogen
Transvaginal ultrasound and/or endometrial biopsy
Polyp
Adenomyosis
Leiomyoma
Ovulatory Dysfunction[2]
Malignancy & Hyperplasia
NSAIDs and/or OCPs in patients without complications. Expectant management, polypectomy
NSAIDs and/or OCPs in patients without complications, hysterectomy
Myomectomy, OCPs
Abnormal
Normal
Progestin therapy, hysterectomy
Coagulopathy
Endometrial Dysfunction
OCPs, referral to endocrinology if indicated
Referral to hematology
OCPs, NSAIDs
Footnotes
1. Examples include IUDs, gonadal steroids, SSRIs, and anticoagulants.
2. Examples include PCOS, hyperprolactinemia, hypothalamic amenorrhea, thyroid disorders, obesity.

FIGURE 25.12

25-12 Abnormal Uterine Bleeding

IATROGENIC CAUSE

A 32-year-old F with a history of IUD placement 6 months ago presents with irregular menstrual bleeding. **Exam** and **labs** are normal.

Management:

1. Reassurance, shared decision-making.

Complications: Dependent on specific etiology.

HYF: For iatrogenic causes of abnormal uterine bleeding (AUB), the most common cause will be medical devices such as IUDs. Medications that may cause AUB include gonadal steroids, drugs that affect gonadal steroid production (aromatase inhibitors, SERMs), anticoagulants, and agents that contribute to disorders of ovulation by interfering with dopamine metabolism or inducing hyperprolactinemia (1st- and 2nd-generation antipsychotics, tricyclic antidepressants, SSRIs).

ENDOMETRIAL POLYPS

A 32-year-old F with unremarkable PMH presents with "spotting in between periods." Pelvic **exam** and **labs** are normal. On **imaging**, transvaginal ultrasound (TVUS) shows endometrial polyps.

Management:

1. If asymptomatic (ie, discovered incidentally): Expectant management.
2. If symptomatic (intermenstrual bleeding): Polypectomy and histologic analysis.

Complications: Recurrence (rare).

HYF: Polyps are caused by the proliferation of endometrial glands and stroma around a vascular core that projects from the surface of the endometrium. In addition to symptomatic AUB, other indications for polyp removal include risk factors for endometrial hyperplasia/cancer, polyp diameter >1.5 cm, multiple polyps, and prolapsed polyps.

ADENOMYOSIS

A 43-year-old F with PMH of heavy, painful periods presents with fatigue. On pelvic **exam**, she has a diffusely enlarged, soft, mobile uterus. **Labs** show anemia. On **imaging**, TVUS shows thickening of the posterior myometrium, myometrial cysts, linear striations from the endometrium, and/or loss of a clear endomyometrial border.

Management:

1. Hysterectomy is the definitive treatment.
2. For patients who have not completed childbearing, levonorgestrel-releasing IUD may alleviate symptoms.

Complications: Dysmenorrhea, chronic pelvic pain.

HYF: Adenomyosis is caused by the proliferation of endometrial glands and stroma within the myometrium, resulting in hypertrophy. Adenomyosis often co-occurs with uterine leiomyomas and endometriosis. Parity is associated with increased risk.

LEIOMYOMA

A 32-year-old F with PMH of heavy menstrual periods lasting >7 days presents with fatigue, constipation, and pelvic pressure. On pelvic **exam**, she has a large, irregularly shaped uterus. **Labs** show anemia. On **imaging**, pelvic US shows uterine fibroids.

Management:

1. Initiate combined oral contraceptives (COCs).
2. If COCs are ineffective at controlling bleeding, proceed to surgical management (uterine artery embolization, hysteroscopic myomectomy).

Complications:

- Urinary and/or bowel symptoms.
- Dysmenorrhea, dyspareunia.
- Infertility, recurrent pregnancy loss.

HYF: Fibroids are caused by the proliferation of smooth muscle cells within the myometrium. Heavy and/or prolonged menstrual bleeding is the most common symptom of fibroids, but they can also present with bulk symptoms and/or reproductive dysfunction. Parity is associated with decreased risk.

OVULATORY DYSFUNCTION

A 17-year-old F with a history of obesity presents with irregular menstrual periods and cystic acne. On **exam**, she has terminal hair growth on the upper lip and cheeks. **Labs** show elevated androgens. On **imaging**, US shows polycystic ovaries.

Management:

1. Weight loss.
2. OCPs for menstrual regulation.
3. Letrozole for ovulation induction.

Complications: Endometrial hyperplasia/malignancy.

HYF: Polycystic ovarian syndrome (PCOS) is a common cause of ovulatory dysfunction and often presents during adolescence. It is the most common cause of infertility in women.

MALIGNANCY AND ENDOMETRIAL HYPERPLASIA

A 43-year-old F with PMH of obesity presents with persistent intermenstrual spotting. Pelvic **exam** and **labs** are normal. Biopsy shows endometrial hyperplasia (EH) with atypia.

Management:

1. Progestin therapy is 1st-line (levonorgestrel-releasing IUD preferred over oral agents) for patients desiring to maintain fertility. In patients who are done with fertility, always perform hysterectomy (the definitive treatment due to risk of endometrial cancer).

25-12 Abnormal Uterine Bleeding

Complications: Endometrial carcinoma.

HYF: Risk factors for endometrial hyperplasia center on conditions that produce excess or unopposed estrogen, including obesity, early menarche/late menopause, nulliparity, chronic anovulation, and tamoxifen use. Compared to EH *without* atypia, patients with EH *with* atypia are 4 times as likely to progress to endometrial cancer.

COAGULOPATHY

A 17-year-old F with PMH of frequent epistaxis presents with heavy menstrual periods that regularly soak through her clothes. Pelvic **exam** is normal. **Labs** show coagulopathy (eg, in the setting of von Willebrand disease, labs often show normal CBC, normal PT, and prolonged aPTT).

Management:

1. Referral to hematology for diagnosis and ongoing management.
2. COCs or IUD to control bleeding.
3. Desmopressin (DDAVP) or antifibrinolytics.

Complications: Dependent on specific coagulopathy.

HYF: von Willebrand disease (VWD) is the most common inherited bleeding disorder. In the OB/GYN context, look for heavy menstrual bleeding in an adolescent that seems excessive (eg, patient awakens multiple times per night to change pads, bleeding soaks through clothes), possibly accompanied by bleeding in other settings (eg, mucocutaneous bleeding).

ENDOMETRIAL DYSFUNCTION

A 32-year-old F with unremarkable PMH presents with heavy menstrual periods and no other symptoms. Pelvic **exam** and **labs** are normal.

Management:

1. Combined oral contraceptives or IUD to control bleeding.
2. NSAIDs to reduce prostaglandin levels.

Complications: Dependent on specific etiology.

HYF: Endometrial dysfunction as a cause of AUB refers to a primary disorder of the endometrium and is a diagnosis of exclusion. Rule out adenomyosis, leiomyoma, and coagulopathy with exam, labs, and imaging.

25-13 Adnexal Mass

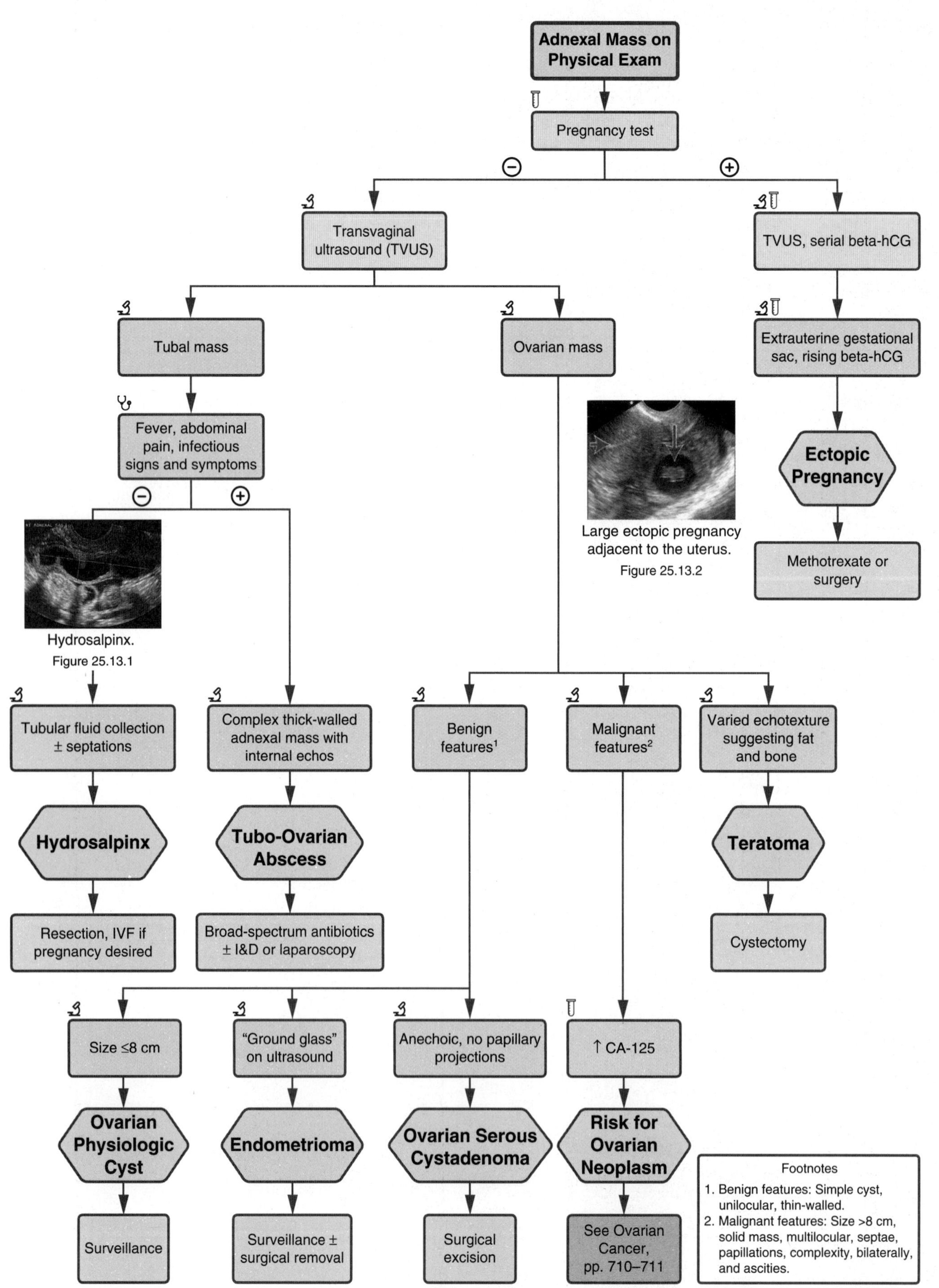

Adnexal Mass on Physical Exam
Pregnancy test
⊖
⊕
Transvaginal ultrasound (TVUS)
TVUS, serial beta-hCG
Tubal mass
Ovarian mass
Extrauterine gestational sac, rising beta-hCG
Fever, abdominal pain, infectious signs and symptoms
Ectopic Pregnancy
Methotrexate or surgery
Large ectopic pregnancy adjacent to the uterus.
Figure 25.13.2
Hydrosalpinx.
Figure 25.13.1
Tubular fluid collection ± septations
Complex thick-walled adnexal mass with internal echos
Benign features[1]
Malignant features[2]
Varied echotexture suggesting fat and bone
Hydrosalpinx
Tubo-Ovarian Abscess
Teratoma
Resection, IVF if pregnancy desired
Broad-spectrum antibiotics ± I&D or laparoscopy
Cystectomy
Size ≤8 cm
"Ground glass" on ultrasound
Anechoic, no papillary projections
↑ CA-125
Ovarian Physiologic Cyst
Endometrioma
Ovarian Serous Cystadenoma
Risk for Ovarian Neoplasm
Surveillance
Surveillance ± surgical removal
Surgical excision
See Ovarian Cancer, pp. 710–711
Footnotes
1. Benign features: Simple cyst, unilocular, thin-walled.
2. Malignant features: Size >8 cm, solid mass, multilocular, septae, papillations, complexity, bilaterally, and ascities.

FIGURE 25.13

25-13 Adnexal Mass

ECTOPIC PREGNANCY

A 28-year-old F with PMH of PID presents with vaginal bleeding and abdominal pain. On bimanual **exam**, she has an adnexal mass. **Labs** show ↑ beta-hCG. On **imaging**, US shows gestational implantation outside the uterus.

Management if unruptured:

1. Methotrexate or surgery.
2. Follow beta-hCG if medically managed.

Management if ruptured:

1. Stabilize patient with fluids, blood products, pressors.
2. Surgery.

Complications: Life-threatening hemorrhage if ruptured.

HYF: Implantation occurs in the fallopian tube 95–99% of the time in ectopic pregnancy.

HYDROSALPINX

A 35-year-old F with PMH of gonorrhea and chlamydia presents with infertility and abdominal pain. On **exam**, she has bilateral adnexal masses. On **imaging**, US shows bilateral distended fallopian tubes.

Management:

1. Hysterosalpingogram can confirm diagnosis.
2. IVF if pregnancy is desired.

Complications: Future ectopic pregnancy.

HYF: Hydrosalpinx is often asymptomatic and only recognized in the setting of infertility.

TUBO-OVARIAN ABSCESS

A 40-year-old F with PMH of PID presents with abdominal pain and fever. **Exam** shows tender adnexal mass. Wet prep shows elevated WBC.

Management:

1. US to confirm diagnosis.
2. Inpatient broad-spectrum antibiotics.
3. If no improvement in 48 hours, drainage by US guidance or laparoscopy may be necessary.

Complications: Sepsis post-rupture.

HYF: Progression from pelvic inflammatory disease to tubo-ovarian abscess is 3–16%.

TERATOMA

A 20-year-old F presents with acute pelvic pain. On bimanual **exam**, she has an adnexal mass. On **imaging**, US shows a cystic mass containing skin, hair, and teeth.

Management:

1. Cystectomy.
2. Histopathology of specimen.

Complications:

- Malignant germ cell tumor.
- Ovarian torsion.
- Ovarian rupture.

HYF: 95% of germ cell tumors are benign.

OVARIAN PHYSIOLOGIC CYST

An 18-year-old F G0 with asymptomatic menstrual history is found on bimanual **exam** to have a unilateral, nontender, mobile, 6-cm adnexal mass. On **imaging**, US shows a simple cyst.

Management:

1. Periodic US surveillance.

Complications:

- <1% of simple cysts are malignant.
- Ovarian torsion.

HYF: Nearly all simple cysts are benign and will resolve spontaneously. Cysts >4 cm are at a greater risk of torsion.

ENDOMETRIOMA

A 25-year-old F with PMH of endometriosis presents with dysmenorrhea. On bimanual **exam**, she has an adnexal mass. On **imaging**, US shows a "ground-glass" ovarian cyst.

Management:

1. Repeat US in 6–12 weeks.
2. Surgical removal or follow yearly with US surveillance.

Complications:

- Infertility.
- Chronic pelvic pain.

HYF: Also called "chocolate cysts" because of the thick, brown, old-blood contents.

OVARIAN SEROUS CYSTADENOMA

A 70-year-old F presents with pelvic pain and bloating. On bimanual **exam**, she has a unilateral adnexal mass. On **imaging**, US shows a small, unilocular cyst.

Management:

1. Labs: CA-125.
2. Surgical excision and histopathology of specimen.

Complications:

- Ovarian torsion.
- Cyst rupture.

HYF: Represents 20% of ovarian neoplasms and is benign.

25-14 Ovarian Cancer

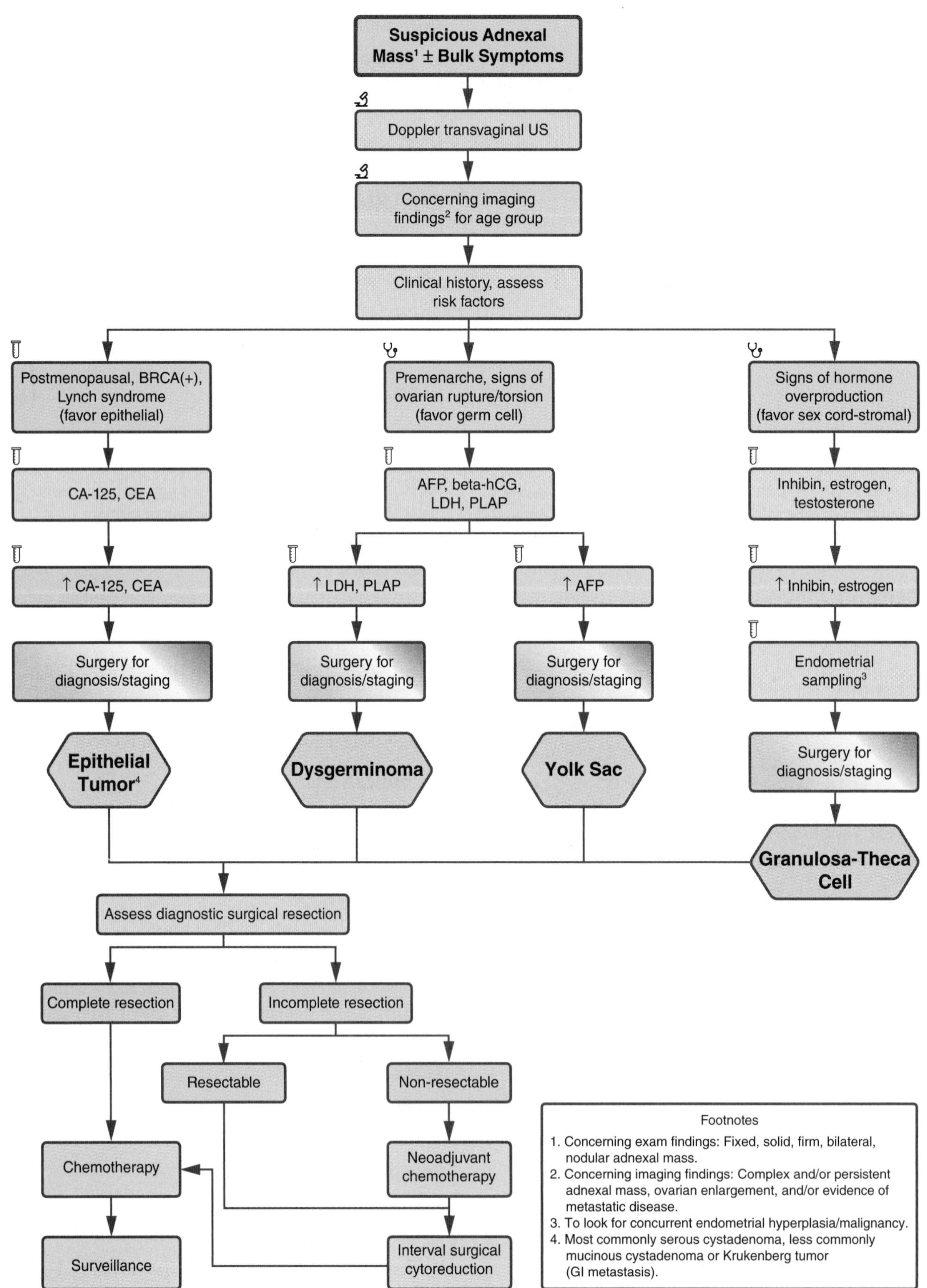

Suspicious Adnexal Mass[1] ± Bulk Symptoms
Doppler transvaginal US
Concerning imaging findings[2] for age group
Clinical history, assess risk factors
Postmenopausal, BRCA(+), Lynch syndrome (favor epithelial)
Premenarche, signs of ovarian rupture/torsion (favor germ cell)
Signs of hormone overproduction (favor sex cord-stromal)
CA-125, CEA
AFP, beta-hCG, LDH, PLAP
Inhibin, estrogen, testosterone
↑ CA-125, CEA
↑ LDH, PLAP
↑ AFP
↑ Inhibin, estrogen
Surgery for diagnosis/staging
Surgery for diagnosis/staging
Surgery for diagnosis/staging
Endometrial sampling[3]
Surgery for diagnosis/staging
Epithelial Tumor[4]
Dysgerminoma
Yolk Sac
Granulosa-Theca Cell
Assess diagnostic surgical resection
Complete resection
Incomplete resection
Resectable
Non-resectable
Chemotherapy
Neoadjuvant chemotherapy
Surveillance
Interval surgical cytoreduction

Footnotes

1. Concerning exam findings: Fixed, solid, firm, bilateral, nodular adnexal mass.
2. Concerning imaging findings: Complex and/or persistent adnexal mass, ovarian enlargement, and/or evidence of metastatic disease.
3. To look for concurrent endometrial hyperplasia/malignancy.
4. Most commonly serous cystadenoma, less commonly mucinous cystadenoma or Krukenberg tumor (GI metastasis).

FIGURE 25.14

25-14 Ovarian Cancer

EPITHELIAL TUMORS

Types: Serous, mucinous, endometrioid.

A 68-year-old, postmenopausal F presents with pelvic pain, a bloating sensation, and increased urinary frequency. Pelvic **exam** is notable for a palpable adnexal mass. **Labs** show elevated CA-125. On **imaging**, TVUS shows complex bilateral cystic masses measuring 15 mL and 12 mL.

Management:

1. Primary surgery to confirm diagnosis with biopsy, assess resectability, debulk, and stage tumor.
   a. Total hysterectomy with bilateral salpingo-oopherectomy, or unilateral salpingo-oopherectomy for those with disease limited to 1 ovary who wish to preserve fertility.
2. Neoadjuvant platinum-based chemotherapy for non-resectable tumors.
3. Interval surgical cytoreduction for advanced disease.
4. Adjuvant platinum-based chemotherapy for advanced disease ± radiation therapy.
5. Post-treatment surveillance: Monitor symptoms, pelvic exams, monitor relevant tumor markers.

Complications:

- Ascites.
- Malignant pleural effusion.
- Bowel obstruction.

HYF: 90% of ovarian cancers, usually in those age ≥50.

GERM CELL TUMORS (GCT)

Types: Dysgerminoma, yolk sac, choriocarcinoma.

An 11-year-old F presents with acute abdominal pain and distension. **Exam** reveals palpable adnexal mass. On **imaging**, Doppler TVUS shows a large solid ovarian mass measuring 6×8×5 cm with prominent blood flow.

Management:

1. Same management as epithelial tumors.

Complications:

- Acute abdomen from ovarian torsion, hemorrhage, or tumor rupture.
- Ascites.

HYF: Usually occur in people age <30. Rapid growth predisposes these tumors to ovarian rupture or torsion. Highly malignant and almost always unilateral, except for dysgerminomas. Most common malignant GCTs:

- **Dysgerminoma (most common):** ↑ LDH and placental alkaline phosphatase (PLAP); AUB. Increased risk in patients with dysgenetic gonads (eg, 46,XY).
- **Yolk sac tumor** (endodermal sinus tumor): ↑ AFP; mixed solid and cystic ovarian mass with a hemorrhagic portion.
- **Choriocarcinoma:** ↑ beta-hCG; precocious puberty, AUB, pregnancy-like symptoms.

SEX CORD-STROMAL TUMORS

Types: Granulosa-theca, Sertoli-Leydig.

A 53-year-old, postmenopausal F with PMH of PCOS presents with vaginal bleeding, breast tenderness, and abdominal pain. Pelvic **exam** reveals a palpable adnexal mass. **Labs** reveal elevated serum inhibin B level. On **imaging**, TVUS shows thickened endometrial stripe and a unilateral solid ovarian mass measuring 24 mL.

Management:

1. Same as epithelial tumors.
2. Pre-operative endometrial biopsy to identify possible concurrent endometrial hyperplasia/carcinoma.

Complications:

- Ascites and hydrothorax.
- Granulosa-theca: Rupture and hemorrhage; concurrent endometrial hyperplasia/carcinoma.

HYF: Least associated with abdominal metastasis. Can occur at any age.

- **Granulosa-theca (most common):** Estradiol overproduction → precocious puberty; cystic breast disease and/or breast tenderness; postmenopausal bleeding and endometrial hyperplasia/carcinoma.
- **Sertoli-Leydig:** Testosterone overproduction → virilization and hirsutism.

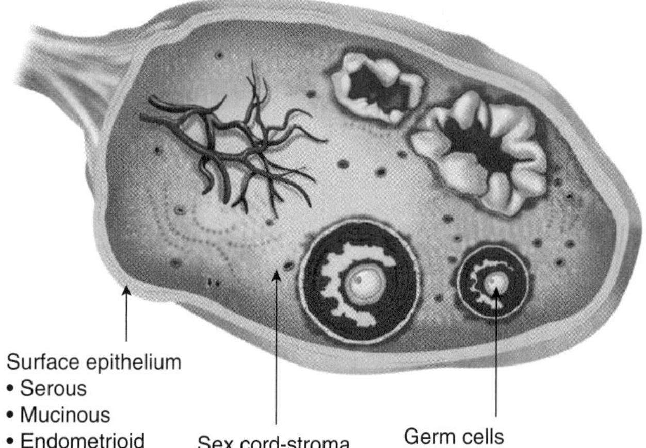
Surface epithelium
• Serous
• Mucinous
• Endometrioid
• Clear cell
• Transitional cell
Sex cord-stroma
• Granulosa cell
• Thecoma
• Fibroma
• Sertoli cell
• Sertoli-Leydig
• Steroid
Germ cells
• Dysgerminoma
• Yolk sac
• Embryonal carcinoma
• Choriocarcinoma
• Teratoma

Origins of 3 main types of ovarian tumors.

25-15 Cervical Pathology

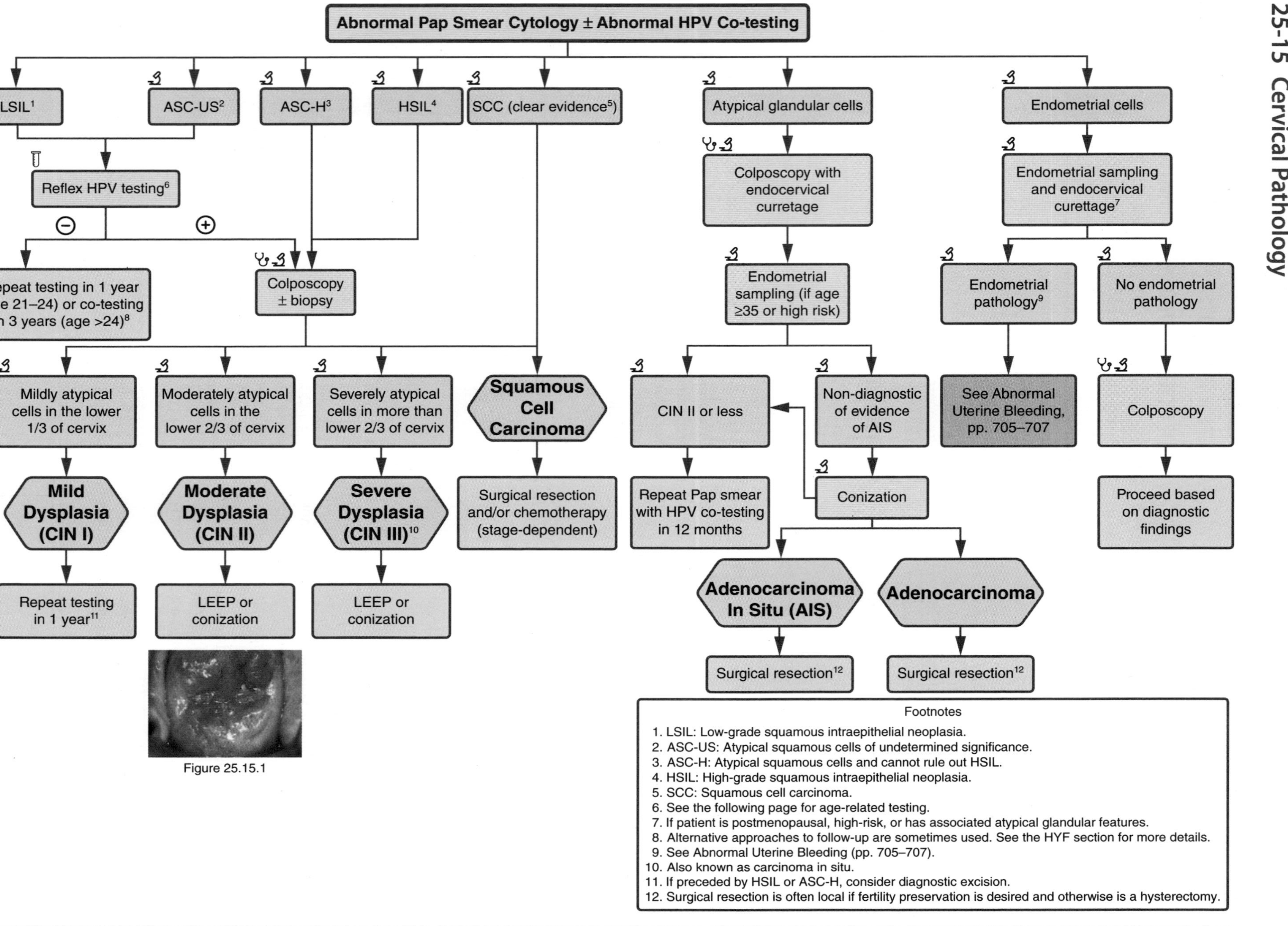
Abnormal Pap Smear Cytology ± Abnormal HPV Co-testing
LSIL[1]
ASC-US[2]
ASC-H[3]
HSIL[4]
SCC (clear evidence[5])
Atypical glandular cells
Endometrial cells
Reflex HPV testing[6]
⊖
⊕
Repeat testing in 1 year (age 21–24) or co-testing in 3 years (age >24)[8]
Colposcopy ± biopsy
Colposcopy with endocervical curretage
Endometrial sampling and endocervical curettage[7]
Endometrial sampling (if age ≥35 or high risk)
Endometrial pathology[9]
No endometrial pathology
Mildly atypical cells in the lower 1/3 of cervix
Moderately atypical cells in the lower 2/3 of cervix
Severely atypical cells in more than lower 2/3 of cervix
Squamous Cell Carcinoma
CIN II or less
Non-diagnostic of evidence of AIS
See Abnormal Uterine Bleeding, pp. 705–707
Colposcopy
Mild Dysplasia (CIN I)
Moderate Dysplasia (CIN II)
Severe Dysplasia (CIN III)[10]
Surgical resection and/or chemotherapy (stage-dependent)
Repeat Pap smear with HPV co-testing in 12 months
Conization
Proceed based on diagnostic findings
Repeat testing in 1 year[11]
LEEP or conization
LEEP or conization
Adenocarcinoma In Situ (AIS)
Adenocarcinoma
Surgical resection[12]
Surgical resection[12]
Figure 25.15.1
Footnotes
1. LSIL: Low-grade squamous intraepithelial neoplasia.
2. ASC-US: Atypical squamous cells of undetermined significance.
3. ASC-H: Atypical squamous cells and cannot rule out HSIL.
4. HSIL: High-grade squamous intraepithelial neoplasia.
5. SCC: Squamous cell carcinoma.
6. See the following page for age-related testing.
7. If patient is postmenopausal, high-risk, or has associated atypical glandular features.
8. Alternative approaches to follow-up are sometimes used. See the HYF section for more details.
9. See Abnormal Uterine Bleeding (pp. 705–707).
10. Also known as carcinoma in situ.
11. If preceded by HSIL or ASC-H, consider diagnostic excision.
12. Surgical resection is often local if fertility preservation is desired and otherwise is a hysterectomy.

FIGURE 25.15

25-15 Cervical Pathology

CERVICAL DYSPLASIA (CIN I–III)

A 25-year-old F with no PMH presents with no complaints for 1st Pap testing. Exam shows no abnormalities. On labs, Pap with HPV co-testing shows atypical cells of unknown significance (ASC-US) with (+)HPV16.

Management:

1. Colposcopy ± biopsy as appropriate.
2. HPV vaccine.
3. Subsequent management based on biopsy findings (see table below).

Complications:

- Recurrence.
- Progression to cervical dysplasia or cervical carcinoma.

HYF: HPV co-testing is important in determining risk after abnormal Pap smear findings. If someone age <26 has not been previously vaccinated against HPV, they should receive the vaccine.

Pap Smear Cytologic Findings and Management

Findings	Management
Negative	Routine screening
ASC-US	**21–24 years:** Repeat cytology in 12 months. - If negative, ASC-US or LSIL: Repeat in 12 months (return to routine screening if negative × 2). - If ASC-H, HSIL, atypical glandular cells: Colposcopy. **>24 years:** Reflex HPV. - If negative: Co-testing in 3 years. - If positive: Colposcopy.
ASC-H	Colposcopy
LSIL	**21–24 years:** See ASC-US. **>24 years:** - If HPV negative: Repeat co-testing in 12 months. - If HPV positive: Colposcopy. - If no HPV test (24–30 years): Colposcopy.
HSIL	**21–24 years:** Colposcopy **>24 years:** Immediate LEEP (if not pregnant) or colposcopy.

Management of Cervical Dysplasia

CIN I	Repeat testing in 1 year
CIN II	LEEP or conization
CIN III	LEEP or conization

CERVICAL SQUAMOUS CELL CARCINOMA (SCC)

A 45-year-old F with PMH of LSIL at age 21 presents with bleeding after intercourse with her husband. On exam, she has a friable lesion on the cervix.

Management:

1. Cervical biopsy; conization or LEEP if non-diagnostic or considering microinvasive surgery.
2. Advanced imaging.
3. Chemoradiation and/or surgery (hysterectomy) depending on staging.

Complications:

- Recurrence.
- Complications of cancer treatment.

HYF: SCC accounts for 70–75% of cervical cancers. Women who develop SCC often had Pap or HPV testing abnormalities many years prior.

CERVICAL ADENOCARCINOMA IN SITU (AIS)

A 42-year-old F presents with atypical glandular cells on Pap smear. She endorses no other symptoms.

Management:

1. Colposcopy with endocervical curettage; endometrial sampling (if age ≥35 or high-risk).
2. Diagnostic excision procedure via conization or LEEP.
3. Surgical resection: Hysterectomy (recommended) or local excision (if fertility preservation is desired).

Complications:

- Recurrence.
- Progression to adenocarcinoma.

HYF: Risk factors for AIS are the same as for invasive cervical adenocarcinoma, including high-risk HPV (16 and 18).

CERVICAL ADENOCARCINOMA

A 43-year-old F presents with atypical glandular cells on Pap smear. She endorses no other symptoms.

Management:

1. Colposcopy with endocervical curettage; endometrial sampling (if age ≥35 or high-risk).
2. Diagnostic excision procedure via conization or LEEP.
3. Chemoradiation and/or surgery (hysterectomy) depending on staging.

Complications:

- Recurrence.
- Complications of cancer treatment.

HYF: Adenocarcinoma accounts for 25% of cervical cancers.

(Continued)

25-15 Cervical Pathology

Cervical Cancer Screening Guidelines

Under age 21	No screening.
Ages 21–29	Cytology alone every 3 years.
Ages 30–65	Cytology alone every 3 years OR High-risk HPV testing every 5 years OR High-risk HPV testing and cytology (co-testing) every 5 years.
Over age 65	No screening with adequate negative prior screening results.

*Those with DES exposure (clear cell cancer risk) and those who are immunocompromised (eg, HIV+) should continue lifelong screening.

HPV Vaccine Guidelines (for Both Females and Males)

Ages 11–12	Routine vaccination should occur.
Ages 13–26	Vaccination should occur if not previously vaccinated.
Ages 27–45	Vaccination based on clinician risk assessment.

26
Neurology

26-1 Weakness/Sensory Loss

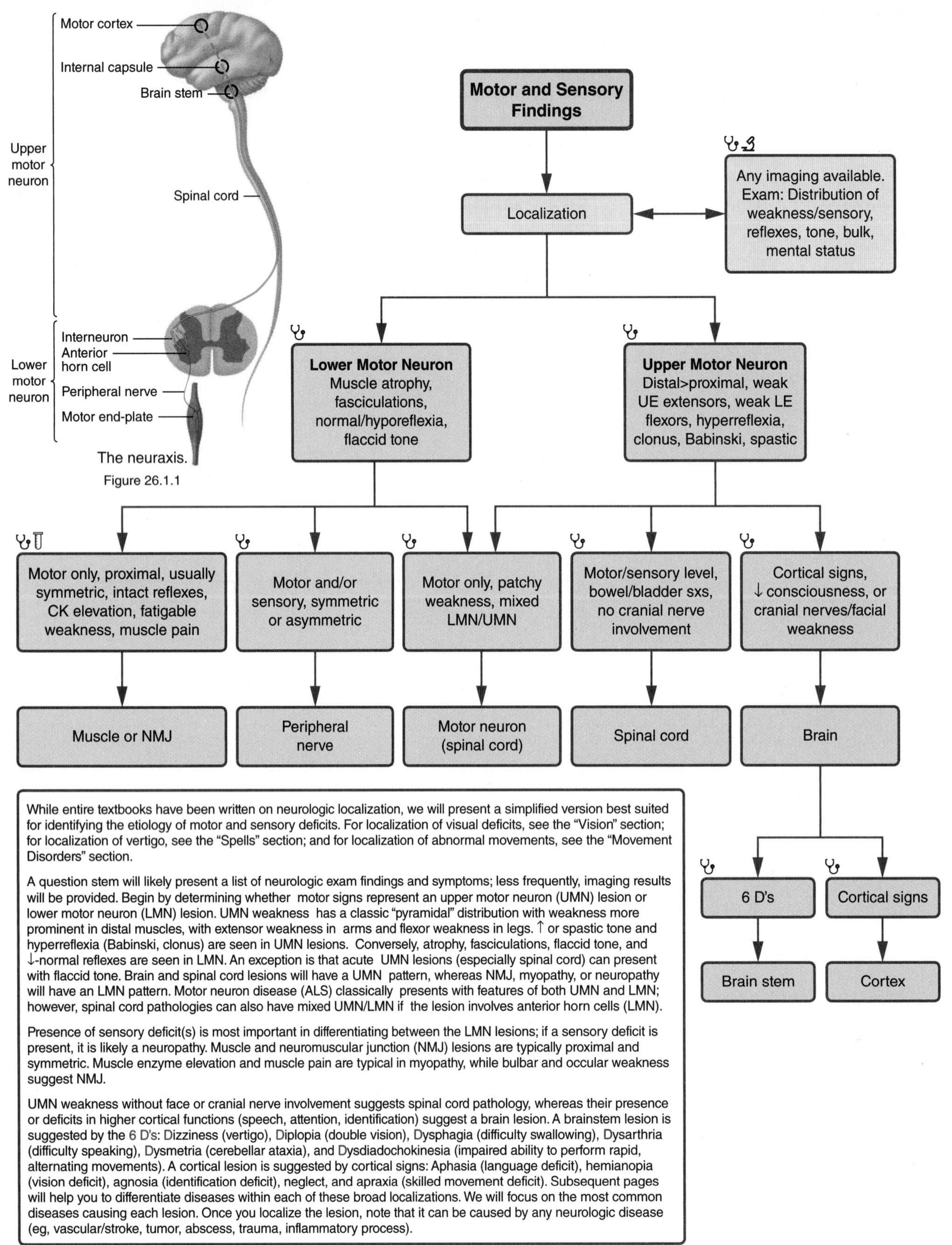
Upper motor neuron
Motor cortex
Internal capsule
Brain stem
Spinal cord
Lower motor neuron
Interneuron
Anterior horn cell
Peripheral nerve
Motor end-plate
The neuraxis.
Figure 26.1.1
Motor and Sensory Findings
Localization
Any imaging available. Exam: Distribution of weakness/sensory, reflexes, tone, bulk, mental status
Lower Motor Neuron Muscle atrophy, fasciculations, normal/hyporeflexia, flaccid tone
Upper Motor Neuron Distal>proximal, weak UE extensors, weak LE flexors, hyperreflexia, clonus, Babinski, spastic
Motor only, proximal, usually symmetric, intact reflexes, CK elevation, fatigable weakness, muscle pain
Motor and/or sensory, symmetric or asymmetric
Motor only, patchy weakness, mixed LMN/UMN
Motor/sensory level, bowel/bladder sxs, no cranial nerve involvement
Cortical signs, ↓ consciousness, or cranial nerves/facial weakness
Muscle or NMJ
Peripheral nerve
Motor neuron (spinal cord)
Spinal cord
Brain
6 D's
Cortical signs
Brain stem
Cortex
While entire textbooks have been written on neurologic localization, we will present a simplified version best suited for identifying the etiology of motor and sensory deficits. For localization of visual deficits, see the "Vision" section; for localization of vertigo, see the "Spells" section; and for localization of abnormal movements, see the "Movement Disorders" section.
A question stem will likely present a list of neurologic exam findings and symptoms; less frequently, imaging results will be provided. Begin by determining whether motor signs represent an upper motor neuron (UMN) lesion or lower motor neuron (LMN) lesion. UMN weakness has a classic "pyramidal" distribution with weakness more prominent in distal muscles, with extensor weakness in arms and flexor weakness in legs. ↑ or spastic tone and hyperreflexia (Babinski, clonus) are seen in UMN lesions. Conversely, atrophy, fasciculations, flaccid tone, and ↓-normal reflexes are seen in LMN. An exception is that acute UMN lesions (especially spinal cord) can present with flaccid tone. Brain and spinal cord lesions will have a UMN pattern, whereas NMJ, myopathy, or neuropathy will have an LMN pattern. Motor neuron disease (ALS) classically presents with features of both UMN and LMN; however, spinal cord pathologies can also have mixed UMN/LMN if the lesion involves anterior horn cells (LMN).
Presence of sensory deficit(s) is most important in differentiating between the LMN lesions; if a sensory deficit is present, it is likely a neuropathy. Muscle and neuromuscular junction (NMJ) lesions are typically proximal and symmetric. Muscle enzyme elevation and muscle pain are typical in myopathy, while bulbar and occular weakness suggest NMJ.
UMN weakness without face or cranial nerve involvement suggests spinal cord pathology, whereas their presence or deficits in higher cortical functions (speech, attention, identification) suggest a brain lesion. A brainstem lesion is suggested by the 6 D's: Dizziness (vertigo), Diplopia (double vision), Dysphagia (difficulty swallowing), Dysarthria (difficulty speaking), Dysmetria (cerebellar ataxia), and Dysdiadochokinesia (impaired ability to perform rapid, alternating movements). A cortical lesion is suggested by cortical signs: Aphasia (language deficit), hemianopia (vision deficit), agnosia (identification deficit), neglect, and apraxia (skilled movement deficit). Subsequent pages will help you to differentiate diseases within each of these broad localizations. We will focus on the most common diseases causing each lesion. Once you localize the lesion, note that it can be caused by any neurologic disease (eg, vascular/stroke, tumor, abscess, trauma, inflammatory process).

FIGURE 26.1

26-2 Myopathy/Neuromuscular Junction

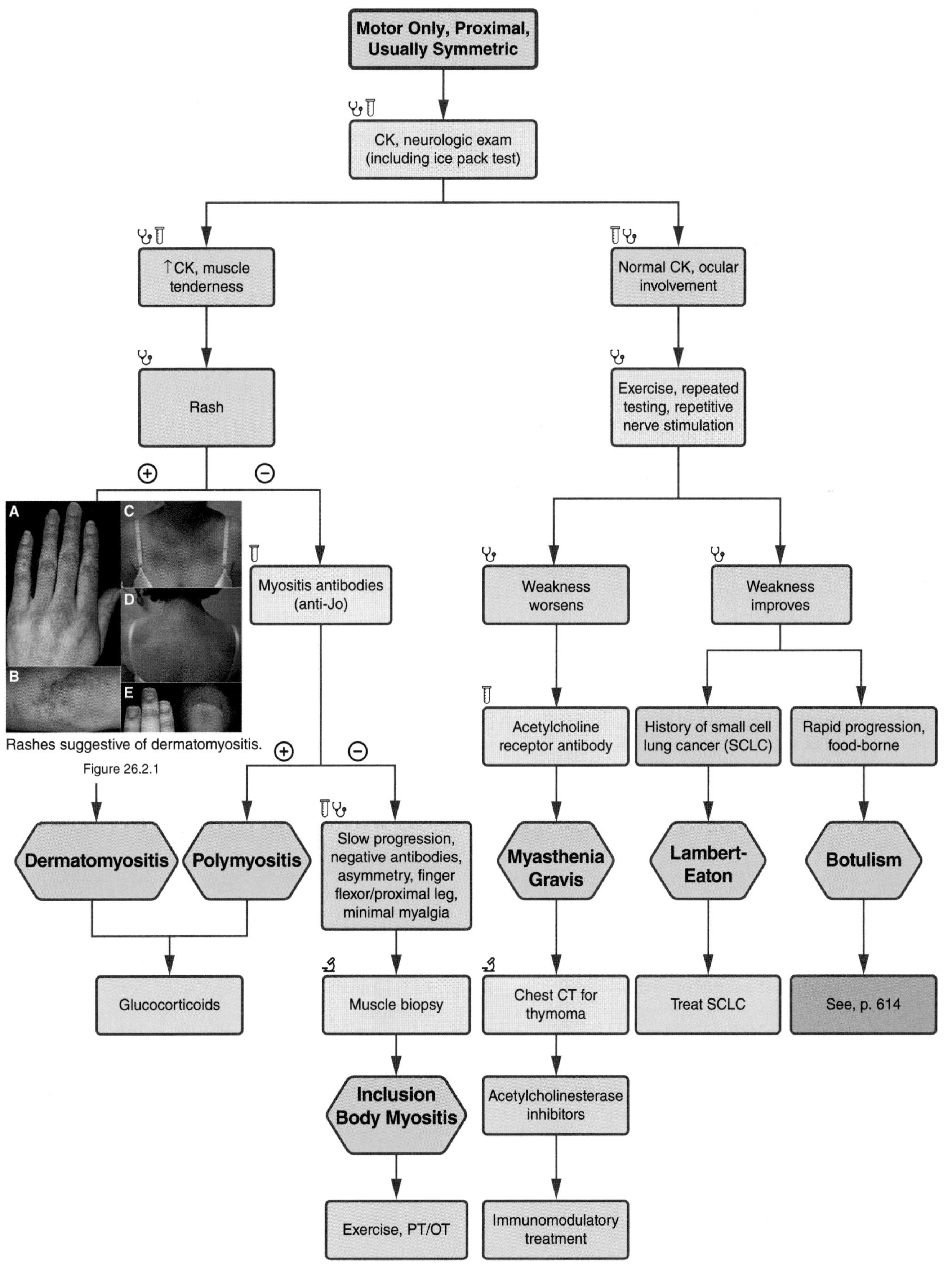
Motor Only, Proximal, Usually Symmetric
CK, neurologic exam (including ice pack test)
↑CK, muscle tenderness
Normal CK, ocular involvement
Rash
Exercise, repeated testing, repetitive nerve stimulation
⊕
⊖
A
B
C
D
E
Myositis antibodies (anti-Jo)
Weakness worsens
Weakness improves
Rashes suggestive of dermatomyositis.
Figure 26.2.1
Acetylcholine receptor antibody
History of small cell lung cancer (SCLC)
Rapid progression, food-borne
Dermatomyositis
Polymyositis
Slow progression, negative antibodies, asymmetry, finger flexor/proximal leg, minimal myalgia
Myasthenia Gravis
Lambert-Eaton
Botulism
Glucocorticoids
Muscle biopsy
Chest CT for thymoma
Treat SCLC
See, p. 614
Inclusion Body Myositis
Acetylcholinesterase inhibitors
Exercise, PT/OT
Immunomodulatory treatment

FIGURE 26.2

26-2 Myopathy/Neuromuscular Junction

POLYMYOSITIS

A 60-year-old F with PMH of malignancy presents with progressive difficulty standing up from the chair or climbing stairs and myalgias. On **exam**, she has symmetric proximal muscle pain or weakness, and **labs/imaging** show elevated serum creatine kinase, positive anti-Jo-1 antibodies, and positive ANA.

Management:

1. Muscle biopsy if needed for confirmation (endomysial CD8/CD4 infiltrate).
2. High-dose steroids with 4–6-week taper.
3. Azathioprine, methotrexate for steroid-sparing.

Complications:

- Myocarditis, cardiac conduction deficits.
- Interstitial lung disease can occur in 10%.

HYF: Anti-Jo-1 is specific for myositis, but many autoantibodies (ANA, SSA, SSB, Smith) are often positive and can suggest overlap with rheumatologic disease.

DERMATOMYOSITIS

See "Polymyositis" PLUS rash: Heliotrope rash (violaceous periorbital), "shawl sign" (rash on shoulders, upper chest, and back), Gottron papules (papular scaling rash over bony prominences dorsa of hands).

INCLUSION BODY MYOSITIS

A 65-year-old M presents with insidious-onset progressive muscle weakness. On **exam**, patient has quad and distal finger flexor weakness, and **labs/imaging** show elevated CK but normal inflammatory markers and no antibodies.

Management:

1. Muscle biopsy for confirmation (inclusion bodies).
2. Exercise, physical therapy, nutrition (creatine).
3. Immune therapy typically not indicated.

Complications: Frailty.

HYF: Less common than above diagnoses but consider in older patients with slow progression and early finger weakness.

MYASTHENIA GRAVIS (MG)

A 30-year-old F with PMH of autoimmune thyroid disease presents with difficulty climbing stairs or standing from a chair, as well as dysphagia and double vision that is worse at the end of the day. On **exam**, she has ptosis and fatigable proximal weakness. **Labs** show positive acetylcholine receptor antibody.

Management:

1. Can confirm diagnosis with single-fiber EMG.
2. Acetylcholinesterase inhibitors (pyridostigmine).
3. IVIG or plasmapharesis, steroids, steroid-sparing agents (azathioprine, MMF, methotrexate, etc.).
4. Thymoma resection if present.

Complications:

- Myasthenic crisis (see below).
- Cholinergic side effects (diarrhea, increased secretions, bradycardia) from pyridostigmine.

HYF: Associated with thymoma. Application of ice pack over eyelids improves ptosis caused by autoantibodies to post-synaptic acetylcholine receptors on the NMJ.

MYASTHENIC CRISIS

A 35-year-old F with PMH of myasthenia gravis post-op day 2 after an appendectomy presents with shortness of breath and dysphagia. On **exam**, she has respiratory distress, and **labs/imaging** show aspiration pneumonia on CXR and abnormal pulmonary function tests (maximal inspiratory pressure, vital capacity).

Management:

1. Secure airway (intubation).
2. Stop offending medications (fluoroquinolones, aminoglycosides, β-blockers).
3. IVIG/plasmapheresis, cautious use of steroids (associated with transient worsening of crisis).

Complications: Aspiration due to dysphagia.

HYF: Potentially lethal secondary to respiratory muscle weakness. Can be precipitated by surgery, trauma, infection, or medications (above). Some patients will not have visible respiratory distress due to weakening of secondary respiratory muscles.

LAMBERT-EATON MYASTHENIC SYNDROME (LEMS)

A 70-year-old M with PMH of small-cell lung cancer (SCLC) presents with proximal muscle weakness. On **exam**, he has depressed deep-tendon reflexes. **Labs/imaging** show lung mass on chest CT, a characteristic incremental response on repetitive nerve stimulation, and autoantibodies to presynaptic calcium channels.

Management:

1. Treat SCLC if present (~50%).
2. 3,4-Diaminopyridine or guanidine +/– acetylcholinesterase inhibitors.
3. Steroids and azathioprine when no cancer identified.

Complications: Respiratory failure can occur in late stages of disease but less commonly than in MG.

HYF: Most often a paraneoplastic disorder with SCLC, but can also be autoimmune (mediated by antibodies to calcium channels). Contrast MG and LEMS: In MG, weakness worsens with repeat stimulation; in LEMS, weakness improves with repeat stimulation.

26-3 Polyneuropathy

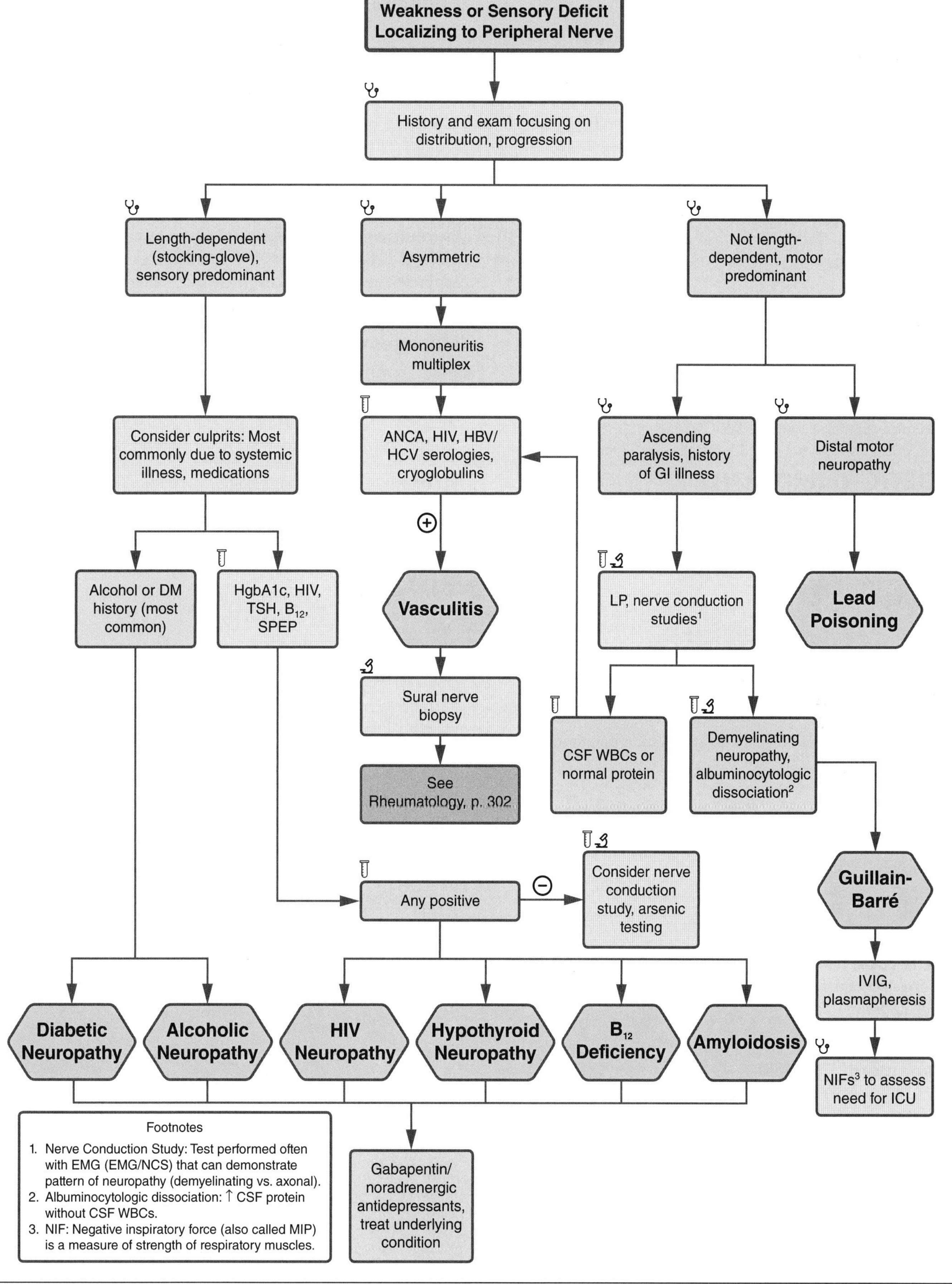
Weakness or Sensory Deficit Localizing to Peripheral Nerve
History and exam focusing on distribution, progression
Length-dependent (stocking-glove), sensory predominant
Asymmetric
Not length-dependent, motor predominant
Mononeuritis multiplex
Consider culprits: Most commonly due to systemic illness, medications
ANCA, HIV, HBV/HCV serologies, cryoglobulins
Ascending paralysis, history of GI illness
Distal motor neuropathy
Alcohol or DM history (most common)
HgbA1c, HIV, TSH, B12, SPEP
Vasculitis
LP, nerve conduction studies1
Lead Poisoning
Sural nerve biopsy
CSF WBCs or normal protein
Demyelinating neuropathy, albuminocytologic dissociation2
See Rheumatology, p. 302
Consider nerve conduction study, arsenic testing
Any positive
Guillain-Barré
IVIG, plasmapheresis
Diabetic Neuropathy
Alcoholic Neuropathy
HIV Neuropathy
Hypothyroid Neuropathy
B12 Deficiency
Amyloidosis
NIFs3 to assess need for ICU
Gabapentin/noradrenergic antidepressants, treat underlying condition

Footnotes

1. Nerve Conduction Study: Test performed often with EMG (EMG/NCS) that can demonstrate pattern of neuropathy (demyelinating vs. axonal).
2. Albuminocytologic dissociation: ↑ CSF protein without CSF WBCs.
3. NIF: Negative inspiratory force (also called MIP) is a measure of strength of respiratory muscles.

FIGURE 26.3

26-3 Polyneuropathy

GUILLAIN-BARRÉ SYNDROME

A 35-year-old with recent GI or viral infection presents with rapidly progressive ascending weakness. On **exam**, the patient has symmetric LE > UE weakness and areflexia. **Labs/imaging** show CSF protein >55 without pleocytosis (albuminocytologic dissociation) and decreased nerve conduction velocity.

Management:

1. NIF/VC monitoring for elective intubation.
2. Plasmapheresis and IVIG.

Complications:

- Respiratory failure.
- Cardiac arrythmias/dysautonomia.
- Mortality is rare; most patients recover fully with PT.

HYF: Classically associated with *Campylobacter* infection. Autoimmune demyelination (molecular mimicry) of peripheral nerves leads to protein in CSF without WBCs.

DIABETIC NEUROPATHY

A 75-year-old with PMH of poorly controlled diabetes presents with progressive loss of sensation from toes to legs to hands. On **exam**, patient has decreased pinprick sensation in bilateral lower extremities, and **labs** show HgbA1c of 9.

Management:

1. Glycemic control (see Endocrine, p. 135).
2. Regular foot inspection.
3. Pain control if needed (SNRIs, TCAs, gabapentin).

Complications: Foot ulcers and amputation due to unnoticed injuries.

HYF: While stocking-glove distribution is most common, many patients will also have autonomic neuropathy with gastroparesis and postural hypotension, less commonly radiculopathy. This presentation also applies to the other axonal neuropathies.

ALCOHOLIC NEUROPATHY

A 55-year-old M with PMH of alcohol use disorder presents with lower extremity burning paresthesias. On **exam**, he has decreased pinprick and vibratory sensation and areflexia. **Labs** show mildly increased LFTs and decreased thiamine level.

Management:

1. Alcohol cessation.
2. Thiamine (although patients often present without nutritional deficiency).
3. Pain control if needed (SNRIs, TCAs, gabapentin).

Complications: "Saturday night palsies": Radial nerve is compressed against the spiral groove of the humerus (while intoxicated); associated with alcohol use but not due to direct toxicity.

HYF: Related to cumulative lifetime alcohol use.

B_{12} DEFICIENCY/SUBACUTE COMBINED DEGENERATION

A 45-year-old with PMH of obesity s/p gastrectomy presents with lower extremity paresthesia, weakness, bowel/bladder dysfunction, and sore tongue. On **exam**, the patient has glossitis, increased tone/spasticity, weakness, and decreased sensation in the lower extremities. **Labs** show low B_{12} and elevated methylmalonic acid.

Management:

1. B_{12} repletion (IV > PO).

Complications: Can progress to altered mental status and dementia.

HYF: Classically, a *combined* neuropathy (distal sensory) and myelopathy causing upper and lower motor neuron signs.

B_{12} deficiency is associated with pernicious anemia, gastrectomy, Crohn's disease, ileal surgery, malnutrition, medications, and toxins (N_2O).

LYME NEUROPATHY

A 30-year-old with recent tick bite presents with erythema migrans and myalgias/arthralgias. On **exam**, the patient has facial and peripheral neuropathy, and **labs/imaging** show abnormal LFTs, positive Lyme IgM titer, and nerve conduction study showing mononeuropathy multiplex.

Management:

1. Doxycycline.

Complications: Meningoencephalitis (CSF pleocytosis would be seen).

HYF: *Borrelia burgdorferi* is endemic in the northeastern United States. Bell's palsy is the classic neuropathy, but peripheral nerves are often involved as well.

Vasculitic Neuropathy: See Rheumatology, p. 302.

Amyloid Neuropathy: See Hematology, p. 127.

Hypothyroid Neuropathy: See Hypothyroidism Endocrine, pp. 137–138.

HIV Neuropathy: See ID, p. 203.

26-4 Myelopathy

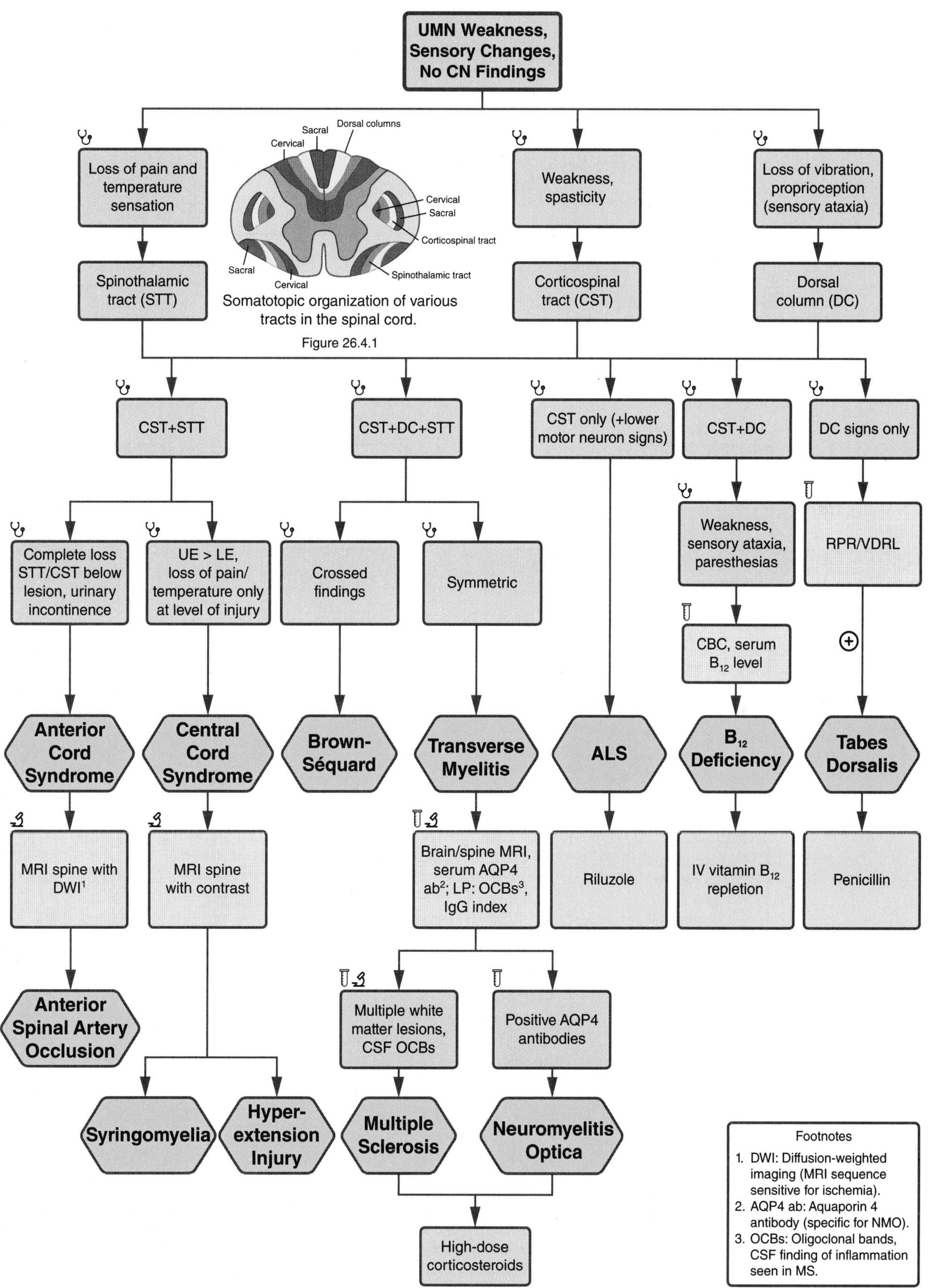
UMN Weakness, Sensory Changes, No CN Findings
Loss of pain and temperature sensation
Spinothalamic tract (STT)
Dorsal columns
Sacral
Cervical
Cervical
Sacral
Corticospinal tract
Spinothalamic tract
Sacral
Cervical
Somatotopic organization of various tracts in the spinal cord.
Figure 26.4.1
Weakness, spasticity
Corticospinal tract (CST)
Loss of vibration, proprioception (sensory ataxia)
Dorsal column (DC)
CST+STT
CST+DC+STT
CST only (+lower motor neuron signs)
CST+DC
DC signs only
Complete loss STT/CST below lesion, urinary incontinence
UE > LE, loss of pain/ temperature only at level of injury
Crossed findings
Symmetric
Weakness, sensory ataxia, paresthesias
RPR/VDRL
CBC, serum B_{12} level
+
Anterior Cord Syndrome
Central Cord Syndrome
Brown-Séquard
Transverse Myelitis
ALS
B_{12} Deficiency
Tabes Dorsalis
MRI spine with DWI[1]
MRI spine with contrast
Brain/spine MRI, serum AQP4 ab[2]; LP: OCBs[3], IgG index
Riluzole
IV vitamin B_{12} repletion
Penicillin
Anterior Spinal Artery Occlusion
Multiple white matter lesions, CSF OCBs
Positive AQP4 antibodies
Syringomyelia
Hyper-extension Injury
Multiple Sclerosis
Neuromyelitis Optica
High-dose corticosteroids
Footnotes
1. DWI: Diffusion-weighted imaging (MRI sequence sensitive for ischemia).
2. AQP4 ab: Aquaporin 4 antibody (specific for NMO).
3. OCBs: Oligoclonal bands, CSF finding of inflammation seen in MS.

FIGURE 26.4

26-4 Myelopathy

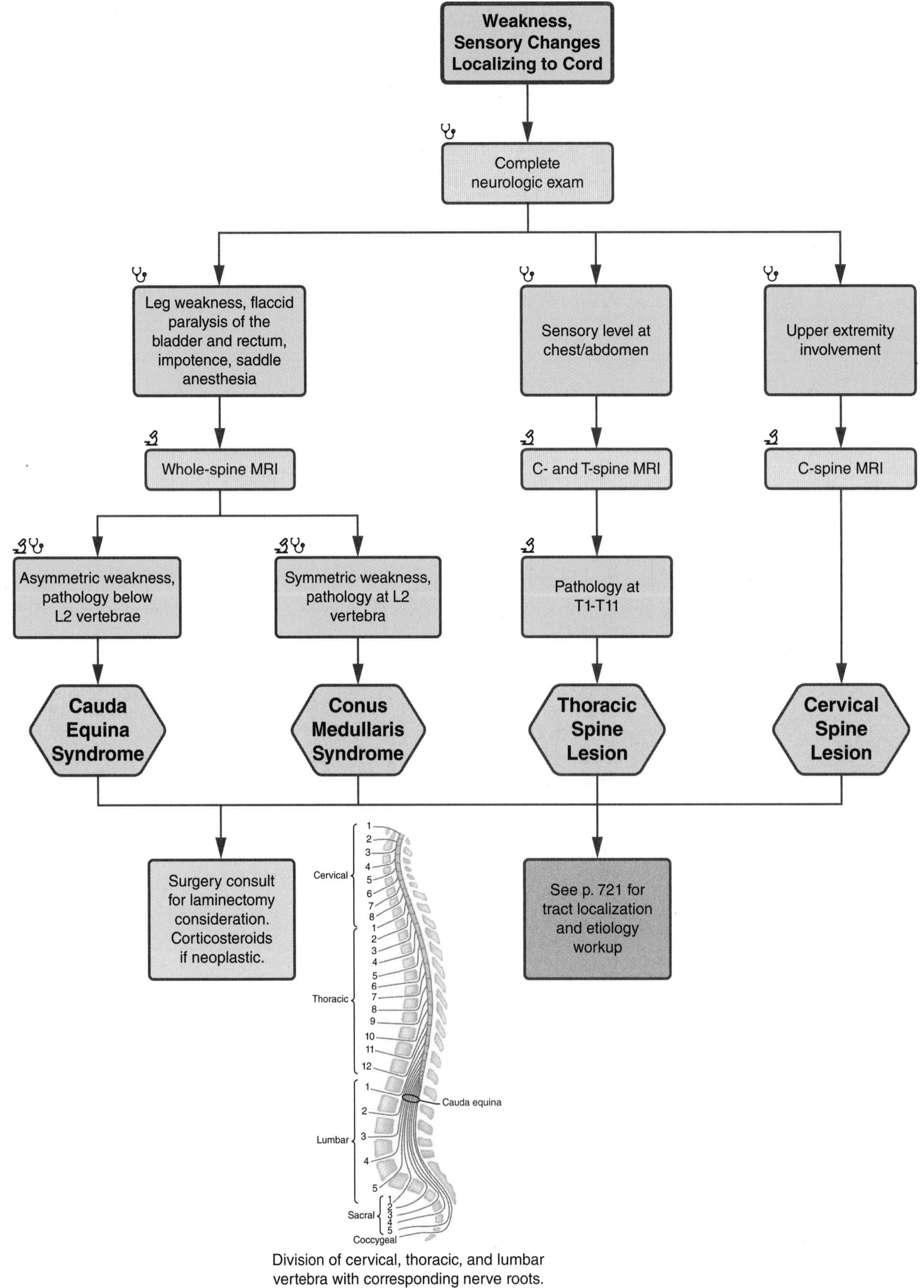
Weakness, Sensory Changes Localizing to Cord
Complete neurologic exam
Leg weakness, flaccid paralysis of the bladder and rectum, impotence, saddle anesthesia
Sensory level at chest/abdomen
Upper extremity involvement
Whole-spine MRI
C- and T-spine MRI
C-spine MRI
Asymmetric weakness, pathology below L2 vertebrae
Symmetric weakness, pathology at L2 vertebra
Pathology at T1-T11
Cauda Equina Syndrome
Conus Medullaris Syndrome
Thoracic Spine Lesion
Cervical Spine Lesion
Surgery consult for laminectomy consideration. Corticosteroids if neoplastic.
See p. 721 for tract localization and etiology workup
Cervical
Thoracic
Lumbar
Sacral
Coccygeal
Cauda equina

Division of cervical, thoracic, and lumbar vertebra with corresponding nerve roots.

Figure 26.4.1

FIGURE 26.4

26-4 Myelopathy

CAUDA EQUINA SYNDROME

A 70-year-old M with PMH of prostate cancer presents with bowel/bladder dysfunction and lower extremity weakness. On **exam**, he has saddle anesthesia and bilateral asymmetric lower extremity weakness with decreased reflexes. **Imaging** shows an epidural mass below L2 causing compression of lumbosacral nerve roots.

Management:

1. MRI whole spine (emergent).
2. High-dose corticosteroids if neoplastic (decrease swelling).
3. Surgery (lumbar laminectomy).

Complications: Permanent neurologic deficits.

HYF: Technically a radiculopathy, not myelopathy (the cauda equina is the bundle of roots present once the cord has terminated), but often on differential for myelopathy given bowel/bladder signs and weakness. Etiology can be any compressive mass (tumor, abscess, trauma, occasionally lumbar stenosis).

CONUS MEDULLARIS SYNDROME

A 70-year-old M with PMH of prostate cancer presents with back pain and bowel/bladder dysfunction. On **exam**, he has bilateral flaccid or spastic weakness and sensory loss (including saddle anesthesia). **Imaging** shows a mass at the L2 vertebral level compressing the cord.

Management:

1. MRI whole spine (emergent).
2. High-dose corticosteroids if neoplastic (decrease swelling).
3. Surgery (lumbar laminectomy).

HYF: Similar presentation to cauda equina syndrome, but weakness is more likely to be symmetric and often presents with early/prominent bowel/bladder symptoms. Typically, the exam is consistent with S2–S5 dysfunction; lesion is at vertebral level L2 (cord ends at vertebral L1 or L2 level). Etiology can be any cause of myelopathy (mass, infection, inflammation).

ANTERIOR CORD SYNDROME/ANTERIOR SPINAL ARTERY OCCLUSION

A 55-year-old with PMH of aortic aneurysm s/p recent surgical repair presents with weakness and bowel/bladder dysfunction. On **exam**, the patient has decreased strength and pain/temperature sensation below lesion, and **imaging** shows cord ischemia on MRI.

Management:

1. See stroke management if ischemic.
2. If due to mass effect or surgery, surgical decompression or lumbar drain.

Complications: Hypotension due to autonomic dysfunction.

HYF: Typically, due to surgery or aneurysm rupture. Initially, patients will present with flaccid tone and areflexia; after weeks, they become spastic and hyperreflexic.

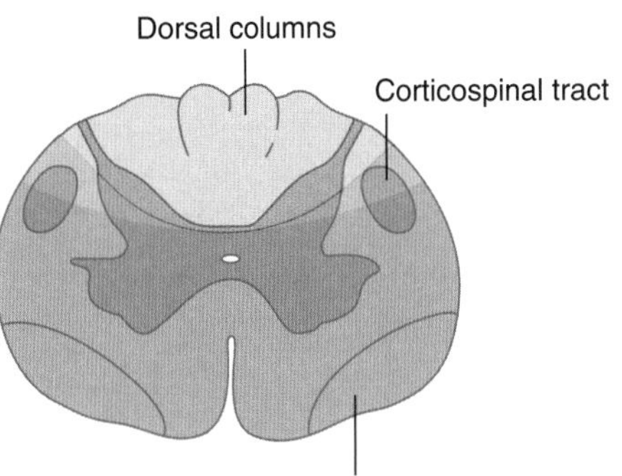
Dorsal columns
Corticospinal tract
Anterolateral (spinothalamic) tract

Territory of an anterior spinal cord infarct.

CERVICAL HYPEREXTENSION/CENTRAL CORD SYNDROME

A 65-year-old with PMH of cervical spondylosis presents with neck pain and weakness after hyperextending the neck in a motor vehicle accident. On **exam**, the patient has UE > LE weakness, and **imaging** shows degeneration and central canal narrowing on C-spine MRI.

Management:

1. C-spine immobilization.
2. Consider surgical decompression.

HYF: Hyperextension is a more common cause of central cord syndrome than syringomyelia, especially in older adults.

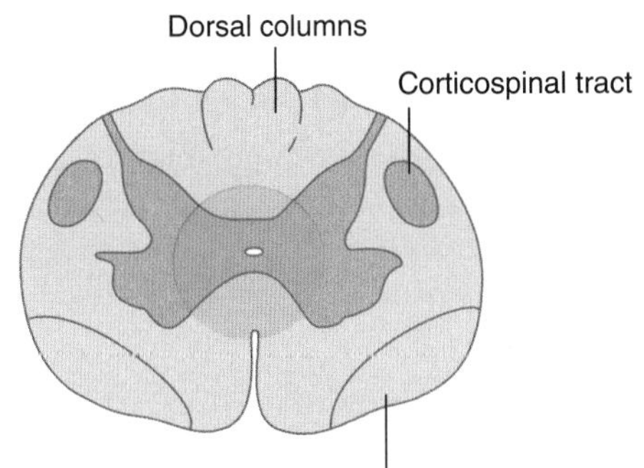
Dorsal columns
Corticospinal tract
Anterolateral (spinothalamic) tract

Spinal cord territory affected by central cord syndrome.

BROWN-SÉQUARD'S SYNDROME

A 35-year-old M with knife wound to the back presents with weakness and loss of sensation. On **exam**, he has weakness and loss of vibration/proprioception on ipsilateral side of lesion and loss of pain/temperature contralateral to the lesion. **Imaging** shows spinal cord hemi-section on MRI.

Management:

1. Depends on etiology (penetrating trauma, demyelination, tumor). See Surgery (p. 391) for management.

HYF: Rare disorder. Classically, the patient experiences weakness/paralysis and proprioceptive deficits on the side of the body ipsilateral to the lesion and loss of pain and temperature sensation on the contralateral side.

(Continued)

26-4 Myelopathy

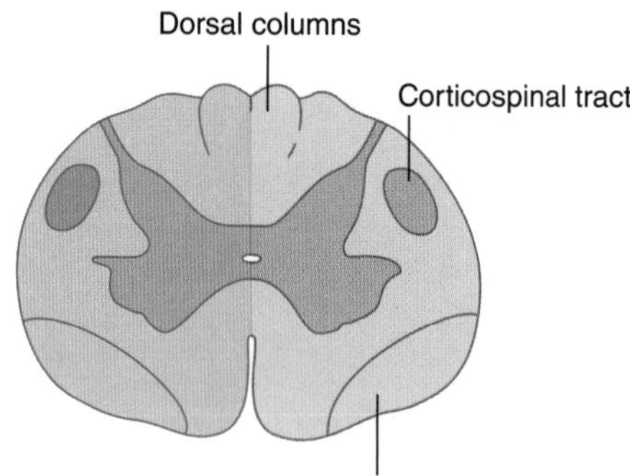
Dorsal columns
Corticospinal tract
Anterolateral (spinothalamic) tract

Spinal cord territory affected by cord hemisection, Brown Sequard's syndrome.

TRANSVERSE MYELITIS

A 35-year-old F with PMH of SLE and recent viral infection presents with LE weakness and loss of sensation. On **exam**, she has a sensory level, and **imaging** shows spinal cord T2 hyperintensity on MRI.

Management:

1. High-dose corticosteroids.
2. Treat underlying rheumatologic disorder if present.

HYF: Typically autoimmune, either post-viral, associated with a systemic rheumatologic disease (eg, lupus), or as a demyelination event of neuromyelitis optica (NMO) or multiple sclerosis (MS) (see below). Most commonly occurs in the thoracic cord so patients typically present with lower extremity weakness.

AMYOTROPHIC LATERAL SCLEROSIS (ALS)

A 55-year-old M presents with slowly progressive weakness in progressive limbs. On **exam**, he has hyperreflexia, fasciculations, and atrophy without bladder disturbance. **Imaging** shows widespread denervation and spontaneous action potentials on EMG/nerve conduction.

Management:

1. Riluzole.
2. Symptomatic management (eg, BiPAP for dyspnea).

Complications:

- Respiratory failure, 2/2 diaphragm weakness.
- Relentlessly progressive, death typically in 5 years.

HYF: Classically presents with UMN (hyperreflexia, stiffness) and LMN (fasciculations, atrophy) features. Bulbar involvement (tongue or oropharyngeal weakness - difficulty swallowing or speaking - from CN IX, X, XII) excludes cervical spondylosis.

TABES DORSALIS

A 40-year-old M with PMH of syphilis and HIV presents with difficulty walking and lancinating pains. On **exam**, he has Argyll-Robertson pupils, areflexia, and decreased vibration/proprioception. **Labs** show VDRL positive in serum and CSF.

Management:

1. Penicillin G (10–14 days).

HYF: A form of tertiary neurosyphilis that occurs years after primary infection. Argyll-Robertson pupils: Small, nonresponsive to light, but contract to accommodation.

SYRINGOMYELIA

A 30-year-old with PMH of type 1 Chiari malformation presents with upper extremity weakness and frequent hand burns. On **exam**, the patient has weakness in UE > LE and "cape-like" loss of pain/temperature sensation in bilateral UE. **Imaging** shows syrinx in central canal between C2–T9.

Management:

1. Surgical decompression.

HYF: Caused by Chiari malformation, tumor, or trauma.

Loss of pain/temperature is caused by compression of crossing CST fibers; therefore, there is only loss at level of injury (suspended sensory level).

MULTIPLE SCLEROSIS (MS)

A 25-year-old F with PMH of vitamin D deficiency presents with multiple neurologic complaints separated in time (~1–2 years between attacks) and space (not localized to single lesion) that are worse with hot showers. On **exam**, she has limb weakness, paresthesias, optic neuritis, internuclear ophthalmoplegia, and nystagmus. **Labs/imaging** show multiple asymmetric white-matter lesions (periventricular or spinal cord) and CSF with elevated IgG index and >2 oligoclonal bands (OCBs).

Management:

1. Acute exacerbations: High-dose IV corticosteroids +/– plasmapheresis.
2. Disease-modifying agents: Glatiramer, ocrelizumab, many newer immunomodulators.
3. Symptomatic therapy: Baclofen for spasticity, antidepressants for depression, TCAs for painful paresthesias, cholinergic/anticholinergics for urinary Retention/incontinence.

Complications:

- Progressive multifocal leukoencephalopathy due to immunosuppression (most associated with natalizumab).
- Deficits can become permanent and accumulate.

HYF: Think MS when there are recurrent attacks of neurologic symptoms that wouldn't otherwise fit together. Pathophysiology: Autoimmune demyelination. Subtypes: relapsing-remitting (most common), primary progressive, secondary progressive, progressive relapsing.

26-4 Myelopathy

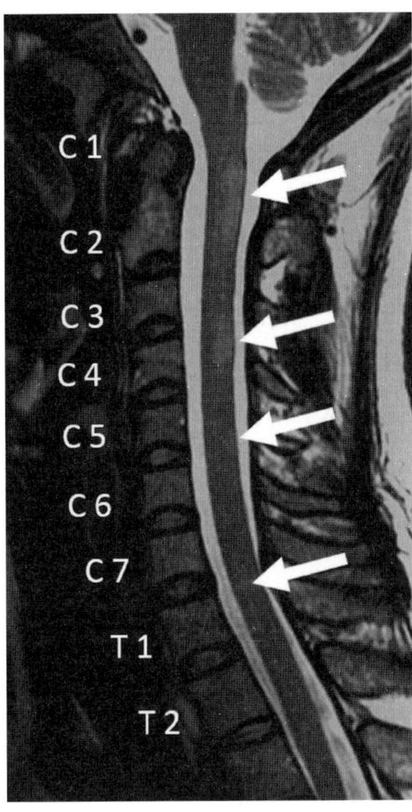
C 1
C 2
C 3
C 4
C 5
C 6
C 7
T 1
T 2

Spinal cord lesions indicated with arrows as seen on MRI in MS.

NEUROMYELITIS OPTICA (NMO)

A 35-year-old F with PMH of rheumatologic disease presents with relapsing course of acute eye pain, vision loss, and weakness/paresthesias. On **exam**, she has evidence of optic neuritis (impaired vision) and myelopathy (sensory level, weakness). **Labs/imaging** show serum AQP4-IgG antibodies and longitudinally extensive transverse myelitis on MRI.

Management:

1. Acute attacks: High-dose IV corticosteroids, plasmapheresis.
2. Long-term therapy: Biologic immunomodulators (eculizumab, rituximab).

Complications: Accumulation of deficits (optic nerve, spinal cord, area postrema).

HYF: While NMO overlaps clinically with MS, typically CSF has significant pleocytosis and no oligoclonal bands (unlike MS).

B_{12} Deficiency/Subacute Combined Degeneration: See Polyneuropathy, pp. 719–720.

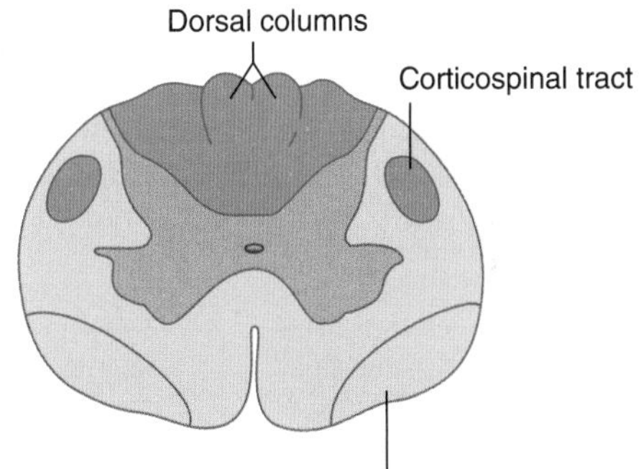
Dorsal columns
Corticospinal tract
Anterolateral (spinothalamic) tract

Territory of cord affected by subacute combined degeneration.

26-5 Stroke Syndrome

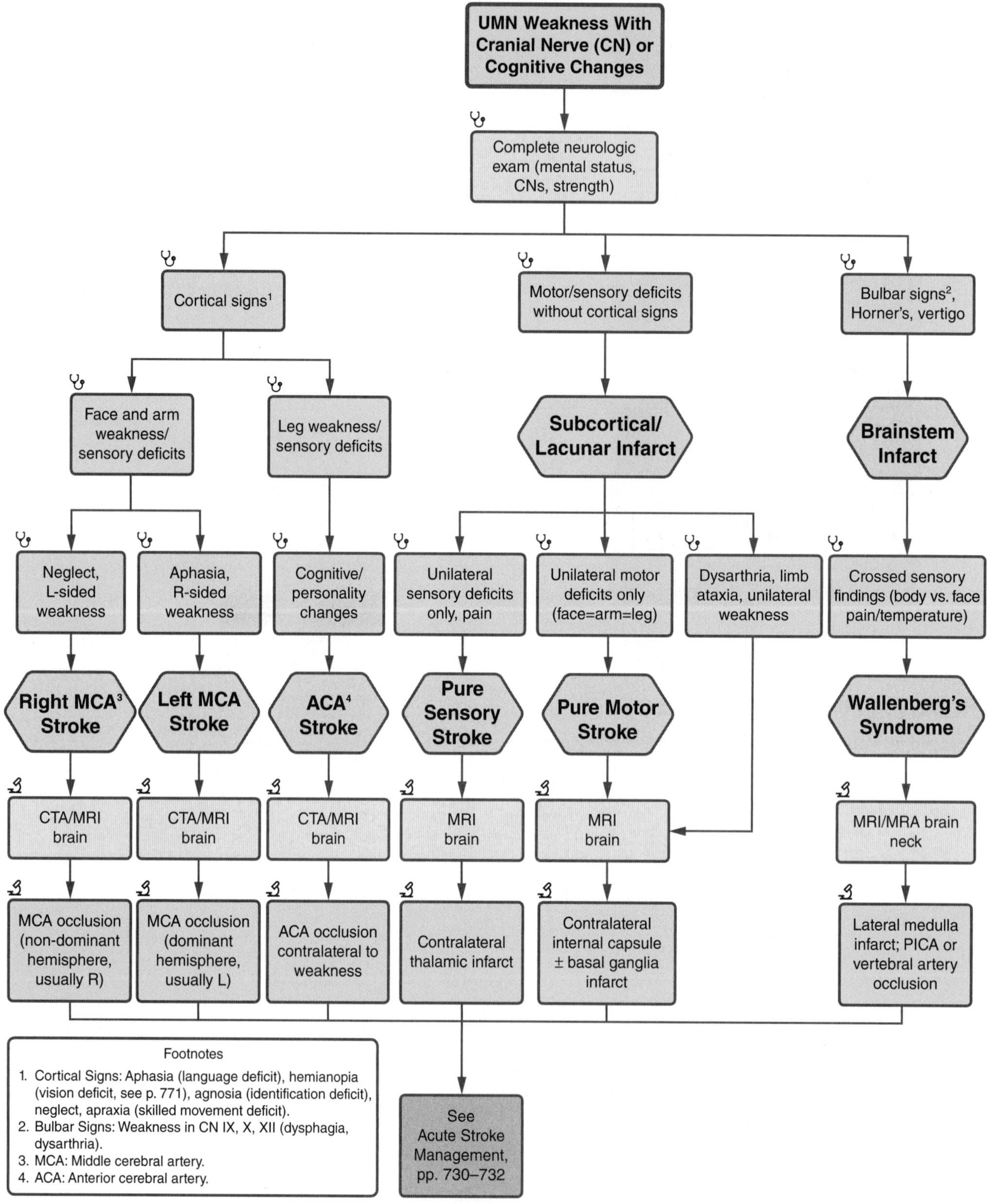
UMN Weakness With Cranial Nerve (CN) or Cognitive Changes
Complete neurologic exam (mental status, CNs, strength)
Cortical signs[1]
Motor/sensory deficits without cortical signs
Bulbar signs[2], Horner's, vertigo
Face and arm weakness/ sensory deficits
Leg weakness/ sensory deficits
Subcortical/ Lacunar Infarct
Brainstem Infarct
Neglect, L-sided weakness
Aphasia, R-sided weakness
Cognitive/ personality changes
Unilateral sensory deficits only, pain
Unilateral motor deficits only (face=arm=leg)
Dysarthria, limb ataxia, unilateral weakness
Crossed sensory findings (body vs. face pain/temperature)
Right MCA[3] Stroke
Left MCA Stroke
ACA[4] Stroke
Pure Sensory Stroke
Pure Motor Stroke
Wallenberg's Syndrome
CTA/MRI brain
CTA/MRI brain
CTA/MRI brain
MRI brain
MRI brain
MRI/MRA brain neck
MCA occlusion (non-dominant hemisphere, usually R)
MCA occlusion (dominant hemisphere, usually L)
ACA occlusion contralateral to weakness
Contralateral thalamic infarct
Contralateral internal capsule ± basal ganglia infarct
Lateral medulla infarct; PICA or vertebral artery occlusion
See Acute Stroke Management, pp. 730–732
Footnotes
1. Cortical Signs: Aphasia (language deficit), hemianopia (vision deficit, see p. 771), agnosia (identification deficit), neglect, apraxia (skilled movement deficit).
2. Bulbar Signs: Weakness in CN IX, X, XII (dysphagia, dysarthria).
3. MCA: Middle cerebral artery.
4. ACA: Anterior cerebral artery.

FIGURE 26.5

26-5 Stroke Syndrome

RIGHT MCA STROKE

A 65-year-old M with PMH of atrial fibrillation not on anticoagulation presents with acute-onset left arm weakness. On **exam**, he has L facial droop, L neglect, R gaze preference, and L arm weakness/decreased sensation. **Imaging** shows occlusion of R MCA on CT angiogram.

Management: See pp. 730–732 for Acute Stroke Management.

Complications:

- Significant brain edema causing mass effect (most common in massive MCA strokes).
- Dysphagia, aspiration.

HYF: Most common etiologies of large-vessel strokes are embolism (atrial fibrillation, intracardiac shunt) and thrombosis (plaque rupture). If a patient is L-handed, the R and L MCA syndromes can be reversed (or occasionally these functions are not lateralized).

LEFT MCA STROKE

A 65-year-old M with PMH of CAD and HLD presents with difficulty speaking and right-sided weakness. On **exam**, he has aphasia, R facial droop, L gaze preference, and R arm weakness/sensory deficit. **Imaging** shows occlusion of L MCA on CT angiogram.

Management: See pp. 730–732 for Acute Stroke Management.

Complications: Same as Right MCA stroke.

HYF: Aphasia (unlike dysarthria, which can be seen with face/bulbar weakness) is characterized by difficulty producing speech (**expressive aphasia** – localizes to inferior frontal lobe) or nonsensical speech with impaired understanding (**receptive aphasia** – localizes to posterior temporal lobe).

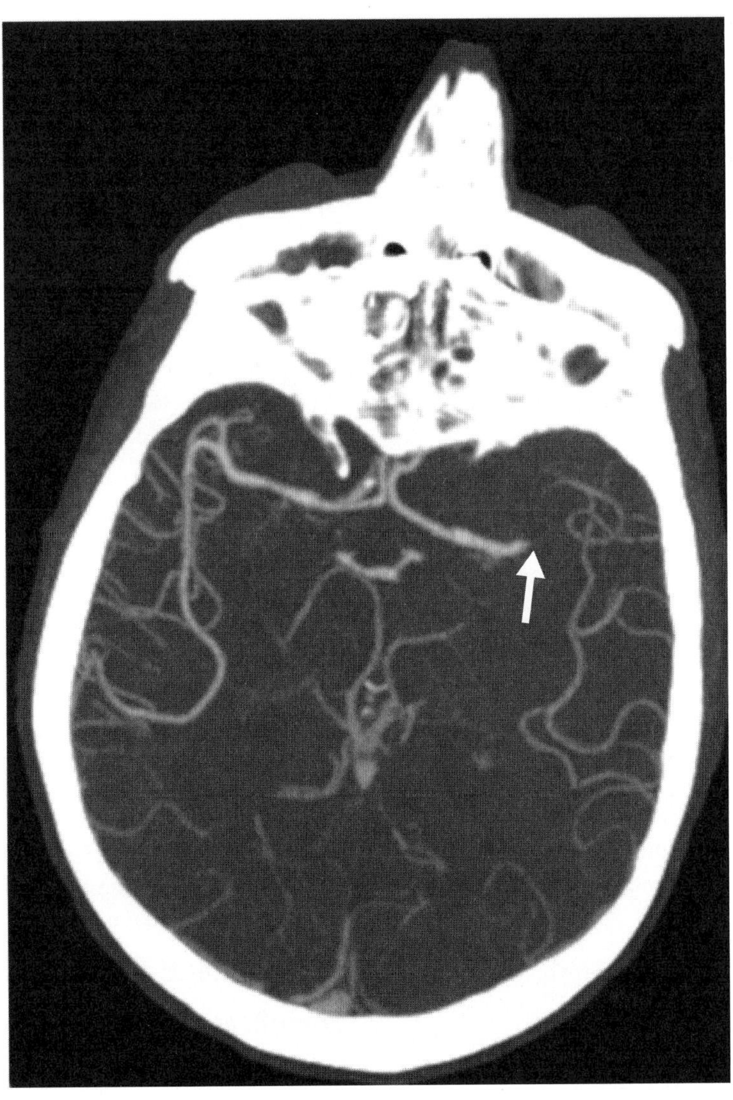

CT angiogram demonstrating a left MCA occlusion (white arrow).

(Continued)

26-5 Stroke Syndrome

ACA STROKE

A 65-year-old M with PMH of CAD and diabetes presents with acute-onset leg weakness. On **exam**, he has unilateral leg weakness and decreased sensation. **Imaging** shows ACA occlusion on CTA and infarct to medial frontal and parietal lobes on MRI.

Management: See pp. 730–732 for Acute Stroke Management.

Complications:

- Personality changes due to frontal lobe involvement.
- Urinary incontinence.

HYF: For anterior circulation strokes (ACA and MCA), it is especially important to image the carotids for source of thrombus.

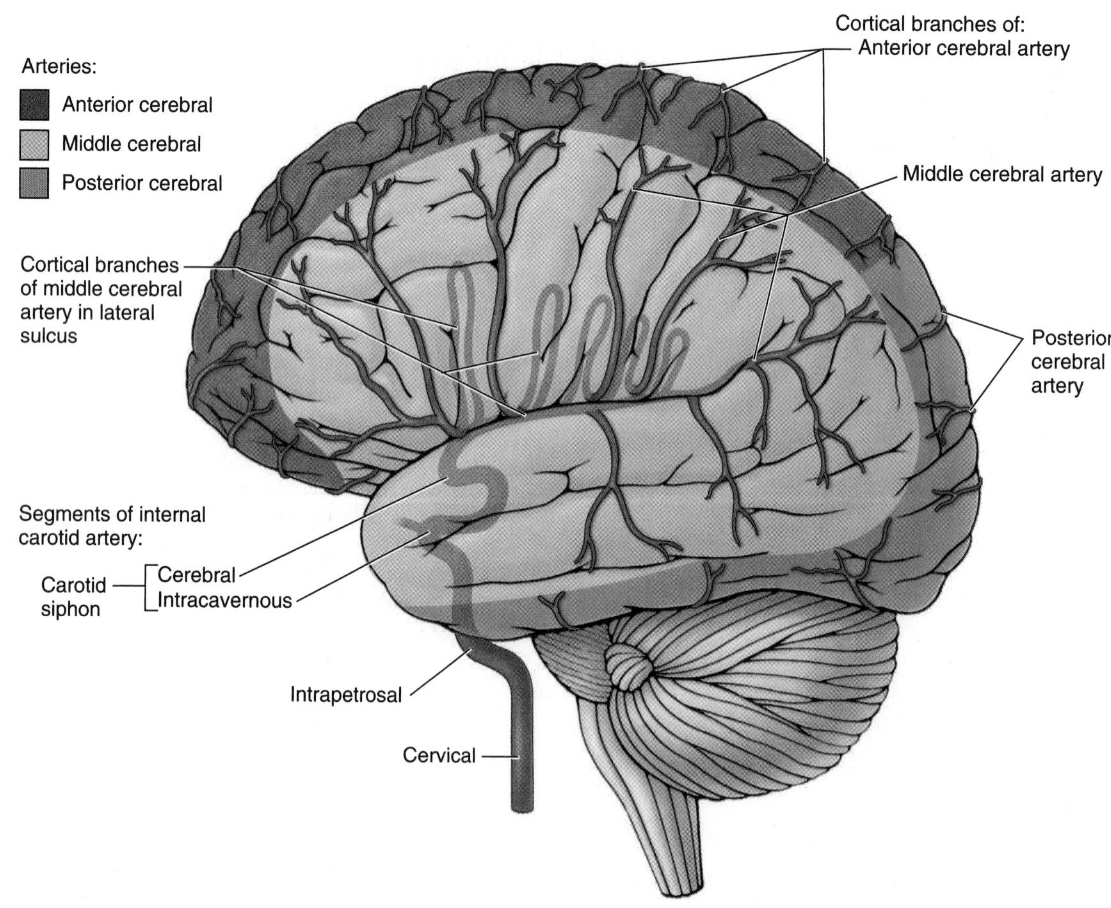
Arteries:
Anterior cerebral
Middle cerebral
Posterior cerebral
Cortical branches of:
Anterior cerebral artery
Middle cerebral artery
Cortical branches of middle cerebral artery in lateral sulcus
Posterior cerebral artery
Segments of internal carotid artery:
Carotid siphon
Cerebral
Intracavernous
Intrapetrosal
Cervical

The major arteries supplying the brain and their vascular territories.

PURE SENSORY STROKE

A 65-year-old with PMH of hypertension, smoking, and diabetes presents with acute-onset face, arm, and leg numbness. On **exam**, the patient has unilateral decreased sensation (vibration, proprioception, and pain/temperature), and **imaging** shows a thalamic infarct on brain MRI.

Management: See pp. 730–732 for Acute Stroke Management

Complications: Post-stroke pain syndrome after thalamic infarct.

HYF: Uncontrolled hypertension is the most important risk factor for lacunar stroke.

PURE MOTOR STROKE

A 65-year-old with PMH of hypertension, smoking, and diabetes presents with weakness of unilateral leg and arm. On **exam**, the patient has equally weak face, and upper and lower extremity without sensory deficit. **Imaging** shows an infarct in internal capsule, corona radiata, or basal ganglia.

Management: See pp. 730–732 for Acute Stroke Management.

Complications: Lacunar infarcts often have better short-term recovery.

HYF: Pure motor stroke is the most common syndrome of lacunar stroke. Other motor lacunar stroke syndromes are ataxic hemiparesis and dysarthria-clumsy hand syndrome.

26-5 Stroke Syndrome

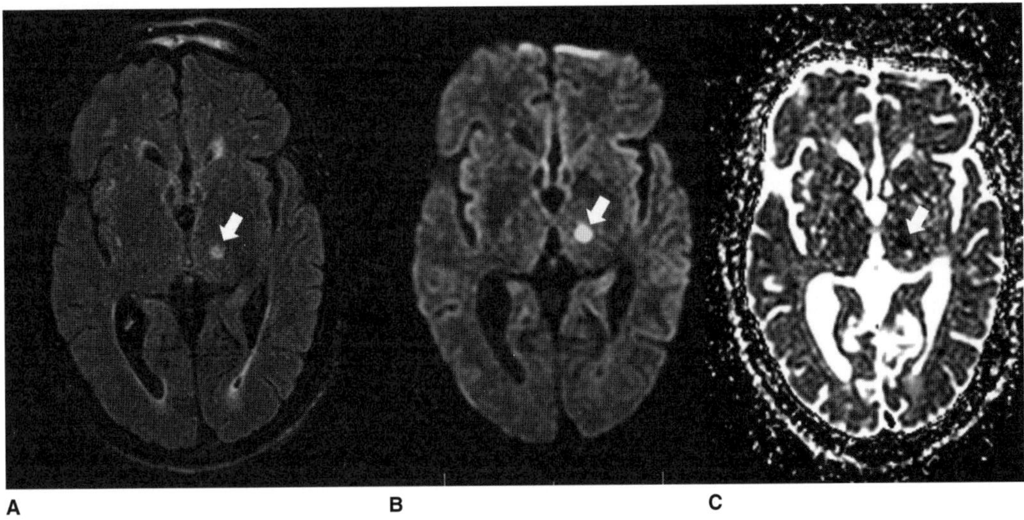
A
B
C

MRI brain including FLAIR sequence (A), diffusion-weighted imaging (B) and ADC sequence (C) demonstrating subacute lacunar infarct.

LATERAL MEDULLARY STROKE/ WALLENBERG STROKE

A 65-year-old with PMH of hypertension, CAD, and diabetes presents with dizziness, hoarseness, and face pain. On **exam**, the patient has loss of pain/temperature on the ipsilateral face and contralateral body, uvula deviation to the contralateral side, and ipsilateral Horner. **Imaging** shows an infarct in the lateral medulla with intracranial vertebral artery occlusion.

Management: See pp. 730–732 for Acute Stroke Management.

Complications:

- Aspiration and pneumonia due to prominent dysphagia.
- Respiratory dysfunction – Ondine's curse (failure to initiate respiration during sleep).

HYF: Think Wallenberg when you see crossed sensory signs with bulbar weakness and vertigo (commonly tested for knowledge of brain stem anatomy).

Can also be caused by vertebral artery dissection. Wallenberg is a PICA stroke that has multiple overlapping signs with other cerebellar strokes (see Vertigo, pp. 759–760). To localize a deficit in the brain stem, determine which cranial nerves are affected.

Rule of 4s: CN 1–4 are above pons (3–4 are midbrain), 5–8 originate in pons, 9–12 in medulla.

26-6 Stroke Management

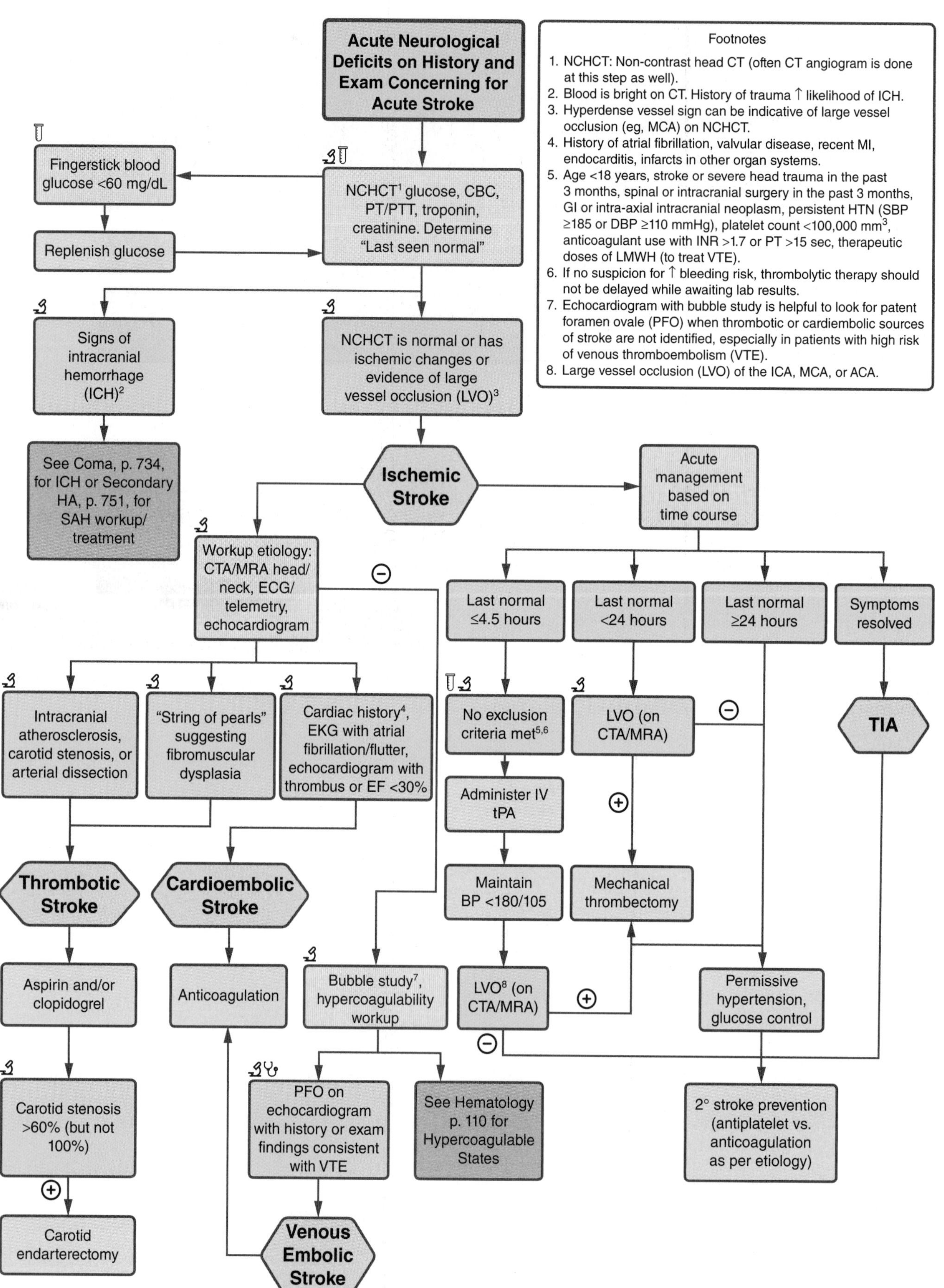

Acute Neurological Deficits on History and Exam Concerning for Acute Stroke
Fingerstick blood glucose <60 mg/dL
Replenish glucose
NCHCT[1] glucose, CBC, PT/PTT, troponin, creatinine. Determine "Last seen normal"
Signs of intracranial hemorrhage (ICH)[2]
See Coma, p. 734, for ICH or Secondary HA, p. 751, for SAH workup/treatment
NCHCT is normal or has ischemic changes or evidence of large vessel occlusion (LVO)[3]
Ischemic Stroke
Acute management based on time course
Workup etiology: CTA/MRA head/neck, ECG/telemetry, echocardiogram
Last normal ≤4.5 hours
Last normal <24 hours
Last normal ≥24 hours
Symptoms resolved
Intracranial atherosclerosis, carotid stenosis, or arterial dissection
"String of pearls" suggesting fibromuscular dysplasia
Cardiac history[4], EKG with atrial fibrillation/flutter, echocardiogram with thrombus or EF <30%
No exclusion criteria met[5,6]
LVO (on CTA/MRA)
TIA
Administer IV tPA
Thrombotic Stroke
Cardioembolic Stroke
Maintain BP <180/105
Mechanical thrombectomy
Aspirin and/or clopidogrel
Anticoagulation
Bubble study[7], hypercoagulability workup
LVO[8] (on CTA/MRA)
Permissive hypertension, glucose control
Carotid stenosis >60% (but not 100%)
PFO on echocardiogram with history or exam findings consistent with VTE
See Hematology p. 110 for Hypercoagulable States
2° stroke prevention (antiplatelet vs. anticoagulation as per etiology)
Carotid endarterectomy
Venous Embolic Stroke
Footnotes
1. NCHCT: Non-contrast head CT (often CT angiogram is done at this step as well).
2. Blood is bright on CT. History of trauma ↑ likelihood of ICH.
3. Hyperdense vessel sign can be indicative of large vessel occlusion (eg, MCA) on NCHCT.
4. History of atrial fibrillation, valvular disease, recent MI, endocarditis, infarcts in other organ systems.
5. Age <18 years, stroke or severe head trauma in the past 3 months, spinal or intracranial surgery in the past 3 months, GI or intra-axial intracranial neoplasm, persistent HTN (SBP ≥185 or DBP ≥110 mmHg), platelet count <100,000 mm3, anticoagulant use with INR >1.7 or PT >15 sec, therapeutic doses of LMWH (to treat VTE).
6. If no suspicion for ↑ bleeding risk, thrombolytic therapy should not be delayed while awaiting lab results.
7. Echocardiogram with bubble study is helpful to look for patent foramen ovale (PFO) when thrombotic or cardiembolic sources of stroke are not identified, especially in patients with high risk of venous thromboembolism (VTE).
8. Large vessel occlusion (LVO) of the ICA, MCA, or ACA.

FIGURE 26.6

26-6 Stroke Management

THROMBOTIC STROKE

A 67-year-old M with PMH of hyperlipidemia, HTN, T2DM, and osteoarthritis presents with sudden-onset weakness. On **exam**, he has R hemiplegia, R hemisensory deficits, and aphasia. **Labs/imaging** show hyperdense vessel sign of the MCA on non-contrast head CT (NCHCT) and significant bilateral atherosclerosis of the MCAs on CTA. Normal serum troponin. No signs of arrhythmia on EKG. Normal ejection fraction with no valvular disorder seen on echocardiogram.

Management:

1. If <4.5 hours since last seen normal, administer IV tPA.
   a. On presentation, draw CBC, PT/PTT, troponin, creatinine. tPA is contraindicated in patients with high bleeding risk: recent stroke/head trauma (3 months), any history of ICH, coagulopathy (INR >1.7 or PTT elevated), including therapeutic heparin or DOAC use, platelets <100, BP >185/110 (can use IV antihypertensives to lower), major surgery in the past 2 weeks, GI or brain neoplasm.
   b. Following administration of IV tPA, keep SBP <180 mmHg and DBP <105 mmHg.
2. If <24 hours since last seen normal with large vessel occlusion on CTA, consider mechanical thrombectomy.
   a. Aspirin if not tPA candidate.
3. If last seen normal >24 hours ago, not eligible for IV tPA or mechanical thrombectomy.
4. Permissive hypertension for the first 24–48 hours after acute stroke onset (≤220/120 mmHg) unless s/p tPA.
5. Continuous telemetry for 24–48 hours to detect paroxysmal Afib.
6. Maintain serum glucose concentrations in the range of 140–180 mg/dL (7.8–10 mmol/L), given that patients with DM are likely to present with hyperglycemia during stroke, which can precipitate brain injury.
7. Long-term secondary prevention: Statin, HTN, and DM management.
8. Antiplatelet treatment: Aspirin and/or clopidogrel.
9. Consider carotid endarterectomy if moderate-severe (but not completely occlusive) carotid stenosis.

Complications:

- Hemorrhagic conversion or other bleed (more likely post-tPA).
- Cerebral edema leading to increased ICP, herniation: Treat with mannitol/hypertonic saline, hyperventilation.
- Seizures (less common than in hemorrhagic stroke but poor prognosis).
- UTIs, pressure ulcers, DVTs, falls due to decreased mobility.
- Aspiration and pneumonia in patients with post-stroke dysphagia.

HYF: Patients with significant atherosclerotic disease can also experience artery-to-artery embolism from a proximal to more distal vascular territory (ie, clot breaks off from ICA to MCA or ACA).

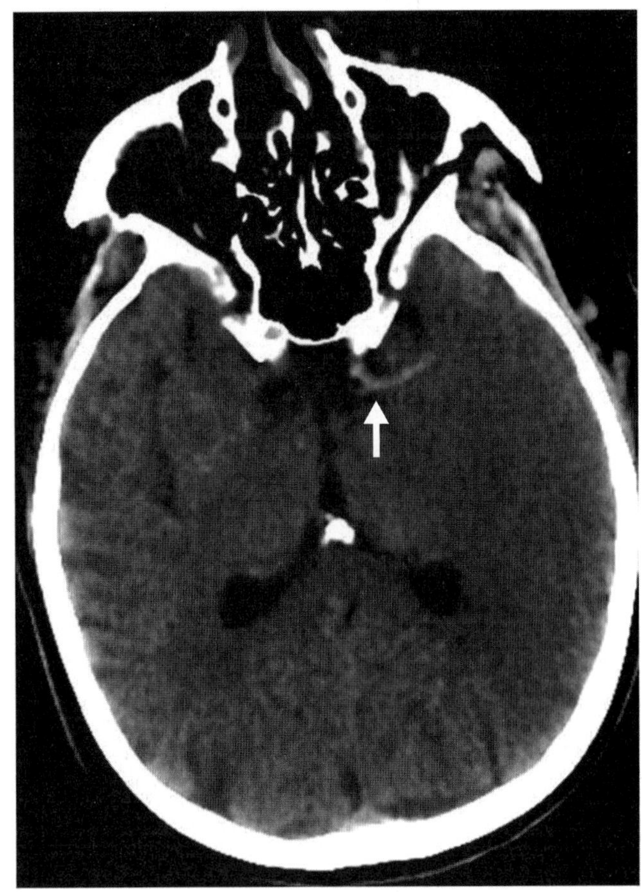

Noncontrast head CT demonstrating "hyperdense vessel sign" suggesting left MCA stroke.

CARDIOEMBOLIC STROKE

A 50-year-old M with PMH of HFrEF <30% presents with sudden-onset left-sided weakness. On **exam**, he has peripheral edema, bilateral crackles on auscultation, and left-sided hemiplegia with right-sided gaze deviation. On **imaging**, NCHCT shows hypointense signal in R MCA vascular territory, and MRI shows old small infarcts in multiple vascular territories.

Management:

1. Acute management as in "Thrombotic Stroke".
2. Obtain troponin, EKG, and echo to assess heart function, given suspicion for cardioembolic source (looking for signs of MI, arrhythmia/Afib, or causes for blood stagnation, such as reduced ejection fraction).
3. Anticoagulation (usually DOAC but if warfarin, goal INR 2–3 in atrial fibrillation, 2.5–3.5 for prosthetic valve).
4. Antiplatelet is not indicated in cardioembolic stroke.

HYF: Use calculators such as $CHADS_2$-VASc to determine risk of stroke in atrial fibrillation. Anticoagulation is essential.

(Continued)

26-6 Stroke Management

TRANSIENT ISCHEMIC ATTACK (TIA)

A 50-year-old M with PMH of atrial fibrillation and peripheral vascular disease presents with difficulty speaking and R-sided weakness that resolves during ambulance transport, with a normal **exam** by time of presentation and head **imaging** without evidence of infarct.

Management:

1. Determine source (embolic vs. thrombotic).
2. Secondary prevention as above.

Complications: Stroke if risk factors not corrected.

HYF: Occurs when a clot is spontaneously thrombolysed prior to any therapy, leaving no deficit. By definition, deficits must resolve within 24 hours, but typically resolve <1 hour.

EMBOLISM FROM VENOUS THROMBOSIS TO BRAIN

A 65-year-old F with PMH of colon adenocarcinoma who is hospitalized POD 2 following L hemicolectomy was last seen normal 3.5 hours ago and now presents with aphasia and R hemiplegia. On **exam**, she has an erythematous and edematous calf. On **imaging**, CTA shows L MCA occlusion without signs of intracranial atherosclerotic disease.

Management:

1. Acute management as in "Thrombotic Stroke".
2. EKG, echocardiogram, and serum troponin should be assessed to look for cardioembolic source.
3. If no cardioembolic source is found, an echocardiogram with bubble study can be obtained to look for PFO (if no other source of stroke is found, this can be a likely cause of stroke in this patient with VTE on exam s/p surgery for neoplasm).
4. If PFO is found, this patient should be treated with anticoagulation therapy for secondary stroke prevention (PFO closure not usually performed on patients age >60).

Complications: In patients in hypercoagulable state (malignancy, SLE, antiphospholipid syndrome) with recurrent DVTs, the risk of recurrent stroke increases.

HYF: Rare occurrence but should be considered in patients with DVT in whom other causes of stroke have been ruled out.

26-7 Coma

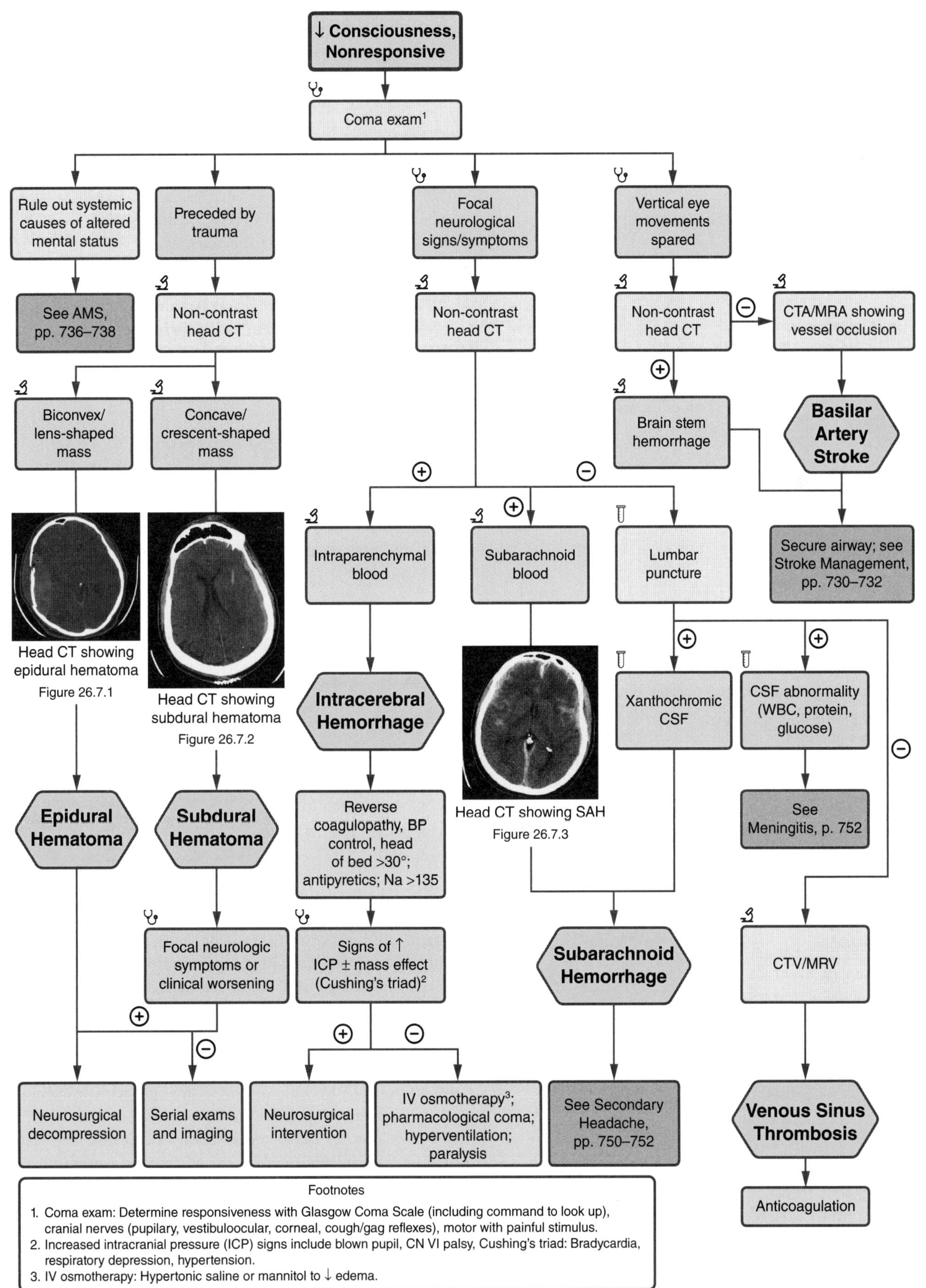
↓ Consciousness, Nonresponsive
Coma exam[1]
Rule out systemic causes of altered mental status
See AMS, pp. 736–738
Preceded by trauma
Non-contrast head CT
Biconvex/ lens-shaped mass
Concave/ crescent-shaped mass
Head CT showing epidural hematoma
Figure 26.7.1
Head CT showing subdural hematoma
Figure 26.7.2
Epidural Hematoma
Subdural Hematoma
Focal neurologic symptoms or clinical worsening
Neurosurgical decompression
Serial exams and imaging
Focal neurological signs/symptoms
Non-contrast head CT
Intraparenchymal blood
Subarachnoid blood
Lumbar puncture
Intracerebral Hemorrhage
Reverse coagulopathy, BP control, head of bed >30°; antipyretics; Na >135
Signs of ↑ ICP ± mass effect (Cushing's triad)[2]
Neurosurgical intervention
IV osmotherapy[3]; pharmacological coma; hyperventilation; paralysis
Head CT showing SAH
Figure 26.7.3
Xanthochromic CSF
CSF abnormality (WBC, protein, glucose)
See Meningitis, p. 752
Subarachnoid Hemorrhage
See Secondary Headache, pp. 750–752
Vertical eye movements spared
Non-contrast head CT
CTA/MRA showing vessel occlusion
Brain stem hemorrhage
Basilar Artery Stroke
Secure airway; see Stroke Management, pp. 730–732
CTV/MRV
Venous Sinus Thrombosis
Anticoagulation

Footnotes

1. Coma exam: Determine responsiveness with Glasgow Coma Scale (including command to look up), cranial nerves (pupilary, vestibuloocular, corneal, cough/gag reflexes), motor with painful stimulus.
2. Increased intracranial pressure (ICP) signs include blown pupil, CN VI palsy, Cushing's triad: Bradycardia, respiratory depression, hypertension.
3. IV osmotherapy: Hypertonic saline or mannitol to ↓ edema.

FIGURE 26.7

26-7 Coma

EPIDURAL HEMATOMA

A 30-year-old M with no PMH presents with multiple traumas after a motor vehicle collision. He was initially awake after the collision but became increasingly unresponsive over the next hour. On **exam**, he has mydriasis and ptosis of the left eye. On **imaging**, CT shows a biconvex-shaped hyperdense mass.

Management:

1. Reverse anticoagulation for anticoagulated patients.
2. Emergent decompression.
3. For asymptomatic patients with small bleeds: Serial neurologic exams and CT scans to ensure stability.

Complications:

- Increased ICP in the setting of arterial bleeding and hematoma expansion, developing headache, vomiting, seizures, coma.
- Uncal herniation with compression of the midbrain and oculomotor nerve, causing mydriasis and ptosis.

HYF: Occurs due to tearing of the middle meningeal artery in the setting of trauma. Brief loss of consciousness followed by a lucid interval. Loss of consciousness occurs due to increased ICP/herniation.

SUBDURAL HEMATOMA

An 80-year-old with PMH of Afib, hypertension, and diabetes presents with 5-day history of decreased consciousness and weakness in the setting of several falls in the past 3 months after increasing dose of anti-hypertensive medications. On **exam**, the patient has weakness greater in the right side with brisk reflexes. On **imaging**, non-contrast CT scan shows a concave hyperdense mass.

Management:

1. Reverse anticoagulation for anticoagulated patients.
2. Emergent decompression if focal neurologic symptoms, brain stem compression, hydrocephalus, or midline shift.
3. For asymptomatic patients with small bleeds: Serial neurologic exams and CT scans to ensure stability.

Complications:

- Compression of brain parenchyma and displacement of the cerebral hemisphere → focal deficits and/or seizures.
- Increased intracranial pressure → vomiting, nausea, headache.
- Herniation with decreased consciousness and posturing.

HYF: Risk factors for subdural hematoma from trauma: Old age, age <2 years, alcohol use disorder, malignancy, and anticoagulation. Associated with rupture of bridging cortical veins.

INTRACEREBRAL HEMORRHAGE

A 70-year-old with PMH of hypertension and diabetes presents with sudden severe headache associated with altered mental status, R-side weakness, conjugate gaze deviation, and vomiting. On **imaging**, non-contrast CT reveals a putamen hemorrhage.

Management:

1. Preventive measures: Strict BP control, head of bed >30°, sedation, serum sodium >135, antipyretics.
2. Serial exams and imaging. Neurosurgery if elevated ICP or mass effect. If no mass effect, hypertonic saline, mannitol, hyperventilation, neuromuscular blockade, hypothermia.

Complications:

- Increased ICP with mydriasis, Cushing's triad.
- Sequelae related to the affected area.

HYF: Most common cause is hypertension with Charcot-Bouchard microaneurysms and hemorrhage of small penetrating arteries, most often in the basal ganglia, putamen, and thalamus. Variable presentations depending upon the affected area. Also caused by amyloid angiopathy (lobar) and arteriovenous malformation in children.

BASILAR ARTERY STROKE

A 50-year-old M with PMH of hypertension and hyperlipidemia presents with L-sided body weakness and numbness, followed by quadriplegia and respiratory distress. On **exam**, he has intact vertical eye movements. On **imaging**, MRI shows acute infarct of the pons and basilar artery thrombosis.

Management:

1. Secure and maintain airway.
2. Treat the cause of basilar artery occlusion: Ischemia with revascularization/thrombolysis, infection with antibiotics, inflammation with steroids.

Complications:

- Sequelae from neurological deficits.
- Locked-in syndrome (which can be mistaken for coma) occurs if patient retains alertness and only vertical eye movements are spared.

HYF: The basilar artery is the only unpaired cerebral artery, so a single occlusion can lead to bilateral dysfunction. The patient retains alertness when the reticular activating system is spared. The initial presentation usually progresses from hemiparesis to quadriplegia, including loss of voluntary facial, mouth, and tongue movements. Vertical eye movements are preserved.

VENOUS SINUS THROMBOSIS

A 40-year-old M with no PMH presents with worsening headache, diplopia, progressive confusion, fever, and bilateral proptosis 10 days after an initial presentation of sinusitis. On **exam**, he is febrile with bilateral periorbital edema and significant drainage. On **labs/imaging**, MRI/MRV shows low signal and lack of flow in cavernous sinus, and blood cultures are positive for *Staphylococcus aureus*.

26-7 Coma

Management:

1. Antibiotics.
2. Heparin infusion.
3. Surgical drainage.

Complications:

- Mortality associated with septic cavernous sinus thrombosis is 30%.
- Sequelae with oculomotor weakness, blindness, pituitary insufficiency.

HYF: Follows an infection or trauma involving the cavernous sinus (eg, sinusitis) and affects cranial nerves that traverse the cavernous sinus (CNs III, IV, V1, V2, and VI). *S. aureus* is the most common pathogen.

Subarachnoid Hemorrhage: See p. 751 in the Neurology section for secondary headaches.

26-8 Altered Mental Status

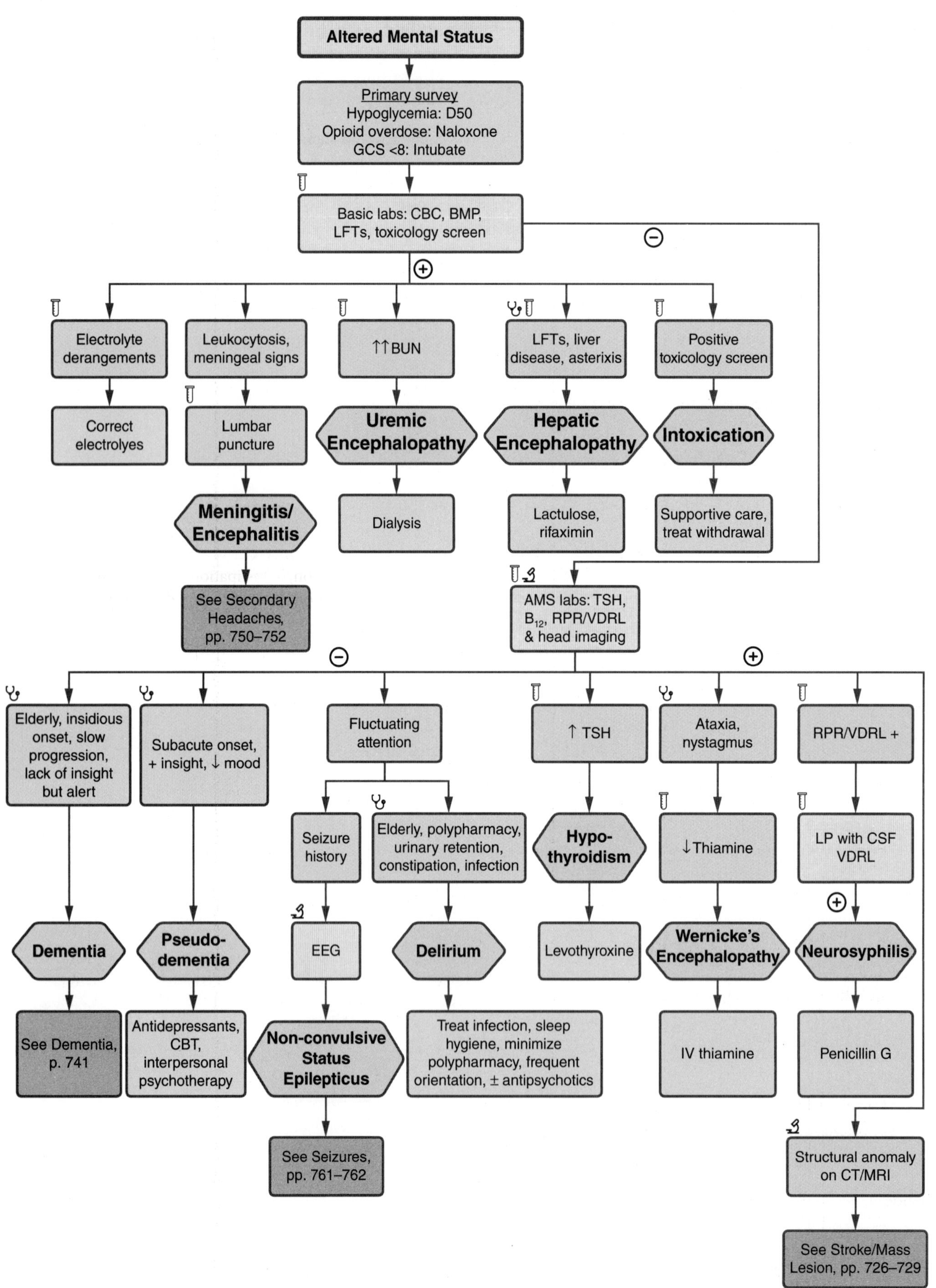
Altered Mental Status
Primary survey
Hypoglycemia: D50
Opioid overdose: Naloxone
GCS <8: Intubate
Basic labs: CBC, BMP, LFTs, toxicology screen
Electrolyte derangements
Leukocytosis, meningeal signs
↑↑BUN
LFTs, liver disease, asterixis
Positive toxicology screen
Correct electrolyes
Lumbar puncture
Uremic Encephalopathy
Hepatic Encephalopathy
Intoxication
Meningitis/ Encephalitis
Dialysis
Lactulose, rifaximin
Supportive care, treat withdrawal
See Secondary Headaches, pp. 750–752
AMS labs: TSH, B12, RPR/VDRL & head imaging
Elderly, insidious onset, slow progression, lack of insight but alert
Subacute onset, + insight, ↓ mood
Fluctuating attention
↑ TSH
Ataxia, nystagmus
RPR/VDRL +
Seizure history
Elderly, polypharmacy, urinary retention, constipation, infection
Hypo-thyroidism
↓Thiamine
LP with CSF VDRL
Dementia
Pseudo-dementia
EEG
Delirium
Levothyroxine
Wernicke's Encephalopathy
Neurosyphilis
See Dementia, p. 741
Antidepressants, CBT, interpersonal psychotherapy
Non-convulsive Status Epilepticus
Treat infection, sleep hygiene, minimize polypharmacy, frequent orientation, ± antipsychotics
IV thiamine
Penicillin G
See Seizures, pp. 761–762
Structural anomaly on CT/MRI
See Stroke/Mass Lesion, pp. 726–729

FIGURE 26.8

26-8 Altered Mental Status

UREMIC ENCEPHALOPATHY (UE)

A 70-year-old with PMH of end-stage renal disease (EGFR <15) presents with altered mental status. On exam, he has a mild tremor and asterixis. Labs show markedly elevated BUN.

Management:

1. Dialysis.
2. Correct electrolyte derangements.
3. Consider renal transplant.

Complications:

- Coma, psychosis, or generalized seizure (rare).
- A higher risk for stroke and adverse cardiac events.
- High uremic state also increases risk for pericarditis and uremic coagulopathy.

HYF: Often due to chronic ESRD but can also occur with AKI. Reversible with dialysis.

HEPATIC ENCEPHALOPATHY (HE)

A 60-year-old M with PMH of alcohol use disorder and alcoholic cirrhosis presents with fatigue and confusion ×2 weeks. On exam, he has abdominal distention with fluid wave and shifting dullness, asterixis, and hemorrhoids and is not oriented to place or time. Labs are unremarkable.

Management:

1. Lactulose is 1st-line. Titrate to 2–3 soft BMs/day.
2. Rifaximin can be added.
3. Evaluate for precipitating causes (dehydration, infection, GI bleed, constipation, hyperkalemia, alcohol intake, etc.) and treat precipitant.

Complications: Coma.

HYF: Important to rule out infection (especially spontaneous bacterial peritonitis) that can trigger HE. Serum ammonia is not needed to make a diagnosis.

PSEUDODEMENTIA

A 70-year-old F with PMH of major depressive disorder presents with 1-month history of forgetfulness, fatigue, and sleep disturbances. On exam, she is disheveled and malodorous and has a flat affect. She is AOx3 but only recalled 0/3 objects after 5 minutes.

Management:

1. Assess for suicidal ideation.
2. Antidepressants (supplemented with CBT).

Complications:

- Suicide

HYF: Neurovegetative and neurocognitive ("pseudodementia") symptoms can result in the elderly due to major depressive disorder, not just as a result of normal aging or sequelae of comorbid medical conditions.

NON-CONVULSIVE STATUS EPILEPTICUS

A 60-year-old with PMH of epilepsy and atrial fibrillation on warfarin presents with headache. The patient was found to have subdural hemorrhage s/p craniotomy and did not wake up after surgery.
See pp. 761–762 in Neurology section for seizures.

DELIRIUM

An 80-year-old F with PMH of Alzheimer's dementia is brought to the ED with acute onset of combativeness and paranoia. On exam, the patient has restless movements and agitation followed by a period of drowsiness and responds to internal stimuli. On labs, she has leukocytosis, and UA shows 3+ leukocyte esterase and WBCs.

Management:

1. Assess for infection with blood culture, urine culture, sputum culture, and CXR. Treat with antibiotics if there is evidence of infection.
2. Frequent reorientation, maintenance of sleep-wake cycles, calm/soothing environment.

HYF: Delirium (hypoactive or hyperactive) is common in elderly patients with underlying dementia who experience a trigger, usually an infection such as a UTI, as in this patient. Other triggers include dehydration, constipation, polypharmacy (anticholinergics), hospitalization, and electrolyte derangements.

WERNICKE ENCEPHALOPATHY (WE)

A 65-year-old M with PMH of alcohol use disorder presents with acute confusion and lethargy. On exam, he appears malnourished and has a disconjugate gaze and broad-based gait.

Management:

1. IV thiamine.

Complications:

- Wernicke-Korsakoff's syndrome.
- Coma, death.

HYF: Classically, a triad of acutely altered mental status, ophthalmoplegia (along with nystagmus), and ataxia in the setting of extreme malnourishment or alcohol use disorder. Korsakoff's syndrome (retrograde and anterograde amnesia, confabulation, horizontal nystagmus) may develop if left untreated. If glucose needs to be administered in patients with alcohol use disorder or alcohol intoxication, it should be done after thiamine repletion or it will precipitate WE.

NEUROSYPHILIS

A 45-year-old M presents with progressive headache, unsteady gait, and worsening reading vision. On exam, he has pupils that accommodate but do not constrict to light, truncal ataxia, decreased vibration sense, and painless, non-pruritic rash across entire body. Labs with +serum RPR/VDRL and +CSF VDRL.

(Continued)

26-8 Altered Mental Status

Management:

1. IV penicillin G (ceftriaxone if penicillin allergy).

Complications:

- Progressive dementia (general paresis).
- Tabes dorsalis (posterior column disease with sensory ataxia and lancinating pains).
- Syphilitic meningitis.
- Ocular and otic involvement common.

HYF: Most commonly presents as meningitis early in disease and tabes dorsalis/general paresis later. LP with CSF studies are important if there is any suspicion for neurosyphilis.

Intoxication: See Psychiatry section for intoxication syndromes pp. 798–799.

Dementia: See Neurology section for dementia pp. 740–741.

Hypothyroidism: See Endocrinology section for thyroid disorders pp. 137–139.

26-9 Movement Disorders and Dementia

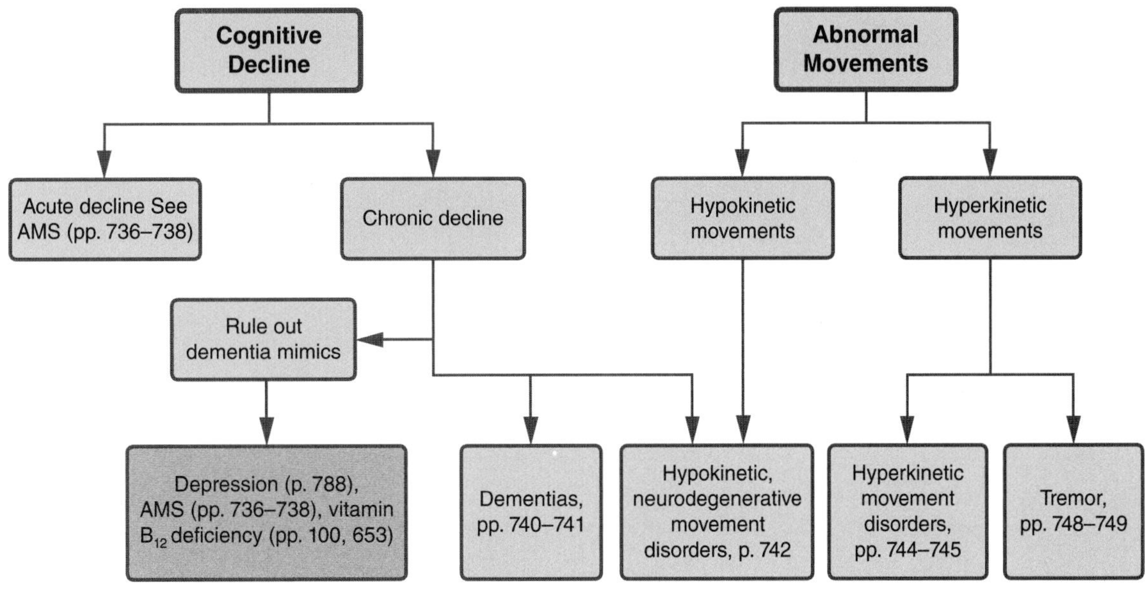
Cognitive Decline
Abnormal Movements
Acute decline See AMS (pp. 736–738)
Chronic decline
Hypokinetic movements
Hyperkinetic movements
Rule out dementia mimics
Depression (p. 788), AMS (pp. 736–738), vitamin B12 deficiency (pp. 100, 653)
Dementias, pp. 740–741
Hypokinetic, neurodegenerative movement disorders, p. 742
Hyperkinetic movement disorders, pp. 744–745
Tremor, pp. 748–749

Neurodegenerative disorders typically present with chronic cognitive decline, abnormal movements, or both. In a patient presenting with cognitive decline, acute causes (covered elsewhere in the Neurology section, especially under altered mental status) and dementia mimics must be first ruled out. The most common disorders mimicking dementia are depression, delirium (both covered in the Psychiatry chapter), B_{12}/thiamine deficiency, and hypothyroidism. Other chronic neurologic disorders such as multiple sclerosis and infection can also lead to cognitive decline, but typically the classic symptoms of those diseases will predominate. Neurodegenerative diseases presenting with only cognitive symptoms will be presented under Dementia while those with prominent movement components will be presented under Hypokinetic Movement Disorders.

When a patient presents with abnormal movements, it is important to first determine whether there is too much movement (tremor, chorea, tics, dystonia) (ie, hyperkinetic) or too little (rigidity, shuffling gait, bradykinesia). Besides Huntington's Disease, which has a hyperkinetic presentation, the neurodegenerative disorders that overlap with dementia are hypokinetic. These often have a component of cognitive decline and therefore overlap heavily with causes of dementia, including Parkinson's Disease and the "Parkinson's Plus" diseases.

FIGURE 26.9

26-10 Dementia

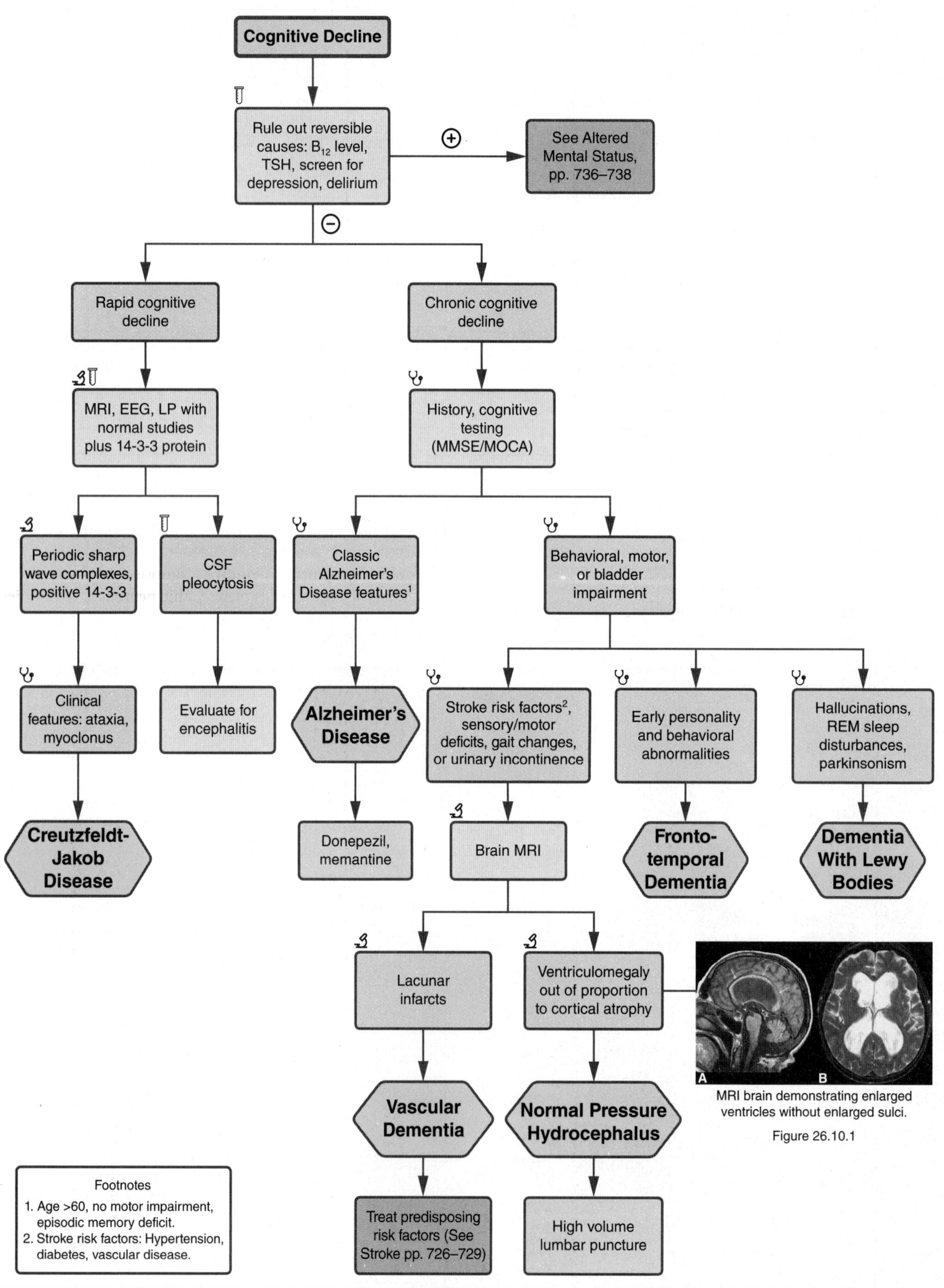

Cognitive Decline
Rule out reversible causes: B12 level, TSH, screen for depression, delirium
⊕
See Altered Mental Status, pp. 736–738
⊖
Rapid cognitive decline
Chronic cognitive decline
MRI, EEG, LP with normal studies plus 14-3-3 protein
History, cognitive testing (MMSE/MOCA)
Periodic sharp wave complexes, positive 14-3-3
CSF pleocytosis
Classic Alzheimer's Disease features¹
Behavioral, motor, or bladder impairment
Clinical features: ataxia, myoclonus
Evaluate for encephalitis
Alzheimer's Disease
Stroke risk factors², sensory/motor deficits, gait changes, or urinary incontinence
Early personality and behavioral abnormalities
Hallucinations, REM sleep disturbances, parkinsonism
Creutzfeldt-Jakob Disease
Donepezil, memantine
Brain MRI
Fronto-temporal Dementia
Dementia With Lewy Bodies
Lacunar infarcts
Ventriculomegaly out of proportion to cortical atrophy
A
B
Vascular Dementia
Normal Pressure Hydrocephalus
Treat predisposing risk factors (See Stroke pp. 726–729)
High volume lumbar puncture
Footnotes
1. Age >60, no motor impairment, episodic memory deficit.
2. Stroke risk factors: Hypertension, diabetes, vascular disease.

MRI brain demonstrating enlarged ventricles without enlarged sulci.

Figure 26.10.1

FIGURE 26.10

26-10 Dementia

CREUTZFELDT-JAKOB DISEASE (CJD)

A 65-year-old presents with subacute (weeks-months) cognitive decline and gait difficulty. On **exam**, the patient has ataxia, nystagmus, and startle myoclonus. **Labs/imaging** show elevated CSF 14-3-3 and tau proteins. EEG shows periodic sharp-wave complexes.

Management:

1. No effective treatment, uniformly fatal (median survival time of 6 months).
2. Can give benzodiazepines or anticonvulsants for myoclonus.

HYF: New-variant CJD (mad cow disease) is seen in younger patients with a history of eating beef or human brains (kuru); progression is slower. CJD is caused by an abnormal protease-resistant prion protein and causes spongiform degeneration. Current practice uses RT-QuIC test for diagnosis.

ALZHEIMER'S DISEASE (AD)

An 80-year-old F with family history of dementia presents with memory deficits regarding new information that has progressed to visuospatial and language deficits. On **exam**, she has impaired memory, and **imaging** shows atrophy in the temporal and parietal lobes on brain MRI.

Management:

1. Cholinesterase inhibitors (donepezil) for symptoms.
2. NMDA receptor antagonist (memantine) may slow decline.

Complications:

- Depression is often comorbid.
- Delirium and agitation (sundowning) are common, especially during hospitalizations.
- Spontaneous lobar hemorrhage (in patients with amyloid angiopathy).

HYF: AD is more common and occurs at younger ages in people with Down syndrome.

Pathology: Neurofibrillary tangles, neuritic plaques with amyloid.

FRONTOTEMPORAL DEMENTIA

A 55-year-old M with family history of dementia presents with behavioral and personality changes, including disinhibition, compulsivity, and apathy. On **exam**, he has inattention and decreased verbal fluency, and **imaging** shows frontal and temporal atrophy on brain MRI.

Management:

1. Supportive care.

Complications:

- Safety: given impulsivity, patients can often endanger themselves, and therefore, behavioral interventions are essential.
- 15–20% of patients also develop motor neuron disease.

HYF: Can often be misdiagnosed as a psychiatric disorder; if patient is age >50, suspect dementia/medical cause for behavioral changes. Think FTD in a younger (age 50–60) patient with dementia and personality changes; rare in patients age >75.

DEMENTIA WITH LEWY BODIES (DLB)

A 65-year-old presents with visual hallucinations and progressive fluctuating decline in attention, visuospatial processing, and executive function, occurring at the same time or earlier than parkinsonism. On **exam**, the patient has bradykinesia, rigidity, and shuffling gait. **Imaging** shows REM sleep behavior disorder on polysomnography.

Management:

1. Supportive care.
2. Cholinesterase inhibitors (donepezil) for cognitive and behavioral symptoms.
3. Less levodopa-responsive than Parkinson's Disease.
4. Quetiapine for psychosis (lowest effective dose).
5. Identify triggers: caffeine, anxiety, hyperthyroidism, fatigue.

Complications:

- Similar to those of Parkinson's Disease; no curative/disease-modifying treatment.
- Median time to severe dementia is 5 years.
- Orthostatic hypotension and urinary incontinence.
- Exquisitely sensitive to medications, so use as low a dose as possible.

HYF: Distinction from Parkinson's disease dementia is somewhat arbitrary: Diagnose PDD if motor symptoms are present >1 year prior to cognitive symptoms. Definitive diagnosis is with autopsy: abnormal clumps of α-synuclein proteins within neurons (Lewy bodies).

VASCULAR DEMENTIA

A 75-year-old with PMH of HTN, DM2, HLD, CAD, and obesity presents with stepwise decline in cognitive function. On **exam**, the patient has focal motor and sensory deficits, and **imaging** shows multiple lacunar infarcts in cortical and subcortical areas on brain MRI.

Management:

1. Management of risk factors (antihypertensives, statins, glucose management).
2. Secondary stroke prevention (aspirin or other antiplatelet agents, see Stroke, p. 731).

Complications: Recurrent stroke.

HYF: Because vascular and Alzheimer's dementia are common, they can often be comorbid in the same patient. Vascular dementia can occur after successive clinically silent strokes seen later on MRI.

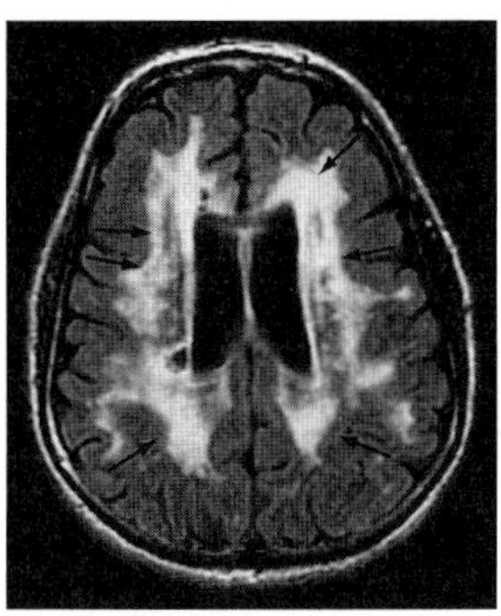

MRI brain (T2 FLAIR sequence) demonstrating white matter hyperintensities suggesting vascular dementia.

Normal Pressure Hydrocephalus: See Gait Disorders, pp. 748–749.

26-11 Neurodegenerative Movement Disorders

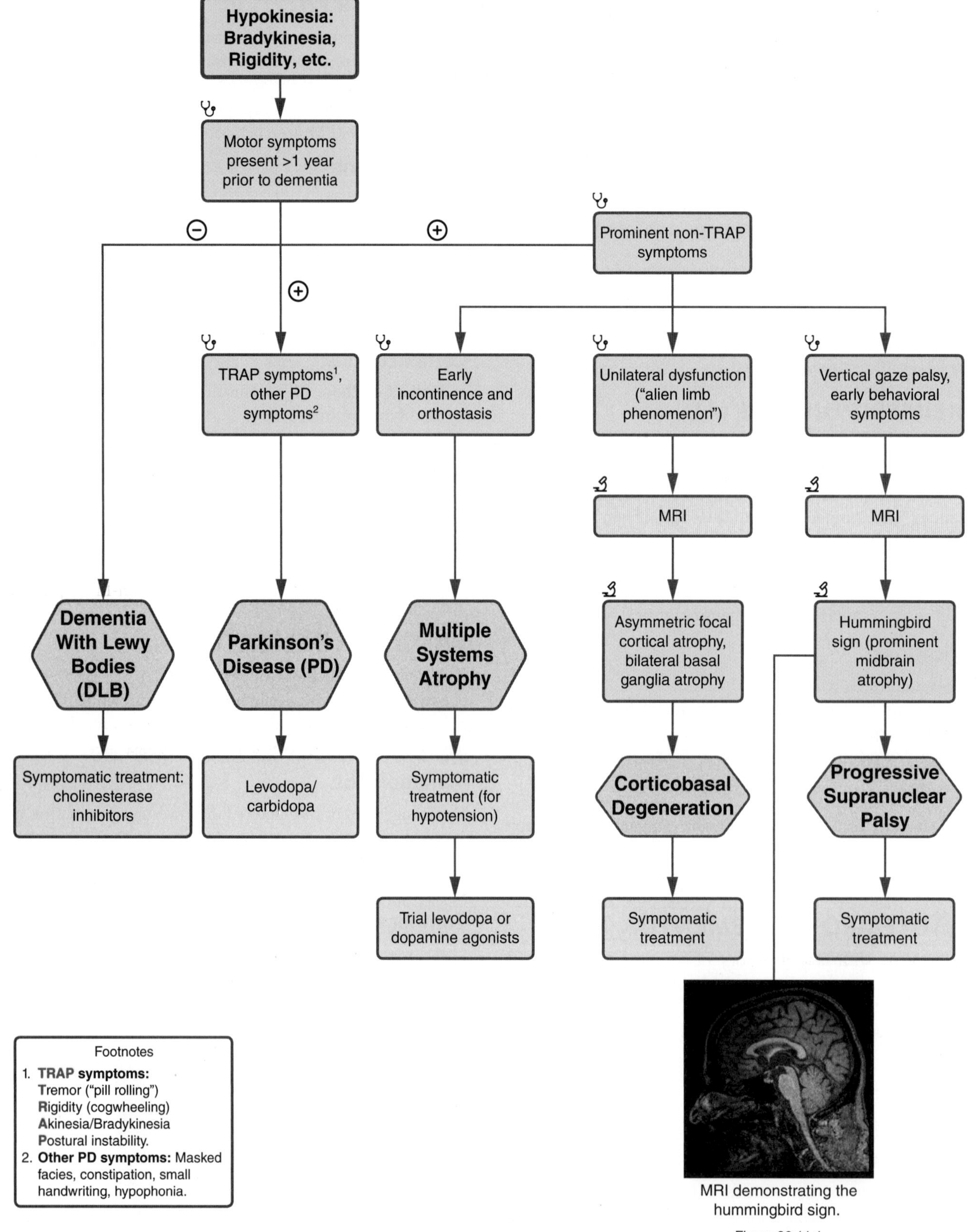
Hypokinesia: Bradykinesia, Rigidity, etc.
Motor symptoms present >1 year prior to dementia
⊖
⊕
Prominent non-TRAP symptoms
⊕
TRAP symptoms¹, other PD symptoms²
Early incontinence and orthostasis
Unilateral dysfunction ("alien limb phenomenon")
Vertical gaze palsy, early behavioral symptoms
MRI
MRI
Asymmetric focal cortical atrophy, bilateral basal ganglia atrophy
Hummingbird sign (prominent midbrain atrophy)
Dementia With Lewy Bodies (DLB)
Parkinson's Disease (PD)
Multiple Systems Atrophy
Corticobasal Degeneration
Progressive Supranuclear Palsy
Symptomatic treatment: cholinesterase inhibitors
Levodopa/ carbidopa
Symptomatic treatment (for hypotension)
Trial levodopa or dopamine agonists
Symptomatic treatment
Symptomatic treatment
Footnotes
1. TRAP symptoms: Tremor ("pill rolling") Rigidity (cogwheeling) Akinesia/Bradykinesia Postural instability.
2. Other PD symptoms: Masked facies, constipation, small handwriting, hypophonia.

MRI demonstrating the hummingbird sign.

Figure 26.11.1

FIGURE 26.11

26-11 Neurodegenerative Movement Disorders

PARKINSON'S DISEASE (PD)

A 60-year-old M with unremarkable PMH presents with recent fall. On **exam**, he has a pill-rolling tremor, limb rigidity, and difficulty starting movements. **Labs/imaging** are unremarkable.

Management:

1. Serial evaluation of symptoms, especially **TRAP** symptoms (**t**remor, **r**igidity, **a**kinesia/bradykinesia, **p**ostural instability).
2. 1st-line: Levodopa/carbidopa (levodopa can cross BBB, and carbidopa prevents peripheral conversion to dopamine to prevent nausea and GI upset).
3. 2nd-line: Dopamine agonists (pramipexole, ropinirole).
4. 3rd-line: Either COMT inhibitor such as entacapone or tolcapone (increases levodopa availability in CNS), MAO-B inhibitor such as selegiline (decreases required levodopa), or anticholinergics in younger patients with primarily tremors.
5. Treat comorbid depression or psychosis (low-potency 2nd-generation antipsychotics, pimavanserin).
6. For patients whose disease does not respond to medications, consider deep-brain stimulator placement.

Complications:

- Progressive, no curative or disease-modifying treatment.
- Patients can develop dementia over time; if within 1 year of parkinsonism, dementia is attributed to Lewy body dementia.
- Use of levodopa/carbidopa can lead to on-off phenomenon due to variable levels of dopamine available in the brain.
- High doses of dopaminergic medications (especially levodopa/carbidopa but including amantadine, MAO-Bi, COMTi) can cause hallucinations/psychotic symptoms.

HYF: Classic TRAP symptoms +/− masked facies, hypophonia, or memory loss. Due to loss of dopaminergic neurons in substantia nigra, resulting in difficulty initiating movements.

MULTIPLE SYSTEMS ATROPHY

A 70-year-old with PMH of hypertension presents with parkinsonism as well as recurrent falls and incontinence. On **exam**, he has orthostatic hypotension and abnormal sweating.

Management:

1. Increase salt intake, use compression stockings for autonomic nervous system (ANS) dysfunction. Midodrine/fludrocortisone for medication support.
2. Oxybutynin or tolterodine for incontinence.
3. MRI shows "**hot cross bun**" (T2 hyperintensity) **in pons**.

Complications: Can develop fatal bulbar dysfunction or laryngeal stridor.

HYF: Combination of parkinsonism and significant ANS dysfunction.

CORTICOBASAL DEGENERATION

A 65-year-old presents with abnormal sensation that their right arm does not belong to them. On **exam**, the patient has difficulty moving the arm and concurrent cognitive impairment. On **imaging**, MRI shows atrophy of the left parietal lobe and bilateral basal ganglia.

Management:

1. May benefit from Botox injections for contractures or pain in limb affected.
2. PT/OT and benzodiazepines show some benefit in some patients.

Complications: Poor prognosis of <10 years.

HYF: Asymmetric motor findings and "alien-limb" phenomenon differentiate this from other neurodegenerative conditions.

PROGRESSIVE SUPRANUCLEAR PALSY

A 78-year-old presents with vertical gaze palsy and disinhibition, as well as frequent falls. On **exam**, the patient has dysarthria and bradykinesia. On **imaging**, MRI shows atrophy of the midbrain but spared pons.

Management:

1. MRI to confirm presence of atrophy.
2. May attempt trial of levodopa to differentiate from PD.
3. Botox injection for blepharospasm, dystonia, sialorrhea.
4. PT, OT, and speech therapy.

Complications: Usually fatal within a decade.

HYF: Consider when a patient has vertical gaze palsy and bradykinesia or postural instability.

Dementia With Lewy Bodies (DLB): See p. 741.

26-12 Hyperkinetic Disorders

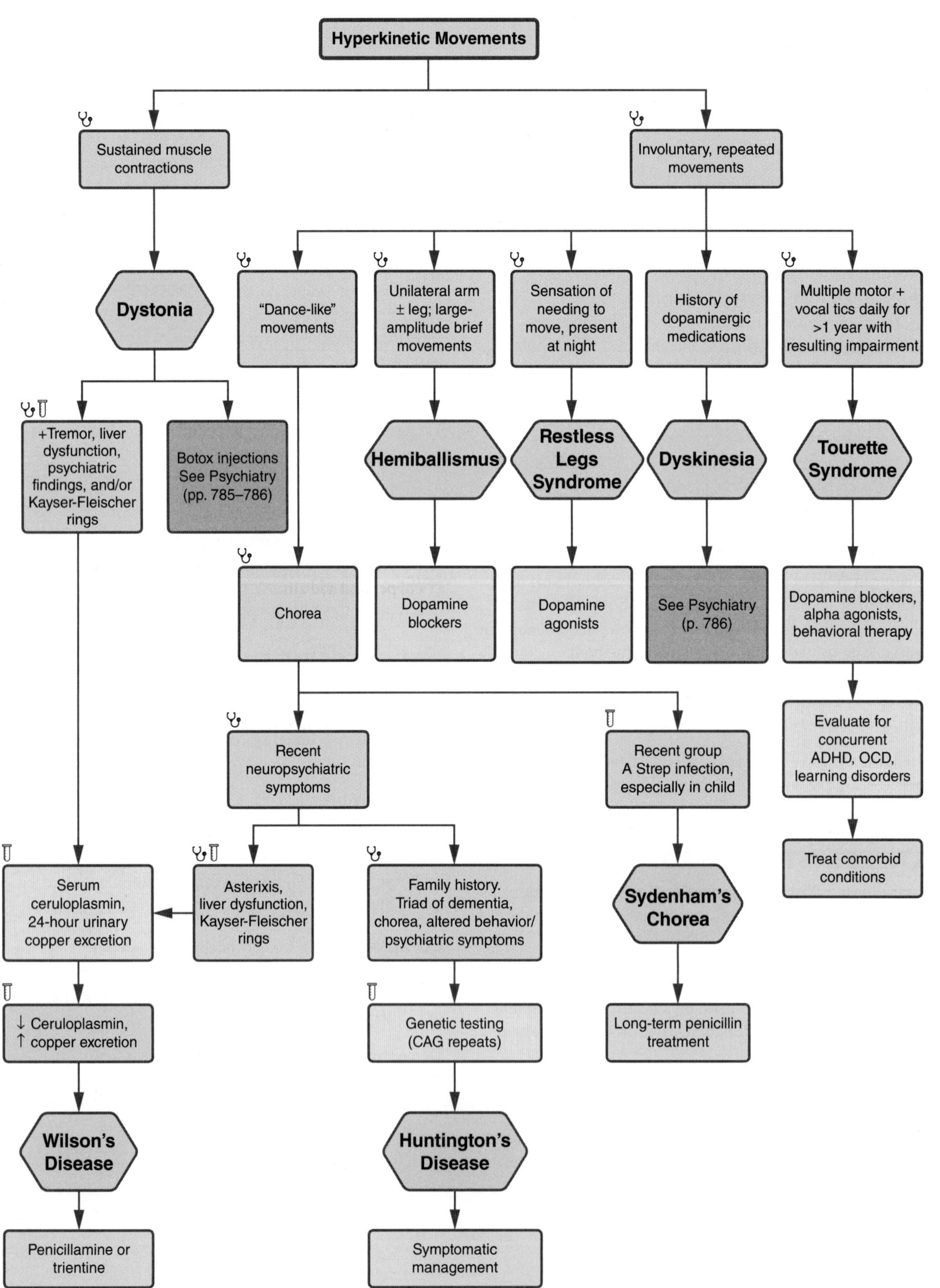
Hyperkinetic Movements
Sustained muscle contractions
Involuntary, repeated movements
Dystonia
+Tremor, liver dysfunction, psychiatric findings, and/or Kayser-Fleischer rings
Botox injections See Psychiatry (pp. 785–786)
"Dance-like" movements
Unilateral arm ± leg; large-amplitude brief movements
Sensation of needing to move, present at night
History of dopaminergic medications
Multiple motor + vocal tics daily for >1 year with resulting impairment
Hemiballismus
Restless Legs Syndrome
Dyskinesia
Tourette Syndrome
Chorea
Dopamine blockers
Dopamine agonists
See Psychiatry (p. 786)
Dopamine blockers, alpha agonists, behavioral therapy
Evaluate for concurrent ADHD, OCD, learning disorders
Treat comorbid conditions
Recent neuropsychiatric symptoms
Recent group A Strep infection, especially in child
Serum ceruloplasmin, 24-hour urinary copper excretion
Asterixis, liver dysfunction, Kayser-Fleischer rings
Family history. Triad of dementia, chorea, altered behavior/ psychiatric symptoms
Sydenham's Chorea
↓ Ceruloplasmin, ↑ copper excretion
Genetic testing (CAG repeats)
Long-term penicillin treatment
Wilson's Disease
Huntington's Disease
Penicillamine or trientine
Symptomatic management

FIGURE 26.12

26-12 Hyperkinetic Disorders

HEMIBALLISMUS

A 57-year-old with PMH of stroke, CAD, and DM2 presents with involuntary flinging movement of the left arm. On **imaging**, MRI shows an ischemic stroke in the right subthalamic nucleus.

Management:

1. CT/MRI to identify responsible lesion. If stroke is suspected, complete stroke workup.
2. Dopamine receptor blocker such as haloperidol or pimozide is 1st-line.
3. If refractory, may require surgical pallidotomy.

Complications: Rare if treated.

HYF: Due to lesion in subthalamic nucleus of basal ganglia (eg, stroke, vasculitis, tumor).

RESTLESS LEGS SYNDROME

A 40-year-old with PMH of CKD and iron deficiency presents with crawling sensation in legs at night, relieved with movement.

Management:

1. Dopamine agonists (pramipexole or ropinirole) and benzodiazepines.
2. Gabapentin if 1st-line treatment insufficient.
3. Treat underlying iron deficiency or kidney disease.

Complications: Insomnia.

HYF: Suspect this diagnosis in a patient with iron deficiency or kidney disease who reports a crawling sensation in their legs at night.

TOURETTE SYNDROME

A 12-year-old with PMH of ADHD and OCD, who is not on any medications, presents with intermittent, daily, brief repetitive movements and repeated grunting ongoing for >1 year, worse with anxiety and better when calm or asleep. Patient also reports sense of tension if not expressed.

Management:

1. Dopamine receptor antagonists, such as haloperidol or pimozide.
2. Some patients benefit from SSRIs and/or behavioral therapy.
3. Treat comorbid psychiatric conditions.

Complications: Generally resolves by the late 20s. However, tics can be embarrassing or impair daily life.

HYF: Diagnosis requires presence of both motor and vocal tics (though can vary in severity of either) several times per day, daily, or intermittently for >1 year prior to age 18 without other causative factor.

SYDENHAM'S CHOREA

A 12-year-old with strep throat infection 2 months prior presents with sudden-onset chorea, hypotonia, mood lability, and decreased verbal output. On **labs**, the patient has +ASO and anti-DNAseB titers. On **imaging**, MRI is normal.

Management:

1. Long-term treatment with penicillin until adulthood to prevent further group A *streptococcal* (GAS) infections and rheumatic heart disease.
2. If required, dopamine receptor blockers to suppress chorea.

Complications: Usually self-resolving within weeks. If not treated, can have long-term sequelae of rheumatic disease.

HYF: Due to molecular mimicry and autoimmune attack on basal ganglia antigens after GAS infection (strep pharyngitis or acute rheumatic fever), especially in children.

WILSON'S DISEASE

An 18-year-old with no notable PMH presents with tremor, jaundice, mood lability, and abnormal discoloration of the eyes. On **exam**, the patient has asterixis. **Labs** show low ceruloplasmin and elevated 24-hour urinary copper excretion.

Management:

1. Check for abnormal LFTs, low ceruloplasmin, and/or high 24-hour urinary copper excretion.
2. Slit-lamp exam to evaluate for Kayser-Fleischer rings (dark gold to green-brown discoloration of peripheral cornea).
3. Penicillamine or trientine for copper chelation. Limit dietary copper and add zinc.

Complications: Can rarely result in severe to fulminant liver failure, especially in young patients.

HYF: Genetic disorder that can cause liver failure in adolescents. Combination of neuropsychiatric symptoms, signs of liver disease, and neurologic findings should raise suspicion for this diagnosis.

HUNTINGTON'S DISEASE (HD)

A 45-year-old M presents with involuntary jerking movements of arms and legs, depressive symptoms, choreiform movements, and new-onset irritability, with family history notable for similar presentation in his father at age 50. On **imaging**, MRI shows atrophy of caudate and putamen.

Management:

1. Genetic testing for CAG repeats. If positive, offer testing for family members.
2. Tetrabenazine or reserpine for chorea. SSRIs or atypical antipsychotics (eg, olanzapine) for mood symptoms.
3. There are currently no treatments that are curative or prevent disease progression.
4. May benefit from psychotherapy, PT/OT, and speech therapy.

Complications:

- Can develop aggression or dementia mistaken for drug intoxication. Suicide is common.
- Anticipation: Phenomenon where disease presents at a younger age and with greater symptoms each generation.

HYF: HD typically presents with insidious onset of psychiatric and cognitive symptoms, with motor symptoms appearing later in the disease course.

26-13 Tremor

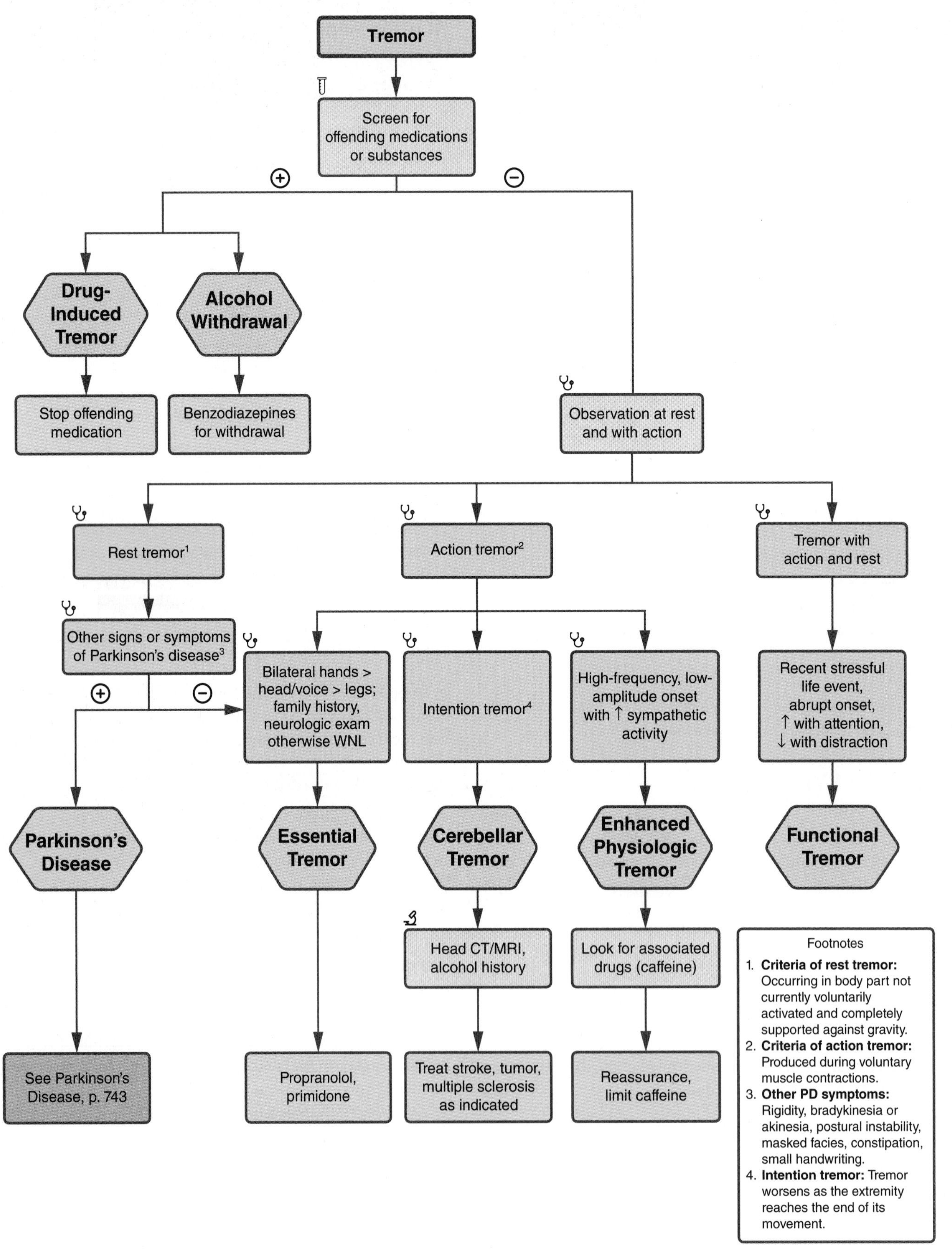
Tremor
Screen for offending medications or substances
⊕
⊖
Drug-Induced Tremor
Alcohol Withdrawal
Stop offending medication
Benzodiazepines for withdrawal
Observation at rest and with action
Rest tremor[1]
Action tremor[2]
Tremor with action and rest
Other signs or symptoms of Parkinson's disease[3]
⊕
⊖
Bilateral hands > head/voice > legs; family history, neurologic exam otherwise WNL
Intention tremor[4]
High-frequency, low-amplitude onset with ↑ sympathetic activity
Recent stressful life event, abrupt onset, ↑ with attention, ↓ with distraction
Parkinson's Disease
Essential Tremor
Cerebellar Tremor
Enhanced Physiologic Tremor
Functional Tremor
Head CT/MRI, alcohol history
Look for associated drugs (caffeine)
See Parkinson's Disease, p. 743
Propranolol, primidone
Treat stroke, tumor, multiple sclerosis as indicated
Reassurance, limit caffeine
Footnotes
1. **Criteria of rest tremor:** Occurring in body part not currently voluntarily activated and completely supported against gravity.
2. **Criteria of action tremor:** Produced during voluntary muscle contractions.
3. **Other PD symptoms:** Rigidity, bradykinesia or akinesia, postural instability, masked facies, constipation, small handwriting.
4. **Intention tremor:** Tremor worsens as the extremity reaches the end of its movement.

FIGURE 26.13

26-13 Tremor

DRUG-INDUCED TREMOR

A 40-year-old who recently started on fluoxetine and atorvastatin presents with new-onset tremor of hands, interfering with daily tasks. **Labs** and **imaging** are unremarkable.

Management:

1. Identify new medications, as many medications are associated with a variety of tremor subtypes (sympathomimetics and psychoactive medications are the most likely culprits).
2. Trial of drug discontinuation for a period.
3. If no culprit medication is identified, investigate for vitamin and electrolyte deficiencies (low Ca, Na, Mg, B_{12}).

HYF: Sympathomimetics and psychoactive substances are most high-yield, but numerous medications are associated with tremor.

ESSENTIAL TREMOR

A 45-year-old M with PMH of HTN presents with chronic shaking or twitching of both his hands that is worse with stress and better with alcohol. There are no other associated symptoms. **Labs** and **imaging** are unremarkable.

Management:

1. Identify other neurologic symptoms, which may suggest other pathology (eg, movement disorder or medication effect).
2. 1st-line: Lifestyle modification (stress management, avoidance of triggers).
3. If severe, can use non-selective β-blocker such as propranolol (especially if comorbid hypertension).
4. Second-line: Primidone.

Complications:

- Not life-threatening but can impair ADLs as it progresses.
- Can present with isolated facial essential tremor, though rare.
- Often runs in families.

HYF: High-frequency action tremor, usually bilateral in nature, worsening with stress and improving with alcohol.

CEREBELLAR TREMOR

A 65-year-old with PMH of HTN and DM2 presents with chronic difficulty doing daily tasks. On **exam**, the patient has difficulty with finger-nose-finger testing due to shaking as finger approaches target. **Labs** and **imaging** are unremarkable.

Management:

1. Evaluate for vascular risk factors: hypertension, diabetes, high cholesterol, alcohol use.
2. Head CT/MRI for stroke/mass/MS. If concern for acute stroke of cerebellum, follow stroke algorithm (p. 730).

HYF: May be described as an intention tremor (ie, the tremor worsens as the extremity reaches the end of its movement). Patients can present with other signs of cerebellar dysfunction (hypotonia, postural tremor). Can also be caused by toxic effects of long-term alcohol use on cerebellum.

PHYSIOLOGIC TREMOR

A 25-year-old with no notable PMH presents with high-frequency, low-amplitude tremor of both hands and rarely the face during periods of stress, without any other neurologic findings. **Labs** and **imaging** are unremarkable.

Management:

1. Identify triggers: Caffeine, anxiety, hyperthyroidism, fatigue.
2. Trigger management and treatment of comorbid conditions that increase sympathetic activity.

HYF: Exacerbated with increased sympathetic activity.

Alcohol Withdrawal Tremor: See Psychiatry section, p. 799.

Parkinson's Disease: See Neurology section, p. 743.

26-14 Gait

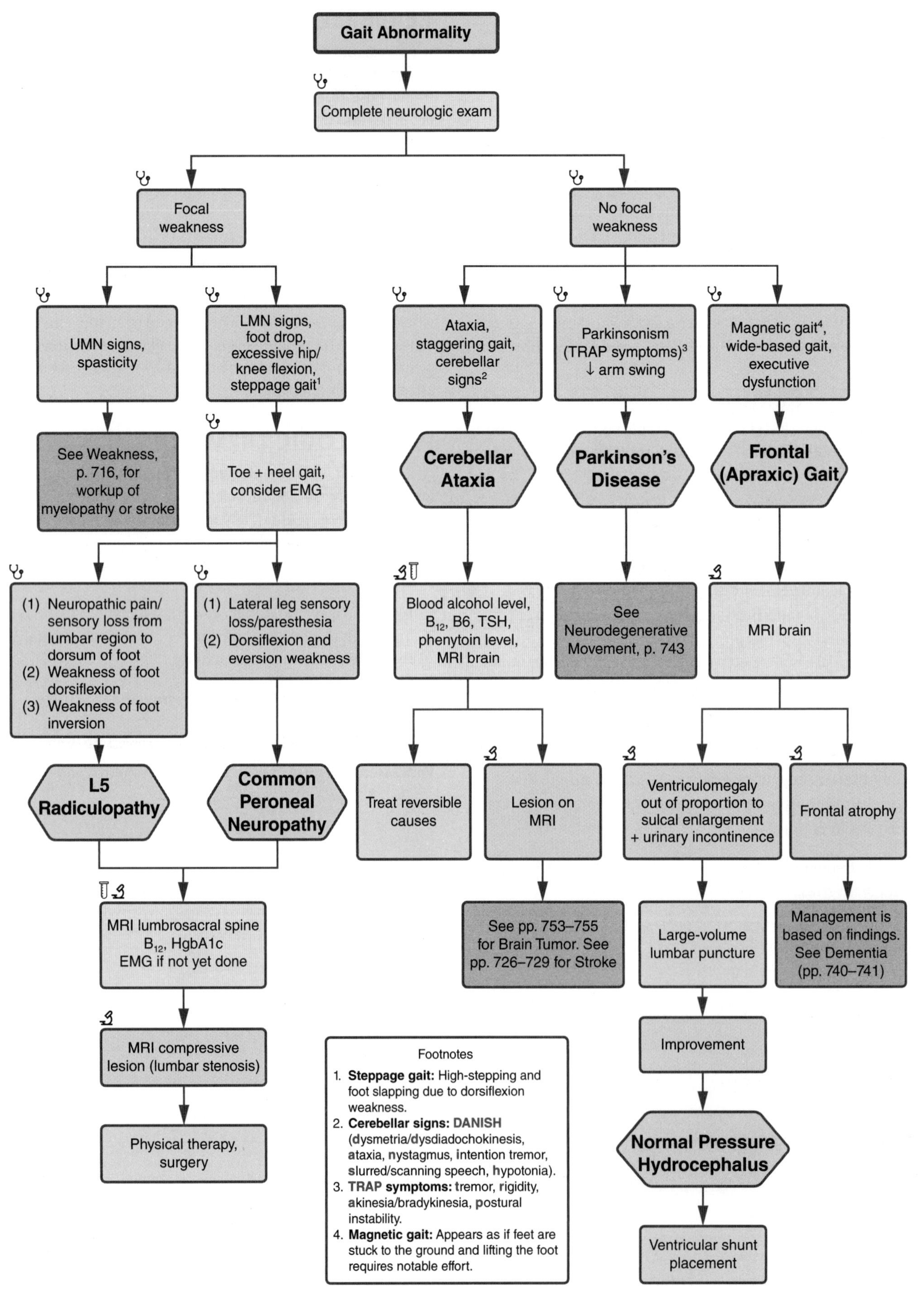
Gait Abnormality
Complete neurologic exam
Focal weakness
No focal weakness
UMN signs, spasticity
LMN signs, foot drop, excessive hip/knee flexion, steppage gait[1]
Ataxia, staggering gait, cerebellar signs[2]
Parkinsonism (TRAP symptoms)[3] ↓ arm swing
Magnetic gait[4], wide-based gait, executive dysfunction
See Weakness, p. 716, for workup of myelopathy or stroke
Toe + heel gait, consider EMG
Cerebellar Ataxia
Parkinson's Disease
Frontal (Apraxic) Gait
(1) Neuropathic pain/sensory loss from lumbar region to dorsum of foot
(2) Weakness of foot dorsiflexion
(3) Weakness of foot inversion
(1) Lateral leg sensory loss/paresthesia
(2) Dorsiflexion and eversion weakness
Blood alcohol level, B_{12}, B6, TSH, phenytoin level, MRI brain
See Neurodegenerative Movement, p. 743
MRI brain
L5 Radiculopathy
Common Peroneal Neuropathy
Treat reversible causes
Lesion on MRI
Ventriculomegaly out of proportion to sulcal enlargement + urinary incontinence
Frontal atrophy
MRI lumbrosacral spine B_{12}, HgbA1c EMG if not yet done
See pp. 753–755 for Brain Tumor. See pp. 726–729 for Stroke
Large-volume lumbar puncture
Management is based on findings. See Dementia (pp. 740–741)
MRI compressive lesion (lumbar stenosis)
Improvement
Physical therapy, surgery
Normal Pressure Hydrocephalus
Ventricular shunt placement
Footnotes
1. Steppage gait: High-stepping and foot slapping due to dorsiflexion weakness.
2. Cerebellar signs: DANISH (dysmetria/dysdiadochokinesis, ataxia, nystagmus, intention tremor, slurred/scanning speech, hypotonia).
3. TRAP symptoms: tremor, rigidity, akinesia/bradykinesia, postural instability.
4. Magnetic gait: Appears as if feet are stuck to the ground and lifting the foot requires notable effort.

FIGURE 26.14

26-14 Gait

CEREBELLAR ATAXIA

A 49-year-old with PMH of CAD, DM2, tobacco use disorder, and alcohol use disorder presents with staggering gait and loss of balance. On **exam**, the patient has an intention tremor. On **imaging**, brain MRI reveals a large unilateral cerebellar lesion.

Management:

1. MRI to identify any vascular/neoplastic lesion that may be present to cause unilateral cerebellar injury.
2. If no vascular lesion found, check for medications (antiepileptics), as well as blood alcohol, B_{12}, B_6, and TSH levels.
3. Treat underlying condition.
4. Physical therapy for ataxia symptoms.

Complications:

- Can progress to immobility if not treated.
- May have emotional and psychological consequences.

HYF: Cerebellar lesions cause ipsilateral symptoms. Can occur following acute febrile illness in age <6 years. Acute-onset cerebellar symptoms require emergent imaging.

NORMAL PRESSURE HYDROCEPHALUS

A 65-year-old F with PMH of hypertension and subarachnoid hemorrhage presents with progressively worsening dementia, incontinence, and difficulty lifting her feet from the floor. On **labs/imaging**, the patient is found to have normal CSF pressure on lumbar puncture (LP). MRI shows ventricular enlargement out of proportion to sulcal atrophy.

Management:

1. Confirmatory testing: improvement in symptoms after high-volume LP, which should show normal CSF pressure.
2. Treatment with LP or lumbar CSF drainage is temporary.
3. Longer-term treatment is ventriculoperitoneal (VP) shunting.

Complications:

- Even with treatment, there may only be minimal improvement in dementia and incontinence.
- If untreated, can progress to death.

HYF: Classic triad of symptoms (dementia, incontinence, gait apraxia) without symptoms of elevated ICP.

L5 RADICULOPATHY

A 45-year-old former construction worker presents with unilateral lateral leg pain radiating down to the foot and difficulty dorsiflexing the same foot. On **exam**, he has a positive straight-leg raise test. On **imaging**, lumbar spine MRI shows a herniated disc.

Management:

1. MRI to identify any disc herniation or nerve root compression.
2. Some utility in spinal x-rays to identify osteoarthritis.
3. EMG if MRI results are negative.
4. Usually self-resolving; use NSAIDs for pain relief and physical therapy.
5. If refractory to above, can consider epidural steroid injections (limited evidence).
6. If refractory to medical therapy, may require surgical intervention to relieve a herniated disc or source of compression.

Complications: Muscle atrophy from nerve damage, chronic pain, physical deconditioning.

HYF: Conservative treatment is usually sufficient for recovery.

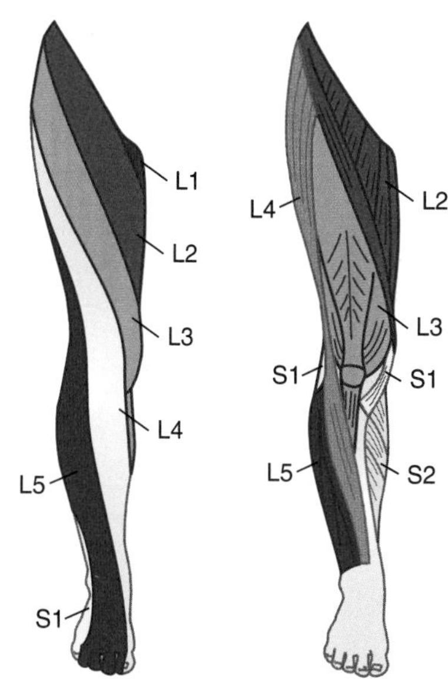
L1
L2
L3
L4
L5
S1
L4
L2
L3
S1
S1
L5
S2

Dermatomes (left) and myotomes (right) corresponding to lumbosacral roots.

COMMON PERONEAL/FIBULAR NEUROPATHY

A 65-year-old with PMH of recent knee injury presents with unilateral isolated ankle dorsiflexion, toe extension weakness, and lateral sensory loss. On **exam**, the patient is found to have a decreased Achilles reflex.

Management:

1. EMG to localize neuropathy.
2. Can treat pain with NSAIDs and disability with physical therapy and moderate exercise.

Complications: Peripheral nerve injury can result in muscle atrophy.

HYF: The pattern of weakness and sensory loss helps differentiate this diagnosis from L5 radiculopathy (foot inversion weakness is present in L5 radiculopathy but not peroneal neuropathy).

Parkinson's Disease: See p. 743.

26-15 Secondary Headache

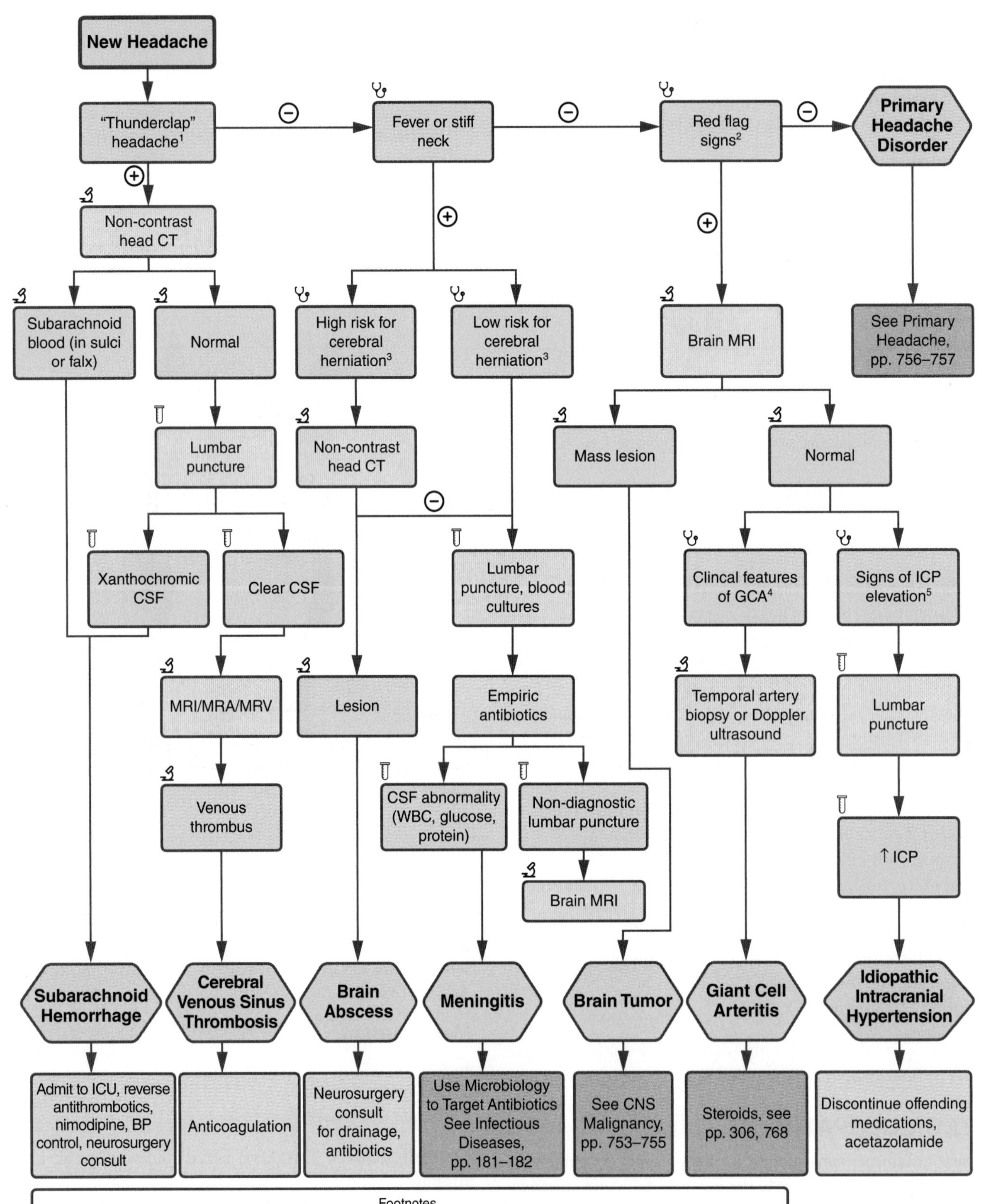
New Headache
"Thunderclap" headache[1]
Fever or stiff neck
Red flag signs[2]
Primary Headache Disorder
Non-contrast head CT
Subarachnoid blood (in sulci or falx)
Normal
High risk for cerebral herniation[3]
Low risk for cerebral herniation[3]
Brain MRI
See Primary Headache, pp. 756–757
Lumbar puncture
Non-contrast head CT
Mass lesion
Normal
Xanthochromic CSF
Clear CSF
Lumbar puncture, blood cultures
Clincal features of GCA[4]
Signs of ICP elevation[5]
MRI/MRA/MRV
Lesion
Empiric antibiotics
Temporal artery biopsy or Doppler ultrasound
Lumbar puncture
Venous thrombus
CSF abnormality (WBC, glucose, protein)
Non-diagnostic lumbar puncture
↑ ICP
Brain MRI
Subarachnoid Hemorrhage
Cerebral Venous Sinus Thrombosis
Brain Abscess
Meningitis
Brain Tumor
Giant Cell Arteritis
Idiopathic Intracranial Hypertension
Admit to ICU, reverse antithrombotics, nimodipine, BP control, neurosurgery consult
Anticoagulation
Neurosurgery consult for drainage, antibiotics
Use Microbiology to Target Antibiotics See Infectious Diseases, pp. 181–182
See CNS Malignancy, pp. 753–755
Steroids, see pp. 306, 768
Discontinue offending medications, acetazolamide

Footnotes

1. **Thunderclap:** Maximal intensity at onset, worst headache of life.
2. **Red Flag signs:** Seizures, focal exam, papilledema, morning headache, headache w/ Valsalva.
3. **Risk for Cerebral Herniation:** Active CNS disease (stroke, mass lesion), immunocompromised, new seizure, papilledema, ↓ consciousness, focal neurologic deficit.
4. **Features of GCA:** New headache, age >50, jaw claudication, abrupt vision loss, known polymyalgia rheumatica, ESR/CRP.
5. **Signs of ↑ Intracranial Pressure (ICP):** Papilledema, nausea, postural headache.

FIGURE 26.15

26-15 Secondary Headache

SUBARACHNOID HEMORRHAGE

A 50-year-old with PMH of smoking and HTN presents with "thunderclap headache" (sudden-onset, worst headache of life). On **exam**, the patient has HTN, neck stiffness, and neurologic deficits (sometimes present based on location of bleed), and **labs/imaging** show xanthochromic CSF and evidence of bleed on CT.

Management:

1. Prevent rebleeding: BP control (SBP <160, use IV agents), reverse antithrombotics.
2. Angiography (traditional or CT) to determine source of bleed.
3. Aneurysm repair (clipping or coiling).
4. Nimodipine calcium channel blocker to prevent vasospasm.

Complications:

- Increased ICP and hydrocephalus: first hours, treat with hyperventilation, raise head of bed, CSF drainage.
- Rebleeding: first 24 hours, worsening neurologic status.
- Vasospasm: can cause ischemia (signs of stroke) 4–10 days after SAH, prevented with nimodipine.
- Hyponatremia (SIADH or cerebral salt wasting), see pp. 206–210.
- Seizure: most often focal, see pp. 761–762.

HYF: Occurs due to ruptured saccular (berry) aneurysms, arteriovenous malformation (AVM), or trauma.

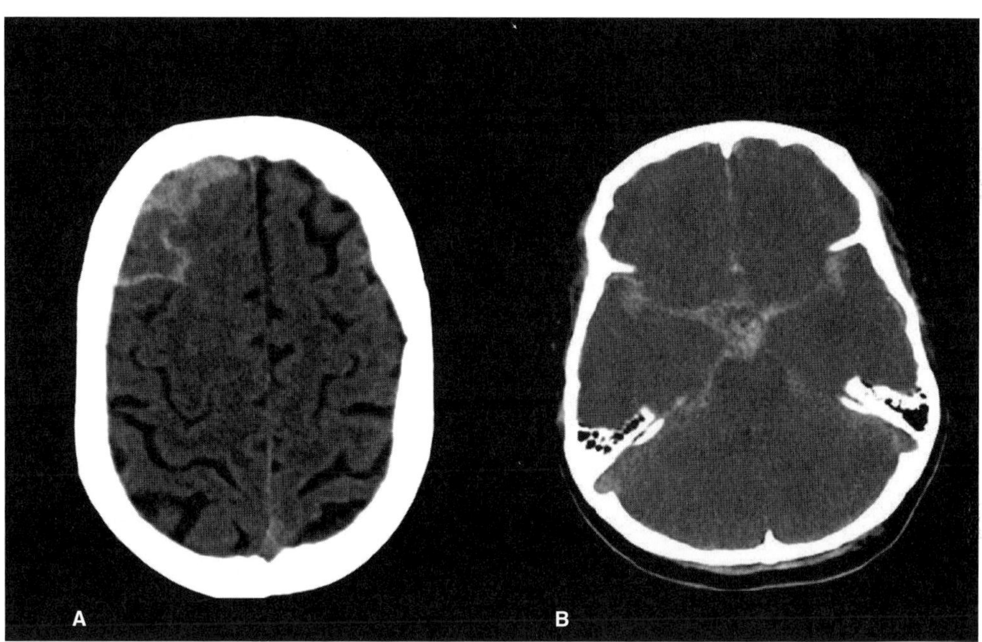
A
B

Examples of subarachnoid hemorrhage: right frontal lobe (A) and circle of Willis (B).

CEREBRAL VENOUS SINUS THROMBOSIS

A 40-year-old F with PMH of prothrombotic risk (eg, antiphosholipid syndrome) presents with headache (gradual or thunderclap). On **exam**, she has evidence of intracranial pressure (papilledema). **Labs/imaging** show "dense triangle sign," "empty triangle sign," or "cord sign" on head CT, confirmed on MR venography.

Management:

1. Anticoagulation: Heparin.
2. If patient was previously already on anticoagulation and failed, consider endovascular treatment.

Complications:

- Elevated ICP, herniation.
- Venous infarction.
- Intraparenchymal hemorrhage.
- Seizures.

HYF: Blood clot in the venous sinuses, part of the brain's blood drainage system. Symptoms can include headache, seizure, nausea, visual changes, or even coma. Anticoagulation with heparin is crucial. Depending on the patient's clinical course, treatment may also include measures to reduce intracranial pressure and antiepileptics to prevent or treat seizures. Potentially fatal. Consider this diagnosis in patients who are hypercoagulable.

BRAIN ABSCESS

A 40-year-old with PMH of endocarditis presents with headache and fever. On **exam**, the patient has focal neurologic findings. **Labs/imaging** show multiple ring-enhancing brain lesions and positive blood cultures.

Management:

1. Antibiotics, surgical drainage.
2. Glucocorticoids if significant mass effect.

(Continued)

26-15 Secondary Headache

HYF: Lumbar puncture is contraindicated in focal lesions such as abscesses.

MENINGITIS

A 20-year-old presents with fever and headache. On **exam**, the patient has neck stiffness and altered mental status. **Labs/imaging** show CSF WBCs >1000, glucose <40, protein >200, and + Gram stain.
Note: presentation differs by microbiology; see Medicine section (pp. 181–182).

Management:

1. Lumbar puncture before broad-spectrum antibiotics (ceftriaxone, vancomycin, acyclovir ± ampicillin).
2. Dexamethasone (empirically, for *Streptococcus pneumoniae*).
3. ICP management.
4. Pathogen-guided antibiotics (see pp. 181–182).

Complications:

- Impaired mental status, intellectual ability.
- Sensorineural hearing loss.
- Seizures, focal neurologic deficits.

HYF: While it is important to obtain CSF for culture before starting antibiotics, delays in obtaining LP should never delay antibiotics, given high mortality.

IDIOPATHIC INTRACRANIAL HYPERTENSION (PSEUDOTUMOR CEREBRII)

A 30-year-old F with PMH of obesity and acne treated with doxycycline presents with headache and vision changes. On **exam**, she has papilledema. On **labs/imaging**, head CT is normal, and LP shows elevated ICP but normal CSF studies.

Management:

1. Weight loss, discontinue associated medications (eg, tetracyclines).
2. Acetazolamide, topiramate.
3. If rapidly progressing vision loss: glucocorticoids, serial LPs.
4. Surgery: Optic nerve sheath fenestration, CSF shunt.

Complications: Vision loss.

HYF: Associated with many medications, but most important is retinoids (vitamin A excess). Pathogenesis poorly understood.

Brain Tumor: See Neurology section, pp. 753–755.

Giant Cell/Temporal Arteritis: See Neurology section, p. 769.

Primary Headache Disorders: See Migraine, Tension Headache, Cluster Headache section, p. 757.

26-16 Brain Tumors

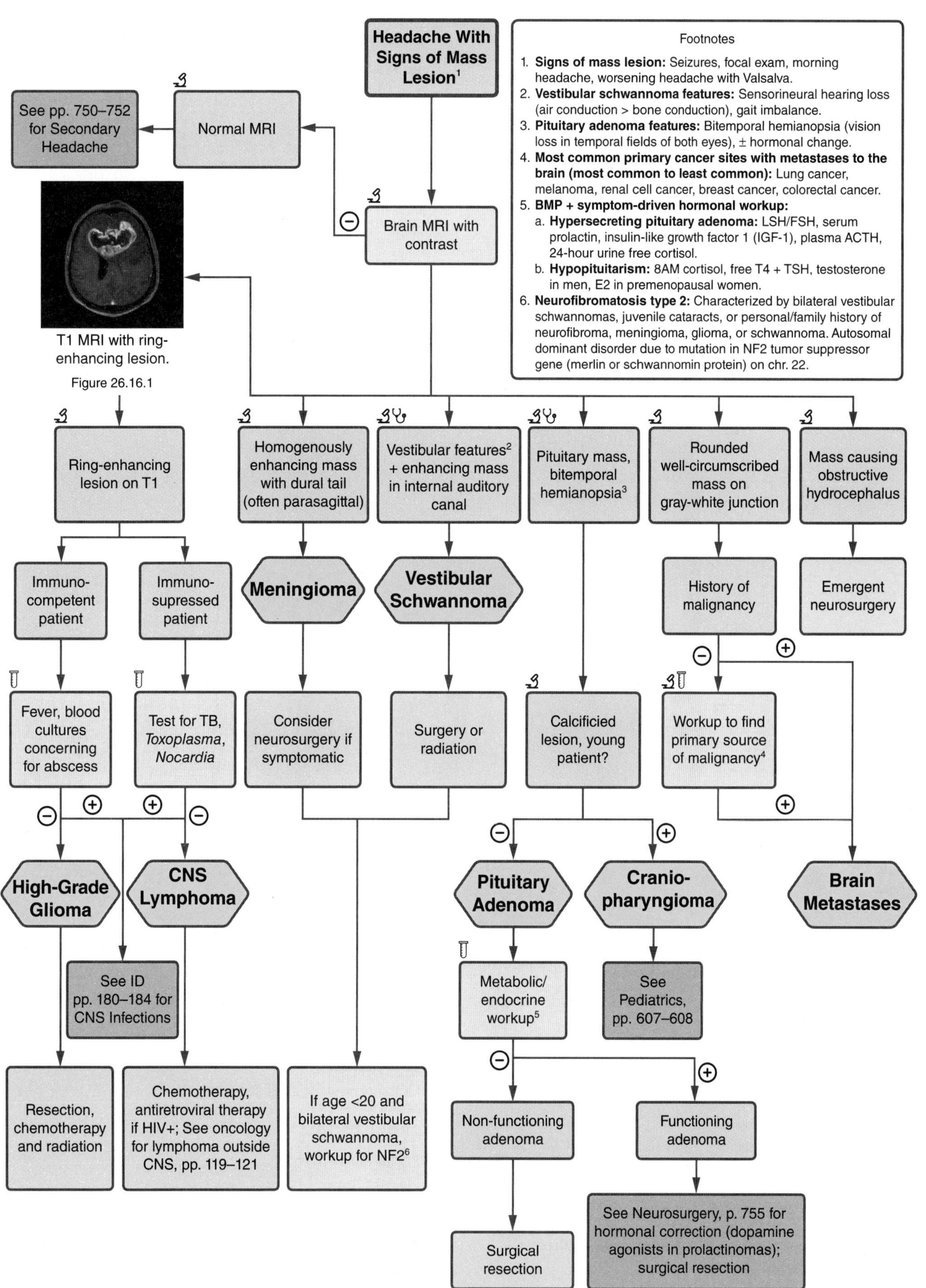
Headache With Signs of Mass Lesion[1]
Brain MRI with contrast
Normal MRI
See pp. 750–752 for Secondary Headache
T1 MRI with ring-enhancing lesion.
Figure 26.16.1
Ring-enhancing lesion on T1
Immuno-competent patient
Immuno-supressed patient
Fever, blood cultures concerning for abscess
Test for TB, *Toxoplasma*, *Nocardia*
High-Grade Glioma
CNS Lymphoma
See ID pp. 180–184 for CNS Infections
Resection, chemotherapy and radiation
Chemotherapy, antiretroviral therapy if HIV+; See oncology for lymphoma outside CNS, pp. 119–121
Homogenously enhancing mass with dural tail (often parasagittal)
Meningioma
Consider neurosurgery if symptomatic
Vestibular features[2] + enhancing mass in internal auditory canal
Vestibular Schwannoma
Surgery or radiation
If age <20 and bilateral vestibular schwannoma, workup for NF2[6]
Pituitary mass, bitemporal hemianopsia[3]
Calcificied lesion, young patient?
Pituitary Adenoma
Cranio-pharyngioma
Metabolic/ endocrine workup[5]
See Pediatrics, pp. 607–608
Non-functioning adenoma
Functioning adenoma
Surgical resection
See Neurosurgery, p. 755 for hormonal correction (dopamine agonists in prolactinomas); surgical resection
Rounded well-circumscribed mass on gray-white junction
History of malignancy
Workup to find primary source of malignancy[4]
Brain Metastases
Mass causing obstructive hydrocephalus
Emergent neurosurgery
Footnotes
1. **Signs of mass lesion:** Seizures, focal exam, morning headache, worsening headache with Valsalva.
2. **Vestibular schwannoma features:** Sensorineural hearing loss (air conduction > bone conduction), gait imbalance.
3. **Pituitary adenoma features:** Bitemporal hemianopsia (vision loss in temporal fields of both eyes), ± hormonal change.
4. **Most common primary cancer sites with metastases to the brain (most common to least common):** Lung cancer, melanoma, renal cell cancer, breast cancer, colorectal cancer.
5. **BMP + symptom-driven hormonal workup:**
a. **Hypersecreting pituitary adenoma:** LSH/FSH, serum prolactin, insulin-like growth factor 1 (IGF-1), plasma ACTH, 24-hour urine free cortisol.
b. **Hypopituitarism:** 8AM cortisol, free T4 + TSH, testosterone in men, E2 in premenopausal women.
6. **Neurofibromatosis type 2:** Characterized by bilateral vestibular schwannomas, juvenile cataracts, or personal/family history of neurofibroma, meningioma, glioma, or schwannoma. Autosomal dominant disorder due to mutation in NF2 tumor suppressor gene (merlin or schwannomin protein) on chr. 22.

FIGURE 26.16

26-16 Brain Tumors

MENINGIOMA

A 65-year-old F with PMH of HTN presents with headache over the past 5 months and 2 falls over the last month. On **exam**, she has LLE > RLE weakness without any other associated neurological symptoms and no signs of papilledema. On **imaging**, non-contrast head CT shows a parasagittal mass with no signs of intracranial bleeding.

Management:

1. Obtain MRI with and without contrast to characterize mass in relation to brain anatomy.
2. Since this meningioma is symptomatic, the next step is surgical resection (surveillance through serial MRIs may be indicated for small asymptomatic meningioma).

Complications: Incomplete resection of benign meningioma can increase risk of recurrence and progression of tumor grade.

HYF: Meningiomas seen in patients age <30 with associated cataracts or vestibular schwannoma are likely due to NF2. Dural tail is often seen on imaging.

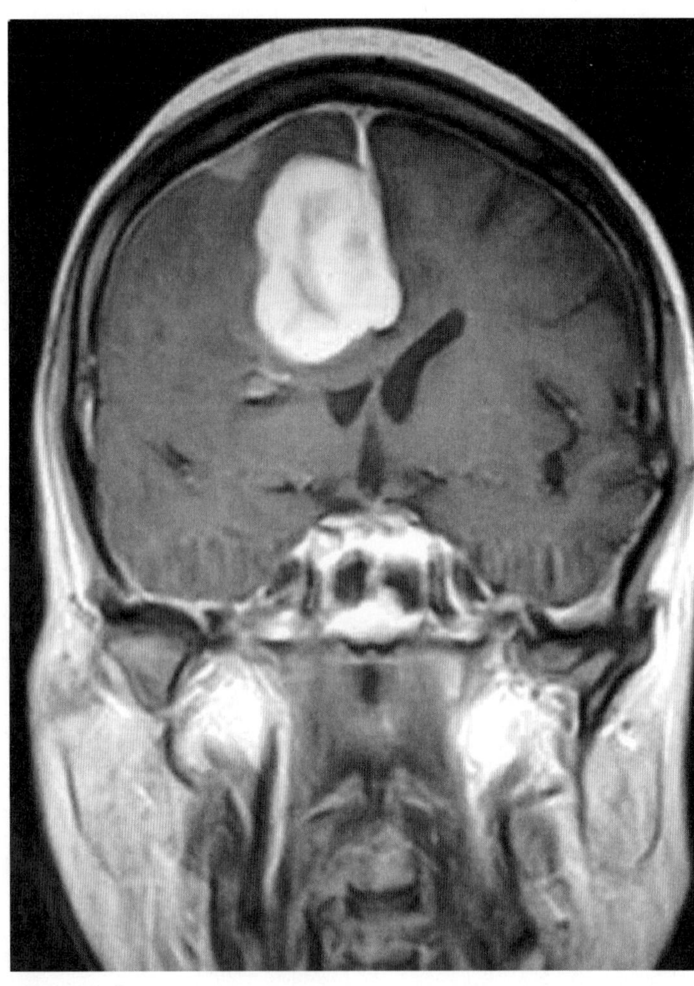

Falcine meningioma with moderate edema and mass effect on the right lateral ventricle.

VESTIBULAR SCHWANNOMA

A 27-year-old M with PMH of multiple asymptomatic meningiomas and no PSH presents with nausea, vomiting, and dizziness. On **exam**, he has right-sided air conduction (AC) > bone conduction (BC) hearing loss. On **imaging**, there is a T2-enhancing mass on CN VIII on the right side.

Management:

1. Obtain MRI of the craniospinal axis to exclude further intracranial or spinal tumors.
2. Audiology, ophthalmologic evaluation, and cutaneous examination.
3. Workup to identify constitutional or mosaic pathogenic *NF2* gene mutation.
4. Consult neurological surgery.

Complications:

- Facial nerve palsy.
- Hearing loss.
- Brain stem compression.

HYF: Bilateral vestibular schwannoma is a characteristic finding in patients with NF2. Cutaneous schwannomas can also be found.

26-16 Brain Tumors

PITUITARY ADENOMA

A 30-year-old F with PMH of irregular menstrual cycles presents with 6-month history of amenorrhea and diffuse headaches. On **exam**, there are no significant findings. **Labs** show serum prolactin level of 180 ng/mL.

Management:

1. See pp. 488–490 for pituitary adenoma workup.
2. 1st-line treatment of prolactinoma is dopamine agonist (cabergoline).
3. Consider surgical resection.

Complications:

- Progression of a microadenoma (<10 mm) to a macroadenoma (≥10 mm) is very uncommon (~2.4%).
- Progression to macroadenoma can lead to compression of the optic chiasm and cause bitemporal hemianopsia and hypopituitarism.

HYF: Pituitary adenomas are common in MEN1 syndrome.

HIGH-GRADE GLIOMA

A 70-year-old M with PMH of osteoarthritis presents with 1-month history of headaches. On **exam**, he has R-sided weakness. On **imaging**, T1 post-contrast MRI shows a ring-enhancing lesion in the left frontal lobe.

Management:

1. Consult neurosurgery for resection/biopsy.
2. Consider steroids.
3. Management of glioblastoma consists of a combination of surgical resection, temozolomide, and radiation therapy.

Complications: Glioblastoma inevitably recurs after treatment and has a high mortality rate.

HYF: Glioblastoma is characterized pathologically as necrotic foci surrounded by "pseudopalisading" cells; it is highly invasive and can involve both hemispheres ("butterfly glioma").

BRAIN METASTASES

A 66-year-old M with PMH of renal-cell carcinoma and 5 months of headaches presents with new-onset generalized tonic-clonic seizure lasting 30 seconds. On **exam**, he has aphasia. On **imaging**, MRI shows multiple hyperintense masses in the temporal lobe.

Management:

1. See pp. 761–762 for new seizure management.
2. MRI of the spine must be obtained as well to evaluate for metastatic disease in the spinal cord.
3. In this patient, RCC metastasis to the brain is highly likely. Treatment involves a combination of surgery, radiation therapy, and systemic chemotherapy.

Complications:

- Intracranial bleeds from aberrant tumor vasculature.
- Recurrent seizures.
- Mass effect.

HYF: Lung, melanoma, renal-cell carcinoma, breast, and colorectal cancer are, respectively, the most common primary sites of malignancy that metastasize to the brain.

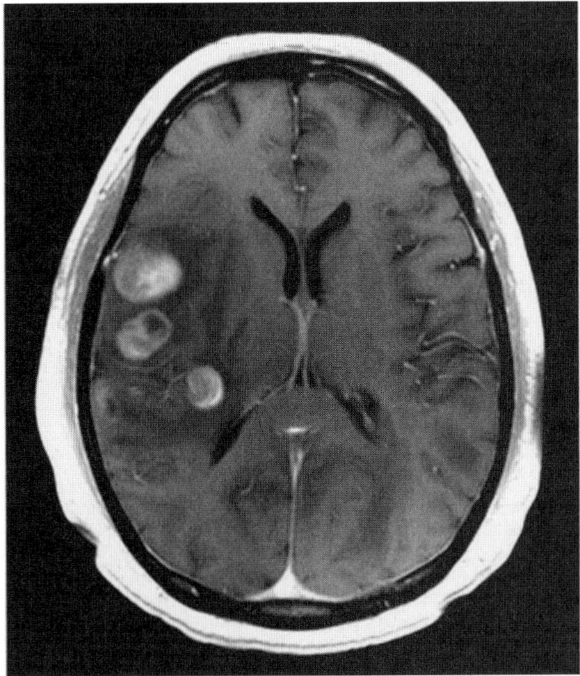
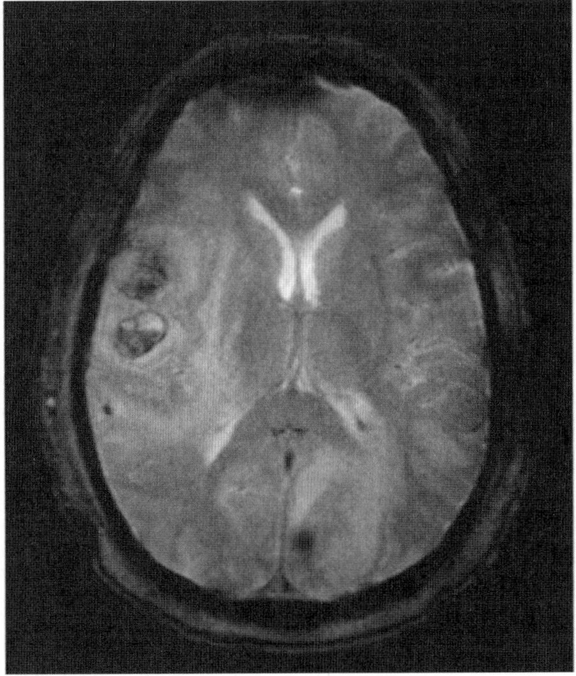

Multiple enhancing lesions at the gray white junction concerning for brain metastases with surrounding edema (left). Hypointesity on GRE sequence corresponds to blood products (right).

26-17 Primary Headache Disorders

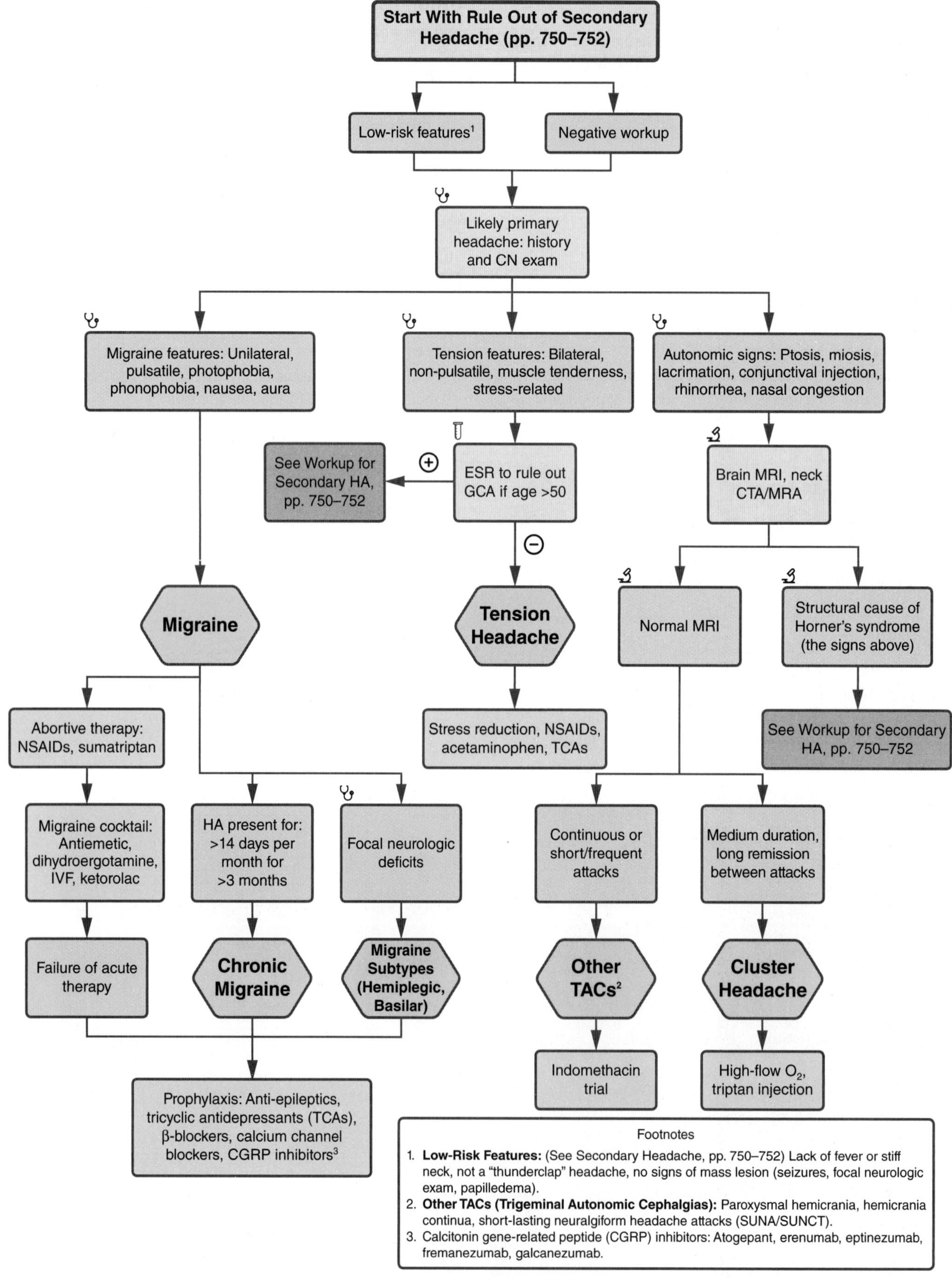
Start With Rule Out of Secondary Headache (pp. 750–752)
Low-risk features[1]
Negative workup
Likely primary headache: history and CN exam
Migraine features: Unilateral, pulsatile, photophobia, phonophobia, nausea, aura
Tension features: Bilateral, non-pulsatile, muscle tenderness, stress-related
Autonomic signs: Ptosis, miosis, lacrimation, conjunctival injection, rhinorrhea, nasal congestion
See Workup for Secondary HA, pp. 750–752
⊕
ESR to rule out GCA if age >50
⊖
Brain MRI, neck CTA/MRA
Migraine
Tension Headache
Normal MRI
Structural cause of Horner's syndrome (the signs above)
Abortive therapy: NSAIDs, sumatriptan
Stress reduction, NSAIDs, acetaminophen, TCAs
See Workup for Secondary HA, pp. 750–752
Migraine cocktail: Antiemetic, dihydroergotamine, IVF, ketorolac
HA present for: >14 days per month for >3 months
Focal neurologic deficits
Continuous or short/frequent attacks
Medium duration, long remission between attacks
Failure of acute therapy
Chronic Migraine
Migraine Subtypes (Hemiplegic, Basilar)
Other TACs[2]
Cluster Headache
Indomethacin trial
High-flow O_2, triptan injection
Prophylaxis: Anti-epileptics, tricyclic antidepressants (TCAs), β-blockers, calcium channel blockers, CGRP inhibitors[3]

Footnotes

1. **Low-Risk Features:** (See Secondary Headache, pp. 750–752) Lack of fever or stiff neck, not a "thunderclap" headache, no signs of mass lesion (seizures, focal neurologic exam, papilledema).
2. **Other TACs (Trigeminal Autonomic Cephalgias):** Paroxysmal hemicrania, hemicrania continua, short-lasting neuralgiform headache attacks (SUNA/SUNCT).
3. Calcitonin gene-related peptide (CGRP) inhibitors: Atogepant, erenumab, eptinezumab, fremanezumab, galcanezumab.

FIGURE 26.17

26-17 Primary Headache Disorders

MIGRAINE

A 35-year-old F with family history of migraine presents with unilateral throbbing headache lasting hours, associated with nausea, vomiting, and aura (visual/sensory/auditory/other). On **exam**, she has photophobia and phonophobia without neurologic deficit, and **labs/imaging** are negative.

Management:

1. Avoid triggers.
2. Abortive therapy (at home): NSAIDs, triptans.
3. Migraine cocktail (at hospital): Varies but often antiemetic, IV fluids, magnesium, ketorolac.
4. Prophylaxis indicated if failed acute therapy, disabling, >4 per month, >12-hour headaches: Anticonvulsants (topiramate, valproate), antidepressants (amitriptyline, venlafaxine), β-blockers, CGRP antagonists.

Complications:

- Status migrainosus (headache >72 hour).
- Migrainous infarction (rare).

HYF: Common triggers: Foods, fasting, stress, weather, menses/OCPs, sleep disruption. Multitude of subtypes and different presentations; the clinical scenario above describes migraine with aura. Most common visual aura is scintillating scotoma (flashing lights) or visual field cut. Other subtypes are below (lower yield).

Chronic Migraine: ≥5 per month for >3 months.

Hemiplegic Migraine: Aura includes weakness.

Basilar Migraine: Aura includes combination of vertigo, dysarthria, tinnitus, diplopia, and ataxia.

Vestibular Migraine: Episodic vertigo in patient with migraines. Must rule out other causes (see Vertigo, pp. 759–760).

TENSION HEADACHE

A 50-year-old M with PMH of anxiety presents with bilateral non-throbbing, band-like headache. On **exam**, he has pericranial muscle tenderness, and **labs/imaging** are normal.

Management:

1. Non-pharmacologic therapy: Stress reduction, avoid triggers.
2. NSAIDs > acetaminophen.
3. TCAs.

Complications: Medication overuse headaches often occur in patients with migraine or tension headache taking excessive abortive medications (especially combination medicines or opioids). Stop offending medications and try preventative therapy.

HYF: Overlaps with migraines, but distinguish through bilaterality, non-throbbing quality, and lack of migraine features (eg, aura, nausea, photophobia).

TRIGEMINAL AUTONOMIC CEPHALGIAS

A 35-year-old F with no PMH presents with unilateral periorbital headache that is either continuous or with very brief (seconds–minutes) attacks. On **exam**, she has lacrimation and Horner's syndrome, and **labs/imaging** are unremarkable.

Management:

1. Paroxysmal hemicrania or hemicrania continua: indomethacin (response is diagnostic).

HYF: If it sounds like a cluster headache but doesn't occur in a "cluster," think of one of the other trigeminal autonomic cephalgias (TACs). Subtypes: Paroxysmal hemicrania, hemicrania continua, short-lasting neuralgiform headache attacks (SUNA/SUNCT).

CLUSTER HEADACHE

A 25-year-old M with PMH of smoking presents with severe periorbital unilateral headache lasting 0.5–3 hours, recurring in a "cluster." On **exam**, the patient has lacrimation, conjunctival injection, nasal congestion, and Horner's syndrome (ptosis/miosis). He has unremarkable **imaging**.

Management:

1. High-flow O_2.
2. Subcutaneous sumatriptan injection.
3. Prophylaxis: Verapamil.

HYF: Cluster headache is the most common (and the most commonly tested) TAC; others are described above.

26-18 Dizziness

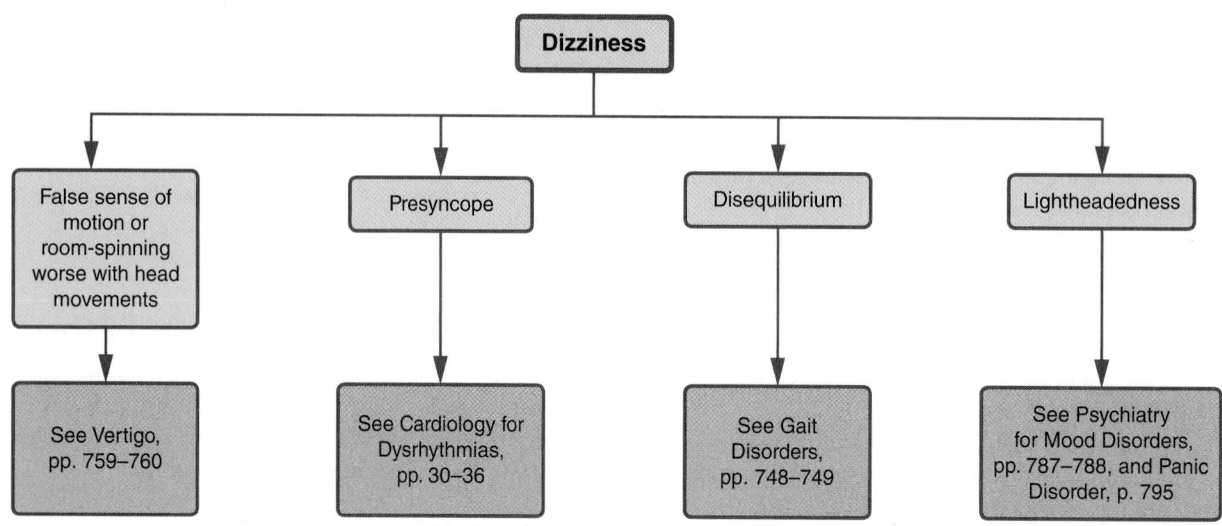
Dizziness
False sense of motion or room-spinning worse with head movements
Presyncope
Disequilibrium
Lightheadedness
See Vertigo, pp. 759–760
See Cardiology for Dysrhythmias, pp. 30–36
See Gait Disorders, pp. 748–749
See Psychiatry for Mood Disorders, pp. 787–788, and Panic Disorder, p. 795

Dizziness is a very common chief complaint with a broad differential. Therefore, the general approach hinges on clarifying exactly what the patient means by "dizziness," as this clues you in to different etiologic clusters. Vertigo is often first considered with complaints of dizziness and will be described as room-spinning or a false sense of motion that is often exacerbated with head movement or changes in position. Within vertigo, it will be important to clarify between peripheral (most common) and central (possibly life-threatening); additionally, attention to the time course will help parse out the various conditions in this bucket. If patients describe a sense of almost "blacking out," this speaks to presyncope that warrants a cardiologic workup. In the question stem, look for cardiac history and/or associated complaints of chest pain, palpitations, pallor, or diaphoresis. Some patients might describe a loss of balance, especially when walking, which evokes gait disorders (eg, Parkinson's Disease) or cerebellar dysfunction, which will often occur in older patients. Finally, non-specific complaints of "lightheadedness" could be associated with psychiatric conditions, especially anxiety or panic disorder (hyperventilation-induced).

FIGURE 26.18

26-19 Vertigo

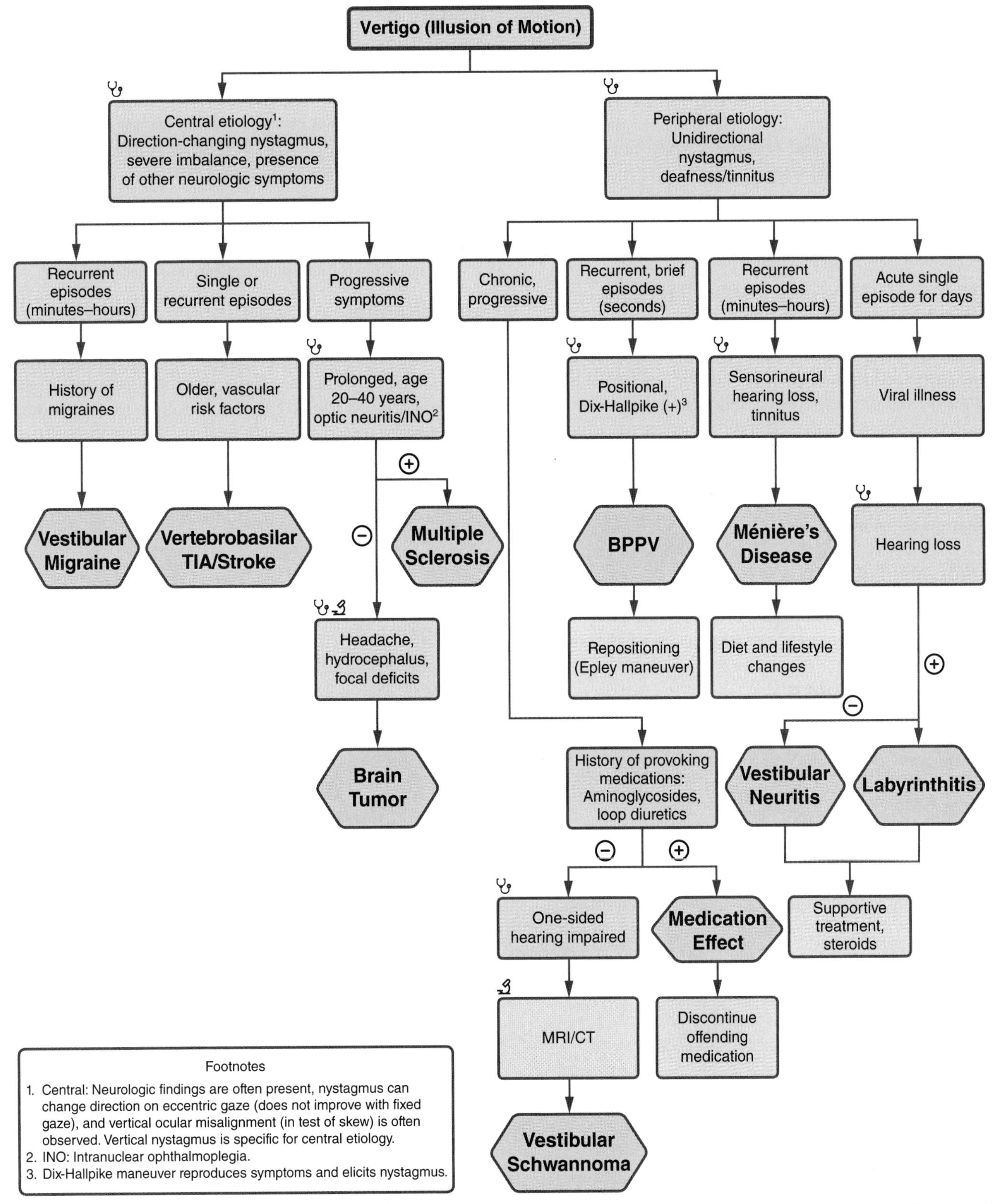
Vertigo (Illusion of Motion)
Central etiology[1]: Direction-changing nystagmus, severe imbalance, presence of other neurologic symptoms
Peripheral etiology: Unidirectional nystagmus, deafness/tinnitus
Recurrent episodes (minutes–hours)
Single or recurrent episodes
Progressive symptoms
Chronic, progressive
Recurrent, brief episodes (seconds)
Recurrent episodes (minutes–hours)
Acute single episode for days
History of migraines
Older, vascular risk factors
Prolonged, age 20–40 years, optic neuritis/INO[2]
Positional, Dix-Hallpike (+)[3]
Sensorineural hearing loss, tinnitus
Viral illness
Vestibular Migraine
Vertebrobasilar TIA/Stroke
Multiple Sclerosis
BPPV
Ménière's Disease
Hearing loss
Headache, hydrocephalus, focal deficits
Repositioning (Epley maneuver)
Diet and lifestyle changes
Brain Tumor
History of provoking medications: Aminoglycosides, loop diuretics
Vestibular Neuritis
Labyrinthitis
One-sided hearing impaired
Medication Effect
Supportive treatment, steroids
MRI/CT
Discontinue offending medication
Vestibular Schwannoma
Footnotes
1. Central: Neurologic findings are often present, nystagmus can change direction on eccentric gaze (does not improve with fixed gaze), and vertical ocular misalignment (in test of skew) is often observed. Vertical nystagmus is specific for central etiology.
2. INO: Intranuclear ophthalmoplegia.
3. Dix-Hallpike maneuver reproduces symptoms and elicits nystagmus.

FIGURE 26.19

26-19 Vertigo

VERTEBROBASILAR TIA/STROKE (INSUFFICIENCY)

A 72-year-old with PMH of HTN, CAD, MI, and DM2 presents with acute-onset diplopia, dizziness, and loss of balance that began 6 hours ago. On **exam**, BP is 160/90 in both arms, and the patient has a carotid bruit and nystagmus. Vessel **imaging** shows atherosclerosis of a vertebral artery.

Management:

1. See pp. 730–732 in Neurology section for Stroke Management.

BENIGN PAROXYSMAL POSITIONAL VERTIGO (BPPV)

A 50-year-old F with no PMH presents with sudden-onset spinning sensation and loss of equilibrium lasting 1 minute numerous times a day ×1 month whenever she rolls over in bed or turns her head to the left. On **exam**, Dix-Hallpike maneuver reproduces the symptoms.

Management:

1. Maneuvers to reposition otolith (eg, Epley).

HYF: BPPV occurs when an otolith becomes dislodged from the utricle and enters semicircular canals during changes in head position, resulting in sudden-onset, brief episodes of symptoms (vertigo, nausea, vomiting, visual disturbance due to nystagmus).

MÉNIÈRE'S DISEASE

A 28-year-old F with no PMH presents with episodes of severe room-spinning dizziness lasting minutes to hours, associated with nausea, ringing of the ears, and decreased hearing in the left ear.

Management:

1. Diet (reduced salt, caffeine) and lifestyle changes (less alcohol).
2. Vestibular rehabilitation, symptom management (meclizine).
3. Diuretics (hydrochlorothiazide, acetazolamide) if refractory.

HYF: Classic triad of episodic vertigo, tinnitus, and sensorineural hearing loss due to pressure from accumulation of endolymph in the inner ear.

MEDICATION EFFECT

A 78-year-old M with recent PMH of pneumonia s/p prolonged treatment with ceftriaxone and gentamicin presents with 1-month history of room-spinning dizziness, tinnitus, deafness, and difficulty with balance. On **exam**, he has severe loss of hearing bilaterally, broad-based gait, and normal Weber and Rinne tests.

Management:

1. Stop offending medication (although changes are typically irreversible).
2. Vestibular rehabilitation, symptom management.

Complications: Permanent hearing loss, vertigo, ataxia.

HYF: Aminoglycosides accumulate in the inner ear and cause cochlear ototoxicity and vestibulotoxicity (in up to 10% of patients) that can occur even after 1 dose. Loop diuretics (eg, furosemide) can also cause ototoxicity.

VESTIBULAR NEURITIS/LABYRINTHITIS

A 24-year-old M with PMH of resolving upper respiratory infection that began 5 days ago presents with room-spinning dizziness and gait instability. On **exam**, he has an ataxic gait, nystagmus, and positive head impulse test.

Management:

1. Steroids during acute period of vertigo.
2. Vestibular rehabilitation, symptom management.

HYF: In pure vestibular neuritis, auditory function is preserved. If there is unilateral hearing loss, it is labyrinthitis. The acute illness lasts a few days–weeks but may have residual symptoms for months. Head Impulse Test: Positive if rapid turning of the head to the affected side results in a catch-up saccade (ie, patient is unable to maintain visual fixation on examiner).

Vestibular Migraine: See Neurology section, p. 757.

Brain Tumor: See Neurology section, pp. 753–755.

Multiple Sclerosis: See Neurology section, p. 724.

Vestibular Schwannoma: See Neurology section, p. 754.

26-20 Seizures

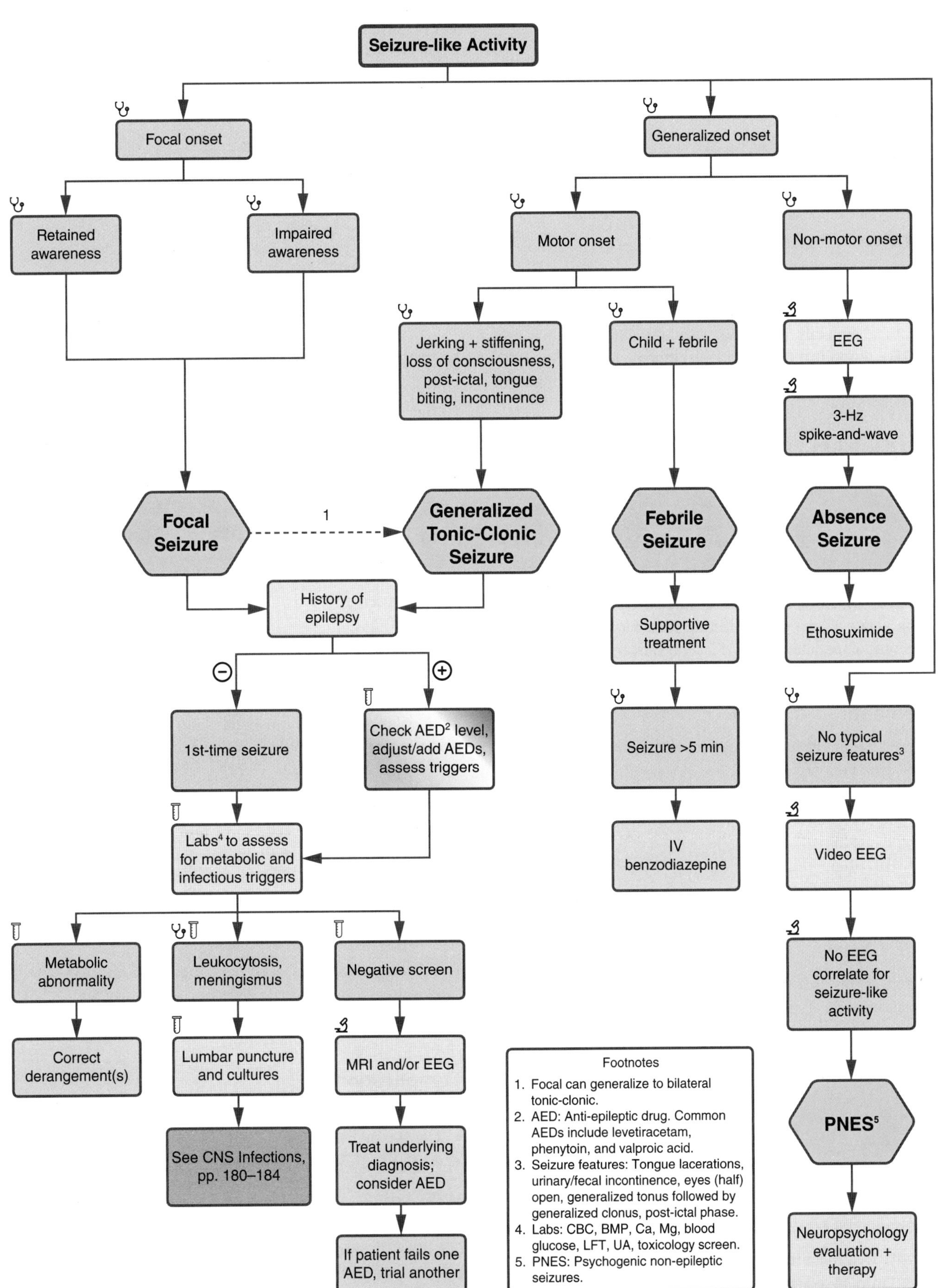

Seizure-like Activity
Focal onset
Generalized onset
Retained awareness
Impaired awareness
Motor onset
Non-motor onset
Jerking + stiffening, loss of consciousness, post-ictal, tongue biting, incontinence
Child + febrile
EEG
3-Hz spike-and-wave
Focal Seizure
1
Generalized Tonic-Clonic Seizure
Febrile Seizure
Absence Seizure
History of epilepsy
Supportive treatment
Ethosuximide
⊖
⊕
1st-time seizure
Check AED[2] level, adjust/add AEDs, assess triggers
Seizure >5 min
No typical seizure features[3]
Labs[4] to assess for metabolic and infectious triggers
IV benzodiazepine
Video EEG
Metabolic abnormality
Leukocytosis, meningismus
Negative screen
No EEG correlate for seizure-like activity
Correct derangement(s)
Lumbar puncture and cultures
MRI and/or EEG
See CNS Infections, pp. 180–184
Treat underlying diagnosis; consider AED
PNES[5]
If patient fails one AED, trial another
Neuropsychology evaluation + therapy
Footnotes
1. Focal can generalize to bilateral tonic-clonic.
2. AED: Anti-epileptic drug. Common AEDs include levetiracetam, phenytoin, and valproic acid.
3. Seizure features: Tongue lacerations, urinary/fecal incontinence, eyes (half) open, generalized tonus followed by generalized clonus, post-ictal phase.
4. Labs: CBC, BMP, Ca, Mg, blood glucose, LFT, UA, toxicology screen.
5. PNES: Psychogenic non-epileptic seizures.

FIGURE 26.20

26-20 Seizures

FOCAL SEIZURE

A 40-year-old M presents with multiple 1–2-min episodes ×1 month of numbness and tingling beginning in R hand and spreading to R arm and face. On exam, he has no focal deficits.

Management:

1. Start antiepileptic drug (AED).
2. If first seizure presentation, MRI and EEG.

Complications: Status epilepticus.

HYF: If a patient has >1 unprovoked seizure and high risk of recurrence, can start AED. It is important to evaluate for an underlying structural anomaly with MRI with and without gadolinium (since a brain lesion can create an epileptogenic focus). Focal seizures can have motor or non-motor onset and can have intact or impaired awareness.

GENERALIZED TONIC-CLONIC SEIZURE (GTCS)

An 80-year-old M with no prior seizure history presents with headache and confusion after a fall with head strike. On exam, he does not have focal neurologic deficits. On **imaging**, he has bilateral subdural hematomas. He proceeded to have a witnessed seizure while under observation, with tonic trunk stiffening and synchronous clonic jerks of extremities lasting 2 min, and concomitant urinary incontinence, lateral tongue lacerations, and unresponsiveness during and after the episode.

Management:

1. If seizure >5 min or multiple seizures without return to baseline, give IV lorazepam.
2. Start AED.
3. Treat underlying cause.

Complications:

- Head trauma.
- Aspiration pneumonia.
- Status epilepticus.

HYF: Often begins as a focal seizure that subsequently generalizes/becomes bilateral. Typically lasts 1–3 min followed by postictal state (lasting up to hours). Lactate is often elevated due to muscle contraction and self-resolves.

FEBRILE SEIZURE

A 3-year-old M with current viral illness presents with generalized tonic-clonic seizure lasting 3 min. On exam, he has a temperature of 40°C.

Management:

1. Supportive treatment (antipyretic), reassurance.
2. If lasts >5 min, IV benzodiazepine.

Complications: Rarely develops into epilepsy in the future.

HYF: Simple febrile seizures are generalized, <15 min long, 1 event within 24 h. Complex febrile seizures are focal, >15 min, and/or >1 event within 24 h. Important to rule out CNS infection if physical exam suggests meningitis.

ABSENCE SEIZURE

An 8-year-old M presents with multiple episodes of transient blank stares in school and at home with 3-Hz spike-and-wave complexes on EEG during episodes.

Management:

1. 1st-line: Ethosuximide.
2. 2nd-line: Valproate (lamotrigine if female of childbearing age).

HYF: Can occur in otherwise healthy child. Leads to loss of consciousness without loss of muscle tone; there is no postictal confusion.

PSYCHOGENIC NON-EPILEPTIC SEIZURES

A 34-year-old F with PMH of depression, PTSD, and chronic pain presents with 5-min episodes of asynchronous movements of the upper and lower extremities with immediate return to baseline. There is no seizure correlation on video EEG.

Management:

1. Neuropsychology evaluation.
2. Psychotherapy.

HYF: Seizure-like activity without typical signs (eg, tongue lacerations, incontinence, postictal state) or EEG correlate. Can also occur in people with proven epilepsy.

STATUS EPILEPTICUS

A 34-year-old M is brought in by EMS after being found down in the bathroom having continuous generalized tonic-clonic seizures. On exam, he has tonic trunk stiffening and synchronous clonic jerks of extremities lasting >7 min. On **labs**, lactate is elevated.

Management:

1. IV benzodiazepine (lorazepam, diazepam) and IV AED (fosphenytoin, valproate, levetiracetam) together.
2. Evaluate for and treat any precipitating factors (CT head, BMP, AED level, toxicology screen).

Complications:

- Non-convulsive status epilepticus (can follow convulsive status).
- Cardiac arrhythmias.
- Aspiration pneumonia, hypoxia.

HYF: Status epilepticus is a neurologic emergency defined as continuous epileptic activity for ≥5 min or ≥2 discrete seizures without interval return to baseline consciousness. Typically occurs in patients with epilepsy or critical illness. Can be convulsive or non-convulsive (ie, with decreased consciousness and subtle signs like aphasia, myoclonus, and abnormal eye movements).

26-21 Visual Complaints

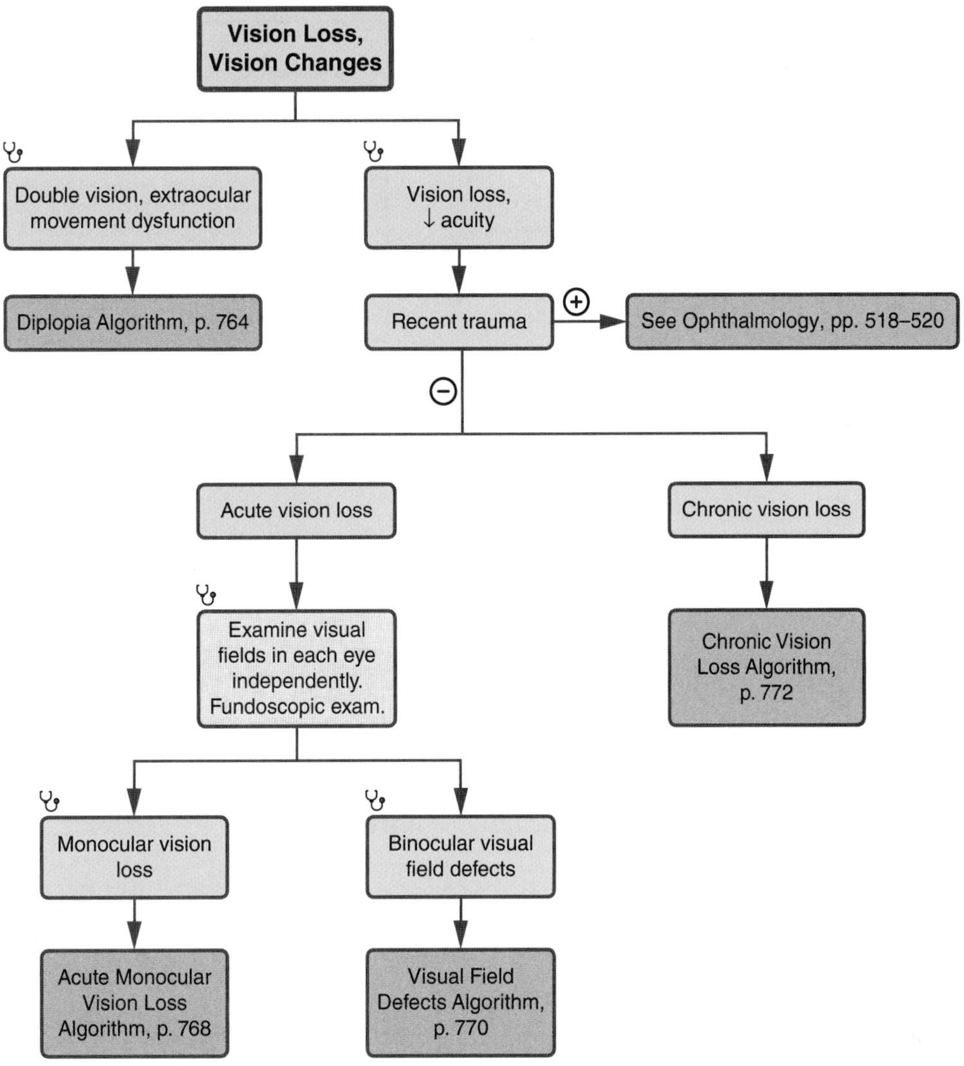
Vision Loss, Vision Changes
Double vision, extraocular movement dysfunction
Vision loss, ↓ acuity
Diplopia Algorithm, p. 764
Recent trauma
⊕
See Ophthalmology, pp. 518–520
⊖
Acute vision loss
Chronic vision loss
Examine visual fields in each eye independently. Fundoscopic exam.
Chronic Vision Loss Algorithm, p. 772
Monocular vision loss
Binocular visual field defects
Acute Monocular Vision Loss Algorithm, p. 768
Visual Field Defects Algorithm, p. 770

Vision loss and visual changes can be due to an array of diseases that fall under the purview of ophthalmology and neurology. One should initially distinguish between vision changes (the most clinically relevant being diplopia) and vision loss, which can present as complete blindness, ↓ visual acuity, or patchy loss of vision that may only be detected on careful exam. A history of recent eye trauma should trigger consideration of traumatic etiologies and an urgent ophthalmology consultation. In a patient without recent trauma, chronic vision loss will be the presentation of a different subset of disorders, which will more likely be seen in an outpatient setting. Acute vision loss is an emergency and should be rapidly delineated as monocular (exam defects only seen in only one eye) or binocular (defects seen when examining each eye). Monocular defects are caused by pathology anterior to the optic chiasm (eye, optic nerve) and are typically ophthalmologic, while binocular defects localize to pathology in the more distal optic pathways or brain and therefore are typically neurologic. Careful examination of the visual fields, extraocular movements, and fundus is essential.

FIGURE 26.21

26-22 Diplopia

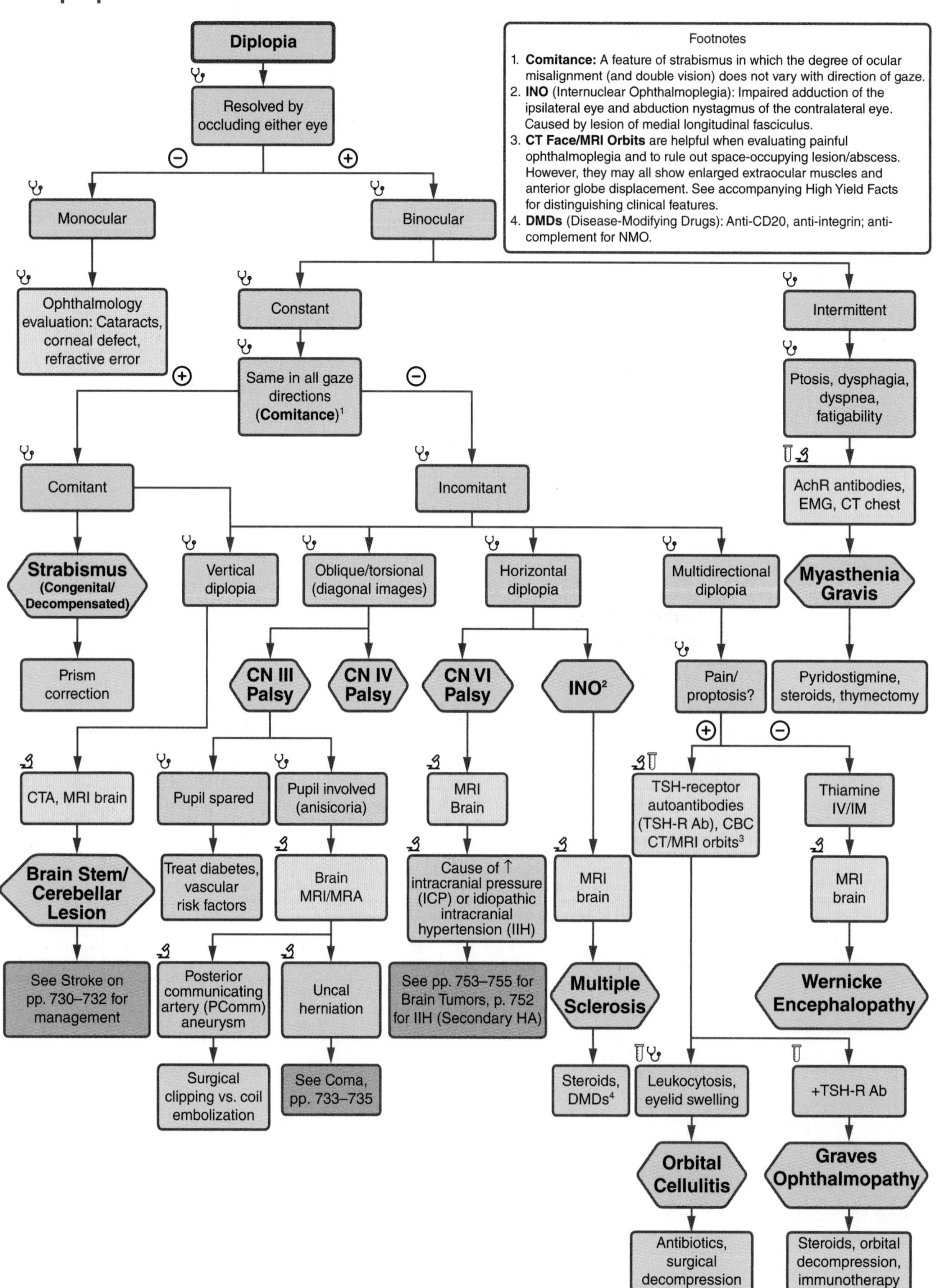
Diplopia
Resolved by occluding either eye
Monocular
Binocular
Ophthalmology evaluation: Cataracts, corneal defect, refractive error
Constant
Intermittent
Same in all gaze directions (Comitance)[1]
Ptosis, dysphagia, dyspnea, fatigability
Comitant
Incomitant
AchR antibodies, EMG, CT chest
Strabismus (Congenital/ Decompensated)
Vertical diplopia
Oblique/torsional (diagonal images)
Horizontal diplopia
Multidirectional diplopia
Myasthenia Gravis
Prism correction
CN III Palsy
CN IV Palsy
CN VI Palsy
INO[2]
Pain/ proptosis?
Pyridostigmine, steroids, thymectomy
CTA, MRI brain
Pupil spared
Pupil involved (anisicoria)
MRI Brain
TSH-receptor autoantibodies (TSH-R Ab), CBC CT/MRI orbits[3]
Thiamine IV/IM
Brain Stem/ Cerebellar Lesion
Treat diabetes, vascular risk factors
Brain MRI/MRA
Cause of ↑ intracranial pressure (ICP) or idiopathic intracranial hypertension (IIH)
MRI brain
MRI brain
See Stroke on pp. 730–732 for management
Posterior communicating artery (PComm) aneurysm
Uncal herniation
See pp. 753–755 for Brain Tumors, p. 752 for IIH (Secondary HA)
Multiple Sclerosis
Wernicke Encephalopathy
Surgical clipping vs. coil embolization
See Coma, pp. 733–735
Steroids, DMDs[4]
Leukocytosis, eyelid swelling
+TSH-R Ab
Orbital Cellulitis
Graves Ophthalmopathy
Antibiotics, surgical decompression
Steroids, orbital decompression, immunotherapy
Footnotes
1. Comitance: A feature of strabismus in which the degree of ocular misalignment (and double vision) does not vary with direction of gaze.
2. INO (Internuclear Ophthalmoplegia): Impaired adduction of the ipsilateral eye and abduction nystagmus of the contralateral eye. Caused by lesion of medial longitudinal fasciculus.
3. CT Face/MRI Orbits are helpful when evaluating painful ophthalmoplegia and to rule out space-occupying lesion/abscess. However, they may all show enlarged extraocular muscles and anterior globe displacement. See accompanying High Yield Facts for distinguishing clinical features.
4. DMDs (Disease-Modifying Drugs): Anti-CD20, anti-integrin; anti-complement for NMO.

FIGURE 26.22

26-22 Diplopia

DECOMPENSATED/CONGENITAL STRABISMUS

An 80-year-old M with PMH of osteoarthritis presents with worsening double vision. He reports he was told he had a lazy eye as a child. He had occasional double vision during adulthood, primarily when he was tired, but in the past few years, his double vision has become constant. The double vision is the same in all directions of gaze. **Exam** is notable for inward deviation of one eye relative to the other (estropia).

Management:

1. Prism correction.

HYF: Strabismus refers to ocular axis misalignment, which may be congenital (hypoplastic extraocular muscle) or acquired (cranial nerve injury). Risk of decompensated strabismus increases with age, as the occipital cortex is increasingly unable to fuse 2 disparate projections into a single image.

CN III (OCULOMOTOR) PALSY

A 70-year-old F with PMH of HTN, HLD, and poorly controlled type 2 diabetes presents with sudden-onset painless double vision upon waking in the morning. Double vision goes away by covering 1 eye. She complains of seeing 2 images next to each other, worst in L gaze. On **exam**, BP 180/87, and pupils are equally round and reactive. Her R eye is turned downward and outward. **Labs** show A1c 9%.

OR

A 70-year-old F with PMH of poorly controlled HTN, HLD, and tobacco use presents with sudden-onset double vision upon waking in the morning. She complains of seeing 2 images next to each other, worst in L gaze. She also noticed her R eyelid is drooping. On **exam**, BP 180/87. There is ptosis on the right. R pupil is 5 mm and unreactive vs. reactive and 3 mm on the L. R eye is deviated downward and outward.

Management:

1. MRI with contrast/MRA/CTA to evaluate for intracranial aneurysm, urgently if pupil involvement.
2. Surgical embolization/clipping if aneurysm.
3. Antiplatelet therapy for isolated ischemic CN III palsy.
4. LP/temporal artery biopsy if persistent deficits.

Complications: Subarachnoid hemorrhage (aneurysm rupture).

HYF: A pupil-involving CN III palsy should immediately raise suspicion for a compressive lesion (most commonly an aneurysm arising from the posterior communicating artery) affecting the parasympathetic fibers that control pupillary constriction and course along the external surface of CN III. ~40% of CN III palsies are caused by microvascular ischemia, which are pupil-sparing, as the parasympathetic nerves that control pupil constriction are unaffected.

CN IV (TROCHLEAR) PALSY

A 27-year-old M with no PMH presents after MVC complaining of double vision. He was the restrained driver and sustained minor injuries. On **exam**, he sits with his head tilted to the L and reports double vision is worst in down and L gaze. R eye is deviated upward and extorted. On **imaging**, non-contrast head CT shows no acute intracranial pathology.

Management:

1. Prism correction if persistent/prolonged diplopia resulting in functional impairment.

Complications: Persistent diplopia.

HYF: Traumatic CN IV is largely self-limiting and should resolve over weeks to months.

CN VI (ABDUCENS) PALSY

A 17-year-old F with PMH of obesity presents with several weeks of HA, tinnitus, and new double vision. She also reports blurry vision. On **exam**, she covers 1 eye with her hand. The L eye is unable to abduct. She has bilateral optic disc swelling and markedly constricted visual fields. On **imaging**, MRI brain is unrevealing. LP OP is 35 cmH_2O.

Management:

1. Treat underyling etiology.

HYF: CN VI palsy from increased intracranial pressure is referred to as a "false localizing sign"; global increases in intracranial pressure cause stretching of the nerve at points of angulation as it travels from the pons to the superior orbital fissure.

INTERNUCLEAR OPHTHALMOPLEGIA

A 22-year-old F presents with 1 week of worsening double vision. On **exam**, both of her eyes are unable to adduct. She has persistent nystagmus in abduction bilaterally. On **imaging**, MRI brain shows scattered flame-shaped T1 hypointensities arising perpendicular to the corpus callosum and a T2 hyperintense lesion in the brain stem, which crosses the midline. LP is notable for + oligoclonal bands.

Management:

1. If MS, give IV corticosteroids to reduce duration of flare.
2. Initiation of disease-modifying drugs (DMDs) to reduce risk of relapse.

Complications: If untreated, accumulation of more disability.

HYF: Multiple sclerosis is the most common etiology for a young patient presenting with bilateral INO. See Myelopathy on pp. 721–725 for more details. INO can also be caused by a brain stem stroke.

26-22 Diplopia

WERNICKE ENCEPHALOPATHY

A 23-year-old F with PMH of anorexia is admitted for severe malnutrition but develops gait difficulty and vision changes. She has just begun total parenteral nutrition. She is confused and unable to provide history. **Exam** is notable for BMI 13.6 kg/m^2, resting nystagmus, impairment of multiple extraocular muscles, and a wide-based and unsteady gait. On **imaging,** MRI brain obtained the next day shows bilateral mamillary-body T2 hyperintensities.

Management:

1. High-dose IV/IM thiamine (vitamin B_1).

Complications:

- Wernicke-Korsakoff's syndrome.
- If untreated, coma/death.

HYF: Wernicke encephalopathy is most commonly associated with chronic alcoholism but is also seen in individuals with chronic malnutrition, including anorexia/prolonged starvation, hyperemesis of pregnancy, and malabsorptive conditions (bariatric surgery).

ORBITAL CELLULITIS

A 12-year-old M with PMH of recurrent sinusitis presents with several days of eye pain and double vision. On **exam,** he has a fever, marked erythema and edema of the L eye, chemosis, and restricted and painful extraocular movements. **Labs** are notable for WBC 20k with 97% neutrophils. On **imaging,** CT face shows edema and fat stranding of extraocular muscles with anterior globe displacement.

Management:

1. Broad-spectrum IV antibiotics.
2. Surgical drainage of abscess if impending vision loss, evidence of intracranial extension, or inadequate response to IV antibiotics.

Complications:

- Vision loss from extension into the orbit.
- Orbital/subperiosteal abscess.
- Brain abscess, meningitis, cavernous sinus thrombosis.

HYF: Pain with eye movement (painful ophthalmoplegia) helps to distinguish orbital (postseptal) cellulitis from preseptal cellulitis, which is limited to the soft tissues anterior to the orbital septum.

GRAVES' OPHTHALMOPATHY

A 34-year-old M with PMH of Graves' disease treated with radioiodine ablation presents with double vision and blurry vision. On **exam,** he has bilateral proptosis with excessive tearing and periorbital edema. Extraocular movements are restricted in all directions of gaze, and visual acuity is decreased. On **labs,** TSH-R Ab is positive. On **imaging,** CT orbits shows markedly enlarged extraocular muscles with increased orbital fat volume compressing the optic nerves.

Management:

1. Treat hyperthyroidism if present: Thionamides, thyroidectomy (radioablative therapy may worsen orbital disease).
2. Glucocorticoids.
3. Surgical decompression if impending vision loss, severe cosmetic defects, or refractory disease.

Complications:

- Proptosis leads to exposure keratitis, corneal ulcerations.
- Compressive optic neuropathy → permanent vision loss.

HYF: Graves ophthalmopathy is characterized by fibroblast proliferation and abnormal deposition of retroorbital connective tissue, leading to muscle swelling, increased intra-orbital pressure, and impaired venous drainage.

Myasthenia Gravis: See p. 718.

Brain Stem/Cerebellar Lesion: See Stroke Syndrome, pp. 726–729.

Multiple Sclerosis: See p. 724.

26-23 Acute Monocular Vision Loss

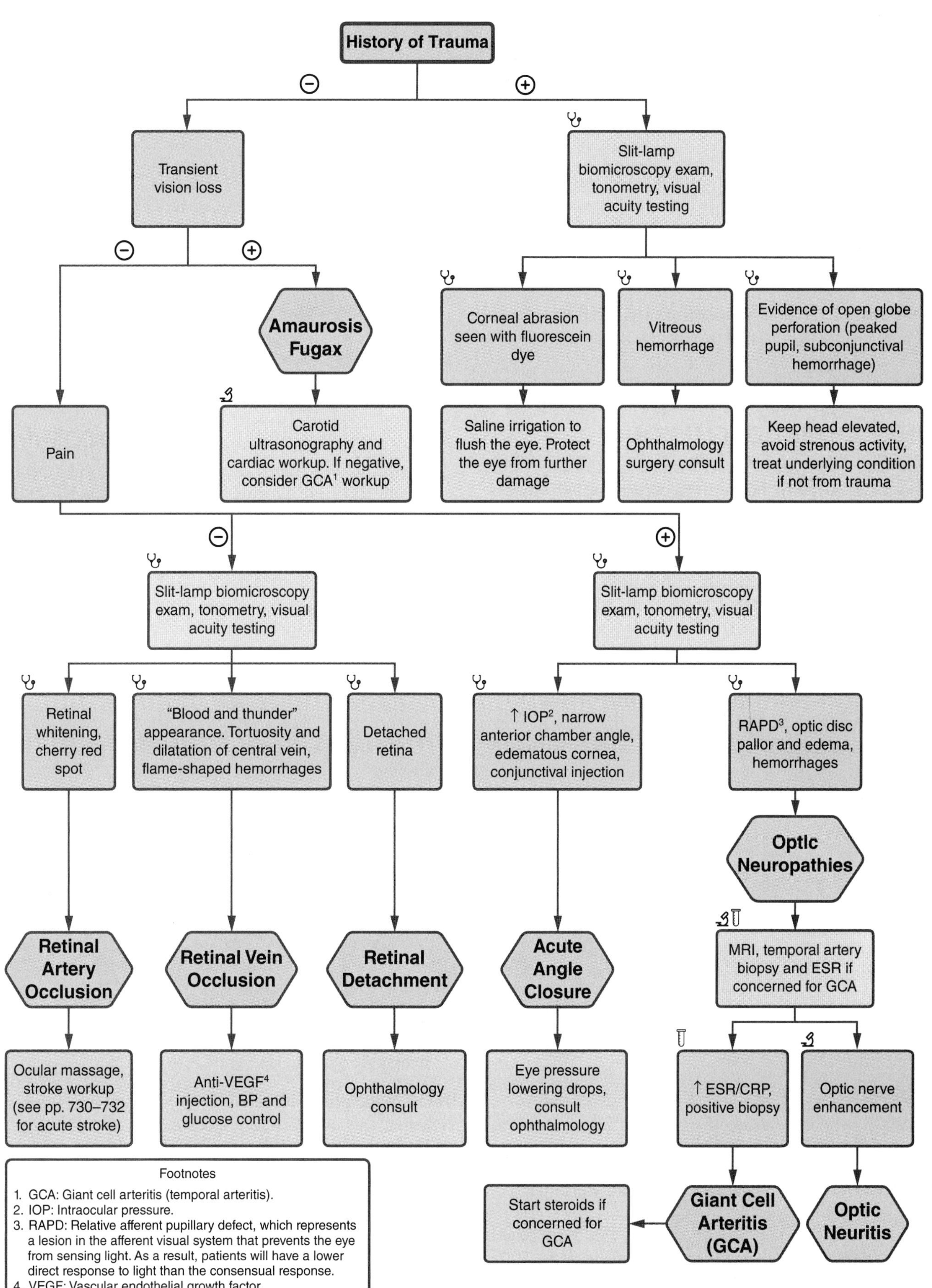

History of Trauma
Transient vision loss
Slit-lamp biomicroscopy exam, tonometry, visual acuity testing
Amaurosis Fugax
Corneal abrasion seen with fluorescein dye
Vitreous hemorrhage
Evidence of open globe perforation (peaked pupil, subconjunctival hemorrhage)
Pain
Carotid ultrasonography and cardiac workup. If negative, consider GCA[1] workup
Saline irrigation to flush the eye. Protect the eye from further damage
Ophthalmology surgery consult
Keep head elevated, avoid strenous activity, treat underlying condition if not from trauma
Slit-lamp biomicroscopy exam, tonometry, visual acuity testing
Slit-lamp biomicroscopy exam, tonometry, visual acuity testing
Retinal whitening, cherry red spot
"Blood and thunder" appearance. Tortuosity and dilatation of central vein, flame-shaped hemorrhages
Detached retina
↑ IOP[2], narrow anterior chamber angle, edematous cornea, conjunctival injection
RAPD[3], optic disc pallor and edema, hemorrhages
Optic Neuropathies
MRI, temporal artery biopsy and ESR if concerned for GCA
Retinal Artery Occlusion
Retinal Vein Occlusion
Retinal Detachment
Acute Angle Closure
Ocular massage, stroke workup (see pp. 730–732 for acute stroke)
Anti-VEGF[4] injection, BP and glucose control
Ophthalmology consult
Eye pressure lowering drops, consult ophthalmology
↑ ESR/CRP, positive biopsy
Optic nerve enhancement
Start steroids if concerned for GCA
Giant Cell Arteritis (GCA)
Optic Neuritis

Footnotes

1. GCA: Giant cell arteritis (temporal arteritis).
2. IOP: Intraocular pressure.
3. RAPD: Relative afferent pupillary defect, which represents a lesion in the afferent visual system that prevents the eye from sensing light. As a result, patients will have a lower direct response to light than the consensual response.
4. VEGF: Vascular endothelial growth factor.

FIGURE 26.22

26-23 Acute Monocular Vision Loss

AMAUROSIS FUGAX

A 73-year-old M with PMH of hypertension and atrial fibrillation presents with transient vision loss in the R eye lasting a few minutes. On **exam**, visual acuity is 20/20. On **imaging**, slit-lamp microscopy exam is unremarkable. Carotid US demonstrates stenosis.

Management:

1. If concerned for cardiovascular/ischemic etiology, start stroke workup and initiate antiplatelet therapy. See pp. 730–732 for acute management of stroke.
2. If GCA suspected, start steroids immediately.

Complications: Delayed treatment for GCA has worse prognosis. Consequently, early steroid treatment is imperative.

HYF: Patients will often have a normal physical exam.

RETINAL ARTERY OCCLUSION

A 82-year-old F with PMH of hypertension and diabetes presents with painless vision loss in the R eye that occurred within seconds. She has had previous episodes of vision loss that resolved after a few minutes. On fundus **exam**, there is retinal whitening with a cherry-red spot, and the blood vessels show sluggish blood flow. On **imaging**, fluorescein angiography shows delay in filling of the retinal arteries. Echocardiogram demonstrates an embolic source in the left atrium.

Management:

1. Ocular massage should be started immediately; consider tPA.
2. Stroke workup (pp. 726, 730).
3. Management of risk factors (anticoagulation, antihypertensive medications).

Complications: Neovascularization of the iris and retina, which may be treated with anti-VEGF agents.

HYF: Lack of quality data for tPA use in CRAO but may have benefit if administered early.

RETINAL VEIN OCCLUSION

A 68-year-old M with PMH of hypertension and hyperlipidemia presents with sudden, painless blurry vision and vision loss in the L eye. On **exam**, the fundus shows hemorrhages with dilated and tortuous veins.

Management:

1. Anti-VEGF injection (bevacizumab, aflibercept) for macular edema.
2. Management of risk factors.

Complications: Neovascularization of the iris and retina.

HYF: >90% of cases occur in patients age >55. Pathogenesis follows the principles of Virchow triad for thrombogenesis.

RETINAL DETACHMENT

A 62-year-old with PMH of pathological myopia presents with sudden increase in flashes, like a snowstorm. On **exam**, the fundus shows retinal detachment.

Management:

1. Ophthalmology consult.
2. Nonsurgical management for serous detachment (from sarcoidosis or malignancy).

Complications:

- Proliferative retinopathy.
- Future retinal detachments.

HYF: Risk factors include pathological myopia (refraction worse than −6.0 D), trauma, previous retinal tears, and family history.

ACUTE ANGLE CLOSURE GLAUCOMA

A 55-year-old F presents with acute onset of ocular pain, halos around lights, and eye redness after watching a movie in the theater. On **exam**, visual acuity is 20/60 with an IOP of 42. Her pupil is mid-dilated, and the cornea is clear with no edema.

Management:

1. Medical treatment to lower IOP: Carbonic anhydrase inhibitors and osmotic agents.
2. Laser iridotomy.
3. Prophylaxis includes laser iridotomy and cataract surgery to increase the anterior chamber angles.

HYF: Mydriatic agents such as anticholinergic and alpha-agonistic medications can induce angle closure.

OPTIC NEUROPATHY

A 32-year-old F presents with painful vision loss in the L eye that worsens after a hot shower. On **exam**, she has a relative afferent pupillary defect (RAPD) and optic disc pallor. On **imaging**, MRI shows periventricular white-matter lesions and enhancement of the L optic nerve, consistent with multiple sclerosis.

Management:

1. See Multiple Sclerosis (p. 724).
2. If GCA suspected, start steroids immediately and obtain temporal artery biopsy. See GCA (p. 769).

HYF: Optic neuropathies can be divided into inflammatory and ischemic. Inflammatory conditions include optic neuritis, which can be secondary to multiple sclerosis, and neuromyelitis optica, which can also present as bilateral eye pain and vision loss. Ischemic etiologies include GCA and nonarteritic anterior ischemic optic neuropathy. An early sign of optic neuropathy is change in color vision (red desaturation).

26-23 Acute Monocular Vision Loss

TRAUMA

An 18-year-old M presents with L eye pain and photophobia after getting hit by a branch while hiking outdoors. He now has excess tearing and foreign body sensation. On **exam**, his visual acuity is 20/40 in the L eye. Further examination does not show any evidence of a ruptured globe, and fluorescein dye demonstrates a corneal epithelial defect. Fundoscopy is normal.

Management:

1. Lubrication ± antibiotic drops.
2. Protect the eye from further damage.
3. Topical anesthetic is typically avoided because it can mask worsening symptoms or infection.

Complications:

- Persistent epithelial defects and recurrent infections.
- Trauma increases the risk of cataract formation, retinal detachments, and vitreous hemorrhage.
- Posttraumatic endophthalmitis.

HYF: Corneal epithelial defects have a variety of etiologies, including mechanical, chemical, and ultraviolet exposure.

GIANT CELL ARTERITIS (TEMPORAL ARTERITIS)

A 20-year-old F with PMH of shoulder and hip pains suggestive of polymyalgia rheumatica presents with new headache along with jaw claudication and transient monocular vision loss. On **exam**, tender and thickened temporal arteries and spots on fundoscopy. **Labs/imaging** show elevated ESR and CRP.

Management:

1. If high suspicion, start empiric high dose glucocorticoids.
2. Confirm diagnosis: Temporal artery ultrasound or biopsy.
3. Taper steroids as able.

Complications:

- Complete vision loss from central retinal artery occlusion.
- Large vessel involvement: Aortic aneurysm.
- Stroke, especially posterior circulation.
- Long-term steroid use complications.

HYF: Strong association with polymyalgia rheumatica. Consider this diagnosis in an older patient age >50 years with new headache. Pathology: granulomatous inflammation of large vessels (slides may show thrombosis, lymphocytes, plasma cells, giant cells).

Optic Neuritis: See p. 516.

26-24 Visual Field Defects

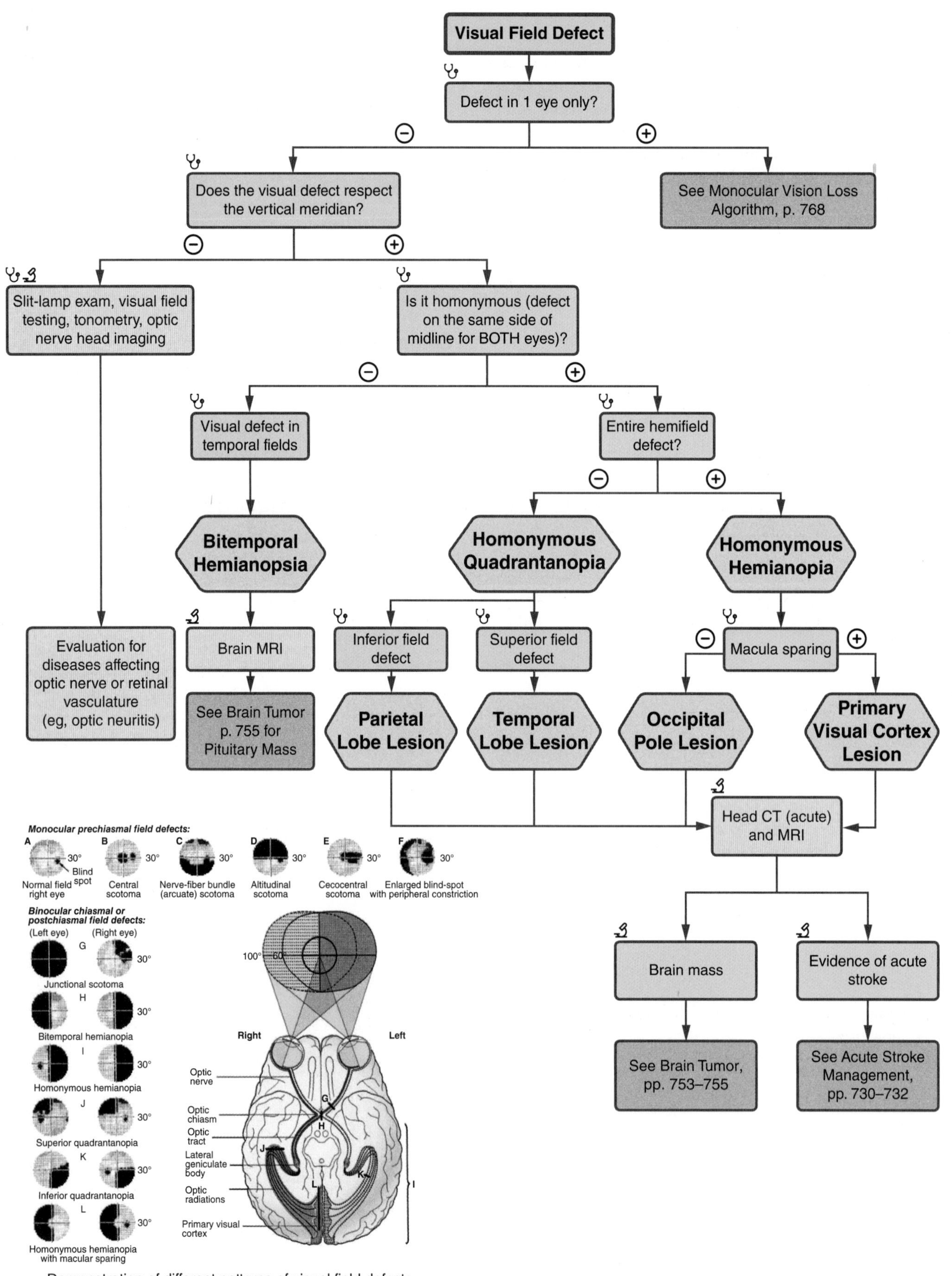
Visual Field Defect
Defect in 1 eye only?
See Monocular Vision Loss Algorithm, p. 768
Does the visual defect respect the vertical meridian?
Slit-lamp exam, visual field testing, tonometry, optic nerve head imaging
Is it homonymous (defect on the same side of midline for BOTH eyes)?
Visual defect in temporal fields
Entire hemifield defect?
Bitemporal Hemianopsia
Homonymous Quadrantanopia
Homonymous Hemianopia
Evaluation for diseases affecting optic nerve or retinal vasculature (eg, optic neuritis)
Brain MRI
See Brain Tumor p. 755 for Pituitary Mass
Inferior field defect
Superior field defect
Macula sparing
Parietal Lobe Lesion
Temporal Lobe Lesion
Occipital Pole Lesion
Primary Visual Cortex Lesion
Head CT (acute) and MRI
Brain mass
Evidence of acute stroke
See Brain Tumor, pp. 753–755
See Acute Stroke Management, pp. 730–732
Monocular prechiasmal field defects:
Normal field right eye
Blind spot
Central scotoma
Nerve-fiber bundle (arcuate) scotoma
Altitudinal scotoma
Cecocentral scotoma
Enlarged blind-spot with peripheral constriction
Binocular chiasmal or postchiasmal field defects:
(Left eye)
(Right eye)
Junctional scotoma
Bitemporal hemianopia
Homonymous hemianopia
Superior quadrantanopia
Inferior quadrantanopia
Homonymous hemianopia with macular sparing
Right
Left
Optic nerve
Optic chiasm
Optic tract
Lateral geniculate body
Optic radiations
Primary visual cortex

Demonstration of different patterns of visual field defects.

Figure 26.24.1

FIGURE 26.24

26-24 Visual Field Defects

BITEMPORAL HEMIANOPIA

A 35-year-old F G1P1 presents with new-onset lactation despite discontinuing breastfeeding 2 years ago and 6 months of amenorrhea. She has had several months of low libido, and she also notes not noticing things in her peripheral vision. On exam, she has papilledema, and she is spontaneously lactating. Visual field testing shows a visual field defect in the temporal visual field of both eyes, consistent with a bitemporal hemianopia. On imaging, brain MRI demonstrates a pituitary adenoma adjacent to the optic chiasm.

Management:

1. See Pituitary Tumors (pp. 488–490).

HYF: The nasal retina fibers, which are responsible for the temporal visual field, decussate at the optic chiasm. As a result, a bitemporal hemianopia visual defect is immediately suspicious for a lesion or mass at the optic chiasm. Often this can be described as tunnel vision.

SUPERIOR HOMONYMOUS QUADRANTANOPIA

A 53-year-old M with PMH of mastoidectomy presents with a worsening headache and new-onset fever. On exam, he has a temperature of 39°C. The patient has right-sided weakness and is unable to identify the number of fingers held in the superior R visual field. Imaging shows an abscess in the L temporal lobe. Additional visual field testing demonstrates a visual defect in the superior, R visual field of both eyes.

Management:

1. See Stroke (pp. 726–732) and Brain Tumor (pp. 753–755).

HYF: Superior homonymous quadrantanopia localizes to the temporal lobe, where the temporal radiations course through. Like any form of homonymous vision loss, the lesion localizes posterior to the optic chiasm, and a differential for this vision loss includes strokes and masses (eg, tumors, infectious causes).

INFERIOR HOMONYMOUS QUADRANTANOPIA

A 78-year-old F with PMH of hypertension and a previous stroke presents for follow-up. On exam, the patient is unable to identify the number of fingers held in the inferior L visual field. Visual field testing corroborates a visual field defect in the inferior L visual field of both eyes consistent with a lesion affecting the R parietal optic radiations.

Management:

1. See Stroke (pp. 726–732) and Brain Tumors (pp. 753–755).

HYF: Posterior to the optic chiasm, the optic radiations travel through the temporal and parietal lobes. The temporal radiations are responsible for superior vision. The parietal radiations are responsible for inferior vision. A lesion in either location would be homonymous because it is posterior to the optic chiasm. This will result in a quadrantanopia because only a portion of that hemifield is affected. A parietal stroke or mass would localize to an inferior homonymous quadrantanopia.

HOMONYMOUS HEMIANOPIA

A 45-year-old M with PMH of hypertension presents with subacute headache and an acute onset of right-sided weakness, aphasia, and L eye gaze deviation. The eyes cannot cross midline. On exam, he has a pyramidal pattern weakness on the R side of the body. Visual field testing demonstrates a defect in the R visual field of both eyes, consistent with a homonymous hemianopia. On imaging, MRI brain is consistent with a mass in the right cerebral hemisphere.

Management:

1. See Stroke (pp. 726–732) and Brain Tumors (pp. 753–755).

HYF: A lesion posterior to the optic chiasm will cause a homonymous defect, which is a defect that affects the same side of the visual field in both eyes. These visual defects will respect the vertical meridian because, posterior to the optic chiasm, the left hemisphere processes the right visual field and the right hemisphere processes the left visual field. Common causes of a homonymous hemianopia include posterior cerebral artery (PCA) strokes and brain masses that affect the visual tract, posterior to the optic chiasm. Of note, a stroke in the primary visual cortex may result in macular sparing, so central visual acuity may be preserved. This is because macular vision is processed in the occipital pole, which is also supplied by collaterals of the middle cerebral artery (MCA).

OPTIC NEUROPATHIES

A 72-year-old F presents with right-sided headache associated with decreased vision in the right eye. On exam, her visual acuity is 20/25, and there is optic pallor. Her temporal region is also tender to palpation. On imaging, MRI does not show any focal lesion. On labs, she has an elevated ESR and CRP, and temporal artery biopsy is consistent with giant-cell arteritis (GCA).

Management:

1. See Monocular Vision Loss (p. 768).
2. If there is concern for optic neuropathy, GCA and optic neuritis should be ruled out. If high likelihood for GCA, start steroids prior to temporal artery biopsy. Additional tests include ESR, CRP, and MRI imaging.

HYF: Optic nerve pathologies include inflammatory and ischemic etiologies (eg, giant cell arteritis). In addition to being monocular, many optic neuropathies will have a visual defect that respects the horizontal meridian (ie, the defect does not cross from the superior to inferior hemifield or vice versa). Some causes of monocular vision loss may also occur bilaterally (eg, neuromyelitis optica, an autoimmune condition that attacks the optic nerve myelin).

MONOCULAR VISION LOSS

A 35-year-old M with PMH of retinal tears presents with sudden change in vision described as flashes of lights and floaters as well as decreased peripheral vision. Funduscopic exam shows a retinal detachment.

Management:

1. See: Monocular Vision Loss (pp. 767–769).

HYF: Vision loss in 1 eye localizes anterior to the optic chiasm. This can occur anywhere from the eye itself to the retina and optic nerve.

26-25 Chronic Vision Loss

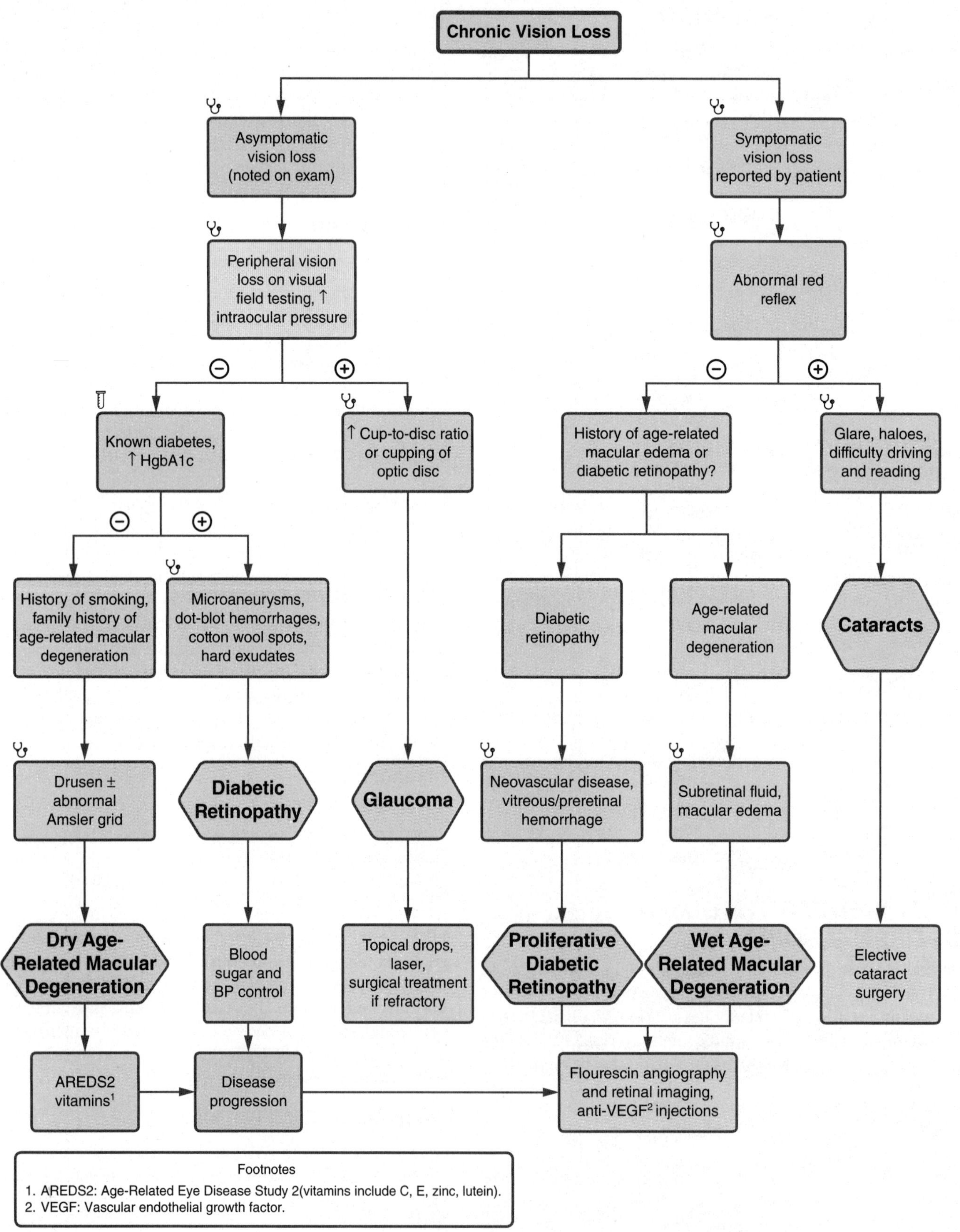
Chronic Vision Loss
Asymptomatic vision loss (noted on exam)
Symptomatic vision loss reported by patient
Peripheral vision loss on visual field testing, ↑ intraocular pressure
Abnormal red reflex
Known diabetes, ↑ HgbA1c
↑ Cup-to-disc ratio or cupping of optic disc
History of age-related macular edema or diabetic retinopathy?
Glare, haloes, difficulty driving and reading
History of smoking, family history of age-related macular degeneration
Microaneurysms, dot-blot hemorrhages, cotton wool spots, hard exudates
Diabetic retinopathy
Age-related macular degeneration
Cataracts
Drusen ± abnormal Amsler grid
Diabetic Retinopathy
Glaucoma
Neovascular disease, vitreous/preretinal hemorrhage
Subretinal fluid, macular edema
Dry Age-Related Macular Degeneration
Blood sugar and BP control
Topical drops, laser, surgical treatment if refractory
Proliferative Diabetic Retinopathy
Wet Age-Related Macular Degeneration
Elective cataract surgery
AREDS2 vitamins[1]
Disease progression
Flourescin angiography and retinal imaging, anti-VEGF[2] injections
Footnotes
1. AREDS2: Age-Related Eye Disease Study 2(vitamins include C, E, zinc, lutein).
2. VEGF: Vascular endothelial growth factor.

FIGURE 26.25

26-25 Chronic Vision Loss

CATARACTS

A 65-year-old F with PMH of hypertension presents with blurry vision that is more noticeable when driving at night and haloes when looking at bright lights. She reports less reliance on glasses for near reading. On **exam**, her visual acuity is 20/40, which does not improve with spectacle correction. Slit-lamp exam is consistent with a medium dense cataract, bilaterally.

Management:

1. Conservative management includes spectacle correction.
2. Cataract extraction with intraocular lens implant.

Complications: Endophthalmitis is a rare but vision-threatening infection that can occur post-cataract surgery.

HYF: Over half of adults age >75 have cataracts. Steroid use, diabetes, and trauma are risk factors for cataract development.

DIABETIC RETINOPATHY

A 73-year-old M with PMH of diabetes with a HgbA1c of 9.8 and followed for non-proliferative diabetic retinopathy presents with worsening vision. **Exam** shows neovascularization of the iris, and fundus shows frank vitreous hemorrhages, consistent with proliferative diabetic retinopathy.

Management:

1. Blood glucose control.
2. Anti-VEGF injection if hemorrhages are present.
3. Can also consider laser to treat hemorrhages.

Complications:

- Injection has a risk for endophthalmitis.
- Neovascular disease can cause glaucoma.
- Cataract formation.

HYF: All patients diagnosed with type 2 diabetes mellitus should undergo annual ophthalmologic screening.

AGE-RELATED MACULAR DEGENERATION

A 55-year-old F with PMH of hypertension and smoking and notable family history of macular degeneration presents for annual eye exam. Patient is taking AREDS2 vitamins. **Exam** is notable for several drusen but no evidence of hemorrhage, consistent with dry ARMD. Retinal **imaging** is consistent with physical exam.

Management:

1. AREDS2 vitamins.
2. Encourage smoking cessation.
3. Anti-VEGF injection or laser to treat hemorrhage for wet ARMD.

HYF: One of the most common causes of vision loss in the population >65. Central vision is typically affected while peripheral vision is preserved.

GLAUCOMA

A 52-year-old M with PMH of myopia, hypertension, and diabetes and a family history of glaucoma presents with normal vision (visual acuity 20/20) but elevated IOP of 24 mmHg. **Exam** is notable for open anterior chamber angles, a cup-to-disc ratio of 0.6, and increased cupping of the optic nerve. Visual field testing demonstrates a superior arcuate defect but preserved central vision. Optic nerve head **imaging** (optical coherence tomography [OCT]) demonstrates thinning of the retina in the inferior portion, corresponding with the superior arcuate defect.

Management:

1. Start IOP-lowering eye drop medications. Common medications include timolol (beta-blocker), brimonidine (alpha-agonist), latanoprost (prostaglandin analogue), and dorzolamide (carbonic anhydrase inhibitor).
2. Laser iridotomy can be done for chronic angle closure glaucoma.
3. Laser trabeculoplasty to reduce IOP in open-angle glaucoma.
4. Cataract surgery can increase the anterior chamber angle.
5. Additional surgical procedures to lower IOP.
6. Patients should be followed regularly with visual fields and optic nerve head imaging to monitor progression.

Complications:

- Vision loss.
- Endophthalmitis from surgery.

HYF: A leading cause of irreversible blindness worldwide. Patients are often asymptomatic because it usually affects peripheral vision before affecting central vision (preserved visual acuity). Patients may have normal IOP in primary open-angle glaucoma.

27
Psychiatry

27-1 Diagnosis of Psychiatric Concerns

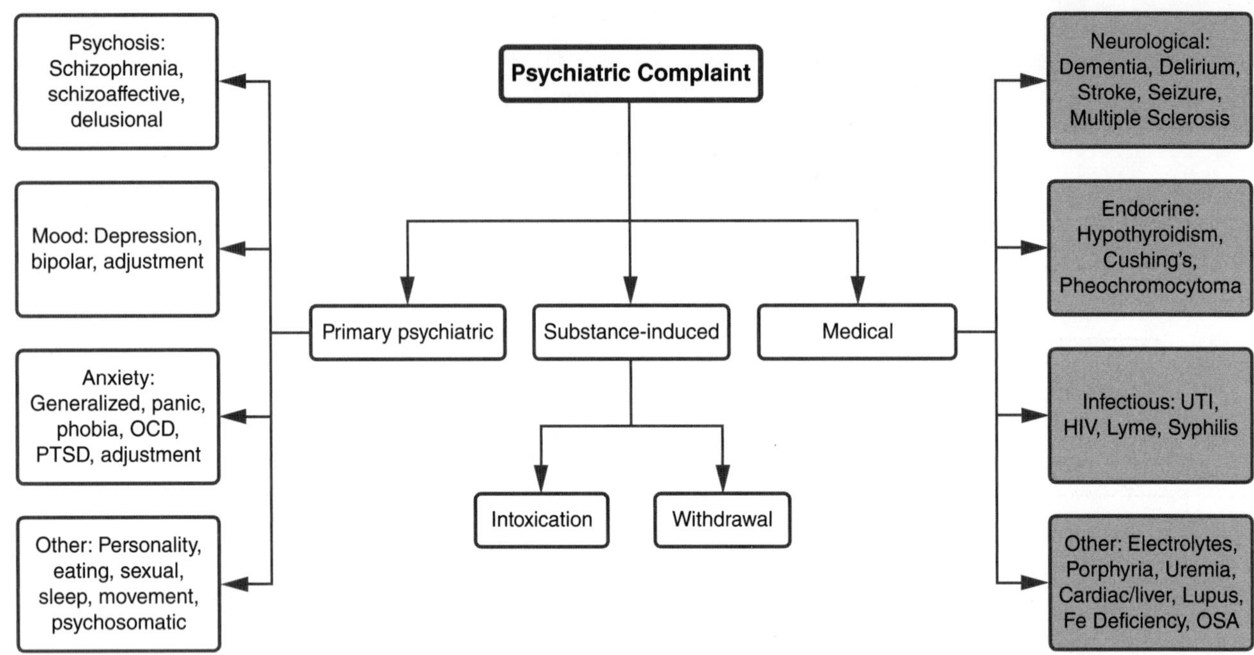
Psychiatric Complaint
Primary psychiatric
Substance-induced
Medical
Psychosis: Schizophrenia, schizoaffective, delusional
Mood: Depression, bipolar, adjustment
Anxiety: Generalized, panic, phobia, OCD, PTSD, adjustment
Other: Personality, eating, sexual, sleep, movement, psychosomatic
Intoxication
Withdrawal
Neurological: Dementia, Delirium, Stroke, Seizure, Multiple Sclerosis
Endocrine: Hypothyroidism, Cushing's, Pheochromocytoma
Infectious: UTI, HIV, Lyme, Syphilis
Other: Electrolytes, Porphyria, Uremia, Cardiac/liver, Lupus, Fe Deficiency, OSA

When presented with a patient complaining of psychiatric issues, the vignette will help to point you toward the set of diseases that should be considered. While this chapter will primarily deal with primary psychiatric pathologies, it is important to rule out substance-induced presentations (both intoxication and withdrawal) and also consider a medical cause. Some clues for substance/medication-induced cases include an acute onset (symptoms develop during or soon after exposure to and/or withdrawal from offending agent) and features that point more toward an "organic" origin (eg, visual and tactile hallucinations). The relevant algorithms for these diagnoses are present in the corresponding chapter. Among psychiatric causes, it is generally possible to decide whether the question is describing acute or chronic illness, which can narrow your differential based on DSM-5 timeline criteria. Demographic information such as age, gender, family history, and other pertinent risk factors may clue you into the correct diagnosis or treatment plan. Finally, pharmacology is heavily tested, so it is essential to not only know the indications for the psychotropics, but also medical monitoring, contraindications, and complications that may arise. There will be medication decision trees grouped with the disorders they are treating for antipsychotics, antidepressants, mood stabilizers, and anxiolytics/sedatives to detail these considerations.

Disorders by Symptom Duration

Anxiety Disorders	Acute stress <1 mo	Post-traumatic stress >1mo	
	Adjustment <6 mo	Generalized anxiety >6 mo	
Psychotic Disorders	Brief psychotic <1 mo	Schizophreniform 1–6 mo	Schizophrenia >6 mo
Mood Disorders	Hypomania >4 days	Mania >7 days	Cyclothymia >2 years
	Major depression >2 weeks	Dysthymia >2 years	

FIGURE 27.1

27-2 Psychology, Psychodynamic & Behavioral Factors

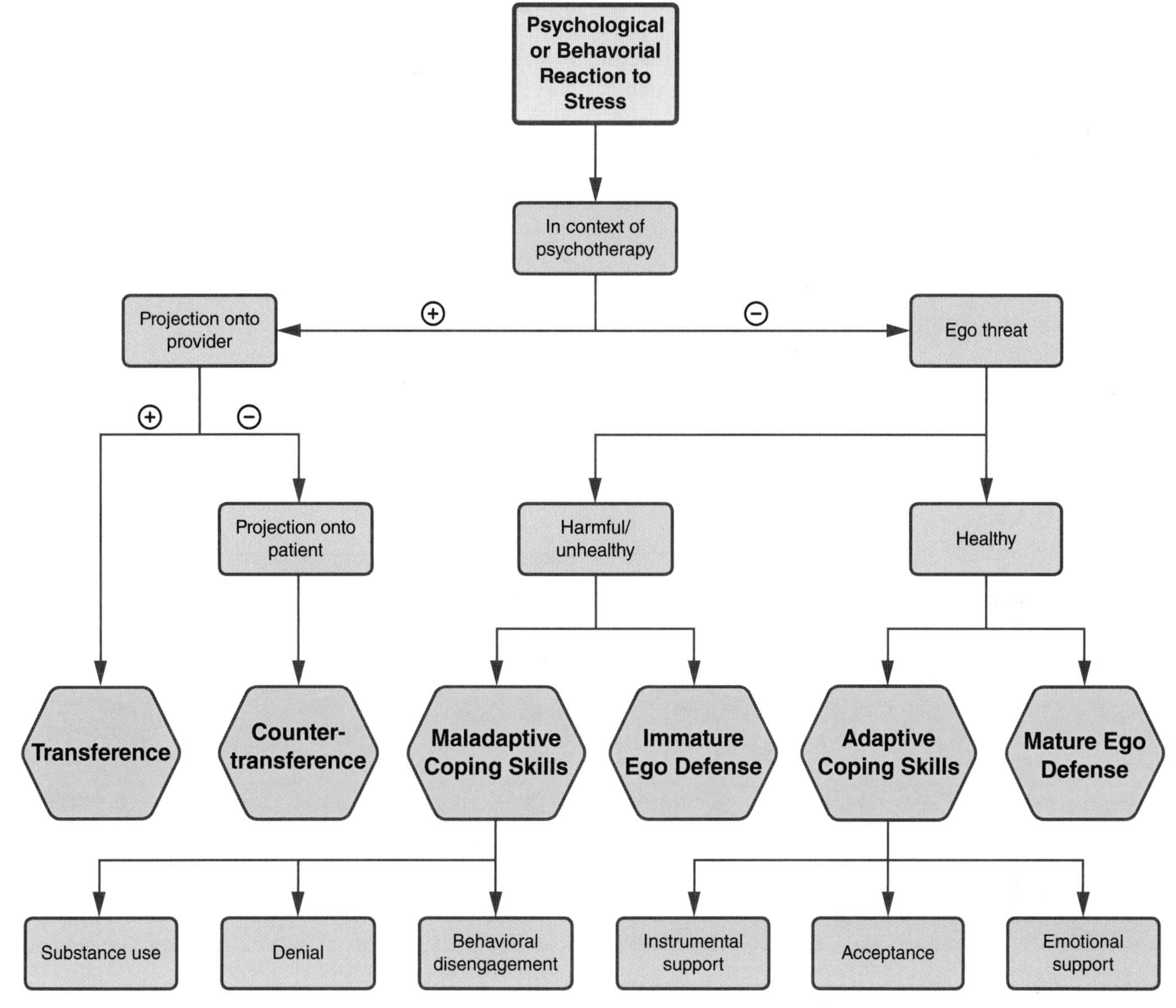
Psychological or Behavorial Reaction to Stress
In context of psychotherapy
Projection onto provider
⊕
⊖
Ego threat
⊕
⊖
Projection onto patient
Harmful/ unhealthy
Healthy
Transference
Counter-transference
Maladaptive Coping Skills
Immature Ego Defense
Adaptive Coping Skills
Mature Ego Defense
Substance use
Denial
Behavioral disengagement
Instrumental support
Acceptance
Emotional support

FIGURE 27.2

27-2 Psychology, Psychodynamic & Behavioral Factors

TRANSFERENCE AND COUNTERTRANSFERENCE

A 45-year-old F is seen in her psychotherapist's office. When discussing her relationship with her father, she becomes angry at the therapist, as she feels he is treating her the same way as her father did, and she recognizes this as transference. Her psychotherapist then experiences countertransference when he becomes quiet, as her angry shouting reminds him of his mother yelling in anger.

HYF:

- Transference = redirection of a patient's feelings for a significant person to the therapist.
- Countertransference = redirection of a therapist's feelings toward a patient, or more generally, a therapist's emotional entanglement with a patient.

COPING SKILLS

A 31-year-old M was recently fired from his job. He is upset about this and drinks several alcoholic drinks until he passes out.

HYF:

- Conscious or unconscious strategies used to reduce unpleasant emotions.
- Adaptive or maladaptive. Adaptive techniques are further divided:
  - Appraisal-focused.
  - Adaptive behavioral.
  - Emotion-focused.

Adaptive	Maladaptive
Active coping	Denial
Positive reframing	Self-distraction
Planning	Substance use
Acceptance	Behavioral disengagement
Religion	Venting
Emotional support	Self-blame
Instrumental support	
Humor	

EGO DEFENSES

A 17-year-old F does not perform as well on a test as she thought she would. She makes a self-deprecating joke about needing to study more in the future.

HYF:

- Initially described by Sigmund Freud and then enumerated by Anna Freud.
- George Eman Vailant introduced a 4-level classification.
  - Level 1: Pathological
  - Level 2: Immature
  - Level 3: Neurotic
  - Level 4: Mature
- More defenses have since been added, including conversion and splitting.

Pathologic	Immature	Neurotic	Mature
Delusion	Acting out	Displacement	Altruism
Denial	Hypochondriasis	Dissociation	Humor
Distortion	Passive aggression	Intellectualization	Suppression
	Projection	Reaction formation	Sublimation
	Fantasy	Repression	Anticipation

- **Displacement:** Redirecting a negative emotion from its original source to a less-threatening recipient.
- **Projection:** Unwanted feelings are ascribed to another person.
- **Fixation:** Stuck at a particular point in psychosexual development.
- **Regression:** Reversion to patterns of behavior used earlier in development.
- **Reaction formation:** Taking up the opposition feeling, impulse, or behavior.
- **Sublimation:** Converting behaviors into a more acceptable form.
- **Repression:** Unconsciously stopping information from rising to level of consciousness.
- **Suppression:** Consciously pushing information from consciousness.

27-3 Personality Disorders

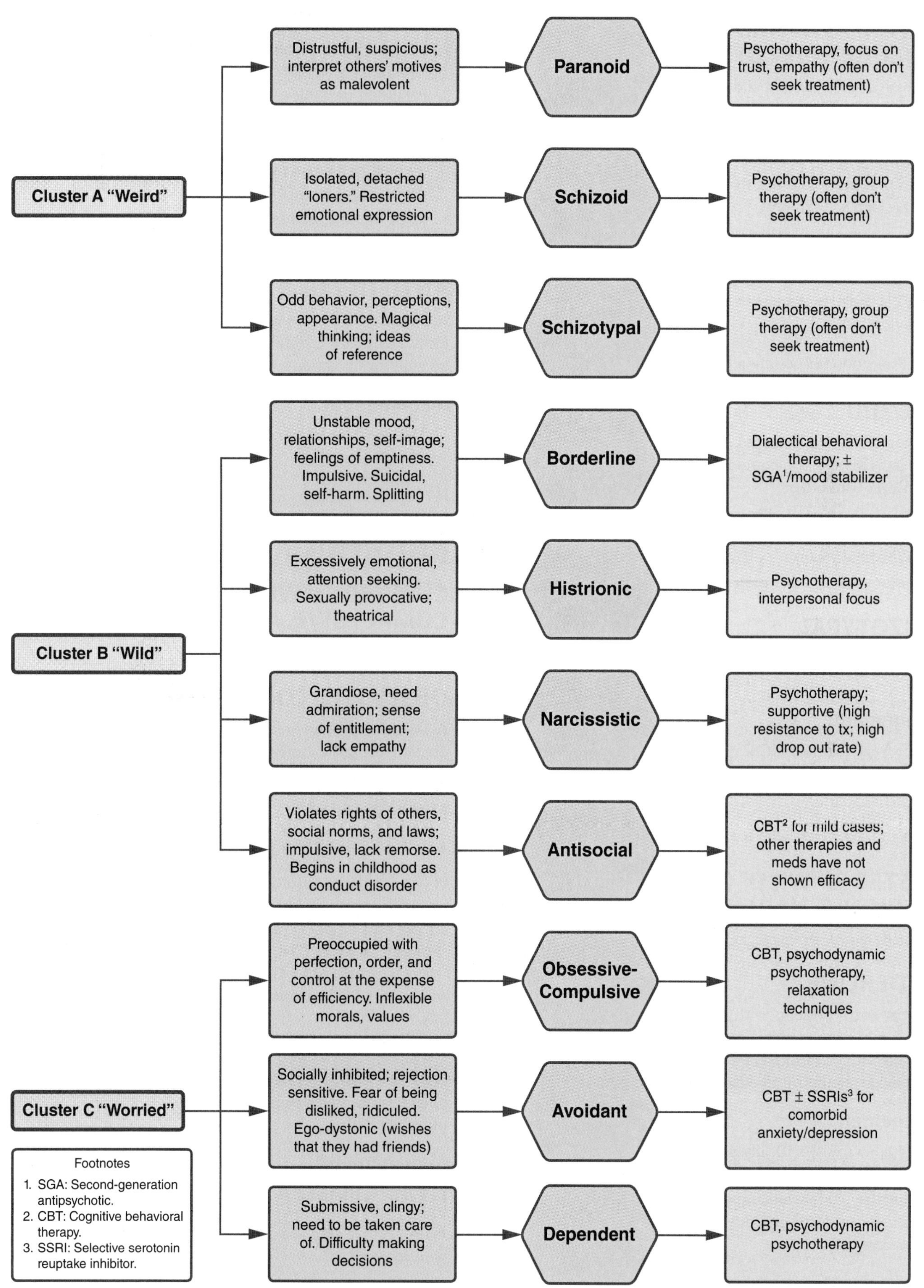
Cluster A "Weird"
Distrustful, suspicious; interpret others' motives as malevolent
Paranoid
Psychotherapy, focus on trust, empathy (often don't seek treatment)
Isolated, detached "loners." Restricted emotional expression
Schizoid
Psychotherapy, group therapy (often don't seek treatment)
Odd behavior, perceptions, appearance. Magical thinking; ideas of reference
Schizotypal
Psychotherapy, group therapy (often don't seek treatment)
Cluster B "Wild"
Unstable mood, relationships, self-image; feelings of emptiness. Impulsive. Suicidal, self-harm. Splitting
Borderline
Dialectical behavioral therapy; ± SGA1/mood stabilizer
Excessively emotional, attention seeking. Sexually provocative; theatrical
Histrionic
Psychotherapy, interpersonal focus
Grandiose, need admiration; sense of entitlement; lack empathy
Narcissistic
Psychotherapy; supportive (high resistance to tx; high drop out rate)
Violates rights of others, social norms, and laws; impulsive, lack remorse. Begins in childhood as conduct disorder
Antisocial
CBT2 for mild cases; other therapies and meds have not shown efficacy
Cluster C "Worried"
Preoccupied with perfection, order, and control at the expense of efficiency. Inflexible morals, values
Obsessive-Compulsive
CBT, psychodynamic psychotherapy, relaxation techniques
Socially inhibited; rejection sensitive. Fear of being disliked, ridiculed. Ego-dystonic (wishes that they had friends)
Avoidant
CBT ± SSRIs3 for comorbid anxiety/depression
Submissive, clingy; need to be taken care of. Difficulty making decisions
Dependent
CBT, psychodynamic psychotherapy
Footnotes
1. SGA: Second-generation antipsychotic.
2. CBT: Cognitive behavioral therapy.
3. SSRI: Selective serotonin reuptake inhibitor.

FIGURE 27.3

27-3 Personality Disorders

CLUSTER A: "WEIRD" (PARANOID, SCHIZOID, SCHIZOTYPAL)

Individuals can appear odd and eccentric.

PARANOID

A 45-year-old M has persistent beliefs that his wife is cheating on him and that his boss is out to get him. He does not demonstrate other psychiatric symptoms.

Management:

1. Early referral to mental health provider.
2. CBT can help recognize destructive thought patterns and behaviors.

HYF: Projection is a common defense mechanism.

SCHIZOID

A 60-year-old M, unpartnered, lives in an isolated village with his computer as his sole companion and does not desire to make close relationships with others.

Management:

1. CBT/psychotherapy.
2. Treat for anxiety/depression if indicated.

SCHIZOTYPAL

A 35-year-old M exhibits eccentric clothing, odd speech, and ideas of reference but without delusions or hallucinations.

Management:

1. Rarely seek treatment; CBT/psychotherapy.

HYF: Both schizotypal and schizoid share the inability to maintain relationships; schizotypals avoid because of deep-seated fear of people vs. schizoids, who see no point in forming relationships.

CLUSTER B: "WILD" (BORDERLINE, HISTRIONIC, NARCISSISTIC, ANTISOCIAL)

Individuals appear dramatic, emotional, erratic.

BORDERLINE

A 25-year-old F presents with history of non-suicidal self-injury due to a relationship with her partner, with whom she is either infatuated with or cannot stand. She has a history of 5 prior non-lethal suicide attempts immediately after a break-up.

Management:

1. Psychotherapy, specifically dialectical behavioral therapy (DBT).
2. Adjunctive pharmacotherapy to target mood instability and transient psychosis (eg, 2nd-generation antipsychotics, mood stabilizers)

HYF: For diagnosis, must have a pervasive pattern of unstable relationships, self-image, impulsivity, and ≥5 of the following:

1. Frantic efforts to avoid abandonment.
2. Unstable personal relationships; alternating between extremes (splitting).
3. Persistent unstable self-image.
4. Impulsivity.
5. Recurrent suicidal behavior.
6. Marked mood reactivity.
7. Chronic feelings of emptiness.
8. Inappropriate intense anger.
9. Stress-related paranoia/dissociation.

ANTISOCIAL

A 25-year-old M presents on court-ordered visit for assault/battery. He has a history of violence toward animals as a child. He displays no guilt for his actions.

Management:

1. Treatment-resistant; patients often lack insight. Extreme cases often end with jail.

HYF: Often presents with evidence of conduct disorder before age 15. Must be >18 for this diagnosis (<18 usually meets criteria for conduct disorder).

CLUSTER C: "WORRIED" (OBSESSIVE-COMPULSIVE, AVOIDANT, DEPENDENT)

Individuals appear anxious, fearful.

OBSESSIVE-COMPULSIVE

A 34-year-old M was recently fired from work for not making production quotas at his factory job because he was consumed with making every widget perfect before moving on to the next.

Management:

1. CBT/psychotherapy.

HYF: Similar to obsessive-compulsive disorder (OCD), obsessive-compulsive personality disorder (OCPD) exhibits rigid behaviors, but patients do not generally feel compelled to repeatedly perform ritualistic actions. They also find pleasure in perfecting a task, whereas people with OCD are often more distressed after their actions. OCPD is *egosyntonic*. OCD is *egodystonic*.

AVOIDANT

A 22-year-old M complains of low self-esteem, loneliness, a sense of emptiness, social isolation, substance abuse, and general unhappiness with life.

Management:

1. CBT/psychotherapy

HYF: People with avoidant PD desire to have friends, unlike those with schizoid PD.

27-4 Psychotic Disorders

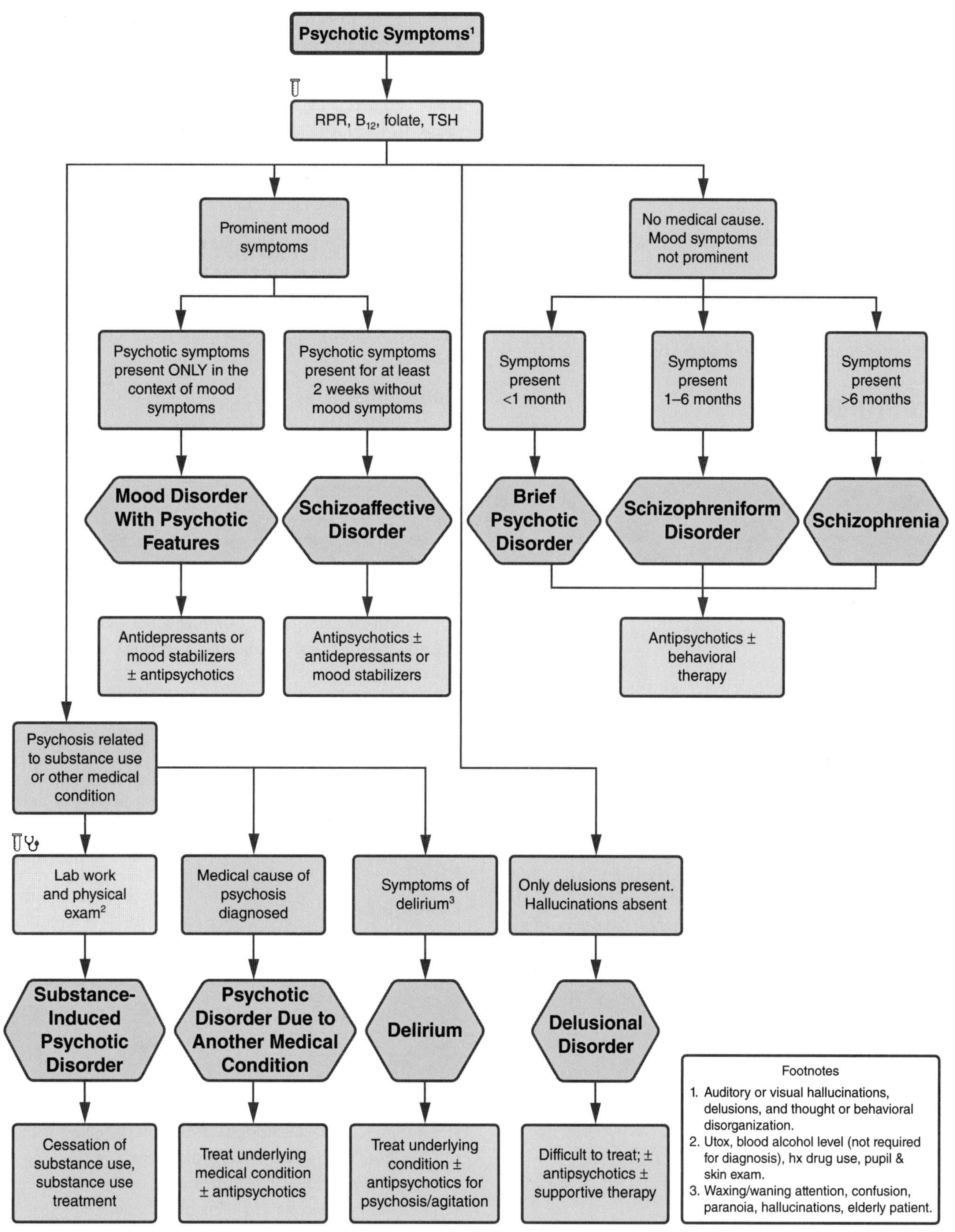
Psychotic Symptoms[1]
RPR, B_{12}, folate, TSH
Prominent mood symptoms
No medical cause. Mood symptoms not prominent
Psychotic symptoms present ONLY in the context of mood symptoms
Psychotic symptoms present for at least 2 weeks without mood symptoms
Symptoms present <1 month
Symptoms present 1–6 months
Symptoms present >6 months
Mood Disorder With Psychotic Features
Schizoaffective Disorder
Brief Psychotic Disorder
Schizophreniform Disorder
Schizophrenia
Antidepressants or mood stabilizers ± antipsychotics
Antipsychotics ± antidepressants or mood stabilizers
Antipsychotics ± behavioral therapy
Psychosis related to substance use or other medical condition
Lab work and physical exam[2]
Medical cause of psychosis diagnosed
Symptoms of delirium[3]
Only delusions present. Hallucinations absent
Substance-Induced Psychotic Disorder
Psychotic Disorder Due to Another Medical Condition
Delirium
Delusional Disorder
Cessation of substance use, substance use treatment
Treat underlying medical condition ± antipsychotics
Treat underlying condition ± antipsychotics for psychosis/agitation
Difficult to treat; ± antipsychotics ± supportive therapy
Footnotes
1. Auditory or visual hallucinations, delusions, and thought or behavioral disorganization.
2. Utox, blood alcohol level (not required for diagnosis), hx drug use, pupil & skin exam.
3. Waxing/waning attention, confusion, paranoia, hallucinations, elderly patient.

FIGURE 27.4

27-4 Psychotic Disorders

SCHIZOAFFECTIVE DISORDER

A 41-year-old presents with auditory hallucinations and grossly disorganized behavior along with 1–2 hours sleep per night for 7 days, grandiosity, distractibility, increased talkativeness, and risk-taking behavior.

Management:

1. Antipsychotic medication.
2. Mood stabilizers.
3. Consider inpatient hospitalization.

HYF: Differentiate schizoaffective disorder (delusions or hallucinations present for 2 weeks in the absence of mood symptoms) from mood disorder with psychotic symptoms (psychotic symptoms ONLY present during mood episode) by time course.

SCHIZOPHRENIA

A 25-year-old M presents with 4 months of flat affect, anhedonia, and apathy on exam he has auditory hallucinations and disorganized speech.

Management:

1. Antipsychotic medications.

HYF:

- For diagnosis, 2 of the following criteria must be present for ≥1 month:
  - Delusions.
  - Hallucinations.
  - Disorganized speech.
  - Grossly disorganized or catatonic behavior.
  - Negative symptoms: Flat affect, alogia, avolition.
- Neuroimaging *may* find enlargement of 3rd and lateral ventricles.
- Brief psychotic disorder (<1 month), schizophreniform disorder (1–6 months), and schizophrenia (>6 months) have similar diagnostic criteria but differ based on duration.
- Schizoid and schizotypal personality disorder have *intact* reality.

SUBSTANCE-INDUCED PSYCHOTIC DISORDER

A 26-year-old M with strong substance abuse history and no history of psychosis presents with agitation, dilated pupils, HR 125, BP 170/110, and prominent paranoid delusions on exam. **Labs** are notable for methamphetamine on urine toxicology.

Management:

1. Benzodiazepines.
2. Antipsychotics, PRN agitation.
3. Fluids if dehydrated.
4. Substance-use treatment.

Complications:

- Severe agitation and violence.
- Withdrawal syndrome: Dysphoria, fatigue, anxiety, etc.

HYF: Drugs that can present with psychosis: adrenergic, **alcohol**/benzo/barbiturate withdrawal, antiarrhythmics, antibiotics, **anticholinergics**, antihistamines, cannabis, ketamine, cocaine, MDMA, **corticosteroids**, dextromethorphan, **antiparkinsonian medications**, heavy metals, organophosphates, thyroid hormones.

PSYCHOTIC DISORDER DUE TO ANOTHER MEDICAL CONDITION

A 68-year-old M with history of shuffling gait, resting tremors, and cogwheel rigidity presents with visual hallucinations and paranoia on exam.

Management:

1. Assess for delirium, dementia, adverse effect of anti-Parkinson drug.
2. May need to lower dopamine agonist drugs.
3. Last resort: Antipsychotic medication (should be used with extreme caution in patients with Parkinson's disease. Prioritize quetiapine or clozapine over other anti-psychotics.).

HYF: Many non-psychiatric disorders can present with psychosis:

- CNS disease: Parkinson's, MS, Alzheimer's, encephalitis, etc.
- Endocrinopathies: Addison's/Cushing's disease, hypo/hyperthyroidism, etc.
- Nutritional: B_{12}/folate deficiency, etc.
- Other: Lupus, porphyria, etc.

DELUSIONAL DISORDER

A 52-year-old M presents with a 6-month history of fixed belief that the government is monitoring his every move. No hallucinations are present. He has a reactive affect and linear thought process on exam.

Management:

1. Difficult to treat; antipsychotics are recommended though efficacy is unclear.
2. Supportive therapy.

Complications:

- ~50% of people have a full recovery.

HYF: Types of delusions:

- Erotomanic type: Delusion that someone is in love with them.
- Grandiose type: Delusions of great talent.
- Somatic type: Physical delusions.
- Persecutory: Delusions of being persecuted.
- Jealous: delusions of unfaithfulness.

Delirium: See p. 737.

27-5 Antipsychotics

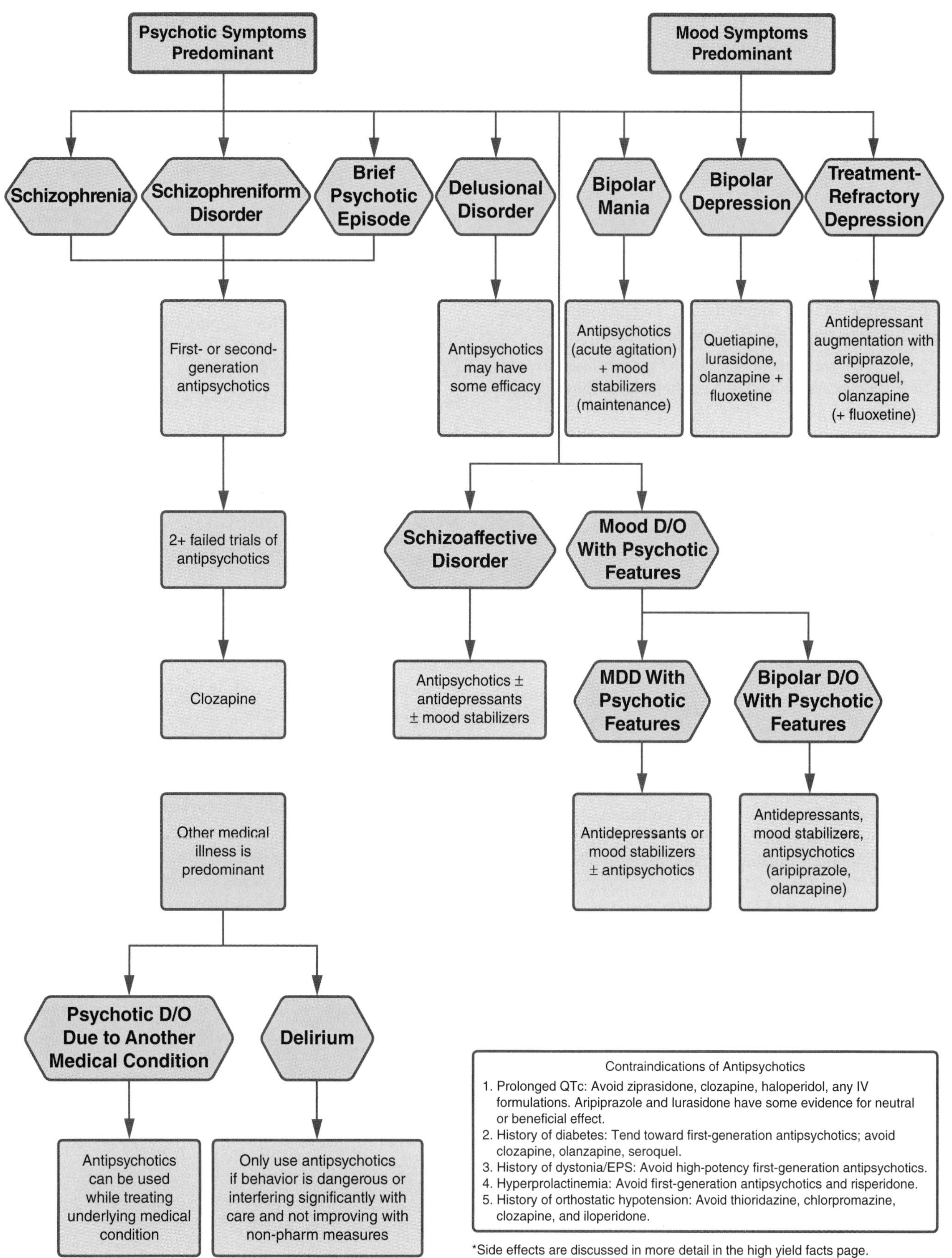
Psychotic Symptoms Predominant
Mood Symptoms Predominant
Schizophrenia
Schizophreniform Disorder
Brief Psychotic Episode
Delusional Disorder
Bipolar Mania
Bipolar Depression
Treatment-Refractory Depression
First- or second-generation antipsychotics
Antipsychotics may have some efficacy
Antipsychotics (acute agitation) + mood stabilizers (maintenance)
Quetiapine, lurasidone, olanzapine + fluoxetine
Antidepressant augmentation with aripiprazole, seroquel, olanzapine (+ fluoxetine)
2+ failed trials of antipsychotics
Schizoaffective Disorder
Mood D/O With Psychotic Features
Clozapine
Antipsychotics ± antidepressants ± mood stabilizers
MDD With Psychotic Features
Bipolar D/O With Psychotic Features
Other medical illness is predominant
Antidepressants or mood stabilizers ± antipsychotics
Antidepressants, mood stabilizers, antipsychotics (aripiprazole, olanzapine)
Psychotic D/O Due to Another Medical Condition
Delirium
Antipsychotics can be used while treating underlying medical condition
Only use antipsychotics if behavior is dangerous or interfering significantly with care and not improving with non-pharm measures
Contraindications of Antipsychotics
1. Prolonged QTc: Avoid ziprasidone, clozapine, haloperidol, any IV formulations. Aripiprazole and lurasidone have some evidence for neutral or beneficial effect.
2. History of diabetes: Tend toward first-generation antipsychotics; avoid clozapine, olanzapine, seroquel.
3. History of dystonia/EPS: Avoid high-potency first-generation antipsychotics.
4. Hyperprolactinemia: Avoid first-generation antipsychotics and risperidone.
5. History of orthostatic hypotension: Avoid thioridazine, chlorpromazine, clozapine, and iloperidone.
*Side effects are discussed in more detail in the high yield facts page.

FIGURE 27.5

27-5 Antipsychotics

Indications: Psychotic spectrum disorders, mood disorders with psychotic features, bipolar disorder, augmentation for antidepressants, and behavioral management.

The decision tree for this topic lists the most common agents used in each disorder. This page will mainly discuss side effects, which also weigh heavily in picking an agent.

FIRST-GENERATION (TYPICAL) ANTIPSYCHOTICS (FGAs)

Mechanism: Postsynaptic blockade of D2 receptors.

High-potency FGAs: Fluphenazine, haloperidol, loxapine, perphenazine, pimozide, thiothixene, trifluoperazine.

- Low activity at histaminic (low sedation) and muscarinic receptors (low anticholinergic activity), but higher risk for extrapyramidal symptoms (EPS).

Low-potency FGAs: Chlorpromazine, thioridazine.

- High activity at histaminic (sedating) and muscarinic (anticholinergic) receptors, but low risk of EPS.
- Adverse effects: Blurred vision, ocular toxicity, orthostatic hypotension, QTc prolongation, urinary retention, retinopathy (thioridazine, specifically); not often used.

Extrapyramidal symptoms include akathisia, rigidity, bradykinesia, tremor, acute dystonia.

- More common with high-potency agents.
- Treatment: Anticholinergic agents.

Tardive dyskinesia: Involuntary choreoathetoid movements of mouth, tongue, face, extremities, trunk (lip-smacking, tongue writhing, jaw movements, facial grimacing, trunk writhing).

- More common among FGAs, even more so among high-potency agents.
- Treatment: Benzodiazepines, VMAT2 inhibitors.

Neuroleptic malignant syndrome: Fever, muscle rigidity, mental status change, autonomic instability, rhabdomyolysis often with elevated CK.

- No differences demonstrated between FGAs.

Prolactin elevation among all FGAs via blockade of tuberoinfundibular dopamine.

SECOND-GENERATION (ATYPICAL) ANTIPSYCHOTICS (SGAs)

Mechanism: Generally, blockade of D2 receptors. Also with 5HT2a antagonism.

Examples: Olanzapine, quetiapine, risperidone. Drugs with different mechanisms include aripiprazole and brexpiprazole (D2-partial agonist), cariprazine (D3-preferring partial agonist), pimavanserin (5HT2A-inverse agonist and antagonist with no dopamine D2 affinity).

Generally, SGAs carry lower risk of EPS than FGAs. These should still be monitored for anyone on antipsychotics.

Clozapine, though the most effective antipsychotic, comes with unique side effects, and use must be monitored. Potential side effects include:

- Myocarditis and cardiomyopathy.
- Agranulocytosis/neutropenia.
- QTc prolongation, PE, metabolic syndrome, seizures, excessive salivation, constipation.
- Monitoring: CBC and ANC (regularly), weight, height, BMI, fasting glucose and HbA1c, lipids, EKG.

OTHER SIDE EFFECTS

Metabolic syndrome: Weight gain, diabetes, dyslipidemia.

- Generally attributed to SGAs, but chlorpromazine carries relatively high risk. Fluphenazine, haloperidol, and pimozide show the lowest risk.
- SGAs: Most common among clozapine and olanzapine; quetiapine also relatively high-risk.
- Management: Routine monitoring of weight, BP, glucose and HbA1c, lipid profile.

Anticholinergic effects (dry mouth, constipation, less commonly urinary retention and blurred vision).

- FGAs: Most prominent with low-potency agents, chlorpromazine, and thioridazine.
- SGAs: Most common with clozapine; intermediate risk with quetiapine and olanzapine.

QT prolongation:

- Sudden cardiac death is reported in 1.5 to 1.8 people per 1000 years' exposure to antipsychotic medication. This is thought to be secondary to QT prolongation leading to torsades de pointes.
- FGAs: Most with chlorpromazine, thioridazine, IV haloperidol.
- SGAs: Most with ziprasidone; less with clozapine, olanzapine, quetiapine, and risperidone; least with aripiprazole, brexpiprazole, cariprazine, and lurasidone.

Orthostatic hypotension:

- Caused by adrenergic blockade.
- FGAs: Most common with thioridazine and chlorpromazine; least common with fluphenazine, haloperidol, and perphenazine.
- SGAs: Most common with clozapine and iloperidone

*All antipsychotics carry a "black box" warning from the FDA of a 1.6- to 1.7-fold increase in mortality from all causes for older adult patients with dementia-related psychosis.

27-6 Psychotropic-Induced Movement Disorders

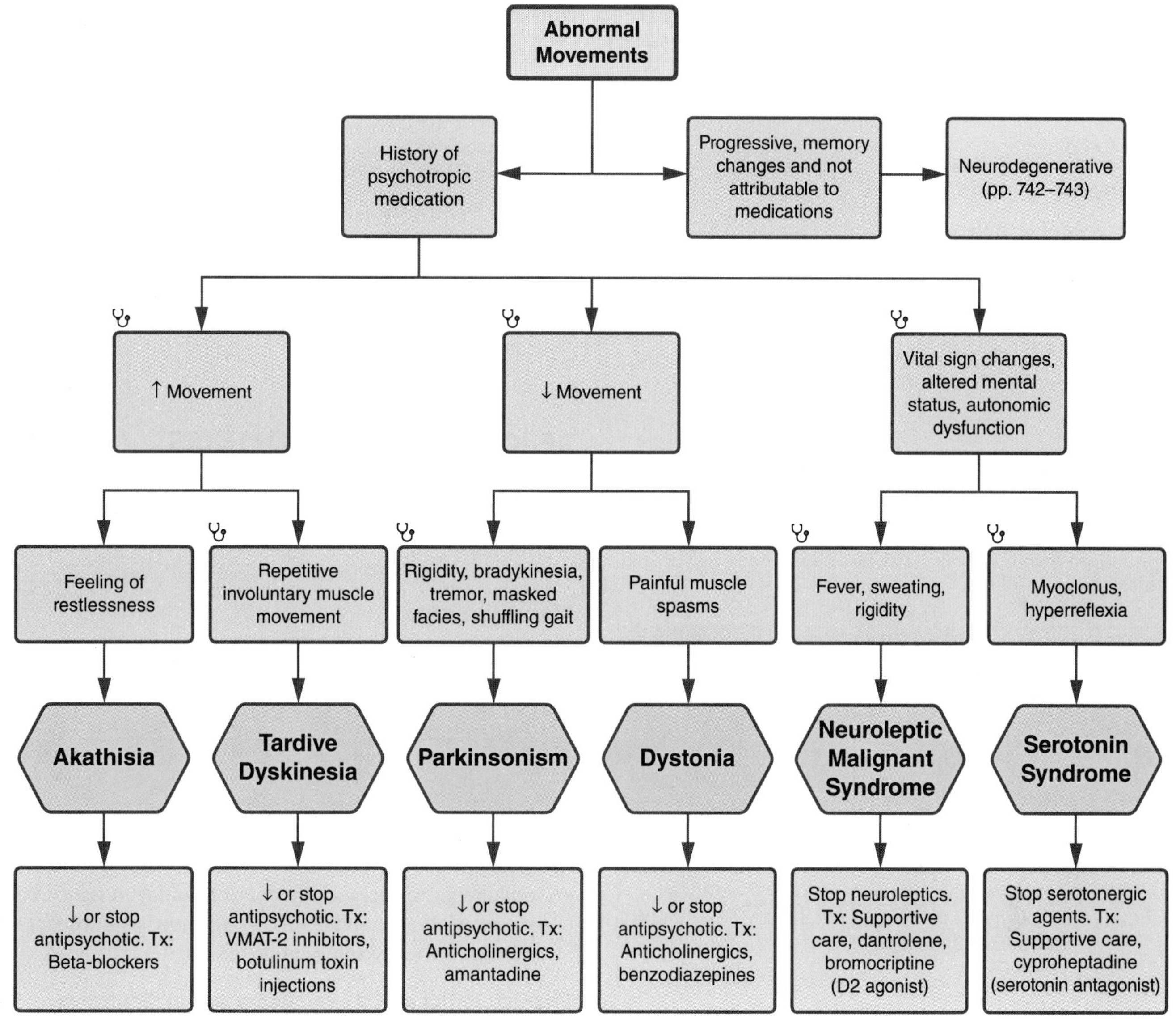
Abnormal Movements
History of psychotropic medication
Progressive, memory changes and not attributable to medications
Neurodegenerative (pp. 742–743)
↑ Movement
↓ Movement
Vital sign changes, altered mental status, autonomic dysfunction
Feeling of restlessness
Repetitive involuntary muscle movement
Rigidity, bradykinesia, tremor, masked facies, shuffling gait
Painful muscle spasms
Fever, sweating, rigidity
Myoclonus, hyperreflexia
Akathisia
Tardive Dyskinesia
Parkinsonism
Dystonia
Neuroleptic Malignant Syndrome
Serotonin Syndrome
↓ or stop antipsychotic. Tx: Beta-blockers
↓ or stop antipsychotic. Tx: VMAT-2 inhibitors, botulinum toxin injections
↓ or stop antipsychotic. Tx: Anticholinergics, amantadine
↓ or stop antipsychotic. Tx: Anticholinergics, benzodiazepines
Stop neuroleptics. Tx: Supportive care, dantrolene, bromocriptine (D2 agonist)
Stop serotonergic agents. Tx: Supportive care, cyproheptadine (serotonin antagonist)

FIGURE 27.6

27-6 Psychotropic-Induced Movement Disorders

EXTRAPYRAMIDAL SYMPTOMS (EPS)

A 66-year-old F is started on a new antipsychotic after she had intolerable side effects from her last medication. A few days later, she complains of extreme restlessness and feels like she must constantly move around.

Management:

1. Decrease dose of neuroleptic.
2. Switch to lower-potency neuroleptic.
3. Pharmacologic:
   a. Anticholinergics.
   b. Beta-blockers.
   c. Vesicular monoamine transporter 2 inhibitors.

HYF:

- Includes akathisia, dystonia, pseudoparkinsonism (drug-induced parkinsonism), and tardive dyskinesia.
- Oculogyric crisis is a kind of acute dystonic reaction that involves the prolonged involuntary upward deviation of the eyes.

Domain	Symptoms	Treatment
Dystonia	Continuous spasms and muscle contractions	Anticholinergics PO or IM
Akathisia	Internal motor restlessness	Beta-blockers, benzodiazepines, clonidine, mirtazapine
Parkinsonism	Rigidity, bradykinesia, tremor	Anticholinergics, amantadine
Tardive dyskinesia	Involuntary muscle movements in the lower face and distal extremities	Vesicular monoamine transporter 2 inhibitors

NEUROLEPTIC MALIGNANT SYNDROME (NMS)

A 25-year-old M is started on haloperidol to treat psychosis in the inpatient psychiatric unit. A few days later, he develops high fever, confusion, rigid muscles, variable blood pressure, sweating, and elevated heart rate on exam.

Management:

1. Stop neuroleptics.
2. Rapid cooling.
3. Supportive care.
4. Pharmacologic:
   a. Dantrolene.
   b. Bromocriptine.
   c. Benzodiazepines.

HYF:

- Typical antipsychotics are more likely to cause NMS than atypicals.
- Catatonia is a risk factor for NMS.

SEROTONIN SYNDROME (SS)

A 40-year-old F presents to the emergency department with palpitations. She is found to have elevated blood pressure, elevated heart rate, fever, hyperreflexia, and myoclonus on exam. She reports that she is cross-titrating from an SSRI to an MAOI.

Management:

1. Stop serotonergic agents.
2. Supportive care.
3. Pharmacologic:
   a. Cyproheptadine.
   b. Benzodiazepines.

HYF:

- Typically caused by the use of 2 or more serotonergic medications.
- Serotonergic agents include not only antidepressants, but also opioids, CNS stimulants, 5-HT_1 agonists, psychedelics, some antipsychotics, and some antibiotics.

Characteristics of NMS versus Serotonin Syndrome

NMS	Serotonin Syndrome
Autonomic dysfunction	Autonomic dysfunction
Rigidity	No rigidity
No myoclonus	Myoclonus
No hyperreflexia	Hyperreflexia
Fever	Fever less prominent

27-7 Mood Disorders

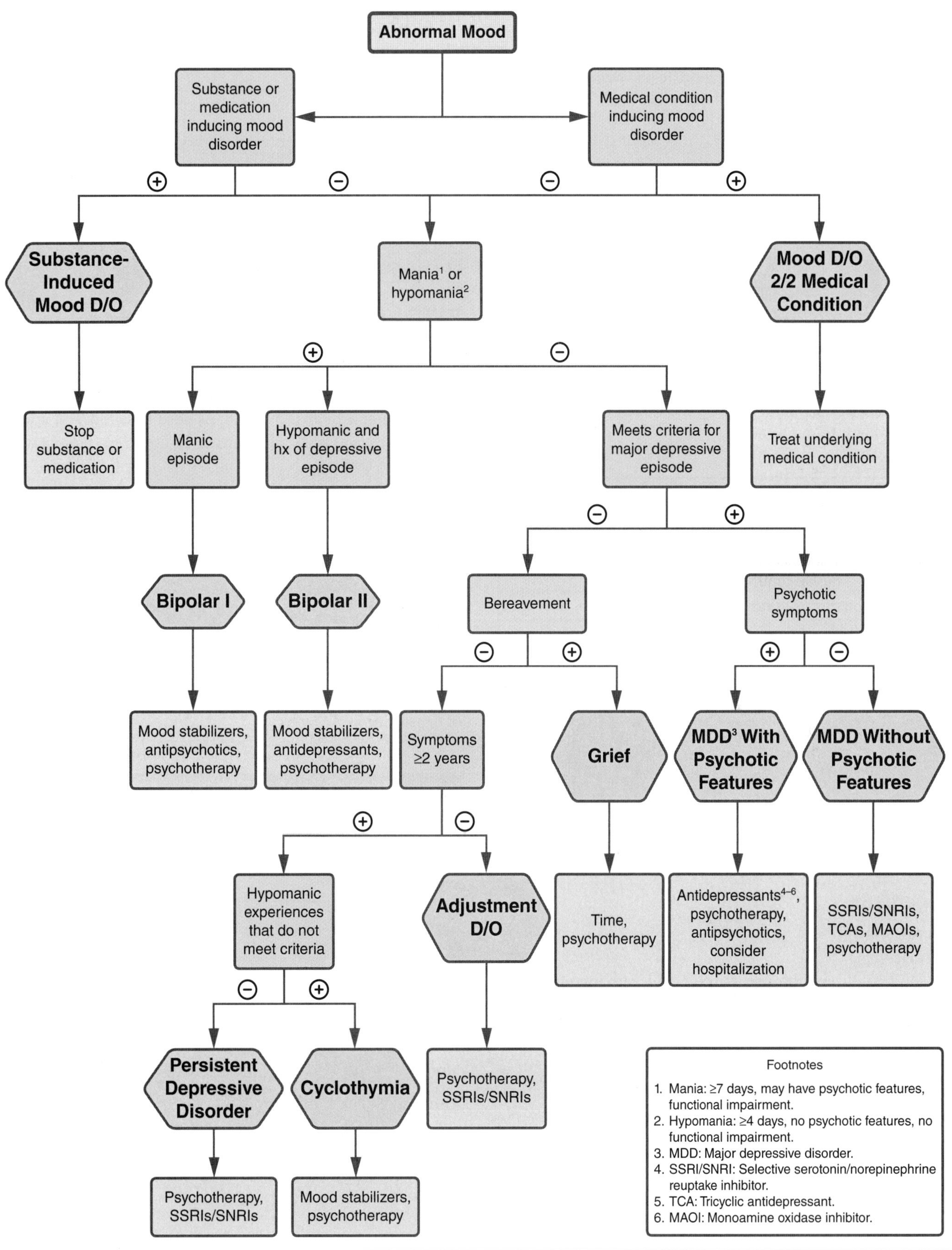
Abnormal Mood
Substance or medication inducing mood disorder
Medical condition inducing mood disorder
⊕
⊖
⊖
⊕
Substance-Induced Mood D/O
Mania[1] or hypomania[2]
Mood D/O 2/2 Medical Condition
⊕
⊖
Stop substance or medication
Manic episode
Hypomanic and hx of depressive episode
Meets criteria for major depressive episode
Treat underlying medical condition
⊖
⊕
Bipolar I
Bipolar II
Bereavement
Psychotic symptoms
⊖
⊕
⊕
⊖
Mood stabilizers, antipsychotics, psychotherapy
Mood stabilizers, antidepressants, psychotherapy
Symptoms ≥2 years
Grief
MDD[3] With Psychotic Features
MDD Without Psychotic Features
⊕
⊖
Hypomanic experiences that do not meet criteria
Adjustment D/O
Time, psychotherapy
Antidepressants[4–6], psychotherapy, antipsychotics, consider hospitalization
SSRIs/SNRIs, TCAs, MAOIs, psychotherapy
⊖
⊕
Persistent Depressive Disorder
Cyclothymia
Psychotherapy, SSRIs/SNRIs
Psychotherapy, SSRIs/SNRIs
Mood stabilizers, psychotherapy
Footnotes
1. Mania: ≥7 days, may have psychotic features, functional impairment.
2. Hypomania: ≥4 days, no psychotic features, no functional impairment.
3. MDD: Major depressive disorder.
4. SSRI/SNRI: Selective serotonin/norepinephrine reuptake inhibitor.
5. TCA: Tricyclic antidepressant.
6. MAOI: Monoamine oxidase inhibitor.

FIGURE 27.7

27-7 Mood Disorders

MAJOR DEPRESSIVE DISORDER (MDD)

A 50-year-old F presents to the outpatient office with 1 month of low mood, anhedonia, fatigue, poor appetite and sleep, and passive death wish. She has had similar episodes in the past.

Management

1. Risk assessment.
2. Psychotherapy.
3. Pharmacologic:
   a. SSRI/SNRI, bupropion or mirtazapine.
   b. TCA.
   c. MAOI.
4. For treatment refractory consider augmentation versus interventional treatments (TMS, ketamine, ECT).

HYF:

- Major depressive episode defined by low mood and 5 SIGECAPS symptoms for at least 2 weeks.

S	Sleep: Either increase or decrease
I	Interest: Loss of interest in activities
G	Guilt: Excessive guilt
E	Energy: Lack of energy, fatigue
C	Concentration: Difficulty concentrating
A	Appetite: Either increase or decrease
P	Psychomotor agitation/retardation
S	Suicidal ideation

BIPOLAR DISORDER I

A 25-year-old M is brought to ED by his girlfriend. For the past week, he has been sleeping 2 hours per night, quit his job to start his own business, and spent $10,000 on sports equipment. On exam, he talks quickly and jumps from one topic to another, sharing his plans to cure cancer and end world hunger.

Management:

1. Risk assessment.
2. Pharmacologic:
   a. Mood stabilizers (lithium, valproic acid, carbamazepine, lamotrigine).
   b. 2nd-generation antipsychotics.
3. ECT for treatment of refractory cases.

HYF: Diagnosis only requires 1 episode of mania.

D	Distractibility
I	Indiscretion/impulsivity: Spending money, sexual promiscuity
G	Grandiosity: Feeling on top of the world
F	Flight of ideas: Racing thoughts
A	Activity increase in goal-directed behavior
S	Sleep deficit: Decreased need for sleep
T	Talkative: Pressured speech

BIPOLAR DISORDER II

A 28-year-old F presents to the outpatient office with a recurrent depressive episode. She reports that before the current episode, she had a week-long period where she felt "on top of the world" and could accomplish anything, felt less need for sleep, and completed all her projects at work. Her partner commented that she was talking more at that time.

Management:

1. Risk assessment.
2. Psychotherapy.
3. Pharmacologic:
   a. Mood stabilizers.
   b. Antidepressants (combine with mood stabilizer to prevent manic switch).

HYF: Diagnosis requires ≥1 episode of hypomania and 1 episode of depression.

Mania	Hypomania
Elevated or irritable mood + 3/7 (4 for irritable mood) DIGFAST symptoms	Elevated or irritable mood + 3/7 (4 for irritable mood) DIGFAST symptoms
≥7 days	≥4 days
Psychotic features	No psychotic features
Hospitalization	No hospitalization
Functional impairment	No functional impairment

Substance-Induced Mood Disorder: See p. 782.

Mood Disorder 2/2 Medical Condition: See p. 782.

Adjustment Disorder: See p. 795.

27-8 Antidepressants

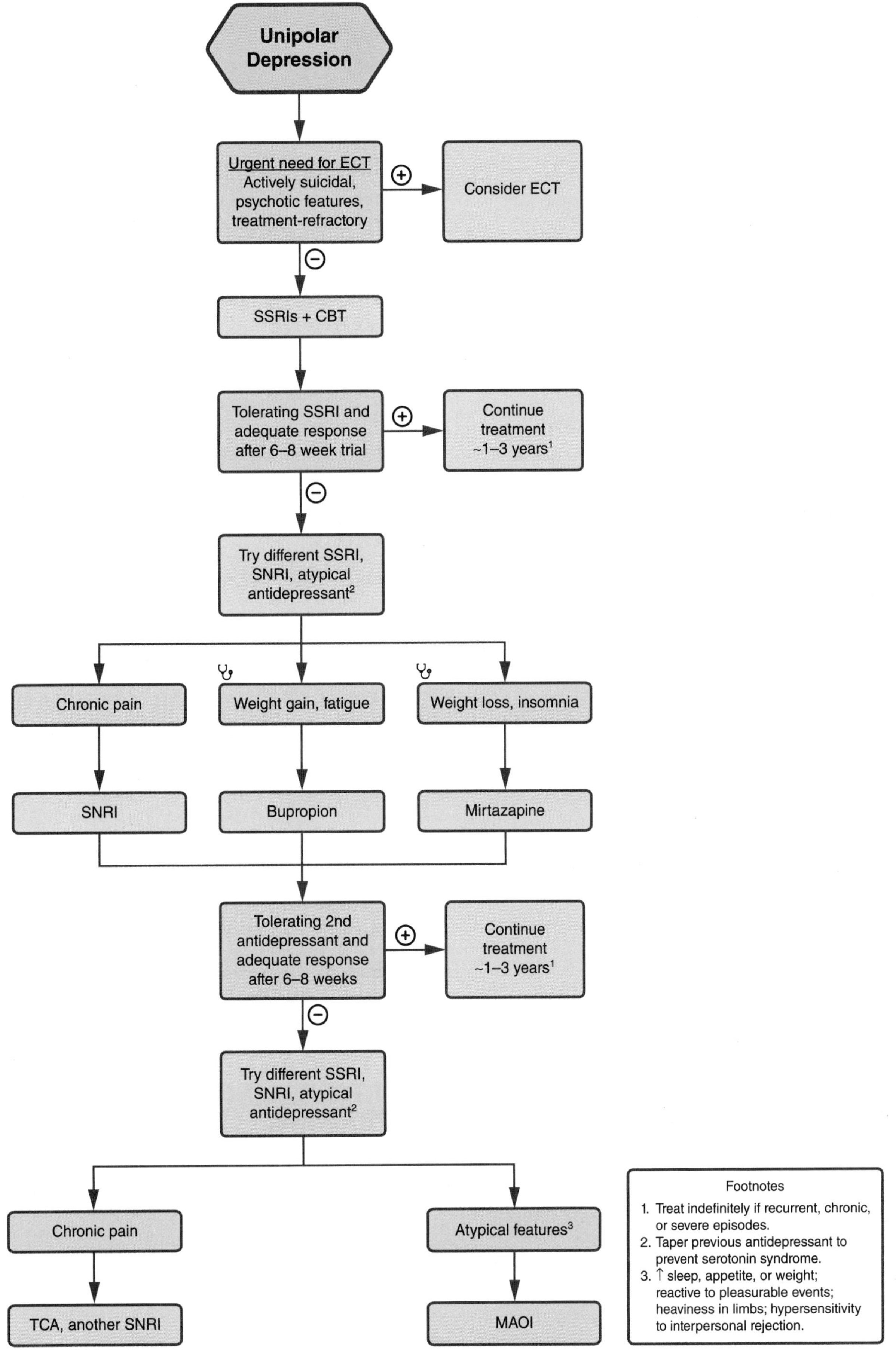
Unipolar Depression
Urgent need for ECT
Actively suicidal, psychotic features, treatment-refractory
⊕
Consider ECT
⊖
SSRIs + CBT
Tolerating SSRI and adequate response after 6–8 week trial
⊕
Continue treatment ~1–3 years[1]
⊖
Try different SSRI, SNRI, atypical antidepressant[2]
Chronic pain
Weight gain, fatigue
Weight loss, insomnia
SNRI
Bupropion
Mirtazapine
Tolerating 2nd antidepressant and adequate response after 6–8 weeks
⊕
Continue treatment ~1–3 years[1]
⊖
Try different SSRI, SNRI, atypical antidepressant[2]
Chronic pain
Atypical features[3]
TCA, another SNRI
MAOI
Footnotes
1. Treat indefinitely if recurrent, chronic, or severe episodes.
2. Taper previous antidepressant to prevent serotonin syndrome.
3. ↑ sleep, appetite, or weight; reactive to pleasurable events; heaviness in limbs; hypersensitivity to interpersonal rejection.

FIGURE 27.8

27-8 Antidepressants

SSRI (FLUOXETINE, SERTRALINE, PAROXETINE, CITALOPRAM, ESCITALOPRAM, FLUVOXAMINE)

Mechanism: Presynaptic serotonin reuptake inhibitor.

Indications:

1. Anxiety, OCD, social anxiety, panic disorder (long-term), PTSD, selective mutism.
2. Depression, adjustment disorder, persistent dysthymic disorder, pseudodementia, complex grief.
3. Premenstrual dysphoric disorder.
4. Bulimia, binge-eating disorder, body dysmorphic disorder.
5. Kleptomania, somatic symptom disorder.

Side Effects:

- Sexual side effects, GI distress, agitation, insomnia, tremor.
- Citalopram: Contraindicated in post-MI patients due to dose-dependent QT prolongation; choose sertraline or escitalopram.
- Paroxetine: Contraindicated in pregnancy due to fetal cardiac defects (1st trimester), pulmonary hypertension (3rd trimester).

HYF:

- SSRIs should be trialed for 6 weeks at full dose; change to a different SSRI or SNRI if inadequate response.
- Abrupt cessation: Discontinuation syndrome (flu-like symptoms, nausea, insomnia, brain zaps).
- Interactions with other serotonergic drugs and herbs (St. John's wort): Serotonin syndrome risk.

ATYPICAL ANTIDEPRESSANT: BUPROPION

A 27-year-old F with MDD has only a partial response to SSRI therapy and complains of weight gain, fatigue, hypersomnia, and sexual side effects. She is requesting an alternative agent.

Mechanism: Presynaptic dopamine and norepinephrine reuptake inhibitor (mild stimulant effect).

Indications:

1. Depression with inadequate response to SSRI, especially those with weight gain, fatigue, difficulty concentrating.
2. Nicotine withdrawal.

Side Effects: Decreased seizure threshold in patients with electrolyte abnormalities (anorexia or bulimia).

HYF: Contraindicated in seizure or eating disorder history. Can also be used for nicotine cessation or off-label for ADHD.

ATYPICAL ANTIDEPRESSANT: MIRTAZAPINE

Mechanism: 5-HT2, 5-HT3 receptor, alpha-2, H1 antagonist.

Indications:

1. Depression with inadequate response to SSRI, especially in those who are underweight or have insomnia.
2. Anxiety.
3. Insomnia.

Side Effects:

- Increased appetite and weight gain.
- Sedation.
- Dry mouth.

ATYPICAL ANTIDEPRESSANT: TRAZODONE

Mechanism: 5-HT2 receptor, alpha-1, H1 antagonist.

Indications:

1. Depression with inadequate response to SSRI, especially for patient with insomnia.
2. Anxiety, insomnia

Side Effects:

- Highly sedating.
- Priapism.
- Antiadrenergic: Orthostatic hypotension.

SNRI (DULOXETINE, VENLAFAXINE, DESVENLAFAXINE, MILNACIPRAN, LEVOMILNACIPRAN)

Mechanism: Presynaptic serotonin and norepinephrine reuptake inhibitor.

Indications:

1. Anxiety, panic disorder (long-term), PTSD.
2. Depression.
3. Neuropathic pain, fibromyalgia.

Side Effects: Venlafaxine: Diastolic hypertension at higher doses. Venlafaxine is also commonly associated with discontinuation syndrome when stopped abruptly. Rare hepatotoxicity with duloxetine.

TRICYCLIC ANTIDEPRESSANTS (NORTRIPTYLINE, DESIPRAMINE, IMIPRAMINE, CLOMIPRAMINE)

Mechanism: Presynaptic serotonin and norepinephrine reuptake inhibitor.

Indications:

1. Anxiety.
2. Depression with inadequate response to SSRI.
3. Migraine.
4. Enuresis.
5. OCD (clomipramine).

27-8 Antidepressants

Side Effects:

- Antihistamine effect: Sedation, weight gain.
- Anticholinergic: Dry mouth, tachycardia, urinary retention.
- Antiadrenergic: Orthostatic hypotension, dizziness.

HYF:

- Overdose can be lethal: Convulsion (seizure), coma, cardiotoxicity, respiratory depression, hyperpyrexia.
- Treat with sodium bicarbonate if QRS >100 msec, hypotensive, or arrhythmic.

MAOI (PHENELZINE, TRANYLCYPROMINE, SELEGILINE)

Mechanism: Inhibit monoamine oxidase, which leads to increased serotonin, dopamine, norepinephrine.

Indications:

1. Treatment-resistant depression.
2. Atypical depression.

Side Effects: Sexual side effects, orthostatic hypotension, weight gain.

HYF:

- Hypertensive crisis with high-tyramine foods (aged cheese, red wine).
- Serotonin syndrome risk.

27-9 Mood Stabilizers

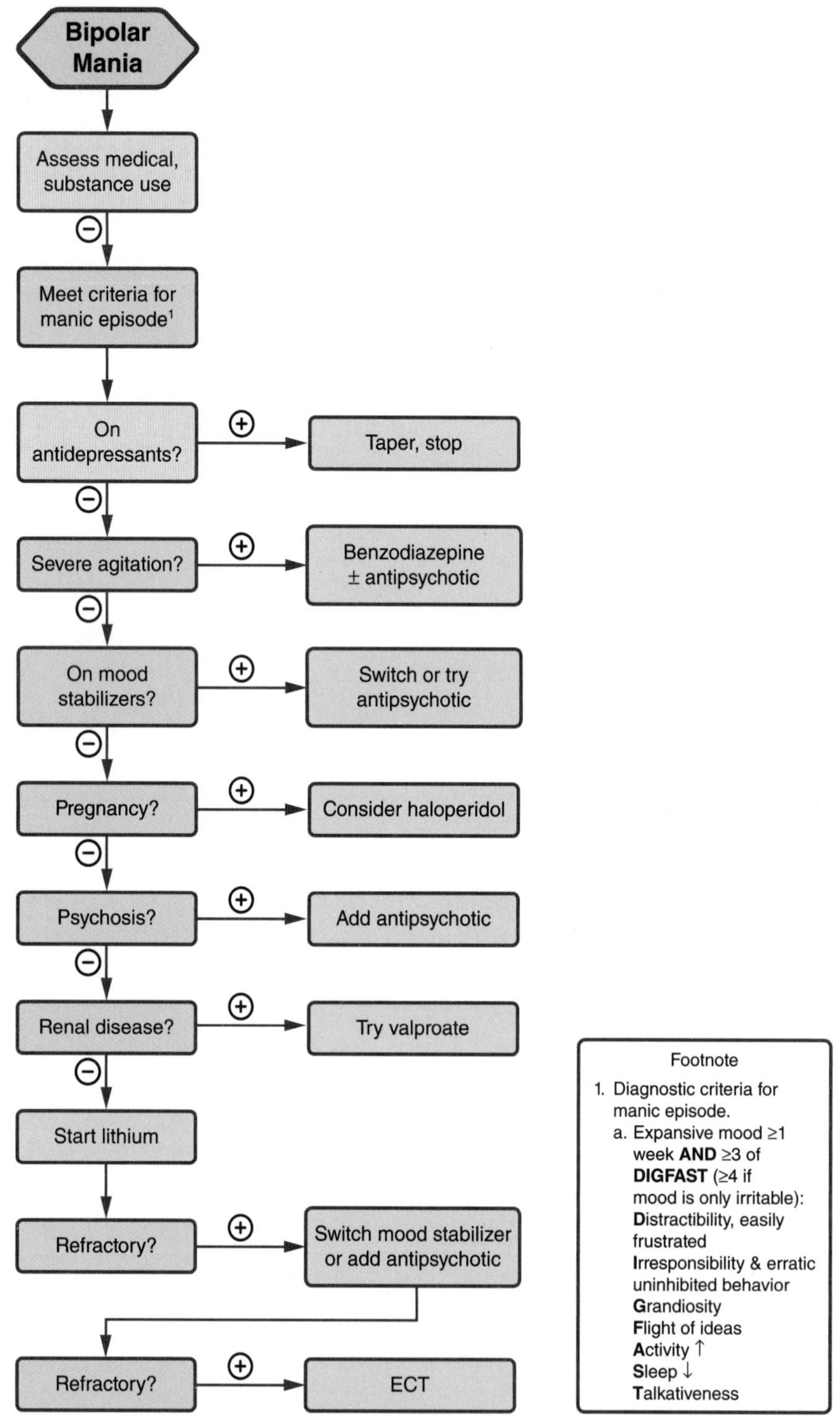
Bipolar Mania
Assess medical, substance use
⊖
Meet criteria for manic episode[1]
On antidepressants?
⊕
Taper, stop
⊖
Severe agitation?
⊕
Benzodiazepine ± antipsychotic
⊖
On mood stabilizers?
⊕
Switch or try antipsychotic
⊖
Pregnancy?
⊕
Consider haloperidol
⊖
Psychosis?
⊕
Add antipsychotic
⊖
Renal disease?
⊕
Try valproate
⊖
Start lithium
Refractory?
⊕
Switch mood stabilizer or add antipsychotic
Refractory?
⊕
ECT
Footnote
1. Diagnostic criteria for manic episode.
a. Expansive mood ≥1 week AND ≥3 of DIGFAST (≥4 if mood is only irritable):
Distractibility, easily frustrated
Irresponsibility & erratic uninhibited behavior
Grandiosity
Flight of ideas
Activity ↑
Sleep ↓
Talkativeness

FIGURE 27.9

27-9 Mood Stabilizers

LITHIUM

Toxicity: A 65-year-old M with PMH of mania and severe aggression presents to the ER with confusion, tremors, ataxia, and seizures on exam after starting thiazide diuretics.

Mechanism: Possibly related to inhibition of phosphoinositol-signaling pathway.

Indications:

1. 1st-line mood stabilizer for acute mania (in combination with antipsychotics if severe).
2. Maintenance therapy in bipolar disorder.
3. Reduces suicide risk.
4. Augmentation in depression treatment.

Side Effects:

- Nephrogenic diabetes insipidus.
- Hypothyroidism.
- Hyperparathyroidism.
- Lithium toxicity (blood level >1.5 mEq/L).
- Acute toxicity: GI distress, nausea, diarrhea, vomiting.
- Chronic toxicity: Confusion, agitation, ataxia, tremors, seizures.

HYF:

- Contraindicated in patients with ↓ renal function.
- Narrow therapeutic window (0.8–1.2 mEq/L).
- Dialysis indicated for lithium toxicity >4.
- Risk to fetus if used in pregnancy (Ebstein anomaly in 1st trimester).
- Drug interactions with thiazide diuretics, NSAIDs (except aspirin), ACE inhibitors, tetracyclines, metronidazole.

VALPROATE

A 35-year-old M with PMH of kidney disease presents to the ER with mania and severe aggression.

Mechanism: Sodium, calcium channel blocker, GABA agonist.

Indications:

1. 1st-line mood stabilizer.
2. 1st-line maintenance therapy for bipolar disorder.
3. Combine with antipsychotic in severe mania (psychotic features, aggression, DTS, DTO).

Side Effects:

- GI (nausea, vomiting), tremor, sedation, alopecia, weight gain, teratogenicity (3–5% risk for neural tube defect), hyperammonemia.
- Pancreatitis, thrombocytopenia, fatal hepatotoxicity, and agranulocytosis (rare).

HYF: Avoid in liver disease, thrombocytopenia and pregnancy.

ATYPICAL ANTIPSYCHOTICS (QUETIAPINE, OLANZAPINE)

Mechanism: Antagonize both 5-HT2A and D2 receptors.

Indications:

1. 2nd line in acute mania.
2. 1st-line maintenance treatment in bipolar disorder.
3. Combined with valproate or lithium for maintenance therapy in bipolar disorder.

Side Effects: See "Antipsychotics," pp. 783–784.

HYF: Quetiapine dosed at nighttime helps with sleep. Other atypicals approved for bipolar maintenance include: Risperidone, Aripiprazole, Cariprazine, Lurasidone, Asenapine.

LAMOTRIGINE

Mechanism: Sodium channel blockade, inhibits glutamate release.

Indications:

1. 2nd-line mood stabilizer for acute mania.
2. 1st line for maintenance treatment in bipolar disorder.

Side Effects: Blurred vision, GI distress, Stevens-Johnson syndrome. ↑ dose slowly to monitor for rashes.

HYF: Primarily an anticonvulsant. If using with valproate, halve the dose of lamotrigine as valproate can double lamotrigine levels.

CARBAMAZEPINE

Mechanism: Sodium channel blocker.

Indications:

1. 3rd line for acute mania.

Side Effects:

- Nausea, skin rash, agranulocytosis, AV block. Teratogenicity (0.5–1% neural tube defect).
- Blood dyscrasias like aplastic anemia.
- DRESS, Stevens-Johnson syndrome (rare).

HYF: Cytochrome P450 inducer.

ECT

Mechanism: Neurophysiological and neurochemical change in the brain modeling and perfusion.

Indications:

- Refractory manic episode, mixed episode in bipolar disorder.
- Schizoaffective disorder.
- Schizophrenia with catatonia.
- Highly suicidal patients.
- Treatment-refractory depression.
- MDD with psychotic features.

Side Effects:

- Reversible retrograde or anterograde memory loss.
- Tension headache.
- Transient muscle loss.

HYF: Generally safe in all populations, including pregnancy.

27-10 Anxiety Disorders

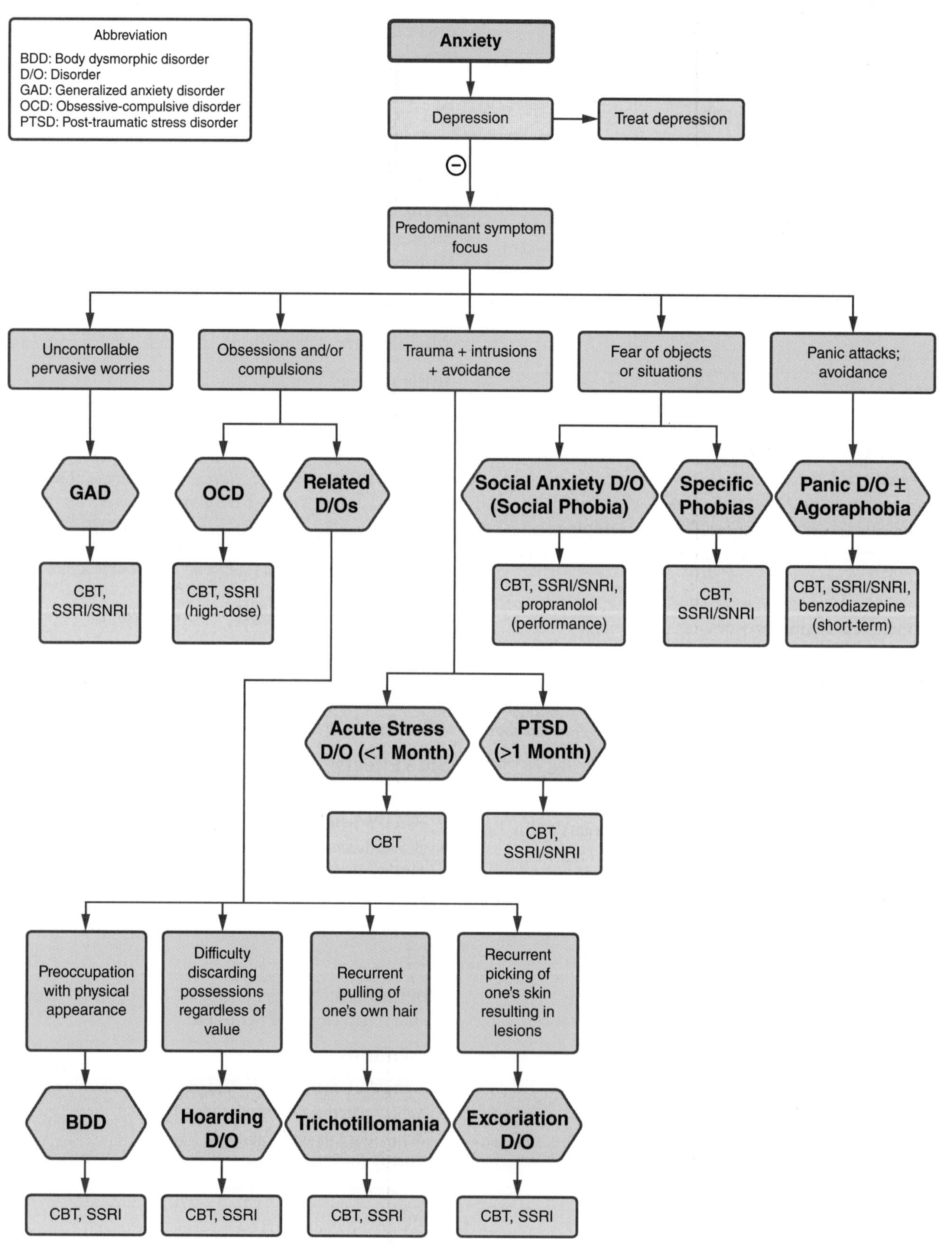
Abbreviation
BDD: Body dysmorphic disorder
D/O: Disorder
GAD: Generalized anxiety disorder
OCD: Obsessive-compulsive disorder
PTSD: Post-traumatic stress disorder
Anxiety
Depression
Treat depression
⊖
Predominant symptom focus
Uncontrollable pervasive worries
Obsessions and/or compulsions
Trauma + intrusions + avoidance
Fear of objects or situations
Panic attacks; avoidance
GAD
OCD
Related D/Os
Social Anxiety D/O (Social Phobia)
Specific Phobias
Panic D/O ± Agoraphobia
CBT, SSRI/SNRI
CBT, SSRI (high-dose)
CBT, SSRI/SNRI, propranolol (performance)
CBT, SSRI/SNRI
CBT, SSRI/SNRI, benzodiazepine (short-term)
Acute Stress D/O (<1 Month)
PTSD (>1 Month)
CBT
CBT, SSRI/SNRI
Preoccupation with physical appearance
Difficulty discarding possessions regardless of value
Recurrent pulling of one's own hair
Recurrent picking of one's skin resulting in lesions
BDD
Hoarding D/O
Trichotillomania
Excoriation D/O
CBT, SSRI
CBT, SSRI
CBT, SSRI
CBT, SSRI

FIGURE 27.10

27-10 Anxiety Disorders

ANXIETY DISORDERS

1. Significant functional impairment.
2. R/O medical condition- or substance/medication-induced.

If indicated (eg, catatonia, panic), benzodiazepines for short-term use only; monitor for withdrawal; avoid in substance use

GENERALIZED ANXIETY DISORDER (GAD)

A 30-year-old F presents with 6+ months of uncontrollable worry about multiple issues and 3+ symptoms (1 in children): Restlessness/on edge, irritability, disturbed sleep, fatigue, difficulty concentrating, muscle tension.

Management:

1. CBT, SSRI/SNRI.
2. Buspirone, benzodiazepines.

OBSESSIVE-COMPULSIVE DISORDER

A 30-year-old F with obsessions and/or compulsions, eg, contamination/cleaning, safety/checking, symmetry/ordering, intrusive sexual/violent thoughts. She spends several hours per day performing her compulsions and is significantly distressed by them.

Management:

1. CBT (exposure & response prevention), SSRI.
2. TCA (clomipramine).
3. Deep brain stimulation for severe or refractory cases.

HYF: Abnormal orbitofrontal cortex and striatum. OCD is ego-dystonic versus OCPD which is ego-syntonic.

SOCIAL ANXIETY DISORDER (SOCIAL PHOBIA)

A 30-year-old F presents with 6+ months of irrational fear of public scrutiny/humiliation in social situations, leading to intense anxiety/avoidance of social situations. Performance-only subtype: Fear of public speaking/presentations.

Management:

1. CBT, SSRI/SNRIs.
2. Beta-blockers (propranolol for performance subtype; avoid in asthma).

SPECIFIC PHOBIAS

A 30-year-old F presents with 6+ months of irrational fear of a certain object/situation, leading to intense anxiety/avoidance of feared object/situation, eg, needles, elevators, snakes, heights.

Management:

1. CBT (exposure techniques/systematic desensitization).
2. SSRI/SNRIs, benzodiazepines.

Complications: Vasovagal syncope in needle injections.

HYF: Panic disorder may present with agoraphobia (fear of being in public where escape may be hard).

PANIC DISORDER ± AGORAPHOBIA

A 25-year-old M presents with recurrent unexpected panic attacks. 1+ month of fear of additional panic attacks and/or avoidance of panic attack triggers.

Management:

1. CBT (graded exposure), SSRI/SNRIs.
2. TCAs (imipramine, clomipramine), benzodiazepines.

HYF: Decreased amygdala volume.

ACUTE STRESS DISORDER

1. Trauma occurred <1 month ago.
2. PTSD symptoms last between 3 days and 1 month.

Management: Same as PTSD management.

ADJUSTMENT DISORDER

1. Onset of depressed mood, anxiety, and/or disturbance of conduct within 3 months of stressor.
2. Resolution within 6 months of stressor termination

Management: Supportive therapy only.

POST-TRAUMATIC STRESS DISORDER (PTSD)

A 20-year-old M presents with direct or witnessed exposure to death, serious injury or sexual violence and 1+ month of intrusions, avoidance, negative thoughts/mood, hyperarousal.

Management:

1. CBT (exposure therapy, cognitive processing therapy), SSRI/SNRI.
2. Alpha-1 receptor antagonist (prazosin, doxazosin) for nightmares.

HYF: Decreased hippocampal volume.

BODY DYSMORPHIC DISORDER (BDD)

Preoccupation with imagined defect in physical appearance → repetitive behaviors to fix appearance concerns.

Management: CBT, SSRIs; avoid surgery.

HOARDING DISORDER

Difficulty discarding possessions regardless of value/distress associated with discarding.

27-11 Anxiolytics

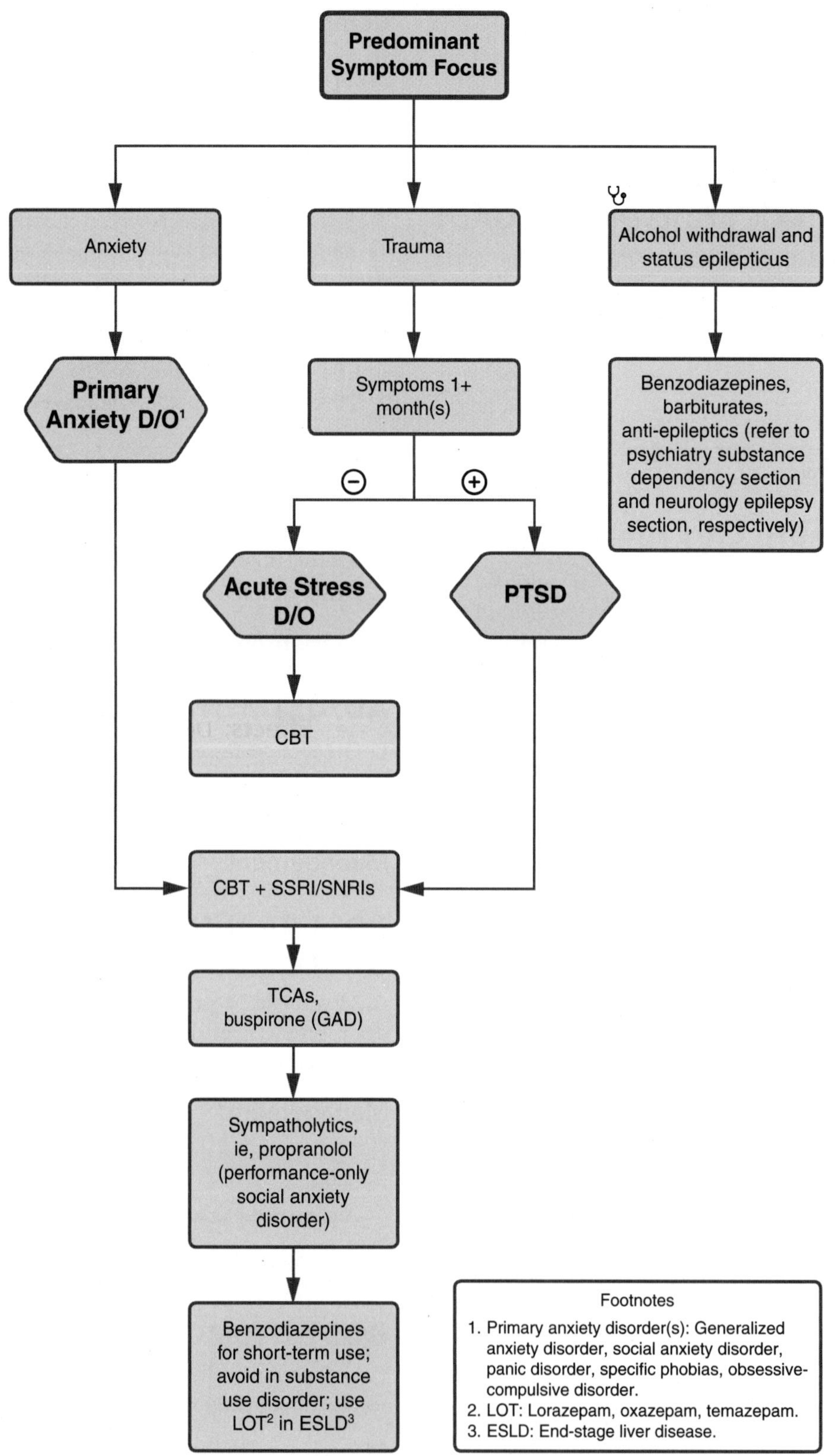

Predominant Symptom Focus
Anxiety
Trauma
Alcohol withdrawal and status epilepticus
Primary Anxiety D/O[1]
Symptoms 1+ month(s)
Benzodiazepines, barbiturates, anti-epileptics (refer to psychiatry substance dependency section and neurology epilepsy section, respectively)
⊖
⊕
Acute Stress D/O
PTSD
CBT
CBT + SSRI/SNRIs
TCAs, buspirone (GAD)
Sympatholytics, ie, propranolol (performance-only social anxiety disorder)
Benzodiazepines for short-term use; avoid in substance use disorder; use LOT[2] in ESLD[3]
Footnotes
1. Primary anxiety disorder(s): Generalized anxiety disorder, social anxiety disorder, panic disorder, specific phobias, obsessive-compulsive disorder.
2. LOT: Lorazepam, oxazepam, temazepam.
3. ESLD: End-stage liver disease.

FIGURE 27.11

27-11 Anxiolytics & Hypnotics

BENZODIAZEPINES

Mechanism: GABA-A receptor agonists act by increasing binding frequency of the Cl^- channel opening.

Indication(s): Anxiety, agitation, panic attacks, performance-only social anxiety disorder (SAD), alcohol withdrawal, catatonia.

Side Effects: Anterograde amnesia, drowsiness, dizziness, confusion, hangover effect, habit-forming potential, paradoxical agitation.

HYF: Antidote for overdose is flumazenil; death from overdose rare without concurrent use of CNS depressant; LOT (lorazepam, oxazepam, temazepam) are NOT metabolized by the liver; ATOM (alprazolam, triazolam, oxazepam, midazolam) have short half-lives.

BENZODIAZEPINE-LIKE SUBSTANCES (Z-DRUGS)

Mechanism: Selective for GABA-A receptors with onset or maintenance α1 subunits.

Indication(s): Primary insomnia.

Side Effects: Ataxia, headaches, confusion, hangover effect, habit-forming potential (lower risk than benzodiazepines).

HYF: Antidote for overdose is flumazenil. Examples includes: zaleplon, eszopiclone, zolpidem.

BARBITURATES

Mechanism: GABA-A receptor agonists (binding site different from that of benzodiazepines) by increasing binding duration Cl^- channel opening.

Indication(s): Seizures/status epilepticus, alcohol withdrawal, general anesthesia.

Side Effects: Hypotension, respiratory depression, habit-forming potential. Examples include: Phenobarbital, primidone.

MELATONIN AGONISTS

Mechanism: Activation of MT1 and MT2 receptors in the suprachiasmatic nuclei of the hypothalamus.

Indication(s): Primary insomnia, circadian rhythm disorders, jet lag.

Side Effects: Headache, dizziness, nausea, fatigue, arthralgias, angioedema (rare). Examples include: Ramelteon, agomelatine.

DUAL OREXIN RECEPTOR ANTAGONISTS

Mechanism: Antagonism of orexin (hypocretin) receptors.

Indication(s): Primary maintenance or mixed insomnia.

Side Effects: Sleep disturbances, suicidal thoughts, headache, somnolence, habit-forming potential (low risk). Examples include: suvorexant, lemborexant, daridorexant).

PROPRANOLOL

Mechanism: Non-selective beta-blocker.

Indication(s): Performance-only SAD, essential tremor, migraine prophylaxis, akathisia.

Side Effects: Decrease heart rate and blood pressure, bronchoconstriction.

PRAZOSIN

Mechanism: Selective α1 antagonist.

Indication(s): PTSD-related nightmares.

Side Effects: Orthostatic hypotension, syncope, priapism.

BUSPIRONE

Mechanism: 5-HT1A receptor stimulation.

Indication(s): GAD.

Side Effects: Nausea, dizziness, headache, somnolence, MI (rare), CVA (rare).

Typical/Atypical Antidepressants: See pp. 789–791.

27-12 Substance Use Disorders

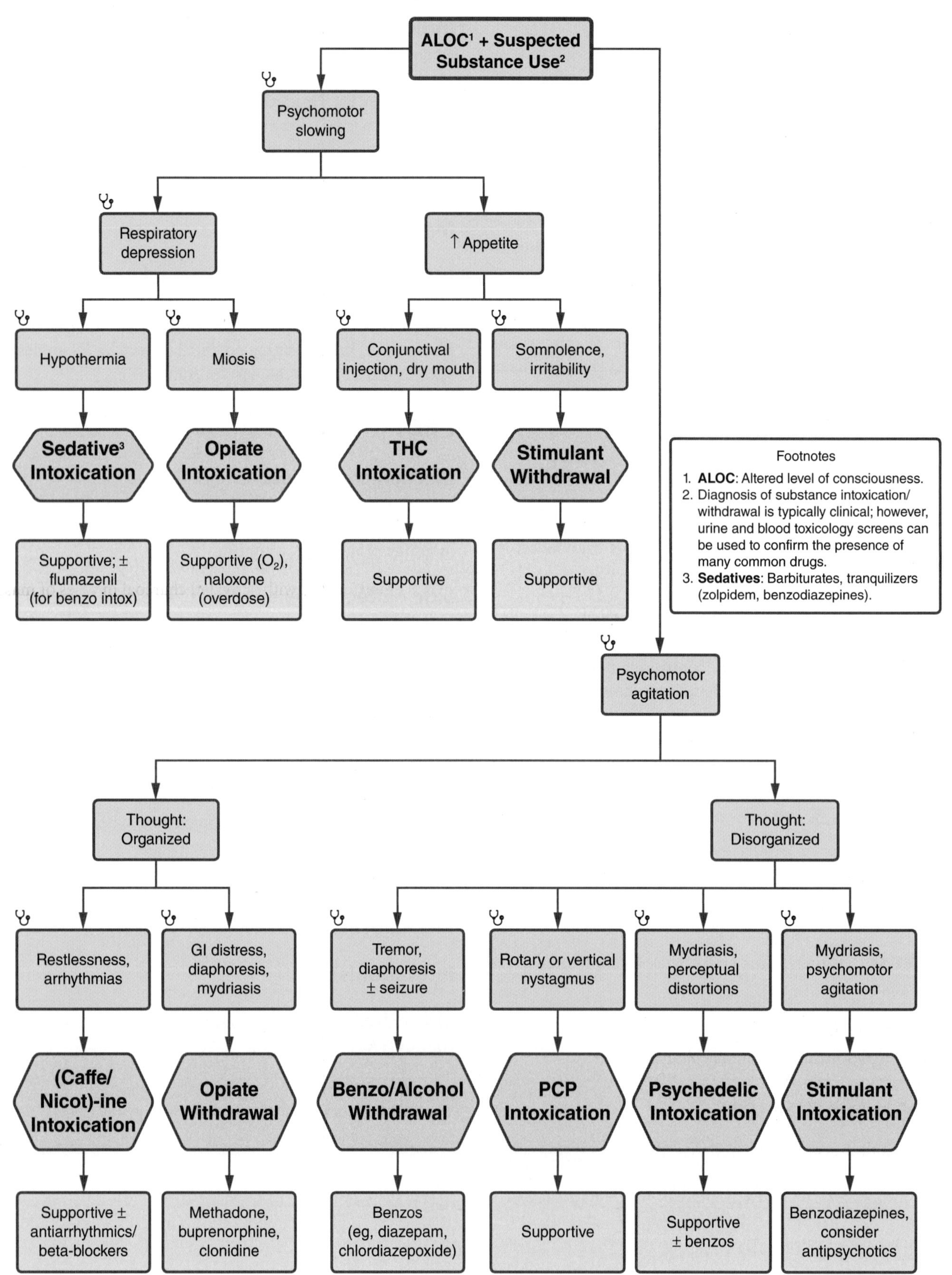

ALOC[1] + Suspected Substance Use[2]
Psychomotor slowing
Respiratory depression
↑ Appetite
Hypothermia
Miosis
Conjunctival injection, dry mouth
Somnolence, irritability
Sedative[3] Intoxication
Opiate Intoxication
THC Intoxication
Stimulant Withdrawal
Supportive; ± flumazenil (for benzo intox)
Supportive (O_2), naloxone (overdose)
Supportive
Supportive
Footnotes
1. **ALOC**: Altered level of consciousness.
2. Diagnosis of substance intoxication/withdrawal is typically clinical; however, urine and blood toxicology screens can be used to confirm the presence of many common drugs.
3. **Sedatives**: Barbiturates, tranquilizers (zolpidem, benzodiazepines).
Psychomotor agitation
Thought: Organized
Thought: Disorganized
Restlessness, arrhythmias
GI distress, diaphoresis, mydriasis
Tremor, diaphoresis ± seizure
Rotary or vertical nystagmus
Mydriasis, perceptual distortions
Mydriasis, psychomotor agitation
(Caffe/Nicot)-ine Intoxication
Opiate Withdrawal
Benzo/Alcohol Withdrawal
PCP Intoxication
Psychedelic Intoxication
Stimulant Intoxication
Supportive ± antiarrhythmics/beta-blockers
Methadone, buprenorphine, clonidine
Benzos (eg, diazepam, chlordiazepoxide)
Supportive
Supportive ± benzos
Benzodiazepines, consider antipsychotics

FIGURE 27.12

27-12 Substance Use Disorders

ALCOHOL WITHDRAWAL – ACUTE (DELIRIUM TREMENS)

A 55-year-old M presents to the ED with BP 180/110, HR 130, disorientation, tremors, and auditory hallucinations on exam. Blood alcohol concentration >0.3. Last known drink was 72 hours ago.

Management:

1. Stabilize electrolytes, vitals.
2. Thiamine (to prevent Wernicke's encephalopathy), glucose, folic acid.
3. Benzodiazepines (eg, lorazepam, chlordiazepoxide if no liver failure) or phenobarbital.
4. Antipsychotics as needed for agitation.
5. Long term: Substance-use treatment.

Complications:

- Severe agitation and violence.
- Seizures, arrhythmias.

HYF: Delirium tremens onset 48–96 hours after last drink vs. alcoholic hallucinosis 12–24 hours.

CHRONIC ALCOHOL USE DISORDER

A 60-year-old M with history of chronic alcohol use presents with abdominal pain and ataxia. On exam they have palmar erythema, telangiectasias and horizontal nystagmus.

Management:

1. Electrolyte repletion, glucose, parenteral thiamine, folic acid, multivitamins.
2. Long term treatment for AUD includes pharmacological and psychosocial interventions.
3. Pharmacological: Naltrexone for cravings, acamprosate, disulfiram, topiramate.
4. Psychosocial: Motivational interviewing, cognitive behavioral therapy, 12-step programs, psychoeducation, contingency management.

Complications:

- GI bleeds, ulcers, varices, Mallory-Weiss tears.
- Pancreatitis, liver failure.
- Fetal alcohol syndrome.
- Cardiomyopathy, anemia.
- Wernicke-Korsakoff syndrome.

HYF: Naltrexone blocks the mu-opioid receptor and helps reduce the craving for alcohol. Patients who continue drinking can still use it. CAGE questionnaire: **C**ut down, **A**nnoyed, **G**uilty, **E**ye opener.

STIMULANT INTOXICATION

A 30-year-old M with polysubstance abuse history and no history of psychosis presents with exam findings of agitation, dilated pupils, elevated HR and BP, and delusions of grandeur. **Labs** are notable for + amphetamine.

Management:

1. Stabilize vitals, fluids.
2. Benzodiazepines.
3. Antipsychotics as needed for agitation.
4. Long term: Substance-use treatment.

Complications:

- Agitation, seizures, acute coronary syndrome, stroke.
- Withdrawal syndrome: Dysphoria, somnolence, anxiety.

HYF: Commonly abused common stimulants that can present with psychosis: Methamphetamine, phencyclidine (PCP), cocaine.

PCP INTOXICATION

A 21-year-old M is brought in by police for assault and hallucinations. On exam, he is noted to have hypertension, tachycardia, and vertical nystagmus.

Management:

1. Stabilize vitals, fluids.
2. Benzodiazepines.
3. Antipsychotics as needed for agitation.
4. Decontamination with activated charcoal in cases of massive ingestion.

HYF: Overdose can be life-threatening. Symptoms can recur after reabsorption of the drug in the GI tract.

BENZODIAZEPINE INTOXICATION

A 44-year-old F with a history of panic attacks is brought in by her husband as she has been stuporous, minimally responsive, and drowsy.

Management:

1. Supportive care. Monitor respiratory status. Naloxone for possible concomitant opioid intoxication.
2. Flumanezil in select patient populations (no seizure hx, no chronic benzo use, requiring intubation).

HYF: In general, benzodiazepine intoxication is benign, and patients can "sleep off" the overdose. Benzodiazepine withdrawal, on the other hand, can be life-threatening (seizures) and necessitates treatment with long-acting benzodiazepines (eg, clonazepam, diazepam) to taper off dose.

27-13 Somatoform, Factitious & Related Disorders

SOMATIC SYMPTOM DISORDER

A 23-year-old M presents with 2 years of multiple chronic complaints including fatigue, nausea, and headache. He spends much of the day worrying about his symptoms and researching them online. Extensive medical/neurological workup is negative.

Management:

1. Establishment with a single provider as designated point of contact (primary team while admitted to hospital, PCP on an outpatient basis) with frequent communication.
2. Setting clear boundaries for not pursuing unnecessary tests or inappropriate medical/surgical treatments.
3. CBT, mindfulness-based therapy, consider SSRIs, TCAs.

Complications: Excessive invasive diagnostic tests and inappropriate medical or surgical treatments.

HYF: One or more symptom(s) must be present for ≥6 months. However, the same symptoms do not have to be constantly present during this period. Associated with excessive thoughts and anxiety and cause significant time and energy devoted to the symptoms.

CONVERSION DISORDER

A 28-year-old F presents with bilateral upper extremity weakness. She reports frequently dropping items. On exam, she has 3/5 strength and give-way weakness in her upper extremities. When she is asked to hold arms outstretched with palms up, her arms drift downward while palms remain face up in supination. She is observed opening and closing doors and using her phone without difficulty.

Management:

1. Psychotherapy and physical therapy with a focus on regaining function even if symptoms persist.

Complications: Excessive invasive diagnostic tests and inappropriate medical or surgical treatments.

HYF:

- Defined as motor or sensory symptoms with clinical findings incompatible with recognized medical conditions. Can occur in tandem with real neurological disease (ie. patient with real seizures and PNES).
- Seizure-like spells = psychogenic non-epileptic spells (PNES).
- Other neurologic symptoms = functional neurological disorder (FND).
- *La belle indifference*: Patients seem unconcerned by their symptoms.

ILLNESS ANXIETY DISORDER

A 38-year-old M presents to his PCP with concerns that he may have cancer for the past 12 months. His uncle died of pancreatic cancer 2 years ago. He frequently worries that he has undetected cancer and spends many hours each week looking up symptoms of cancer. He denies any symptoms. Exam and screening labs are normal. He requests a full body CT to look for occult cancer.

Management:

1. Regular follow up and therapeutic alliance. Limit diagnostic testing and referrals.
2. Psychotherapy: CBT, ACT or mindfulness therapy.
3. If refractory, SSRIs/SNRIs.

Complications: Excessive invasive diagnostic tests and inappropriate medical or surgical treatments.

HYF:

- Differs from somatic symptoms disorder in that minimal or no symptoms are present in illness anxiety disorder.
- The anxiety may resemble obsessions but differs from OCD because no anxiety-relieving compulsions are present.
- Patients may perform excessive health-related behaviors (eg, weighing self daily to ensure no abnormal weight loss) or develop maladaptive avoidance patterns (eg, avoiding doctors' appointments for fear of bad health news).

FACTITIOUS DISORDER

A 25-year-old F in nursing school presents via EMS after a witnessed seizure at the mall. She is hospitalized and started on levetiracetam (Keppra). EEG and brain MRI are unremarkable. She is stable throughout admission. On day of discharge, patient has a tonic-clonic seizure. An empty insulin syringe is found in her bed. Insulin to C-peptide ratio is >1.

Management:

1. Sitter to observe patient behavior and intervene if potentially harmful behavior is observed.
2. If factitious disorder is imposed on another, legal services (eg, child protective services) may need to be involved.
3. Psychotherapy is the only known treatment, though engagement is often poor.

Complications: Significant bodily harm or death from induced symptoms.

HYF:

- Higher frequency in individuals who work in healthcare.
- Driven by primary gain of taking the sick role.
- Can be imposed on self or another (Munchausen by proxy).

MALINGERING

A 38-year-old M presents with depression and suicidal ideation with plan to jump off a bridge. He is unhoused and unemployed. He is admitted to the inpatient psychiatric unit where he declines medications. He is pleasant euthymic and engaged on the unit. The treatment team discusses his positive progress and suggests discharge the following day. Later that day, he attempts to cut his wrist with a plastic knife in front of the nursing station.

Management:

1. Avoid reinforcement of behavior. Careful and thorough risk assesment and documentation.

Complications: Misuse of medical system for secondary gain.

HYF: Examples of secondary gain: Time off from work, gifts, housing, disability benefits, improved chances of success in a lawsuit, avoidance of incarceration, shelter.

27-14 Eating Disorders

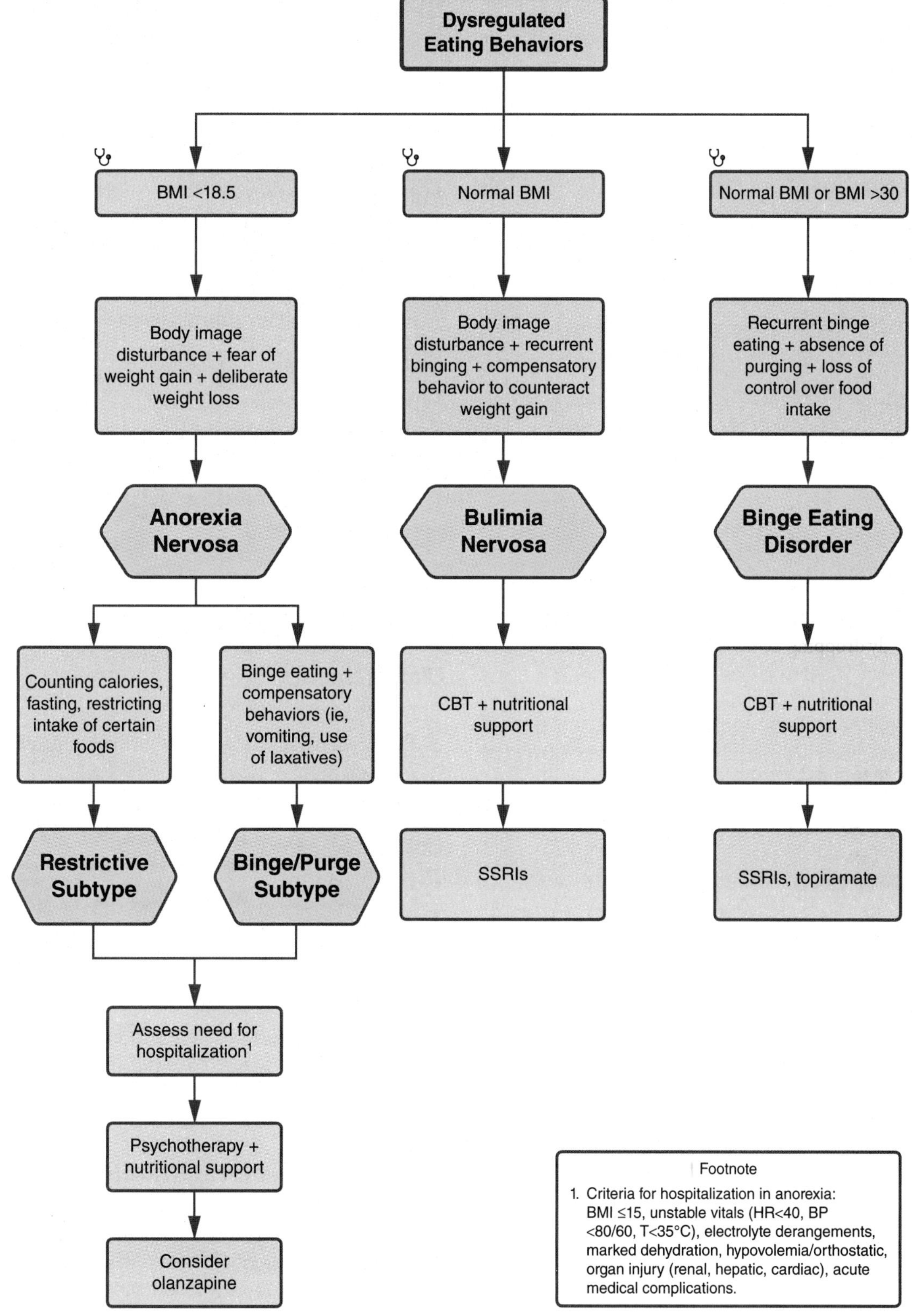
Dysregulated Eating Behaviors
BMI <18.5
Normal BMI
Normal BMI or BMI >30
Body image disturbance + fear of weight gain + deliberate weight loss
Body image disturbance + recurrent binging + compensatory behavior to counteract weight gain
Recurrent binge eating + absence of purging + loss of control over food intake
Anorexia Nervosa
Bulimia Nervosa
Binge Eating Disorder
Counting calories, fasting, restricting intake of certain foods
Binge eating + compensatory behaviors (ie, vomiting, use of laxatives)
CBT + nutritional support
CBT + nutritional support
Restrictive Subtype
Binge/Purge Subtype
SSRIs
SSRIs, topiramate
Assess need for hospitalization1
Psychotherapy + nutritional support
Consider olanzapine
Footnote
1. Criteria for hospitalization in anorexia: BMI ≤15, unstable vitals (HR<40, BP <80/60, T<35°C), electrolyte derangements, marked dehydration, hypovolemia/orthostatic, organ injury (renal, hepatic, cardiac), acute medical complications.

FIGURE 27.14

27-14 Eating Disorders

ANOREXIA NERVOSA

A 20-year-old F with BMI <18.5, body image disturbance/fear of weight gain, deliberate reduction in body mass.

- Restricting subtype: Counting calories, fasting, restricting intake of certain foods.
- Binge/purge subtype: Binge eating or purging behaviors such as vomiting, use of laxatives.

Management:

1. Hospitalize if needed.
2. 1st line: CBT + nutritional support.
3. Adjunctive pharmacotherapy (olanzapine, treat comorbid diagnoses).

Complications:

- Secondary amenorrhea.
- Secondary osteoporosis.
- Euthyroid sick syndrome.
- Lanugo body hair.
- Cardiovascular remodeling, gastroparesis, Wernicke-Korsakoff syndrome.
- Russell sign/dental caries/metabolic alkalosis (binge/purge subtype).

HYF:

- Refeeding syndrome (increase in glucose intake → excessive insulin release → hypomagnesemia, hypokalemia, hypophosphatemia → arrhythmias, seizures).
- Antidepressant bupropion lowers seizure threshold and is contraindicated.

BULIMIA NERVOSA

A 20-year-old M with normal BMI, presents with recurrent binge eating and compulsive exercise and laxative use to counteract weight gain.

Management:

1. 1st line: CBT + nutritional support.
2. SSRIs.

Complications:

- Cardiac arrhythmias.
- Seizures.
- Hypotension.
- Sialadenosis.
- Esophagitis/gastritis.
- Mallory-Weiss syndrome.
- Russell sign/dental caries/metabolic alkalosis.

BINGE EATING DISORDER

A 30-year-old obese M presents with recurrent binge eating without purging behavior, loss of control over food intake with 3+ symptoms: Faster-than-normal eating, eating until uncomfortably full, eating large amounts when not hungry, eating alone due to shame, feeling of disgust/guilt after eating.

Management:

1. 1st line: Guided self-help (CBT-based), interpersonal psychotherapy, nutritional support.
2. Adjunctive pharmacotherapy: SSRIs, topiramate, can consider lisdexamfetamine, methylphenidate.

Complications:

- Metabolic syndrome (HTN, HLD, DM2).
- Cardiovascular disease.

HYF: Emotional distress centers around binge eating but not about weight/physical appearance.

PICA

A 30-year-old pregnant F presents with 1+ month of appetite for and ingestion of non-nutritive substances (ie, hair, ice, clay, paint).

Management:

1. CBC, ferritin.
2. Harm reduction strategies, behavioral interventions, nutritional support.
3. Consider SSRIs.

Complications:

- Lead poisoning 2/2 ingested paint.
- GI infections/obstruction/perforation.

AVOIDANT RESTRICTIVE FOOD INTAKE DISORDER (ARFID)

A 10-year-old F with disinterest in eating/avoidance of food (ie, dislikes texture of food), resulting in persistent failure to meet nutritional needs (significant weight loss, nutritional deficiency, dependence on enteral feeding or oral nutritional supplementation).

RUMINATION DISORDER

A 20-year-old F with 1+ month of repeated regurgitation of ingested food during/after meal (regurgitated food can be rechewed/swallowed or spit out).

OTHER SPECIFIED FEEDING AND EATING DISORDER (OSFED)

A 20-year-old M with eating disorder characteristics (ie, body image disturbances, dysregulated eating behaviors) NOT meeting DSM criteria for other eating disorders.

27-15 Sleep Disorders

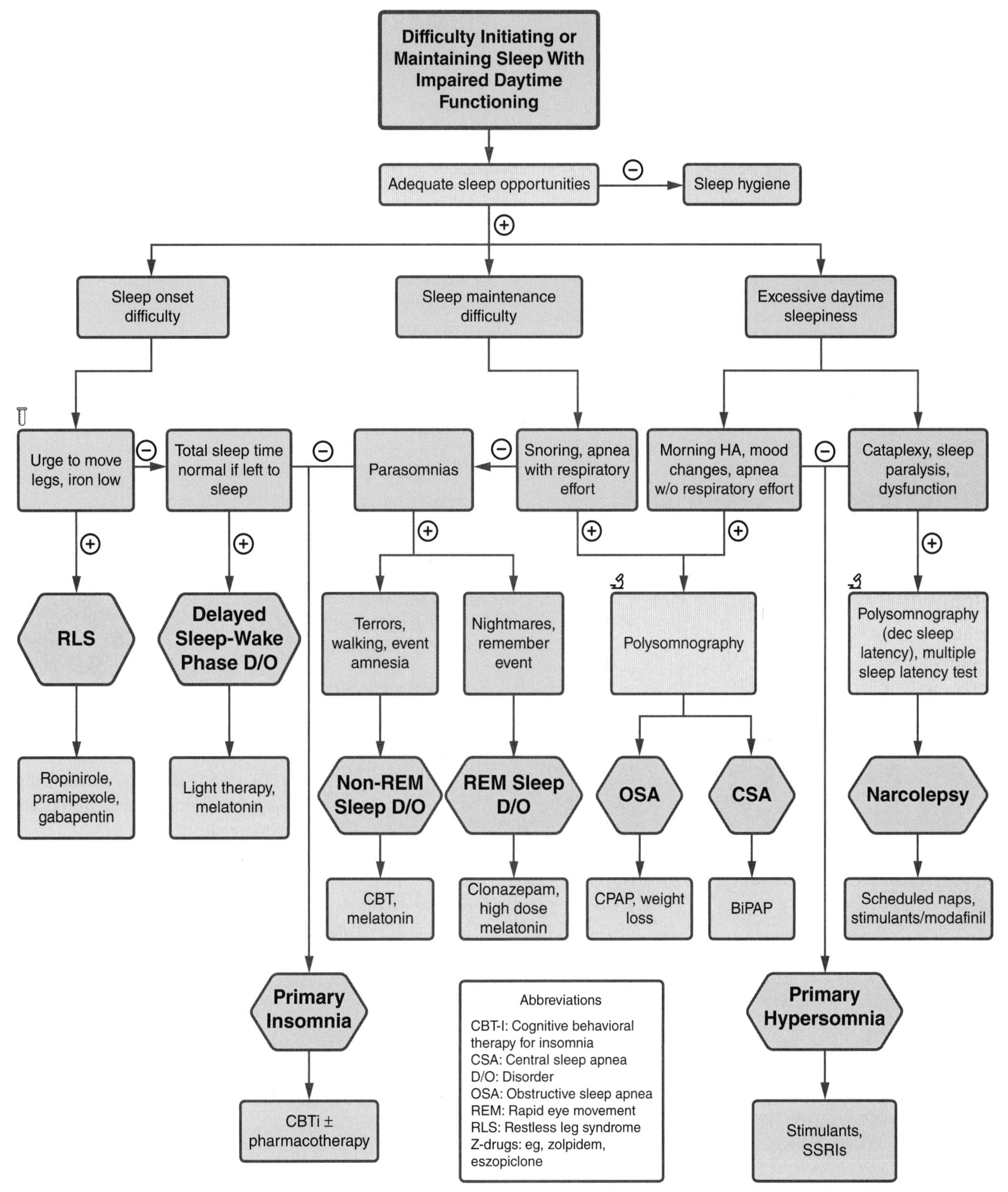
Difficulty Initiating or Maintaining Sleep With Impaired Daytime Functioning
Adequate sleep opportunities
Sleep hygiene
Sleep onset difficulty
Sleep maintenance difficulty
Excessive daytime sleepiness
Urge to move legs, iron low
Total sleep time normal if left to sleep
Parasomnias
Snoring, apnea with respiratory effort
Morning HA, mood changes, apnea w/o respiratory effort
Cataplexy, sleep paralysis, dysfunction
RLS
Delayed Sleep-Wake Phase D/O
Terrors, walking, event amnesia
Nightmares, remember event
Polysomnography
Polysomnography (dec sleep latency), multiple sleep latency test
Ropinirole, pramipexole, gabapentin
Light therapy, melatonin
Non-REM Sleep D/O
REM Sleep D/O
OSA
CSA
Narcolepsy
CBT, melatonin
Clonazepam, high dose melatonin
CPAP, weight loss
BiPAP
Scheduled naps, stimulants/modafinil
Primary Insomnia
CBTi ± pharmacotherapy
Abbreviations
CBT-I: Cognitive behavioral therapy for insomnia
CSA: Central sleep apnea
D/O: Disorder
OSA: Obstructive sleep apnea
REM: Rapid eye movement
RLS: Restless leg syndrome
Z-drugs: eg, zolpidem, eszopiclone
Primary Hypersomnia
Stimulants, SSRIs

FIGURE 27.15

27-15 Sleep Disorders

RESTLESS LEGS SYNDROME (RLS)

A 67-year-old M presents with intolerable sensation of restlessness in legs, especially when lying down for sleep. Symptoms resolve when he stands up or takes a few steps. His wife also complains that he often kicks her during sleep.

Management:

1. Replete iron if deficient.
2. Dopamine agonists (eg, ropinirole, pramipexole), pregabalin, gabapentin
3. Avoid caffeine, antihistamines, antidepressants, dopamine antagonists (eg, antipsychotics).

Complications:

- Insomnia.
- Excessive daytime sleepiness.

HYF: Always check iron studies first when suspecting RLS!

OBSTRUCTIVE SLEEP APNEA (OSA)

A 50-year-old M with BMI 36 presents with depression and daytime sleepiness. His wife complains that he snores loudly.

Management:

1. Polysomnography, CPAP.
2. Self-care (side sleep, weight loss).
3. Surgery (eg, tonsillectomy).

Complications:

- Hypertension.
- Pulmonary hypertension.
- Sudden death 2/2 cardiac arrhythmias.

HYF: Differentiate OSA: Upper airway blocked during sleep vs. central sleep apnea (cessation of respiratory drive → lack of respiration).

NARCOLEPSY

A 25-year-old M presents with irresistible attacks of sleep during the day. On intense emotion, he loses muscle tone (cataplexy).

Management:

1. Scheduled naps.
2. Stimulants (modafinil, amphetamines).
3. SSRIs, SNRIs, TCAs, or sodium oxybate for cataplexy.

HYF:

- HypnaGOgic hallucinations occur when you GO to sleep.
- **Hypno**POMPic hallucinations occur when you are getting up and POMPed in the morning.
- Caused by **L**ow **Hypo**cretin (orexin) in **L**ateral **Hypo**thalamus.

PRIMARY INSOMNIA

A 45-year-old F presents with trouble falling asleep and staying asleep, causing functional impairment at work. Polysomnography is negative. Other medical issues are ruled out.

Management:

1. CBT for insomnia, sleep hygiene, treat comorbid psychiatric disorders.
2. Isolated onset insomnia: Non-benzo hypnotics, ramelteon, 1st generation antihistamines, trazodone, mirtazapine.
3. Maintenance or mixed insomnia: Dual orexin receptor antagonists, low dose doxepin, non-benzo hypnotics, trazodone, mirtazapine.

Complications:

- Depression, anxiety, substance use.
- Caution: Can develop high dependence on sleep aids.

HYF: Sleep hygiene measures: ASLEEP

A: Alcohol, caffeine, nicotine avoidance
S: Sleep and sex only in bed
L: Leave electronics out of bedroom
E: Exercise early in the day
E: Early rise rather than sleeping in, avoid naps.
P: Plan a regular sleep schedule and routine (bath, meditate, sleep only when tired)

NIGHT TERRORS (NON-REM SLEEP DISORDER)

A 6-year-old M presents with parents who remark he has several episodes of aggressive thrashing while sleeping, occasionally yelling or even walking in his sleep. He is inconsolable upon awakening but does not remember the events the next day.

Management:

1. Reduce stress.
2. Anticipatory awakening.
3. Strong bedtime routine.

Complications:

- Injury to self or others.
- Daytime sleepiness.

HYF: Sleep/night terror: Non-REM, non-REMembered, boys > girls, 3–12 years.

Nightmare: REM, REMembered, boys = girls, 2 years–adolescence.

27-16 Sexual & Gender Identity Disorders

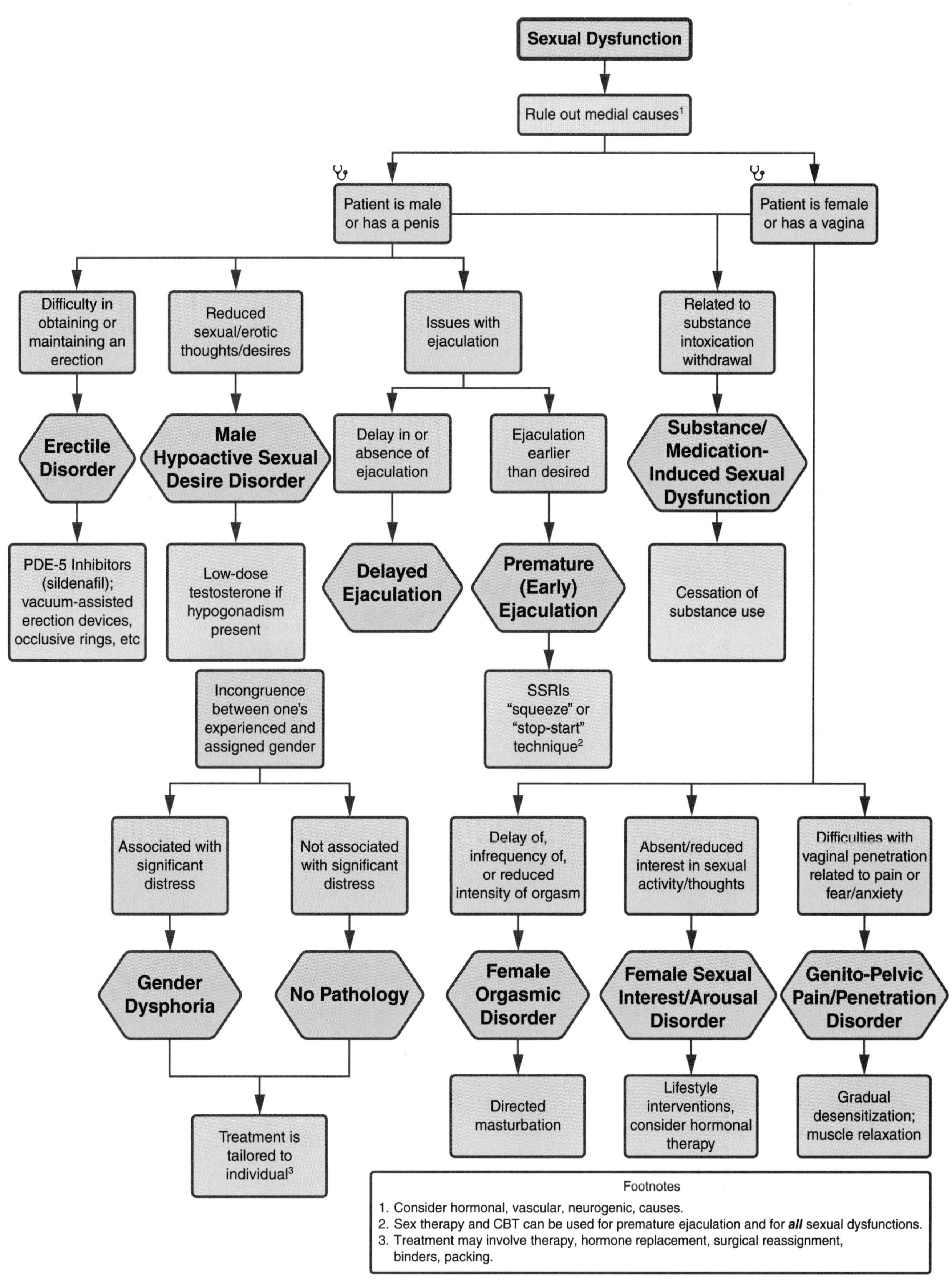
Sexual Dysfunction
Rule out medial causes[1]
Patient is male or has a penis
Patient is female or has a vagina
Difficulty in obtaining or maintaining an erection
Reduced sexual/erotic thoughts/desires
Issues with ejaculation
Related to substance intoxication withdrawal
Erectile Disorder
Male Hypoactive Sexual Desire Disorder
Delay in or absence of ejaculation
Ejaculation earlier than desired
Substance/ Medication-Induced Sexual Dysfunction
PDE-5 Inhibitors (sildenafil); vacuum-assisted erection devices, occlusive rings, etc
Low-dose testosterone if hypogonadism present
Delayed Ejaculation
Premature (Early) Ejaculation
Cessation of substance use
Incongruence between one's experienced and assigned gender
SSRIs "squeeze" or "stop-start" technique[2]
Associated with significant distress
Not associated with significant distress
Delay of, infrequency of, or reduced intensity of orgasm
Absent/reduced interest in sexual activity/thoughts
Difficulties with vaginal penetration related to pain or fear/anxiety
Gender Dysphoria
No Pathology
Female Orgasmic Disorder
Female Sexual Interest/Arousal Disorder
Genito-Pelvic Pain/Penetration Disorder
Directed masturbation
Lifestyle interventions, consider hormonal therapy
Gradual desensitization; muscle relaxation
Treatment is tailored to individual[3]
Footnotes
1. Consider hormonal, vascular, neurogenic, causes.
2. Sex therapy and CBT can be used for premature ejaculation and for ***all*** sexual dysfunctions.
3. Treatment may involve therapy, hormone replacement, surgical reassignment, binders, packing.

FIGURE 27.16

27-16 Sexual & Gender Identity Disorders

ERECTILE DISORDER

A 56-year-old M with PMH of HTN and HLD presents to his PCP complaining of difficulty achieving erection, which has caused significant strain on his sex life and relationship.

Management:

1. PDE-5 inhibitors (eg, sildenafil).
2. Vacuum-assisted erection devices.
3. Occlusive rings.

HYF:

- This should be contrasted with *performance anxiety*. This can lead to decreased libido, decreased ability to obtain or maintain an erection, or issues with ejaculation. Patients who experience sexual dysfunction secondary to performance anxiety often typically continue to experience nocturnal tumescence. Patients with erectile disorder, on the other hand, do not have erections during the night.
- Concomitant urinary symptoms (such as polyuria, dribbling, or incomplete bladder emptying) may suggest a diagnosis of BPH.

PREMATURE EJACULATION

A 35-year-old M comes to his PCP complaining of dissatisfaction with his sex life. He will often ejaculate in one minute or less after initiating intercourse and has been unsuccesful at multiple attempts to delay ejaculation.

Management:

1. SSRIs/TCAs (clomipramine), topical anesthetics.
2. "Squeeze" or "stop/start technique."

SUBSTANCE-INDUCED SEXUAL DYSFUNCTION

A 61-year-old M with alcohol use disorder presents with inability to achieve erection. He notes that he is often intoxicated when attempting sexual intercourse with this wife.

Management:

1. Treat underlying substance use disorder

HYF: Many medications (both recreational and prescription) can interfere with sexual function:

- Psychiatric: SSRIs, TCAs, MAOIs, benzodiazepines, antipsychotics.
- Antihypertensives.
- Hormonal drugs and chemotherapeutics.
- Recreational: Alcohol, amphetamines, barbiturates, cocaine, marijuana, opioids, nicotine.
- Antihistamines.

GENDER DYSPHORIA

A 19-year-old who grew up as M comes in after 4 years identifying as F only to close friends. This identity is causing her significant distress and fear of being in public.

Management:

1. Highly personalized: Can range from no treatment to changes in clothing, hormones, and/or surgery.

FEMALE SEXUAL INTEREST/AROUSAL DISORDER

A 53-year-old F presents around 4 years after menopause with significantly decreased interest in sexual intercourse, which is causing a strain on her relationship with her partner.

Management:

Multifaceted and can include: Lifestyle changes, couples therapy, individual psychotherapy, pelvic physical therapy, hormone therapy.

GENITO-PELVIC PAIN/PENETRATION DISORDER

A 22-year-old F comes into the office several years after her first sexual encounter, which was very painful. She tried several other times, which also caused significant pain. The last time she tried to engage in sexual intercourse, she was in so much pain that she now has marked fear and anxiety just thinking about vaginal penetration.

Management:

1. Gradual desensitization.
2. Muscle relaxation techniques.
3. Sexual therapy can be helpful.

PARAPHILIC DISORDERS (ATYPICAL SEXUAL INTEREST)

Voyeuristic Disorder: Observing as an unsuspecting person is naked, disrobing, or engaging in sexual activity.

Exhibitionistic Disorder: Exposure of one's genitals to an unsuspecting person.

Frotteuristic Disorder: Touching or rubbing against a non-consenting person.

Sexual Masochism Disorder: Being humiliated, beaten, bound, or otherwise made to suffer.

Sexual Sadism Disorder: Physical or psychological suffering of another person.

Pedophilic Disorder: Prepubescent children.

Fetishistic Disorder: Non-living objects or non-genital body parts.

27-17 Self-Harm/Suicide

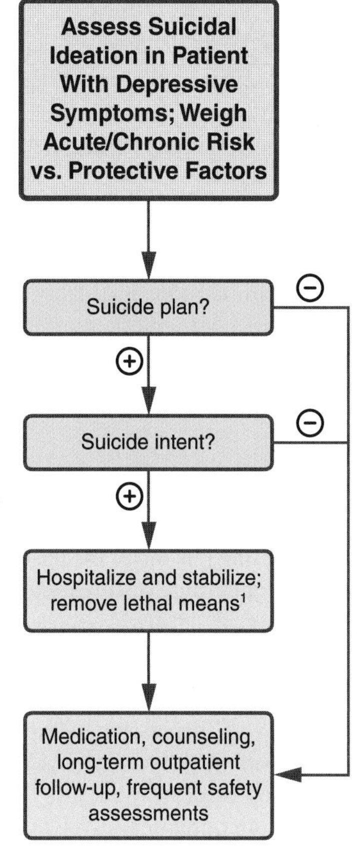
Assess Suicidal Ideation in Patient With Depressive Symptoms; Weigh Acute/Chronic Risk vs. Protective Factors
Suicide plan?
⊖
⊕
Suicide intent?
⊖
⊕
Hospitalize and stabilize; remove lethal means[1]
Medication, counseling, long-term outpatient follow-up, frequent safety assessments

Protective Factors
Coping skills
Religion or cultural beliefs
Social support
Connection to mental health provider
Limited access to lethal means

Acute Risk Factors
Acute symptoms of mental disorder
Hopelessness, lack of purpose or meaning
Impulsivity
Recent loss or disruption of relationships
Anniversary of loss of relationships
Preparation for suicide (giving away possessions)

Chronic Risk Factors
S Sex – females attempt more, **males succeed more**
A Age – <19 or >45 years
D **Depression, hopelessness, other mental illness**
P **Previous attempts**
E Ethanol/substance use
R Rational thinking loss (psychosis)
S Separated/divorced/widowed
O Organized or serious attempt
N No social support
S Stated future intent/Sickness (chronic or terminal)

Footnote
1. Lethal means: Guns, sharp objects, medications that patient could overdose on, supplies for hanging.

FIGURE 27.17

27-17 Self-Harm/Suicide

SUICIDAL IDEATION AND BEHAVIOR

Overall Management:

1. Conduct suicide risk assessment and assure immediate safety.
   a. Assess suicide ideation, intent, and lethality of plan.
   b. Assess acute risk factors.
   c. Assess chronic risk factors.
   d. Coach/Sitter in room at all times for elevated risk.
2. Determine level of care:
   a. Voluntary or involuntary hospitalization.
   b. Partial hospitalization, intensive outpatient program.
   c. Outpatient clinic
3. Address modifiable risk factors:
   a. Non-pharmacologic:
      i. Counseling and therapy, social interventions (housing, basic income and access to food).
      ii. Electroconvulsive therapy.
   b. Pharmacologic: Treat underlying disorder.
      i. Antidepressants.
      ii. Antipsychotics.
      iii. Mood stabilizers (eg, lithium).

HYF:

- 2nd leading cause of death in 15–24-year-olds.
- Most suicides in the United States involve firearms.
- Major risk factors for suicide: Prior suicide attempts, prior psychiatric illness, hopelessness, male gender.

ACTIVE SUICIDALITY WITH PLAN AND INTENT

A 25-year-old M with amphetamine use, schizoaffectice disorder, and homelessness presents with command auditory hallucinations and plan with intent to jump off of a bridge.

Management:

1. High acute risk.
2. Consider voluntary or involuntary hospitalization
3. Antipsychotic, mood stabilizer and connection with social support and long-term outpatient psychiatric care.

ACTIVE SUICIDALITY WITH NO INTENT OR NO PLAN

A 50-year-old F with chronic suicidality, past amphetamine use, and recent loss of her boyfriend presents and states, "I want to join him in heaven," but doesn't think she will follow through with the plan due to her morals and her family's support.

Management:

1. Intermediate acute risk.
2. Consider partial hospitalization or day program.
3. Consider addressing risk factor of substance use, psychotherapy for chronic suicidality, and long-term outpatient care.

PASSIVE SUICIDALITY

A 53-year-old M with depression with psychotic features self-presents to the inpatient service, stating, "I'm better off dead. I'm hopeless and just gonna rot away because I'm a horrible person." He lives alone and has an outpatient psychiatrist, but his medications aren't helping.

Management:

1. High acute risk.
2. Consider inpatient hospitalization.
3. Address refractory depression (consider ECT) and connect him with social support and outpatient psychiatric care.

27-18 Pediatric Psychiatry

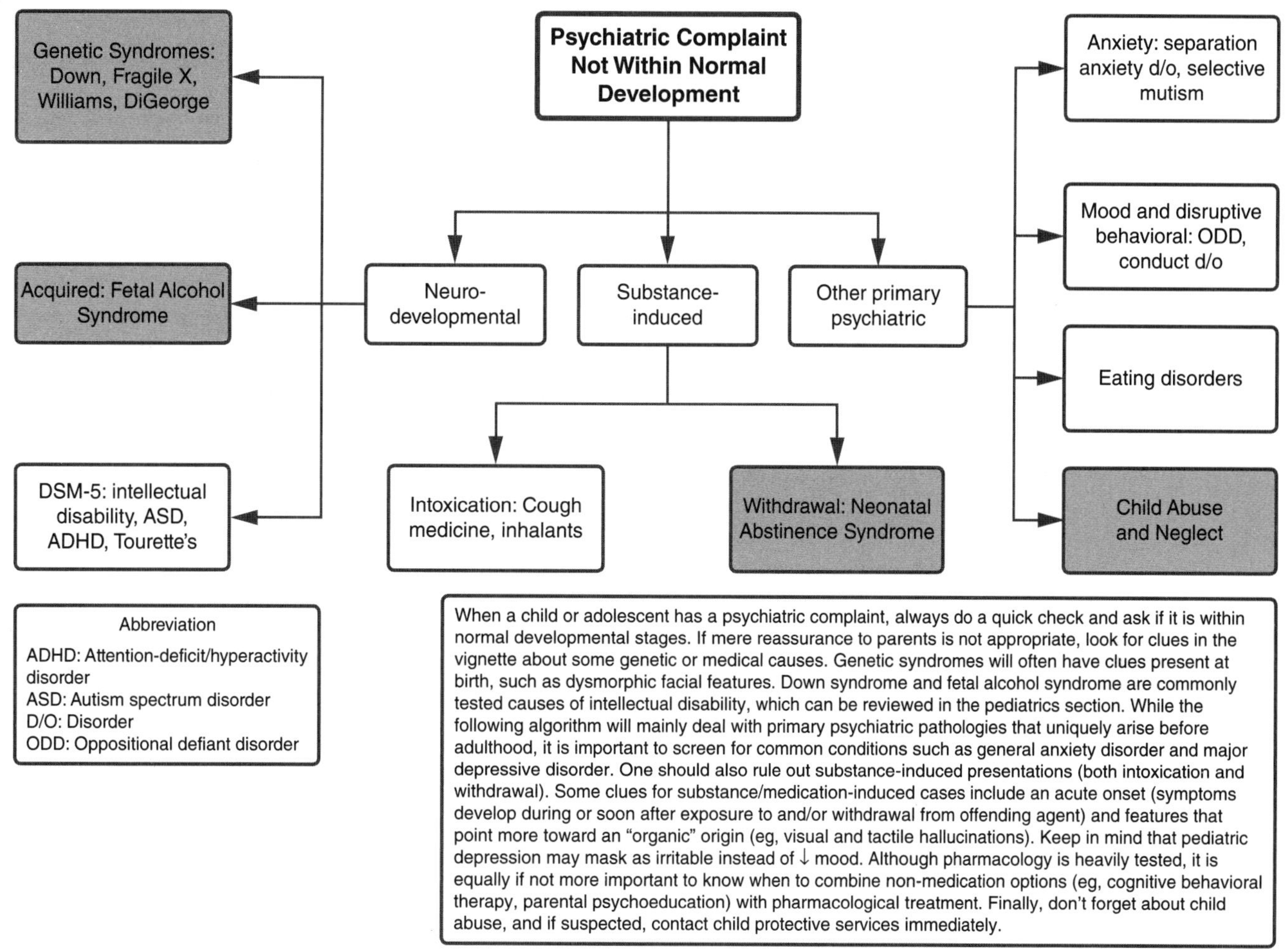
Psychiatric Complaint Not Within Normal Development
Neuro-developmental
Substance-induced
Other primary psychiatric
Genetic Syndromes: Down, Fragile X, Williams, DiGeorge
Acquired: Fetal Alcohol Syndrome
DSM-5: intellectual disability, ASD, ADHD, Tourette's
Intoxication: Cough medicine, inhalants
Withdrawal: Neonatal Abstinence Syndrome
Anxiety: separation anxiety d/o, selective mutism
Mood and disruptive behavioral: ODD, conduct d/o
Eating disorders
Child Abuse and Neglect
Abbreviation
ADHD: Attention-deficit/hyperactivity disorder
ASD: Autism spectrum disorder
D/O: Disorder
ODD: Oppositional defiant disorder
When a child or adolescent has a psychiatric complaint, always do a quick check and ask if it is within normal developmental stages. If mere reassurance to parents is not appropriate, look for clues in the vignette about some genetic or medical causes. Genetic syndromes will often have clues present at birth, such as dysmorphic facial features. Down syndrome and fetal alcohol syndrome are commonly tested causes of intellectual disability, which can be reviewed in the pediatrics section. While the following algorithm will mainly deal with primary psychiatric pathologies that uniquely arise before adulthood, it is important to screen for common conditions such as general anxiety disorder and major depressive disorder. One should also rule out substance-induced presentations (both intoxication and withdrawal). Some clues for substance/medication-induced cases include an acute onset (symptoms develop during or soon after exposure to and/or withdrawal from offending agent) and features that point more toward an "organic" origin (eg, visual and tactile hallucinations). Keep in mind that pediatric depression may mask as irritable instead of ↓ mood. Although pharmacology is heavily tested, it is equally if not more important to know when to combine non-medication options (eg, cognitive behavioral therapy, parental psychoeducation) with pharmacological treatment. Finally, don't forget about child abuse, and if suspected, contact child protective services immediately.

FIGURE 27.18

27-19 Pediatric Psychiatry Presentations

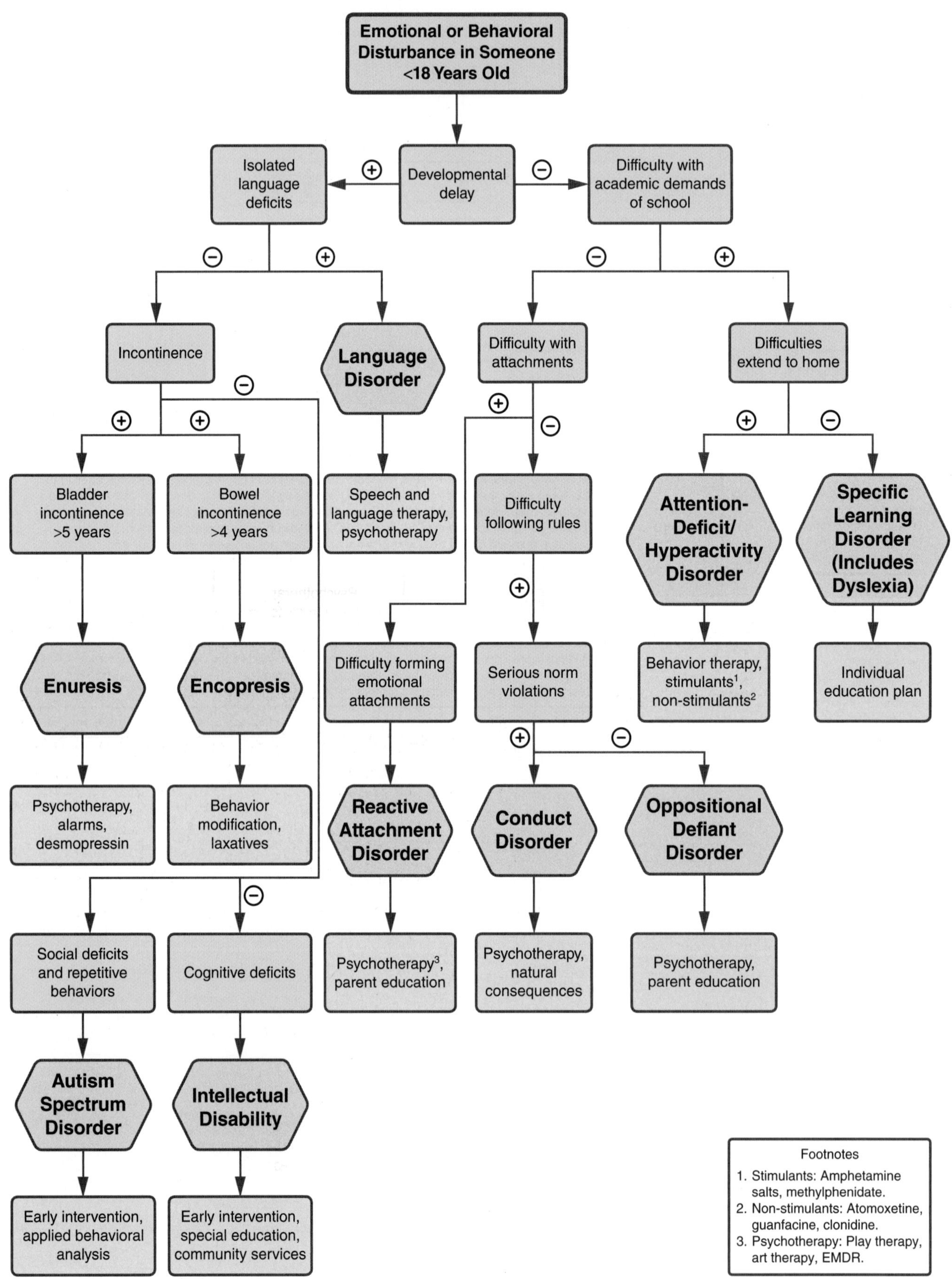
Emotional or Behavioral Disturbance in Someone <18 Years Old
Developmental delay
Isolated language deficits
Difficulty with academic demands of school
Incontinence
Language Disorder
Difficulty with attachments
Difficulties extend to home
Bladder incontinence >5 years
Bowel incontinence >4 years
Speech and language therapy, psychotherapy
Difficulty following rules
Attention-Deficit/ Hyperactivity Disorder
Specific Learning Disorder (Includes Dyslexia)
Enuresis
Encopresis
Difficulty forming emotional attachments
Serious norm violations
Behavior therapy, stimulants[1], non-stimulants[2]
Individual education plan
Psychotherapy, alarms, desmopressin
Behavior modification, laxatives
Reactive Attachment Disorder
Conduct Disorder
Oppositional Defiant Disorder
Social deficits and repetitive behaviors
Cognitive deficits
Psychotherapy[3], parent education
Psychotherapy, natural consequences
Psychotherapy, parent education
Autism Spectrum Disorder
Intellectual Disability
Early intervention, applied behavioral analysis
Early intervention, special education, community services
Footnotes
1. Stimulants: Amphetamine salts, methylphenidate.
2. Non-stimulants: Atomoxetine, guanfacine, clonidine.
3. Psychotherapy: Play therapy, art therapy, EMDR.

FIGURE 27.19

27-19 Pediatric Psychiatry Presentations

AUTISM SPECTRUM DISORDER (ASD)

A 2-year-old M presents to the pediatrician's office after his mother noticed that he had delays in social communication skills, lack of conversational speech, poor eye contact, and repetitive and stereotyped behaviors, including hand flapping and toe walking.

Management

1. Autism diagnostic observation schedule (ADOS).
2. Early intervention.
3. Behavior and communication approaches:
   a. Applied behavioral analysis (ABA).
4. Assistive technology.
5. Developmental, individual differences, relationship-based approach.
6. Occupational therapy.
7. Social skills therapy.
8. Speech therapy.
9. Pharmacology for comorbid disorders.

HYF:

- ASD is frequently comorbid with other psychiatric conditions such as ADHD, mood disorders, and anxiety disorders.
- ASD and intellectual disability (ID) are sometimes comorbid but are distinct disorders with distinct symptoms.

ATTENTION-DEFICIT/HYPERACTIVITY DISORDER (ADHD)

An 8-year-old M is brought to the pediatrician by his mother. Both at home and at school, he has been restless, overly talkative, unable to stay seated, intruding on conversations, impulsively blurting answers, and seems to "be driven by a motor."

Management:

1. Vanderbilt assessment, Conners assessment, SNAP assessment.
2. Behavioral therapy.
3. Pharmacologic:
   a. Stimulants (methylphenidate, amphetamine salts).
   b. Non-stimulants (guanfacine, clonidine).

HYF:

- Symptoms must be present age <12.
- Inattentive type, hyperactive type, or combined type.

Inattentive	Hyperactive
Poor listening skills	Squirms or fidgets
Loses or misplaces items	Restlessness
Sidetracked by stimuli	Driven by a motor
Forget daily activities	Overly talkative
Diminished attention span	Unable to stay seated
No follow-through	Difficulty waiting turn
Avoids tasks with concentration	Intrudes on others
Thoughtless mistakes	Impulsively blurts answers

OPPOSITIONAL DEFIANT DISORDER (ODD)

A 10-year-old M is brought to the counselor's office because parents have noticed that he has been more angry and that he becomes argumentative or defiant when they are imposing limitations or boundaries.

Management:

1. Psychotherapy:
   a. Parent training.
   b. Parent-child interaction therapy (PCIT).
   c. Family therapy.
   d. Cognitive problem-solving training.
   e. Social skills training.
2. Pharmacology for comorbid disorders.

HYF: ODD is frequently comorbid with other psychiatric conditions such as ADHD, mood disorders, and anxiety disorders. Differentiate from conduct disorder, adjustment disorder, ADHD and trauma reaction.

ODD	Conduct Disorder
Angry or Irritable mood, argumentative or defiant, and vindictiveness	Aggression, destruction, deceitfulness/theft, serious rule violations
Less physical violence	More physical violence
≥ 6 months	≥ 12 months
Severity = number of settings	Severity = frequency and extent of misconduct

28
Biostatistics, Epidemiology, and Medical Ethics

28-1 Biostatistics and Epidemiology

Description of Study Designs

Study Design	Description	Advantages	Disadvantages	Measures
Cross-sectional	Measures prevalence of disease and risk factors at 1 time point.	Shows risk factor association with disease.	Cannot establish causality.	Prevalence
Case reports, case series	Tracks ≥1 subject with a known exposure and reports characteristics of a disease.	Provides insight into rare conditions that are poorly understood.	No comparison group, so cannot show association between risk factor and disease.	Descriptive
Case control	Selects participants based on outcome status (disease vs. no disease) and asks about past risk factors. Assesses if odds of prior risk factor (eg, exposure) differ by disease state.	Can examine small group sizes (eg, rare diseases) and multiple risk factors.	Subject to recall bias, selection bias.	Odds ratio (**OR**) **Control** the **case** in the **OR**.
Prospective cohort	Ongoing observation of a group of people until they develop the outcome of interest.	Can examine rare exposures and multiple effects of exposures, can determine temporality and incidence.	Loss to follow-up.	Relative risk (RR). Also OR, incidence, prevalence.
Retrospective cohort	Often database studies, uses stored records to evaluate the association of risk factors and outcomes in a group.	Can examine rare exposures and multiple effects of exposures, can determine temporality and incidence.	Only as good as the database, which was often created for another purpose; selection bias.	Relative risk (RR) Coho**r**t**: R**ela**t**ive risk.
Randomized controlled trial	Participants are randomly assigned to interventions and followed prospectively. Clinical trials: **I SWIM**. -Phase 0: **I**f/how the new treatment works in people, compared to laboratory studies. Preliminary assessment of pharmacologic and pharmacokinetic properties. <15 participants receive a tiny dose of the drug. Not a required step in testing a new drug. -Phase I: Is the treatment **S**afe? Evaluate safety, toxicity, proper dose, and pharmacologic and pharmacokinetic properties. 15–50 participants. -Phase II: "Does the treatment **W**ork?" Evaluate treatment efficacy and adverse effects. <100 participants. -Phase III: "Is the treatment an **I**mprovement to what's already available?" Compare new treatment to standard of care. Hundreds of patients are randomly assigned either to the treatment group or standard of care (or placebo) group. -Phase IV: "Can the treatment remain on the **M**arket?" After drug approval, assess long-term adverse effects, impact on quality of life, and cost effectiveness. Thousands of patients.	Gold standard for establishing cause and effect. Can be double-blinded (neither participant nor researcher knows which intervention the participant is receiving) or triple-blinded (researcher analyzing the data also does not know which intervention the participant is receiving) to minimize bias.	Expensive, potentially unethical to deny treatment to 1 group.	Depends on the study.

28-1 Biostatistics and Epidemiology

Description of Study Designs

Study Design	Description	Advantages	Disadvantages	Measures
Meta-analysis	Pool multiple studies that examine a disease or exposure.	Larger study size.	Limited by factors in original studies.	Depends on original studies.
Crossover study	Participants are randomly assigned to a series of ≥2 interventions (eg, treatments A and B). The order in which participants receive the interventions is randomized (A then B vs. B then A). There is a washout period between interventions. There are 2 important methods for comparing the treatment groups: *Per-protocol analysis:* Includes only patients who completed the study based on study protocol. Risk of attrition bias (comparison groups no longer have similar characteristics in the end due to nonrandom noncompliance). *Intention-to-treat analysis:* Includes all patients as if they had received the intervention they were supposed to receive, regardless of adherence to study protocol. Minimizes misleading bias due to loss to follow-up.	Participants serve as their own control, so risk of confounding is minimized and fewer study participants are required.	Effects of 1st intervention may "carry over" and alter the response to the subsequent intervention. To prevent aliasing, there is a washout (no treatment) period between interventions to allow the effects of the 1st treatment to wear off.	Depends on the study.

28-1 Biostatistics and Epidemiology

Forms of Bias in Study Designs

Type of bias	Definition
Participant Recruitment	
Selection bias	Error in how subjects are enrolled in a study.
The healthy worker effect	Working populations appear to be healthier when compared with the general population due to out-migration of sick people from the workforce.
Volunteer bias	Subjects who agree to participate in a study differ from those who refuse, generally by being healthier.
Admission rate (Berkson's bias)	Admission rates of exposed and unexposed cases and controls differ, resulting in a distortion of odds of exposure in hospital-based studies.
Nonresponse bias	Nonrespondents may exhibit exposures or outcomes that differ from respondents, resulting in over- or underestimation of odds or risk.
Prevalence-incidence (Neyman) bias	Timing of exposure identification causes some cases to be missed.
Unmasking bias	An innocent exposure causes a sign or symptom that precipitates search for a disease but does not itself cause the disease.
Performing Study	
Recall bias	Participants differ in the accuracy and/or completeness of their recollections. For example, participants who are sick tend to recall more past exposures, independent of any causal role.
Measurement bias	Systematic (ie, non-random) error that occurs in data collection.
Procedure bias	Participants allocated to different groups are not treated the same (apart from the variable being studied). Methods of control: Blinding of participants/investigators, use of placebo.
Attention bias (Hawthorn effect)	Participants change their behavior because they know they are being observed.
Observer-Expectancy bias (Pygmalion effect)	Investigators may err in measuring data towards the outcome they expect.
Interviewer bias	Investigators may preferentially elicit information about exposure or outcomes if aware of the subject's status in a study.
Misclassification bias	Putting an individual, value, or characteristic into a category other than the one originally assigned. This could lead to erroneous associations that are observed between different groups and the outcome of interest.
Lag time bias	The time period before the enrollment or start date of the study was not taken into consideration before evaluating exposure.
Exposure suspicion bias	Knowledge of a subject's disease status may influence both intensity and outcome of a search for exposure.
Surveillance bias	Increased possibility for a study outcome to be detected with more diagnostic tests or follow-up methods.
Loss to follow-up	Error introduced if loss to follow-up in a study is related to outcome under investigation.
Data analysis	
Post hoc significance bias	When decisions regarding level of significance are selected *a posteriori*, conclusion may be biased.
Significance bias	Confusing statistical significance with clinical significance.
Correlation bias	Correlation does not equal causation.
Interpreting Results	
Confounding bias	A systematic distortion in the measure of the association between outcome and exposure due to an extraneous third variable, called a confounder.
Lead-time bias	Early diagnosis of a disease through screening leads to overestimation of survival duration. For example, patient A is diagnosed with lung cancer at age 69 and dies at age 70 (1-year survival), whereas patient B is diagnosed with lung cancer at age 65 after undergoing lung cancer screening and dies at age 70 (5-year survival). The survival time appears longer for the latter, but the patient did not actually live longer.
Length-time bias	Relative excess of slowly progressing cases detected through screening leads to overestimation of survival duration. Often discussed in the context of disease screening. For example, Patient A has a slow-growing tumor and is more likely to be diagnosed with cancer through screening (before their disease has become severe enough to present symptomatically) compared to Patient B who has a rapidly growing tumor (which more often presents with symptoms that require immediate clinical attention). Patients with slowly progressing disease have longer survival times, which is falsely attributed to early detection via screening but is actually due to the slow rate of disease progression.

28-1 Biostatistics and Epidemiology

RATES OF DISEASE

- **Incidence** is the number of *new* cases of a disease that occur in a population during a specific time period (**incidence** looks at **incidents**).
  - Incidence

$$=\frac{\text{number of new cases of a disease in a specific time period}}{\text{total population at risk}}$$

- **Prevalence** is the number of *existing* cases at a specific time. (Prevalence looks at **all** current cases.)
  - Prevalence $=\frac{\text{number of existing cases}}{\text{total population}}$
- **Case fatality rate** is the proportion of cases who die within a specific time period.
  - Case fatality rate

$$=\frac{\text{patients who die from disease in a specific time period}}{\text{total number of cases in a specific time period}}$$

EVALUATION OF DIAGNOSTIC TESTS

2×2 Table Comparing Test Results with Presence of Disease

	Condition Present	Condition Absent
⊕ test	TP	FP
⊖ test	FN	TN

- **Sensitivity** = true positive rate (the proportion of persons with the disease who test positive) = TP/(TP + FN) = 1 – FN rate.
  - A high-sensitivity test is used for *screening* in diseases with low prevalence (SN-N-OUT = highly SeNsitive test. When Negative, rules OUT disease).
- **Specificity** = true negative rate (the proportion of persons without the disease who test negative) = TN/(TN + FP) = 1 – FP rate.
  - A high-specificity test is used for *confirmation* after a positive screening test (SP-P-IN = highly SPecific test. When Positive, rules IN disease).
- **Positive predictive value (PPV)** = the proportion of persons with a positive test who have the disease: TP/(TP + FP).
  - Prevalence, sensitivity, and specificity determine PPV:

$$\text{PPV}=\frac{\text{prevalence}\times\text{sensitivity}}{(\text{prevalence}\times\text{sensitivity})+(1\text{-prevalence})(1\text{-specificity})}$$

  - PPV varies directly with prevalence or pretest probability.
- **Negative predictive value (NPV)** = the proportion of persons with a negative test who do not have the disease = TN/(TN + FN).
  - NPV varies inversely with prevalence or pretest probability.

Compromise between Specificity and Sensitivity

- **Likelihood ratio** = odds that a given test result is expected in a patient with the disease compared to the odds that the same test result is expected in a patient without the disease.
  - Positive likelihood ratio (LR+) = sensitivity/(1-specificity) = TP/FP.
  - Negative likelihood ratio (LR–) = (1-sensitivity)/specificity = FN/TN.
  - Post-test odds = pretest odds × LR.
- **Accuracy** = performance of tests based on only the number of true results = (TP + TN)/(TP + TN + FP + FN).

MEASURING RISK

2×2 Contingency Table

	Disease	No Disease
⊕ Exposure or Risk Factor	*a*	*b*
⊖ Exposure or Risk Factor	*c*	*d*

- **Odds ratio (OR)** = odds of exposure in patients with disease compared with odds of exposure in patients without disease =

$$\frac{a/c}{b/d}=\frac{ad}{bc}.$$

  - Estimates relative risk if prevalence is low.
- **Relative risk (RR)** = Probability of developing disease in the exposed group compared to probability of developing disease in the unexposed group $=\frac{a/(a+b)}{c/(c+d)}$
  - RR <1: Negative relationship between exposure and disease occurrence.
  - RR=1: No association between exposure and disease occurrence.
  - RR >1: Positive relationship between exposure and disease occurrence.
- **Attributable risk (AR)** = *difference* in rates of disease between exposed and unexposed groups $=\frac{a}{a+b}-\frac{c}{c+d}$
- **Absolute risk reduction (ARR)** = *difference* in risk attributable to specific intervention $=\frac{c}{c+d}-\frac{a}{a+b}$

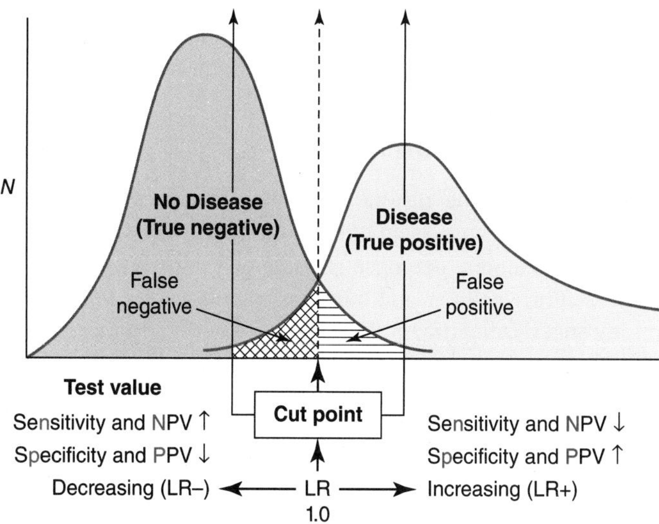
N
No Disease
(True negative)
Disease
(True positive)
False
negative
False
positive
Test value
Cut point
Sensitivity and NPV ↑
Specificity and PPV ↓
Decreasing (LR–)
LR
1.0
Sensitivity and NPV ↓
Specificity and PPV ↑
Increasing (LR+)

(Continued)

28-1 Biostatistics and Epidemiology

- **Relative risk reduction (RRR)** = *proportion* of risk reduction attributable to specific intervention = 1-RR.
- **Number needed to treat (NNT)** = number of patients that need to be treated to benefit 1 patient = 1/ARR.
- **Number needed to harm (NNH)** = number of patients that need to have an exposure for 1 patient to be harmed = 1/AR.

TYPES OF ERROR

- **Null hypothesis (Ho)** states there is no association between exposure and disease.
- **Alternative hypothesis (H_1)** states there is a relationship between exposure and disease.
- **Type 1 error (α):** False positive; **Ho** is rejected even though it is true.
- **Type 2 error (β):** False negative; **Ho** is not rejected even though it is false.
- **Power** = a study's ability to detect a difference between 2 groups = 1 – β.
  - ↑ sample size, ↑ power (there is power in numbers).

PRECISION AND ACCURACY

- **Precision (reliability)** is the reproducibility of a test (ie, absence of random variation).
  - Random error → ↓ precision.
  - ↓ standard deviation → ↑ precision.
  - ↑ power → ↑ precision.
- **Accuracy (validity)** is the trueness of the measurements of a test (ie, absence of systematic error in a test).
  - Systemic error → ↓ accuracy.

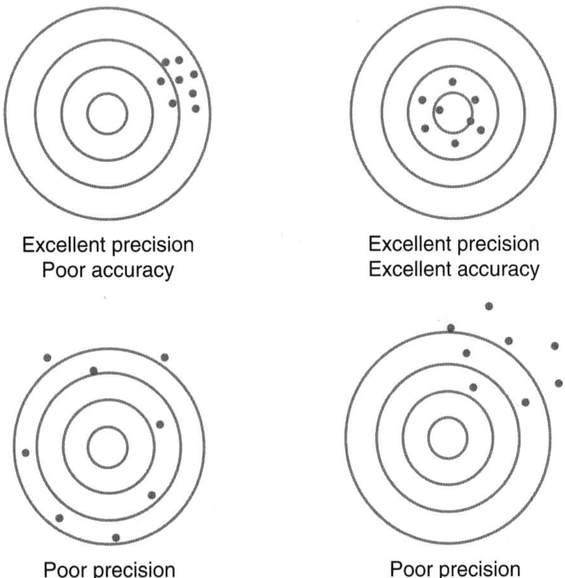
Excellent precision
Poor accuracy
Excellent precision
Excellent accuracy
Poor precision
Excellent accuracy
Poor precision
Poor accuracy

28-2 Disease Prevention

There are 4 levels of prevention:

- **1° Prevention:** Prevents disease occurrence (eg, vaccinations).
- **2° Prevention:** Early disease detection to prevent and/or ↓ morbidity before onset of symptoms. Includes screening tests to identify subclinical disease (eg, colonoscopies).
- **3° Prevention:** Measures to ↓ morbidity or mortality after symptom onset (eg, blood pressure medications to treat hypertension).
- **4° Prevention:** Methods of reducing harm from unnecessary and/or excessive new medical interventions (eg, obtaining unnecessary imaging that will not change a patient's treatment plan).
- Disease prevention at the community level (**primordial prevention**) involves population-level health promotion and avoidance of health risks, which can include social and economic policy-making (eg, taxes on cigarettes, smoke-free buildings, reducing pollution), investing in health education (eg, risks associated with smoking and alcohol use), and addressing healthcare disparities.

28-3 Vaccinations

Vaccines are among the most effective measures of preventive medicine. There are 4 main types of vaccines:

- **Live-attenuated:** Pathogen is rendered nonpathogenic but can still induce cellular and humoral responses (eg, MMR, BCG, intranasal influenza, polio—Sabin, rotavirus). Induces lifelong immunity. Contraindicated in pregnant and immunodeficient patients.
- **Inactivated:** Pathogen is inactivated but retains the epitope structure on surface antigens, inducing a humoral response (eg, HAV, rabies, intramuscular influenza, polio—Salk). Booster shots are usually necessary.
- **Subunit:** Contains only the antigen(s) that optimally induce an immune response (eg, HBV, HPV, *Neisseria meningitidis*, *Streptococcus pneumoniae*, HiB).
- **Toxoid:** Bacterial toxoid is denatured but retains an intact receptor binding site, stimulating antibody production (eg, tetanus, diphtheria). Booster shots are usually necessary.

28-4 Immunization Schedules

Recommended Child and Adolescent Immunization Schedule for Ages 18 Years or Younger, United States, 2022

These recommendations must be read with the notes that follow. For those who fall behind or start late, provide catch-up vaccination at the earliest opportunity as indicated by the green bars. To determine minimum intervals between doses, see the catch-up schedule (Table 2).

Vaccine	Birth	1 mo	2 mos	4 mos	6 mos	9 mos	12 mos	15 mos	18 mos	19–23 mos	2–3 yrs	4–6 yrs	7–10 yrs	11–12 yrs	13–15 yrs	16 yrs	17–18 yrs
Hepatitis B (HepB)	1st dose	←2nd dose→			←3rd dose→												
Rotavirus (RV): RV1 (2-dose series), RV5 (3-dose series)			1st dose	2nd dose	See Notes												
Diphtheria, tetanus, acellular pertussis (DTaP <7 yrs)			1st dose	2nd dose	3rd dose			←4th dose→				5th dose					
Haemophilus influenzae type b (Hib)			1st dose	2nd dose	See Notes		←3rd or 4th dose, See Notes→										
Pneumococcal conjugate (PCV13)			1st dose	2nd dose	3rd dose		←4th dose→										
Inactivated poliovirus (IPV <18 yrs)			1st dose	2nd dose	←3rd dose→							4th dose					
Influenza (IIV4)					Annual vaccination 1 or 2 doses									Annual vaccination 1 dose only			
or													or				
Influenza (LAIV4)											Annual vaccination 1 or 2 doses			Annual vaccination 1 dose only			
Measles, mumps, rubella (MMR)					See Notes		←1st dose→					2nd dose					
Varicella (VAR)							←1st dose→					2nd dose					
Hepatitis A (HepA)					See Notes		2-dose series, See Notes										
Tetanus, diphtheria, acellular pertussis (Tdap ≥7 yrs)														1 dose			
Human papillomavirus (HPV)														See Notes			
Meningococcal (MenACWY-D ≥9 mos, MenACWY-CRM ≥2 mos, MenACWY-TT ≥ 2 years)			See Notes											1st dose		2nd dose	
Meningococcal B (MenB-4C, MenB-FHbp)																See Notes	
Pneumococcal polysaccharide (PPSV23)														See Notes			
Dengue (DEN4CYD; 9–16 yrs)															Seropositive in endemic areas only (See Notes)		

- Range of recommended ages for all children
- Range of recommended ages for catch-up vaccination
- Range of recommended ages for certain high-risk groups
- Recommended vaccination can begin in this age group
- Recommended vaccination based on shared clinical decision-making
- No recommendation/ not applicable

28-4 Immunization Schedules

Recommended Child and Adolescent Immunization Schedule by Medical Indication, United States, 2022

Always use this table in conjunction with Table 1 and the Notes that follow.

VACCINE	INDICATION									
	Pregnancy	Immunocompromised status (excluding HIV infection)	HIV infection CD4+ count[1]: <15% or total CD4 cell count of <200/mm³	HIV infection CD4+ count[1]: ≥15% and total CD4 cell count of ≥200/mm³	Kidney failure, end-stage renal disease, or on hemodialysis	Heart disease or chronic lung disease	CSF leak or cochlear implant	Asplenia or persistent complement component deficiencies	Chronic liver disease	Diabetes
Hepatitis B										
Rotavirus		SCID[2]								
Diphtheria, tetanus, and acellular pertussis (DTaP)										
Haemophilus influenzae type b										
Pneumococcal conjugate										
Inactivated poliovirus										
Influenza (IIV4)										
or										
Influenza (LAIV4)						Asthma, wheezing: 2–4 yrs[3]				
Measles, mumps, rubella	*									
Varicella	*									
Hepatitis A										
Tetanus, diphtheria, and acellular pertussis (Tdap)										
Human papillomavirus	*									
Meningococcal ACWY										
Meningococcal B										
Pneumococcal polysaccharide										
Dengue										

- Vaccination according to the routine schedule recommended
- Recommended for persons with an additional risk factor for which the vaccine would be indicated
- Vaccination is recommended, and additional doses may be necessary based on medical condition or vaccine. See Notes.
- Precaution—vaccine might be indicated if benefit of protection outweighs risk of adverse reaction
- Contraindicated or not recommended—vaccine should not be administered
  *Vaccinate after pregnancy
- No recommendation/not applicable

1 For additional information regarding HIV laboratory parameters and use of live vaccines, see the *General Best Practice Guidelines for Immunization*, "Altered Immunocompetence," at www.cdc.gov/vaccines/hcp/acip-recs/general-recs/immunocompetence.html and Table 4-1 (footnote J) at www.cdc.gov/vaccines/hcp/acip-recs/general-recs/contraindications.html.
2 Severe Combined Immunodeficiency.
3 LAIV4 contraindicated for children 2–4 years of age with asthma or wheezing during the preceding 12 months.

28-4 Immunization Schedules

Recommended Adult Immunization Schedule by Age Group, United States, 2022

Vaccine	19–26 years	27–49 years	50–64 years	≥65 years
Influenza inactivated (IIV4) or **Influenza recombinant** (RIV4)	1 dose annually			
or				
Influenza live, attenuated (LAIV4)	1 dose annually			
Tetanus, diphtheria, pertussis (Tdap or Td)	1 dose Tdap each pregnancy; 1 dose Td/Tdap for wound management (see notes)			
	1 dose Tdap, then Td or Tdap booster every 10 years			
Measles, mumps, rubella (MMR)	1 or 2 doses depending on indication (if born in 1957 or later)			
Varicella (VAR)	2 doses (if born in 1980 or later)		2 doses	
Zoster recombinant (RZV)	2 doses for immunocompromising conditions (see notes)		2 doses	
Human papillomavirus (HPV)	2 or 3 doses depending on age at initial vaccination or condition	27 through 45 years		
Pneumococcal (PCV15, PCV20, PPSV23)	1 dose PCV15 followed by PPSV23 OR 1 dose PCV20 (see notes)			1 dose PCV15 followed by PPSV23 OR 1 dose PCV20
Hepatitis A (HepA)	2 or 3 doses depending on vaccine			
Hepatitis B (HepB)	2, 3, or 4 doses depending on vaccine or condition			
Meningococcal A, C, W, Y (MenACWY)	1 or 2 doses depending on indication, see notes for booster recommendations			
Meningococcal B (MenB)	19 through 23 years; 2 or 3 doses depending on vaccine and indication, see notes for booster recommendations			
***Haemophilus influenzae* type b** (Hib)	1 or 3 doses depending on indication			

Legend:

- Recommended vaccination for adults who meet age requirement, lack documentation of vaccination, or lack evidence of past infection
- Recommended vaccination for adults with an additional risk factor or another indication
- Recommended vaccination based on shared clinical decision-making
- No recommendation/Not applicable

28-4 Immunization Schedules

Recommended Adult Immunization Schedule by Medical Condition or Other Indication, 2022

Vaccine	Pregnancy	Immuno-compromised (excluding HIV infection)	HIV infection CD4 percentage and count: <15% or <200 mm[3]	HIV infection CD4 percentage and count: ≥15% and ≥200 mm[3]	Asplenia, complement deficiencies	End-stage renal disease, or on hemodialysis	Heart or lung disease; alcoholism[1]	Chronic liver disease	Diabetes	Health care personnel[2]	Men who have sex with men
IIV4 or RIV4	1 dose annually										
or										or	
LAIV4	Contraindicated					Precaution				1 dose annually	
Tdap or Td	1 dose Tdap each pregnancy	1 dose Tdap, then Td or Tdap booster every 10 years									
MMR	Contraindicated*	Contraindicated		1 or 2 doses depending on indication							
VAR	Contraindicated*	Contraindicated			2 doses						
RZV		2 doses at age ≥19 years			2 doses at age ≥50 years						
HPV	Not Recommended*	3 doses through age 26 years			2 or 3 doses through age 26 years depending on age at initial vaccination or condition						
Pneumococcal (PCV15, PCV20, PPSV23)		1 dose PCV15 followed by PPSV23 OR 1 dose PCV20 (see notes)									
HepA	2 or 3 doses depending on vaccine										
HepB	3 doses (see notes)	2, 3, or 4 doses depending on vaccine or condition									
MenACWY	1 or 2 doses depending on indication, see notes for booster recommendations										
MenB	Precaution	2 or 3 doses depending on vaccine and indication, see notes for booster recommendations									
Hib		3 doses HSCT[3] recipients only			1 dose						

- Recommended vaccination for adults who meet age requirement, lack documentation of vaccination, or lack evidence of past infection
- Recommended vaccination for adults with an additional risk factor or another indication
- Recommended vaccination based on shared clinical decision-making
- Precaution—vaccination might be indicated if benefit of protection outweighs risk of adverse reaction
- Contraindicated or not recommended—vaccine should not be administered.
- No recommendation/ Not applicable

*Vaccinate after pregnancy.

1. Precaution for LAIV4 does not apply to alcoholism. **2.** See notes for influenza; hepatitis B; measles, mumps, and rubella; and varicella vaccinations. **3.** Hematopoietic stem cell transplant.

28-5 Screening Recommendations

Health Screening Recommendations for Women by Age

	Recommendations		
Age	Screening for Metabolic Syndrome	Recommended Cancer Screenings	Other Screenings
20-39	Hypertension: Blood pressure screening every 3-5 years if not at increased risk for hypertension. Dyslipidemia: Lipid screening starting at age 30 if higher cardiovascular risk[2]. Type 2 diabetes: Screen for prediabetes and type 2 diabetes with A1c in overweight or obese adults starting at age 35.	Cervical cancer: In women age 21-29, pap smear alone every 3 years. Starting at age 30, screening with pap smear alone every 3 years, hrHPV[1] testing alone every 5 years, or pap smear in combination with hrHPV testing (cotesting) every 5 years.	Chlamydia and gonorrhea: Annual screening in all sexually active women until age 24. Screen women age ≥ 25 only if they are at increased risk for infection. Syphilis: Screen women only if at increased risk for infection. HIV and HCV screening at least once. Offer PrEP[1] to persons with high risk of HIV infection[3]. Depression. Intimate partner violence. Tobacco smoking cessation. Unhealthy alcohol use. Unhealthy drug use.
40-49	Hypertension: Annual blood pressure screening. Cholesterol: Lipid screening. A statin is indicated for the primary prevention of CVD[1] in adults age >40 with CVD risk factor(s) and an estimated 10-year risk of a cardiovascular event ≥10%. Type 2 diabetes: Screen for prediabetes and type 2 diabetes with A1c in overweight or obese adults.	Cervical cancer: Screening with pap smear alone every 3 years, hrHPV testing alone every 5 years, or pap smear in combination with hrHPV testing (cotesting) every 5 years. Colorectal cancer: Screening starting at age 45 with fecal occult blood testing yearly, multi-target stool DNA testing every 3 years, flexible sigmoidoscopy every 5 years, or colonoscopy every 10 years.	Chlamydia, gonorrhea, syphilis: Screen women only if at increased risk for infection. HIV and HCV screening at least once. Offer PrEP to persons with high risk of HIV infection. Depression. Intimate partner violence. Tobacco smoking cessation. Unhealthy alcohol use. Unhealthy drug use.
50-64	Hypertension: Annual blood pressure screening. Cholesterol: Lipid screening. A statin is indicated for the primary prevention of CVD in patients with CVD risk factor(s) and an estimated 10-year risk of a cardiovascular event ≥10%. Type 2 diabetes: Screen for prediabetes and type 2 diabetes with A1c in overweight or obese adults.	Cervical cancer: Screening with pap smear alone every 3 years, hrHPV testing alone every 5 years, or pap smear in combination with hrHPV testing (cotesting) every 5 years until age 65. Breast cancer: Screening mammogram once every 1–2 years (patients can choose to start at age 40). Colorectal cancer: Screening with fecal occult blood testing yearly, multi-target stool DNA testing every 3 years, flexible sigmoidoscopy every 5 years, or colonoscopy every 10 years. Lung cancer: Annual screening with low-dose computed tomography in adults starting at age 55 who have a 20 pack-year smoking history and currently smoke or have quit within the past 15 years.	Chlamydia, gonorrhea, syphilis: Screen women only if at increased risk for infection. HIV and HCV screening at least once. Offer PrEP to persons with high risk of HIV infection. Depression. Intimate partner violence. Tobacco smoking cessation. Unhealthy alcohol use. Unhealthy drug use.
≥65	Hypertension: Annual blood pressure screening. Cholesterol: Lipid screening. A statin is indicated for the primary prevention of CVD in patients with CVD risk factor(s) and an estimated 10-year risk of a cardiovascular event ≥10%. Type 2 diabetes: Screen for prediabetes and type 2 diabetes with A1c in overweight or obese adults.	Breast cancer: Screening mammogram once every 1–2 years until age 74. Colorectal cancer: Screening with fecal occult blood testing yearly, multi-target stool DNA testing every 3 years, flexible sigmoidoscopy every 5 years, or colonoscopy every 10 years until age 75. Lung cancer: Annual screening with low-dose computed tomography in adults who have a 20 pack-year smoking history and currently smoke or have quit within the past 15 years until age 80.	Chlamydia, gonorrhea, syphilis: Screen women only if at increased risk for infection. HIV and HCV screening at least once. Offer PrEP to persons with high risk of HIV infection. Osteoporosis: DEXA[1] scan to measure bone density at least once. AAA[1]: One-time screening with ultrasonography in patients age 65–75 years who have ever smoked. Depression. Intimate partner violence. Tobacco smoking cessation. Unhealthy alcohol use. Unhealthy drug use.

1. hrHPV: High-risk human papillomavirus. PrEP: HIV preexposure prophylaxis. CVD: Cardiovascular disease. DEXA: Dual x-ray absorptiometry. AAA: Abdominal aortic aneurysm.
2. Risk factors for cardiovascular disease: Hypertension, dyslipidemia, diabetes, tobacco smoking, and positive family history.
3. Risk factors for HIV infection: Multiple sexual partners, inconsistent use of barrier protection during sexual activity, and IV drug use.

28-5 Screening Recommendations

Health Screening Recommendations for Men by Age

Age	Recommendations		
	Screening for Metabolic Syndrome	Recommended Cancer Screenings	Other Screenings
20-39	Hypertension: Blood pressure screening every 3-5 years if not at increased risk for hypertension. Dyslipidemia: Lipid screening starting at age 25 if higher cardiovascular risk[2]. Type 2 diabetes: Screen for prediabetes and type 2 diabetes with A1c in overweight or obese adults starting at age 35.	N/A	Chlamydia, gonorrhea, syphilis: Screen men only if at increased risk for infection. HIV and HCV screening at least once. Offer PrEP[1] to persons with high risk of HIV infection[3]. Depression. Intimate partner violence. Tobacco smoking cessation. Unhealthy alcohol use. Unhealthy drug use.
40-49	Hypertension: Annual blood pressure screening. Cholesterol: Lipid screening. A statin is indicated for the primary prevention of CVD[1] in adults age >40 with CVD risk factor(s) and an estimated 10-year risk of a cardiovascular event ≥10%. Type 2 diabetes: Screen for prediabetes and type 2 diabetes with A1c in overweight or obese adults.	Colorectal cancer: Screening starting at age 45 with fecal occult blood testing yearly, multi-target stool DNA testing every 3 years, flexible sigmoidoscopy every 5 years, or colonoscopy every 10 years.	Chlamydia, gonorrhea, syphilis: Screen men only if at increased risk for infection. HIV and HCV screening at least once. Offer PrEP to persons with high risk of HIV infection. Depression. Intimate partner violence. Tobacco smoking cessation. Unhealthy alcohol use. Unhealthy drug use.
50-64	Hypertension: Annual blood pressure screening. Cholesterol: Lipid screening. A statin is indicated for the primary prevention of CVD[1] in patients with CVD risk factor(s) and an estimated 10-year risk of a cardiovascular event ≥10%. Type 2 diabetes: Screen for prediabetes and type 2 diabetes with A1c in overweight or obese adults.	Colorectal cancer: Screening with fecal occult blood testing yearly, multi-target stool DNA testing every 3 years, flexible sigmoidoscopy every 5 years, or colonoscopy every 10 years. Lung cancer: Annual screening with low-dose computed tomography in adults starting at age 55 who have a 20 pack-year smoking history and currently smoke or have quit within the past 15 years. Prostate cancer: Screening with PSA[1] based on shared decision-making.	Chlamydia, gonorrhea, syphilis: Screen men only if at increased risk for infection. HIV and HCV screening at least once. Offer PrEP to persons with high risk of HIV infection. Depression. Intimate partner violence. Tobacco smoking cessation. Unhealthy alcohol use. Unhealthy drug use.
≥65	Hypertension: Annual blood pressure screening. Cholesterol: Lipid screening. A statin is indicated for the primary prevention of CVD[1] in patients with CVD risk factor(s) and an estimated 10-year risk of a cardiovascular event ≥10%. Type 2 diabetes: Screen for prediabetes and type 2 diabetes with A1c in overweight or obese adults.	Colorectal cancer: Screening with fecal occult blood testing yearly, multi-target stool DNA testing every 3 years, flexible sigmoidoscopy every 5 years, or colonoscopy every 10 years until age 75. Lung cancer: Annual screening with low-dose computed tomography in adults who have a 20 pack-year smoking history and currently smoke or have quit within the past 15 years until age 80. Prostate cancer: Screening with PSA until age 75 based on shared decision-making.	Chlamydia, gonorrhea, syphilis: Screen men only if at increased risk for infection. HIV and HCV screening at least once. Offer PrEP to persons with high risk of HIV infection. AAA[1]: One-time screening with ultrasonography in patients age 65-75 years who have ever smoked. Depression. Intimate partner violence. Tobacco smoking cessation. Unhealthy alcohol use. Unhealthy drug use.

1. PrEP: HIV preexposure prophylaxis. CVD: Cardiovascular disease. DEXA: Dual x-ray absorptiometry. PSA: Prostate-Specific Antigen. AAA: Abdominal aortic aneurysm.
2. Risk factors for cardiovascular disease: Hypertension, dyslipidemia, diabetes, tobacco smoking, and positive family history.
3. Risk factors for HIV infection: Multiple sexual partners, inconsistent use of barrier protection, and IV drug use.

28-6 Medical Ethics

Four Principles of Medical Ethics

Non-maleficence: Do no harm.
Beneficence: Do good and promote patients' well-being.
Autonomy: Respect adult patients' right to self-determination.
Justice: Provide care and allocate resources fairly and equitably to all patients. Protect vulnerable populations.

Patient Rights

- **Confidentiality**: All information about the patient should be kept confidential between the physician and the patient. Exceptions include the following: 1. A patient may waive their right to privacy (eg, communication with family, insurance companies) with verbal and/or written consent, 2. Communicable diseases (eg, STIs; HIV; TB; diseases affecting unvaccinated patients; and water/foodborne, zoonotic, mosquito-borne, and tick-borne diseases), 3. A patient poses a danger to self or others (Tarasoff decision), 4. Child or elder abuse, and 5. Gunshot and/or other penetrating wounds (report to police).
- **Informed Consent:** Before a procedure or therapy, the patient must be adequately informed about the intervention and its indications, its risks and benefits, and risks and benefits of other options, including no intervention. Patients can change their mind at any point. Exceptions include 1. The patient requires emergency intervention, and 2. The patient lacks decision-making capacity, in which case a surrogate decision-maker must provide consent.
- **Minors:** Minors (age <18 years) usually cannot provide consent for their own medical care, and consent must be obtained from a surrogate decision-maker (eg, parent). Exceptions include the following: 1. Emergencies (eg, blood transfusions in the setting of trauma), 2. Substance use disorder treatment, 3. Sexual or reproductive health (STI screening and treatment, contraception, prenatal care except for abortion services); laws vary by state, and 4. Legally emancipated minors (eg, married, in the military, financially self-sufficient).
  - A surrogate decision-maker has the right to refuse medical intervention for a minor in non-life-threatening situations. (eg, declining vaccinations). If their decision may endanger the patient's life, a physician may provide treatment based on either legal precedent in emergencies or a court order in non-emergencies.
- **Disclosure:**
  - **Full disclosure:** Patients have the right to full medical disclosure. Exceptions include if the patient requests that information be withheld from them or if a physician determines that disclosure would harm the patient (therapeutic privilege).
  - **Medical errors:** It is mandatory for doctors to notify patients of any errors that have occurred during their medical treatment.
  - **Physician conflict of interest:** Occurs when physicians are at risk of providing biased care due to personal interests (eg, owning stock in a pharmaceutical company). Physicians should report all potential conflicts of interest.

Patient Decision-Making

- **Capacity** is a patient's ability to make decisions about their care. Capacity can be assessed by the physician and can be situation-dependent. For example, a patient may have capacity to refuse their daily medications, yet lack capacity to consent for a major surgery. Patients with decision-making capacity have the right to refuse medical intervention unless their decision endangers public health (eg, a patient with active TB cannot refuse treatment). Capacity is based on the patient's ability to 1. demonstrate comprehension of the pertinent information, 2. compare risks and benefits of different options, 3. appreciate how the situation relates to themselves, and 4. make a clear, consistent choice with rationale.
- **Competence** is the ability of an individual to participate in legal proceedings. Legal competence is presumed; lack of competence is determined by a judge after presentation of evidence during a court hearing.

End-of-Life Issues

- **Advance directives:**
  - **Written advance directive:** Addresses a patient's wishes regarding life-sustaining treatment in the event that the patient loses decision-making capacity (eg, persistent vegetative state). It can include decisions on CPR, intubation, and specific therapies (eg, antibiotics, dialysis). A living will is an example.
  - **Durable medical power of attorney**: Legally appoints a surrogate decision-maker to make medical decisions if a patient loses decision-making capacity.
  - In the event that a patient loses decision-making capacity and has no written advance directive or durable power of attorney, medical decisions are made by loved ones. Order of precedence depends on the state but is often the spouse, adult children, parents, adult siblings, grandchildren/grandparents, other relatives, and friends.
- **Withdrawal of care:** Patients and their surrogate decision-makers have the right to decline or withdraw life-sustaining treatment (eg, ventilation, medications).
  - **Hospice** focuses on palliative medicine (eg, pain management, quality of life) in patients with an estimated life expectancy of <6 months.
  - **Medical futility**: In cases where further intervention is deemed medically futile, a physician is not ethically obligated to provide treatment in spite of a patient's wishes under any of these circumstances: 1. The intervention will not be effective in achieving the patient's goals of care, 2. Maximal intervention has failed or is failing, and 3. The intervention lacks basis in medical evidence or rationale.

Abbreviations

AAA: Abdominal aortic aneurysm
ABA: Applied behavioral analysis
ABCs: Airway, breathing, circulation
ABG: Arterial blood gases
AC: Acromioclavicular
AC: Air conduction
AC: Anti-coagulation
ACD: Allergic contact dermatitis
ACE: Angiotensin converting enzyme
ACEI: Angiotensin converting enzyme inhibitor
ACLS: Advanced cardiovascular life support
ACT: Acceptance and commitment therapy
ACTH: Adrenocorticotropin hormone
AD: Alzheimer's disease
AD: Atopic dermatitis
ADH: Alcohol dehydrogenase
ADHD: Attention-deficit/hyperactivity disorder
ADOS: Autism diagnostic observation schedule
AED: Antiepileptic drug
AFB: Acid-fast bacillus
AFib: Atrial fibrillation
AFP: Alpha fetoprotein
AG: Anion gap
AGMA: Anion gap metabolic acidosis
AIP: Acute interstitial pneumonia
AIS: Adenocarcinoma in situ
AKI: Acute kidney injury
ALL: Acute lymphoblastic leukemia
ALP: Alkaline phosphatase
ALS: Amyotrophic lateral sclerosis
ALT: Alanine aminotransferase
AMP: Adenosine monophosphate
ANC: Absolute neutrophil count
ANCA: Antibodies against cytoplasmic antigens
ANS: Autonomic nervous system
APL: Acute promyelocytic leukemia
APLS: Antiphospholipid syndrome
AR: Aortic regurgitation
AR: Attributable risk
ARB: Angiotensin II receptor blockers
ARDS: Acute respiratory distress syndrome
ARFID: Avoidant restrictive food intake disorder
ARN: Acute retinal necrosis
ARNI: Angiotensin receptor/neprilysin inhibitor
ARR: Absolute risk reduction
ART: Antiretroviral therapy
AS: Aortic stenosis
ASA: Aspirin
ASD: Autism spectrum disorder
AST: Aspartate aminotransferase
ATIII: Antithrombin III
ATRA: All-trans-retinoic acid
AUB: Abnormal uterine bleeding
AVM: Arteriovenous malformation
AVNRT: Atrioventricular nodal reentrant tachycardia
AVP: Arginine vasopressin
AVRT: Atrioventricular reentrant tachycardia
AXR: Abdominal x-ray
BC: Bone conduction
BCC: Basal cell carcinoma
BDD: Body dysmorphic disorder
BMI: Body mass index
BMP: Basic metabolic panel
BNP: B-type natriuretic peptide
BP: Blood pressure
BPD: Bronchopulmonary dysplasia
BPH: Benign prostatic hypertrophy
BPP: Biophysical profile
BPPV: Benign paroxysmal positional vertigo
BSA: Body surface area
BUN: Blood urea nitrogen
CAD: Coronary artery disease
CAH: Congenital adrenal hyperplasia
CBC: Complete blood count
CBT: Cognitive-behavioral therapy
CBT-I: Cognitive behavioral therapy for insomnia
CCB: Calcium channel blocker
CDH: Congenital diaphragmatic hernia
CF: Cystic fibrosis
CFTR: Cystic fibrosis transmembrane conductance regulator
CGD: Chronic granulomatous disease
CHF: Congestive heart failure
CJD: Creutzfeldt-Jakob's disease
CK-MB: Creatine kinase–MB isoenzyme
CMV: Cytomegalovirus
CN: Cyanide
CNS: Central nervous system
CO: Carbon monoxide
COP: Cryptogenic organizing pneumonia
COPD: Chronic obstructive pulmonary disease
CP: Cerebral palsy
CPAM: Congenital pulmonary airway malformation
CPAP: Continuous positive airway pressure
CPPD: Calcium pyrophosphate dihydrate
CPR: Cardiopulmonary resuscitation
CRH: Corticotropin releasing hormone
CRRP: Closed reduction percutaneous pinning
CSA: Central sleep apnea
CSF: Cerebrospinal fluid
CT: Computed tomography
CT: Cross-sectional imaging
CTA: Computed tomography angiography
CTEPH: Chronic thromboembolic pulmonary hypertension
CTX: CefTriaXone
CVA: Cerebrovascular accident
CVA: Costovertebral angle
CVD: Cardiovascular disease
CVID: Common variable immunodeficiency
Cx: Culture
CXR: Chest x-ray
D&C: Dilatation and curettage
D5NS: Dextrose 5% in normal saline
DAPT: Dual antiplatelet therapy
Dbili: Direct bilirubin
DBP: Diastolic blood pressure
DBT: Dialectical behavioral therapy
DCIS: Ductal carcinoma in situ
DDAVP: Desmopressin

DDH: Developmental dysplasia of the hip
DEXA: Dual x-ray absorptiometry
DIC: Disseminated intravascular coagulation
DJS: Dubin-Johnson syndrome
DKA: Diabetic ketoacidosis
DLB: Dementia with Lewy bodies
DLCO: Diffusion capacity of carbon monoxide
DM: Dermatomyositis
DM1: Type 1 diabetes
DM2: Type 2 diabetes
DMSA: Dimercaptosuccinic acid
DOE: Dyspnea on exertion
DRE: Digital rectal exam
DRUJ: Distal radioulnar joint
DTRs: Deep tendon reflexes
DVT: Deep vein thrombosis
EAC: External auditory canal
EBV: Epstein-Barr virus
ECV: External cephalic version
ED: Erectile dysfunction
EEG: Electroencephalogram
EGD: Esophagogastroduodenoscopy
EH: Endometrial hyperplasia
EHEC: *Escherichia coli* O157:H7
EKG/ECG: Electrocardiogram
ELISA: Enzyme-linked immunoassay
EMDR: Eye movement desensitization and reprocessing
EMG: Electromyography
EPS: Extrapyramidal symptoms
ERCP: Endoscopic retrograde cholangiopancreatography
ESRD: End stage renal (kidney) disease
ET: Endotracheal
ET: Erythrotelangectatic
ETOH: Ethanol (alcohol)
ETT: Epithelioid trophoblastic tumor
EUS: Endoscopic ultrasound
FAP: Familial adenomatous polyposis
FEV1: Forced expiratory volume in 1 second
FFP: Fresh frozen plasma
FHH: Familial hypocalciuric hypercalcemia
FHR: Fetal heart rate
FLC: Free light chain
FLG: Filaggrin
FNA: Fine needle aspiration
FND: Functional neurological disorder
FNH: Focal nodular hyperplasia
FOOSH: Fall on an outstretched hand
FSH: Follicle-stimulating hormone
fT4: Free T4
FVC: Forced vital capacity
GAD: Generalized anxiety disorder
GAS: Group A streptococci
GCA: Giant cell arteritis
GCT: Germ cell tumors
GDMT: Guideline-directed medical therapy
GERD: Gastroesophageal reflux disease
GFR: Glomerular filtration rate
GGT: Gamma-glutamyl transferase
GH: Growth hormone
GHRH: GH-releasing hormone
GIST: GI stromal tumor
GKS: Gamma-knife radiosurgery
GPA: Granulomatosis with polyangiitis
GPC: Gram positive cocci
GSW: Gunshot wound
GTCS: Generalized tonic-clonic seizures
GTT: Glucose tolerance test
GVHD: Graft versus host disease
H/H: Hemoglobin and hematocrit
H2R: Histamine 2 receptor
HAV: Hepatitis A virus
HBV: Hepatitis B virus
HCC: Hepatocellular carcinoma
HCL: Hairy cell leukemia
HCM: Hypertrophic cardiomyopathy
HCN: Hyperpolarization-activated, cyclic nucleotide-gated
HCT: Hematopoietic cell transplantation
HCTZ: Hydrochlorothiazide
HCV: Hepatitis C virus
HD: Hemodialysis
HD: Huntington's disease
HE: Hepatic encephalopathy
HepA: Hepatitis A
HepB: Hepatitis B
HES: Hypereosinophilic syndrome
Hgb: Hemoglobin
HHS: Hyperosmolar hyperglycemic syndrome
HHT: Hereditary hemorrhagic telangiectasias
Hib: Haemophilus influenzae type b
HIE: Hypoxic ischemic encephalopathy
HIT: Heparin-induced thrombocytopenia
HIV: Human immunodeficiency virus
HL: Hodgkin lymphomas
HLA: Human leukocyte antigens
HLD: Hyperlipidemia
HLHS: Hypoplastic left heart syndrome
HOCM: Hypertrophic obstructive cardiomyopathy
HPTH: Hyperparathyroidism
HPV: Human papillomavirus
HR: Heart rate
hrHPV: High-risk human papillomavirus
HRS: Hepatorenal syndrome
HSCT: Hematopoietic stem cell transplant
HSP: Henoch-Schonlein purpura
HSV: Herpes simplex virus
HTN: Hypertension
HUS: Hemolytic uremic syndrome
HVA: Homovanillic acid
IBD: Inflammatory bowel disease
IBS: Irritable bowel syndrome
ICD: Implantable cardiac defibrillator
ICD: Irritant contact dermatitis
ICP: Intracranial pressure
ICS: Inhaled corticosteroid
ID: Intellectual disability
IDA: Iron deficiency anemia
IF: Immunofluorescence
IGRA: Interferon-gamma release assay

IIV4: Influenza inactivated
ILD: Interstitial lung disease
Infxn: Infection
INH: Isoniazid
Intest Isch: Intestinal ischemia
IOP: Intraocular pressure
IPF: Idiopathic pulmonary fibrosis
ITP: Immune thrombocytopenic purpura
IVC: Inferior vena cava
IVF: Intravenous fluid
IVH: Intraventricular hemorrhage
IVIG: IV immunoglobulin
JIA: Juvenile idiopathic arthritis
JVP: Jugular venous pulse
KS: Kaposi sarcoma
LA: Lactic acidosis
LA: Left atrium
LABA: Long-acting beta agonist
LAD: Lymphadenopathy
LAIV4: Influenza live: attenuated
LAMA: Long-acting muscarinic agonist
LAP: Leukocyte alkaline phosphatase
LARC: Long-acting reversible contraception
LCHAD: Long-chain 3-hydroxyacyl-CoA dehydrogenase
LCIS: Lobular carcinoma in situ
LCP: Legg-Calvé-Perthes
LDH: Lactate dehydrogenase
LEEP: Loop electrosurgical excision procedure
LEMS: Lambert-Eaton myasthenic syndrome
LGA: Large for gestational age
LH: Luteinizing hormone
LLQ: Left lower quadrant
LM: Lentigo maligna
LMWH: Low-molecular-weight heparin
LOAF: Lumbricals, opponens pollicis, abductor pollicis brevis, flexor pollicis brevis
LP: Lumbar puncture
LUQ: Left upper quadrant
LVOT: Left ventricular outflow tract
LVOTO: Left ventricular outflow tract obstruction
MAC: *Mycobacterium avium* complex
MAHA: Microangiopathic hemolytic anemia
MALT: Mucosa-associated lymphoid tissue
MAOI: Monoamine oxidase inhibitor
MAS: Milk-alkali syndrome
MAT: Multifocal atrial tachycardia
MCA: Middle cerebral artery
MCV: Mean corpuscular volume
MDD: Major depressive disorder
MDS: Myelodysplastic syndrome
MEN: Multiple endocrine neoplasia
MenACWY: Meningococcal A, C, W, Y
MenB: Meningococcal B
MG: Myasthenia gravis
MGUS: Monoclonal gammopathy of undetermined significance
MI: Myocardial infarction
MM: Multiple myeloma
MMR: Measles, mumps, rubella
MPA: Microscopic polyangiitis
MPO: Myeloperoxidase
MR: Mitral regurgitation
MRSA: Methicillin-resistant *Staphylococcus aureus*
MS: Mitral stenosis
MS: Multiple sclerosis
MSU: Monosodium urate
NAAT: Nucleic acid amplification test
NAC: N-acetylcysteine
NAFLD: Non-alcoholic fatty liver disease
NAGMA: Non-anion gap metabolic acidoses
NAPQI: N-acetyl-p-benzoquinone imine
NASH: Non-alcoholic steatohepatitis
NCHCT: Non-contrast head CT
NEC: Necrotizing enterocolitis
NGT: Nasogastric tube
NHL: Non-Hodgkin lymphomas
NMO: Neuromyelitis optica
NMS: Neuroleptic malignant syndrome
NNH: Number needed to harm
NNT: Number needed to treat
NPV: Negative predictive value
NRP: Neonatal resuscitation program
NSAIDs: Non-steroidal anti-inflammatory drugs
NSTEMI: Non-ST-segment elevation myocardial infarction
NVE: Native valve endocarditis
OA: Osteoarthritis
OCD: Obsessive-compulsive disorder
OCPD: Obsessive-compulsive personality disorder
OCPs: Oral contraceptives
ODD: Oppositional defiant disorder
OME: Otitis media with effusion
OR: Odds ratio
ORIF: Open reduction and internal fixation
OSA: Obstructive sleep apnea
OSFED: Other specified feeding and eating disorder
OTC: Over the counter
PAC: Premature atrial contraction
PAD: Peripheral arterial disease
PAH: Pulmonary arterial hypertension
PAN: Polyarteritis nodosa
PBC: Primary biliary cholangitis
PCA: Posterior cerebral artery
PCC: Prothrombin complex concentrate
PCH: Paroxysmal cold hemoglobinuria
PCIT: Parent-child interaction therapy
PCOS: Polycystic ovarian syndrome
PCP: Pneumocystis pneumonia
PCT: Porphyria cutanea tarda
PCWP: Pulmonary capillary wedge pressure
PD: Parkinson's disease
PD: Programmed death
PE: Pulmonary embolism
PEA: Pulseless electrical activity
PFPS: Patellofemoral pain syndrome
PFT: Pulmonary function test
PGE: Prostaglandin E1
PH: Pulmonary hypertension
PID: Pelvic inflammatory disease
PKU: Phenylketonuria

PLAP: Placental alkaline phosphatase
PLT: Platelets
PMR: Polymyalgia rheumatica
PNES: Psychogenic non-epileptic spells
PPI: Proton pump inhibitor
PPROM: Preterm prelabor rupture of membranes
PPS: Peripheral pulmonic stenosis
PRCA: Pure red cell aplasia
PrEP: Preexposure prophylaxis
PRES: Posterior reversible (leuko) encephalopathy syndrome
PRL: Prolactin
PROM: Prelabor rupture of membranes
PSA: Prostate-specific antigen
PSC: Primary sclerosing cholangitis
PSTT: Placental site trophoblastic tumor
PSVT: Paroxysmal supraventricular tachycardia
PTH: Parathyroid hormone
PTHrP: PTH related protein
PTSD: Post-traumatic stress disorder
PTU: Propylthiouracil
PUD: Peptic ulcer disease
RA: Rheumatoid arthritis
RAIU: Radioactive iodine uptake test
RAP: Right atrial pressure
RAPD: Relative afferent pupillary defect
RAST: Radioallergosorbent test
RBUS: Renal and bladder ultrasound
RCL: Radial collateral ligament
RDS: Respiratory distress syndrome
REM: Rapid eye movement
Rh: Rhesus
Rhabdo: Rhabdomyolysis
RHC: Right heart catheterization
RIPE: Rifampin, isoniazid, pyrazinamide, ethambutol
RIV4: Influenza recombinant
RLQ: Right lower quadrant
RLS: Restless leg syndrome
ROM: Range of motion
RPR: Rapid plasma reagin
RR: Relative risk
RR: Respiratory rate
RRR: Relative risk reduction
RTA: Renal tubular acidosis
RUQ: Right upper quadrant
RZV: Zoster recombinant
SABA: Short-acting beta agonist
SAD: Social anxiety disorder
SBO: Small bowl obstruction
SBP: Spontaneous bacterial peritonitis
SBP: Systolic blood pressure
SCAPE: Sympathetic crashing acute pulmonary edema
SCC: Squamous cell carcinoma
SCFE: Slipped capital femoral epiphysis
SCID: Severe-combined immunodeficiency
SCLC: Small-cell lung cancer
SIADH: Syndrome of inappropriate antidiuretic hormone secretion
SIBO: Small intestinal bacterial overgrowth
SIDS: Sudden infant death syndrome
SLE: Systemic lupus erythematosus
SOB: Shortness of breath (can change "shortness of breath" to "dyspnea" to save space)
SPEP: Sending serum protein electrophoresis
SPEP: Serum protein electrophoresis
SRS: Stereotactic radiosurgery
SS: Serotonin syndrome
SSC: Scleroderma/systemic sclerosis
SSRI/SNRI: Selective serotonin/norepinephrine reuptake inhibitor
SSSS: Staphylococcal scalded skin syndrome
STEC: Shiga toxin–producing *Escherichia coli*
STEMI: ST-segment elevation myocardial infarction
STI/STD: Sexually transmitted infection/disease
SVCS: Superior vena cava syndrome
SVR: Sustained virologic response
SVT: Supraventricular tachycardia
T: Temperature
TACE: Trans-arterial chemoembolization
TACO: Transfusion-associated circulatory overload
TAPVR: Total anomalous pulmonary venous return
TAVR: Transaortic valve replacement
TB: Tuberculosis
TBI: Traumatic brain injury
Tbili: Total bilirubin
TCA: Tricyclic antidepressant
Tdap: Tetanus:diphtheria:pertussis
TEE: Transesophageal echocardiogram
TEF: Tracheoesophageal fistula
TIA: Transient ischemic attack
TIPS: Trans-jugular intra-hepatic portosystemic shunts
TLC: Total lung capacity
TMP-SMX: Trimethoprim and sulfamethoxazole
TOF: Train-of-four
TRALI: Transfusion-associated lung injury
TRAP: Tartrate-resistant acid phosphatase
TRH: Thyrotropin-releasing hormone
TS: Tuberous sclerosis
TSH: Thyroid-stimulating hormone
TSS: Tay-Sachs syndrome
TTE: Transthoracic echocardiogram
TTN: Transient tachypnea of the newborn
TTP: Tenderness to palpation
TTP: Thrombotic thrombocytopenic purpura
TTR: Transthyretin
TURP: Transurethral resection of the prostate
TVUS: Transvaginal ultrasound
Tx: Treat/treatment
UA: Urinalysis
U_{AG}: Urine anion gap
UC: Ulcerative colitis
UCL: Ulnar collateral ligament
UE: Uremic encephalopathy
UFH: Unfractionated heparin
Uosm: Urine osmolality
UPEP: Urine protein electrophoresis
UPJ: Ureteropelvic junction
URI: Upper respiratory tract infection
UROD: Uroporphyrinogen decarboxylase
US: Ultrasound

UTI: Urinary tract infection
VAR: Varicella
VBG: Venous blood gases
VCUG: Voiding cystourethrogram
VEGF: Vascular endothelial growth factor
VFib: Ventricular fibrillation
VMA: Vanillylmandelic acid
VP: Ventriculoperitoneal
VT/VTach: Ventricular tachycardia
VTE: Venous thromboembolism
VUR: Vesicoureteral reflux
VWD: Von Willebrand disease
WAS: Wiskott-Aldrich's syndrome
WASP: Wiskott-Aldrich's syndrome protein
WBC: White blood cell
WBRT: Whole brain radiation therapy
WE: Wernicke encephalopathy
WNL: Within normal limits
WPW: Wolff-Parkinson-White's syndrome
X-ray: XR

Image and Table Acknowledgments

Chapter 1

5 **ST-segment elevation myocardial infarction.** Reproduced with permission from J. Stephan Stapczynski, Maricopa Medical Center.

31 **Sinus rhythm with 1st-degree atrioventricular block.** Reproduced with permission from Tintinalli JE, Ma OJ, Yealy DM, et al, eds. *Tintinalli's Emergency Medicine: A Comprehensive Study Guide*, 9th ed. New York: McGraw Hill; 2020.

31 **Second-degree AV block: Mobitz type I AV block with Wenckebach phenomenon.** Reproduced with permission from Elmoselhi A. *Cardiology: An Integrated Approach.* New York: McGraw Hill; 2018.

31 **Second-degree AV block: Mobitz type II with a 2:1 to 3:1 AV block.** Reproduced with permission from Elmoselhi A. *Cardiology: An Integrated Approach.* New York: McGraw Hill; 2018.

31 **Complete or third-degree AV block.** Reproduced with permission from McKean SC, Ross JJ, Dressler DD, Scheurer DB, eds. *Principles and Practice of Hospital Medicine*, 2nd ed. New York: McGraw Hill; 2017.

34 **Atrial fibrillation.** Reproduced with permission from Elmoselhi A. *Cardiology: An Integrated Approach.* New York: McGraw Hill; 2018.

34 **Re-entrant tachyarrhythmia resulting from Wolff-Parkinson-White syndrome.** Reproduced with permission from Cardiovascular Disorders: Heart Disease In: Hammer GD, McPhee SJ. Pathophysiology of Disease: *An Introduction to Clinical Medicine*, 8e, New York: McGraw Hill, 2019.

34 **Atrial flutter with variable block.** Reproduced with permission from McKean SC, Ross JJ, Dressler DD, Scheurer DB, eds: *Principles and Practice of Hospital Medicine*, 2nd ed. New York, McGraw Hill, 2017.

34 **Multifocal atrial tachycardia (MAT) with varying P-wave morphologies and P-P intervals.** Courtesy of Jason E. Roediger, CCT, CRAT.

34 **Atrioventricular nodal reentrant tachycardia (AVNRT).** Reproduced with permission from McKean SC, Ross JJ, Dressler DD, Scheurer DB, eds. *Principles and Practice of Hospital Medicine*, 2nd ed. New York: McGraw Hill; 2017.

36 **Torsade de Pointes ventricular tachycardia (VT).** Reproduced with permission from Hall JB, Schmidt GA, Kress JP. *Principles of Critical Care*, 4th ed. New York: McGraw Hill; 2015.

36 **Ventricular fibrillation. After 6 beats, sinus rhythm degenerates into ventricular fibrillation.** Reproduced with permission from Stone CK, Humphries RL. *Current Diagnosis & Treatment: Emergency Medicine*, 7th ed. New York: McGraw Hill; 2011.

36 **Multifocal PVCs: 2nd, 6th, and 9th beats are PVCs.** Reproduced with permission from Cardiac rhythm disturbances. In: Tintinalli JE, Ma O, Yealy DM, et al, eds. *Tintinalli's Emergency Medicine: A Comprehensive Study Guide*, 9th ed. New York: McGraw Hill; 2020.

41 **Acute pericarditis.** Reproduced with permission from Loscalzo J, Fauci AS, Kasper DL, et al, eds. *Harrison's Principles of Internal Medicine*, 21st ed. New York: McGraw Hill; 2022.

41 **Electrical alternans in the setting of cardiac tamponade.** Reproduced with permission from Loscalzo J, Fauci AS, Kasper DL, et al, eds. *Harrison's Principles of Internal Medicine*, 21st ed. New York: McGraw Hill; 2022.

43 **Timing and intensity of cardiac murmurs.** Reproduced with permission from Cardiovascular disorders: heart disease. In: Hammer GD, McPhee SJ. *Pathophysiology of Disease: An Introduction to Clinical Medicine*, 8th ed. New York: McGraw Hill; 2019.

43 **Heart auscultation points.** Used with permission from Artemida-psy/Shutterstock.

49 **Table. Summary of Antihypertensive Drugs.** Reproduced with permission from Tintinalli JE, Ma OJ, Yealy DM, et al, eds. *Tintinalli's Emergency Medicine: A Comprehensive Study Guide*, 9th ed. New York: McGraw Hill; 2020.

Chapter 2

56 **Eosinophilic esophagitis with mucosal lacerations.** Reproduced with permission from Greenberger NJ, Blumberg RS, Burakoff R, eds. *Current Diagnosis & Treatment: Gastroenterology, Hepatology, & Endoscopy*, 3rd ed. New York: McGraw Hill; 2016.

66 **"Beads on a string" appearance of intrahepatic and extrahepatic ducts in primary sclerosing cholangitis.** From Papadakis MA, McPhee SJ, Rabow MW, McQuaid KR, eds. *Current Diagnosis & Treatment 2022.* New York: McGraw Hill; 2022, eFigure 16-57. Reproduced with permission from Nicholas Fidelman, MD.

70 **Timeline of HBV infection with serologic markers.** Reproduced with permission from Hollinger FB, Dienstag JL. Hepatitis B and D viruses. In Murray PR, ed. *Manual of Clinical Microbiology*, 7th ed. Washington, DC: ASM Press, 1999.

70 **Kayser-Fleischer rings seen in Wilson's disease.** Reproduced by permission from Schaefer GB, Thompson JN Jr. *Medical Genetics: An Integrated Approach.* New York: McGraw-Hill; 2014.

72 **Figure 2.7.1.** Reproduced with permission from Huppert LA, Dyster TG. *Huppert's Notes: Pathophysiology and Clinical Pearls for Internal Medicine.* New York: McGraw Hill; 2021.

74 **Esophageal varices on EGD in a patient with liver cirrhosis.** Reproduced with permission from Loscalzo J, Fauci AS, Kasper DL, et al, eds. *Harrison's Principles of Internal Medicine*, 21st ed. New York: McGraw Hill; 2022.

76 **Differential diagnosis for abdominal pain based on area of pain.** Reproduced with permission from Huppert LA, Dyster TG. *Huppert's Notes: Pathophysiology and Clinical Pearls for Internal Medicine.* New York: McGraw Hill; 2021.

76 **Barrett's esophagus.** Reproduced with permission from Loscalzo J, Fauci AS, Kasper DL, et al, eds. *Harrison's Principles of Internal Medicine*, 21st ed. New York: McGraw Hill; 2022.

76 **Esophageal adenocarcinoma with Barrett's esophagus.** Reproduced with permission from Loscalzo J, Fauci AS, Kasper DL, et al, eds. *Harrison's Principles of Internal Medicine*, 21st ed. New York: McGraw Hill; 2022.

86 **Colon adenocarcinoma on colonoscopy.** Reproduced with permission from Loscalzo J, Fauci AS, Kasper DL, et al, eds. *Harrison's Principles of Internal Medicine*, 21st ed. New York: McGraw Hill; 2022.

87 **Table 2-11A: Vitamin Deficiencies.** Reproduced with permission from Peter J. Kennelly, Kathleen M. Botham, et al. *Harper's Illustrated Biochemistry*, 32nd ed. New York: McGraw Hill; 2023.

87 Table 2-11B: Mineral Deficiencies. Reproduced with permission from Lee W. Janson, Marc E. Tischler. The Big Picture: *Medical Biochemistry.* New York: McGraw Hill, 2012.

Chapter 3

93 Hypochromic microcytic anemia. Reproduced with permission from Lichtman M, et al, eds. *Williams Hematology*, 7th ed. New York: McGraw Hill; 2005; Hillman RS, Ault KA. *Hematology in General Practice*, 4th ed. New York: McGraw Hill; 2005, Figure 62-3.

93 Target cells. Reproduced with permission from Lichtman M, et al, eds. *Williams Hematology*, 7th ed. New York: McGraw Hill; 2005; Hillman RS, Ault KA. *Hematology in General Practice*, 4th ed. New York: McGraw Hill; 2005, Figure 62-13.

93 Ringed sideroblasts in bone marrow. Reproduced with permission from Loscalzo J, Fauci AS, Kasper DL, et al, eds. *Harrison's Principles of Internal Medicine*, 21st ed. New York: McGraw Hill; 2022, Figure A6-9.

98 Sickled red blood cells. Reproduced with permission from Kemp WL, Burns DK, Brown TG. *Pathology: The Big Picture.* New York: McGraw Hill; 2008, Figure 12-8.

98 Spherocytes. Reproduced with permission from Lichtman MA, Shafer MS, Felgar RE, Wang N. *Lichtman's Atlas of Hematology.* New York: McGraw Hill; 2017, Figure I.A.054.

98 Schistocytes. Reproduced with permission from Kemp WL, Burns DK, Brown TG. *Pathology: The Big Picture.* New York: McGraw Hill; 2008, Figure 12-24.

98 Bite cells. Reproduced with permission from Lichtman MA, Shafer MS, Felgar RE, Wang N. *Lichtman's Atlas of Hematology.* New York: McGraw Hill; 2017, Figure I.A.007.

104 Purpuric lesions in DIC. Reproduced with permission from Wolff K, Johnson R. *Fitzpatrick's Color Atlas & Synopsis of Clinical Dermatology*, 6th ed. New York: McGraw Hill; 2009, Figure 79–2.

104 Coagulation cascade. Reproduced with permission from Reisner HM. *Pathology: A Modern Case Study*, 2nd ed. New York: McGraw Hill; 2020.

108 Atopic dermatitis in Wiskott-Aldrich syndrome. Reproduced with permission from Kang S, Amagai M, Bruckner AL, Enk AH, Margolis DJ, McMichael AJ, Orringer JS, eds. *Fitzpatrick's Dermatology*, 9th ed. New York: McGraw Hill; 2019, Figure 132-71.

108 Thrombocytopenia. Reproduced with permission from Lichtman MA, Shafer MS, Felgar RE, Wang N. *Lichtman's Atlas of Hematology.* New York: McGraw Hill; 2017, Figure IV.A.021.

112 Acute DVT. From Knoop KJ, Stack LB, Storrow AB, Thurman RJ, eds. *The Atlas of Emergency Medicine*, 5th ed. New York: McGraw Hill; 2021, Figure 12.45. Reproduced with permission from photo contributor: Kevin J. Knoop, MD, MS.

114 Table: Types of Immunological (Hypersensitivity) Reactions. Reproduced with permission from DiPiro JT, Yee GC, Posey LM, et al, eds. *Pharmacotherapy: A Pathophysiologic Approach*, 11th ed. New York: McGraw Hill; 2020.

121 Reed-Sternberg cell. Reproduced with permission from Loscalzo J, Fauci AS, Kasper DL, et al, eds. *Harrison's Principles of Internal Medicine*, 21st ed. New York: McGraw Hill; 2022, Figure A6-23.

121 Follicular lymphoma. Reproduced with permission from Loscalzo J, Fauci AS, Kasper DL, et al, eds. *Harrison's Principles of Internal Medicine*, 21st ed. New York: McGraw Hill; 2022, Figure A6-19.

121 Burkitt lymphoma. Reproduced with permission from Loscalzo J, Fauci AS, Kasper DL, et al, eds. *Harrison's Principles of Internal Medicine*, 21st ed. New York: McGraw Hill; 2022, Figure A6-21.

121 Diffuse large B-cell lymphoma. Reproduced with permission from Loscalzo J, Fauci AS, Kasper DL, et al, eds. *Harrison's Principles of Internal Medicine*, 21st ed. New York: McGraw Hill; 2022, Figure A6-20.

124 Hypergranular cells. Can occur in all AML subtypes. Reproduced with permission from Jameson J, Fauci AS, Kasper DL, Hauser SL, Longo DL, Loscalzo J, eds. *Harrison's Principles of Internal Medicine*, 20th ed. New York: McGraw Hill; 2018, Figure A5-11.

124 Acute lymphoblastic leukemia. Reproduced with permission from Jameson J, Fauci AS, Kasper DL, Hauser SL, Longo DL, Loscalzo J, eds. *Harrison's Principles of Internal Medicine*, 20th ed. New York: McGraw Hill; 2018, Figure A5-13.

124 Acute promyelocytic leukemia. Reproduced with permission from Jameson J, Fauci AS, Kasper DL, Hauser SL, Longo DL, Loscalzo J, eds. *Harrison's Principles of Internal Medicine*, 20th ed. New York: McGraw Hill; 2018, Figure A5-10.

124 Smudge cells in chronic lymphocytic leukemia. Reproduced with permission from Jameson J, Fauci AS, Kasper DL, Hauser SL, Longo DL, Loscalzo J. eds. *Harrison's Principles of Internal Medicine*, 20th ed. New York: McGraw Hill; 2018, Figure A5-16.

127 Rouleaux formation in multiple myeloma. Reproduced with permission from Lichtman M et al, eds. *Williams Hematology*, 7th ed. New York: McGraw-Hill; 2005; Hillman RS, Ault KA. *Hematology in General Practice*, 4th ed. New York: McGraw Hill; 2005, Figure 62-9.

127 Apple-green birefringence with Congo red staining in AL amyloidosis. Reproduced with permission from Lichtman MA, Shafer MS, Felgar RE, Wang N. *Lichtman's Atlas of Hematology.* New York: McGraw Hill; 2017, Figure VII.C.080.

128 Mediastinal teratoma containing a tooth. Reproduced with permission from Yuh DD, Vricella LA, Yang SC, Doty JR, eds. *Johns Hopkins Textbook of Cardiothoracic Surgery*, 2nd ed. New York: McGraw-Hill; 2014, Figure 17-4.

Chapter 4

132 Figure 4.1.1. CT - Insulinoma. Reproduced with permission from Elsayes KM, Oldham SAA. *Introduction to Diagnostic Radiology.* New York: McGraw Hill; 2014.

134 Figure 4.2.1. Acanthosis nigricans in diabetes. Reproduced with permission from Loscalzo J, Fauci AS, Kasper DL, et al, eds. *Harrison's Principles of Internal Medicine*, 21st ed. New York: McGraw Hill; 2022.

142 Goiter. Reproduced, with permission from Usatine RP, Smith MA, Mayeaux EJ Jr, Chumley HS. *The Color Atlas and Synopsis of Family Medicine*, 3rd ed. Copyright 2019 by McGraw Hill. All rights reserved. Figure 236-3. Reproduced with permission from Richard P. Usatine, MD.

142 **Thyroid eye disease in a patient with Graves'.** Reproduced with permission from Greenspan FS, Strewler GJ, eds. *Basic & Clinical Endocrinology*, 5th ed. New York: McGraw-Hill; 1997.

142 **Radioactive iodine uptake test (RAIU) findings.** Reproduced with permission from Elsayes KM, Oldham SAA. *Introduction to Diagnostic Radiology*. New York: McGraw Hill; 2014.

143 **Figure 4.6.1.** Reproduced with permission from Jameson J, Fauci AS, Kasper DL, Hauser SL, Longo DL, Loscalzo J, eds. *Harrison's Principles of Internal Medicine*, 20th ed. New York: McGraw Hill; 2018.

146 **Right proximal femur and pelvis radiograph of a man with Paget's disease of bone involving both the femur and ilium.** Reproduced with permission from Halter JB, Ouslander JG, Studenski S, et al, eds. *Hazzard's Geriatric Medicine and Gerontology*, 7th ed. New York: McGraw Hill; 2017.

147 **Control of blood calcium and phosphate levels.** Reproduced with permission from Lee W. Janson, Marc E. Tischler, *The Big Picture: Medical Biochemistry*. New York: McGraw Hill; 2012, and reproduced with permission from Katzung BG, et al. *Basic and Clinical Pharmacology*, 11th ed. New York: McGraw Hill; 2009.

151 **Table.** Reproduced with permission from Khan AR, Geraghty JR. *First Aid® Clinical Pattern Recognition for the USMLE® Step 1*. New York: McGraw Hill; 2022.

151 **Lytic lesions in the skull of a patient with multiple myeloma.** Reproduced with permission from Chapter 11 Multiple myeloma and other plasma cell dyscrasias. In: Kantarjian HM, Wolff RA. *The MD Anderson Manual of Medical Oncology*, 3rd ed. New York: McGraw Hill; 2016.

154 **Figure 4.10.1.** Reproduced with permission from Fitzpatrick TB, Johnson RA, Polano MK, et al. *Fitzpatrick's Color Atlas and Synopsis of Clinical Dermatology: Common and Serious Diseases*, 2nd ed. New York: McGraw-Hill; 1992.

155 **Pituitary adenoma.** Reproduced with permission from Loscalzo J, Fauci AS, Kasper DL, et al, eds. *Harrison's Principles of Internal Medicine*, 21st ed. New York: McGraw Hill; 2022.

159 **Classic findings in Cushing's syndrome.** Reproduced with permission from Hammer GD, McPhee SJ. *Pathophysiology of Disease: An Introduction to Clinical Medicine*, 8th ed. New York: McGraw Hill; 2019.

Chapter 5

165 **Figure 5.2.1. Bacterial lobar pneumonia.** Reproduced with permission from Jameson J, Fauci AS, Kasper DL, Hauser SL, Longo DL, Loscalzo J, eds. *Harrison's Principles of Internal Medicine*, 20th ed. New York: McGraw Hill; 2018.

168 **Figure 5.3.1. Distribution of endemic mycoses in the United States.** Reproduced with permission from Grippi MA, Elias JA, Fishman JA, et al, eds. *Fishman's Pulmonary Diseases and Disorders*. 5th ed. New York: McGraw Hill; 2015.

168 **Figure 5.3.2. Blastomyces yeast.** From Loscalzo J, Fauci AS, Kasper DL, et al, eds. *Harrison's Principles of Internal Medicine*, 21st ed. New York: McGraw Hill; 2022, Figure 214-1. Reproduced with permission from Gregory M. Gauthier, MD, MS.

168 **Figure 5.3.3. Histoplasmosis.** Reproduced with permission from Lichtman MA, Shafer MS, Felgar RE, Wang N. *Lichtman's Atlas of Hematology*. New York: McGraw Hill; 2017.

168 **Figure 5.3.4. Coccidioides.** Reproduced with permission from Riedel S, Hobden JA, Miller S, et al. *Jawetz, Melnick, & Adelberg's Medical Microbiology*, 28th ed. New York: McGraw Hill; 2019.

168 **Figure 5.3.5. Paracoccidioides.** Reproduced with permission from Riedel S, Hobden JA, Miller S, et al. *Jawetz, Melnick, & Adelberg's Medical Microbiology*, 28th ed. New York: McGraw Hill; 2019.

170 **Erythema nodosum.** Nodules on the legs are usually very tender. Reproduced with permission from Maxine A. Papadakis, Stephen J. McPhee, Michael W. Rabow, Kenneth R. McQuaid. *Current Medical Diagnosis & Treatment 2023*. New York: McGraw Hill; 2023. Figure 6–20. Used, with permission, from TG Berger, MD, Dept Dermatology, UCSF.

171 **Figure 5.4.1.** Reproduced with permission from Soutor C, Hordinsky MK. *Clinical Dermatology: Diagnosis and Management of Common Disorders*, 2nd ed. New York: McGraw Hill; 2022.

171 **Figure 5.4.2.** Reproduced with permission from Soutor C, Hordinsky MK. *Clinical Dermatology: Diagnosis and Management of Common Disorders*, 2nd ed. New York: McGraw Hill; 2022.

171 **Figure 5.4.3.** Reproduced with permission from Soutor C, Hordinsky MK. *Clinical Dermatology: Diagnosis and Management of Common Disorders*, 2nd ed. New York: McGraw Hill; 2022.

171 **Figure 5.4.4.** Reproduced with permission from Aster JC, Bunn HF, eds. *Pathophysiology of Blood Disorders*, 2nd ed. New York: McGraw Hill; 2017.

175 **Thumbprint sign seen in epiglottitis.** Reproduced with permission from Stone CK, Humphries RL. *Current Diagnosis & Treatment: Emergency Medicine*, 8th ed. New York: McGraw Hill; 2017.

175 **Peritonsillar abscess.** From Knoop KJ, Stack LB, Storrow AB, Thurman RJ, eds. *The Atlas of Emergency Medicine*, 5th ed. New York: McGraw Hill; 2021, Figure 5.53. Reproduced with permission from photo contributor: Kevin J. Knoop, MD, MS.

182 **MRI/CT showing temporal lobe involvement in HSV encephalitis.** Reproduced with permission from Jameson J, Fauci AS, Kasper DL, Hauser SL, Longo DL, Loscalzo J, eds. *Harrison's Manual of Medicine*, 20th ed. New York: McGraw Hill; 2020.

198 **Figure 5.16.1. RMSF rash.** From Knoop KJ, Stack LB, Storrow AB, Thurman RJ, eds. *The Atlas of Emergency Medicine*, 5th ed. New York: McGraw Hill; 2021, Figure 13.27. Reproduced with permission from photo contributor: Daniel Noltkamper, MD.

198 **Figure 5.16.2. Babesia blood smear.** Reproduced with permission from Centers for Disease Control and Prevention. U.S. Department of Health & Human Services. DPDx—Laboratory Identification.

199 **Babesia spp. parasitizes RBCs as shown in this blood film.** Reproduced with permission from Centers for Disease Control and Prevention. U.S. Department of Health & Human Services. DPDx—Laboratory Identification of Parasites of Public Health Concern, Babesiosis. October, 2017.

200 Figure 5.17.1. From Steven Glenn, Laboratory & Consultation Division, Public Health Image Library, CDC.

200 Figure 5.17.2. From Usatine RP, Smith MA, Mayeaux EJ Jr, Chumley HS. *The Color Atlas and Synopsis of Family Medicine*, 3rd ed. New York: McGraw Hill; 2019, Figure 56-7. Reproduced with permission from Richard P. Usatine, MD.

201 Figure 5.18.1. Reproduced with permission from Papadakis MA, McPhee SJ, Rabow MW, McQuaid KR. *Current Medical Diagnosis & Treatment 2022.* New York: McGraw Hill; 2022.

201 Figure 5.18.2. Reproduced with permission from Southwick FS. *Infectious Diseases: A Clinical Short Course*, 4th ed. New York: McGraw Hill; 2020.

201 Figure 5.18.3. Reproduced with permission from Levinson W, Chin-Hong P, Joyce EA, Nussbaum J, Schwartz B. *Review of Medical Microbiology & Immunology: A Guide to Clinical Infectious Diseases*, 17th ed. Figure 52-7. Reproduced with permission from Ropper AH, Samuels M, Klein J. *Adams and Victor's Principles of Neurology*, 11th ed. New York: McGraw Hill; 2019.

201 Figure 5.18.4. Reproduced with permission from Jameson J, Fauci AS, Kasper DL, Hauser SL, Longo DL, Loscalzo J, eds. *Harrison's Principles of Internal Medicine*, 20th ed. New York: McGraw Hill; 2018.

201 Figure 5.18.5. Reproduced with permission from Jameson J, Fauci AS, Kasper DL, Hauser SL, Longo DL, Loscalzo J, eds. *Harrison's Principles of Internal Medicine*, 20th ed. New York: McGraw Hill; 2018.

201 Figure 5.18.6. Reproduced with permission from Claasens S, Schwartz IS, Jordaan HF, et al. Bacillary angiomatosis presenting with polymorphic skin lesions. IDCases. 2016;6:77-78.

Chapter 6

214 Figure 6.4.1. Arrow points to U wave. Reproduced from Van Beers EJ, Stam J, van den Bergh WM. Licorice consumption as a cause of posterior reversible encephalopathy syndrome: a case report. *Crit Care.* 2011;15(1):R64.

217 EKG changes in hyperkalemia and progressive changes in hypokalemia. Reproduced with permission from Lerma EV, Rosner MH, Perazella MA. *Current Diagnosis & Treatment: Nephrology & Hypertension*, 2nd ed. New York: McGraw Hill; 2018.

236 White blood cell casts suggest a diagnosis of acute interstitial nephritis (AIN) or acute pyelonephritis. Reproduced with permission from Mohsenin V. Practical approach to detection and management of acute kidney injury in critically ill patient. *J Intensive Care.* 2017;5:57. Figure 1C.

236 Red cell casts denote glomerular disease (eg, glomerulonephritis, small vessel vasculitis). Reproduced with permission from Mohsenin V. Practical approach to detection and management of acute kidney injury in critically ill patient. *J Intensive Care.* 2017;5:57. Figure 1D.

236 Muddy brown granular casts suggest acute tubular injury/necrosis (ATN) as the etiology of AKI. Reproduced with permission from Mohsenin V. Practical approach to detection and management of acute kidney injury in critically ill patient. *J Intensive Care.* 2017;5:57, Figure 1B.

248 Figure 6.22.1. Hypopigmented macules. Reproduced with permission from Taylor SC, Kelly AP, Lim HW, Serrano AMA, eds. *Taylor and Kelly's Dermatology for Skin of Color*, 2nd ed. New York: McGraw Hill; 2016, Figure 72-7.

248 Figure 6.22.2. Angiofibroma. Reproduced with permission from Taylor SC, Kelly AP, Lim HW, Serrano AMA, eds. *Taylor and Kelly's Dermatology for Skin of Color*, 2nd ed. New York: McGraw Hill; 2016, Figure 72-8.

Chapter 7

253 Figure 7.2.1. Reproduced with permission from Jameson J, Fauci AS, Kasper DL, Hauser SL, Longo DL, Loscalzo J, eds. *Harrison's Principles of Internal Medicine*, 20th ed. New York: McGraw Hill; 2018.

253 Figure 7.2.2. Reproduced with permission from Grippi MA, Elias JA, Fishman JA, et al, eds. *Fishman's Pulmonary Diseases and Disorders*, 5th ed. New York: McGraw Hill; 2015.

254 Figure 7.3.1. Reproduced with permission from Grippi MA, Elias JA, Fishman JA, et al, eds. *Fishman's Pulmonary Diseases and Disorders*, 5th ed. New York: McGraw Hill; 2015.

263 Figure 7.8.1. Diffuse alveolar opacities in ARDS. Reproduced with permission from McKean SC, Ross JJ, Dressler DD, Scheurer DB, eds. *Principles and Practice of Hospital Medicine*, 2nd ed. New York: McGraw Hill; 2017.

265 Figure 7.9.1. Atelectasis in the RUL. Reproduced with permission from Chen MM, Pope TL, Ott DJ, eds. *Basic Radiology*, 2nd ed. New York: McGraw Hill; 2011.

264 Figure 7.9.2. Acute pulmonary emboli in the RLL segmental arteries and LLL anterior segmental artery. Reproduced with permission from Grippi MA, Elias JA, Fishman JA, et al, eds. *Fishman's Pulmonary Diseases and Disorders*, 5th ed. New York: McGraw Hill; 2015.

264 Figure 7.9.3. Idiopathic pulmonary fibrosis (IPF). Classic findings include traction bronchiectasis (*black arrow*) and honeycombing (*red arrows*). Reproduced with permission from Jameson J, Fauci AS, Kasper DL, Hauser SL, Longo DL, Loscalzo J, eds. *Harrison's Principles of Internal Medicine*, 20th ed. New York: McGraw Hill; 2018.

272 Axial and coronal CT images of interstitial pulmonary fibrosis, depicting symmetric, basilar- and peripheral-predominant reticular opacities, traction bronchiectasis, and honeycombing. Reproduced with permission from Grippi MA, Elias JA, Fishman JA, et al, eds. *Fishman's Pulmonary Diseases and Disorders*, 5th ed. New York: McGraw Hill; 2015.

273 Lung hyperinflation with flattened hemidiaphragms and increased bronchovascular markings seen in COPD. Reproduced with permission from Tintinalli JE, Ma OJ, Yealy DM, et al, eds. *Tintinalli's Emergency Medicine: A Comprehensive Study Guide*, 9th ed. New York: McGraw Hill; 2020.

273 PFT flow volume loops. Reproduced with permission from Huppert LA, Dyster TG. *Huppert's Notes: Pathophysiology and Clinical Pearls for Internal Medicine*. New York: McGraw Hill; 2021.

274 Figure 7.13.1. Reproduced with permission from Elsayes KM, Oldham SAA. *Introduction to Diagnostic Radiology*. New York: McGraw Hill; 2014.

274 **Figure 7.13.2.** Reproduced with permission from Jameson J, Fauci AS, Kasper DL, Hauser SL, Longo DL, Loscalzo J, eds. *Harrison's Principles of Internal Medicine*, 20th ed. New York: McGraw Hill; 2018.

277 **Figure 7.14.1. PA and lateral chest X-ray demonstrate bilateral hilar adenopathy in sarcoidosis.** Reproduced with permission from Elsayes KM, Oldham SAA. *Introduction to Diagnostic Radiology*. New York: McGraw Hill; 2014.

278 **Table. Initial Asthma Treatment: Recommended Options for Adults and Adolescents.** Reproduced with permission from Hay Jr WW, Levin MJ, Abzug MJ, Bunik M, eds. *Current Diagnosis & Treatment: Pediatrics*, 25th ed. New York: McGraw Hill; 2020.

279 **Table. Pharmacologic Therapy for COPD.** Reproduced with permission from Walter LC, Chang A, Chen P, et al, eds. *Current Diagnosis & Treatment Geriatrics*, 3rd ed. New York: McGraw Hill; 2021.

280 **Table. Management of COPD Based on Clinical Severity.** Reproduced with permission from Usatine RP, Smith MA, Mayeaux EJ Jr, Chumley HS. *The Color Atlas and Synopsis of Family Medicine*, 3rd ed. New York: McGraw Hill; 2019.

281 **Figure 7.15.1.** Reproduced with permission from Grippi MA, Elias JA, Fishman JA, et al, eds. *Fishman's Pulmonary Diseases and Disorders*, 5th ed. New York: McGraw Hill; 2015.

281 **Figure 7.15.2.** Reproduced with permission from Jameson J, Fauci AS, Kasper DL, Hauser SL, Longo DL, Loscalzo J, eds. *Harrison's Principles of Internal Medicine*, 20th ed. New York: McGraw Hill; 2018.

282 **CT scan of diffuse, cystic bronchiectasis (red arrows).** Reproduced with permission from Jameson J, Fauci AS, Kasper DL, Hauser SL, Longo DL, Loscalzo J, eds. *Harrison's Principles of Internal Medicine*, 20th ed. New York: McGraw Hill; 2018.

284 **Biopsy-proven lung adenocarcinoma on CT chest.** Reproduced with permission from Elsayes KM, Oldham SAA. *Introduction to Diagnostic Radiology*. New York: McGraw Hill; 2014.

284 **Biopsy-proven small cell carcinoma of the lung on (A) CXR, and (B) CT chest.** Reproduced with permission from Elsayes KM, Oldham SAA. *Introduction to Diagnostic Radiology*. New York: McGraw Hill; 2014.

285 **"S1Q3T3" pattern in a patient with pulmonary embolism.** Reproduced from Islamoglu MS, Dokur M, Ozdemir E, Unal OF. Massive pulmonary embolism presenting with hemoptysis and S1Q3T3 ECG findings. *BMC Cardiovasc Disord.* 2021;21(1):224.

286 **CT showing bilateral ground-glass infiltrates due to alveolar hemorrhage, which can occur in granulomatosis with polyangiitis, microscopic polyangiitis, or eosinophilic granulomatosis with polyangiitis.** Reproduced with permission from Loscalzo J, Fauci AS, Kasper DL, et al, eds. *Harrison's Principles of Internal Medicine*, 21st ed. New York: McGraw Hill; 2022.

288 **Asbestosis.** Reproduced with permission from Loscalzo J, Fauci AS, Kasper DL, et al, eds. *Harrison's Principles of Internal Medicine*, 21st ed. New York: McGraw Hill; 2022.

288 **Pleural effusion in the context of mesothelioma.** Reproduced with permission from Loscalzo J, Fauci AS, Kasper DL, et al, eds. *Harrison's Principles of Internal Medicine*, 21st ed. New York: McGraw Hill; 2022.

289 **Figure 7.19.1. Lung abscesses. Note the areas of cavitation with air-fluid levels.** From Loscalzo J, Fauci AS, Kasper DL, et al, eds. *Harrison's Principles of Internal Medicine*, 21st ed. New York: McGraw Hill; 2022, Figure 127-1B. Reproduced with permission from Dr. Ritu Gill, Division of Chest Radiology, Brigham and Women's Hospital, Boston.

291 **Aspergilloma.** Reproduced with permission from Grippi MA, Elias JA, Fishman JA, et al, eds. *Fishman's Pulmonary Diseases and Disorders*, 5th ed. New York: McGraw Hill; 2015.

291 **Reactivation TB with patchy airspace opacities in the right upper lung.** Reproduced with permission from Elsayes KM, Oldham SAA. *Introduction to Diagnostic Radiology*. New York: McGraw Hill; 2014.

291 **"Halo" sign in angioinvasive aspergillosis.** Reproduced with permission from Grippi MA, Elias JA, Fishman JA, et al, eds. *Fishman's Pulmonary Diseases and Disorders*, 5th ed. New York: McGraw Hill; 2015.

Chapter 8

294 **Figure 8.1.1. Joint space narrowing and loss of articular cartilage seen in osteoarthritis.** Reproduced with permission from Kasper DL, Fauci AS, Hauser SL, Longo DL, Jameson J, Loscalzo J, eds. *Harrison's Principles of Internal Medicine*, 19th ed. New York: McGraw Hill; 2015.

294 **Figure 8.1.2. Positively birefringent, rhomboid crystals seen in pseudogout.** Reproduced with permission from Kasper DL, Fauci AS, Hauser SL, Longo DL, Jameson J, Loscalzo J, eds. *Harrison's Principles of Internal Medicine*, 19th ed. New York: McGraw Hill; 2015.

294 **Figure 8.1.3. Negatively birefringent, needle-shaped crystals seen in gout.** Reproduced with permission from Kasper DL, Fauci AS, Hauser SL, Longo DL, Jameson J, Loscalzo J, eds. *Harrison's Principles of Internal Medicine*, 19th ed. New York: McGraw Hill; 2015.

296 **Figure 8.2.1. Sites of hand or wrist involvement and their potential disease associations.** Reproduced with permission from Laura A. Huppert, Timothy G. Dyster eds. *Huppert's Notes: Pathophysiology and Clinical Pearls for Internal Medicine*. New York: McGraw Hill; 2021.

296 **Figure 8.2.2. Ulnar deviation of MCP joints in rheumatoid arthritis.** From Usatine RP, Smith MA, Mayeaux EJ Jr, Chumley HS. *The Color Atlas and Synopsis of Family Medicine*, 3rd ed. New York: McGraw Hill; 2019, Figure 97-5. Reproduced with permission from Richard P. Usatine, MD.

296 **Figure 8.2.3. Classic "bamboo" appearance of the spine in ankylosing spondylitis resulting from fusion of the vertebral bodies and posterior elements.** Reproduced with permission from Chen MM, Pope TL, Ott DJ, eds. *Basic Radiology*, 2nd ed. New York: McGraw Hill; 2011.

305 **Malar rash of acute lupus erythematosus.** Reproduced with permission from Soutor C, Hordinsky MK. *Clinical Dermatology*, 2nd ed. New York: McGraw Hill; 2022.

305 **Sclerodactyly in systemic sclerosis.** Reproduced with permission from Soutor C, Hordinsky MK. *Clinical Dermatology*, 2nd ed. New York: McGraw Hill; 2022.

306 **Figure 8.6.1. Cutaneous manifestations of dermatomyositis. A. Macular erythema plaques (Gottron sign) and erythematous papules (Gottron papules) on extensor surface of fingers and B. elbow. C. Macular erythematous plaques over the anterior neck and chest (V-sign) and D. the posterior neck, shoulder, and upper back (Shawl sign). E. Nail bed changes with dilated capillaries.** Reproduced with permission from Jameson J, Fauci AS, Kasper DL, Hauser SL, Longo DL, Loscalzo J, eds. *Harrison's Principles of Internal Medicine*, 20th ed. New York: McGraw Hill; 2018.

Chapter 9

310 **Figure 9.1.1.** Reproduced with permission from Kang S, Amagai M, Bruckner AL, Enk AH, Margolis DJ, McMichael AJ, Orringer JS, eds. *Fitzpatrick's Dermatology*, 9th ed. New York: McGraw Hill; 2019.

310 **Figure 9.1.2.** Reproduced with permission from Kang S, Amagai M, Bruckner AL, Enk AH, Margolis DJ, McMichael AJ, Orringer JS, eds. *Fitzpatrick's Dermatology*, 9th ed. New York: McGraw Hill; 2019.

310 **Figure 9.1.3.** Reproduced with permission from Kang S, Amagai M, Bruckner AL, Enk AH, Margolis DJ, McMichael AJ, Orringer JS, eds. *Fitzpatrick's Dermatology*, 9th ed. New York: McGraw Hill; 2019.

310 **Figure 9.1.4.** Reproduced with permission from Kang S, Amagai M, Bruckner AL, Enk AH, Margolis DJ, McMichael AJ, Orringer JS, eds. *Fitzpatrick's Dermatology*, 9th ed. New York: McGraw Hill; 2019.

313 **Figure 9.2.1.** Reproduced with permission from Wolff K, Johnson RA, Saavedra AP, Roh EK. *Fitzpatrick's Color Atlas and Synopsis of Clinical Dermatology*, 8th ed. New York: McGraw Hill; 2017.

313 **Figure 9.2.2.** Reproduced with permission from Kang S, Amagai M, Bruckner AL, Enk AH, Margolis DJ, McMichael AJ, Orringer JS, eds. *Fitzpatrick's Dermatology*, 9th ed. New York: McGraw Hill; 2019.

313 **Figure 9.2.3.** Reproduced with permission from Kang S, Amagai M, Bruckner AL, Enk AH, Margolis DJ, McMichael AJ, Orringer JS, eds. *Fitzpatrick's Dermatology*, 9th ed. New York: McGraw Hill; 2019.

313 **Figure 9.2.4.** Reproduced with permission from Kang S, Amagai M, Bruckner AL, Enk AH, Margolis DJ, McMichael AJ, Orringer JS, eds. *Fitzpatrick's Dermatology*, 9th ed. New York: McGraw Hill; 2019.

315 **Figure 9.3.1.** Reproduced with permission from Kang S, Amagai M, Bruckner AL, Enk AH, Margolis DJ, McMichael AJ, Orringer JS, eds. *Fitzpatrick's Dermatology*, 9th ed. New York: McGraw Hill; 2019.

316 **Figure 9.4.1. Squamous cell carcinoma.** Reproduced with permission from Kang S, Amagai M, Bruckner AL, Enk AH, Margolis DJ, McMichael AJ, Orringer JS, eds. *Fitzpatrick's Dermatology*, 9th ed. New York: McGraw Hill; 2019.

316 **Figure 9.4.2. Basal cell carcinoma.** From Usatine RP, Smith MA, Mayeaux EJ Jr, Chumley HS. *The Color Atlas and Synopsis of Family Medicine*, 3rd ed. New York: McGraw Hill; 2019, Figure 177-2. Reproduced with permission from Richard P. Usatine, MD.

319 **Figure 9.5.1.** From Usatine RP, Smith MA, Mayeaux EJ Jr, Chumley HS. *The Color Atlas and Synopsis of Family Medicine*, 3rd ed. New York: McGraw Hill; 2019, Figure 114-1. Reproduced with permission from Richard P. Usatine, MD.

319 **Figure 9.5.2.** Reproduced with permission from Wolff K, Johnson RA, Saavedra AP, Roh EK. *Fitzpatrick's Color Atlas and Synopsis of Clinical Dermatology*, 8th ed. New York: McGraw Hill; 2017.

320 **Figure 9.6.1.** Reproduced with permission from Jameson J, Fauci AS, Kasper DL, Hauser SL, Longo DL, Loscalzo J, eds. *Harrison's Principles of Internal Medicine*, 20th ed. New York: McGraw Hill; 2018.

320 **Figure 9.6.2.** Used with permission Claudio Divizia/500px/Getty Images.

320 **Figure 9.6.3.** From Usatine RP, Smith MA, Mayeaux EJ Jr, Chumley HS. *The Color Atlas and Synopsis of Family Medicine*, 3rd ed. New York: McGraw Hill; 2019, Figure 115-1. Reproduced with permission from Richard P. Usatine, MD.

320 **Figure 9.6.4.** From Usatine RP, Smith MA, Mayeaux EJ Jr, Chumley HS. *The Color Atlas and Synopsis of Family Medicine*, 3rd ed. New York: McGraw Hill; 2019, Figure 211-3. Reproduced with permission from Richard P. Usatine, MD.

323 **Figure 9.7.1.** Reproduced with permission from Jameson J, Fauci AS, Kasper DL, Hauser SL, Longo DL, Loscalzo J, eds. *Harrison's Principles of Internal Medicine*, 20th ed. New York: McGraw Hill; 2018.

325 **Figure 9.8.1.** From Jameson J, Fauci AS, Kasper DL, Hauser SL, Longo DL, Loscalzo J, eds. *Harrison's Principles of Internal Medicine*, 20th ed. New York: McGraw Hill; 2018, Figure 52-9. Reproduced with permission from the Yale Resident's Slide Collection.

325 **Figure 9.8.2.** Reproduced with permission from Kaushansky K, Prchal JT, Burns LJ, Lichtman MA, Levi M, Linch DC, eds. Williams Hematology, 10th ed. New York; McGraw Hill; 2021.

325 **Figure 9.8.3.** Reproduced, with permission, from Bondi EE, Jegasothy BV, Lazarus GS, eds. *Dermatology: Diagnosis & Treatment.* Originally published by Appleton & Lange. McGraw-Hill; 1991.

325 **Figure 9.8.4.** Reproduced with permission from Oropello JM, Pastores SM, Kvetan V, eds. *Critical Care*. New York: McGraw Hill; 2017.

325 **Figure 9.8.5a.** Reproduced with permission from Division of STD Prevention, National Center for HIV/AIDS, Viral Hepatitis, STD, and TB Prevention, Center for Disease Control and Prevention.

325 **Figure 9.8.5b.** Reproduced with permission from Usatine RP, Smith MA, Mayeaux EJ, et al. *The Color Atlas of Family Medicine*, 3rd ed. New York: McGraw Hill Education; 2019, Figure 5-8. Photo contributor: Jonathan B. Karnes, MD.

325 **Figure 9.8.6.** From Jameson J, Fauci AS, Kasper DL, Hauser SL, Longo DL, Loscalzo J, eds. *Harrison's Principles of Internal Medicine*, 20th ed. New York: McGraw Hill; 2018, Figure A4-43. Reproduced with permission from Robert Swerlick, MD.

327 **Figure 9.9.1.** Reproduced with permission from Kang S, Amagai M, Bruckner AL, Enk AH, Margolis DJ, McMichael AJ, Orringer JS, eds. *Fitzpatrick's Dermatology*, 9th ed. New York: McGraw Hill; 2019.

327 **Figure 9.9.2.** Reproduced with permission from Soutor C, Hordinsky MK. *Clinical Dermatology*. New York: McGraw Hill; 2013.

327 **Figure 9.9.3.** From Usatine RP, Smith MA, Mayeaux EJ Jr, Chumley HS. *The Color Atlas and Synopsis of Family Medicine*, 3rd ed. New York: McGraw Hill; 2019, Figure 119-13. Reproduced with permission from Richard P. Usatine, MD.

327 **Figure 9.9.4.** From Usatine RP, Smith MA, Mayeaux EJ Jr, Chumley HS. *The Color Atlas and Synopsis of Family Medicine*, 3rd ed. New York: McGraw Hill; 2019, Figure 133-4. Reproduced with permission from Richard P. Usatine, MD.

327 **Figure 9.9.5.** Reproduced with permission from Grippi MA, Elias JA, Fishman JA, et al, eds. *Fishman's Pulmonary Diseases and Disorders*, 5th ed. New York: McGraw Hill; 2015.

329 **Figure 9.10.1. Scarlet fever exanthem.** Reproduced with permission from K Wolff, RA Johnson: *Color Atlas and Synopsis of Clinical Dermatology*, 6th ed. New York: McGraw-Hill; 2009.

329 **Figure 9.10.2. Cherry-red lips with hemorrhagic fissures in Kawasaki disease. Note the erythema and edema of fingertips.** Reproduced with permission from Wolff K, Johnson RA, Saavedra AP, Roh EK. *Fitzpatrick's Color Atlas and Synopsis of Clinical Dermatology*, 8th ed. New York: McGraw Hill; 2017.

329 **Figure 9.10.3. Rubella exanthem.** Used with permission of the Centers for Disease Control and Prevention.

329 **Figure 9.10.4. Classic measles exanthem on the trunk.** From Usatine RP, Smith MA, Mayeaux EJ Jr, Chumley HS. *The Color Atlas and Synopsis of Family Medicine*, 3rd ed. New York: McGraw Hill; 2019, Figure 132-2. Reproduced with permission from Richard P. Usatine, MD.

331 **Figure 9.11.1.** Photo courtesy Medicina Oral S.L.

331 **Figure 9.11.2.** Reproduced with permission from Jameson J, Fauci AS, Kasper DL, Hauser SL, Longo DL, Loscalzo J, eds. *Harrison's Principles of Internal Medicine*, 20th ed. New York: McGraw Hill; 2018.

331 **Figure 9.11.3.** Reproduced with permission from Soutor C, Hordinsky MK. *Clinical Dermatology: Diagnosis and Management of Common Disorders*, 2nd ed. New York: McGraw Hill; 2022.

331 **Figure 9.11.4.** Reproduced with permission from Jameson J, Fauci AS, Kasper DL, Hauser SL, Longo DL, Loscalzo J, eds. *Harrison's Principles of Internal Medicine*, 20th ed. New York: McGraw Hill; 2018.

331 **Figure 9.11.5.** Reproduced with permission from Jameson J, Fauci AS, Kasper DL, Hauser SL, Longo DL, Loscalzo J, eds. *Harrison's Principles of Internal Medicine*, 20th ed. New York: McGraw Hill; 2018.

334 **Figure 9.12.1.** From Jameson J, Fauci AS, Kasper DL, Hauser SL, Longo DL, Loscalzo J, eds. *Harrison's Principles of Internal Medicine*, 20th ed. New York: McGraw Hill; 2018, Figure 55-2. Reproduced with permission from the Yale Resident's Slide Collection; with permission.

334 **Figure 9.12.2.** Reproduced with permission from Soutor C, Hordinsky MK. *Clinical Dermatology*. New York: McGraw Hill; 2013.

334 **Figure 9.12.3.** Reproduced with permission from Jameson J, Fauci AS, Kasper DL, Hauser SL, Longo DL, Loscalzo J, eds. *Harrison's Principles of Internal Medicine*, 20th ed. New York: McGraw Hill; 2018.

334 **Figure 9.12.4.** From Knoop KJ, Stack LB, Storrow AB, Thurman RJ, eds. *The Atlas of Emergency Medicine*, 5th ed. New York: McGraw Hill; 2021, Figure 16.135. Reproduced with permission from photo contributor: Alan B. Storrow, MD.

336 **Figure 9.13.1.** Reproduced with permission from Kang S, Amagai M, Bruckner AL, Enk AH, Margolis DJ, McMichael AJ, Orringer JS, eds. *Fitzpatrick's Dermatology*, 9th ed. New York: McGraw Hill; 2019.

336 **Figure 9.13.2.** Reproduced with permission from Kang S, Amagai M, Bruckner AL, Enk AH, Margolis DJ, McMichael AJ, Orringer JS, eds. *Fitzpatrick's Dermatology*, 9th ed. New York: McGraw Hill; 2019.

336 **Figure 9.13.3.** From Jameson J, Fauci AS, Kasper DL, Hauser SL, Longo DL, Loscalzo J, eds. *Harrison's Principles of Internal Medicine*, 20th ed. New York: McGraw Hill; 2018, Figure 53-8. Reproduced with permission from Robert Swerlick, MD.

338 **Figure 9.14.1.** Reproduced with permission from Taylor SC, Kelly AP, Lim HW, Serrano AMA, eds. *Taylor and Kelly's Dermatology for Skin of Color*, 2nd ed. New York: McGraw Hill; 2016.

338 **Figure 9.14.2.** Reproduced with permission from Kang S, Amagai M, Bruckner AL, Enk AH, Margolis DJ, McMichael AJ, Orringer JS, eds. *Fitzpatrick's Dermatology*, 9th ed. New York: McGraw Hill; 2019.

340 **Figure 9.15.1.** From Knoop KJ, Stack LB, Storrow AB, Thurman RJ, eds. *The Atlas of Emergency Medicine*, 5th ed. New York: McGraw Hill; 2021, Figure 13.111. Reproduced with permission from photo contributor: David Effron, MD.

340 **Figure 9.15.2.** Reproduced with permission from Wolff K, Johnson RA, Saavedra AP, Roh EK. *Fitzpatrick's Color Atlas and Synopsis of Clinical Dermatology*, 8th ed. New York: McGraw Hill; 2017.

340 **Figure 9.15.3.** Reproduced with permission from Wolff K, Johnson RA, Saavedra AP, Roh EK. *Fitzpatrick's Color Atlas and Synopsis of Clinical Dermatology*, 8th ed. New York: McGraw Hill; 2017.

340 **Figure 9.15.4.** Reproduced with permission from Wolff K, Johnson RA, Saavedra AP, Roh EK. *Fitzpatrick's Color Atlas and Synopsis of Clinical Dermatology*, 8th ed. New York: McGraw Hill; 2017.

340 **Figure 9.15.5.** National Cancer Institute.

342 **Figure 9.16.1.** Reproduced with permission from Taylor SC, Kelly AP, Lim HW, Serrano AMA, eds. *Taylor and Kelly's Dermatology for Skin of Color*, 2nd ed. New York: McGraw Hill; 2016.

342 **Figure 9.16.2.** Reproduced with permission from Dean SM, Satiani B, Abraham WT. *Color Atlas and Synopsis of Vascular Diseases*. New York: McGraw-Hill; 2014.

342 **Figure 9.16.3.** Reproduced with permission from Kang S, Amagai M, Bruckner AL, Enk AH, Margolis DJ, McMichael AJ, Orringer JS, eds. *Fitzpatrick's Dermatology*, 9th ed. New York: McGraw Hill; 2019.

342 **Figure 9.16.4.** Reproduced with permission from Kang S, Amagai M, Bruckner AL, Enk AH, Margolis DJ, McMichael AJ, Orringer JS, eds. *Fitzpatrick's Dermatology*, 9th ed. New York: McGraw Hill; 2019.

342 **Figure 9.16.5.** Reproduced with permission from Kang S, Amagai M, Bruckner AL, Enk AH, Margolis DJ, McMichael AJ, Orringer JS, eds. *Fitzpatrick's Dermatology*, 9th ed. New York: McGraw Hill; 2019.

344 **Figure 9.17.1.** Reproduced with permission from Wolff K, Johnson RA, Saavedra AP, Roh EK. *Fitzpatrick's Color Atlas and Synopsis of Clinical Dermatology*, 8th ed. New York: McGraw Hill; 2017.

344 **Figure 9.17.2.** Reproduced with permission from Reisner HM. *Pathology: A Modern Case Study*, 2nd ed. New York: McGraw Hill; 2020.

344 **Figure 9.17.3.** Reproduced with permission from Soutor C, Hordinsky MK. *Clinical Dermatology*. New York: McGraw Hill; 2013.

344 **Figure 9.17.4.** Reproduced with permission from Soutor C, Hordinsky MK. *Clinical Dermatology*. New York: McGraw Hill; 2013.

346 **Figure 9.18.1.** Reproduced with permission from Hamm R, Carey JN. *Essential Elements of Wound Diagnosis*. New York: McGraw Hill; 2021.

346 **Figure 9.18.2.** Used with permission TisforThan/Shutterstock

350 **Figure 9.20.1.** Reproduced with permission from Kang S, Amagai M, Bruckner AL, Enk AH, Margolis DJ, McMichael AJ, Orringer JS, eds. *Fitzpatrick's Dermatology*, 9th ed. New York: McGraw Hill; 2019.

350 **Figure 9.20.2a.** From Usatine RP, Smith MA, Mayeaux EJ Jr, Chumley HS. *The Color Atlas and Synopsis of Family Medicine*, 3rd ed. New York: McGraw Hill; 2019, Figure 158-4. Reproduced with permission from Richard P. Usatine, MD.

350 **Figure 9.20.2b.** From Usatine RP, Smith MA, Mayeaux EJ Jr, Chumley HS. *The Color Atlas and Synopsis of Family Medicine*, 3rd ed. New York: McGraw Hill; 2019, Figure 143-6. Reproduced with permission from Richard P. Usatine, MD.

352 **Figure 9.21.1.** From Knoop KJ, Stack LB, Storrow AB, Thurman RJ, eds. *The Atlas of Emergency Medicine*, 5th ed. New York: McGraw Hill; 2021, Figure 5.33. Reproduced with permission from photo contributor: Kevin J. Knoop, MD, MS.

352 **Figure 9.21.2.** From Usatine RP, Smith MA, Mayeaux EJ Jr, Chumley HS. *The Color Atlas and Synopsis of Family Medicine*, 3rd ed. New York: McGraw Hill; 2019, Figure 44-3. Reproduced with permission from Ellen Eisenberg, DMD.

352 **Figure 9.21.3.** Reproduced with permission from Kang S, Amagai M, Bruckner AL, Enk AH, Margolis DJ, McMichael AJ, Orringer JS, eds. *Fitzpatrick's Dermatology*, 9th ed. New York: McGraw Hill; 2019.

352 **Figure 9.21.4.** Reproduced with permission from Wolff K, Johnson RA, Saavedra AP, Roh EK. *Fitzpatrick's Color Atlas and Synopsis of Clinical Dermatology*, 8th ed. New York: McGraw Hill; 2017.

352 **Figure 9.21.5.** Reproduced with permission from Wolff K, Johnson RA, Saavedra AP, Roh EK. *Fitzpatrick's Color Atlas and Synopsis of Clinical Dermatology*, 8th ed. New York: McGraw Hill; 2017.

352 **Figure 9.21.6.** Used with permission from Gabdrakipova Dilyara/Shutterstock.

352 **Figure 9.21.7.** Reproduced with permission from Kang S, Amagai M, Bruckner AL, Enk AH, Margolis DJ, McMichael AJ, Orringer JS, eds. *Fitzpatrick's Dermatology*, 9th ed. New York: McGraw Hill; 2019.

352 **Figure 9.21.8.** Reproduced with permission from Kang S, Amagai M, Bruckner AL, Enk AH, Margolis DJ, McMichael AJ, Orringer JS, eds. *Fitzpatrick's Dermatology*, 9th ed. New York: McGraw Hill; 2019.

354 **Figure 9.22.1.** Used with permission from TisforThan/Shutterstock.

354 **Figure 9.22.2.** Reproduced with permission from Taylor SC, Kelly AP, Lim HW, Serrano AMA, eds. *Taylor and Kelly's Dermatology for Skin of Color*, 2nd ed. New York: McGraw Hill; 2016.

354 **Figure 9.22.3.** From Usatine RP, Smith MA, Mayeaux EJ Jr, Chumley HS. *The Color Atlas and Synopsis of Family Medicine*, 3rd ed. New York: McGraw Hill; 2019, Figure 152-6. Reproduced with permission from Richard P. Usatine, MD.

356 **Figure 9.23.1.** Reproduced with permission from Taylor SC, Kelly AP, Lim HW, Serrano AMA, eds. *Taylor and Kelly's Dermatology for Skin of Color*, 2nd ed. New York: McGraw Hill; 2016.

356 **Figure 9.23.2.** From Usatine RP, Smith MA, Mayeaux EJ Jr, Chumley HS. *The Color Atlas and Synopsis of Family Medicine*, 3rd ed. New York: McGraw Hill; 2019, Figure 203-2. Reproduced with permission from Richard P. Usatine, MD.

Chapter 10

362 **Tension pneumothorax.** Reproduced with permission from Schwartz DT, ed. *Emergency Radiology, Case Studies*. McGraw-Hill Inc.; 2008.

362 **Large pericardial effusion.** Reproduced with permission from Imazio M: Contemporary management of pericardial diseases. *Curr Opin Cardiol*. 2012;27(3):308-317.

369 **Pulmonary contusion**. Reproduced with permission from Tintinalli JE, Ma OJ, Yealy DM, et al, eds. *Tintinalli's Emergency Medicine: A Comprehensive Study Guide*, 9th ed. New York: McGraw Hill; 2020.

369 **Hemothorax.** Reproduced with permission from Block J, Jordanov MI, Stack LB, Thurman RJ, eds. *The Atlas of Emergency Radiology*. McGraw-Hill, Inc.; 2013.

369 **Pneumothorax.** Reproduced with permission from Tintinalli JE, Ma OJ, Yealy DM, et al, eds. *Tintinalli's Emergency Medicine: A Comprehensive Study Guide*, 9th ed. New York: McGraw Hill; 2020.

369 **Pneumomediastinum.** Reproduced with permission from Tintinalli JE, Ma OJ, Yealy DM, et al, eds. *Tintinalli's Emergency Medicine: A Comprehensive Study Guide*, 9th ed. New York: McGraw Hill; 2020.

390 **Figure 10.13.1.** Redrawn from https://uihc.org/health-topics/what-happens-spinal-cord.

Chapter 11

395 **Bowel obstruction with air-fluid levels and a dilated portion of colon with transition point to decompressed bowel.** Reproduced with permission from Elsayes KM, Oldham SAA. *Introduction to Diagnostic Radiology*. New York: McGraw Hill; 2014.

398 Infographic: Postoperative fever. Reproduced with permission from Shah N. *The Infographic Guide to Medicine.* New York: McGraw Hill; 2021.

Chapter 12

404 Zenker's diverticula. Reproduced with permission from Loscalzo J, Fauci AS, Kasper DL, et al, eds. *Harrison's Principles of Internal Medicine*, 21st ed. New York: McGraw Hill; 2022.

404 Achalasia. Reproduced with permission from Loscalzo J, Fauci AS, Kasper DL, et al, eds. *Harrison's Principles of Internal Medicine*, 21st ed. New York: McGraw Hill 2022.

413 Sigmoid volvulus. Note the characteristic "coffee bean" sign. Reproduced with permission from Jameson J, Fauci AS, Kasper DL, Hauser SL, Longo DL, Loscalzo J, eds. *Harrison's Principles of Internal Medicine*, 20th ed. New York: McGraw Hill; 2018.

416 Amoebic abscesses of the liver. Used with permission from Creative Endeavors/Shutterstock

417 Figure 12.6.1. Gallbladder ultrasound in cholecystitis. Reproduced with permission from Chen MM, Pope TL, Ott DJ, eds. *Basic Radiology*, 2nd ed. New York: McGraw Hill; 2011.

421 Table. Causes of Acute Pancreatitis. Reproduced with permission from Tintinalli JE, Ma OJ, Yealy DM, et al, eds. *Tintinalli's Emergency Medicine: A Comprehensive Study Guide*, 9th ed. New York: McGraw Hill; 2020.

422 Figure 12.8.1. Reproduced with permission from Knoop KJ, Stack LB, Storrow AB, Thurman RJ, eds. *The Atlas of Emergency Medicine*, 5th ed. New York: McGraw Hill; 2021.

Chapter 14

441 Figure 14.6.1. Reproduced with permission from Lerma EV, Rosner MH, Perazella MA. *Current Diagnosis & Treatment: Nephrology & Hypertension*, 2nd ed. New York: McGraw Hill; 2018.

447 Osteoblastic lesions in metastatic prostate cancer. Reproduced with permission from Elsayes KM, Oldham SAA. *Introduction to Diagnostic Radiology*. New York: McGraw Hill; 2014.

Chapter 16

458 Table. Radiculopathies. Reproduced with permission from Jameson JL, Fauci AS, Kasper DL, et al, *Harrison's Manual of Medicine*, 20th ed. New York: McGraw Hill, 2020.

462 ACL tear. Reproduced with permission from Tehranzadeh J, ed. *Basic Musculoskeletal Imaging*, 2nd ed. New York; McGraw Hill; 2021.

466 Hand injuries. Reproduced with permission from Suneja M, Szot JF, LeBlond RF, Brown DD. *DeGowin's Diagnostic Examination*, 11th ed. New York: McGraw Hill; 2020.

468 Gout (podagra). The left 1st MTP joint is swollen, erythematous, and tender. Reproduced with permission from Suneja M, Szot JF, LeBlond RF, Brown DD. *DeGowin's Diagnostic Examination*, 11th ed. McGraw Hill; 2020.

472 Skull with "cotton wool" areas of fluffy sclerosis and skull base thickening (arrowheads) in a patient with Paget's disease of bone. Reproduced with permission from Tehranzadeh J, ed. *Basic Musculoskeletal Imaging*, 2nd ed. New York: McGraw Hill; 2021.

472 Lucent lytic lesion (arrowheads) in distal femoral diaphysis with adjacent cortical thinning (arrow). Reproduced with permission from Tehranzadeh J, ed. *Basic Musculoskeletal Imaging*, 2nd ed. New York: McGraw Hill; 2021.

473 Extensive sclerotic (osteoblastic) metastases in lower lumbar spine, pelvis, and bilateral femurs. Reproduced with permission from Tehranzadeh J, ed. *Basic Musculoskeletal Imaging*, 2nd ed. New York: McGraw Hill; 2021.

473 Osteoid matrix (black arrow) and "sunburst" soft tissue ossifications (white arrows). Reproduced with permission from Tehranzadeh J, ed. *Basic Musculoskeletal Imaging*, 2nd ed. New York: McGraw Hill; 2021.

473 Codman's triangle periosteal reaction seen in various bone lesions, including osteosarcoma (most common) and Ewing's sarcoma. Reproduced with permission from Tehranzadeh J, ed. *Basic Musculoskeletal Imaging*, 2nd ed. New York: McGraw Hill; 2021.

474 Erb Palsy. Reproduced with permission from Socolovsky M, Costales JR, et al, Obstetric brachial plexus palsy: reviewing the literature comparing the results of primary versus secondary surgery. *Childs Nerv Syst.* 2016;32(3):415-425, Springer Nature.

474 Winged scapula. Used with permission from Chu KyungMin/Shutterstock.

474 Klumpke palsy. Used with permission from Ilina93/Shutterstock.

476 Superior gluteal. Used with permission from Chu KyungMin/Shutterstock.

478 Cutaneous innervation of the upper extremity. Used with permission from Chu KyungMin/Shutterstock.

478 Cutaneous innervation of the lower extremity. Used with permission from Chu KyungMin/Shutterstock.

478 Dermatomes (anterior and posterior views). Used with permission from stihii/Shutterstock.

Chapter 17

482 Lumbar disc herniation. Reproduced with permission from Parks E. *Practical Office Orthopedics*. McGraw Hill; 2017.

482 Ankylosing spondylosis. Reproduced with permission from Tehranzadeh J, ed. *Basic Musculoskeletal Imaging*, 2nd ed. New York; McGraw Hill; 2021.

482 Leptomeningeal metastases. Reproduced with permission from Loscalzo J, Fauci AS, Kasper DL, et al, eds. *Harrison's Principles of Internal Medicine*, 21st ed. New York: McGraw Hill; 2022.

486 Figure 17.3.1. Reproduced with permission from Loscalzo J, Fauci AS, Kasper DL, et al, eds. *Harrison's Principles of Internal Medicine*, 21st ed. New York: McGraw Hill; 2022.

486 Figure 17.3.2. Reproduced with permission from Loscalzo J, Fauci AS, Kasper DL, et al, eds. *Harrison's Principles of Internal Medicine*, 21st ed. New York: McGraw Hill; 2022.

488 Table. Summary of Pituitary Hormones. Reproduced with permission from Reisner HM. *Pathology: A Modern Case Study*, 2nd ed. New York: McGraw Hill; 2020.

489 Diagram of pituitary axes. Reproduced with permission from Loscalzo J, Fauci AS, Kasper DL, et al, eds. *Harrison's Principles of Internal Medicine*, 21st ed. New York: McGraw Hill; 2022.

Chapter 18

497 Thoracic aortic aneurysm. Reproduced with permission from Loscalzo J, Fauci AS, Kasper DL, et al, eds. *Harrison's Principles of Internal Medicine*, 21st ed. New York: McGraw Hill; 2022.

497 Classification of aortic dissections. Reproduced with permission from Doroghazi RM, Slater EE, eds. *Aortic Dissection.* New York: McGraw-Hill; 1983.

500 Acute ischemia of distal lower extremities. Reproduced with permission from Fuster V, Narula J, Vaishnava P, et al, eds. *Fuster and Hurst's The Heart*, 15th ed. New York: McGraw Hill 2022.

Chapter 19

504 Table. Common and serious side effects of breast cancer therapies. Reproduced with permission from Kantarjian HM, Wolff RA, Rieber AG, eds. *The MD Anderson Manual of Medical Oncology*, 4th ed. New York: McGraw Hill; 2022.

Chapter 20

511 Hemorrhages and exudates ("cheese pizza" appearance) seen with CMV retinitis. Reproduced with permission Jameson J, Fauci AS, Kasper DL, Hauser SL, Longo DL, Loscalzo J, eds. *Harrison's Principles of Internal Medicine*, 20th ed. New York: McGraw Hill; 2018.

511 Hypopyon. Reproduced, with permission, from Papadakis MA, McPhee SJ, Rabow MW, McQuaid KR, eds. *Current Diagnosis & Treatment 2022.* New York: McGraw Hill; 2022.

512 Diffuse anterior scleritis. Note the deep, dark vessels. Reproduced, with permission from Nevares A, Raut R, Libman B, et al. Noninfectious autoimmune scleritis: recognition, systemic associations, and therapy. *Curr Rheumatol Rep.* 2020;22:11.

513 Scattered flame hemorrhages and macular exudates in non-proliferative diabetic retinopathy. From Usatine RP, Smith MA, Mayeaux EJ Jr, Chumley HS. *The Color Atlas and Synopsis of Family Medicine*, 3rd ed. New York: McGraw Hill; 2019.

514 Blurred optic disc, scattered hemorrhages, cotton-wool spots, and foveal exudate can be seen in a patient with hypertensive retinopathy. Reproduced with permission from Jameson J, Fauci AS, Kasper DL, Hauser SL, Longo DL, Loscalzo J, eds. *Harrison's Principles of Internal Medicine*, 20th ed. New York: McGraw Hill; 2018.

514 Glaucoma results in destruction of the neural rim and an enlarged, excavated cup, leading to "cupping." Reproduced with permission from Paul D. Comeau.

515 An elevated sheet of retinal tissue with folds can be seen in retinal detachment. Reproduced with permission from Jameson J, Fauci AS, Kasper DL, Hauser SL, Longo DL, Loscalzo J, eds. *Harrison's Principles of Internal Medicine*, 20th ed. New York: McGraw Hill; 2018.

515 A central cherry red spot, Hollenhorst plaques, diffuse macular edema, and thready residual arterial flow can be visualized in this patient with central retinal artery occlusion. Reproduced with permission from Suneja M, Szot JF, LeBlond RF, Brown DD. *DeGowin's Diagnostic Examination*, 11th ed. New York: McGraw Hill; 2020.

516 Disc swelling, retinal hemorrhages, and suffusion of the veins can be seen in central retinal vein occlusion. Reproduced with permission from Maxine A. Papadakis, Stephen J. McPhee, Michael W. Rabow, Kenneth R. McQuaid. *Current Medical Diagnosis & Treatment 2023.*

519 Subconjunctival hemorrhage that completely surrounds the eye. Reproduced with permission from Riordan-Eva P, Augsburger JJ, eds. *Vaughan & Asbury's General Ophthalmology*, 19th ed. New York: McGraw Hill; 2017.

519 Traumatic hyphema with associated subconjunctival hemorrhage. Used with permission from ARZTSAMUI/Shutterstock.

Chapter 23

534 Tanner staging of pubertal development. Reproduced with permission from Hoffman BL, Schorge JO, Halvorson LM, et al, eds. *Williams Gynecology*, 4th ed. New York: McGraw Hill; 2020.

538 Figure 23.4.1. Reproduced with permission from Cunningham FG, Leveno KJ, Bloom SL, Hauth JC, Rouse DJ, Spong CY, eds. *Williams Obstetrics.* 23rd ed. New York: McGraw-Hill; 2010.

540 Steroidogenesis pathway. Reproduced with permission from Nicoll D, Lu CM, McPhee SJ. *Guide to Diagnostic Tests*, 7th ed. New York: McGraw Hill; 2017.

543 Neonatal extremity with classic erythema toxicum. Photo contributor: Robert W. Hickey, MD.

545 Figure 23.7.1. Used with permission from Craig W. Lillehei, MD.

545 Figure 23.7.2. Used with permission from Craig W. Lillehei, MD.

545 Figure 23.7.3. Reproduced with permission from Brunicardi FC, Andersen DK, Billiar TR, et al, eds. *Schwartz's Principles of Surgery*, 11th ed. New York: McGraw Hill; 2019.

545 Figure 23.7.4. Reproduced with permission from Schaefer GB, Thompson JN Jr. *Medical Genetics: An Integrated Approach.* New York: McGraw Hill; 2014.

547 Figure 23.8.1. Reproduced with permission from McMahon PJ, Skinner HB. *Current Diagnosis & Treatment in Orthopedics*, 6th ed. New York: McGraw Hill; 2021.

557 Unilateral purulent discharge with associated periorbital edema and erythema. Photo contributor: David Effron, MD.

557 Mild crusting noted along lashline. Photo contributor: Kevin J. Knoop, MD, MS.

559 Congenital pneumonia. Reproduced with permission from Elsayes KM, Oldham SAA. *Introduction to Diagnostic Radiology.* New York: McGraw Hill; 2014.

559 Respiratory distress syndrome. Reproduced with permission from Cunningham FG, Leveno KJ, Dashe JS, et al, eds. *Williams Obstetrics*, 26th ed. New York: McGraw Hill; 2022.

559 Transient tachypnea of the newborn. Reproduced with permission from Elsayes KM, Oldham SAA. *Introduction to Diagnostic Radiology.* New York: McGraw Hill; 2014.

560 Tracheoesophageal fistula. A coiled NG tube can be visualized in the esophagus. Reproduced with permission from Brunicardi FC, Andersen DK, Billiar TR, et al, eds. *Schwartz's Principles of Surgery*, 11th ed. New York: McGraw Hill; 2019.

560 Congenital diaphragmatic hernia. Reproduced with permission from Brunicardi FC, Andersen DK, Billiar TR, et al, eds. *Schwartz's Principles of Surgery*, 11th ed. New York: McGraw Hill; 2019.

563 Diagram illustrating a left-to-right shunt from the descending aorta to the main pulmonary artery via the patent ductus arteriosus. Reproduced with permission from Jameson J, Fauci AS, Kasper DL, Hauser SL, Longo DL, Loscalzo J, eds. *Harrison's Principles of Internal Medicine*, 20th ed. New York: McGraw Hill; 2018.

565 Right ventricular outflow tract obstruction leads to a right-to-left shunt via the ventricular septal defect (VSD). Reproduced with permission from Jameson J, Fauci AS, Kasper DL, Hauser SL, Longo DL, Loscalzo J, eds. *Harrison's Principles of Internal Medicine*, 20th ed. New York: McGraw Hill; 2018.

565 Transposition of the great arteries. Reproduced with permission from Fuster V, Narula J, Vaishnava P, et al, eds. *Fuster and Hurst's The Heart*, 15th ed. New York: McGraw Hill; 2022.

567 Figure 23.15.1. Reproduced with permission from Wyllie R. Pyloric stenosis and congenital anomalies of the stomach. In: Behrman RE, Kliegman RM, Jensen HB, eds. *Nelson Textbook of Pediatrics*, 17th ed. Philadelphia: WB Saunders; 2004:1230.

567 Figure 23.15.2. Reproduced with permission from Zinner MJ, Ashley SW, Hines OJ. Maingot's *Abdominal Operations*, 13th ed. New York: McGraw Hill; 2019.

567 Figure 23.15.3. Reproduced with permission from Kline MW, ed. *Rudolph's Pediatrics*, 23rd ed. New York: McGraw Hill; 2018.

569 Cherry red spot on macula. Used with permission from Kateryna Kon/Shutterstock.

572 Brushfield spots. Reproduced with permission from Schaefer GB, Thompson JN Jr. *Medical Genetics: An Integrated Approach*. New York: McGraw Hill; 2014.

572 Rocker bottom feet. Reproduced with permission from Schaefer GB, Thompson JN Jr. *Medical Genetics: An Integrated Approach*. New York: McGraw Hill; 2014.

573 Cutis aplasia of the neonatal scalp. Reproduced with permission from Schaefer GB, Thompson JN Jr. *Medical Genetics: An Integrated Approach*. New York: McGraw Hill; 2014.

574 Intracranial calcifications. Reproduced with permission from Ropper AH, Samuels MA, Klein JP, Prasad S, eds. *Adams and Victor's Principles of Neurology*, 11th ed. New York: McGraw Hill; 2019.

574 "Blueberry muffin" rash. Reproduced with permission from Lichtman MA, Shafer MS, Felgar RE, Wang N. *Lichtman's Atlas of Hematology*. New York: McGraw Hill; 2017.

575 Periventricular calcifications. Reproduced with permission from Cunningham FG, Leveno KJ, Bloom SL, et al, eds. *Williams Obstetrics*, 25th ed. New York: McGraw Hill; 2018.

575 Vesicular lesions. Reproduced with permission from Wolff K, Johnson RA, Saavedra AP, Roh EK. *Fitzpatrick's Color Atlas and Synopsis of Clinical Dermatology*, 8th ed. New York: McGraw Hill; 2017.

576 Hutchinson teeth. Reproduced with permission from Kang S, Amagai M, Bruckner AL, Enk AH, Margolis DJ, McMichael AJ, Orringer JS, eds. *Fitzpatrick's Dermatology*, 9th ed. New York: McGraw Hill; 2019.

576 Skin peeling rash. Photo contributor: Daniel M. Lindberg, MD.

577 Hydrops fetalis. Reproduced with permission from Kemp WL, Burns DK, Brown TG. *Pathology: The Big Picture*. New York: McGraw Hill; 2008.

582 Notable erythema of tympanic membrane with visible meniscus of effusion. Reproduced with permission from Knoop KJ, Stack LB, Storrow AB, Thurman RJ. *The Atlas of Emergency Medicine*, 5th ed. New York: McGraw Hill; 2021, Figure 5.3. Photo contributor: Richard A. Chole, MD, PhD.

584 Honey crusted lesions seen in impetigo. Reproduced with permission from Wolff K, Johnson RA, Saavedra AP, Roh EK. *Fitzpatrick's Color Atlas and Synopsis of Clinical Dermatology*, 8th ed. New York: McGraw Hill; 2017.

584 Erythematous papules on palms characteristic of hand-foot-mouth disease. Reproduced with permission from Kang S, Amagai M, Bruckner AL, Enk AH, Margolis DJ, McMichael AJ, Orringer JS, eds. *Fitzpatrick's Dermatology*, 9th ed. New York: McGraw Hill; 2019.

584 Classic sandpaper rash in scarlet fever. Reproduced with permission from Richard P. Usatine, MD.

585 Staphylococcal scalded skin syndrome. Flaccid blisters have sloughed, leaving denuded areas of "scalded skin." Reproduced with permission from Soutor C, Hordinsky MK. *Clinical Dermatology: Diagnosis and Management of Common Disorders*, 2nd ed. New York: McGraw Hill; 2022.

585 "Slapped-cheek" rash of face along with rash on torso. Photo contributor: Anne W. Lucky, MD.

589 Types of craniosynostosis. Reproduced with permission from Brunicardi FC, Andersen DK, Billiar TR, et al, eds. *Schwartz's Principles of Surgery*, 11th ed. New York: McGraw Hill; 2019.

591 Tram-tracking along bowel wall indicative of pneumatosis intestinalis. Reproduced with permission from Brunicardi FC, Andersen DK, Billiar TR, et al, eds. *Schwartz's Principles of Surgery*, 11th ed. New York: McGraw Hill; 2019.

591 Target sign. Reproduced with permission from Elsayes KM, Oldham SAA. *Introduction to Diagnostic Radiology*. New York: McGraw Hill; 2014.

593 Figure 23.26.1. Reproduced with permission from Elsayes KM, Oldham SAA. *Introduction to Diagnostic Radiology*. New York: McGraw Hill; 2014.

594 Steeple sign. Reproduced with permission from Elsayes KM, Oldham SAA. *Introduction to Diagnostic Radiology*. New York: McGraw Hill; 2014.

595 Epiglottic edema (thumbprint sign) in epiglottitis. Reproduced with permission from Stone CK, Humphries RL. *Current Diagnosis & Treatment: Emergency Medicine*, 8th ed. New York: McGraw Hill; 2017.

606 Round lucent lesion of osteoid osteoma. Reproduced with permission from Elsayes KM, Oldham SAA. *Introduction to Diagnostic Radiology*. New York: McGraw Hill; 2014.

606 Arrow showing pedunculated lesion of distal femur. Reproduced with permission from Tehranzadeh J, ed. *Basic Musculoskeletal Imaging*, 2nd ed. New York; McGraw Hill; 2021.

607 Ewing sarcoma. Reproduced with permission from Tehranzadeh J, ed. *Basic Musculoskeletal Imaging*, 2nd ed. New York: McGraw Hill; 2021.

608 Craniopharyngioma as seen on MRI. Reproduced with permission from Riordan-Eva P, Augsburger JJ, eds. *Vaughan & Asbury's General Ophthalmology*, 19th ed. New York: McGraw Hill; 2017.

611 Prominent follicles under the upper eyelid seen in trachoma. Reproduced with permission from Richard P. Usatine, MD.

612 Esotropia of left eye in comparison to right eye that is midline. Reproduced with permission from Riordan-Eva P, Augsburger JJ, eds. *Vaughan & Asbury's General Ophthalmology*, 19th ed. New York: McGraw Hill; 2017.

612 Leukocoria (white pupil) is seen in this child with retinoblastoma. Used with permission ARZTSAMUI/Shutterstock.

613 Lisch nodules. Reproduced with permission from Usatine RP, Smith MA, Mayeaux EJ Jr, Chumley HS. *The Color Atlas and Synopsis of Family Medicine*, 3rd ed. New York: McGraw Hill; 2019, Figure 245-10. Reproduced with permission from Richard P. Usatine, MD.

616 Positive Gower sign seen in Duchenne and Becker muscular dystrophies. Reproduced with permission from Loscalzo J, Fauci AS, Kasper DL, et al, eds. *Harrison's Principles of Internal Medicine*, 21st ed. New York: McGraw Hill; 2022.

625 Transillumination of hydrocele. Reproduced with permission from photo contributor: Kevin J. Knoop, MD, MS.

632 Displaced femoral epiphysis in SCFE. Reproduced with permission from Bailey J, Gu Y, Olufade A, Maitin IB, Weinik M. Rehabilitation of common musculoskeletal conditions. In: Maitin IB, Cruz E, eds. *Current Diagnosis & Treatment: Physical Medicine & Rehabilitation*. New York: McGraw-Hill; 2014.

635 Fragmentation of the tibial tubercle in Osgood-Schlatter disease. Reproduced with permission from Elsayes KM, Oldham SAA. *Introduction to Diagnostic Radiology*. New York: McGraw-Hill; 2014.

637 Figure 23.44.1. Reproduced with permission from Hay Jr WW, Levin MJ, Abzug MJ, Bunik M, eds. *Current Diagnosis & Treatment: Pediatrics*, 25th ed. New York: McGraw Hill; 2020.

637 Figure 23.44.2. Reproduced with permission from Tehranzadeh J, ed. *Basic Musculoskeletal Imaging*, 2nd ed. New York; McGraw Hill; 2021.

637 Figure 23.44.3. Used with permission of Karen Black, BC Children's Hospital, Vancouver.

639 Figure 23.45.1. Reproduced with permission from Caserta MP, Chaudhry F, Bechtold RE. Liver, biliary tract, and pancreas. In: Chen MM, Pope TL, Ott DJ, eds. *Basic Radiology*, 2nd ed. New York: McGraw Hill; 2011.

640 Arrows pointing to type 4 Salter-Harris fracture of the distal tibia. Used with permission of Karen Black, BC Children's Hospital, Vancouver.

642 Patterned bruising of cheek in the impression of a handprint. Reproduced with permission from photo contributor: Kathi L. Makoroff, MD.

Chapter 24

663 A complete hydatidiform mole with the characteristic "snowstorm" appearance on ultrasound. From Cunningham FG, Leveno KJ, Bloom SL, et al, eds. *Williams Obstetrics*, 25th ed. New York: McGraw Hill; 2018, Figure 20-4A. Reproduced with permission from Dr. Elysia Moschos.

663 A partial hydatidiform mole on ultrasound. From Cunningham FG, Leveno KJ, Bloom SL, et al, eds. *Williams Obstetrics*, 25th ed. New York: McGraw Hill; 2018, Figure 20-4A. Reproduced with permission from Dr. Elysia Moschos.

664 Trophoblastic disease. Transverse scan of the pelvis with a hydatidiform mole (M) and ovarian theca lutein cysts (*arrowheads*). Reproduced with permission from Krebs CA, Giyanani VL, Eisenberg RL. *Ultrasound Atlas of Disease Processes*. Originally published by Appleton & Lange. New York: McGraw-Hill; 1993.

669 Figure 24.13.1. Reproduced with permission from Cunningham FG, Leveno KJ, Bloom SL, et al, eds. *Williams Obstetrics*, 25th ed. New York: McGraw Hill; 2018.

669 Figure 24.13.2. Reproduced with permission from Cunningham FG, Leveno KJ, Bloom SL, et al, eds. *Williams Obstetrics*, 25th ed. New York: McGraw Hill; 2018.

669 Figure 24.12.3. Reproduced with permission from Cunningham FG, Leveno KJ, Bloom SL, et al, eds. *Williams Obstetrics*, 25th ed. New York: McGraw Hill; 2018.

669 Figure 24.13.4. Reproduced with permission from Cunningham FG, Leveno KJ, Bloom SL, et al, eds. *Williams Obstetrics*, 25th ed. New York: McGraw Hill; 2018.

673 Figure 24.15.1. Reproduced with permission from Cunningham FG, Leveno KJ, Bloom SL, et al, eds. *Williams Obstetrics*, 25th ed. New York: McGraw Hill; 2018.

673 Figure 24.15.2. Reproduced with permission from Cunningham FG, Leveno KJ, Bloom SL, et al, eds. *Williams Obstetrics*, 25th ed. New York: McGraw Hill; 2018.

673 Figure 24.15.3. Reproduced with permission from Cunningham FG, Leveno KJ, Bloom SL, et al, eds. *Williams Obstetrics*, 25th ed. New York: McGraw Hill; 2018.

Chapter 25

687 A patient with stage 3 vulvar intraepithelial neoplasia and adjacent exophytic condyloma. From Usatine RP, Smith MA, Mayeaux EJ Jr, Chumley HS. *The Color Atlas and Synopsis of Family Medicine*, 3rd ed. New York: McGraw Hill; 2019, Figure 89-1. Reproduced with permission from Hope Haefner, MD.

690 Figure 25.5.1. Reproduced with permission from Hoffman BL, Schorge JO, Halvorson LM, et al, eds. *Williams Gynecology*, 4th ed. New York: McGraw Hill; 2020.

690 Figure 25.5.2. Reproduced with permission from Soutor C, Hordinsky MK. *Clinical Dermatology*. New York: McGraw Hill; 2013.

692 Figure 25.6.1. Large, mononuclear cell with multiple Donovan bodies. Reproduced with permission from O'Farrell N. Donovanosis. In: Longo, DL, Fauci AS, Kasper DL, et al, eds. *Harrison's Principles of Internal Medicine*, 18th ed. New York: McGraw-Hill; 2012.

692 **Figure 25.6.2. Multiple superficial ulcerations of primary genital herpes.** Reproduced with permission from Wolf K, Johnson RA, Saavedra AP, Roh EK. *Fitzpatrick's Color Atlas and Synopsis of Clinical Dermatology*, 8th ed. New York: McGraw Hill; 2017.

692 **Figure 25.6.3.** Reproduced with permission from Kang S, Amagai M, Bruckner AL, Enk AH, Margolis DJ, McMichael AJ, Orringer JS, eds. *Fitzpatrick's Dermatology*, 9th ed. New York: McGraw Hill; 2019.

692 **Figure 25.6.4.** Reproduced with permission from Kang S, Amagai M, Bruckner AL, Enk AH, Margolis DJ, McMichael AJ, Orringer JS, eds. *Fitzpatrick's Dermatology*, 9th ed. New York: McGraw Hill; 2019.

692 **Figure 25.6.5**. Reproduced with permission from Jameson J, Fauci AS, Kasper DL, Hauser SL, Longo DL, Loscalzo J, eds. *Harrison's Principles of Internal Medicine*, 20th ed. New York: McGraw Hill; 2018.

692 **Figure 25.6.6.** Reproduced with permission from Hoffman BL, Schorge JO, Halvorson LM, Hamid CA, Corton MM, Schaffer JI. *Williams Gynecology*, 4th ed. New York: McGraw Hill; 2020.

695 **Clue cells.** From Knoop KJ, Stack LB, Storrow AB, Thurman RJ, eds. *The Atlas of Emergency Medicine*, 5th ed. New York: McGraw Hill; 2021, Figure 25-16. Reproduced with permission from Curatek Pharmaceuticals.

695 ***Candida albicans.*** From Handsfield HH, ed. *Atlas of Sexually Transmitted Diseases*, 3rd ed. New York: McGraw Hill; 2011. Figure 25-19. Reproduced with permission from photo contributor: David A. Eschenbach, MD.

701 **Figure 25.10.1.** Reproduced with permission from Jameson J, Fauci AS, Kasper DL, Hauser SL, Longo DL, Loscalzo J, eds. *Harrison's Principles of Internal Medicine*, 20th ed. New York: McGraw Hill; 2018.

708 **Figure 25.13.1. Hydrosalpinx.** From Hoffman BL, Schorge JO, Halvorson LM, et al, eds. *Williams Gynecology*, 4th ed. New York: McGraw Hill; 2020, Figure 10-12A. Reproduced with permission from Dr. Elysia Moschos.

708 **Figure 25.13.2. Large ectopic pregnancy adjacent to the uterus.** Reproduced with permission from Ma OJ, Mateer JR, Reardon RF, Joing SA. *Ma & Mateer's Emergency Ultrasound*, 3rd ed. New York: McGraw Hill; 2014.

711 **Origins of 3 main types of ovarian tumors.** Reproduced with permission from Hoffman BL, Schorge JO, Halvorson LM, et al, eds. *Williams Gynecology*, 4th ed. New York: McGraw Hill; 2020.

712 **Figure 25.15.1.** From Public Health Image Library, CDC.

Chapter 26

716 **The neuraxis.** Reproduced with permission from Waxman SG. *Clinical Neuroanatomy*, 26th ed. New York: McGraw Hill; 2010.

717 **Rashes suggestive of dermatomyositis.** Reproduced with permission from Jameson J, Fauci AS, Kasper DL, Hauser SL, Longo DL, Loscalzo J, eds. *Harrison's Principles of Internal Medicine*, 20th ed. New York: McGraw Hill; 2018.

721 **Figure 26.4.1. Somatotopic organization of various tracts in the spinal cord.** Reproduced with permission from Waxman S. *Clinical Neuroanatomy*, 27th ed. New York: McGraw Hill; 2013.

722 **Figure 26.4.1. Division of cervical, thoracic, and lumbar vertebra with corresponding nerve roots.** Reproduced with permission from Waxman SG. *Correlative Neuroanatomy*, 24th ed. New York: McGraw Hill; 2000.

723 **Territory of an anterior spinal cord infarct.** Reproduced with permission from Aminoff M, Greenberg D, Simon R. *Clinical Neurology*, 9th ed. New York: McGraw Hill Education; 2015.

723 **Spinal cord territory affected by central cord syndrome.** Reproduced with permission from Aminoff M, Greenberg D, Simon R. *Clinical Neurology*, 9th ed. New York: McGraw Hill Education; 2015.

724 **Spinal cord territory affected by cord hemisection, Brown-Sequard's syndrome.** Reproduced with permission from Aminoff M, Greenberg D, Simon R. *Clinical Neurology*, 9th ed. New York: McGraw Hill Education; 2015.

725 **Spinal cord lesions indicated with arrows as seen on MRI in MS.** Reproduced with permission from Jameson J, Fauci AS, Kasper DL, Hauser SL, Longo DL, Loscalzo J, eds. *Harrison's Principles of Internal Medicine*, 20th ed. New York: McGraw Hill; 2018.

725 **Territory of cord affected by subacute combined degeneration.** Reproduced with permission from Aminoff M, Greenberg D, Simon R. *Clinical Neurology*, 9th ed. New York: McGraw Hill Education; 2015.

727 **CT angiogram demonstrating a left MCA occlusion (white arrow).** Reproduced with permission from Berkowitz AL. *Clinical Neurology and Neuroanatomy: A Localization-Based Approach*. New York: McGraw Hill; 2017.

728 **The major arteries supplying the brain and their vascular territories.** Reproduced with permission from Berkowitz AL. *Clinical Neurology and Neuroanatomy: A Localization-Based Approach*. New York: McGraw Hill; 2017.

729 **MRI brain including FLAIR sequence (A), diffusion-weighted imaging (B) and ADC sequence (C) demonstrating subacute lacunar infarct.** Reproduced with permission from Jameson J, Fauci AS, Kasper DL, Hauser SL, Longo DL, Loscalzo J, eds. *Harrison's Principles of Internal Medicine*, 20th ed. New York: McGraw Hill; 2018.

731 **Noncontrast head CT demonstrating "hyperdense vessel sign" suggesting left MCA stroke.** Reproduced with permission from Berkowitz AL. *Clinical Neurology and Neuroanatomy: A Localization-Based Approach*. New York: McGraw Hill; 2017.

733 **Figure 26.7.1. Head CT showing epidural hematoma.** Reproduced with permission from Oropello JM, Pastores SM, Kvetan V, eds. *Critical Care*. New York: McGraw Hill; 2017.

733 **Figure 26.7.2. Head CT showing subdural hematoma.** Reproduced with permission from Oropello JM, Pastores SM, Kvetan V, eds. *Critical Care*. New York: McGraw Hill; 2017.

733 **Figure 26.7.3. Head CT showing SAH.** Reproduced with permission from Oropello JM, Pastores SM, Kvetan V, eds. *Critical Care*. New York: McGraw Hill; 2017.

740 **Figure 26.10.1. MRI brain demonstrating enlarged ventricles without enlarged sulci.** Reproduced with permission from Jameson J, Fauci AS, Kasper DL, Hauser SL, Longo DL, Loscalzo J, eds. *Harrison's Principles of Internal Medicine*, 20th ed. New York: McGraw Hill; 2018.

741 **MRI brain (T2 FLAIR sequence) demonstrating white matter hyperintensities suggesting vascular dementia.** Reproduced with permission from Jameson J, Fauci AS, Kasper DL, Hauser SL, Longo DL, Loscalzo J, eds. *Harrison's Principles of Internal Medicine*, 20th ed. New York: McGraw Hill; 2018.

742 **Figure 26.11.1. MRI demonstrating the hummingbird sign.** Reproduced with permission from Berkowitz AL. *Clinical Neurology and Neuroanatomy: A Localization-Based Approach*. New York: McGraw Hill; 2017.

749 **Dermatomes (left) and myotomes (right) corresponding to lumbosacral roots.** Reproduced with permission from Waxman SG. *Clinical Neuroanatomy*, 29th ed. New York: McGraw Hill; 2020.

751 **Examples of subarachnoid hemorrhage: right frontal lobe (A) and circle of Willis (B).** Reproduced with permission from Berkowitz AL. *Clinical Neurology and Neuroanatomy: A Localization-Based Approach*. New York: McGraw Hill; 2017.

753 **Figure 26.16.1. T1 MRI with ring-enhancing lesion.** Reproduced with permission from Reisner HM. *Pathology: A Modern Case Study*, 2nd ed. New York: McGraw Hill; 2020.

754 **Falcine meningioma with moderate edema and mass effect on the right lateral ventricle.** Reproduced with permission from Brunicardi FC, Andersen DK, Billiar TR, et al, eds. *Schwartz's Principles of Surgery*, 11th ed. New York: McGraw Hill; 2019.

755 **Multiple enhancing lesions at the gray white junction concerning for brain metastases with surrounding edema (left). Hypointesity on GRE sequence corresponds to blood products (right).** Reproduced with permission from Ropper AH, Samuels MA, Klein JP, Prasad S, eds. *Adams and Victor's Principles of Neurology*, 11th ed. New York: McGraw Hill; 2019.

770 **Demonstration of different patterns of visual field defects.** Reproduced with permission from Jameson J, Fauci AS, Kasper DL, eds. *Harrison's Principles of Internal Medicine*, 20th ed. New York: McGraw Hill; 2018.

Chapter 28

814 **Description of Study Designs.** Reproduced with permission from Mazer LM, Lagisetty K, Butler KL, eds. *Pocket Journal Club: Essential Articles in General Surgery*. New York: McGraw Hill; 2017.

817 **2×2 Contingency Table.** Reproduced with permission from White SE. *Basic & Clinical Biostatistics*, 5th ed. New York: McGraw Hill; 2020.

817 **Compromise between Specificity and Sensitivity.** Reproduced with permission from Suneja M, Szot JF, et al, *DeGowin's Diagnostic Examination*, 11th ed. New York: McGraw Hill; 2020.

818 **Precision and Accuracy.** Reproduced with permission from Laposata M. *Laposata's Laboratory Medicine: Diagnosis of Disease in the Clinical Laboratory*, 3rd ed. New York: McGraw Hill; 2019.

819 **Recommended Child and Adolescent Immunization Schedule for Ages 18 Years or Younger, United States, 2022.** https://www.cdc.gov/vaccines/schedules/downloads/child/0-18yrs-child-combined-schedule.pdf.

821 **Recommended Adult Immunization Schedule by Age Group, United States, 2022.** https://www.cdc.gov/vaccines/schedules/downloads/adult/adult-combined-schedule.pdf.

822 **Recommended Adult Immunization Schedule by Medical Condition or Other Indication, 2022.** https://www.cdc.gov/vaccines/schedules/downloads/adult/adult-combined-schedule.pdf.

825 **Four Principles of Medical Ethics.** Reproduced with permission from Mitra R, ed. *Principles of Rehabilitation Medicine*. New York: McGraw Hill; 2019.

Index

Note: Page numbers in *italics* indicate figures or tables.